NITRIC OXIDE AND THE CARDIOVASCULAR SYSTEM

CONTEMPORARY ◊ CARDIOLOGY

Christopher P. Cannon, Series Editor

NITRIC OXIDE AND THE CARDIOVASCULAR SYSTEM

Edited by

JOSEPH LOSCALZO, MD, PHD
JOSEPH A. VITA, MD

Boston University Medical Center, Boston, MA

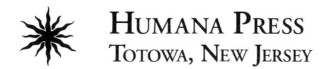

HUMANA PRESS
TOTOWA, NEW JERSEY

© 2000 Humana Press Inc.
999 Riverview Drive, Suite 208
Totowa, New Jersey 07512

For additional copies, pricing for bulk purchases, and/or information about other Humana titles, contact Humana at the above address or at any of the following numbers: Tel.: 973-256-1699; Fax: 973-256-8341, E-mail: humana@humanapr.com; or visit our Website: http://humanapr.com

Due diligence has been taken by the publishers, editors, and authors of this book to assure the accuracy of the information published and to describe generally accepted practices. The contributors herein have carefully checked to ensure that the drug selections and dosages set forth in this text are accurate and in accord with the standards accepted at the time of publication. Notwithstanding, as new research, changes in government regulations, and knowledge from clinical experience relating to drug therapy and drug reactions constantly occurs, the reader is advised to check the product information provided by the manufacturer of each drug for any change in dosages or for additional warnings and contraindications. This is of utmost importance when the recommended drug herein is a new or infrequently used drug. It is the responsibility of the treating physician to determine dosages and treatment strategies for individual patients. Further it is the responsibility of the health care provider to ascertain the Food and Drug Administration status of each drug or device used in their clinical practice. The publisher, editors, and authors are not responsible for errors or omissions or for any consequences from the application of the information presented in this book and make no warranty, express or implied, with respect to the contents in this publication.

Cover design by Patricia F. Cleary.

This publication is printed on acid-free paper. ∞
ANSI Z39.48-1984 (American National Standards Institute) Permanence of Paper for Printed Library Materials.

Printed in the United States of America.   10 9 8 7 6 5 4 3 2 1

Library of Congress Cataloging-in-Publication Data

Nitric oxide and the cardiovascular system/edited by Joseph Loscalzo, Joseph A. Vita.
    p.   cm.—(Contemporatry cardiology)
  Includes bibliographical references and index.
  ISBN 0-89603-620-0 (alk. paper)
    1. Cardiovascular system—Pathophysiology.   2. Cardiovascular system—Physiology.   3. Nitric oxide—Pathophysiology.   4. Nitric oxide—Physiological effect. I. Loscalzo, Joseph. II. Vita, Joseph A. III. Contemporary cardiology (Totowa, NJ)
    [DNLM: 1. Cardiovascular System—physiopathology. 2. Nitric Oxide—physiology. WG 120 N731 2000]
  RC669.9.N58 2000
  616.1'07—dc21
                                                                                    99-054493

PREFACE

The field of nitric oxide biology has expanded considerably over the past decade with a growing appreciation of its many roles in a variety of cell and organ systems. Nitric oxide was first discovered in the cardiovascular system, and the importance of this discovery led to the award of the 1998 Nobel Prize in Physiology or Medicine to Robert Furchgott, Louis Ignarro, and Fred Murad, well-known cardiovascular investigators. With this history, it should come as no surprise that our understanding of the role of nitric oxide in biology and pathobiology is, perhaps, best developed as it relates to cardiovascular biology and disease. For this reason, we felt it would be both timely and relevant to review in detail the role of nitric oxide in cardiovascular biomedicine. To this end, we assembled a group of contributing authors with expertise in areas that include the chemistry of nitric oixide, the biochemistry of its synthesis, the molecular biology of nitric oxide synthases, the pharmacology of nitrovasodilators, and the role of nitric oxide in vascular diseases.

With the recent expansion of the field in directions that range from the development of novel nitric oxide donors for the treatment of myocardial ischemia and thrombosis to the development of gene therapy approaches for the restoration of endothelial function in atherosclerosis, the application of nitric oxide biology to investigative and clinical arenas in cardiovascular medicine is, indeed, rapidly evolving. This comprehensive overview should prove useful for basic and clinical investigators alike, as well as practicing clinicians in the fields of cardiology, hematology, and vascular medicine. With a balanced presentation of basic and clinically relevant subject matter, this text will provide a compendium of information that may guide the reader through the foundations of the most recent developments in this rich and exciting field.

ACKNOWLEDGMENT

We thank Stephanie Tribuna for her assistance throughout the many phases of the development of this text, and Jalna Ross for her assistance in reference verification.

Joseph Loscalzo, MD, PHD
Joseph A. Vita, MD

To Anita, Julia, Alex, Gina, Olivia, and Sam

CONTENTS

CONTRIBUTORS

JEAN-LUC BALLIGAND, MD, PHD • *Department of Medicine, Pharmacology Unit, University of Louvain Medical School, Brussels, Belgium*

ELIZABETH M. BATTINELLI, MSC • *Whitaker Cardiovascular Institute and Evans Department of Medicine, Boston University School of Medicine, Boston, MA*

KENNETH D. BLOCH, MD • *Cardiology Division and the Cardiovascular Research Center, Department of Medicine, Massachusetts General Hospital, Harvard Medical School, Boston, MA*

VICTORIA BOLOTINA, PHD • *Vascular Biology Unit, Evans Department of Medicine, Boston University School of Medicine, Boston, MA*

PETER BRECHER, PHD • *Whitaker Cardiovascular Institute, Boston University School of Medicine, Boston, MA*

PAUL J. CANNON , MD • *Department of Medicine, Division of Cardiology, Columbia University College of Physicians and Surgeons, New York, NY*

WOLFGANG CERWINKA, MD • *Department of Molecular and Cellular Physiology, Louisiana State University Medical Center, Shreveport, LA*

RICHARD A. COHEN, MD • *Vascular Biology Unit, Evans Department of Medicine, Boston University School of Medicine, Boston, MA*

WILSON S. COLUCCI, MD, FACC • *Myocardial Biology Unit, Boston University School of Medicine, and Cardiovascular Division, Department of Medicine, Boston University Medical Center, Boston, MA*

JOHN P. COOKE, MD, PHD • *Section of Vascular Medicine, Division of Cardiovascular Medicine, Stanford University School of Medicine, Stanford, CA*

AMI A. DEORA, PHD • *Department of Biochemistry, Cornell University Medical College, New York, NY*

GERARD DILLON, MD • *Evans Department of Medicine and Whitaker Cardiovascular Institute, Boston University School of Medicine, Boston, MA*

STEFANIE DIMMELER, PHD • *Molecular Cardiology, Department of Internal Medicine IV, University of Frankfurt, Germany*

ROBERT T. EBERHARDT, MD • *Whitaker Cardiovascular Institute and Evans Department of Medicine, Boston University School of Medicine, Boston, MA*

LÜ FEI, MD, PHD • *Krannert Institute of Cardiology, Department of Medicine, Indiana University School of Medicine, and the Roudebush Veterans Administration Medical Center, Indianapolis, IN*

OLIVIER FERON, PHD • *Pharmacology and Therapeutic Unit, Department of Medicine, University of Louvain Medical School, Brussels, Belgium*

ANTHONY L. FITZHUGH, MD • *Intramural Research Support Program, SAIC Frederick, National Cancer Institute, Frederick Cancer Research and Development Center, Frederick, MD*

JOHN D. FOLTS, PHD, FACC • *Coronary Thrombosis Research Laboratory, Department of Cardiology, University of Wisconsin Medical School, Madison, WI*

JANE E. FREEDMAN, MD • *Department of Clinical Pharmacology, Georgetown University, Washington, DC*

D. NEIL GRANGER, PHD • *Department of Molecular and Cellular Physiology, Louisiana State University Medical Center, Shreveport, LA*

REID HAYWARD, PHD • *Department of Physiology, Jefferson Medical College, Thomas Jefferson University, Philadelphia, PA*

STANLEY HEYDRICK, PHD • *Boston University School of Medicine, Boston, MA*

JOHN D. HOROWITZ, MBBS, PHD • *Cardiology Unit, The Queen Elizabeth Hospital, Woodville, Australia*

ANNONG HUANG, PHD • *Evans Memorial Department of Medicine and Whitaker Cardiovascular Institute, Boston University School of Medicine, Boston, MA*

PAUL L. HUANG, MD, PHD • *Cardiovascular Research Center and Cardiology Division, Massachusetts General Hospital and Harvard Medical School, Charlestown, MA*

WILLIAM E. HURFORD, MD • *Department of Anesthesia and Critical Care, Massachusetts General Hospital, Boston, MA*

JOHN F. KEANEY, JR., MD • *Evans Memorial Department of Medicine and Whitaker Cardiovascular Institute, Boston University School of Medicine, Boston, MA*

LARRY K. KEEFER, PHD • *Chemistry Section, Laboratory of Comparative Carcinogenesis, National Cancer Institute, Frederick Cancer Research and Development Center, Frederick, MD*

HARRY M. LANDER, PHD • *Department of Biochemistry, Cornell University Medical College, New York, NY*

ALLAN M. LEFER, PHD • *Department of Physiology, Jefferson Medical College, Thomas Jefferson University, Philadelphia, PA*

JANE A. LEOPOLD, MD • *Whitaker Cardiovascular Institute and Evans Department of Medicine, Boston University School of Medicine, Boston, MA*

JOHN J. LEPORE, MD • *Cardiology Division and the Cardiovascular Research Center, Department of Medicine, Massachusetts General Hospital, Harvard Medical School, Boston, MA*

JOSEPH LOSCALZO, MD, PHD • *Whitaker Cardiovascular Institute and Evans Department of Medicine, Boston University School of Medicine, Boston, MA*

ANDREW J. MAXWELL, MD • *Cooke Pharma, Belmont, CA*

THOMAS MICHEL, MD, PHD • *Cardiology Division, West Roxbury VA Medical Center, Brigham and Women's Hospital, Harvard Medical School, Boston, MA*

DAVID J. PINSKY, MD • *Divisions of Cardiology and Circulatory Physiology, Department of Medicine, College of Physicians and Surgeons, Columbia University, New York, NY*

M. AUDREY RUDD, PHD • *Whitaker Cardiovascular Institute and Evans Department of Medicine, Boston University School of Medicine, Boston, MA*

HARTMUT RUETTEN, MD • *The William Harvey Research Institute, St. Bartholomew's and the Royal London School of Medicine and Dentistry, London, UK*

JOESPH E. SAAVEDRA, PHD • *Intramural Research Support Program, SAIC Frederick, National Cancer Institute, Frederick Cancer Research and Development Center, Frederick, MD*

DOUGLAS B. SAWYER, MD • *Myocardial Biology Unit, Boston University School of Medicine, and Cardiovascular Division, Department of Medicine, Boston University Medical Center, Boston, MA*

NANCY E. STAGLIANO, PHD • *Cardiovascular Research Center and Cardiology Division, Massachusetts General Hospital and Harvard Medical School, Charlestown, MA*

DAVID M. STERN, MD • *Divisions of Cardiology and Circulatory Physiology, Department of Medicine, College of Physicians and Surgeons, Columbia University, New York, NY*

CHRISTOPH THIEMERMANN, MD • *The William Harvey Research Institute, St. Bartholomew's and the Royal London School of Medicine and Dentistry, London, UK*

MARÍA R. TROLLIET, PHD • *Whitaker Cardiovascular Institute and Evans Department of Medicine, Boston University School of Medicine, Boston, MA*

JOSEPH A. VITA, MD • *Evans Department of Medicine and Whitaker Cardiovascular Institute, Boston University School of Medicine, Boston, MA*

HEIKO E. VON DER LEYEN, MD, PHD • *Cardiogene AG, Erkrath, Germany, and Department Innere Medizin, Medizinische Hochschule, Hannover, Germany*

WARREN M. ZAPOL, MD • *Department of Anesthesia and Critical Care, Massachusetts General Hospital, Boston, MA*

ANDREAS M. ZEIHER, MD • *Molecular Cardiology, Department of Internal Medicine IV, University of Frankfurt, Germany*

DOUGLAS P. ZIPES, MD • *Krannert Institute of Cardiology, Department of Medicine, Indiana University School of Medicine, and the Roudebush Veterans Administration Medical Center, Indianapolis, IN*

I BIOLOGY OF NITRIC OXIDE

1

The Biological Chemistry of Nitric Oxide

Joseph Loscalzo

INTRODUCTION

Nitric oxide (NO•) is a heterodiatomic free radical that can participate in a wide range of biochemically relevant reactions to evoke a panoply of biological responses. In order to understand the biochemistry of NO•, we must first consider its chemistry. This introductory chapter provides an overview of the relevant chemistry of NO• and its derivative biochemical reactions, both with respect to normal biological actions and pathophysiological effects.

CHEMICAL PROPERTIES OF NO•

In contrast to other biological free radicals, NO• is a free radical of limited reactivity. As one measure of this important property, NO• can diffuse over distances as great as several microns in aqueous solvent before engaging in collision-dependent reactions; superoxide anion radicals and hydroxyl radicals, in comparison, are much more reactive, diffusing over very much shorter reaction distances. The relative stability of NO• is a consequence of its unpaired electron being localized to a 2p-π-antibonding orbital. The bond order of NO• is 2.5 (defined by three bonds gained from the filled σ_x, π_x, and π_y molecular orbitals minus half a bond from the partially filled π^* antibonding orbital), and this order does not change appreciably on dimerization (approx 5), again supporting the relatively low reactivity of the molecule.

At room temperature, NO• is a colorless gas (boiling point, 151.7°C at 1 atm). The solubility of NO• is 1.9 mM/atm in aqueous solution *(1,2)*, which is comparable to that of molecular oxygen. Because of its somewhat nonpolar nature and relative stability, NO• can diffuse at a rate of approx 50 μm/s *(14)* in aqueous solution; its half-life in vivo is approximately 10 s *(4)*.

The broad range of reactions in which NO• can participate is largely attributable to the variety of nitrogen oxide (NO_x) species found in aqueous systems. NO• can undergo one-electron oxidation (to nitrosonium, NO^+) or reduction (to nitroxyl anion, NO^-) with the following estimated half-cell potentials *(5)*:

$$NO^\bullet \rightarrow NO^+ + e^- \qquad E_{1/2} = -1.2 \text{ V} \qquad (1)$$

$$NO^\bullet + e^- \rightarrow NO^- \qquad E_{1/2} = -0.33 \text{ V} \qquad (2)$$

These reactions are analogous to oxidation and reduction reactions of superoxide radical to molecular oxygen and to hydroxyl radical/hydrogen peroxide, respectively. Yet the analogy is imperfect, as nitrosonium is isoelectronic to carbon monoxide, whereas nitroxyl anion is isoelectronic to molecular oxygen. The susceptibility of NO• to oxidation is consonant with

From: *Contemporary Cardiology, vol. 4: Nitric Oxide and the Cardiovascular System*
Edited by: J. Loscalzo and J. A. Vita © Humana Press Inc., Totowa, NJ

the fact that the highest occupied molecular orbital is an antibonding orbital. In support of this view, the ionization potential of $NO^{\bullet}$ is low (9.25 eV) compared with that of N_2 (15.56 eV), and the N–O bond length decreases by only 0.09 Å when $NO^{\bullet}$ is oxidized to nitrosonium (6).

$NO^{\bullet}$ is central to the overall redox scheme for nitrogen oxides. This scheme begins with ammonia and ends with nitrate by way of a series of intermediates as shown in Eq. 3 with the nitrogen valence states indicated beneath each species:

$$NH_3 \leftrightarrows NH_2OH \leftrightarrows HNO \leftrightarrows NO^{\bullet} \leftrightarrows NO_2^- \leftrightarrows NO_3^- \quad (3)$$

ammonia	hydroxyl amine	hydrogen nitride (nitroxyl)	nitric oxide	nitrite	nitrate
−3	−1	+1	+2	+3	+5

REACTIONS WITH OXYGEN

$NO^{\bullet}$ reacts readily with oxygen, largely as a consequence of the diradical nature of the triplet species of molecular oxygen (with two unpaired electrons occupying degenerate π^{*} antibonding molecular orbitals, formally given as $^3O_2$). The product of this reaction is nitrogen dioxide (NO_2), and the kinetics of its formation are second order in $NO^{\bullet}$ and first order in O_2, consistent with the third-order equation:

$$d[NO^{\bullet}]/dt = k[NO^{\bullet}]^2[O_2] \quad (4)$$

where $k = 7 \times 10^6\,M^{-2} \cdot s^{-1}$ (7–10). Interestingly, this reaction is virtually unaffected by normal physiological ranges of pH and temperature. The importance of this rate process rests on its second-order dependence on $NO^{\bullet}$, indicating that the oxidative decomposition of the molecule is a strict function of its concentration: the higher the concentration, the more rapid its autooxidation. This property of $NO^{\bullet}$ indicates that the further $NO^{\bullet}$ diffuses from its source of synthesis, the more likely it is to be available to exert its biological effects.

In aqueous environments, the terminal oxidation product of $NO^{\bullet}$ is nitrite (NO_2^-), into which NO_2 stoichiometrically decomposes by the following mechanism:

$$2NO^{\bullet} + O_2 \rightarrow 2NO_2 \quad (5)$$

$$NO^{\bullet} + NO_2 \rightarrow N_2O_3 \quad (6)$$

$$N_2O_3 + H_2O \rightarrow 2NO_2^- + 2H^+ \quad (7)$$

REACTIONS WITH OXYGEN-DERIVED RADICALS

Nitric oxide can react readily with superoxide anion at a rate that is essentially diffusion controlled ($k = 6.7 \times 10^9\,M^{-1}/s^{-1}$) (11) to form the oxidant peroxynitrite (^-OONO):

$$NO^{\bullet} + O_2^{-\bullet} \rightarrow {}^-OONO \quad (8)$$

Importantly, this reaction is approximately fivefold faster than the dismutation of superoxide by superoxide dismutase. Peroxynitrite has a $pK_a = 6.8$ and is a relatively stable species under alkaline conditions, slowly undergoing dismutation spontaneously to nitrite and molecular oxygen (12). Protonation destabilizes the molecule and facilitates anion isomerization to NO_3^-:

$$^-OONO + H^+ \leftrightarrows HOONO \rightarrow [{}^{\bullet}OH + NO_2] \rightarrow NO_3^- + 2H^+ \quad (9)$$

The formation of ^-OONO has two important consequences in biological systems: loss of bioactive $NO^{\bullet}$ and oxidation of a wide variety of biological molecules. One of the principal stable oxidation products results from the reaction of ^-OONO with the amino acid tyrosine:

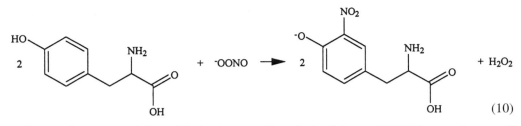

$$+ \, H_2O_2 \tag{10}$$

The precise nature of the oxidative intermediate derived from ^-OONO has not been well characterized to date. In addition, recent data from Pryor's group *(14)* suggest that in carbonate-enriched buffer systems, CO_2 reacts with ^-OONO rapidly to form the nitrosoperoxycarbonate anion adduct $O = N - OOCO_2^-$, which then rearranges to yield a nitrocarbonate anion $O_2N - OCO_2^-$. The latter species may, in turn, serve as an oxidant in biological systems (by one- or two-electron oxidation reactions), engage in electrophilic nitration reactions, such as nitrotyrosine formation,

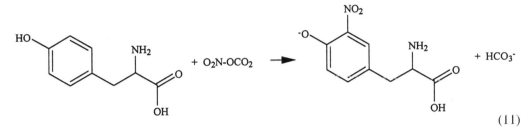

$$\tag{11}$$

or undergo hydrolysis to yield nitrate and bicarbonate *(13,14)*:

$$O_2N - OCO_2^- + H_2O \rightarrow NO_3^- + HCO_3^- + H^+ \tag{12}$$

Peroxynitrite also reacts with $NO^\bullet$ to form nitrogen dioxide radical ($NO_2^{-\bullet}$) and nitrite in an exothermic reaction. An analogous reaction between ^-OONO and H_2O_2 leads to the energetically favorable formation of nitrite and water; however, the physiological relevance of this reaction has yet to be demonstrated. There has also been some debate in the literature as to the possibility that HOONO undergoes homolytic cleavage to generate a hydroxyl radical; however, Koppenol and colleagues *(12)* have argued that the rate constant for homolysis is too slow to compete meaningfully with the rate of isomerization.

In addition to superoxide, other peroxyl radicals react readily with $NO^\bullet$ to form lipid peroxynitrite compounds (LOONO) *(15)*:

$$NO^\bullet + LOO^\bullet \rightarrow LOONO \tag{13}$$

This reaction is, again, near diffusion-limited ($k = 2 \times 10^9 \, M^{-1} \cdot s^{-1}$), and likely explains the effect of $NO^\bullet$ on lipid peroxidation in cellular systems *(16)*.

Recent data suggest that $NO^\bullet$ can react with H_2O_2 to form $^\bullet OH$ *(17)*. The mechanism for this reaction is as yet unknown, but may involve either a direct reaction between $NO^\bullet$ and H_2O_2 or the formation of an intermediate that undergoes homolysis to yield $^\bullet OH$.

Nitric oxide reacts with $^\bullet OH$ at a diffusion-controlled rate ($k = 1 \times 10^{10} \, M^{-1} \cdot s^{-1}$) *(18)* in aqueous solution by the following reaction:

$$NO^\bullet + {}^\bullet OH \rightarrow HNO_2 \tag{14}$$

In addition, $NO^\bullet$ reacts with NO_2 to form the nitrosating species N_2O_3 (written as $^{\delta-}OON\text{-}NO^{\delta+}$) with a rate constant that is near diffusion-limited ($k = 1 \times 10^9 \, M^{-1} \cdot s^{-1}$), and this species can undergo hydrolysis to nitrite as shown in reactions (6) and (7). The rate constant for the latter reaction is only 1000 s^{-1}, and this slow rate becomes important when we consider the nitrosation of thiols under physiological conditions (*vide infra*).

REACTIONS WITH THIOLS

Although NO· does not directly react with the functional groups of biological molecules, oxidized derivatives of NO· with nitrosating capacity, such as N_2O_3, react with thiols to form S-nitrosothiols *(19)*:

$$N_2O_3 + RSH \rightarrow RSNO + HNO_2 \tag{15}$$

This reaction competes favorably with reaction (7) in the intracellular milieu where glutathione concentrations in the millimolar range react 5–10-fold faster with N_2O_3 than does water *(20)*. The formation of S-nitrosothiols occurs under normal physiological conditions *(21,22)*, and the parent thiol can either be a low-molecular-weight species or a cysteinyl side chain of a protein.

S-Nitrosation of proteins can modify protein function, and this form of posttranslational modification has been shown to have wide-ranging biological effects. The S-nitrosation of serum albumin's single free cysteinyl group (cys 83) represents a special situation that yields a stable pool of −NO· equivalents. S-Nitroso-albumin is the most abundant extracellular −NO· pool *(21)*, serving as a buffer for −NO· and stabilizing it from further oxidation in the comparatively oxidative extracellular space.

S-Nitrosothiols also engage in *trans-S*-nitrosation reactions *(23)*, which are thermodynamically and mechanistically equivalent to thiol–disulfide exchange reactions:

$$RS - NO· + R'SH \leftrightarrows RSH + R'SNO \tag{16}$$

The transfer of −NO· between low-molecular-weight thiols and serum albumin is supported by this chemistry *(24)*.

Under anaerobic conditions, NO· reacts with low-molecular-weight thiols to produce the corresponding disulfide:

$$2RSH + 2NO· \rightarrow RSSR + N_2O + H_2O \tag{17}$$

At pHs near or above the pK_a of the thiol, this reaction is accelerated *(24)*. Cysteinyl side chains of proteins, in contrast, can undergo oxidation to sulfenic acids when reacted with NO· under anerobic conditions *(25)*; however, the relevance of this reaction to physiological conditions is questionable.

S-Nitrosation of the cysteinyl side chains of proteins may lead to disulfide formation even under aerobic conditions when two thiols are vicinal, or in close proximity. It has been argued that the "activity" of the thiols, or their effective local molarity, sustains this reaction, and, in part, depends on the relative pK_a of the two thiols. Thiols with anomalously low pK_as can attack the sulfur involved in the −S–H bond by a nucleophilic mechanism:

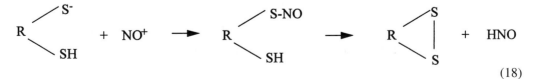

$$\tag{18}$$

This type of mechanism has been postulated as the basis for NO·-mediated inactivation of the *N*-methyl-D-aspartate receptor in neurons *(26)* and for the NO·-mediated inactivation of Ca^{2+}-dependent potassium channels *(27)*.

Importantly, S-nitrosation reactions are quenched by $O_2^-{}^\bullet$, and oxidation of thiols by $O_2^-{}^\bullet$ to the disulfide form mediated by peroxynitrite is quenched by excess flux of either $NO^\bullet$ or $O_2^-{}^\bullet$. Thus, nitrosation and oxidation of thiols by $O_2^-{}^\bullet/^-OONO$ and NO_x are dependent on their relative flux rates with peak oxidation occurring when fluxes are equivalent (28).

Recently, a novel mechanism for the formation of S-nitrosothiols was identified that may have relevance to their formation in vivo. This mechanism involves the direct reaction of $NO^\bullet$ with the thiol to produce the radical intermediate, $RSN^\bullet - OH$, which, in turn, reacts with an electrophile to yield the S-nitrosothiol; under aerobic conditions, molecular oxygen is the electron acceptor and is reduced to $O_2^-{}^\bullet$ in the process (29). As yet another potential S-nitrosating mechanism of physiological relevance, dinitrosyl–iron complexes (vide infra), which have been detected in tissues, can serve as direct nitrosating species that react with the thiolate functionality of serum albumin (30).

REACTIONS WITH OTHER NUCLEOPHILIC CENTERS

In addition to thiols, biological systems contain a variety of other nucleophilic centers that are potentially susceptible to nitrosative attack, including amines, amides, carboxyl groups, and hydroxyl groups. Primary amine deamination and N-nitrosation of secondary or tertiary amines may occur in acidic environments and the latter species have been studied as mediators of carcinogenesis (31,32). In contrast, the biological relevance of the reaction of $NO^\bullet$ with amides, carboxyl groups, and hydroxyl groups is speculative (33). Recently, we demonstrated that the indole group of tryptophan can undergo N-nitrosation, and that this derivative can engage in transnitrosation reactions that evoke biological responses (34). Aromatic rings also undergo nitrosation in a process that involves the formation of charge-transfer complexes between NO^+ and aromatic electron donors (35):

$$Ar - NO^+ \leftrightarrows Ar^{\bullet +} - NO^\bullet \qquad (19)$$

This type of one-electron transfer may provide a mechanism by which to interconvert the redox-related forms of $NO^\bullet$ (36).

REACTIONS WITH METALS

$NO^\bullet$ reacts both with heme iron as well as nonheme iron. In contradistinction to other heme iron ligands, including O_2 and CO, $NO^\bullet$ can bind to both ferric [Fe(III)] and ferrous [Fe(II)] iron. The binding of $NO^\bullet$ to Fe(III) leads to the formation of a charge-transfer complex that can be represented either as $Fe(III) - NO^\bullet$ or $Fe(II) - {}^+NO$ (37). This latter complex can serve as a nitrosating species since the complex renders the nitrosyl moiety susceptible to nucleophilic attack:

$$[Fe(III) - NO \leftrightarrow Fe(II) - {}^+NO] + Nucleophile \rightarrow Fe(II) + Nucleophile - NO \qquad (20)$$

In addition, $NO^\bullet$ can react readily with Fe(II) to form a strong ligand complex through donation of electrons from $NO^\bullet$ to the metal as well as donation of electrons from the metal to $NO^\bullet$ by a backbonding interaction between the d-orbitals of the metal and the antibonding orbitals of $NO^\bullet$ (38).

Recent X-ray crystallographic studies of the ferrous nitric oxide form of sperm whale myoglobin shows that the nitric oxide ligand is bent with respect to the heme plane with an Fe(II)-N-O angle of 112°. This angle appears to be influenced by the both the proximal bond strength and hydrogen-bonding interactions between the distal histidine and the bound nitrosyl moiety. The ring nitrogen atom of histidine 64 is located 2.8 Å from the $-NO^\bullet$ group's nitrogen atom, suggesting that electrostatic interactions stabilize the $Fe(II) - NO^\bullet$ complex (39), as shown in structure (21).

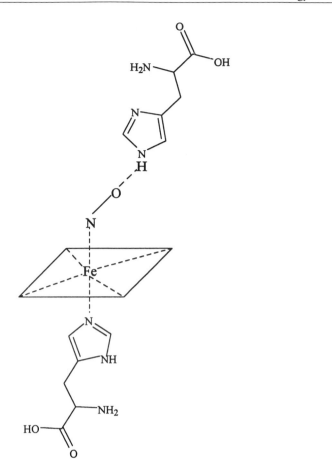

(21)

In the heme-binding site of guanylyl cyclase, the ligation of NO$^\bullet$ to heme iron liberates the transaxial ligand, histidine, which leads to enzyme activation *(40)*. Other heme ligands, such as O_2 and CO, do not render the transaxial histidine ligand labile, and thus do not activate guanylyl cyclase. In the heme-binding site of oxyhemoglobin or oxymyoglobin, NO$^\bullet$ binding leads to the formation of methemoglobin or metmyoglobin, respectively, by the following reaction scheme that involves the resonance forms of $Fe(II) - O_2$ and $Fe(III) - O_2^-$ *(41)*:

$$[Fe(II) - O_2 \leftrightarrow Fe(III) - O_2^-] + NO^\bullet \rightarrow Fe(III) + NO_3^- \tag{22}$$

This reaction is quite rapid and can serve as the basis of a spectroscopic assay for NO$^\bullet$.

NO$^\bullet$ also forms charge–transfer complexes with nonheme transition metals. In particular, NO$^\bullet$ can complex with iron–sulfur centers in proteins or within cell membranes *(42,43)*, often to form iron-dinitrosyl-dithiolate complexes of the following form, as shown in scheme (23).

$$\begin{array}{c} \text{ON} \diagdown \qquad \diagup \text{SR} \\ \qquad \text{Fe} \\ \text{ON} \diagup \qquad \diagdown \text{SR} \end{array} \tag{23}$$

Many of these nitrosyl complexes are effective electrophilic nitrosating species, having the general formula, $Me - {}^+NO$, whereas others behave principally as nucleophilic nitroxylating species, having the general formula, $Me - NO^-$. The unique chemistry of these metal–nitrosyl charge–transfer complexes offers another mechanism by which the redox states of NO$^\bullet$ can be modulated *(36)*.

CONCLUSIONS

The chemistry of NO$^\bullet$ is quite varied in physiological environments, and accounts for a rich and complex array of reactions. This chemistry serves as the basis for an equally broad range of biological effects, and these are discussed in turn throughout the first section of this book.

REFERENCES

1. Dean JA. Table 10-17: molecular elevation of the boiling point (ebullioscopic constants). In: Dean JA, ed. Lange's Handbook of Chemistry (13th ed.). McGraw-Hill, New York, 1985, pp. 10–73.
2. Armor JN. Influence of pH and ionic strength upon solubility of nitric oxide in aqueous solution. J Chem Eng Data 1974;19:82–84.
3. Gally JA, Montague PR, Reeke GN Jr, Edelman GM. The NO hypothesis: possible effects of a short-lived, rapidly diffusible signal in the development and function of the nervous system. Proc Natl Acad Sci USA 1990;87:3547–3551.
4. Moncada S, Palmer RM, Higgs EA. Nitric oxide: physiology, pathophysiology, and pharmacology. Pharm Rev 1991;43:109–142.
5. Stanbury DM. Reduction potentials involving inorganic free radicals in aqueous solution. Adv Org Chem 1989;33:69–138.
6. Cotton FA, Wilkinson G. The chemistry of the main group elements. In: Advanced Organic Chemistry, 5th ed. Wiley, New York, 1988, pp. 585–597.
7. Ford PC, Wink DA, Stanbury DM. Autoxidation kinetics of aqueous nitric oxide. FEBS Lett 1993; 326:1–3.
8. Wink DA, Darbyshire JF, Nims RW, Saavedra JE, Ford PC. Reactions of the bioregulatory agent nitric oxide in oxygenated aqueous media: determination of the kinetics for oxidation and nitrosation by intermediates generated in the NO/O2 reaction. Chem Res Toxicol 1993;6:23–27.
9. Kharitonov VG, Sundquist AR, Sharma VS. Kinetics of nitric oxide autoxidation in aqueous solution. J Biol Chem 1994;269:5881–5883.
10. Lewis RS, Deen WM. Kinetics of the reaction of nitric oxide with oxygen in aqueous solutions. Chem Res Toxicol 1994;7:568–574.
11. Huie RE, Padmaja S. The reaction of NO with superoxide. Free Rad Res Commun 1993;18:195–199.
12. Koppenol WH, Moreno JJ, Pryor WA, Ischiropoulos H, Beckman JS. Peroxynitrite, a cloaked oxidant formed by nitric oxide and superoxide. Chem Res Toxicol 1992;5:834–842.
13. Uppu RM, Squadrito GL, Pryor WA. Acceleration of peroxynitrite oxidations by carbon dioxide. Arch Biochem Biophys 1996;327:335–343.
14. Pryor WA, Lemercier JN, Zhang H, Uppu RM, Squadrito GL. The catalytic role of carbon dioxide in the decomposition of peroxynitrite. Free Rad Biol Med 1997;23:331–338.
15. Padmaja S, Huie RE. The reaction of nitric oxide with organic peroxyl radicals. Biochem Biophys Res Commun 1993;195:539–544.
16. Rubbo H, Radi R, Trujillo M, Telleri R, Kalyanaraman B, Barnes S, Kirk M, Freeman BA. Nitric oxide regulation of superoxide and peroxynitrite-dependent lipid peroxidation. Formation of novel nitrogen-containing oxidized lipid derivatives. J Biol Chem 1994;269:26,066–26,075.
17. Nappi AJ, Vass E. Hydroxyl radical formation resulting from the interaction of nitric oxide and hydrogen peroxide. Biochim Biophys Acta 1998;1380:55–63.
18. Buxton BF, Greenstock CL, Helman WP, Ross AB. Critical review of rate constants for reactions of hydrated electrons. Hydrogen atoms and hydroxyl radicals in aqueous solution. J Phys Chem Ref Data 1988;17:513–886.
19. Wink DA, Ford PC. Nitric oxide reactions important to biological systems: a survey of some kinetics investigations. Methods 1995;7:14–20.
20. Kharitonov VG, Sundquist AR, Sharma VS. Kinetics of nitrosation of thiols by nitric oxide in the presence of oxygen. J Biol Chem 1995;270:28,158–28,164.
21. Stamler JS, Simon DI, Osborne JA, Mullins ME, Jaraki O, Michel T, Singel DJ, Loscalzo J. S-nitrosylation of proteins with nitric oxide: synthesis and characterization of biologically active compounds. Proc Natl Acad Sci USA 1992;89:444–448.
22. Stamler JS, Jaraki O, Osborne JA, Simon DI, Keaney JF Jr, Vita JA, Singel DJ, Valeri CR, Loscalzo J. Nitric oxide circulates in mammalian plasma primarily as an S-nitroso adduct of serum albumin. Proc Natl Acad Sci USA 1992;89:7674–7677.

23. Scharfstein JS, Keaney JF Jr, Slivka A, Welch GN, Vita JA, Stamler JS, Loscalzo J. In vivo transfer of nitric oxide between a plasma protein-bound reservoir and low molecular weight thiols. J Clin Invest 1994;94:1432–1439.

24. Pryor WA, Church DF, Govindan CK, Crank G. Oxidation of thiols by nitric oxide and nitrogen dioxide: synthetic utility and toxicological implications. J Org Chem 1982;47:156–159.

25. DeMaster EG, Quast BJ, Redfern B, Nagasawa HT. Reaction of nitric oxide with the free sulfhydryl group of human serum albumin yields a sulfenic acid and nitrous oxide. Biochemistry 1995;34: 11,494–11,499.

26. Lei SZ, Pan ZH, Aggarwal SK, Chen HS, Hartman J, Sucher NJ, Lipton SA. Effect of nitric oxide production on the redox modulatory site of the NMDA receptor-channel complex. Neuron 1992;8: 1087–1099.

27. Bolotina VM, Najibi S, Palacino JJ, Pagano PJ, Cohen RA. Nitric oxide directly activates calcium-dependent potassium channels in vascular smooth muscle. Nature 1994;368:850–853.

28. Wink DA, Cook JA, Kim SY, Vodovotz Y, Pacelli R, Krishna MC, Russo A, Mitchell JB, Jourd'heuil D, Miles AM, Grisham MB. Superoxide modulates the oxidation and nitrosation of thiols by nitric oxide-derived reactive intermediates. Chemical aspects involved in the balance between oxidative and nitrosative stress. J Biol Chem 1997;272:11,147–11,151.

29. Gow AJ, Buerk DG, Ischiropoulos H. A novel reaction mechanism for the formation of S-nitrosothiol in vivo. J Biol Chem 1997;272:2841–2845.

30. Boese M, Mordvintcev PI, Vanin AF, Busse R, Mulsch A. S-nitrosation of serum albumin by dinitrosyl-iron complex. J Biol Chem 1995;270:29,244–29,249.

31. Mirvish SS. Formation of N-nitroso compounds: chemistry, kinetics, and in vivo occurrence. Toxicol Appl Pharm 1975;31:325–351.

32. Challis BC, Fernandes MH, Glover BR, Latif F. Formation of diazopeptides by nitrogen oxides. IARC Sci Pub 1987;84:308–314.

33. Ridd JH. Diffusion control and pre-association of nitrosation, nitration and halogenation. Adv Phys Org Chem 1978;16:1–49.

34. Zhang YY, Xu AM, Nomen M, Walsh M, Keaney JF Jr, Loscalzo J. Nitrosation of tryptophan residue(s) in serum albumin and model dipeptides. Biochemical characterization and bioactivity. J Biol Chem 1996;271:14,271–14,279.

35. Stamler JS, Singel DJ, Loscalzo J. Biochemistry of nitric oxide and its redox-activated forms. Science 1992;258:1898–1902.

36. Wayland BB, Olson LW. Spectroscopic studies and bonding model for nitric oxide complexes of iron porphyrins. J Am Chem Soc 1974;96:6037–6041.

37. Jameson GB, Ibers JA. Biological and synthetic dioxygen carriers. In: Bertini I, Gray HB, Lippard SJ, Valentine JS, eds. Bioinorganic Chemistry. University Science Books, Mill Valley, CA, 1994, pp. 167–252.

38. Traylor TG, Sharma VS. Why NO? Biochemistry 1992;31:2847–2849.

39. Brucker EA, Olson JS, Ikeda-Saito M, Phillips GN Jr. Nitric oxide myoglobin: crystal structure and analysis of ligand geometry. Proteins 1998;30:352–356.

40. Doyle MP, Hoekstra JW. Oxidation of nitrogen oxides by bound dioxygen in hemoproteins. J Inorg Chem 1981;14:351–358.

41. Henry Y, Ducrocq C, Drapier JC, Servent D, Pellat C, Guissani A. Nitric oxide, a biological effector. Electron paramagnetic resonance detection of nitrosyl-iron-protein complexes in whole cells. Eur Biophys J 1991;20:1–15.

42. Vanin AF. [EMR identification of ferro-cysteine complexes in biological systems.] Identifikatsiia metodom EPR kompleksov dvukhvalentnogo zheleza s tsisteinom v biologischeskihk sistemakh. Biokhimiia 1967;32:277–282.

43. Drapier JC. Interplay between NO and [Fe-S] clusters: relevance to biological systems. Methods 1997; 11:319–329.

2

Cell and Molecular Biology of Nitric Oxide Synthases

Olivier Feron and Thomas Michel

THE MAMMALIAN NO SYNTHASE ISOFORMS

This chapter focuses on the factors influencing cellular and molecular regulation of the three known mammalian nitric oxide synthase (NOS) isoforms in the cardiovascular system. It is now known that the different NOS isoforms can be found in numerous different human tissues, including diverse locales within the cardiovascular system. The overall amino acid sequence identity for the three human NOS isoforms is approx 50–55%, with particularly strong sequence conservation in regions of the proteins involved in catalysis *(1)*. Alignment of the amino acid sequences of the different NOS isoforms reveals two domains of amino acid sequence similarity along the length of the proteins. The NOS C-terminal domain, comprising nearly half the molecule, has been termed the "reductase domain," as it bears striking sequence similarity to the mammalian cytochrome P450 reductase, and even shows significant sequence similarities to archetypal reductases from plants and bacteria. The N terminal domain, variably termed the heme or oxygenase domain, shows significant sequence similarities only among the three members of the NOS family, and contains the site for binding of the enzymes' heme prosthetic group. These striking similarities in the proteins' primary structure are likely to be reflected in homologies in their tertiary structure, but three-dimensional structural data currently exist only for the iNOS isoform *(2,3)*.

The three NOS enzyme isoforms are commonly denoted by prefixes that reflect the tissues of origin for the original isolation of their protein and cDNA: the nomenclature of nNOS, iNOS, and eNOS enzymes reflect their initial characterizations in neuronal tissue, immuno-activated macrophages, and endothelial cells, respectively *(4)*. The official nomenclature of the corresponding human NOS genes reflects instead the order of isolation and characterization of human genomic clones: the human genes encoding nNOS, iNOS, and eNOS are thus termed *NOS1*, *NOS2*, and *NOS3*, respectively. The three NOS genes share many features in their overall genomic structure, with striking similarity in the size of the exons and the location of the splice junctions, suggesting that the three NOS isoforms derive from a common ancestral gene. However, as might be anticipated from their distinct modes of transcriptional regulation and tissue-specific expression, there are significant divergences in the putative promoter regions among members of the NOS gene family.

The different NOS isoforms share a similar overall catalytic scheme, in which the homodimeric enzyme catalyzes the formation of NO° plus L-citrulline by oxidizing one of the two guanido nitrogens of the amino acid L-arginine. NOS catalysis involves the reduced form of nicotimamide adenine dinucleotide phosphate (NADPH) and molecular oxygen as cosubstrates, with the flavins adenine dinucleotide (FAD) and mononucleotide (FMN) representing key cofactors in promoting electron transfer to the NOS heme moiety; tetrahydrobiopterin

From: *Contemporary Cardiology, vol. 4: Nitric Oxide and the Cardiovascular System*
Edited by: J. Loscalzo and J. A. Vita © Humana Press Inc., Totowa, NJ

represents another key cofactor, but the role of this compound in NOS catalysis remains less well understood. For all three mammalian NOS isoforms, binding of the ubiquitous Ca^{2+}-binding regulatory protein calmodulin (CaM) appears to be required for efficient electron transfer between the reductase and oxygenase domain of NOSs (5,6). The dependence of the different NOS isoforms on Ca^{2+}/CaM constitutes, however, a major difference in the regulatory mechanisms of NO· production. Both nNOS and eNOS bind CaM in a reversible and Ca^{2+}-dependent manner, but iNOS avidly binds CaM even at the low ambient intracellular Ca^{2+} concentration characteristic of resting cells. iNOS activity in the cell is therefore largely independent of changes in intracellular Ca^{2+} (7), whereas the temporal pattern of nNOS or eNOS activation is closely regulated by transient changes in intracellular Ca^{2+}. The level of cellular iNOS activity appears to be closely related to the amount of iNOS protein, which, as a first approximation, is determined by mRNA abundance, which is in turn governed by the rate of iNOS gene transcription and by the stability of its mRNA. The principal form of iNOS regulation does appear to be at the level of genetic induction, hence its common appellation as an "inducible" enzyme. However, iNOS may be constitutively expressed under physiological conditions in some tissues, including pulmonary and bladder epithelia, and renal medulla (8,9). The eNOS and nNOS enzymes are often found expressed at stable levels in their characteristic tissues, and were originally denoted as "constitutive" enzymes. However, it has become clear that the expression of eNOS and nNOS genes can be regulated under different physiological and pathophysiological conditions (e.g., hemodynamic shear stress, nerve injury). In addition, posttranscriptional and posttranslational modifications importantly modulate the structure and function of all three NOS isoforms, as we discuss in detail in the following sections.

Neuronal NOS

GENOMIC STRUCTURE AND mRNA PROCESSING

The gene encoding nNOS (*NOS1*) includes 29 exons scattered over a region of 200 kb located on the human chromosome 12 (10,11). The full-length open reading frame of *NOS1* encodes a protein of 1434 amino acids with a predicted molecular mass of 160 kDa (12,13). Two major transcriptional clusters, denoted as neuronal- and testis-specific, have been identified for human *NOS1* (11,14); the identification of three potential polyadenylation sites adds to the complexity of *NOS1* posttranscriptional processing (14).

In the neuronal transcriptional cluster of the *NOS1* gene, distinct first exons of nNOS appear to splice to a common exon 2, which contains the initiator ATG codon. These different mRNA species, therefore, each encode the full-length nNOS protein, but the existence of distinct transcription initiation sites in different first exons may reflect the existence of tissue-specific or developmentally regulated NOS1 promoters. By contrast to the neuronal transcription cluster, the site for transcription initiation from the testis-specific cluster is located between exons 3 and 4, and the predicted site for initiation of translation lies within exon 5. Translation at this site would yield a truncated protein of 125 kDa, which has been termed TnNOS. The existence of the TnNOS protein is inferred from the isolation of its cognate transcript by highly sensitive reverse transcriptase–polymerase chain reaction techniques (RT-PCR), and its corresponding cDNA can be expressed in heterologous cell systems, but the naturally occurring TnNOS protein has not itself been identified (15). The truncated TnNOS would lack key sequences at the protein's extreme N-terminal (PDZ domain) thought to be important for nNOS targeting and protein–protein interactions in the full-length nNOS isoform. In the mouse, additional alternatively spliced nNOS transcripts have been identified: NOSβ and NOSγ appear to be analogous to the human TnNOS in that they lack exon 2 and would encode truncated nNOS without the N-terminal PDZ domain (16). Indeed, NOSγ and β were shown to account for the residual nNOS activity in nNOS knockout mice in which gene targeting inactivated the first coding exon but still allowed processing of transcripts starting downstream from the site of *NOS1* gene disruption *(17)*. Other exon deletions (exons 9/10) and insertions (between exon 16 and 17) have also been documented *(11,18,19)*. Although it remains to be demonstrated that the exon 9/10 deleted transcript is actually translated in vivo, some of the nNOS splice variants appear to be differentially regulated in cellular models of morphine tolerance *(20)*. Another alternatively processed nNOS transcript has been termed μNOS, which is formed by the insertion of 102 bp between exons 16 and 17. Expression of the μNOS protein has been established in rat and human penis as well as in rat skeletal muscle and heart *(18,19)*, and μNOS represents the only alternatively spliced nNOS transcript that has clearly been shown to correspond to a naturally occurring novel nNOS protein. The functional role of μNOS remains less well understood, but the presence of a distinct nNOS enzyme generated by differential mRNA processing identifies another potential point of regulation.

CELLULAR EXPRESSION AND (POST-)TRANSCRIPTIONAL REGULATION

To date, nNOS expression has been identified in diverse neurons throughout the central and peripheral nervous systems *(20)*, and nNOS has also been found in numerous nonneuronal tissues including skeletal muscle *(13,18)*, lung *(21)*, and the genitourinary tract *(15,19)*. Increases in the abundance of nNOS mRNA have been noted following physical and mechanical stresses, including spinal cord and nerve injuries *(22)*, ischemia *(23)*, hypoxia *(21)*, as well as changes in plasma osmolarity *(24)*. Neurotransmitters and hormones also influence the spatial and temporal pattern of *NOS1* expression: upregulation has been reported in various tissues during pregnancy *(25)* and in cerebellar granule cells following inhibition of glutaminergic transmission *(26)*; a development switch to μNOS *(see above)* was recently shown to occur in skeletal muscle in the process of myotube fusion *(18)*. Downregulation of *NOS1* expression is documented in rat brain following corticosterone treatment *(27)* and is also generally observed following bacterial lipopolysaccharide (LPS) and interferon-γ *(28,29)*.

Functional characterization of the *NOS1* gene transcriptional regulatory regions has yet to be established despite the identification of several *cis*-acting and *cis*-regulatory elements in the neuronal and testis transcriptional clusters *(11,14)*. Consensus sequences located in the putative *NOS1* promoter region suggest a possible role for diverse regulatory elements, including AP-1, AP-2, Sp-1, transcriptional enhancer factor-1/M-CAT binding factor, CREB, ATF, c*Fos*, Ets, NF-1, NF-κB motifs, GATA sites, p53 half-element, myocyte-specific enhancer factor 2 motif, and an insulin-responsive element. The presence of these putative regulatory motifs does not, in itself, establish their biological relevance, and the role, if any, of these diverse sequences for *NOS1* gene regulation remains to be defined.

"Inducible" Nitric Oxide Synthase

GENOMIC STRUCTURE AND MRNA PROCESSING

The iNOS gene (*NOS2*) is located on the human chromosome 17 and contains 26 exons spanning a region of 37 kb *(30)*. The full-length open reading frame encodes a protein of 1153 amino acids with a predicted molecular mass of 130 kDa. Alternatively spliced iNOS transcripts have been identified using RT-PCR chain reaction techniques *(31)*. Although they were using recombinant iNOS mutants, these authors showed that alternative splicing of exons 8 and 9 is critical for the enzyme dimerization, the endogenous expression of novel iNOS proteins derived from these transcripts has not yet been detected in tissues or cells.

CELLULAR EXPRESSION AND (POST-)TRANSCRIPTIONAL REGULATION

Since the prototypical iNOS enzyme was first characterized expressed in murine macrophages, numerous studies have documented that the *NOS2* gene can be induced in many different cell types. In human tissues, the initial report of iNOS expression in human hepatocytes *(32)* was followed by a plethora of studies showing iNOS expression following immunoactivation of macrophages, monocytes, myocytes, epithelial and endothelial cells, astrocytes, fibroblasts, keratinocytes, osteoblasts, and neutrophils/eosinophils (for review *see* ref. *33*). Although iNOS induction may generally reflect a pathophysiological cellular response to immunoactivation, it has been recently found that iNOS may be constitutively expressed in some tissues without any known antecedent exposure to pathological immunoactivating stimuli *(8,9)*, suggesting that iNOS may be subserving a physiological role in some tissues.

Most commonly, however, transcriptional induction of iNOS appears to be a consequence of immunoactivation, and numerous reports in a wide variety of cell types have explored iNOS induction in response to bacterial endotoxin or following stimulation by cytokines such as interferon-gamma (IFN-γ), tumor necrosis factor-alpha (TNF-α), and interleukin-1 (IL-1). It should be emphasized that even though a large number of different cell types have been found to express iNOS under different conditions of gene induction, one must use caution in extrapolating the transcriptional regulatory mechanisms characterized for one cellular system to another. For example, in some cell types the *NOS2* gene may be induced in response to cyclic adenosine monophosphate (cAMP)-elevating agents, by activation of protein kinase C (PKC), or by the action of various growth factors including platelet-derived growth factor (PDGF) and fibroblast growth factor (FGF) *(33)*. Comparison of the rodent and human *NOS2* gene promoter indicates that although only 1 kb of the proximal 5' flanking region of the murine promoter is required to confer endotoxin and cytokine inducibility, other critical cytokine-responsive elements are present between 3.8 and 16 kb upstream the initiation codon of the human gene *(34–36)*. Three γ-IRE as well as NF-κB, NF-IL6, and TNF-RE sites have however been identified in the very proximal 5'-flanking region of the human *NOS2* gene *(37–40)*. Among these elements, a functional role in transcriptional regulation of *NOS2* gene has been demonstrated for γ-IRE and NF-κB sites, and these elements appear to be involved in IFN-γ- and endotoxin-stimulated gene expression, respectively *(37,38)*. Shortly after the characterization of *NOS2* gene induction in macrophages and hepatocytes, several groups provided evidence for a similar glucocorticoid- and TGF-β-sensitive induction of iNOS by cytokine and lipopolysaccharide (LPS) in cardiac myocytes and microvascular endothelial cells *(41)*. As reported in other cell types, induction of the *NOS2* gene by IL-1β and IFN-γ in cardiac myocytes appears to be preceded by activation of MAPK (ERK1/ERK2) and STAT1α phosphorylation, a finding compatible with the presence of AP-1 and GAS sequences in the *NOS2* promoter *(42)*. Downregulation of *NOS2* gene induction is characteristically observed in various cell types following treatment with glucocorticoids or TGF-β *(33)*. The mechanisms involved in the deactivation of iNOS are less well understood: depending on the cell type, plausible regulatory pathways might include the repression of *NOS2* transcription, alterations in iNOS mRNA stability and/or processing, as well posttranslational mechanisms.

Endothelial Nitric Oxide Synthase

GENOMIC STRUCTURE AND mRNA PROCESSING

The gene encoding for eNOS (*NOS3*) is located on human chromosome 7 and contains 26 exons spanned on a region of 22 kb *(43–45)*. The full-length open reading frame codes for a protein of 1205 residues with a predicted molecular mass of 135 kDa. Alternative polyadenylation sites have been identified in the 3' untranslated region of the eNOS mRNA (K. Sase and T. Michel, unpublished observations; *see* ref. *46*), and may influence the differential stability or subcellular targeting of eNOS transcripts. Alternatively spliced transcripts encoding novel eNOS proteins have not been described.

CELLULAR EXPRESSION AND (POST-)TRANSCRIPTIONAL REGULATION

Immunohistochemical studies have located eNOS in various types of venous and arterial endothelial cells *(47)*, and significant endogenous expression was also reported in myocytes *(48)*, in neuronal cells *(49)*, in platelets *(50)*, and in various other tissues (*see* ref. *51*).

Present in the putative TATA-less promoter region of the eNOS gene are consensus sequences that potentially may serve as sites of binding for transcription/nuclear factors such as AP-1, AP-2, NF-1, IL6, as well as several putative NF-κB sites and several half-palindromic estrogen response elements *(43–45)*. Recently, two tightly clustered *cis*-regulatory regions were identified in the proximal enhancer of the human eNOS promoter using deletion analysis and linker-scanning mutagenesis *(52)*: positive regulatory domains I (–104/–95 relative to transcription initiation) and II (–144/–115). Analysis of *trans*-factor binding and functional expression studies revealed a surprising degree of cooperativity and complexity. The nucleoprotein complexes that form upon these regions in endothelial cells contained Ets family members, Sp1, variants of Sp3, MAZ, and YY1. Functional domain studies in *Drosophila* Schneider cells and endothelial cells revealed examples of positive and negative protein–protein cooperativity involving Sp1, variants of Sp3, Ets-1, Elf-1, and MAZ *(52)*. Therefore, multiprotein complexes are formed on the activator recognition sites within this 50-bp region of the human eNOS promoter in vascular endothelium.

Hemodynamic shear-stress and chronic exercise are among the stimuli that are associated with an increased abundance of the eNOS transcript *(53,54)*. Consensus sequences present in the eNOS 5' flanking region may represent *cis*-regulatory elements responsive to shear stress, and the presence of several half-palindromic estrogen-responsive elements may provide the means for transcriptional regulation of the eNOS gene in response to physiological or pathophysiological perturbations.

Hypoxia appears to influence eNOS abundance in cultured endothelial cells, causing a decrease in steady-state eNOS transcript levels associated with a decrease in eNOS mRNA stability *(55)*. However, in animal models, chronic hypoxia appears to be associated with an *increase* in eNOS mRNA abundance *(21)*. Cell proliferation also profoundly influences the expression of eNOS in cultured endothelial cells: eNOS transcript and protein abundance diminishes significantly when cells reach confluence *(56)*. Thus, any factors that influence endothelial cell growth rate may confound the interpretation of primary effects on eNOS gene expression. The nature, magnitude, and physiological relevance of studies showing altered eNOS transcript abundance analyzed in cultured endothelial cell model systems continue to be actively investigated. Among many other perturbations, sex steroids *(57,58)* or lipoproteins *(59–61)* may also influence the abundance of the eNOS transcript; findings in different experimental models have yielded mutually contradictory results and must be interpreted with caution.

Cytokines such as TNF-α are associated with a decrease in eNOS message and protein abundance in aortic endothelial cells, whereas paradoxically, NO synthesis increases (likely due to influences of the cytokine on NOS cofactor levels) *(62–64)*. The TNF-α-induced decrease in the abundance of the eNOS mRNA in bovine aortic endothelial cells appears to be due to a decrease in eNOS mRNA stability *(65)*; in contrast, transforming growth factor-β appears to increase the abundance of the eNOS transcript *(66)*.

POLYMORPHISMS IN THE *NOS3* GENE

The central role of NO in blood pressure homeostasis has led to studies exploring whether polymorphisms in any of the three NOS genes, or abnormalities in NOS cellular regulation, may be associated with hypertension. To date, there have been compelling experimental or population-based studies in support of a relationship between human *NOS1* polymorphism and hypertension. Although the *NOS2* gene maps to a region in the rat genome linked to hypertension in Dahl salt-sensitive rats *(67)*, disease association, and/or the relevance of this finding to human disease has yet to be established. Numerous studies have failed to link polymorphisms in introns of the human *NOS3* gene with cardiovascular diseases *(68)*; yet recent studies have documented the association of the missense variant Glu298Asp in exon 7 of the eNOS gene with essential hypertension and acute myocardial infarction in two independent populations of Japanese patients *(69,70)*. Interestingly, the same missense variant Glu298Asp was shown to be an independent risk factor for vasospastic angina pectosis *(71)* in Japanese populations. In contrast, other authors failed to find a relationship between the Glu298Asp polymorphism and ischemic cerebral disease in Caucasian populations *(72)*. Taken together, these results seem to indicate that, at least in Japanese populations, the missense variant Glu298Asp polymorphism is associated with, and could predispose to, various cardiovascular diseases. However, the functional consequences of the conservative amino acid change encoded by this eNOS genetic polymorphism have yet to be established.

Cardiovascular Phenotype of NOS Gene Knockout Mice

The characterization of mice with targeted disruption of NOS genes (NOS "knockout" mice) has provided important insights into the physiological and pathophysiological roles of the individual NOS isoforms in the cardiovascular system. Despite the ubiquitous expression of the NOS and their striking evolutionary conservation (and contrary to some expectations), mice with homozygous deletions of individual NOS isoforms are entirely viable. The roles of NO in diverse physiological processes can apparently be largely supplanted or compensated by other regulatory pathways in the cardiovascular system and elsewhere. For example, the nNOS knockout mice do not show any gross neuroanatomic abnormalities or even alteration of long-term potentiation (LTP) processes *(73)*, but do exhibit pyloric stenosis, and have been reported to display abnormal sexual and aggressive behavior *(74)*. iNOS knockout mice are grossly normal, but show increased susceptibility to infection *(75,76)*. From the standpoint of cardiovascular homeostasis, it is the eNOS knockout mice that document a most dramatic phenotype: eNOS$^{-/-}$ mice are hypertensive and show a mean arterial blood pressure approx 30% higher than wild-type littermates *(77)*. This is a key finding: despite the wide array of compensatory mechanisms controlling vascular tone, the genetic abrogation of eNOS cannot be overcome and leads to hypertension. However, treatment of eNOS null mice with pharmacological NOS inhibitors led to a paradoxical decrease in blood pressure *(77)*, suggesting perhaps a role for nNOS in the maintenance of blood pressure (note that nNOS –/– mice present a tendency toward hypotension under anesthesia *[78]*). Actually, the critical role of NO• produced by eNOS in the regulation of vascular tone was recently specifically addressed by the generation of transgenic mice overexpressing eNOS in the vascular wall (using murine preproendothelin-1 promoter) *(79)*. These authors reported that in agreement with the observed increase in basal NO• release and cGMP levels in transgenic aorta, blood pressure was significantly lower in eNOS-overexpressing mice than in control littermates.

The central role of NOS isoforms becomes much more evident when NOS knockout mice are subjected to pathophysiological perturbations. For example, a murine model of operatively induced hindlimb ischemia was recently used to investigate the impact of targeted disruption of the eNOS gene on angiogenesis *(80)*. Laser Doppler flow analysis and capillary measurements revealed that angiogenesis was impaired and was not improved by vascular endothelial growth factor (VEGF) administration in eNOS –/– mice versus wild-type. Moreover, in cerebral ischemia, NO• is known to rise dramatically associated with tissue damage, but the cellular source of NO• and its biological role were less well understood. Analyses of nNOS –/– mice with experimental cerebral infarcts documented reduced infarct size when compared with age-matched wild-type animals; these changes occur independently of alternations in blood flow *(81)*. The nNOS –/– mice are also resistant to ischemic injuries *(82)*, indicating that nNOS is importantly involved in neurotoxic damages. Interestingly, nonspecific NOS inhibitors appear to attenuate the reduced infarct size found in nNOS –/– mice, plausibly by inhibiting the eNOS-mediated relaxation of pial vessels. Indeed, transgenic mice that lack eNOS show, after middle cerebral artery (MCA) occlusion, increased infarct volume and reduced cerebral blood flow *(83)*. Furthermore, nonspecific NOS inhibitors decrease the infarct size in eNOS –/– mice but not in wild-type animals, confirming both that eNOS plays a protective role by maintaining regional cerebral blood flow in the setting of ischemia and that nNOS contributes to neurotoxicity. iNOS also appears to be involved in late neuronal injury following experimental stroke: iNOS null mice show reduced infarct volumes when compared with wild-type animals *(84)*.

COVALENT MODIFICATIONS OF NOS ISOFORMS

Phosphorylation

The three NOS isoforms can be phosphorylated in vitro by purified protein kinases and can be isolated as phosphoproteins in cultured cell systems. However, to date, the roles of specific protein kinases and phosphatases have not been specifically delineated any of the isoforms and the role and regulation of NOS phosphorylation remain incompletely understood. For example, although nNOS has been shown to serve as a substrate for a variety of protein kinases in vitro *(49,85,86)*, phosphorylation of nNOS in neurons has not been definitively demonstrated. In addition, different studies have observed variable effects of nNOS phosphorylation on enzymatic activity, and these in vitro analyses have not yet been clearly correlated with the enzyme's phosphorylation in native cells *(85,86)*. Phosphorylation of iNOS has been even less extensively characterized *(7)*, although a recent report suggests that tyrosine phosphorylation of the enzyme may serve to increase its activity *(87)*. Serine phosphorylation of eNOS was shown to occur in endothelial cells subsequent to agonist-induced translocation of the enzyme to the cytosol *(88)*, suggesting that eNOS deactivation may be regulated by phosphorylation. Treatment of endothelial cells with phorbol esters has also been shown to diminish NO• production, suggesting that phosphorylation may be associated with inhibition of eNOS activity *(89)*. Possible clinical significance for these findings was suggested by studies reported by Craven et al. *(90)*, who correlated increased PKC activity with decreased NO• production in glomeruli isolated from diabetic rats. These investigators further demonstrated that inhibition of PKC restored normal NO• production, suggesting that changes in eNOS phosphorylation may modulate the alterations in NO• signaling observed in diabetic vascular disease. Additionally, several groups have reported that the activation of eNOS by hemodynamic shear stress in cultured endothelial cells is influenced by reagents that modulate protein tyrosine kinase activity *(91–93)*. Tyrosine phosphorylation of eNOS has been explored in several studies with contradictory results: several investigators failed to document any tyrosine phosphorylation of eNOS *(92,94)* whereas others reported either tyrosine phosphorylation *(95)* or dephosphorylation *(93)* of eNOS following incubation of endothelial cells with high concentrations of protein tyrosine phosphatase inhibitors. To date, no physiological agonists promoting the tyrosine phosphorylation of eNOS have been identified, although many agonists that modulate eNOS clearly affect tyrosine phosphorylation pathways, as well.

Acylation

MYRISTOYLATION AND PALMITOYLATION

eNOS is unique among the NOS isoforms in its being dually acylated by myristate and palmitate 14- and 16-carbon saturated fatty acids, respectively (for review *see* ref. *50*), and importantly, both modifications are required for an efficient targeting of the enzyme to plasmalemmal caveolae *(96)*. Myristoylation occurs cotranslationally on an N-terminal glycine residue within a specific consensus sequence (MGXXXS) *(97)* and is essentially irreversible, precluding its dynamic regulation by agonists or other stimuli *(98)*. Moreover, the stable membrane association of myristoylated proteins often requires hydrophobic or electrostatic interactions in addition to those between myristate and membrane lipids; for eNOS, several lines of evidence *(99,100)* suggest that this membrane-targeting role is subserved by palmitoylation.

Palmitoylation of eNOS takes place on two cysteine residues near the protein's N-terminus (Cys-15 and Cys-26) that define a novel motif for protein palmitoylation *(99,101)*. No general consensus sequence for protein palmitoylation has been identified *(98,102)*, although some dually acylated G protein α subunits and members of the Src family of tyrosine kinases are palmitoylated at a cysteine residue within a conserved N-terminal sequence not found in the NOS isoforms. The two palmitoylated cysteines in eNOS flank an unusual Gly–Leu repeat [(Gly–Leu)$_5$] not otherwise described in the protein sequence database. Mutagenesis of the palmitoylation site cysteine residues (to serine) markedly attenuates the association of eNOS with the particulate subcellular fraction, documenting a key role for this posttranslational modification in eNOS targeting *(99)*. The myristoylation-deficient mutant eNOS also fails to undergo palmitoylation *(100)*, plausibly because the mutant is not targeted to the plasma membrane, the presumed site for protein palmitoylation *(98)*. The myristoylation-deficient eNOS is thus de facto an acylation-deficient enzyme, undergoing neither of the fatty acid modifications characteristic of the wild-type eNOS; this acylation-deficient enzyme is entirely cytosolic. The palmitoylation-deficient mutant eNOS still undergoes myristoylation, and, as noted earlier, its membrane targeting is reduced but not completely abrogated. Dual acylation of eNOS is thus required for efficient membrane localization, with cotranslational *N*-myristoylation and posttranslational thiopalmitoylation playing key roles in enzyme targeting.

DYNAMIC REGULATION OF PALMITOYLATION

Palmitoylation is a reversible posttranslational modification that has been shown to modulate the interaction of signaling proteins with the membrane *(103)*. For example, agonist regulation of protein palmitoylation has previously been described for G protein-coupled receptors, such as the β-adrenergic receptor *(104)*. For some peripheral membrane proteins, the loss of palmitate may correlate with protein redistribution to the cytosolic subcellular fraction. Agonists activating G protein α$_s$ appear to stimulate α$_s$ palmitate turnover, specifically accelerating depalmitoylation *(102,105)*. There are striking parallels for eNOS: pulse-chase experiments in endothelial cells biosynthetically labeled with [^{3}H]palmitate showed that bradykinin treatment may promote eNOS depalmitoylation *(100)*. However, it must be noted that another study *(101)* failed to document agonist modulation of eNOS palmitoylation; interpretation of the negative results of this latter study are confounded by the challenges of studying intracellular modulation of biosynthetically labeled proteins under non-steady-state conditions. This controversy aside, reversible palmitoylation of eNOS represents a plausible mechanism for modulating the binding of a large hydrophilic protein such as eNOS to membranes. Depalmitoylation could therefore be part of a cellular mechanism for the release of (myristoylated) eNOS from the plasma membrane and translocation to other cellular structures in response to agonist stimulation. Conversely, repalmitoylation could then facilitate the process of retargeting to specialized compartments such as caveolae (*see* following).

The palmitoylation of several signaling proteins has been shown to influence their signaling activities as well as their subcellular localization *(98,102)*. However, important differences have been noted in the regulatory roles of palmitoylation, even among closely related proteins. The receptor-mediated processes that regulate reversible palmitoylation of signaling proteins are not well understood, and few enzymes involved in the formation or hydrolysis of palmitoyl–protein thioesters have been extensively characterized. A protein palmitoylthioesterase was recently isolated and cloned from bovine brain *(106)*. This palmitoylthioesterase is expressed in diverse cell types, including vascular endothelial cells *(107)*, but its regulatory characteristics are not fully defined, and its relationship to eNOS palmitoylation is completely unknown. Another palmitoylthioesterase has been isolated that appears to be involved in the depalmitoylation of the G protein alpha$_s$ *(108)*, but the role of this enzyme in the regulation of eNOS depalmitoylation remains to be established. Another possibility is that eNOS activation itself could influence depalmitoylation, with NO production itself playing a role. It has recently been shown that NO reduces [^{3}H]palmitate labeling of two nerve growth cone-associated proteins *(109)*. NO might also regulate palmitoyl thioesterase activity or directly influence eNOS palmitoylation via nitrosothiol formation at the site(s) of palmitoylation.

An understanding of the regulation of eNOS palmitoylation/depalmitoylation cycles has been facilitated by the development of heterologous cellular expression systems that permit the reconstitution of endogenous signaling pathways by cotransfecting cDNAs encoding wild-type and acylation-deficient eNOS along with constructs encoding specific cell surface receptors. Using this approach, it was shown that muscarinic cholinergic agonist stimulation rapidly induced the reversible dissociation of eNOS from caveolin. These studies revealed further that enzyme repalmitoylation markedly accelerated eNOS retargeting to caveolae following prolonged agonist stimulation *(110)*.

FUNCTIONAL ROLE OF eNOS TARGETING

The importance of eNOS myristoylation was recently illustrated in an elegant study examining the implication of eNOS in a form of synaptic plasticity termed long-term potentiation (LTP). Kantor and colleagues *(111)* showed that LTP can be attenuated in brain slices by pretreating them with the myristoylation inhibitor, hydroxymyristic acid (HMA). To rule out the possibility than a myristoylated protein other than eNOS was involved, they infected brain slices with a recombinant adenovirus vector encoding a chimeric eNOS protein wherein the N-terminal glycine required for myristoylation is replaced by the extracellular and trans-membrane domain of CD8. Using this fusion protein, they showed that the chimeric eNOS could be targeted to plasma membrane by the CD8 transmembrane sequence (independently of eNOS acylation), and importantly, that the HMA-induced inhibition of LTP was fully rescued by the CD8–eNOS construct. The plasma membrane targeting of eNOS therefore appears necessary for NO to fulfill its proposed role of retrograde messenger, probably by promoting its release into the extrasynaptic region and also by facilitating the enzyme activation by plasmalemmal Ca^{2+} influx.

eNOS acylation also appears to play a vital role in coupling the muscarinic cholinergic NO-mediated regulation of heart rate *(112)*. Cardiac myocytes isolated from mice lacking a functional eNOS gene have proven valuable for the study of eNOS in myocyte function. Cardiac myocytes isolated from these eNOS gene-targeted mice lack the muscarinic cholinergic attenuation in beating rate seen in wild-type mice. The muscarinic cholinergic response can be reconstituted in these cells by the transfection of cDNA constructs encoding wild type eNOS, but not by plasmids encoding the myristoylation-deficient eNOS mutant. In transfected cardiac myocytes expressing wild-type eNOS, the muscarinic cholinergic agonist carbachol completely abrogated the spontaneous beating rate and induced a fourfold elevation of the cyclic guanosine monophosphate (cGMP) level. By contrast, in the myr⁻ eNOS myocytes, carbachol failed to exert its negative chronotropic effect and to increase cGMP levels. These data document an obligatory role for acylated eNOS, which is endogenously expressed in cardiac myocytes, and suggest an important role for eNOS in the modulation of heart rate control.

Although nNOS is not acylated, nNOS directly interacts with two palmitoylated proteins, i.e., PSD-95 in neurons *(113)* and caveolin-3 in skeletal muscle *(114)*. In both cases, the protein–protein association was shown to account for the targeting of the enzyme in these specialized cell compartments (*see* following) and it can, therefore, be postulated that any change in the palmitoylation of nNOS partners could have, as for the eNOS protein, dramatic effects on the location and functional activity of the enzyme.

SUBCELLULAR LOCALIZATION OF NOSs

Criteria

Almost every conceivable intracellular organelle has been postulated as a possible site for NO synthesis, from the plasma membrane to the cell nucleus. There is considerable

NOS in the Cytoskeleton

There are suggestive studies that indicate eNOS may associate with cytoskeletal proteins *(93,114)*. Intuitively, the targeting or association of eNOS with the cytoskeleton may provide a mechanism for mechanochemical coupling of changes in cell shape (e.g., with hemodynamic shear stress or cardiac myocyte contraction) to regulation of the enzyme. However, whether eNOS undergoes direct interactions with cytoskeletal proteins remains to be established by rigorous methodology. By contrast, the cytoskeleton association is much more clearly established for nNOS by virtue of its association with the cytoskeletal dystrophin complex in skeletal muscle *(16,132)* (*see* following). Furthermore, members of the postsynaptic-density 95 family of cytoskeletal proteins, which are known to interact with nNOS, have been shown to mediate receptor clustering at excitatory synapses in the brain *(133)*.

NOS in Specialized Intracellular Organelles

In primary macrophages, subcellular fractionation and immunohistochemical approaches have established the presence of iNOS in intracellular vesicles (phagosomes?), possibly reflecting a locale for NO•-dependent killing of opsonized intracellular microorganisms *(134)*. The molecular mechanisms whereby iNOS is targeted to these macrophage vesicles is not clear, and it remains to be established whether iNOS is similarly targeted in other cells.

REGULATION OF NOS BY PROTEIN-PROTEIN ASSOCIATIONS

Calmodulin: The First NOS-Associated Protein

The requirement for calmodulin in nitric oxide synthesis is an essential characteristic of all three NOS isoforms, although this ubiquitous Ca^{2+} regulatory protein demonstrates important isoform-specific differences in its role as an allosteric activator. Indeed, nNOS and eNOS are low-output NOS whose activity is regulated by Ca^{2+}/calmodulin, increasing as Ca^{2+} rises and decreasing as Ca^{2+} falls. By contrast, iNOS is a high-output NOS whose activity is essentially Ca^{2+}-independent, as calmodulin is very tightly bound to the enzyme.

Moreover, in the case of eNOS, and probably for nNOS in skeletal muscle, calmodulin activation of the enzyme involves not only the binding to the calmodulin binding motif within the NOS sequence but also the allosteric displacement of caveolin from NOS, thereby reversing the inhibitory effect of the scaffolding protein.

nNOS, PSD-93/95, and the Dystrophin Complex

The sarcolemma of skeletal muscle contains a family of intracellular and transmembrane glycoproteins associated with dystrophin, linking the extracellular matrix with the actin-based cytoskeleton. The N-terminus of nNOS interacts with α1-syntrophin, a binding partner of dystrophin through a PDZ/GLGF protein motif of approx 100 amino acids present in both proteins *(132)*. The PDZ-containing domain of nNOS also binds to PDZ repeats in postsynaptic density 95 (PSD-95). In certain nonneuronal cells, including developing chromaffin cells of the adrenal gland and secretory cells of salivary gland, nNOS is coexpressed with the related protein PSD-93 *(16)*. Binding interaction between PDZ domains are selective. Though nNOS binds to the PDZ motif in α1-syntrophin and to the second PDZ motif of PSD-95, nNOS does not associate with the first and third PDZ motifs in PSD-95 *(16)*. Certain PDZ domains are capable of binding to the extreme C-terminus of a family of receptors and ion channels, including *N*-methyl-D-aspartate (NMDA) receptors, Shaker-type K^+ channels, and FAS. Brenman and colleagues found that nNOS and NMDA receptors compete for common or nearby binding sites within the second PDZ repeat of a PSD-95 subunit. The PDZ consensus sequence is present in a diverse family of enzymes and structural proteins. Many of these proteins are found concentrated at specialized cell–cell junctions, such as neuronal synapses, epithelial zona occludens, and septate junctions. PDZ domains may therefore be important elements of interactions required for signal transduction at the membrane. Furthermore, the finding that PDZ/GLGF is present in a heterogeneous family of enzymes has motivated suggestions that the Gly-Leu-Gly-Phe (GLGF) domain may regulate enzyme activities. However, Bredt and colleagues (12) found that deletion of the GLGF domain of nNOS does not alter NOS catalytic activity in transfected cells.

PIN and CAPON

By means of yeast two-hybrid system screening, a 10-kDa protein was identified that physically interacts with and specifically inhibits the activity of nNOS (135). These authors named this protein PIN (for protein inhibitor of neuronal NOS) and presented evidence that the PIN/nNOS interaction leads to the destabilization of the nNOS dimer. Contradictory results (136; I. Rodriguez-Crespo, personal communication) were recently reported according which PIN inhibits all isoforms of NOS and has no effect on nNOS dimerization; stoichiometric analysis also shows that an approx 300-fold molar excess of PIN are required to inhibit nNOS by 50%. Moreover, PIN was simultaneously discovered as a light chain (LC) of dynein and myosin, with a highly conserved sequence over a wide spectrum of different organisms (137), and the role of the NOS inhibitor therefore appears as secondary to its other functions in myosin and dynein complexes. Clearly, the relevance of the PIN/nNOS remains to be rigorously established and considering that the stoichiometry represents a limiting factor, it may be most interesting to explore physiological or pathological conditions where high levels of PIN/dynein LC expression are observed. In this perspective, Gillardon and colleagues (138) recently reported that following global ischemia, mRNA expression of PIN/dynein LC was rapidly induced in pyramidal neurons of the hippocampal CA3 region and granule cell of the dentate gyrus which are resistant to ischemic damage. In vulnerable CA1 pyramidal neurons however, PIN/dynein LC remained at basal level after global ischemia and was associated to neuronal cell death.

CAPON (for carboxyl-terminal PDZ ligand of nNOS) is a recently identified cytosolic protein highly enriched in brain that competes with particulate PSD95 for interaction with nNOS (139). The interaction CAPON/nNOS is highly specific, and although CAPON does not inhibit nNOS activity by itself, CAPON is thought to reduce the accessibility of nNOS to NMDA receptor-mediated calcium influx, thus diminishing the capacity of nNOS to acutely produce NO•. Although phosphorylation of nNOS by various kinases failed to alter the CAPON/nNOS interaction, phosphorylation of CAPON in its C-terminal region could be involved through disruption of its specific β-sheet conformation sequence in the regulation of the interaction (139). Clearly, more needs to be learned and studies are, no doubt, underway to examine the native CAPON/nNOS association in its physiological environment and to address specific questions such as the stoichiometry of the protein–protein interaction.

ENAP-1 or Hsp90

Stimulation of aortic endothelial cells with bradykinin produces cycles of tyrosine phosphorylation/dephosphorylation of a 90-kDa protein, termed ENAP-1 (for eNOS-associated protein-1) by Venema and colleagues (94). This protein, recently identified as the heat-shock protein 90 (Hsp90), appears to facilitate eNOS activation in endothelial cells by forming a heterocomplex with the enzyme following stimulation with a Ca^{2+}-mobilizing agonist or shear stress (140). In the specific case of shear stress, the eNOS/Hsp90 association appears to be somewhat delayed relative to that seen following agonist stimulation (94) and may correspond with the slower change in detergent solubility of eNOS seen in endothelial cells following exposure to shear stress (93).

Caveolin-1, Caveolin-3 and Their Regulatory Cycles

Following the original observation of the caveolar localization of eNOS in plasmalemmal caveolae *(96)*, several lines of evidence in endothelial cells and cardiac myocytes revealed that eNOS is quantitatively associated with caveolin, the structural protein within caveolae *(141)*. Further experiments revealed that this association leads to the inhibition of the enzyme activity, and that a stable protein–protein interaction takes place between both proteins *(142–146)*. Consensus sequences were identified within both proteins: the *scaffolding domain of caveolin*, a juxtamembrane region of 20 amino acids in the C-terminal moiety of caveolin *(143,145)*, and a putative *caveolin-binding motif*, a peptide sequence rich in aromatic residues localized in the oxygenase domain of eNOS *(114,144,146)*; more recently, sites for caveolin inhibition of eNOS have been identified within the reductase domain of the enzyme *(147)* and within the caveolin N-terminal region *(145)*. Like other modular protein domains, the scaffolding domain of caveolin appears to function by providing frameworks for the assembly of preassembled oligomeric signaling proteins, but, in addition, these structures maintain these diverse signaling proteins in their "off" state. The caveolin/eNOS interaction constitutes a new biological framework within which to understand the regulation of eNOS, yet many details still remain to be addressed to attribute to each interaction level the corresponding effect on the catalytic properties and/or targeting of eNOS.

In order for eNOS to be fully activated, caveolin must dissociate from the enzyme. The ubiquitous Ca^{2+} regulatory protein calmodulin (CaM) disrupts the heteromeric complex formed between eNOS and caveolin in a Ca^{2+}-dependent fashion *(142)*: caveolin serves as a competitive inhibitor of CaM-dependent eNOS activation *(143)*. The CaM binding consensus sequence is located at the border of the NOS reductase and heme domains, and CaM binding to this site activates NO synthesis by enabling the reductase domain to transfer electrons to the heme domain. Caveolin appears to attenuate this electron transfer, and CaM apparently rescues the caveolin-inhibited eNOS at this level, probably by binding to sequences in the eNOS reductase domain *(147)*. This close control of enzyme activity may be particularly important for eNOS in caveolae, where CaM is also largely enriched *(96)* and could thus lead to undesired enzyme activation if the interaction of caveolin with eNOS was not keeping the system in check. The relevance of the caveolin/CaM reciprocal regulation of eNOS was recently demonstrated in intact cells wherein transient increase in $[Ca^{2+}]_i$ consequent to agonist activation was shown to promote the dissociation of eNOS from caveolin, associated with translocation of eNOS from caveolae *(110,144)*. Such agonist-induced disruption of the caveolin/eNOS heterocomplex promotes the dissociation of the enzyme from proximity to the transporter of arginine *(119)* and thus, may serve as a feedback mechanism for eNOS activation (*see* earlier).

An obvious question raised by the findings of the counterbalancing modulation of eNOS by caveolin and CaM is related to the cellular regulation of eNOS/caveolin interaction in the context of enzyme acylation. We have observed that the myr⁻ and palm⁻ eNOS mutants may both interact with caveolin in the cytosol *(110,148)*; this association also leads to a marked inhibition of enzyme activity, which is completely reversed by addition of CaM *(144)*. The regulatory caveolin/eNOS association therefore appears independent of the state of eNOS acylation, indicating that agonist-evoked Ca^{2+}/CaM-dependent disruption of the caveolin–eNOS complex, rather than agonist-promoted depalmitoylation of eNOS, relieves caveolin's tonic inhibition of enzyme activity. Thus, we propose that caveolin may serve as an eNOS chaperone regulating NO• production independently of the enzyme's residence within caveolae or its state of acylation *(110,148)*.

These data suggest a dynamic cycle of eNOS–caveolin interactions initiated by agonist-promoted increases in $[Ca^{2+}]_i$ that disrupt the caveolin–eNOS complex, leading to enzyme activation. Following more prolonged agonist stimulation, eNOS is likely to be depalmitoylated, and is no longer selectively sequestered in caveolae. The translocated enzyme then partitions into noncaveolar plasma membrane and also in the perinuclear region of the cell *(131)*, the precise identity of which has not yet been established. Furthermore, several lines of evidence indicate that subsequently to the enzyme's translocation, and following the decline in $[Ca^{2+}]_i$ to basal levels, eNOS may once again interact with caveolin and is then retargeted to caveolae, a process accelerated (or stabilized) by enzyme palmitoylation *(110, 144)*. The reassociation of eNOS with caveolin could occur either at the plasma or perinuclear membrane levels or even in the cytosol through which caveolin complexes may shuttle between caveolae and an internalized caveolar vesicle/*trans*-Golgi network.

G-Protein-Coupled Receptors

A direct interaction between eNOS and seven-transmembrane-segment receptors has recently been described by Ju and colleagues *(149)*: the bradykinin B2 receptor appears to be able to physically associate, through its fourth intracellular domain, with eNOS. Similar results were obtained using peptides derived from the angiotensin II receptor AT-1. This intriguing signaling paradigm was explored principally by studying purified proteins and synthetic peptides, and the role of these protein–peptide interactions remains to be established in intact cell systems. Although a small fraction of cellular eNOS appears to be physically associated with the B2 receptor (<5%), the agonist dependence of this reversible interaction increases the likelihood that these interactions may have physiological relevance. Clearly, more experiments need to be done to understand the role of this nonconventional model of direct receptor–effector coupling.

THE BASEBALL CATCHER'S MITT

Recently published analyses of the crystal structure analysis of NOS have begun to reveal how enzyme dimerization and cofactor/substrate binding combine to form the catalytic center for $NO^{\bullet}$ synthesis *(2,3)*. The structure of the NOS oxygenase dimer has been compared to a left-handed baseball catcher's mitt, with heme clasped in the palm. Interestingly, dimerization creates a 3-nm-deep, funnel-shaped, active-center channel by refolding and recruiting the pterin, thereby exposing a heme edge and the adjacent Trp residue for reductase domain interactions. This Trp residue may form part of the caveolin binding motif, and it can therefore be hypothesized that caveolin binding may biologically regulate NOS by blocking the reductase domain of NOS from supplying electrons to the heme. This finding provides an excellent example of how crystal structure determination may help dissecting the regulatory mechanisms of NOS activation. Perhaps even more exciting is the unexpected finding revealed by crystallography of a Zn^{2+} atom bound at the protein–protein interface of the eNOS dimer *(150)*, a finding that opens intriguing perspectives of investigations for the biochemist, the pathologist, and the drug designer.

REFERENCES

1. Michel T, Xie Q-W, Nathan C. Molecular biological analysis of nitric oxide synthases. In: Feelisch M, Stamler JS, eds. Methods in Nitric Oxide Research. Wiley, Chichester, UK, 1995, pp. 161–175.
2. Crane BR, Arvai AS, Gachhui R, Wu C, Ghosh DK, Getzoff ED, et al. The structure of nitric oxide synthase oxygenase domain and inhibitor complexes. Science 1997;278:425–431.
3. Crane BR, Arvai AS, Ghosh DK, Wu C, Getzoff ED, Stuehr J, et al. Structure of nitric oxide synthase oxygenase dimer with pterin and substrate. Science 1998;279:2121–2125.
4. Moncada S, Higgs A, Furchgott R. International Union of Pharmacology nomenclature in nitric oxide research. Pharmacol Rev 1997;49:137–142.
5. Fukuto JM, Mayer B. The enzymology of nitric oxide synthase. In: Feelisch M, Stamler JS, eds. Methods in Nitric Oxide Research. Wiley, Chichester, UK, 1996, pp. 147–160.
6. Stuehr DJ. Structure-function aspects in the nitric oxide synthases. Ann Rev Pharmacol Toxicol 1997; 37:339–359.

7. Nathan C, Xie Q-W. Regulation of biosynthesis of nitric oxide. J Biol Chem 1994;269:13,725–13,728.
8. Guo FH, De Raeve HR, Rice TW, Stuehr DJ, Thunnissen FB, Erzurum SC. Continuous nitric oxide synthesis by inducible nitric oxide synthase in normal human airway epithelium in vivo. Proc Natl Acad Sci USA 1995;92:7809–7813.
9. Morrissey JJ, McCracken R, Kaneto H, Vehaskari M, Montani D, Klahr S. Location of an inducible nitric oxide synthase mRNA in the normal kidney. Kidney Int 1994;45:998–1005.
10. Kishimoto J, Spurr N, Liao M, Lizhi L, Emson P, Xu W. Localization of brain nitric oxide synthase (NOS) to human chromosome 12. Genomics 1992;14:802–804.
11. Hall AV, Antoniou H, Wang Y, Cheung AH, Arbus AM, Olson SL, et al. Structural organization of the human neuronal nitric oxide synthase gene (NOS1). J Biol Chem 1994;269:33,082–33,090.
12. Bredt DS, Hwang PM, Glatt CE, Lowenstein C, Reed RR, Snyder SH. Cloned and expressed nitric oxide synthase structurally ressembles cytochrome P-450 reductase. Nature 1991;351:714–718.
13. Nakane M, Schmidt HH, Pollock JS, Förstermann U, Murad F. Cloned human brain nitric oxide synthase is highly expressed in skeletal muscle. FEBS Lett 1993;316:175–180.
14. Xie J, Roddy P, Rife TK, Murad F, Young AP. Two closely linked but separable promoters for human neuronal nitric oxide synthase gene transcription. Proc Natl Acad Sci USA 1995;92:1242–1246.
15. Wang Y, Goligorsky MS, Lin M, Wilcox JN, Marsden PA. A novel, testis-specific mRNA transcript encoding an NH2-terminal truncated nitric-oxide synthase. J Biol Chem 1997;272:11,392–11,401.
16. Brenman JE, Chao DS, Gee SH, McGec AW, Craven SE, Santillano DR, et al. Interaction of nitric oxide synthase with the postsynaptic density potein PSD-95 and alpha1-syntrophin mediated by PDZ domains. Cell 1996;84:757–767.
17. Eliasson MK, Blackshaw S, Scheil MJ, Snyder SH. Neuronal nitric oxide synthase alternatively spliced forms: prominent functional localizations in the brain. Proc Natl Acad Sci USA 1997;94: 3396–3401.
18. Silvagno F, Xia H, Bredt DS. Neuronal nitric-oxide synthase-μ, an alternatively spliced isoform expressed in differentiated skeletal muscle. J Biol Chem 1996;271:11,204–11,208.
19. Magee T, Fuentes AM, Garban H, Rajavashisth T, Marquez D, Rodriguez JA, et al. Cloning of a novel neuronal nitric oxide synthase expressed in penis and lower urinary tract. Biochem Biophys Res Commun 1996;226:145–151.
20. Chao DS, Hwang PM, Huang F, Bredt DS. Localization of neuronal nitric oxide synthase. Methods Enzymol 1996;268:488–496.
21. Lin LH, Sandra A, Boutelle S, Talman WT. Up-regulation of nitric oxide synthase and its mRNA in vagal motor nuclei following axotomy in rat. Neurosci Lett 1997;221:97–100.
22. Samdani AF, Dawson TM, Dawson VL. Nitric oxide synthase in models of focal ischemia. Stroke 1997;28:1283–1288.
23. Shaul PW, North AJ, Brannon TS, Ujiie K, Wells LB, Nisen PA, et al. Prolonged in vivo hypoxia enhances nitric oxide synthase type I and type III gene expression in adult rat lung. Am J Respir Cell Mol Biol 1995;13:167–174.
24. O'Shea RD, Gundlach AL. Food or water deprivation modulate nitric oxide synthase (NOS) activity and gene expression in rat hypothalamic neurones: correlation with neurosecretory activity? J Neuroendocrinol 1996;8:417–425.
25. Luckman SM, Huckett L, Bicknell RJ, Voisin DL, Herbison AE. Up-regulation of nitric oxide synthase messenger RNA in an integrated forebrain circuit involved in oxytocin secretion. Neuroscience 1997; 77:37–48.
26. Baader SL, Schilling K. Glutamate receptors mediate dynamic regulation of nitric oxide synthase expression in cerebellar granule cells. J Neurosci 1996;16:1440–1449.
27. Weber CM, Eke BC, Maines MD. Corticosterone regulates heme oxygenase-2 and NO synthase transcription and protein expression in rat brain. J Neurochem 1994;63:953–962.
28. Gath I, Gödtel-Armbrust U, Förstermann U. Expressional downregulation of neuronal-type NO synthase I in guinea pig skeletal muscle in response to bacterial lipopolysaccharide. FEBS Lett 1997;410: 319–323.
29. Bandyopadhyay A, Chakder S, Rattan S. Regulation of inducible and neuronal nitric oxide synthase gene expression by interferon-gamma and VIP. Am J Physiol 1997;272:C1790–C1797.
30. Chartrain N, Geller DA, Koty PP, Sintrin NF, Nussler AK, Hoffman EP, et al. Molecular cloning structure, and chromosomal mapping of the human inducible nitric oxide synthase gene. J Biol Chem 1994;269:6765–6772.
31. Eissa NT, Yuan JW, Haggerty CM, Choo EK, Palmer CD, Moss J. Cloning and characterization of human inducible nitric oxide synthase splice variants: a domain, encoded by exons 8 and 9, is critical for dimerization. Proc Natl Acad Sci USA 1998;95:7625–7630.

32. Nussler AK, DiSilvio M, Billiar TR, Hoffman RA, Geller DA, Selby R, et al. Stimulation of the nitric oxide synthase pathway in human hepatocytes by cytokines and endotoxin. J Exp Med 1992;176: 261–264.
33. Geller DA, Billiar TR. Molecular biology of nitric oxide synthases. Cancer Metastasis Rev 1998; 17:7–23.
34. de Vera ME, Shapiro RA, Nussler AK, Mudgett JS, Simmons RI, Morris SM Jr, et al. Transcriptional regulation of human inducible nitric oxide synthase (NOS2) gene by cytokines: initial analysis of the human NOS2 promoter. Proc Natl Acad Sci USA 1996;93:1054–1059.
35. Xie QW, Whisnan R, Nathan C. Promoter of the mouse gene encoding calcium-independent nitric oxide synthase confers inducibility by interferon-γ and bacterial lipopolysaccharide. J Exp Med 1993; 177:1779–1784.
36. Lowenstein CJ, Alley EW, Raval P, Snowman AM, Snyder SH, Russel SW, et al. Macrophage nitric oxide synthase gene: two upstream regions mediate induction by interferon-γ and lipopolysaccharide. Proc Natl Acad Sci USA 1993;90:9730–9734.
37. Pearse RN, Feinman R, Ravetch JV. Characterization of the promoter of the human gene encoding the high-affinity IgC receptor: transcriptional induction by γ-interferon is mediated through common DNA response elements. Proc Natl Acad Sci USA 1991;88:11,305–11,309.
38. Libermann TA, Baltimore D. Activation of interleukin-6 gene expression through the NF-κB transcription factor. Mol Cell Biol 1990;10:2327–2334.
39. Leitman DC, Ribeiro RC, Mackow ER, Baxter JD, West BL. Identification of a tumor necrosis factor-responsive element in the tumor necrosis factor-α gene. J Biol Chem 1991;266:9343–9346.
40. Nunokawa Y, Ishida H, Tanaka S. Promoter analysis of human inducible nitric oxide synthase gene associated with cardiovascular homeostasis. Biochem Biophys Res Commun 1994;100:802–807.
41. Kelly RA, Balligand JL, Smith TW. Nitric oxide and cardiac function. Circ Res 1996;79:363–380.
42. Chu SC, Wu H-P, Banks TC, Eissa NT, Moss J. Structural diversity in the 5'-untranslated region of cytokine-stimulated human iNOS mRNA. J Biol Chem 1995;270:10,625–10,630.
43. Marsden PA, Heng HH, Scherer SW, Stewart RJ, Hall AV, Shi XM, et al. Structure and chromosomal localization of the human constitutive endothelial nitric oxide synthase gene. J Biol Chem 1993;268: 17,478–17,488.
44. Robinson LJ, Weremowicz S, Morton CC, Michel T. Isolation and chromosomal localization of the human endothelial nitric oxide synthase (NOS3) gene. Genomics 1994;19:350–357.
45. Miyahara K, Kawamoto T, Sase K, Yui Y, Toda K, Yang LX, et al. Cloning and structural characterization of the human endothelial nitric-oxide-synthase gene. Eur J Biochem 1994;223:719–726.
46. Searles CD, Miwa Y, Harrison DG, Ramasamy S. Role of the 3' untranslated region in the regulation of eNOS gene expression. Circulation 1997;96:I–48:259.
47. Pollock JS, Nakane M, Buttery LK, Martinez A, Springall D, Polak JM, et al. Characterization and localization of endothelial nitric oxide synthase using specific monoclonal antibodies. Am J Physiol 1993;265:C1379–C1387.
48. Balligand J-L, Kobzik L, Han X, Kaye DM, Belhassen L, O'Hara D, et al. Nitric oxide-dependent parasympathetic signaling is due to activation of constitutive endothelial (type III) nitric oxide synthase in cardiac myocytes. J Biol Chem 1995;270:14,582–14,586.
49. Dinerman JL, Dawson TM, Schell MJ, Snowman A, Snyder SH. Endothelial nitric oxide synthase localized to hippocampal pyramidal cells: implications for synaptic plasticity. Proc Natl Acad Sci USA 1994;91:4214–4218.
50. Sase K, Michel T. Expression and regulation of endothelial nitric oxide synthase. Trends Cardiovasci Med 1997;7:25–34.
51. Förstermann U, Boissel JP, Kleinert H. Expressional control of the "constitutive" isoforms of nitric oxide synthase (NOS I and NOS III). FASEB J 1998;12:773–790.
52. Karantzoulis-Fegaras F, Antoniou H, Lai SL, Kulkarni G, D'Abreo C, Wong GK, Miller TL, Chan Y, Atkins J, Wang Y, Marsden PA. Characterization of the human endothelial nitric-oxide synthase promoter. J Biol Chem 1999;274:3076–3093.
53. Nishida K, Harrison DG, Navas JP, Fisher AA, Dockery SP, Uematsu M, et al. Molecular cloning and characterization of the constitutive bovine aortic endothelial cell nitric oxide synthase. J Clin Invest 1992;90:2092–2096.
54. Sessa WC, Pritchard K, Seyedi N, Wang J, Hintze TH. Chronic exercise in dogs increases coronary vascular nitric oxide production and endothelial cell nitric oxide synthase gene expression. Circ Res 1994;74:349–353.
55. McQuillan LP, Leung GK, Marsden PA, Kostyk SK, Kourembanas S. Hypoxia inhibits expression of eNOS via transcriptional and posttranscriptional mechanisms. Am J Physiol 1994;267:H1921–H1927.

56. Arnal JF, Yamin J, Dockery S, Harrison DG. Regulation of endothelial nitric oxide synthase mRNA, protein, and activity during cell growth. Am J Physiol 1994;267:C1381–C1388.
57. Hishikawa K, Nakaki T, Marumo T, Suzuki H, Kato R, Saruta T. Up-regulation of nitric oxide synthase by estradiol in human aortic endothelial cells. FEBS Lett 1995;360:291–293.
58. Weiner WP, Lizasoian I, Baylis SA, Knowles RG, Charles IG, Moncada S. Induction of calcium-dependent nitric oxide synthases by sex hormones. Proc Natl Acad Sci USA 1994;91:5212–5216.
59. Liao JK, Shin WS, Lee WY, Clark SL. Oxidized low-density lipoprotein decreases the expression of endothelial nitric oxide synthase. J Biol Chem 1995;270:319–324.
60. Zembowicz A, Tang JL, Wu KK. Transcriptional induction of endothelial nitric oxide synthase type III by lysophosphatidylcholine. J Biol Chem 1995;270:17,006–17,010.
61. Hirata K-I, Miki N, Kuroda Y, Sakoda T, Kawashima S, Yokoyama M. Low concentration of oxidized LDL and lysophosphatidylcholine upregulate constitutive NOS mRNA expression in bovine aortic endothelial cells. Circ Res 1995;76:958–962.
62. Lamas S, Michel T, Brenner B, Marsden P. Nitric oxide synthesis in endothelial cells: evidence for a pathway inducible by tumor necrosis factor-alpha. Am J Physiol 1991;261:C634–C641.
63. Lamas S, Marsden PA, Li GK, Tempst P, Michel T. Endothelial nitric oxide synthase: molecular cloning and characterization of a distinct constitutive enzyme isoform. Proc Natl Acad Sci USA 1992; 89:6348–6352.
64. Werner-Felmayer G, Werner ER, Fuchs D, Hausen A, Reibnegger G, Schmidt K, et al. Pteridine biosynthesis in human endothelial cells. Impact on nitric oxide-mediated formation of cGMP. J Biol Chem 1993;268:1842–1846.
65. Yoshizumi M, Perrella MA, Burnett JC, Lee M-E. Tumor necrosis factor downregulates an endothelial nitric oxide synthase mRNA by shortening its half-life. Circ Res 1993;73:205–209.
66. Inoue N, Venema RC, Sayegh HS, Ohara Y, Murphy TJ, Harrison DG. Molecular regulation of the bovine endothelial cell nitric oxide synthase by transforming growth factor-beta$_1$. Arterioscler Thromb Vasc Biol 1995;15:1255–1261.
67. Deng AY, Rapp JP. Locus for inducible, but not a constitutive, nitric oxide synthase cosegregates with blood pressure in the Dahl salt-sensitive rat. J Clin Invest 1995;95:2170–2177.
68. Bonnardeaux A, Nadaud S, Charru A, Jeunemaitre X, Corvol P, Soubrier F. Lack of evidence for linkage of the endothelial cell nitric oxide synthase gene to essential hypertension. Circulation 1995;91: 96–102.
69. Miyamoto Y, Saito Y, Kajiyama N, Yoshimura M, Shimasaki Y, Nakayama M, et al. Endothelial NOS gene is positively associated with essential hypertension. Hypertension 1998;32:3–8.
70. Hibi K, Ishigami T, Tamura K, Mizushima S, Nyui N, Fujita T, et al. Endothelial nitric oxide synthase gene polymorphism and acute myocardial infarction. Hypertension 1998;32:521–526.
71. Yoshimura M, Yasue H, Nakayama M, Shimasaki Y, Sumida H, Sugiyama S, et al. A missense Glu298Asp variant in the endothelial nitric oxide synthase gene is associated with coronary spasm in the Japanese. Hum Genet 1998;103:65–69.
72. Markus HS, Ruigrok Y, Ali N, Powell JF. Endothelial nitric oxide synthase exon 7 polymorphism, ischemic cerebrovascular disease, and carotid atheroma. Stroke 1998;29:1908–1911.
73. O'Dell TJ, Huang PL, Dawson TM, Dinerman JL, Snyder SH, Kandel ER, et al. Endothelial NOS and the blockade of LTP by NOS inhibitors in mice lacking neuronal NOS. Science 1994;265:542–546.
74. Huang PL, Dawson TM, Bredt DS, Snyder SH, Fishman MC. Targeted disruption of the neuronal nitric oxide synthase gene. Cell 1993;75:1273–1286.
75. MacMicking JD, Nathan C, Hom G, Chartrain N, Fletcher DS, et al. Altered responses to bacterial infection and endotoxic shock in mice lacking inducible nitric oxide synthase. Cell 1995;81:641–650.
76. Wei XQ, Charles IG, Smith A, Ure J, Feng GJ, Huang FP, et al. Altered immune responses in mice lacking iNOS. Nature 1995;375:408–411.
77. Huang PL, Huang Z, Mashimo H, Bloch KD, Moskowitz MA, Bevan JA, et al. Hypertension in mice lacking the gene for endothelial nitric oxide synthase. Nature 1995;377:239–242.
78. Irikura K, Huang PL, Ma J, Lee WS, Dalkara T, Fishman MC, et al. Cerebrovascular alterations in mice lacking neuronal nitric oxide synthase gene expression. Proc Natl Acad Sci USA 1995;92:6823–6827.
79. Ohashi Y, Kawashima S, Hirata K, Yamashita T, Ishida T, Inoue N, Sakoda T, Kurihara H, Yazaki Y, Yokoyama M. Hypotension and reduced nitric oxide-elicited vasorelaxation in transgenic mice over-expressing endothelial nitric oxide synthase. J Clin Invest 1998;102:2061–2071.
80. Murohara T, Asahara T, Silver M, Bauters C, Masuda H, Kalka C, et al. Nitric oxide synthase modulates angiogenesis in response to tissue ischemia. J Clin Invest 1998;101:2567–2578.
81. Huang Z, Huang PL, Panahian N, Dalkara T, Fishman MC, Moskowitz MA. Effects of cerebral ischemia in mice deficient in neuronal nitric oxide synthase. Science 1994;265:1883–1885.

82. Panahian N, Yoshida T, Huang PL, Hedley-Whyte ET, Fishman M, Moskowitz MA. Attenuated hippocampal damage after global cerebral ischemia in mice mutant in neuronal nitric oxide synthase. Neuroscience 1996;72:343–354.

83. Huang Z, Huang PL, Ma J, Meng W, Ataya C, Fishman MC, et al. Enlarged infarcts in endothelial nitric oxide synthase knockout mice are attenuated by nitro-L-arginine. J Cereb Blood Flow Metab 1996; 16:981–987.

84. Iadecola C, Zhang F, Casey R, Nagayama M, Ross ME. Delayed reduction of ischemic brain injury and neurological deficits in mice lacking the inducible nitric oxide synthase gene. J Neurosci 1997;17: 9157–9164.

85. Nakane M, Mitchell J, Forstermann U, Murad F. Phosphorylation by calcium calmodulin-dependent protein kinase II and protein kinase C modulates the activity of nitric oxide synthase. Biochem Biophys Res Commun 1991;180:1396–1402.

86. Bredt DS, Ferris CD, Snyder SH. Nitric oxide synthase regulatory sites. Phosphorylation by cyclic AMP-dependent protein kinase, protein kinase C, and calcium/calmodulin protein kinase; identification of flavin and calmodulin binding sites. J Biol Chem 1992;267:10,976–10,981.

87. Pan J, Burgher KL, Szcepanik AM, Ringhcim GE. Tyrosine phosphorylation of inducible nitric oxide synthase: implications for potential post-translational regulation. Biochem J 1996;314:889–894.

88. Michel T, Li GK, Busconi L. Phosphorylation and subcellular translocation of endothelial nitric oxide synthase. Proc Natl Acad Sci USA 1993;90:6252–6256.

89. Tsukahara H, Gordienko DV, Goligorsky MS. Continuous monitoring of nitric oxide release from human umbilical vein endothelial cells. Biochem Biophys Res Commun 1993;193:722–729.

90. Craven PA, Studer RK, DeRubertis FR. Impaired nitric oxide-dependent cyclic guanosine monophosphate generation in glomeruli from diabetic rats. Evidence for protein kinase C-mediated suppression of the cholinergic response. J Clin Invest 1994;93:311–320.

91. Ayajiki K, Kindermann M, Hecker M, Fleming I, Busse R. Intracellular pH and tyrosine phosphorylation but not calcium determine shear stress induced nitric oxide production in native endothelial cells. Circ Res 1995;78:750–758.

92. Corson MA, James NL, Latta SE, Nerem RM, Berk BC, Harrison DG. Phosphorylation of endothelial nitric oxide synthase in response to fluid shear stress. Circ Res 1996;79:984–991.

93. Fleming I, Bauersachs J, Fisslthaler B, Busse R. Ca^{2+}-independent activation of the endothelial nitric oxide synthase in response to tyrosine phosphatase inhibitors and fluid shear stress. Circ Res 1998; 82:686–695.

94. Venema VJ, Marrero MB, Venema RC. Bradykinin-stimulated protein tyrosine phosphorylation promotes endothelial nitric oxide synthase translocation to the cytoskeleton. Biochem Biophys Res Commun 1996;226:703–710.

95. Garcia-Cardena G, Fan R, Stern DF, Liu J, Sessa WC. Endothelial nitric oxide synthase is regulated by tyrosine phosphorylation and interacts with caveolin-1. J Biol Chem 1996;271:27,237–27,240.

96. Shaul PW, Smart EJ, Robinson LJ, German Z, Yuhanna IS, Ying Y, et al. Acylation targets endothelial nitric-oxide synthase to plasmalemmal caveolae. J Biol Chem 1996;271:6518–6522.

97. Boutin JA. Myristoylation. Cell Signal 1997;9:15–31.

98. Resh MD. Myristylation and palmitylation of Src family members: the fats of the matter. Cell 1994;76: 411–413.

99. Robinson LJ, Michel T. Mutagenesis of palmitoylation sites in endothelial nitric oxide synthase identifies a novel motif for dual acylation and subcellular targeting. Proc Natl Acad Sci USA 1995;92: 11,776–11,780.

100. Robinson LJ, Busconi L, Michel T. Agonist-modulated palmitoylation of endothelial nitric oxide synthase. J Biol Chem 1995;270:995–998.

101. Liu J, Garcia-Cardena G, Sessa WC. Biosynthesis and palmitoylation of endothelial nitric oxide synthase: mutagenesis of palmitoylation sites, cysteines-15 and/or -26, argues against depalmitoylation-induced translocation of the enzyme. Biochemistry 1995;34:12,333–12,340.

102. Wedegaertner PB, Bourne HR. Activation and depalmitoylation of Gs alpha. Cell 1994;77: 1063–1070.

103. Milligan G, Parenti M, Magee AI. The dynamic role of palmitoylation in signal transduction. Trends Biochem Sci 1995;20:181–187.

104. O'Dowd BF, Hnatowich M, Caron MG, Lefkowitz RJ, Bouvier M. Palmitoylation of the human beta 2-adrenergic receptor. Mutation of Cys341 in the carboxyl tail leads to an uncoupled nonpalmitoylated form of the receptor. J Biol Chem 1989;264:7564–7569.

105. Wedegaertner PB, Wilson PT, Bourne HR. Lipid modifications of trimeric G proteins. J Biol Chem 1995;270:503–506.

106. Camp LA, Verkruyse LA, Afendis SJ, Slaughter CA, Hofmann SL. Molecular cloning and expression of palmitoyl-protein thioesterase. J Biol Chem 1994;269:23,212–23,219.
107. Michel JB, Michel T. The role of palmitoyl-protein thioesterase in the palmitoylation of endothelial nitric oxide synthase. FEBS Lett 1997;405:356–362.
108. Duncan JA, Gilman AG. A cytoplasmic acyl-protein thioesterase that removes palmitate from G protein alpha subunits and p21^{RAS}. J Biol Chem 1998;273:15,830–15,837.
109. Hess DT, Patterson SI, Smith DS, Skene JH. Neuronal growth cone collapse and inhibition of protein fatty acylation by nitric oxide. Nature 1993;366:562–565.
110. Feron O, Saldana F, Michel JB, Michel T. The endothelial nitric oxide synthase-caveolin regulatory cycle. J Biol Chem 1998;273:3125–3128.
111. Kantor DB, Lanzrein M, Stary SJ, Sandoval GM, Smith WB, Sullivan BM, et al. A role for endothelial NO synthase in LTP revealed by adenovirus-mediated inhibition and rescue. Science 1996;274:1744–1748.
112. Feron O, Dessy C, Opel DJ, Arstall MA, Kelly RA, Michel T. Modulation of the endothelial nitric oxide synthase-caveolin interaction in cardiac myocytes: implications for the autonomic regulation of heart rate. J Biol Chem 1998;273:30,249–30,254.
113. Topinka JR, Bredt DS. N-terminal palmitoylation of PSP-95 regulates association with cell membranes and interaction with K$^+$ channel K$_v$ 1.4. Neuron 1998;20:125–134.
114. Venema VJ, Ju H, Zou R, Venema RC. Interaction of neuronal nitric-oxide synthase with caveolin-3 in skeletal muscle. Identification of a novel caveolin scaffolding/inhibitory domain. J Biol Chem 1997;272:28,187–28,190.
115. Yamada E. The fine structure of the gall bladder epithelium of the mouse. J Biophys Biochem Cytol 1955;1:445–457.
116. Okamoto T, Schlegel A, Scherer P, Lisanti MP. Caveolins, a family of scaffolding proteins for organizing "preassembled signaling complexes" at the plasma membrane. J Biol Chem 1998;273:5419–5422.
117. Feron O, Smith TW, Michel T, Kelly RA. Dynamic targeting of the agonist-stimulated m2 muscarinic acetylcholine receptor to caveolae in cardiac myocytes. J Biol Chem 1997;272:17,744–17,748.
118. de Weerd WF, Leeb-Lundberg LM. Bradykinin sequesters B2 bradykinin receptors and the receptor-coupled Gα subunits G$_{αq}$ and G$_{αi}$ in caveolae in DDT1 MF-2 smooth muscle cells. J Biol Chem 1997;272:17,858–17,866.
119. McDonald KK, Zharikov S, Block ER, Kilberg MS. A caveolar complex between the cationic amino acid transporter 1 and endothelial nitric oxide synthase may explain the "arginine paradox." J Biol Chem 1997;272:31,213–31,216.
120. Beckman JS, Koppenol WH. Nitric oxide, superoxide, and peroxynitrite: the good, the bad, and ugly. Am J Physiol 1996;271:C1424–C1437.
121. Galbiati F, Volonté D, Gil O, Zanazzi G, Salzer JL, Sargiacomo M, et al. Expression, of caveolin-1 and -2 in differentiating PC12 cells and dorsal root ganglion neurons: caveolin-2 is up-regulated in response to cell injury. Proc Natl Acad Sci USA 1998;95:10,257–10,262.
122. Kröncke KD, Fehsel K, Kolb-Bachofen V. Nitric oxide, cytotoxicity versus cytoprotection: how, why, when and where ? Nitric Oxide 1997;1:107–120.
123. Tamir S, deRojas-Walker T, Wishnok JS, Tannenbaum SR. DNA damage and genotoxicity by nitric oxide. Methods Enzymol 1996;269:230–243.
124. Buchwalow IB, Schulze W, Kostic MM, Wallukat G, Morwinski R. Intracellular localization of inducible nitric oxide synthase in neonatal rat cardiomyocytes in culture. Acta Histochem 1997;99:231–240.
125. Xia H, Bredt DS. Cloned and expressed nitric oxide synthase proteins. Methods Enzymol. 1996;268:427–436.
126. Tatoyan A, Giulivi C. Purification and characterization of a nitric-oxide synthase from rat liver mitochondria. J Biol Chem 1998;273:11,044–11,048.
127. Giulivi C, Poteroso JJ, Boveris A. Production of nitric oxide by mitochondria. J Biol Chem 1998;273:11,038–11,043.
128. Clementi E, Brown GC, Feelisch M, Moncada S. Persistent inhibition of cell respiration by nitric oxide: crucial role of S-nitrosylation of mitochondrial complex I and protective action of glutathione. Proc Natl Acad Sci USA 1998;95:7631–7636.
129. Sessa WC, Garcia-Cardena G, Liu J, Keh A, Pollock JS, Bradley J, et al. The Golgi association of endothelial nitric oxide synthase is necessary for the efficient synthesis of nitric oxide. J Biol Chem 1995;270:17,541–17,644.
130. Liu J, Hughes TE, Sessa WC. The first 35 amino acids and fatty acylation sites determine the molecular targeting of endothelial nitric oxide synthase into the Golgi region of cells: a green fluorescent protein study. J Cell Biol 1997;137:1525–1535.

131. Prabhakar P, Thatte HS, Goetz RM, Cho MR, Golan DE, Michel T. Receptor-regulated translocation of endothelial nitric-oxide synthase. J Biol Chem 1998;273:27,383–27,388.

132. Brenman JE, Chao DS, Xia H, Aldape K, Bredt DS. Nitric oxide synthase complexed with dystrophin and absent from skeletal muscle sarcolemma in Duchenne muscular dystrophy. Cell 1995;82: 743–752.

133. Sheng M. PDZs and receptor/channel clustering: rounding up the latest suspects. Neuron 1996;17: 575–578.

134. Vodovotz Y, Russell D, Xie Q-W, Bogdan C, Nathan C. Vesicle membrane association of nitric oxide synthase in primary mouse macrophages. J Immunol 1995;154:2914–2925.

135. Jaffrey SR, Snyder SH. PIN: an associated protein inhibitor of neuronal nitric oxide synthase. Science 1996;274:774–777.

136. Hemmens B, Woschitz S, Pitters E, Klösch B, Völker C, Schmidt K, et al. The protein inhibitor of neuronal nitric oxide synthase (PIN): characterization of its action on pure nitric oxide synthases. FEBS Lett 1998;430:397–400.

137. King SM, Barbarese E, Dillman JF, Patel-King RS, Carson JH, Pfister KK. Brain cytoplasmic and flagellar outer arm dyneins share a highly conserved M_r 8,000 light chain. J Biol Chem 1996;271: 19,358–19,366.

138. Gillardon F, Krep H, Brinker G, Lenz C, Bottiger B, Hossmann KA. Induction of protein inhibitor of neuronal nitric oxide synthase/cytoplasmic dynein light chain following cerebral ischemia. Neuroscience 1998;84:81–88.

139. Jaffrey SR, Snowman AM, Eliasson MJ, Cohen NA, Snyder SH. CAPON: a protein associated with neuronal nitric oxide synthase that regulates its interactions with PSD95. Neuron 1998;20:115–124.

140. Garcia-Cardena G, Fan R, Shah V, Sorrentino R, Cirino G, Papapetropoulos A, et al. Dynamic activation of endothelial nitric oxide synthase by Hsp90. Nature 1998;392:821–824.

141. Feron O, Belhassen L, Kobzik L, Smith TW, Kelly RA, Michel T. Endothelial nitric oxide synthase targeting to caveolae. Specific interactions with caveolin isoforms in cardiac myocytes and endothelial cells. J Biol Chem 1996;271:22,810–22,814.

142. Michel JB, Feron O, Sacks D, Michel T. Reciprocal regulation of endothelial nitric-oxide synthase by Ca^{2+}-calmodulin and caveolin. J Biol Chem 1997;272:15,583–15,586.

143. Michel JB, Feron O, Sase K, Prabhakar P, Michel T. Caveolin versus calmodulin: counterbalancing allosteric modulators of nitric oxide synthase. J Biol Chem 1997;272:25,907–25,912.

144. Feron O, Michel JB, Sase K, Michel T. Dynamic regulation of endothelial nitric oxide synthase: complementary roles of dual acylation and caveolin interactions. Biochemistry 1998;37:193–200.

145. Ju H, Zou R, Venema VJ, Venema RC. Direct interaction of endothelial nitric-oxide synthase and caveolin-1 inhibits synthase activity. J Biol Chem 1997;272:18,522–18,525.

146. Garcia-Cardena G, Martasek P, Siler Masters BS, Skidd PM, Couet J, Li S, Lisanti MP, Sessa WC. Dissecting the interaction between nitric oxide synthase and caveolin. J Biol Chem 1997;272: 25,437–25,440.

147. Ghosh S, Gachhui R, Crooks C, Wu C, Lisanti MP, Stuehr DJ. Interaction between caveolin-1 and the reductase domain of endothelial nitric oxide synthase. Consequences for catalysis. J Biol Chem 1998; 273:22,267–22,271.

148. Michel T, Feron O. Nitric oxide synthases: which, where, how and why? J Clin Invest 1997;100: 2146–2152.

149. Ju H, Venema VJ, Marrero MB, Venema RC. Inhibitory interactions of the bradykinin B2 receptor with endothelial nitric-oxide synthase. J Biol Chem 1998;273:24,025–24,029.

150. Raman CS, Li H, Martasek P, Kral V, Masters BS, Poulos TL. Crystal structure of constitutive endothelial nitric oxide synthase: a paradigm for pterin function involving a novel metal center. Cell 1998; 95:939–950.

3

Cellular Signal Transduction and Nitric Oxide

Overview

Stanley Heydrick

Nitric oxide (NO•) is an important regulatory determinant of vascular tissue homeostasis that evokes its functional effects through a broad range of signaling elements, including the phospholipase C/calcium signaling systems, tyrosine kinase signaling pathways, G-protein-linked receptors, ion channels, cyclic guanosine monophosphate (cGMP) and cyclic adenosine monophosphate (cAMP)-dependent pathways, and the apoptotic pathway. Traditionally, nitric oxide was thought to signal exclusively via its stimulation of guanylyl cyclase, inducing an increase in intracellular cGMP levels and, in turn, the allosteric activation of cGMP-dependent kinase (protein kinase G [PKG]). However, more recent work has revealed that some of NO•'s signaling effects can also be transduced by S-nitros(yl)ation and tyrosine nitrosation. Moreover, in addition to the activation of PKG, the cGMP-dependent effects can also be mediated by other proteins whose activities are allosterically modified by cGMP (e.g., phosphodiesterases and ion channels), and via cross-activation of cAMP-dependent kinase (protein kinase A [PKA]). This chapter will cover NO•'s specific effects on signaling pathways in vascular smooth muscle cells, cardiomyocytes, endothelial cells, and platelets.

VASCULAR SMOOTH MUSCLE

Vascular smooth muscle has been considered to be the prototypical NO• target tissue since NO• was first identified as the endothelium-derived relaxing factor (EDRF). Its principal effects include relaxation, growth inhibition, and the promotion of apoptosis.

Smooth Muscle Relaxation

The most extensively studied effect of NO• on vascular smooth muscle is relaxation. Physiologically, relaxation triggered by NO• requires cGMP-dependent kinase (PKG) activation, as little NO•-mediated relaxation is observed in mice in which the PKG gene has been eliminated by targeted disruption (1). This observation, however, does not rule out contributory effects by effectors other than PKG. NO•'s specific targets in the contractile signaling pathways are considered below.

One key event in the contractile signaling pathway is an elevation of intracellular calcium. NO• has long been known to lower basal calcium levels and antagonize agonist-mediated increases in intracellular calcium (2,3). This, in turn, promotes relaxation because calmodulin-calcium-dependent enzymes such as myosin light chain kinase are less active (4). Changes in cytosolic calcium levels are brought about by alterations in the net flux of calcium between the cytosol, plasma membrane (sarcolemma), and endoplasmic reticulum (sarcoplasmic

From: *Contemporary Cardiology, vol. 4: Nitric Oxide and the Cardiovascular System*
Edited by: J. Loscalzo and J. A. Vita © Humana Press Inc., Totowa, NJ

reticulum). Flux across both membranes is modulated by NO• such that there is a net exodus of calcium from the cytosol. NO• facilitates calcium removal across the sarcolemma by activating the sarcolemma calcium ATPase (adenosine triphosphate) and blunting calcium entry through L-type voltage-dependent calcium channels while it promotes net calcium uptake into the sarcoplasmic reticulum by stimulating sarcoplasmic reticulum calcium ATPases and blunting the activation of phospholipase C (PLC).

The sarcolemma calcium ATPase, which pumps calcium out of the cytosol into the extracellular space, is activated by NO• as well as by membrane receptors, calmodulin, and negatively charged phospholipids. There is some evidence indicating that a PKG-mediated stimulation of phosphatidylinositol 4-kinase (PI4-kinase) is responsible for the activation of this pump by NO• donors (5). Interestingly, enhanced production of peroxynitrite can lead to inactivation of the sarcolemma calcium ATPase via tyrosine nitration in exhaustively exercised skeletal muscle (6). Because high levels of peroxynitrite are also associated with atherosclerotic plaque formation, this phenomenon may prove to be relevant to vascular responses in atherothrombosis. In contrast, L-type voltage-dependent calcium channels, which permit the inward flow of calcium when cells become depolarized, are inhibited by NO• by what is apparently a PKG-independent mechanism. This conclusion has been reached because both nitroglycerin and 8-Br-cGMP are able to able to inhibit the inward calcium flux through these channels in the presence of the nonspecific serine/threonine kinase inhibitor H8 (7,8).

The net flux of calcium in and out of the sarcoplasmic reticulum is determined by the balance between the release of calcium through the IP_3 receptor calcium channel and its reuptake via calcium ATPases. IP_3, which activates the channel, is produced as a result of the cleavage of phosphatidylinositol 4,5-bisphosphate by PLC. Of the three isoforms of PLC (β,γ,δ), agonist-induced smooth muscle contraction is mediated through G protein-linked receptors (e.g., the bradykinin and muscarinic m_2 receptors) that activate PLCβ. There is abundant evidence demonstrating that NO• inhibits PLCβ in vascular smooth muscle and numerous other cell types, leading to a reduction in intracellular inositol–trisphosphate (IP_3) levels. However, at least one study indicates that the direct NO• target appears to be the coupling G protein rather than PLC per se (9). In this study, addition of cGMP plus ATP to homogenates from aortic smooth muscle completely suppressed the formation of IP_3 evoked by vasopressin or GTPγS, but had no effect on the formation of IP_3 resulting from direct activation of PLC with calcium (9). Because ATP was found to be necessary for cGMP to have its inhibitory effect, it is likely that the effect is mediated by a PKG-dependent mechanism. A similar conclusion was reached in a study conducted with PC12 neural cells, in which the stable cGMP analog 8-Br-cGMP mimicked, and the PKG inhibitor KT-5823 blocked, the inhibitory effect that NO• has on the accumulation of IP_3 induced by ATP, acetylcholine, and bradykinin (10).

In addition to its effects on PLC, NO• also appears to have a stimulatory effect on the phosphorylation state of vascular smooth muscle cell IP_3 receptors (11). The increased phosphorylation is apparently mediated by both PKG and PKA that has been crossactivated by cGMP. The effect of this phosphorylation on IP_3 receptor activity has yet to be determined, although indirect evidence suggests that it may be inhibitory (4).

In concert with diminishing the release of calcium through the IP_3 receptor channel, NO• activates the sarcoplasmic reticulum calcium ATPase. The mechanism by which this effect occurs has not been conclusively established. Early studies in some laboratories indicated that NO• regulation is mediated by phospholamban, which can stimulate the ATPase in vitro after it is phosphorylated by PKG or PKA (3,12–14). However, other work failed to demonstrate a change in the in vivo phosphorylation state of phospholamban with increased cGMP (15).

A second major mechanism by which NO• promotes smooth muscle relaxation is via hyperpolarization. This effect is attributable in large part to a stimulation of the outward potassium current through calcium-dependent potassium channels in the sarcolemma (16–21).

In pharmacological studies, NO·'s effects on these channels were mimicked by 8-Br-cGMP and the NO·/peroxynitrite donor SIN-1, and blocked by cGMP antagonists and PKG inhibitors. In a more direct experiment, administration of purified PKG to isolated membranes in patch clamp experiments activated the channels directly. A PKG-independent mechanism is further supported by studies in smooth muscle *(19)* and mesangial cells *(22)* showing that the phosphatase 1 and 2A inhibitors okadaic acid and calycylin, respectively, cause an even greater and more sustained channel response to NO· and dibutyryl cGMP. Taken together, this data overwhelmingly indicate that NO·'s effects require PKG activation, although the target protein(s) have yet to be identified. Another contributory factor to NO·-induced hyperpolarization is NO·'s stimulatory effect on voltage-dependent potassium channels *(20)*. The mechanism underlying this stimulation has not been examined.

Finally, chronic pharmacological administration of NO· may actually reduce the smooth muscle cell's responsiveness to NO·. This effect, which results from the upregulation of smooth muscle endothelin receptors *(23)*, has been reported for three different NO· donors, all administered over several hours. Based on pharmacological evidence, the receptor upregulation seems to be mediated by the cGMP-dependent activation of PKA *(23)*.

Inhibition of Vascular Smooth Muscle Growth

NO· can either stimulate or inhibit growth, depending on the cell type. It is a potent growth inhibitor in smooth muscle cells. This effect, which is mediated by both cGMP-dependent and cGMP-independent mechanisms, involves the specific modulation of multiple sites in receptor tyrosine kinase pathways, including upstream kinases and downstream transcriptional activators. Later steps in growth cycling, such as ribonucleotide reductase, are also affected.

Major targets for cGMP-dependent inhibition of growth factor signaling include the PDGF receptor, raf-1, MAP kinases, PLC, protein kinase C (PKC), and the AP-1 transcriptional activation complex. PDGF's activation of its receptor tyrosine kinase (PDGFR) in cultured smooth muscle cells is inhibited by the elevated cGMP resulting from prior treatment with atrial natriuretic peptide (ANP), whereas normal PDGFR activation is restored when guanylyl cyclase inhibitors are included in the medium *(24)*. It is not known whether this is an effect of cGMP per se or a consequence of the activation of PKG.

In addition to the activation of the receptor tyrosine kinase per se, another prominent signal generated at growth factor receptors is the stimulation of PLCγ. PLCγ differs from PLC's β and δ in that it is activated by an interaction between its SH2 domains and phosphotyrosine moieties on growth factor receptors rather than by an interaction with G protein βγ subunits. Although the effect of NO· on smooth muscle PLCγ has yet to be examined in cultured fibroblasts and epithelial cells, NO· donors will block, and NOS inhibitors will stimulate, PLCγ-mediated phosphoinositide hydrolysis. These effects are mimicked by cGMP and are blocked by the PKG inhibitor KT5823 *(26)*. Thus PLC is likely to be inhibited by NO· regardless of the isoform.

It should be noted that PLC inhibition by PKG results in an indirect inhibition of total PKC activity owing to the reduced accumulation of the PKC activators diacylglycerol and calcium *(27)*. Indeed, a direct effect of PKG on any PKC isoform has not been observed *(28)*. In contrast, direct PKC inhibition by *S*-nitrosation has been suggested based on the observation that partially purified PKC and PKC in macrophages are inherently less active in the presence of NO· or NO· donors, and activity can be restored by simultaneously adding the NO· scavenger oxyhemoglobin or the reducing agent dithiothreitol (DTT) *(29)*. Of potential interest is the observation that ANP, whose major signaling effect is an activation of its receptor's guanylyl cyclase and subsequent elevation in cGMP, will also modulate PKC such that it is unresponsive to phorbol ester (i.e., direct) activation. The pathway by which ANP evokes this effect has yet to be defined *(27)*. Taken together, these results indicate that NO· may blunt the activation of PKC by multiple mechanisms.

Finally, a recent report *(25)* has made a compelling case for NO• acting via PKG to block the ras-dependent activation of raf-1 by epidermal growth factor (EGF). In this study the authors demonstrate that EGF's stimulation of raf kinase activity is blocked in vivo by agonists that raise cGMP despite normal association of ras with GTP. A similar inactivation of raf was seen when raf was preincubated with recombinant PKG.

At least some of the foregoing growth-inhibitory effects may be mediated by the cross-activation of cyclic AMP-dependent kinase (PKA). Smooth muscle cells express phosphodiesterase III, which will hydrolyze both cAMP and cGMP and is allosterically inhibited by cGMP, but lack phosphodiesterase II, which will also hydrolyze both cyclic nucleotides but is stimulated by cGMP. Hence, agents that induce an increase in cGMP in smooth muscle cells will not only increase cGMP but also often induce an increase in cAMP, leading to activation of PKA. Cyclic GMP itself can also directly activate PKA under some circumstances. For example, when stimulated by IL-1, which raises intracellular cGMP but not cAMP, smooth muscle cells display a blunted growth response to serum and EGF *(30)*. Paradoxically, there is an increase in both PKA and PKG activity in these cells. This effect is mimicked by the NO• donor *S*-nitro-*N*-acetylpenicillamine (SNAP) and blocked by inhibitors of NO• and cGMP production. Using selective PKA and PKG inhibitors, it was demonstrated that the growth-inhibitory effect is mediated via PKA, although growth inhibition was only observed at cGMP levels 10-fold greater than baseline levels.

Although less studied, cGMP-independent mechanisms are also critical for the inhibition of smooth muscle cell growth. In EGF-stimulated fibroblasts, NO•'s growth-inhibitory effects are mediated, at least in part, by the cGMP-independent inhibition of ribonucleotide reductase and a prolongation of the G1 and S phases *(31)*. As shown recently, growth inhibition occurs despite the cGMP-dependent stimulation of AP-1-directed transcription, indicating that the cGMP-independent effects predominate. This conclusion is supported by experiments in which PKG-deficient smooth muscle cells were transfected with PKG *(31)*, where expression of PKG resulted in a blunted migratory response to PDGF, but did not affect PDGF's stimulation of cell growth *(32)*.

Although the sites of these PKG-independent NO• actions remain to be elucidated in smooth muscle cells, some clues can be gleaned from other cell types. For example, the NO• donors SNAP, diethylamine-nitric oxide (DEA-NO•), and diethylenetriamine-nitric oxide (DETA-NO•) all inhibit EGF-mediated EGF receptor autophosphorylation and tyrosine kinase activity *(33)* in fibroblasts transfected with EGF receptors. The inhibitory activity of DEA-NO• is negated by the NO• scavenger hemoglobin or by subsequent incubation with DTT. Interestingly, SIN-1, which generates predominantly peroxynitrite rather than NO•, had no effect on EGF receptor activation. Because peroxynitrite is unable to carry out a nucleophilic attack on free thiols, these results strongly implicate *S*-nitrosation of the EGF receptor or some closely associated regulatory protein as the mechanism of inhibition. Another study examining NO•'s inhibitory effect on tumor cell growth has implicated ribonucleotide reductase as a site of cGMP-independent NO• action *(34)*. Ribonucleotide reductase has a tyrosyl radical at its active site that is lost when it is exposed to NO• and peroxynitrite. Because ribonucleotide reductase can be reactivated by thiol reagents when previously inactivated by NO•, a strong case can be made for a mechanism in which inactivation by the active site is caused by *S*-nitrosation. In contrast, the irreversible loss of its active site with peroxynitrite is likely to result from the formation of nitrotyrosine *(34)*. Thus, in this case the nature of the nitric oxide species determines the final signaling outcome.

Paradoxically, in some cell types, NO• *stimulates* MAP kinase signaling. All three MAP kinase pathways, extracellular signal-regulated kinase (ERK1/2), c-*jun* NH2-terminal kinase (JNK), and p38, seem to be affected. Regulation occurs by both cGMP-dependent and -independent mechanisms.

NO•'s effect on the ERK1/2 pathway involves the upstream activation of ras *(35,36)*, the activation of ERK1/2 itself *(37–39)*, and downstream activation of the AP-1 *(31)* and NFκB *(35)* transcription complexes. Direct NO•-mediated ras activation, which has been observed in Jurkat T lymphocytes in vivo, results from the *S*-nitrosation of Cys 118 of the ras protein *(36)*. In T cells transfected with a mutant ras in which Cys 118 was replaced with serine, there is no stimulation of guanine nucleotide exchange on the mutant ras and no downstream stimulation of ERK1/2. ERK activation by NO• has been observed in endothelial cells *(39)* and hippocampal brain slices *(38)*, in addition to Jurkat T cells *(37)*. Although the activation of ERK in endothelial cells was originally observed in response to sodium nitroprusside (SNP), an NO•- and cGMP-dependent activation ERK was also observed in response to vascular endothelium growth factor (VEGF) *(38)*. Interestingly, NO•-activated ERK1/2 can be further stimulated by glutathione depletion, indicating that, if anything, *S*-nitrosation of ERK1/2 is inhibitory in this cell type *(37)*. In addition to these upstream effectors, NO• donors also appear to stimulate the AP-1 and NFκB transcriptional activation complexes. NO• may mediate AP-1 activation by multiple pathways. There is a cGMP-dependent activation of AP-1-directed transcription in EGF-stimulated fibroblasts, whereas in vitro nitrosation of the AP-1 complex leads to an increase in its ability to bind DNA *(40)*. Similarly, NFκB-dependent transcription is also stimulated by NO• donors in vivo *(35)*, even though binding this factor to DNA can be inhibited in vitro by direct *S*-nitrosation of its p50 subunit *(41)*. In this case, *S*-nitrosation may serve to as a feedback inhibitor of NFκB signaling, although this action remains to be demonstrated in vivo.

Similarly conflicting observations have been made for c-Jun-N-terminal kinase (JNK). Treatment of T cells with NO• donors strongly stimulates JNK, but, in vitro, *S*-nitrosation of both JNK and stress-activated protein kinase (SAPK) results in their inactivation *(42)*. These in vitro NO•-induced inhibitory effects, obtained using S-NO•-glutathione as a donor, were reversed by coincubation of the purified proteins with either DTT or reduced glutathione. Their relevance to in vivo states remains to be explored.

The significance of these stimulatory effects on MAP kinase signaling is uncertain. Because it is clear that NO•'s inhibitory effect on other growth-promoting pathways predominate, the most straightforward hypothesis would be that enhanced MAP kinase signaling is required for NO•'s other effects.

Induction of Apoptosis

Chronic exposure to high levels of NO• or transfection of inducible NOS can promote apoptosis (programmed cell death) of smooth muscle cells *(43–44)*. This proapoptotic effect in smooth muscle differentiates it from cell types such as vascular endothelial cells, hepatocytes, and neurons, where NO• has an antiapoptotic effect. The apoptotic effect is neither mimicked by the stable cGMP analog dibutyryl cGMP nor inhibited by the PKG inhibitor KT-5823, indicating that it does not require cGMP/PKG *(43)*. One contributory cGMP-independent mechanism may be the *S*-nitrosation/ADP-ribosylation protein inactivation pathway. This pathway is typified by the inactivation of glyceraldehyde 3-phosphate dehydrogenase (GAPDH). Initially there is a reversible inactivation of GAPDH via *S*-nitrosation of critical cysteine residues *(45)*, which allows its subsequent irreversible modification by adenosine diphosphate (ADP)-ribosylation *(46)*. ADP-ribosylation inactivates the enzyme, and probably leads to its proteolytic degradation *(47)*.

The ADP-ribosylation pathway is not, however, the only mechanism by which NO• promotes smooth muscle apoptosis, as inhibition of ADP-ribosylation with nicotinamide or phylloquinone only slightly attenuates the apoptotic effect *(43)*. Indeed, one signaling event known to be critical for NO•-induced apoptosis in many tissues is the increased expression of the p53 tumor suppressor protein. For example, there is a direct correlation between the potency of NO• donors, p53 accumulation, and apoptosis in macrophages *(48)*. Moreover, in smooth muscle cells, overexpression of inducible nitric oxide synthase (iNOS) is sufficient to increase p53 expression and cause apoptosis *(44)*. Mechanistically, NO•'s effect is likely to involve the modulation of the cellular thiol redox state, as apoptosis is characterized by a decrease in intracellular glutathione in conjunction with an increase in p53 expression in smooth muscle cells exposed to NO• donors *(49)*. Interestingly, the increase in p53 expression and ensuing apoptosis can be blocked if glutathione levels are maintained by adding glutathione monoethylester to the cells *(49)*. Given that glutathione is one of the primary cellular sulfhydryl-reducing agents, these results would suggest that protein *S*-nitrosation at one or more critical regulatory sites may lead to an increase in p53 transcription.

CARDIOMYOCYTES

NO•'s most prominent effect on cardiac muscle is its negative ionotropic effect. Cyclic GMP analogs mimic, and NOS inhibitors blunt, the negative ionotropic response induced by the m2 muscarinic receptor agonist carbachol, whose actions require NOS activation *(50,51)*. The opposite response can be observed with β-adrenergic stimulation. Perfusion of cardiac tissue with the NOS inhibitor N^G-monomethyl-L-argine (L-NMMA) further enhances the increased contractility induced by the β-adrenergic agonist isoproterenol, indicating that NO• is produced in response to isoproterenol and attenuates isoproterenol action *(52)*. A 10-fold higher concentration, however, has the opposite effect *(53)*. Finally, transfection of cardiomyocytes with iNOS results in decreases in contraction, spontaneous beating rate, and peak cytosolic calcium concentration *(54)*. These effects, which are mostly cGMP-dependent, are, for the most part, mediated indirectly by the elevated cAMP levels that are induced because of cGMP's inhibitory effects on phosphodiesterases. Similar to the regulation of contractility in smooth muscle cells, the cellular targets for these signaling events are proteins involved in calcium regulation and myofilaments. However, unlike smooth muscle cells, NO• apparently has no effect on cardiac muscle potassium channels *(55,56)*.

Effects on Calcium-Dependent Pathways

Known NO•-dependent alterations in intracellular calcium in the heart are mediated via the coordinated regulation of plasma membrane calcium channels. For example, the total inward calcium current is inhibited by high (100 μM) concentrations of the NO•/peroxynitrite donor SIN-1 *(55,57)*. This effect is blocked by KT-5823, indicating PKG-dependency. The regulation of the portion of this current due to the L-type calcium channel activity in cardiomyocytes is complex and controversial. Carbachol inhibits the L-type calcium current in isopreterenol-stimulated cardiomyocytes from adult wild-type, but not eNOS −/−, mice, indicating that the effect is NO•-dependent *(56)*. Pharmacological administration of NO• via SIN-1 and the NO• donor SNAP were able to increase cGMP and inhibit the current even in eNOS null myocytes. Another group of investigators found that inhibition of NOS and PKG inhibits the voltage-dependent calcium current in ventricular cells from newborn animals but have no effect on this current in ventricular cells from adult animals *(58)*. In still another report, NO• and 8-Br-cGMP inhibited the L-type current, but the NO•/peroxynitrite donor SIN-1 stimulated it *(59)*. One explanation for these varied results may be the differential regulation of phosphodiesterases by cGMP *(60)*. For example, low concentrations of SIN-1 enhance cAMP's activation of the L-type calcium current, but higher concentrations of SIN-1 inhibit cAMP-dependent current stimulation *(60)*. Although both effects are blocked by NO• scavengers, neither effect is observed when the nonhydrolyzable cAMP analog 8-Br-cAMP is used to stimulate the L-type current, indicating that NO•'s effect is mediated by cGMP-dependent effects on the cGMP-activatable phosphodiesterase II (PDE II) and the cGMP-inhibitable PDE III, respectively. Taken together, these data indicate that NO•'s effect on this channel could potentially depend on the relative abundance of NO[•] and superoxide, and the types and sensitivities of the phosphodiesterases that are expressed in that tissue.

Similar complex, phosphodiesterase-linked effects have been described in AV nodal cells (61). Treatment of AV-nodal cells with acetylcholine reduces the basal calcium current by lowering cAMP levels, primarily via stimulation of types III and IV PDE. When cAMP is pharmacologically elevated to maximum levels by globally inhibiting phosphodiesterase activity III and the acetylcholine effect is somewhat blunted by L-NMMA and methylene blue, indicating that NO[•] may contribute to acetylcholine's actions. Interestingly, cGMP also blunted acetylcholine's effect on calcium currents under these conditions, whereas the PKG-inhibitor KT-5823 had no effect. Thus NO[•] per se and PDE II both may contribute to the regulation of this current.

Finally, there are also purely cGMP-independent mechanisms by which NO[•] can influence intracellular calcium fluxes. There is some evidence indicating S-nitrosation may play a role in the regulation of the L-type calcium channel, as S-nitrosothiols activate the L-type current in a manner that is independent of cGMP, kinase activation, phosphatase inhibition, and modulation of sarcoplasmic reticulum calcium handling (59). Moreover, recent work has established that the cardiac calcium-release channel (ryanodine receptor) can be activated by NO[•], and that this effect is mediated by S-nitrosation (62). Finally, there is also evidence that the m2 muscarinic receptor can undergo inhibitory S-nitrosation (63), which may provide one means by which feedback inhibition of receptor activity can be achieved.

NO[•] also has effects on cardiac fibroblast calcium handling. In this cell type, NO[•]-dependent changes in calcium are likely to be part of the mechanism by which NO[•] blunts MAP kinase activation by angiotensin II and EGF (64). One of its potential targets is the PYK tyrosine kinase (D. Wang and P. Brecher, personal communication), although this remains to be demonstrated conclusively.

Effects Not Related to Calcium

In addition to changes in calcium handling, NO[•] appears to induce a blunted myofilament response to calcium (twitch amplitude, time to peak shortening, and myocyte resting length) at all calcium concentrations (7). This effect is due, at least in part, to PKG, as the blunted myofilament responses were all observed with the administration of 8-Br-cGMP and were blocked by the PKG inhibitor KT-5823 (7).

ENDOTHELIAL CELLS

Endothelial cells are the primary source of NO[•] in the vasculature, releasing it in response to vasodilatory stimuli such as acetylcholine or shear stress. However, NO[•] is not without effect on endothelial signaling per se. Indeed, in addition to several homeostatic roles, NO[•] appears to block apoptosis and to enhance significantly the mitogenic effects of VEGF and bFGF during endothelial wound healing and angiogenesis.

Homeostatic Effects

At least two of NO[•]'s homeostatic functions are related to the modulation of other pathways that contribute to the regulation of smooth muscle relaxation. First, NO[•] seems to blunt signaling by endothelin, the principal peptide responsible for vascular smooth muscle cell contraction, by slowing its release. Treatment of stationary endothelial cell cultures with 8-Br-cGMP is sufficient to mediate this effect, although the potential involvement of PKG is unknown (65). Physiologically, NO[•] appears to be a critical mediator of the decrease in endothelin release observed with chronic shear stress (65), as the decrease in endothelin release is abrogated by the NOS inhibitors methylene blue and N^{ω}-nitro-L-arginine (L-NNA) and potentiated by the phosphodiesterase inhibitor 3-isobutyl-1-methylxanthine (IBMX).

NO•'s second modulatory effect on the maintenance of smooth muscle tone is its multifaceted regulation of the release vasodilatory prostaglandins. In cultured endothelial cells stimulated with the calcium-mobilizing agonists bradykinin (66) and angiotensin II (67), or the calcium ionophore A23187 (68), NO• inhibits the release of prostacyclins by roughly 30%. This inhibitory effect involves cGMP (66), whose levels rise after NO• release as a result of paracrine stimulation of endothelial guanylyl cyclase (69). Consistent with these models, the peroxynitrite-mediated inhibition of purified prostacyclin synthase has also been described (70), although the relevance of this mechanism to in vivo models has not yet been established. In contrast, NO• has a stimulatory effect on prostacyclin release in the absence of calcium-mobilizing agents (68,71). Under these conditions, NO• donors *stimulate*, and NOS inhibitors *inhibit* the release of prostacyclins (71). Since the same study demonstrated that guanylyl cyclase inhibitors (i.e., diminished cGMP) also stimulate prostacyclin release, it is likely that NO• has a direct stimulatory effect on one or more enzymes in the prostacyclin synthetic pathway in the absence of elevated intracellular calcium levels. Interestingly, NO• does not appear to have an inhibitory effect on its own synthesis, as SNP and agonist-induced increases in cyclic GMP have little effect on NO• synthesis in endothelial cells (72).

NO• also appears to be critical for the maintenance of endothelial barrier function. Pharmacological administration of NO• donors or 8-Br-cGMP can either increase (73) or decrease (74) basal fluid permeability, but both consistently attenuate the enhanced permeability that occurs after stimulation with agonists such as thrombin (75), histamine (76), and VEGF (74). NO• affects agonist-induced changes in endothelial barrier function by at least two mechanisms (75). The first, enhanced PKA signaling, is typified by the responses in umbilical vein endothelial cells. In these cells, cGMP inhibits phosphodiesterase (PDE III), leading to a secondary increase in cAMP and activation of PKA (77). The second, typified by aortic endothelial cells, involves abrogation of the thrombin-induced increase in intracellular calcium, most likely by the PKG-dependent inhibition of PLC and the stimulation of plasma membrane calcium channels (75). The first mechanism is not operational in aortic endothelial cells because they lack PDE III, the cGMP-inhibitable isoform.

It must be noted that, although NO• donors at high doses inhibit VEGF-mediated increases in vascular permeability, NO• is produced as a result of VEGF stimulation, and this event is critical for VEGF-mediated *increases* in permeability (78,79). In this case, NO•, in synergy with prostacyclin, activates the ERK 1 and 2 pathway upstream of MEK (probably at ras) to induce the disaggregation of adherens and occludens junctions (39,80).

Other NO• target signaling systems that may be involved in stimulating venule endothelial cell hyperpermeability are the kinases and phosphatases that mediate myosin light-chain phosphorylation and dephosphorylation, respectively. Thus, inhibition of myosin light-chain phosphorylation with the myosin light-chain kinase inhibitor H7 decreases permeability, whereas stimulation of phosphorylation with the phosphatase inhibitor calyculin increases permeability (73). Still another downstream NO• target protein that may be involved in maintaining endothelial barrier function is vasodilator-stimulated phosphoprotein (VASP). VASP, a well-recognized substrate of both PKG and PKA, is present in all vascular tissue and is concentrated at focal adhesions, stress fibers, and surface protrusions rich in actin (81). VASP has recently been found to be a ligand for profilins, which form complexes with G-actin and phosphoinositides (82), indicating that it may transduce signals between the cytoskeleton and the plasma membrane.

In the absence of vasoactive stimuli (hormones, cytokines, and the like), NO• donors may induce a slight elevation in intracellular calcium in endothelial cells due to a net increase in the release from stores in the endoplasmic reticulum. For example, cultured human endothelial cells respond to the NO• donors SNAP and SNP with a transient, cGMP-independent, oscillatory stimulation of intracellular calcium release from IP_3-dependent stores (83). Because NO• donors inhibit PLC activity and would presumably lower IP_3 levels, these results imply that there is at least one protein at the endoplasmic reticulum that undergoes either S-nitrosation or tyrosine nitration, presumably closely associated with either the IP3 receptor or calcium ATPase. These cGMP-independent effects on calcium handling may reflect the action of peroxynitrite rather than NO• itself. In a carefully conducted study, SIN-1, which generates predominantly peroxynitrite as a result of its spontaneous release of NO• and superoxide, was found to inhibit the bradykinin-stimulated influx of calcium and to stimulate the net release of calcium from internal stores in vascular endothelial cells (84). SIN-1's effects were mimicked neither by the exclusive NO• donors spermine NONOate (a diazenium-diolate) and SNAP, nor 8-Br-cGMP. Studies using gastric smooth muscle have produced similar results (85), although in this tissue the effect is cGMP-dependent but PKA- and G-inde-pendent since NO• donors, 8-Br-cGMP, and the guanylyl cyclase stimulator VIP all increased net calcium release from internal stores in the presence of effective concentrations of PKG and PKA inhibitors. When considered with results in vascular smooth muscle, these results indicate that NO• can have opposite effects on the regulation of internal calcium stores in different tissues.

Growth Stimulation

Another difference between the effects of NO• on endothelial cells and smooth muscle cells is that NO• can stimulate endothelial cell growth. This stimulatory effect can be observed in vivo during angiogenesis and wound healing and in subconfluent endothelial cell cultures. Indeed, VEGF, interleukin-1 (IL-1), and substance P all stimulate endothelial cell growth by pathways requiring the production of NO• (86–88). The NO• requirement for VEGF signal-ing has been correlated to its ability to stimulate ERK1/2, the MAP kinases that are preferen-tially regulated by growth factors (39). ERK1/2 activity increases following the administration of both VEGF and SNP to endothelial cells, and in the case of VEGF, the increased activity is blocked when the cells are preincubated with the NOS inhibitor L-NMMA or the guanylyl cyclase inhibitor ODQ. These results indicate that the activation of ERK1/2 in VEGF-stimulated cells requires an elevation of cGMP. Interleukin-1 (IL-1) and substance P exerts their down-stream effects on endothelial cells via an NO•-dependent induction of basic fibroblast growth factor (bFGF), which in turn promotes growth by binding to and activating FGF receptors on the surface of the endothelial cell (86,89). Substance P can induce NO•-dependent bFGF production by endothelial cells, resulting in paracrine growth stimulation, whereas IL-1 works indirectly by stimulating bFGF release from associated smooth muscle cells, possibly as a result of NO•-mediated apopotosis. Thus in these systems NO• would indirectly stimulate a number of downstream tyrosine kinase-activated pathways, and potentially directly activate ERK1/2.

Closely related to NO•'s stimulatory effect on growth promotion by VEGF is its permis-sive effect on VEGF- and endothelin-1-induced motility of venular endothelial cells (90). The sites at which NO• acts have yet to be identified, but in other cells types motility often involves stimulation of the small G protein rac and one or more PKC isoforms. This effect is not observed in all types of endothelial cells, as SNAP and sodium nitroprusside both inhibit migration by human umbilical vein endothelial cells via a mechanism that at least partially involves cGMP (91). Again, the specific target proteins remain to be identified.

Cell Survival (Antiapoptosis)

At least one report has indicated that NO• plays a central role in the suppression of endothelial cell apoptosis by shear stress (92) i.e., in promoting cell survival. TNF-induced apoptosis was completely blocked by shear stress in an NO•-dependent manner. Moreover, the shear stress effect could be mimicked by NO• donors, indicating that NO• signaling is sufficient to elicit the antiapoptotic response. It is likely that cysteine proteases are important NO• targets in this system, as cysteine protease activity, which is required for TNF-mediated apoptosis, is completely inhibited by NO• *(92)*. Mechanistically, NO• has been demonstrated to directly inhibit cysteine protease-32 *(92)*, caspase 3 *(92,93)*, and six other caspases *(94)* via *S*-nitrosation of a critical active site cysteine in tissues where it has an antiapoptotic effect. Because all cysteine proteases have this critical active site cysteine, *S*-nitrosation is likely to be a universal means of inhibiting their enzymatic activity.

PLATELETS

Among the earliest effects attributed to NO• was its inhibitory effect on platelet activation, as evidenced by blunted responses to agonist-induced aggregation, fibrinogen binding, degranulation, and adherence to matrix *(95)*. Platelet aggregation induced with agonists such as thrombin, ADP, and arachidonic acid involves the activation of phospholipase C (with the ensuing release of calcium from intracellular stores and stimulation of PKC), plasma membrane calcium channels, components of the tyrosine kinase cascade, and a number of cytoskeletal rearrangements. There is also a secondary reinforcement of the aggregatory stimulus by activation of the fibrinogen receptor GPIIb–IIIa and the release of vasoactive substances (e.g., ADP, thromboxane A2) via degranulation and phospholipase activation.

As with other tissues, NO• stimulates platelet guanylyl cyclase, resulting in an increase intracellular cGMP and activation of PKG *(95,96)*. There is also a parallel increase in cAMP because platelets express primarily the cGMP-inhibitable isoform of phosphodiesterase (phosphodiesterase III), which hydrolyzes both cGMP and cAMP, and the cGMP-specific phosphodiesterase V *(97,98)*. The parallel activation of PKG and PKA has traditionally been thought to mediate NO•'s effects on platelets. However, recent work showing that the NO• donor *S*-NO-glutathione has some anti-aggregation activity in the presence of the guanylyl cyclase inhibitor ODQ has led to the suggestion that PKG-independent pathways may also make a contribution *(99)*.

The NO•-mediated inhibition of PLC activation in platelets appears to be similar to that in other tissues. Thus, NO• donors blunt the agonist-evoked rise in intracellular calcium and the accumulation of diacylglycerol, phosphatidic acid (the product resulting from both PLD activation and diacylglycerol rephosphorylation), or inositol trisphosphate *(100–102)*. These effects are mimicked by 8-Br-cGMP; based on analogy with other tissues they are likely to be PKG-dependent.

The blunted production of IP3 that results from NO•-mediated PLC inhibition in turn contributes to a blunted release of calcium from internal stores *(103)*, as evidenced by the inhibition of thrombin, thromboxane, and ADP-induced calcium mobilization from internal stores by SIN-1, 8-Br-cGMP, the cAMP-dependent prostaglandin PGE-1, and 8-Br-cAMP *(103)*. As in smooth muscle, this effect may be amplified by a direct NO•-dependent decrease in the intrinsic flux of calcium out of internal stores responsive to the endoplasmic reticulum calcium ATPase inhibitor thapsigargin *(103)*, although in platelets the target protein(s) have not been identified. NO• also inhibits the secondary influx of calcium due to store depletion (capacitive influx), but only indirectly, i.e., it inhibits capacitive influx because it inhibits store depletion. Indeed, capacative influx per se is regulated independently of changes in NO• or cyclic nucleotides *(104,105)*. Similarly, NO• has little effect on the rapid influx of extracellular calcium promoted by ADP *(103)*. The latter results indicate that, unlike calcium fluxes across smooth muscle cell plasma membranes, calcium fluxes across platelet plasma membranes are not directly modulated by NO•.

Platelet PKC activation, as measured by the phosphorylation of its primary substrate, p47 pleckstrin, is also inhibited by NO•. The NOS inhibitor N^G-nitro arginine methylester (L-NAME) increases membrane PKC activity in a manner similar to that of phorbol esters, and L-NAME's inhibitory effect can be overcome by L-arginine, SNP, or 8-Br-cGMP *(101)*. However, as in smooth muscle cells, the inhibition of platelet PKC is probably achieved primarily via the combination of S-nitrosation and the PKG-dependent inhibition of phospholipase C, as direct inhibition of PKC activity by PKG has not been demonstrated (101).

NO•'s inhibitory effects on platelet activation are not limited to effects mediated by calcium and PKC. SNP and 8-Br-cGMP will both attenuate phorbol-ester and calcium ionophore-stimulated platelet aggregation and degranulation (106). Because phorbol esters and calcium directly activate classical and novel type PKC's, and calcium ionophores bypass the biochemical steps needed to raise cytosolic calcium, these results indicate that NO• has inhibitory signaling effects downstream of PKC and calcium (104–108).

Together, these inhibitory effects lead to a dampening of cytoskeletal rearrangements in conjunction with enhanced phosphorylation of the cytoskeletal protein VASP (109–111). They also lead to a blunted expression of the GPIIb–IIIa fibrinogen receptor, P-selectin, and the lysosomal protein CD63 on the membrane surface following thrombin stimulation (112,113). The decrease in fibrinogen receptor number is associated with a decreased receptor affinity for fibrinogen (93), resulting in a substantially reduced capacity for "outside-in" signaling via this receptor. Interestingly, endogenous NO• production may be a significant downregulator of the increased P-selectin expression, which results from the fusion of P-selectin-rich A granules with the platelet plasma membrane. The NO• synthase inhibitor L-NAME significantly increases platelet surface P-selectin expression in concert with membrane-associated PKC activity. The enhanced P-selectin expression seen with the inhibition of NO• synthesis is additive to that observed after thrombin stimulation and can be attenuated by 8-Br-cGMP, SNP, and the NO• precursor L-arginine.

In addition to phospholipase C-dependent pathways, NO• donors can also effect downstream tyrosine kinase pathways in thrombin stimulated platelets. Two recently identified targets are the pool of activated PI3-kinase and the src family kinase lyn (114). The most prevalent means of PI3-kinase activation is when the SH2 domains in its regulatory subunit interact with phosphotyrosine moieties in other proteins. PI3-kinase associated with tyrosine-phosphorylated proteins and that specifically in lyn signaling complexes, are both stimulated by thrombin, and this effect is blocked by the NO• donors diethylamine NONOate and S-NO-glutathione. In the case of lyn-associated PI3-kinase, NO•'s effect appears to be on lyn, rather than PI3-kinase per se, as (1) total PI3-kinase activity is unaffected by S-NO-glutathione, (2) PI3-kinase activation in lyn complexes requires src-family tyrosine kinase activation, and (3) S-NO-glutathione blocks lyn tyrosine kinase activation by thrombin.

Finally, NO• has recently been demonstrated to antagonize thromboxane A2-mediated platelet activation by inhibiting the GTPase activity associated with the thromboxane A2 receptor (102). As determined in peptide mapping studies, the inhibitory effect seems to be due to the direct phosphorylation of the A2 receptor by PKG, rendering the receptor incapable of hydrolyzing GTP (115). In contrast, receptor-associated G-proteins do not appear to be affected (115). A similar inhibition of thromboxane A2 function has also been observed in mesangial cells (116).

SUMMARY

In conclusion, NO• and its downstream signaling systems impinge on a multitude of other signaling pathways, often at multiple sites within the same pathway. These effects are summarized in Table 1. The specific effects it has on a given tissue depend on what signaling pathways are present (e.g., cGMP-activatable vs. -inhibitable phosphodiesterases), as well as what function a given common pathway may have (e.g., tyrosine-kinase-mediated growth in smooth muscle cells and aggregation in platelets). Moreover, an increasing body of literature supports the hypothesis that the specific NO•-mediator (NO•, peroxynitrite, S-nitroso-thiols) also plays an important role in determining NO•'s effects on a given tissue's signaling pathways. A more complete understanding of these processes will clearly enhance our understanding of NO•'s multifaceted cardiovascular actions.

Table 1
NO• Signaling Targets

Tissue	Effect	Known targets
Smooth muscle	Relaxation	Phospholipase C, calcium channels, calcium ATPases, potassium channels, phosphodiesterases, PKA, myofilaments
	MAP kinase	ERK 1/2, p38, JNK, ras, AP-1, NFκB
	Growth inhibition	Receptor tyrosine kinases, ribonucletoide reductase, phospholipase C, PKC, phosphodiesterases, PKA
	Apoptosis	p53, ADP ribosylation pathway
Cardiac muscle	Negative inotrophy	Calcium channels, calcium ATPases, myofilaments, phosphodiesterases, PKA
Endothelial cells	Feedback inhibition of other vasoactive substances	Unknown
	Decreased water permeability	Phosphodiesterases, PKA, VASP?, other cytoskeletal elements
	Growth, growth factor release	Ras, ERK 1/2, AP-1
	Antiapoptosis	Caspases
Platelets	Activation	Phospholipase C, PKC, src family kinases, phosphodiesterases, PKA, VASP?, other cytoskeletal elements

REFERENCES

1. Pfeifer A, Klatt P, Massberg S, Ny L, Sausbier M, Hirneiss C, et al. Defective smooth muscle regulation in cGMP kinase I-deficient mice. EMBO J 1998;17:3045–3051.
2. Kai H, Kanaide H, Matsumoto T, Nakamura M. 8-Bromoguanosine 3':5'-cyclic monophosphate decreases intracellular free calcium concentrations in cultured vascular smooth muscle cells from rat aorta. FEBS Lett 1987;221:284–288.
3. Rashatwar SS, Cornwell TL, Lincoln TM. Effects of 8-bromo-cGMP on Ca^{2+} levels in vascular smooth muscle cells: possible regulation of Ca^{2+} ATPase by cGMP-dependent protein kinase. Proc Natl Acad Sci USA 1987;84:5685–5689.
4. Andriantsitohaina R, Lagaud GJ, Andre A, Muller B, Stoclet JC. Effects of cGMP on calcium handling in ATP-stimulated rat resistance arteries. Am J Physiol 1995;268:H1223–H1231.
5. Vrolix M, Raeymaekers L, Wuytack F, Hofmann F, Casteels R. Cyclic GMP-dependent protein kinase stimulates the plasmalemmal Ca^{2+} pump of smooth muscle via phosphorylation of phosphatidylinositol. Biochem J 1988;255:855–863.
6. Klebl BM, Ayoub AT, Pette D. Protein oxidation, tyrosine nitration, and inactivation of sarcoplasmic reticulum Ca^{2+}-ATPase in low-frequency stimulated rabbit muscle. FEBS Lett 1998;422:381–384.
7. Blatter LA, Wier WG. Nitric oxide decreases $[Ca^{2+}]$ in vascular smooth muscle by inhibition of the calcium current. Cell Calcium 1994;15:122–131.
8. Taguchi K, Ueda, M, Kubo T. Effects of cAMP and cGMP on L-type calcium channel currents in rat mesenteric artery cells. Jpn J Pharmacol 1997;74:179–186.
9. Hirata M, Kohse KP, Chang CH, Ikebe T, Murad F. Mechanism of cyclic GMP inhibition of inositol phosphate formation in rat aorta segments and cultured bovine aortic smooth muscle cells. J Biol Chem 1990;265:1268–1273.
10. Clementi E, Vecchio I, Sciorati C, Nistico G. Nitric oxide modulation of agonist-evoked intracellular Ca^{2+} release in neurosecretory PC-12 cells: inhbition of phospholipase C activity via cyclic GMP-dependent protein kinase I. Mol Pharm 1995;47:517–524.

11. Komalavilas P, Lincoln TM. Phosphorylation of the inositol 1,4,5-trisphosphate-receptor. Cyclic GMP-dependent protein kinase mediates cAMP and cGMP dependent phosphorylation in the intact rat aorta. J Biol Chem 1996;271:21,933–21,938.

12. Raeymaekers L, Hofmann F, Casteels R. Cyclic GMP-dependent protein kinase phosphorylates phospholamban in isolated sarcoplasmic reticulum from cardiac and smooth muscle. Biochem J 1988;252: 269–273.

13. Eggermont JA, Raeymaekers L, Casteels R. Ca^{2+} transport by smooth muscle membranes and its regulation. Biomed Biochim Acta 1989;48:S370–S381.

14. Sarcevic B, Brookes V, Martin TJ, Kemp BE, Robinson PJ. Atrial natriuretic peptide-dependent phosphorylation of smooth muscle cell particulate fraction proteins is mediated by cGMP-dependent protein kinase. J Biol Chem 1989;264:20,648–20,654.

15. Huggins JP, Cook EA, Piggott JR, Mattinsley TJ, England PJ. Phospholamban is a good substrate for cyclic GMP-dependent protein kinase in vitro, but not in intact cardiac or smooth muscle. Biochem J 1989;260:829–835.

16. Robertson BE, Schubert R, Hescheler J, Nelson MT. cGMP-dependent protein kinase activates Ca-activated K channels in cerebral artery smooth muscle cells. Am J Physiol 1993;265:C299–C303.

17. Bolotina VM, Najibi S, Palacino JJ, Pagano PJ, Cohen RA. Nitric oxide directly activates calcium-dependent potassium channels in vascular smooth muscle. Nature 1994;368:850–853.

18. Archer SL, Huang JMC, Hampl V, Nelson DP, Shultz PJ, Weir EK. Nitric oxide and cGMP cause vasorelaxation by activation of a charybdotoxin-sensitive K channel by cGMP-dependent protein kinase. Proc Natl Acad Sci USA 1994;91:7583–7587.

19. Peng W, Hoidal JR, Farrukh IS. Regulation of Ca^{2+}-activated K^+ channels in pulmonary vascular smooth muscle cells: role of nitric oxide. J Appl Physiol 1996;81:1264–1272.

20. Carrier GO, Fuchs LC, Winecoff AP, Giulumian AD, White RE. Nitrovasodilators relax mesenteric microvessels by cGMP-induced stimulation of Ca-activated K channels. Am J Physiol 1997;273: H76–H84.

21. Hampl V, Huang JM, Weir EK, Archer SL. Activation of the cGMP-dependent protein kinase mimics the stimulatory effect of nitric oxide and cGMP on calcium-gated potassium channels. Physiol Res 1995;44:39–44.

22. Sansom SC, Stockand JD, Hall D, Williams B. Regulation of large calcium-activated potassium channels by protein phosphatase 2A. J Biol Chem 1997;272:9902–9906.

23. Redmond EM, Cahill PA, Hodges R, Zhang S, Sitzmann JV. Regulation of endothelin receptors by nitric oxide in cultured rat vascular smooth muscle cells. J Cell Physiol 1996;166:469–479.

24. Awazu M. Inhibition of platelet-derived growth factor receptor tyrosine kinase by atrial natriuretic peptide. Kidney Int 1997;52:356–362.

25. Yu SM, Hung LM, Lin CC. cGMP-elevating agents suppress proliferation of vascular smooth muscle cells by inhibiting the activation of epidermal growth factor signaling pathway. Circulation 1997;95: 1269–1277.

26. Clementi E, Sciorati C, Riccio M, Miloso M, Meldolesi J, Nistico G. Nitric oxide on growth factor-elicited signals. Phosphoinositide hydrolysis and Ca^{2+} responses are negatively modulated via a cGMP-dependent protein kinase I pathway. J Biol Chem 1995;270:22,277–22,282.

27. Sauro MD, Fitzpatrick DF. Atrial natriuretic peptides inhibit protein kinase C activation in rat aortic smooth muscle. Peptide Res 1990;3:138–141.

28. Nguyen BL, Saitoh M, Ware JA. Interaction of nitric oxide and cGMP with signal transduction in activated platelets. Am J Physiol 1991;261:H1043–H1052.

29. Gopalakrishna R, Chen ZH, Gundimeda U. Nitric oxide and nitric oxide-generating agents induce a reversible inactivation of protein kinase C activity and phorbol ester binding. J Biol Chem 1993;268: 27,180–27,185.

30. Cornwell TL, Soff GA, Traynor AE, Lincoln TM. Regulation of the expression of cyclic GMP-dependent protein kinase by cell density in vascular smooth muscle cells. J Vasc Res 1994;31:330–337.

31. Sciorati C, Nistico G, Meldolesi J, Clementi E. Nitric oxide effects on cell growth: GMP-dependent stimulation of the AP-1 transcription complex and cyclic GMP-independent slowing of cell cycling. Br J Pharmacol 1997;122:687–697.

32. Boerth NJ, Dey NB, Cornwell TL, Lincoln TM. Cyclic GMP-dependent protein kinase regulates vascular smooth muscle cell phenotype. J Vasc Res 1997;34:245–259.

33. Estrada C, Gomez C, Martin-Nieto J, De Frutos T, Jimenz A, Villalobo A. Nitric oxide reversibly inhibits the epidermal growth factor receptor tyrosine kinase. Biochem J 1997;326:369–376.

34. Guittet O, Ducastel B, Salem JS, Henry Y, Rubin H, Lemaire G, et al. Differential sensitivity of the tyrosyl radical of mouse rebonucleotide reductase to nitric oxide and peroxynitrite. J Biol Chem 1998; 273:22,136–22,144.

35. Lander HM, Ogiste JS, Pearce SF, Levi R, Novogrodsky A. Nitric oxide-stimulated guanine nucleotide exchange on p21 ras. J Biol Chem 1995;270:7017–7020.
36. Lander HM, Hajjar DP, Hempstead BL, Mirza UA, Chait BT, Campbell S, et al. A molecular redox switch on p21 ras. Structural basis for nitric oxide-p21 (ras) interaction. J Biol Chem 1997;272:4323–4326.
37. Lander HM, Jacovina AT, Davis RJ, Tauras JM. Differential activation of mitogen-activated protein kinases by nitric oxide-related species. J Biol Chem 1996;271:19,705–19,709.
38. Kanterewicz BI, Knapp LT, Klann E. Stimulation of p42 and p44 mitogen-activated protein kinases by reactive oxygen species and nitric oxide in hippocampus. J Neurochem 1998;70:1009–1016.
39. Parenti A, Morbidell C, Cui XL, Douglas JG, Hood JD, Granger HJ, et al. Nitric oxide is an upstream signal of vascular endothelial growth factor-induced extracellular signal-regulated kinase 1/2 activation in postcapillary endothelium. J Biol Chem 1998;273:4220–4226.
40. Tabuchi A, Sano K, Oh E, Tsuchiya T, Tsuda M. Modulation of AP-1 activity by nitric oxide (NO) in vitro: NO-mediated modulation of AP-1. FEBS Lett 1994;351:123–127.
41. DelaTorre A, Schroeder RA, Kuo PC. Alteration of NF-kappa B p50 DNA binding kinetics by S-nitrosylation. Biochem Biophys Res Commun 1997;238:703–706.
42. So HS, Park RK, Kim MS, Lee SR, Jung BH, Chung SY, et al. Nitric oxide inhibits c-Jun N-terminal kinase 2 (JNK2) via S-nitrosylation. Biochem Biophys Res Commun 1998;247:809–813.
43. Nishio E, Fukushima K, Shiozaki M, Watanabe Y. Nitric oxide donor SNAP induces apoptosis in smooth muscle cells through cGMP-independent mechanism. Biochem Biophys Res Commun 1996; 221:163–168.
44. Iwashina M, Shichiri M, Marumo F, Hirata Y. Transfection of inducible nitric oxide synthase gene causes apoptosis in vascular smooth muscle cells. Circulation 1998;98:1212–1218.
45. Molina Y, Molina y Verdia L, McDonald B, Reep B, Brune B, DiSilvio M, Billiar TR, et al. Nitric oxide-induced S-nitrosylation of glyceraldehyde-3-phosphate dehydrogenase inhibits enzymatic activity and increases endogenous ADP-rebisylation. J Biol Chem 1992;267:24,929–24,932.
46. Mohr S, Stamler JS, Brune B. Mechanism of covalent modification of glyceraldehyde-3-phosphate dehydrogenase at its active site thiol by nitric oxide, peroxynitrite and related nitrosating agents. FEBS Lett 1994;348:223–227.
47. Mohr S, Stamler JS, Brune B. Posttranslational modification of glyceraldehyde-3-phosphate dehydrogenase by S-nitrosylation and subsequent NADH attachment. J Biol Chem 1996;271:4209–4214.
48. Messmer UK, Brune B. Nitric oxide-induced apoptosis: p53-dependent and p53-independent signalling pathways. Biochem J 1996;319:299–305.
49. Zhao Z, Francis CE, Welch G, Loscalzo J, Ravid K. Reduced glutathione prevents nitric oxide-induced apopotosis in vascular smooth muscle cells. Biochim Biophys Acta 1997;1359:143–152.
50. Vila Echague A, Genaro AM, Sterin-Borda L. Negative inotropic effect of carbachol on rat atria mediated by nitric oxide. Acta Physiol Pharm Ther Latinoam 1994;44:100–107.
51. Sterin-Borda L, Echague AV, Leiros CP, Genaro A, Borda E. Endogenous nitric oxide signalling system and the cardiac muscarinic acetylcholine receptor-inotropic response. Br J Pharmacol 1995;115: 1525–1531.
52. Sterin-Borda L, Genaro A, Perez Leiros C, Cremaschi G, Vila Echague A, Borda E. Role of nitric oxide in cardiac beta-adrenoceptor-inotropic response. Cell Signal 1998;10:253–257.
53. Klabunde RE, Kimber ND, Kuk JE, Helgren MC, Forstermann U. NG-methyl-L-arginine decreases contractility, cGMP and cAMP in isoproterenol-stimulated rat hearts in vitro. Eur J Pharmacol 1992; 223:1–7.
54. Kinugawa KI, Kohmoto O, Yao A, Serizawa T, Takahashi T. Cardiac inducible nitric oxide synthase negatively modulates myocardial function in cultured rat myocytes. Am J Physiol 1997;272:H35–H47.
55. Han X, Shimoni Y, Giles WR. A cellular mechanism for nitric oxide-mediated cholinergic control of mammalian heart rate. J Gen Physiol 1995;106:45–65.
56. Han X, Kubota I, Feron O, Opel DJ, Arstall MA, Zhao YY, et al. Muscarinic cholinergic regulation of cardiac myocyte ICa-L is absent in mice with targeted disruption of endothelial nitric oxide synthase. Proc Natl Acad Sci USA 1998;95:6510–6515.
57. Wahler GM, Dollinger SJ. Nitric oxide donor SIN-1 inhibits mammalian cardiac calcium current through cGMP-dependent protein kinase. Am J Physiol 1995;268:C45–C54.
58. Kumar R, Namiki T, Joyner RW. Effects of cGMP on L-type calcium current of adult and newborn rabbit ventricular cells. Cardiovasc Res 1997;33:573–582.
59. Campbell DL, Stamler JS, Strauss HC. Redox modulation of L-type calcium channels in ferret ventricular myocytes. Dual mechanism regulation by nitric oxide and S-nitrosothiols. J Gen Physiol 1996; 108:277–293.

60. Mery PF, Pavoine C, Belhassen L, Pecker F, Fischmeister R. Nitric oxide regulates cardiac Ca^{2+} current. Involvement of cGMP-inhibited and cGMP-stimulated phosphodiesterases through guanylyl cyclase activation. J Biol Chem 1993;268:26,286–26,295.

61. Habuchi Y, Nishio M, Tanaka H, Yamamoto T, Lu LL, Yoshimura M. Regulation by acetylcholine of Ca^{2+} current in rabbit atrioventricular node cells. Am J Physiol 1996;271:H2274–H2282.

62. Xu L, Eu JP, Meissner G, Stamler JS. Activation of the cardiac calcium release channel (ryonadine receptor) by poly-S-nitrosylation. Science 1998;279:234–237.

63. Aronstam RS, Martin DC, Dennison RL, Cooley HG. S-nitrosylation of m2 muscarinic receptor thiols disrupts receptor-G-protein coupling. Ann NY Acad Sci 1995;757:215–217.

64. Wang D, Yu X, Brecher P. Nitric oxide and N-acetylcysteine inhibit the activation of mitogen-activated protein kinases by angiotensin II in rat cardiac fibroblasts. J Biol Chem 1998;273:33,027–33,034.

65. Kuchan MJ, Frangos JA. Shear stress regulates endothelin-1 release via protein kinase C and cGMP in cultured endothelial cells. Am J Physiol 1993;264:H150–H156.

66. Doni MG, Whittle BJ, Palmer RM, Moncada S. Actions of nitric oxide on the release of prostacyclin from bovine endothelial cells in culture. Eur J Pharmacol 1988;151:19–25.

67. Barker JE, Bakhle YS, Anderson J, Treaure T, Piper PJ. Reciprocal inhibition of nitric oxide and prostacyclin synthesis in human saphenous vein. Br J Pharmacol 1996;118:643–648.

68. Alanko J, Sievi E, Lahteenmaki T, Mucha I, Ruitta A, Vapaatalo H. Effects of NO-donors, SIN-1 and GEA 3175 on prostacyclin and cGMP synthesis in cultured rat. Agents Actions 1995;45:195–199.

69. Schroder H, Strobach H, Schror K. Nitric oxide but not prostacyclin is an autocrine endothelial mediator. Biochem Pharmacol 1992;43:533–537.

70. Zou M, Martin C, Ullrich V. Tyrosine nitration as a mechanism of selective inactivation of prostacyclin synthase by peroxynitrite. Biol Chem 1997;378:707–713.

71. Sievi E, Lahteenmaki TA, Alanko J, Vuorinen P, Vapaatalo H. Nitric oxide as a regulator of prostacyclin synthesis in cultured rat heart endothelial cells. Arzneimittel-Forschung 1997;47:1093–1098.

72. Kuhn M, Otten A, Frolich JC, Forstermann U. Endothelial cyclic GMP and cyclic AMP do not regulate the release of endothelium-derived relaxing factor/nitric oxide from bovine aortic endothelial cells. J Pharmacol Exp Ther 1991;256:677–682.

73. Yuan Y, Huang Q, Wu HM. Myosin light chain phosphorylation: modulation of basal and agonist-stimulated venular permeability. Am J Physiol 1997;272:H1437–H1443.

74. Wu HM, Huang Q, Yuan Y, Granger HJ. VEGF induces NO-dependent hyperpermeability in coronary venules. Am J Physiol 1996;271:H2735–H2739.

75. Draijer R, Atsma DE, van der Laarse A, van Hinsbergh VW. cGMP and nitric oxide modulate thrombin-induced endothelial permeability. Regulation via different pathways in human aortic and umbilical vein endothelial cells. Circ Res 1995;76:199–208.

76. Huang Q, Yuan Y. Interaction of PKC and NOS in signal transduction of microvascular hyperpermeability. Am J Physiol 1997;273:H2442–H2451.

77. Lugnier C, Komas N. Modulation of vascular cyclic nucleotide phosphodiesterases by cyclic GMP: role in vasodilation. Eur Heart J 1993;14:141–148.

78. Wu HM, Huang Q, Yuan Y, Granger HJ. VEGF induces NO-dependent hyperpermeability in coronary venules. Am J Physiol 1996;271:H2735–H2739.

79. Fujii E, Irie K, Ohba K, Ogawa A, Yoshioka T, Yamakawa M, et al. Role of nitric oxide prostaglandins and tyrosine kinase in vascular endothelial growth factor—induced increase in vascular permeability in mouse skin. Naunyn-Schmiedbergs Arch Physiol 1997;356:475–480.

80. Murohara T, Horowitz JR, Silver M, Tsurumi Y, Chen D, Sullivan A, et al. Vascular endothelial growth factor/vascular permeability factor enhances permeability via nitric oxide and prostacyclin. Circulation 1988;97:99–107.

81. Haffner C, Jarchau T, Reinhard M, Hoppe J, Lohmann SM, Walter U. Molecular cloning, structural analysis and functional expression of the proline-rich focal adhesion and microfilament-associated protein VASP. EMBO J 1995;14:19–27.

82. Reinhard M, Giehl K, Abel K, Haffner C, Harchau T, Hoppe V, et al. The proline-rich focal adhesion and microfilamine protein VASP is a ligand for profilins. EMBO J 1995;14:1583–1589.

83. Volk T, Mading K, Hensel M, Kox WJ. Nitric oxide induces transient Ca^{2+} changes in endothelial cells independent of cGMP. J Cell Physiol 1997;172:296–305.

84. Elliott SJ. Peroxynitrite modulates receptor-activated Ca^{2+} signaling in vascular endothelial cells. Am J Physiol 1996;270:L954–L961.

85. Murthy KS, Makhlouf GM. cGMP-mediated Ca^{2+} release from IP3-insenstive Ca^{2+} stores in smooth muscle. Am J Physiol 1998;274:C1199–C1205.

86. Fukuo K, Inoue T, Morimoto S, Nakahashi T, Yasuda O, Kitano S, et al. Nitric oxide mediates cyto-toxicity and basic fibroblast growth factor release in cultured vascular smooth muscle cells. A possible mechanism of neovascularization in atherosclerotic plaques. J Clin Invest 1995;95:669–676.
87. Papapetropoulos A, Garcia-Cardena G, Madri JA, Sessa WC. Nitric oxide production contributes to the angiogenic properties of vascular endothelial growth factor in human endothelial cells. J Clin Invest 1997;100:3131–3139.
88. Morbidelli L, Chang CH, Douglas JG, Granger HJ, Ledda F, Ziche M. Nitric oxide mediates mitogenic effect of VEGF on coronary venular endothelium. Am J Physiol 1996;270:H411–H415.
89. Ziche M. Parenti A, Ledda F, Dell'Era P, Granger HS, Maggi CA, et al. Nitric oxide promotes prolif-eration and plasminogen activator production by coronary venular endothelium through endogenous bFGF. Circ Res 1997;80:845–852.
90. Noiri E, Hu Y, Bahou WF, Keese CR, Giaever I, Goligorsky MS. Permissive role of nitric oxide in endothelin-induced migration of endothelial cells. J Biol Chem 1997;272:1747–1753.
91. Lau YT, Ma WC. Nitric oxide inhibits migration of cultured endothelikal cells. Biochem Biophys Res Commun 1996;221:670–674.
92. Dimmeler S, Haendeler J, Nehls M, Zeiher AM. Suppression of apoptosis by nitric oxide via inhibition of interleukin-1β-converting enzyme (ICE)-like and cysteine protease protein (CPP)-32-like pro-teases. J Exp Med 1997;185:601–607.
93. Kim YM, Talanian RV, Billiar TR. Nitric oxide inhibits apoptosis by preventing increases in caspase-3-like activity via two distinct mechanisms. J Biol Chem 1997;272:31,138–31,148.
94. Li J, Billiar TR, Talanian RV, Kim YM. Nitric oxide reversibly inhibits seven members of the caspase family via S-nitrosylation. Biochem Biophys Res Commun 1997;240:419–424.
95. Lieberman EH, O'Neill S, Mendelsohn ME. S-nitrosocysteine inhibition of human platelet secretion is correlated with increases in platelet cGMP levels. Circ Res 1991;68:1722–1728.
96. Mendelsohn ME, O'Neill S, George D, Loscalzo J. Inhibition of fibrinogen binding to human platelets by S-nitroso-N-acetylcysteine. J Biol Chem 1990;265:19,028–19,034.
97. Macphee CH, Harrison SA, Beavo JA. Immunological identification of the major platelet low-Km cAMP phosphodiesterase: probable target for anti-thrombotic agents. Proc Natl Acad Sci USA 1986; 83:6660–6663.
98. Maurice DH, Haslam RJ. Molecular basis of the synergistic inhibition of platelet function by nitro-vasodilators and activators of adenylate cyclase: inhibition of cyclic AMP breakdown by cyclic GMP. Mol Pharmacol 1990;37:671–681.
99. Gordge MP, Hothersall JS, Noronha-Dutra AA. Evidence for a cyclic GMP-independent mechanism in the anti-platelet action of S-nitrosoglutathione. Br J Pharmacol 1998;124:141–148.
100. Waldmann R, Walter U. Cyclic nucleotide elevating vasodilators inhibit platelet aggregation at an early step of the activation cascade. Eur J Pharmacol 1989;159:317–320.
101. Nguyen BL, Saitoh M, Ware JA. Interaction of nitric oxide and cGMP with signal transduction in activated platelets. Am J Physiol 1991;30:H1043–H1052.
102. Azula FJ, Alzola ES, Conde M, Trueba M, Macarulla JM, Marino A. Thrombin-stimulated phospho-lipase C activity is inhibited without visible delay by a rapid increase in the cyclic GMP levels induced by sodium nitroprusside. Mol Pharmacol 1996;50:367–379.
103. Geiger J, Nolte C, Walter U. Regulation of calcium mobilization and entry in human platelets by endothelium-derived factors. Am J Physiol 1994;267:C236–C244.
104. Okamoto Y, Ninomiya H, Miwa S, Masaki T. Capacitative Ca^{2+} entry in human platelets is resistant to nitric oxide. Biochem Biophys Res Commun 1995;212:90–96.
105. Heemskerk JW, Feijge MA, Sage SO, Walter U. Indirect regulation of Ca^{2+} entry by cAMP-dependent and cGMP-dependent protein kinases and phospholipase C in rat platelets. Eur J Biochem 1994;223: 543–551.
106. Doni MG, Alexandre A, Padoin E, Bertoncello S, Deana R. Nitrovasodilators and cGMP inhibit human platelet activation. Cardioscience 1991;2:161–165.
107. Halbrugge M, Friedrich C, Eigenthaler M, Schanzenbacher P. Walter U. Stoichiometric and reversible phosphorylation of a 46-kDa protein in human platelets in response to cGMP- and cAMP-elevating vasodilators. J Biol Chem 1990;265:3088–3093.
108. Nolte C, Eigenthaler M, Schanzenbacher P, Walter U. Endothelial cell-dependent phosphorylation of a platelet protein mediated by cAMP- and cGMP-elevating factors. J Biol Chem 1991;266:14,808–14,812.
109. Reinhard M, Halbrugge M, Scheer U, Wiegand C, Jockusch BM, Walter U. The 46/50 kDa phospho-protein VASP purified from human platelets is a novel protein associated with actin filaments and focal contacts. EMBO J 1992;11:2063–2070.

110. Horstrup K, Jablonka B, Honig-Liedl P, Just M, Kochsiek K, Walter U. Phosphorylation of focal adhesion vasodilator-stimulated phosphoprotein at Ser157 in intact human platelets correlates with fibrinogen receptor inhibition. Eur J Biochem 1994;225:21–27.

111. Nolte C, Eigenthaler M, Horstrup K, Honig-Liedl P, Walter U. Synergistic phosphorylation of the focal adhesion-associated vasodilator-stimulated phosphoprotein in intact human platelets in response to cGMP- and cAMP-elevating platelet inhibitors. Biochem Pharmacol 1994;48:1569–1575.

112. Michelson AD, Benoit SE, Furman MI, Brechwoldt WL, Rohrer MJ, Barnard MR, et al. Effects of nitric oxide/EDRF on platelet surface glycoproteins. Am J Physiol 1996;270:H1640–H1648.

113. Murohara T, Parkinson SJ, Waldman SA, Lefer AM. Inhibition of nitric oxide biosynthesis promotes P-selectin expression in platelets. Role of protein kinase C. Arterioscler Thromb Vasc Biol 1995;15: 2068–2075.

114. Pigazzi A, Heydrick S, Folli F, Benoit S, Michelson A, Loscalzo J. Nitric oxide inhibits thrombin receptor-activating peptide-induced P13-kinase activity in human platelets. J Biol Chem 1999; 274: 14,368–14,375.

115. Wang GR, Zhu Y, Halushka PV, Lincoln TM, Mendelsohn ME. Mechanism of platelet inhibition by nitric oxide: in vivo phosphorylation of thromboxane receptor by cyclic GMP-dependent protein kinase. Proc Natl Acad Sci USA 1998;95:4888–4893.

116. Studer RK, DeRubertis FR, Craven PA. Nitric oxide suppresses increases in mesangial cell protein kinase C, transforming growth factor beta, and fibronectin synthesis induced by thromboxane. J Am Soc Nephrol 1996;7:999–1005.

4

Regulation of Gene Expression by Nitric Oxide

Ami A. Deora and Harry M. Lander

INTRODUCTION

Nitric oxide (NO•) and related chemical species have emerged as ubiquitous cellular messengers. This smallest known mammalian biological signaling molecule plays a crucial role in human physiology. NO• is synthesized by the enzyme nitric oxide synthase (NOS) and can assume several chemical forms, each of which has its own reactive specificity toward cellular targets. The resulting interaction initiates many signaling events in the cell. NO•-induced signal transduction and gene expression influences various physiological events including vasodilation, cytotoxicity, inflammation, and synaptic plasticity.

The pivotal role of nitric oxide in cardiovascular biology was clearly demonstrated by the fact that eNOS knockout mice have increased blood pressure, a reduced heart rate, and a defect in vascular remodeling *(1,2)*. Thus, aberrant NO• signaling may promote pathophysiological changes such as hypertension and atherosclerosis. A mechanistic understanding of NO•-triggered signaling will have far-reaching implications in the treatment of cardiovascular diseases.

Here we provide an overview of the interaction of various redox forms of NO• with cellular targets and resulting gene expression and discuss its significance in the cardiovascular system.

Localization of Different Isoforms of NOS in Cardiac Tissue

NO• is derived enzymatically by the oxidation of one of the terminal guanidino-nitrogen atoms of L-arginine *(3)* by nitric oxide synthase (NOS), which exists in three isoforms. nNOS (type I, ref. *4*) and eNOS (type III, ref. *5*), which were initially cloned from neuronal and endothelial cells respectively, are calcium–calmodulin dependent and expressed constitutively. iNOS (type II), which was first identified in macrophages, is calcium independent and inducible *(6)*. The regulation of these enzymes is complex and requires five cofactors (flavin adenine dinucleotide [FAD], flavin adenine mononucleotide [FMN], heme, calmodulin, and tetrahydrobiopterin) and three cosubstrates (L-arginine, NADPH, and O_2) *(7)*.

The different cells of cardiac tissue express one or more of these three isoforms. eNOS is constitutively expressed in endothelial cells of arteries, veins, and capillaries, the atrioventricular node, and atrial and ventricular myocytes *(8–12)*. nNOS is expressed in cholinergic, sympathetic, and nonadrenergic, noncholinergic nerve terminals *(13–15)*. iNOS protein expression can be triggered in many cells in response to inflammatory cytokines, including cells of the cardiovascular system, such as endothelial cells, cardiac myocytes, vascular smooth cells, and fibroblasts *(16–19)*. NO• synthesized by different isoforms of NOS regulate various important cardiac functions, which are listed in Table 1.

From: *Contemporary Cardiology, vol. 4: Nitric Oxide and the Cardiovascular System*
Edited by: J. Loscalzo and J. A. Vita © Humana Press Inc., Totowa, NJ

Table 1
Cardiac Functions Regulated by Different Isoforms of NOS

NOS isoform	Cells expressing NOS	Autocrine and paracrine responses
1. eNOS	Endothelial cells	*Autocrine*: proliferation *(61)* *Paracrine*: inhibition of contractile tone, vascular smooth muscle proliferation, platelet adhesion and aggregation, monocyte adhesion, and oxygen consumption; promotes diastolic relaxation *(110,122–129)*
	Cardiac myocytes	*Autocrine*: opposes inotropic action of catecholamines on muscarinic cholinergic and β-adrenergic receptor stimulation *(130)*
2. nNOS	Sympathetic nerve terminals	*Autocrine*: regulates norepinephrine release *(15)*
3. iNOS	All cardiac cell types on stimulation with inflammatory cytokines	*Autocrine and paracrine*: vasoplegia and myocardial depression, enhances cell death by inducing apoptosis *(121)*

Chemistry of Reactive Nitrogen Species and Their Interaction with Cellular Targets

NO• has an unpaired electron making it highly reactive. Its reaction with redox modulators yields many reactive species. The term "NO•" does not provide any information regarding its different redox forms; hence the term "reactive nitrogen species" (RNS) is used in this chapter and refers to species whose origin is the free radical NO•, but whose final chemical nature depends on its interaction with local redox modulators and the redox milieu of the cell *(20)*. Chemically, NO• can exist in three redox forms: nitrosonium (NO^+), nitric oxide (NO•), and nitroxyl anion (NO^-). In the presence of superoxide anion ($O_2^{-•}$), NO• combines to form peroxynitrite ($OONO^-$), a strong pro-oxidant species *(21)*. In aqueous aerobic solutions, NO• predominantly forms nitrite (NO_2^-). In the presence of oxyhemoglobin and oxymyoglobin, NO• is readily oxidized to nitrate (NO_3^-) *(22)*.

Covalent interactions of RNS with cellular macromolecules are responsible for various physiological and pathological consequences. Proteins containing iron and thiol groups are the major cellular targets of RNS. Extensive studies have been performed characterizing the RNS–iron interaction. The iron, as an Fe^{2+} or Fe^{3+}, can be targeted when either in a heme group or in an iron–sulfur cluster *(23,24)*. The physiological significance of *S*-nitrosothiol adduction is now widely accepted. *S*-nitrosothiols at critical active site thiol residues are reported to regulate the function of several proteins *(25–27)*. Under more extreme conditions, such as severe oxidative and nitrosative stress, RNS react at other targets such as amino groups on DNA and tyrosine residues on proteins. RNS modification of target proteins results in modulation of their functional properties and can propagate downstream signals *(25)*.

Many of the studies discussed here use an exogenous source of RNS in the form of RNS donors. These are structurally different compounds and are metabolized by enzymes or undergo spontaneous hydrolysis to release RNS *(28)*. Inhibitors of NOS are also very useful in experimental studies. They include flavoprotein, calmodulin, or heme binders; tetrahydrobiopterin-depleting agents; and the commonly used substrate analogs *(29)*. These compounds have greatly aided pharmacological, biochemical, and molecular studies to elucidate the role of NO• in physiological processes.

Table 2
Cellular Events Regulated by the RNS/cGMP Signaling Pathway in Cardiovascular System

Cell type	Cellular event	Reference
Smooth muscle cells	Vasodilation	32
Platelets	Inhibition of adhesion and aggregation	33, 123
Human myocardium	Negative inotropic effect	131
Rat smooth muscle cells, myocytes, pinealocytes, alveolar epithelial cells	Inhibits spontaneous depolarization of L-type Ca^{2+} channels	132
Rat aorta	Inhibition of α1 adrenergic receptor-induced c-fos and c-jun mRNA	111
Coronary venular endothelial cells	Involved in VEGF-induced endothelial cell proliferation	61

SIGNALING PATHWAYS TRIGGERED BY RNS LEADING TO GENE EXPRESSION

RNS serve as extraordinarily widespread effectors of cellular functions. Generally, RNS-responsive targets serve sensory and regulatory roles in signal transduction. The target recognizes RNS and transduces the chemical signal into a functional response. RNS utilize means of communication used both by protein kinases, which control function by covalent modification (i.e., phosphorylation), and reactive oxygen species, which signal through redox events and coordinative interactions with metals. Some of the signaling pathways involving RNS are next discussed and depicted in Fig. 1.

Interaction with Heme Iron

The redox sensitive heme groups of metalloproteins located at catalytic or allosteric sites of proteins are natural sensors of redox reactive species such as RNS. A variety of heme-containing proteins exhibit RNS-responsive regulation.

GUANYLYL CYCLASE

Guanosine 3',5'-cyclic monophosphate (cGMP) is utilized as an intracellular amplifier and second messenger by a wide spectrum of ligands to elicit diverse physiological responses. cGMP synthesis is catalyzed by multiple types of soluble and particulate guanylyl cyclases (30).

Soluble guanylyl cyclase is a family of heterodimeric heme proteins exhibiting a pyridine hemochrome visual absorption spectrum typical for ferroprotoporphyrin IX and containing copper and iron as transition metals (31). The activation of soluble guanylyl cyclase by RNS is the principal mechanism of action in RNS-induced cellular events, such as smooth muscle relaxation (32) and inhibition of platelet adhesion (33). Many cardiovascular consequences of RNS-induced guanylyl cyclase activation are listed in Table 2. RNS bind to the heme moiety of guanylyl cyclase and, by disrupting the plane of the heme–iron, induce a conformational change that allosterically activates the enzyme (34). The cGMP further modulates an array of mediators, including ion channels, phosphodiesterases, and protein kinases (30). Activation of guanylyl cyclase was the first RNS-induced signaling mechanism reported. To date, it remains the most important physiological pathway by which eNOS regulates cardiac function.

NO• SYNTHASE

NOS is a homodimer with a molecular weight of approx 300 kDa. Its regulation is intricate with checkpoints at transcriptional, posttranscriptional, and posttranslational levels (35). Interestingly, RNS can inhibit the enzyme activity of NOS itself by posttranslational modification.

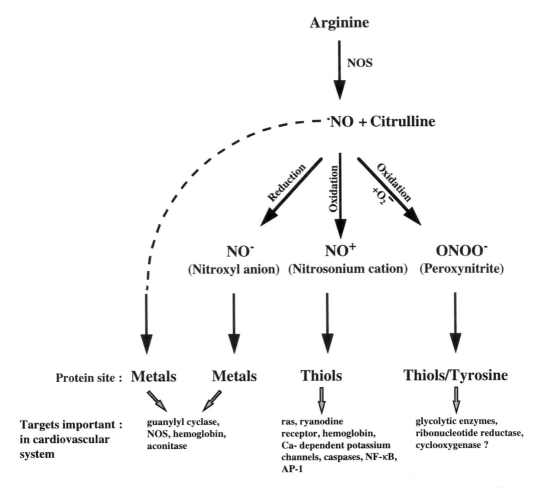

Fig. 1. Posttranslational modification of proteins important in cardiovascular function by different congeners of nitric oxide.

Unlike guanylyl cyclase, this enzyme uses the heme prosthetic group in catalysis. The binding of RNS to either Fe(II) or Fe(III) heme may interfere with the conversion of ferric to ferrous iron required for catalysis and result in attenuation of enzyme activity; thus, negative feedback inhibition is achieved *(36–39)*. This is likely to be a critical event in turning off NO$^{\bullet}$ synthesis and crucial for maintaining redox homeostasis.

Interaction with Fe–S Proteins

Iron–sulfur proteins (Fe–S) are polymetallic structures whose iron atoms are linked to inorganic sulfides and are usually liganded to proteins by cysteine thiolates. These proteins are sensitive to oxidoreduction and have long been known as targets of $O_2^{-\bullet}$ and H_2O_2. In in vitro models, RNS were shown to yield complexes with [Fe–S] clusters *(40)*. It is thought that peroxynitrite may react with iron–sulfur clusters and, in contrast to the reversible reaction of RNS with heme, its reaction with iron–sulfur clusters results in dissolution of the cluster *(41,42)*.

ACONITASE

In addition to its participation in the citric acid cycle, the mammalian [4Fe–4S] cytoplasmic aconitase is also a regulator of iron homeostasis. RNS inhibit aconitase activity by disrupting the [Fe–S] clusters. This disruption exposes its RNA binding site permitting binding of this protein, now called the iron regulatory-binding protein, to the iron-responsive element on the mRNA of the transferrin receptor and ferritin. When bound to the iron-responsive element at the 3' end of transferrin receptor mRNA, it stabilizes the mRNA. However, when bound to the iron-responsive element at the 5' end of ferritin mRNA, it inhibits translation *(43–45)*. Thus, RNS signal through the proteins involved in iron metabolism and regulate iron homeostasis. Inhibiting the enzyme involved in the citric acid cycle is one of the mechanism by which iNOS injures cells.

Interaction with Thiol

Cysteine residues are known to be important for maintaining the native conformation of proteins, are critical residues at the active sites of enzymes, and are the most reactive residues to RNS at physiologic pH. Furthermore, cysteine residues are sites for covalent attachment of other regulatory molecules, e.g., lipid and adenosine diphosphate (ADP)–ribose; hence any modification at this site may have implications extending to other signaling pathways. RNS react with thiols to form a variety of oxidized thiol species including sulfenic acids *(46)*, disulfides *(47)*, mixed disulfides *(48)*, S-nitrosothiols *(49)*, and covalent nicotinamide adenine dinucleotide (NAD)–thiol linkages *(50)*. Modification of protein thiols by RNS alters the function and activity of various proteins, ion channels, receptors, and transcription factors, which will be discussed in detail.

Under physiological aerobic conditions, oxidation of NO$^•$ yields NO$^+$-like species that have a high propensity for nucleophilic centers such as thiols and forms S-nitrosothiol derivatives (RSNO) *(25,49,51)*. Thiol nitrosation may also be mediated by the oxidative activation of NO$^•$ through binding to transition metals. S-nitrosothiol formation by metal ion-mediated formation of NO$^+$ is likely to be faster than via reactions of NO$^•$ and O_2 *(52)*. Also, peroxynitrite anion is capable of nitrosating thiols *(53,54)*. S-nitrosothiols have a longer half-life than free NO$^•$ and are an important pool from which redox signals can be generated. The S-nitrosation of protein thiols represents a form of posttranslational modification and may either activate or inactivate protein function.

PROTEINS ACTIVATED BY S-NITROSOTHIOL FORMATION

Ras. The monomeric G protein Ras is a key element of various signaling pathways. It is implicated in the regulation of proliferation and differentiation by tyrosine kinase- and G-protein-coupled receptors. Activation of Ras involves guanine nucleotide exchange factor-mediated exchange of guanosine diphosphate (GDP) for guanosine triphosphate (GTP) and subsequent interaction with effector proteins. Effector proteins transduce signals via several pathways and induce cellular responses *(55–57)*.

RNS were found to activate Ras in human T cells, rat pheochromocytoma cells, and human endothelial cells. S-nitrosothiol formation at a single cysteine residue, Cys[118] of Ras was found to trigger GDP/GTP exchange *(26,58,59)*. Thus, RNS activate Ras by a mechanism akin to that of growth factors. However, it differs in that it bypasses the requirement for guanine nucleotide exchange factors by directly modifying Ras and triggering GDP/GTP exchange.

Mitogen-activated protein kinases are important components of the Ras-dependent signal transduction pathway. S-nitrosated Ras was found to trigger activation of all three mitogen-activated protein kinases (MAPK), which include extracellular signal-regulated kinase, c-Jun NH$_2$-terminal kinase, and p38 MAPK *(60)*. Interestingly, RNS transduce vascular endothelial growth factor (VEGF)-induced mitogenic signaling in endothelial cells by activating extracellular signal-regulated kinase *(61)*. Moreover, c-Jun NH$_2$-terminal kinase and p38 MAPK are also activated by proinflammatory cytokines and environmental stress *(62)*. Further downstream, RNS were found to activate the transcription factor NF-κB. This activation was observed in human peripheral blood mononuclear cells, T cells, and pheochromocytoma cells and depended on S-nitrosothiol formation at the Cys^{118} residue of Ras *(58,63,64)*. Identifying the signals immediately downstream to RNS-induced Ras activation (which includes Ras effectors such as phosphoinositide 3-kinase, Raf-1, and protein kinase C-ζ) and downstream intermediate signals leading to NF-κB activation will help in deciphering the RNS-induced Ras pathway. Because Ras is also activated by various other redox modulators like hemin, mercuric chloride, and hydrogen peroxide *(64)*, it may serve as a sensor of cellular redox stress and enable the cell to respond appropriately to the external milieu.

Calcium-Release Channel (Ryanodine Receptor). Ryanodine receptors belong to a multigene family of channel proteins. They are localized at the junctional sarcoplasmic reticulum in muscle and the endoplasmic reticulum in epithelial and neuronal cells. These receptors are sensitive to the muscle-paralyzing alkaloid ryanodine and are responsible for release of Ca^{2+} ions from intracellular stores, which activates contraction *(65)*. Ion channels are reported to be redox-regulated via their sulfhydryl groups *(66,67)*. Stoyanovsky et al. *(68)* and Xu et al. *(27)* reported RNS-induced ryanodine receptor channel opening and Ca^{2+} release from skeletal and cardiac sarcoplasmic reticulum into the cytoplasm. They observed that polynitrosation of up to 12 free thiols of the cardiac calcium-release channel reversibly activated the channel, which then released Ca^{2+} from the sarcoplasmic reticulum in response to a muscle action potential. The channel activity was monitored by incorporating calcium-release channels into proteoliposomes. Interestingly, in contrast to S-nitrosation, the oxidation of thiol groups has no effect on channel function, suggesting a specificity of nitrosothiol-induced activation. Thus, direct interaction of RNS with thiols of the cardiac calcium-release channel regulates force in the contracting muscle and controls excitation–contraction coupling.

Tissue-Type Plasminogen Activator. The normal endothelium secretes cardioprotective mediators such as RNS and tissue-type plasminogen activator (t-PA), which is involved in the activation of the fibrinolytic system *(69)*. S-nitrosation of t-PA at Cys^{83} endows the enzyme with vasodilatory and antiplatelet properties and enhances the catalytic efficiency of plasminogen activation in the presence of fibrin *(70)*. S-nitrosated t-PA was also able to attenuate cardiac necrosis after myocardial ischemia/reperfusion and inhibited neutrophil–endothelium interaction. The latter effect may involve a decrease in expression of the adhesion molecule, P-selectin *(71)*. Hence, S-nitrosation of t-PA converts a simple protease to a pleiotropic antithrombotic agent and plays a significant role in the functional regulation of the cardiovascular system.

Calcium-Dependent Potassium Channels. The endothelium controls vascular smooth muscle tone by secreting relaxing and contracting factors. RNS activate calcium-dependent potassium channels leading to hyperpolarization of the vascular smooth muscle cell and is one mechanism of vasodilation. The mechanism of activation involves S-nitrosation of thiols and eventual disulfide formation of vicinal thiols accompanied by the release of NO^- *(72)*. Hence, RNS may regulate vascular tone by activation of calcium-dependent potassium channels in addition to activation of guanylyl cyclase.

PROTEINS INACTIVATED BY S-NITROSOTHIOL FORMATION

Glyceraldehyde-3-Phosphate. RNS react with an active site cysteine of glyceraldehyde-3-phosphate (Cys^{149}), a key enzyme of the glycolytic pathway. This promotes subsequent direct binding of NADH to Cys^{149} and inhibition of glyceraldehyde-3-phosphate catalytic activity, resulting in depression of glycolysis. The first modification step of S-nitrosation is reversible, unlike the irreversible inactivation by subsequent NADH modification. Hence, S-nitrosation of glyceraldehyde-3-phosphate may also be a means to protect it from irreversible inhibition by oxidative damage triggered by inflammatory cytokines *(73)*. Bereta and Bereta *(74)* reported an increase in glyceraldehyde-3-phosphate mRNA levels in murine microvascular endothelial cells stimulated with tumor necrosis factor-α and interferon-γ. This increase in mRNA levels depended on $NO^{\bullet}$ synthesis. This effect may be an RNS-induced adaptive mechanism to compensate for inhibition of glyceraldehyde-3-phosphate enzyme activity and to prevent cell injury.

Caspases. Caspases are a family of at least 10 proteases that cleave at a specific nucleotide consensus sequence and are important effectors in apoptotic signaling. All caspases contain a conserved cysteine residue in the active site *(75)*. Mohr et al. *(76)* demonstrated that caspase-3 activity was attenuated in the actinomycin D-induced leukemic cell line U937 by S-nitrosation and oxidation of a critical thiol group. A similar observation was made by Li et al. *(77)*. They reported reversible inhibition of seven members of the caspase family in vitro by exposing human recombinant caspases to RNS donors. Hence, by inhibiting proapoptotic enzymes, RNS may play a role in rescuing cells from the apoptotic machinery. Moreover, inhibition of caspase-1 by RNS will also affect processing and maturation of the proinflammatory cytokines, IL-1β and IL-18. Therefore, RNS may also control secretion of these cytokines, which play important roles in cardiac inflammation.

Transcription Factors. Transcription factors transduce signals to the transcriptional apparatus by binding to specific DNA sequences of the genes they regulate. Recent studies suggest that mammalian transcription factors can be regulated by S-nitrosation.

NF-κB. The classical, inactive cytoplasmic form of NF-κB exists as a trimer of three subunits—p65, p50, and IκBα. On activation with a stimulus, the inhibitory subunit, IκBα, dissociates and the dimer of p50/p65 translocates to the nucleus. In addition to NF-κB binding sites in the immunoglobulin κ- chain gene, this site has been identified in many other genes including cytokines, cytokine receptors, cell adhesion molecules, genes of the HIV provirus *(78)*, and in the iNOS gene itself *(79,80)*.

RNS were implicated to play an indirect role in the activation of NF-κB in human peripheral mononuclear cells *(63)*. Subsequently, NF-κB activation in human T cells and rat pheochromocytoma cells was found to be dependent on RNS-induced S-nitrosation and activation of Ras *(58,64)*. These studies were the first to demonstrate that RNS can trigger an NF-κB response, and may provide a mechanistic basis by which RNS trigger NF-κB-dependent gene expression.

In contrast, in nonlymphoid astroglial cells, Park et al. *(81)* observed that RNS derived from a spermine NONOate inhibits formation of an NF-κB-DNA complex. Matthews et al. *(82)* studied the direct interaction of RNS with recombinant p50 and p65 subunits, and found that RNS donors inactivated DNA-binding activity of the recombinant subunits. The p50 subunit was S-nitrosated at Cys[62] residue and this modification seemed to be responsible for inhibition of DNA binding. The Cys[62] residue of the p50 subunit is conserved in the NF-κB transcription factor family. Moreover, it is located in the peptide loop, which makes specific contacts with the DNA consensus sequence. This residue is redox sensitive, as its oxidation and subsequent intersubunit disulfide linkage also abrogate DNA binding activity *(83,84)*. Because the promoter of the iNOS gene contains an NF-κB binding motif, RNS can inhibit iNOS gene expression by inhibiting NF-κB activation, and thus regulate the enzyme by feedback inhibition *(85)*.

As with oxidative stress, in some settings nitrosative stress activates NF-κB and may evoke an inflammatory response. In other settings, RNS can downregulate its own synthesis, likely through a direct modification of the NF-κB subunits. This dual functionality of RNS highlights the complex signaling behavior of free radicals.

AP-1. The AP-1 transcription factor mainly controls the expression of genes involved in cell proliferation. It is a heterodimer of Fos and Jun proteins, products of the proto-oncogenes, *c-fos* and *c-jun*. AP-1 interacts with the DNA regulatory element known as the AP-1 binding site.

Like NF-κB, both Jun and Fos possess a conserved cysteine residue in their DNA-binding domain that is sensitive to redox changes *(86,87)*. Nikitovic et al. *(88)* reported inhibition of AP-1 DNA binding by RNS in vitro. The inhibition was mediated by RNS-induced modification of Fos-Cys[154] and Jun-Cys[272] and the effect was abolished by dithiothreitol. Tabuchi et al.

(89) observed that RNS inhibited AP-1 DNA binding in mice cerebellar granule cells. In contrast to inhibition, RNS were found to activate AP-1 DNA binding via a cGMP-dependent mechanism *(90)*. Thus, similar to NF-κB, AP-1 can also be activated or inhibited depending on the cellular setting. Clearly, in vivo studies are badly needed to determine the physiological relevance of the cell culture studies.

Interaction with Heme and Thiol

HEMOGLOBIN

When administered systemically, cell-free hemoglobin leads to hypertension. This effect is thought to be caused by scavenging of RNS by hemoglobin via its heme–iron. Hence, many experimental studies use hemoglobin to determine RNS specific effects. Nevertheless, direct interaction of hemoglobin with RNS was not found to modulate any functional properties of hemoglobin. Recently, Stamler and colleagues demonstrated that hemoglobin can be *S*-nitrosated *(91,92)*. They elucidated a new reaction highlighting the importance of RNS in the respiratory cycle and dynamic properties of hemoglobin in vasoregulation. According to their observation, in the microcirculation and venous system, RNS reside predominantly on the T-state (deoxy) α-chain heme iron of hemoglobin. The β-chain of hemoglobin possess a highly reactive thiol group at Cys^{93}, which is conserved among mammalian species. When venous blood enters the lungs, oxygen favors an allosteric transition with RNS group exchange from α-chain heme to the β-chain (Cys^{93}) thiol and O_2 attaches to the heme. This R-state (oxy) structure of hemoglobin then reenters the circulation and when faced with an O_2 gradient in resistance vessels, releases both O_2 and RNS. The RNS released may bind to the abundant glutathione present in erythrocytes and the *S*-nitrosoglutathione formed dilates the blood vessels; this augments O_2 delivery to the peripheral tissues. This study highlights how redox-regulated residues are conserved at a strategic site and the allosteric changes in protein conformation control dynamic functions of the protein.

CYCLOOXYGENASE

Cyclooxygenase catalyzes the oxidation of arachidonic acid to prostaglandin H_2, the precursor for prostacyclin and thromboxane A_2. The effect of RNS on cyclooxygenase is controversial. It has been reported to inhibit *(93,94)*, activate *(95–97)*, or have no effect *(98)* on cyclooxygenase enzymatic activity. Like hemoglobin, both heme–iron and cysteine residues are potential targets. Heme–iron is present in the active site of the enzyme and is essential for catalytic function, whereas three cysteine residues are present in the catalytic domain. Hajjar et al. *(96)* reported an increase in enzyme activity due to allosteric changes induced by *S*-nitrosothiol formation. However, Tsai et al. *(98)* and Karthein et al. *(99)* reported interaction of RNS at the heme moiety of the enzyme.

The variable effect of RNS on cyclooxygenase activity may be due to the different cell types and experimental settings used. More studies are needed to gain a mechanistic understanding of this interaction.

Cytotoxic Consequences

At high concentrations, RNS are cytotoxic. This action of RNS is utilized as a defense mechanism against pathogens and tumor cells and is responsible for some of the pathophysiological consequences of high output NO• production.

RNS inactivate several mitochondrial iron–sulfur enzymes involved in ATP synthesis. These include NADH:ubiquinone oxidoreductase, NADH:succinate oxidoreductase, and *cis*-acotinase *(29,100)*. Inactivation of glyceraldehyde-3-phosphate dehydrogenase by *S*-nitrosation inhibits glycolysis *(73)*. RNS bind the nonheme–iron of ribonucleotide reductase, attenuating its activity and inhibiting DNA synthesis. Quenching tyrosyl radical with RNS may be another mechanism involved in inactivation of this important enzyme. Iron of the iron-storage protein ferritin is also a target of RNS. This interaction leads to the release of free iron, which may cause lipid peroxidation *(29)*. In the cardiovascular system, the foregoing discussed cytotoxic mechanisms become relevant in pathophysiological conditions such as myocardial infarction and cardiac allograft rejection. Although the vasodilatory properties of RNS impart cardioprotection after myocardial ischemia and reperfusion, overproduction of NO$^\bullet$ and superoxide radicals results in injury to the endothelium and myocytes. In vivo, NO$^\bullet$ derived from cytokine-induced iNOS is thought to be involved in the pathogenesis of these clinical syndromes *(101–105)*. Like other free radicals, RNS can damage DNA by base deamination, resulting in neurotoxicity and suppression of contractile activity in vascular smooth muscle *(106,107)*.

GENE EXPRESSION BY RNS

For over a century, nitroglycerin has been taken by patients with impaired cardiovascular function. The discovery of endogenous NO$^\bullet$, the active species of nitroglycerin, was a watershed event. This observation provided a mechanistic understanding of many physiological processes in the cardiovascular system. Extensive studies in the field of RNS-induced signaling has helped us to appreciate the sophistication as well as simplicity of this protean molecule. In response to environmental cues, RNS can posttranscriptionally modify proteins. This leads to allosteric or catalytic modulation and specific signaling. This section discusses the ultimate outcome of RNS-induced signal transduction.

Cell signaling involves moving information from the extracellular milieu to the nucleus. As discussed previously, RNS propagate many signaling pathways that convey information about environmental changes. The posttranscriptional modification of proteins by RNS may lead to alteration in gene expression. We explore the genes whose expression are known to be regulated by RNS as follows.

Inhibition of Cell Proliferation

VASCULAR SMOOTH MUSCLE

Abnormal proliferation of vascular smooth muscle is implicated in various pathological situations including atherosclerotic lesions, restenosis after balloon angioplasty, and vascular wall thickening in hypertension *(108,109)*. RNS may play a protective role by inhibiting proliferation of vascular smooth muscle cells (VSMC). Mechanisms underlying this reversible inhibition involves regulation at the genetic level and has been elucidated by Ishida et al. *(110)*. VSMC, when treated with the RNS-donor *S*-nitroso-*N*-acetylpenicillamine, had enhanced mRNA levels of the p21 protein, a cyclin-dependent kinase (Cdk) inhibitor, and maintained it for 30 h, resulting in increased p21 protein levels. This led to increased association with one of its substrates Cdk2, thus attenuating its activity. Retinoblastoma protein (pRb) is hyperphosphorylated by Cdk2, facilitating a G_1–S phase transition. Hence, RNS-induced increases of p21 protein results in inhibition of Cdk2 activity and ultimately decreases the phosphorylation of pRb protein. This hinders cell cycle progression and cell division. Whether cGMP is involved in this antiproliferative pathway is not yet known.

Okazaki et al. *(111)* observed that RNS released from endothelial cells inhibited expression of *c-fos* and *c-jun* mRNA induced by α_1 adrenergic receptors in rat aorta. This inhibition was cGMP-dependent. These receptors play important roles in the regulation of blood vessel contraction and smooth muscle proliferation. Hence, RNS-induced inhibition of VSMC proliferation may, in part, involve inhibition of the proto-oncogenes *c-fos* and *c-jun*.

Thus, RNS can protect against atherogenesis by regulating VSMC proliferation in several ways (Fig. 2).

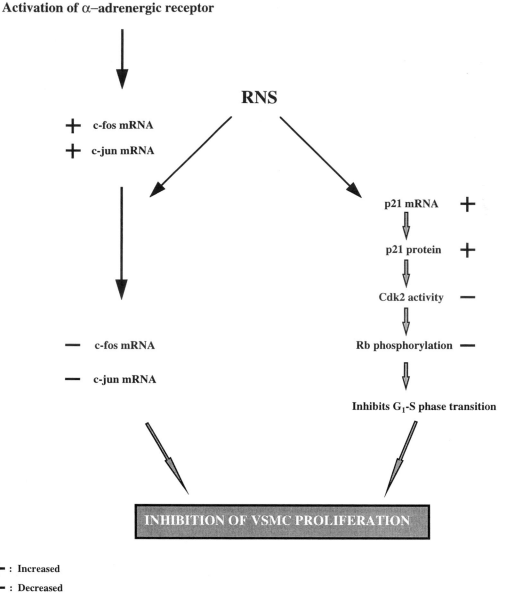

Activation of α–adrenergic receptor

RNS

\+ c-fos mRNA

\+ c-jun mRNA

p21 mRNA \+

p21 protein \+

Cdk2 activity —

— c-fos mRNA

Rb phosphorylation —

— c-jun mRNA

Inhibits G$_1$-S phase transition

INHIBITION OF VSMC PROLIFERATION

\+ : Increased

— : Decreased

VSMC : Vascular smooth muscle cell.

Fig. 2. RNS induced vascular smooth muscle cell proliferation.

ENDOTHELIAL CELLS

VEGF is synthesized by smooth muscle cells and acts as a mitogen for endothelial cells. Arterial injury was found to upregulate VEGF gene expression. This increased expression is due to PKC-induced binding of AP-1 to the VEGF promoter. Van der Zee et al. *(112)* reported that VEGF increases NO• synthesis in endothelial cells. However, RNS released from regenerating endothelial cells were found to downregulate VEGF expression to basal levels. This attenuation was due to RNS-induced inhibition of AP-1 DNA binding *(113)*. Thus, the regenerated endothelium regulates proliferation by negative feedback inhibition and utilizes RNS-induced signaling.

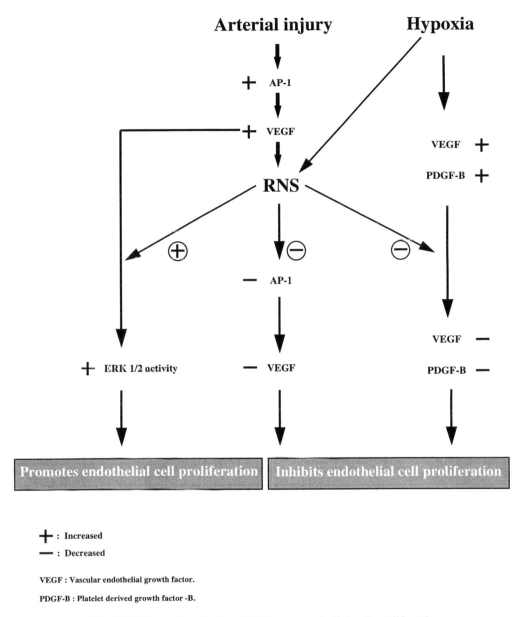

Fig. 3. Differential effects of RNS on endothelial cell proliferation.

Chronic hypoxia leads to pulmonary hypertension and remodeling of pulmonary arteries, concomitant with vascular cell proliferation. Hypoxia increases gene expression of vascular endothelial cell growth factor *(114)* and platelet-derived growth factor *(115)*. Interestingly, RNS prevent this increase and, therefore, inhibit vascular cell proliferation in this setting (Fig. 3).

Inflammatory Response

In the process of atherogenesis, adhesion molecules, such as vascular cell adhesion molecule-1 (VCAM-1), intracellular adhesion molecule-1 (ICAM-1), and endothelial-leukocyte adhesion molecule-1 (E-selectin), play pivotal roles in the recruitment of leukocytes to the site of lesion formation *(108)*. In human saphenous vein endothelial cells, RNS-donors inhibit VCAM-1 gene expression induced by the cytokines IL-1α, IL-1β, IL-4, and tumor necrosis factor-α. In an in vitro assay, reduced VCAM-1 levels were associated with reduced monocyte adhesion. RNS were also found to regulate negatively gene expression of E-selectin, ICAM-1, and the inflammatory cytokines IL-6 and IL-8 *(116)*. Each of these genes have NF-κB-specific DNA binding motifs in their promoters and the mechanism of RNS-induced gene repression seems to be via inhibition of NF-κB. Peng et al. *(117)* observed that RNS prevent NF-κB activation by stabilizing its inhibitor, IκB, and augmenting its mRNA levels. These studies provide insight into the antiatherogenic properties of RNS. In contrast to the foregoing reports, RNS have been implicated in endothelial cell activation. For example, Villarete and Remick *(118)* found that RNS increased cytokine-induced IL-8 expression in endothelial cells.

Polyinosinic-polycytidylic acid [poly(I-C)] is a double-stranded RNA and mimics a virally infected state in cells; it induces an inflammatory response by enhancing adherence of leukocytes to activated endothelial cells. This effect is achieved by activating the transcription factor NF-κB and gene expression of the adhesion molecules, VCAM-1 and E-selectin *(119)*. Faruqi et al. *(120)* observed that NO• synthesized by eNOS was essential for a poly(I-C)-induced inflammatory response since the NOS inhibitor N^G-monomethyl-L-arginine abrogated the inflammatory response.

The apparent conflict between these studies may be due to the experimental settings used. Because RNS can take many forms depending on the redox environment, its ultimate action is equally variable. In vivo studies are awaited to determine the actual role of RNS in the progression of artherogenesis.

Extensive studies in the field of NO• chemistry and signaling that we have discussed and in other chapters have made invaluable contributions in the mechanistic understanding of cardiovascular function. Impaired endothelial NO• synthesis and signaling is implicated in atherosclerosis, hypertension, reperfusion injury, and diabetic angiopathy. Paradoxically, high levels of NO• produced by iNOS have been implicated in viral myocarditis, myocardial infarction, and cardiac allograft rejection *(121)*. These studies have provided an important starting point for intervention in cardiac dysfunction. However, the field of NO• and redox signaling is still in its infancy and future in-depth studies will yield better targets for drug development.

REFERENCES

1. Huang PL, Huang Z, Mashimo H, Block KD, Moskowitz MA, Bevan JA, et al. Hypertension in mice lacking the gene for endothelial nitric oxide synthase. Nature 1995;377:196,197.
2. Rudic RD, Shesely EG, Maeda N, Smithies O, Segal SS, Sessa WC. Direct evidence for the importance of endothelium-derived nitric oxide in vascular remodeling. J Clin Invest 1998;101:731–736.
3. Palmer RM, Rees DD, Ashton DS, Moncada S. L-arginine is the physiological precursor for the formation of nitric oxide in endothelium dependent relaxation. Biochem Biophys Res Commun 1988; 153:1251–1256.
4. Bredt DS, Hwang PM, Glatt CE, Lowenstein C, Reed RR, Synder SH. Cloned and expressed nitric oxide synthase structurally resembles cytochrome P-450 reductase. Nature 1991;351:714–718.
5. Lamas S, Marsden PA, Li GK, Tempst P, Michel T. Endothelial nitric oxide synthase: molecular cloning and characterization of a distinct constitutive enzyme isoform. Proc Natl Acad Sci USA 1992; 89:6348–6352.
6. Xie QW, Cho HJ, Calaycay J, Mumford RA, Swiderek KM, Lee TD, et al. Cloning and characterization of inducible nitric oxide synthase from mouse macrophages. Science 1992;256:225–228.
7. Nathan C, Xie QW. Nitric oxide synthases: roles, tolls and controls. Cell 1994;78:915–918.
8. Balligand JL, Kobzik L, Han X, Kaye DM, Belhassen L, O'Hara DS, et al. Nitric oxide-dependent parasympathetic signaling is due to activation of constitutive endothelial (type III) nitric oxide synthase in cardiac myocytes. J Biol Chem 1995;270:14,582–14,586.
9. Han X, Kobzik L, Balligand JL, Kelly RA, Smith TW. Nitric oxide synthase (NOS3)-mediated cholinergic modulation of Ca2+ current in adult rabbit atrioventricular nodal cells. Circ Res 1996;78:998–1008.

10. Seki T, Hagiwara H, Naruse K, Kadowaki M, Kashiwagi M, Demura H, et al. In situ identification of messenger RNA of endothelial type nitric oxide synthase in rat cardiac myocytes. Biochem Biophys Res Commun 1996;218:601–605.

11. Balligand JL, Smith TW. Molecular regulation of NO synthase in the heart. In: Shah AM, Lewis MS, eds. Endothelial Modulation of Cardiac Contraction. Harwood Academic Publishers, London, UK, 1997, pp. 53–70.

12. Wei C, Jiang S, Lust JA, Daly RC, MacGregor CG. Genetic expression of endothelial nitric oxide synthase in human atrial myocardium. Mayo Clin Proc 1996;71:346–350.

13. Schmidt HH, Gagne GD, Nakane M, Pollock JS, Miller MF, Murad F. Mapping of neural nitric oxide synthase in the rat suggests frequent co-localization with NADPH diaphorase but not with soluble guanylyl cyclase and novel paraneural functions for nitrinergic signal transduction. J Histochem Cytochem 1992;40: 1439–1456.

14. Tanaka K, Hassall CJ, Burnstock G. Distribution of intracardiac neurones and nerve terminals that contain a marker for nitric oxide, NADPH-diaphorase, in the guinea-pig heart. Cell Tissue Res 1993; 273:293–300.

15. Schwarz P, Diem R, Dun NJ, Forstermann U. Endogenous and exogenous nitric oxide inhibits norepinephrine release from rat heart sympathetic nerves. Circ Res 1995;77:841–848.

16. Schulz R, Nava E, Moncada S. Induction and potential biological relevance of a Ca^{2+}-independent nitric oxide synthase in the myocardium. Br J Pharmacol 1992;105:575–580.

17. Roberts AB, Roche NS, Winokur TS, Burmester JK, Sporn MB, Nathan CF. Role of nitric oxide in antagonistic effects of transforming growth factor β and interleukin-1β on the beating rate of cultured cardiac myocytes. J Clin Invest 1992;89:2045–2062.

18. Shindo T, Ikeda U, Ohkawa F, Kawahara Y, Yokoyama M, Shimada K. Nitric oxide synthesis in cardiac myocytes and fibroblasts by inflammatory cytokines. Cardiovasc Res 1995;29:813–819.

19. Nathan C, Xie QW. Regulation of biosynthesis of nitric oxide. J Biol Chem 1994;269:13,725–13,728.

20. Lander HM. An essential role for free radicals and derived species in signal transduction. FASEB J 1997;11:118–124.

21. Stamler JS, Singel DJ, Loscalzo J. Biochemistry of nitric oxide and its redox-activated forms. Science 1992;258:1898–1902.

22. Ignarro LJ, Fukuto JM, Griscavage JM, Rogers NE, Byrns RE. Oxidation of NO in aqueous solution to nitrite but not nitrate: comparison with enzymatically formed nitric oxide from L-arginine. Proc Natl Acad Sci USA 1993;90:8103–8107.

23. Ignarro LJ. Signal transduction mechanisms involving nitric oxide. Biochem Pharmacol 1991;41: 485–490.

24. Bredt DS, Synder SH. Nitric oxide: a physiologic messenger molecule. Ann Rev Biochem 1994;63: 175–195.

25. Stamler JS. Redox signaling: nitrosylation and related target interactions of nitric oxide. Cell 1994;78: 931–936.

26. Lander HM, Milbank AJ, Tauras JM, Hajjar DP, Hempstead BL, Schwartz GD, et al. Redox regulation of cell signalling. Nature 1996;381:380,381.

27. Xu L, Eu JP, Meissner G, Stamler JS. Activation of cardiac calcium release channel (ryanodine receptor) by poly-S-nitrosylation. Science 1998;279:234–237.

28. Bauer JA, Booth BP, Fung HL. Nitric oxide donors: biochemical pharmacology and therapeutics. Adv Pharmacol 1995;34:361–381.

29. Nathan C. Nitric oxide as a secretory product of mammalian cells. FASEB J 1992;6:3051–3064.

30. Schmidt HH, Lohmann SM, Walter U. The nitric oxide and cGMP signal transduction system: regulation and mechanism of action. Biochim Biophys Acta 1993;1178:153–175.

31. Gerzer R, Bohme E, Hofmann F, Schultz G. Soluble guanylate cyclase purified from bovine lung contains heme and copper. FEBS Lett 1981;132:71–74.

32. Ignarro LJ, Kadowitz PJ. The pharmacological and physiological role of cyclic GMP in vascular smooth muscle relaxation. Annu Rev Pharmacol Toxicol 1985;25:171–191.

33. Radomski MW, Palmer RM, Moncada S. The anti-aggregating properties of vascular endothelium; interactions between prostacyclin and nitric oxide. Br J Pharmacol 1987;92:639–646.

34. Ignarro LJ, Wood KS, Wolin MS. Regulation of purified soluble guanylate cyclase by porphyrins and metalloporphrins: a unifying concept. Adv Cyclic Nucleotide Protein Phosphorylation Res 1984;17: 267–274.

35. Forstermann U, Kleinert H. Nitric oxide synthase: expression and expressional control of the three isoforms. Naunyn Schmiedebergs Arch Pharmacol 1995;352:351–364.

36. Buga GM, Griscavage JM, Rogers NE, Ignarro LJ. Negative feedback regulation of endothelial cell function by nitric oxide. Circ Res 1993;73:808–812.
37. Griscavage JM, Fukuto JM, Komori Y, Ignarro LJ. Nitric oxide inhibits neuronal nitric oxide synthase by interacting with their heme prosthetic group. Role of tetrahydrobiopterin in modulating inhibitory action of nitric oxide. J Biol Chem 1994;269:21,644–21,649.
38. Abu-Soud HM, Wang J, Rousseau DL, Fukuto JM, Ignarro LJ, Stuehr DJ. Neuronal nitric oxide synthase self-inactivates by forming a ferrous-nitrosyl complex during aerobic catalysis. J Biol Chem 1995;270:22,997–23,006.
39. Hurshman AR, Marletta MA. Nitric oxide complexes of inducible nitric oxide synthase: spectral characterization and effect on catalytic activity. Biochemistry 1995;34:5627–5634.
40. Butler AR, Glidewell C, Li MS. Nitrosyl complexes of iron-sulfur clusters. Adv Inorg Chem 1988;32: 335–392.
41. Castro L, Rodriguez M, Radi R. Aconitase is readily inactivated by peroxynitrite, but not by its precursor, nitric oxide. J Biol Chem 1994;269:29,409–29,415.
42. Henry Y, Lepoivre M, Drapier JC, Ducrocq C, Boucher JL, Guissani A. EPR characterization of molecular targets for NO in mammalian cells and organelles. FASEB J 1993;7:1124–1134.
43. Drapier JC, Hirling H, Wietzerbin J, Kaldy P, Kuhn LC. Biosynthesis of nitric oxide activates iron regulatory factor in macrophages. EMBO J 1993;12:3643–3649.
44. Weiss G, Goossen B, Doppler W, Fuchs D, Pantopoulos K, Werner-Felmayer G, et al. Translational regulation via iron-responsive elements by the nitric oxide/NO-synthase pathway. EMBO J 1993; 12:3651–3657.
45. Jaffrey SR, Cohen NA, Rouault TA, Klausner RD, Synder SH. The iron-responsive element binding protein: a target for synaptic actions of nitric oxide. Proc Natl Acad Sci USA 1994;91:12,994–12,998.
46. Becker K, Savvides SN, Keese M, Schirmer RH, Karplus PA. Enzyme inactivation through sulfhydryl oxidation by physiologic NO-carriers. Nat Struct Biol 1998;5:267–271.
47. Lei SZ, Pan ZH, Aggarwal SK, Chen HS, Hartman J, Sucher NJ, et al. Effect of nitric oxide production on the redox modulatory site of the NMDA receptor-channel complex. Neuron 1992;8:1087–1099.
48. Luperchio S, Tamir S, Tannenbaum SR. NO-induced oxidative stress and glutathione metabolism in rodent and human cells. Free Radic Biol Med 1996;21:513–519.
49. Williams DLH. S-nitrosation and the reactions of S-nitrosocompounds. Chem Soc Rev 1985;14: 171–196.
50. McDonald LJ, Moss J. Stimulation by nitric oxide of an NAD linkage to glyceraldehyde-3-phosphate dehydrogenase. Proc Natl Acad Sci USA 1993;90:6238–6241.
51. Stamler JS, Simon DI, Osborne JA, Mullins ME, Jaraki O, Michel T, et al. S-nitrosylation of proteins with nitric oxide: synthesis and characterization of biologically active compounds. Proc Natl Acad Sci USA 1992;89:444–448.
52. Kharitonov VG, Sundquist AR, Sharma VS. Kinetics of nitrosation of thiols by nitric oxide in the presence of oxygen. J Biol Chem 1995;270:28,158–28,164.
53. Radi R, Beckman JS, Bush KM, Freeman BA. Peroxynitrite oxidation of sulfhydryls. The cytotoxic potential of superoxide and nitric oxide. J Biol Chem 1991;266:4244–4250.
54. Wu M, Pritchard KA Jr, Kaminski PM, Fayngersh RP, Hintze TH, Wolin MS. Involvement of nitric oxide and nitrosothiols in relaxation of pulmonary arteries to peroxynitrite. Am J Physiol 1994;266: H2108–H2113.
55. Khosravi-Far R, Der CJ. The Ras signal transduction pathway. Cancer Metastasis Rev 1994;13: 67–89.
56. Overbeck AF, Brtva TR, Cox AD, Graham SM, Huff SY, Khosravi-Far R, et al. Guanine nucleotide exchange factors: activators of Ras superfamily proteins. Mol Reprod Dev 1995;42:468–476.
57. Denhardt DT. Signal transducing protein phosphorylation cascades mediated by Ras/Rho proteins in the mammalian cell: the potential for miltiplex signalling. Biochem J 1996;318:729–747.
58. Lander HM, Ogiste JS, Pearce SF, Levi R, Novogrodsky A. Nitric oxide-stimulated guanine nucleotide exchange on p21^{ras}. J Biol Chem 1995;270:7017–7020.
59. Lander HM, Hajjar DP, Hempstead BL, Mirza UA, Chait BT, Campbell S, et al. A molecular redox switch on p21^{ras}. Structural bases for the nitric oxide-p21^{ras} interaction. J Biol Chem 1997;272: 4323–4326.
60. Lander HM, Jacovina AT, Davis RJ, Tauras JM. Differential activation of mitogen-activated protein kinases by nitric oxide-related species. J Biol Chem 1996;271:19,705–19,709.
61. Parenti A, Morbidelli L, Cui XL, Douglas JG, Hood JD, Granger HJ, et al. Nitric oxide is an upstream signal of vascular endothelial growth factor-induced extracellular signal-regulated kinase$_{1/2}$ activation in postcapillary endothelium. J Biol Chem 1998;273:4220–4226.

62. Cano E, Mahadevan LC. Parallel signal processing among mammalian MAPKs. Trends Biochem Sci 1995;20:117–122.

63. Lander HM, Sehajpal P, Levine DM, Novogrodsky A. Activation of human peripheral blood mononuclear cells by nitric oxide-generating compounds. J Immunol 1993;150:1509–1516.

64. Lander HM, Ogiste JS, Teng KK, Novogrodsky A. p21^{ras} as a common signaling target of reactive free radicals and cellular redox stress. J Biol Chem 1995;270:21,195–21,198.

65. Coronado R, Morrissette J, Sukhareva M, Vaughan DM. Structure and function of ryanodine receptors. Am J Physiol 1994;266:C1485–C1504.

66. Abramson JJ, Salama G. Sulfhydryl oxidation and Ca^{2+} release from sarcoplasmic reticulum. Mol Cell Biochem 1988;82:81–84.

67. Oba T, Yamaguchi M, Wand S, Johnson JD. Modulation of the Ca^{2+} channel voltage sensor and excitation-contraction coupling by silver. Biophys J 1992;63:1416–1420.

68. Stoyanovsky D, Murphy T, Anno PR, Kim YM, Salama G. Nitric oxide activates skeletal and cardiac ryanodine receptors. Cell Calcium 1997;21:19–29.

69. Lijnen HR, Collen D. Endothelium in hemostasis and thrombosis. Prog Cardiovasc Dis 1997;39: 343–350.

70. Stamler JS, Simon DI, Jaraki O, Osborne JA, Francis S, Mullins M, et al. S-nitrosylation of tissue-type plasminogen activator confers vasodilatory and antiplatelet properties on the enzyme. Proc Natl Acad Sci USA 1992;89:8087–8091.

71. Delyani JA, Nossuli TO, Scalia R, Thomas G, Garvey JS, Lefer AM. S-nitrosylated tissue-type plasminogen activator protects against myocardial ischemia/reperfusion injury in cats: role of endothelium. J Pharmacol Exp Ther 1996;279:1174–1180.

72. Bolotina VM, Najibi S, Palacino JJ, Pagano PJ, Cohen RA. Nitric oxide directly activates calcium-dependent potassium channels in vascular smooth muscle. Nature 1994;368:850–853.

73. Mohr S, Stamler JS, Brune B. Posttranslational modification of glyceraldehyde-3-phosphate dehydrogenase by S-nitrosylation and subsequent NADH attachment. J Biol Chem 1996;271:4209–4214.

74. Bereta J, Bereta M. Stimulation of glyceraldehyde-3-phosphate dehydrogenase mRNA levels by endogenous nitric oxide in cytokine-activated endothelium. Biochem Biophys Res Commun 1995;217: 363–369.

75. Alnemri ES, Livingston DJ, Nicholson DW, Salvesen G, Thornberry NA, Wong WW, et al. Human ICE/CED-3 protease nomenclature. Cell 1996;87:171.

76. Mohr S, Zech B, Lapetina EG, Brune B. Inhibition of caspase-3 by S-nitrosation and oxidation caused by nitric oxide. Biochem Biophys Res Commun 1997;238:387–391.

77. Li J, Billiar TR. Talanian RV, Kim YM. Nitric oxide reversibly inhibits seven members of the caspase family via S-nitrosylation. Biochem Biophys Res Commun 1997;240:419–424.

78. Baldwin AS Jr. The NF-κB and IκB proteins: new discoveries and insights. Annu Rev Immunol 1996; 14:649–683.

79. Xie QW, Kashiwabara Y, Nathan C. Role of transcription factor NF-kappa B/Rel in induction of nitric oxide synthase. J Biol Chem 1994;269:4705–4708.

80. Chartrain NA, Geller DA, Koty PP, Sitrin NF, Nussler AK, Hoffman EP, et al. Molecular cloning, structure, and chromosomal localization of the human inducible nitric oxide synthase gene. J Biol Chem 1994;269:6765–6772.

81. Park SK, Lin HL, Murphy S. Nitric oxide regulates nitric oxide synthase-2 gene expression by inhibiting NF-kappaB binding to DNA. Biochem J 1997;322:609–613.

82. Matthews JR, Botting CH, Panico M, Morris HR, Hay RT. Inhibition of NF-κB DNA binding by nitric oxide. Nucleic Acids Res 1996;24:2236–2242.

83. Ghosh G, van Duyne G, Ghosh S, Sigler PB. Structure of NF-kappa B p50 homodimer bound to a kappa B site. Nature 1995;373:303–310.

84. Muller CW, Rey FA, Sodeoka M, Verdine GL, Harrison SC. Structure of the NF-kappa B p50 homodimer bound to DNA. Nature 1995;373:311–317.

85. Togashi H, Sasaki M, Frohman E, Taira E, Ratan RR, Dawson TM, et al. Neuronal (type I) nitric oxide synthase regulates nuclear factor (B activity and immunologic (type II) nitric oxide synthase expression. Proc Natl Acad Sci USA 1997;94:2676–2680.

86. Abate C, Patel L, Rauscher FJ 3rd, Curan T. Redox regulation of fos and jun DNA-binding activity in vitro. Science 1990;249:1157–1161.

87. Xanthoudakis S, Curran T. Identification and characterization of Ref-1, a nuclear protein that facilitates AP-1 DNA-binding activity. EMBO J 1992;11:653–665.

88. Nikitovic D, Holmgren A, Spyrou G. Inhibition of AP-1 DNA binding by nitric oxide involving conserved cysteine residues in Jun and Fos. Biochem Biophys Res Commun 1998;242:109–112.

89. Tabuchi A, Oh E, Taoka A, Sakurai H, Tsuchiya T, Tsuda M. Rapid attenuation of AP-1 transcriptional factors associated with nitric oxide (NO)-mediated neuronal death. J Biol Chem 1996;271:31,061–31,067.

90. Pilz RB, Suhasini M, Idriss S, Meinkoth JL, Boss GR. Nitric oxide and cGMP analogs activate transcription from AP-1-responsive promoters in mammalian cells. FASEB J 1995;9:552–558.

91. Jia L, Bonaventura C, Bonaventura J, Stamler JS. S-nitrosohaemoglobin: a dynamic activity of blood involved in vascular control. Nature 1996;380:221–226.

92. Gow AJ, Stamler JS. Reactions between nitric oxide and haemoglobin under physiological conditions. Nature 1998;391:169–173.

93. Matthews JS, McWilliams PJ, Key BJ, Keen M. Inhibition of prostacyclin release from cultured endothelial cells by nitrovasodilator drugs. Biochim Biophys Acta 1995;1269:237–242.

94. Habib A, Bernard C, Lebret M, Creminon C, Esposito B, Tedgui A, et al. Regulation of the expression of cyclooxygenase-2 by nitric oxide in rat peritoneal macrophages. J Immunol 1997;158:3845–3851.

95. Salvemini D, Misko TP, Masferrer JL, Seibert K, Currie MG, Needleman P. Nitric oxide activates cyclooxygenase enzymes. Proc Natl Acad Sci USA 1993;90:7240–7244.

96. Hajjar DP, Lander HM, Pearce SF, Upmacis RK, Pomerantz KB. Nitric oxide enhances prostaglandin-H synthase-1 activity by a heme-independent mechanism: evidence implicating nitrosothiols. J Am Chem Soc 1995;117:3340–3346.

97. Salvemini D. Regulation of cyclooxygenase enzyme by nitric oxide. Cell Mol Life Sci 1997;53:576–582.

98. Tsai AL, Wei C, Kulmacz RJ. Interaction between nitric oxide and prostaglandin H synthase. Arch Biochem Biophys 1994;313:367–372.

99. Karthein R, Nastainczyk W, Ruf HH. EPR study of ferric native prostaglandin H synthase and its ferrous NO derivative. Eur J Biochem 1987;166:173–180.

100. Lowenstein CJ, Dinerman JL, Synder SH. Nitric oxide: a physiologic messenger. Ann Intern Med 1994;120:227–237.

101. Yang X, Chowdhury N, Cai B, Brett J, Marboe C, Sciacca RR, et al. Induction of myocardial nitric oxide synthase by cardiac allograft rejection. J Clin Invest 1994;94:714–721.

102. Suzuki H, Wildhirt SM, Dudek RR, Narayan KS, Bailey AH, Bing RJ. Induction of apoptosis in myocardial infarction and its possible relationship to nitric oxide synthase in macrophages. Tissue Cell 1996;28:89–97.

103. Haywood GA, Tsao PS, von der Leyen HE, Mann MJ, Keeling PF, Trindade PT, et al. Expression of inducible nitric oxide synthase in human heart failure. Circulation 1996;93:1087–1094.

104. Lancaster JR Jr, Langrehr JM, Bergonia HA, Murase N, Simmons RL, Hoffman RA. EPR detection of heme and nonheme iron-containing protein nitrosylation by nitric oxide during rejection of rat heart allograft. J Biol Chem 1992;267:10,994–10,998.

105. Dusting GJ. Nitric oxide in the coronary artery disease: roles in atherosclerosis, myocardial reperfusion and heart failure. EXS 1996;76:33–55.

106. Bredt DS, Synder SH. Nitric oxide: a physiologic messenger molecule. Ann Rev Biochem 1994;63:175–195.

107. Szabo C, Zingarelli B, Salzman AL. Role of poly-ADP ribosyl-transferase activation in the vascular contractile and energetic failure elicited by exogenous and endogenous nitric oxide and peroxynitrite. Circ Res 1996;78:1051–1063.

108. Ross R. The pathogenesis of artherosclerosis: a perspective of the 1990s. Nature 1993;362:801–809.

109. Schwartz SM, deBlois D, O'Brien ER. The intima: soil for artherosclerosis and restenosis. Circ Res 1995;77:445–465.

110. Ishida A, Sasaguri T, Kosaka C, Nojima H, Ogata J. Induction of the cyclin-dependent kinase inhibitor p21 (sdi1/cip1/Waf1) by nitric oxide-generating vasodilator in vascular smooth muscle cells. J Biol Chem 1997;272:10,050–10,057.

111. Okazaki M, Hu ZW, Fujinaga M, Hoffman BB. Alpha1 adrenergic receptor activation of proto-oncogene expression in arterial smooth muscle. Recept Signal Transduct 1996;6:165–178.

112. van der Zee R, Murohara T, Luo Z, Zollman F, Passeri J, Lekutat C, et al. Vascular endothelial growth factor/vascular permeability factor augments nitric oxide release from quiescent rabbit and human vascular endothelium. Circulation 1997;95:1030–1037.

113. Tsurumi Y, Murohara T, Krasinski K, Chen D, Witzenbichler B, Kearney M, et al. Reciprocal relation between VEGF and NO in the regulation of endothelial integrity. Nat Med 1997;3:879–886.

114. Tuder RM, Flook BE, Voelkel NF. Increased gene expression for VEGF and the VEGF receptors KDR/FIK and Flt in lungs exposed to acute or to chronic hypoxia. Modulation of gene expression by nitric oxide. J Clin Invest 1995;95:1798–1807.

115. Kourembanas S, McQuillan LP, Leung GK, Faller DV. Nitric oxide regulates the expression of vasoconstrictors and growth factors by vascular endothelium under both normoxia and hypoxia. J Clin Invest 1993;92:99–104.

116. De Caterina R, Libby P, Peng HB, Thannickal VJ, Rajavashisth TB, Gimbrone MA Jr, et al. Nitric oxide decreases cytokine-induced endothelial activation. Nitric oxide selectively reduces endothelial expression of adhesion molecules and proinflammatory cytokines. J Clin Invest 1995;96:60–68.

117. Peng H, Libby P, Liao JK. Induction and stabilization of IκBα by nitric oxide mediates inhibition of NFκB. J Biol Chem 1995;270:14,214–14,219.

118. Villarete LH, Remick DG. Nitric oxide regulation of IL-8 expression in human endothelial cells. Biochem Biophys Res Commun 1995;211:671–676.

119. Sedmak DD, Knight DA, Vook NC, Waldman JW. Divergent patterns of ELAM-1, ICAM-1 and VCAM-1 expression in cytomegalovirus-infected endothelial cells. Transplantation 1994;58:1379–1385.

120. Faruqi TR, Erzurum SC, Kaneko FT, Dicorleto PE. Role of nitric oxide in poly(I-C)-induced endothelial cell expression of leukocyte adhesion molecules. Am J Physiol 1997;273:2490–2497.

121. Balligand JL, Cannon PJ. Nitric oxide synthases and cardiac muscle. Autocrine and paracrine influences. Arterioscler Thromb Vasc Biol 1997;17:1846–1858.

122. Brady AJ, Warren JB, Poole-Wilson PA, Williams TJ, Harding SE. Nitric oxide attenuates cardiac myocyte contraction. Am J Physiol 1993;265:H176–H182.

123. Radomski MW, Palmer RM, Moncada S. The role of nitric oxide and cGMP in platelet adhesion to vascular endothelium. Biochem Biophys Res Commun 1987;148:1482–1489.

124. Kubes P, Suzuki M, Granger DN. Nitric oxide: an endogenous modulator of leukocyte adhesion. Proc Natl Acad Sci USA 1991;88:4651–4655.

125. Bath PM, Hassall DG, Gladwin AM, Palmer RM, Martin JF. Nitric oxide and prostacyclin. Divergence of inhibitory effects on monocyte chemotaxis and adhesion to endothelium in vitro. Arterioscler Thromb 1991;11:254–260.

126. Tsao PS, Lewis NP, Alpert S, Cooke JP. Exposure to shear stress alters endothelial adhesiveness. Role of nitric oxide. Circulation 1995;92:3513–3519.

127. Zeiher AM, Fisslthaler B, Schray-Utz B, Busse R. Nitric oxide modulates the expression of monocyte chemoattractant protein 1 in cultured human endothelial cells. Circ Res 1995;76:980–986.

128. Grocott-Mason R, Fort S, Lewis MJ, Shah AM. Myocardial relaxant effect of exogenous nitric oxide in isolated ejecting hearts. Am J Physiol 1994;266:H1699–H1705.

129. Xie YW, Shen W, Zhao G, Xu X, Wolin MS, Hintze TM. Role of endothelium-derived nitric oxide in the modulation of canine myocardial respiration in vitro. Implications for the development of heart failure. Circ Res 1996;79:381–387.

130. Balligand JL, Kelly RA, Marsden PA, Smith TW, Michel T. Control of cardiac muscle cell function by an endogenous nitric oxide signaling system. Proc Natl Acad Sci USA 1993;90:347–351.

131. Flesch M, Kilter H, Cremers B, Lenz O, Sudkamp M, Kuhn-Regnier F, et al. Acute effects of nitric oxide and cyclic GMP on human myocardial contractility. J Pharmacol Exp Ther 1997;281:1340–1349.

132. Schobersberger W, Friedrich F, Hoffmann G, Volkl H, Dietl P. Nitric oxide donors inhibit spontaneous depolarizations by L-type Ca2+ currents in alveolar epithelial cells. Am J Physiol 1997;272:L1092–L1097.

5

Cytotoxicity, Apoptosis, and Nitric Oxide

Stefanie Dimmeler and Andreas M. Zeiher

MECHANISMS OF CELL DEATH

Cell death plays an important physiological role during development and the turnover of cells in the tissue. However, the induction of excessive cell death by injury also contributes to various pathophysiological disorders. Toxic insults or ischemic injury can lead to the destruction of cells. Such cytotoxic effects are often the consequence of necrotic cell death. Necrotic processes are characterized by the disruption of cell homeostasis, energy depletion, organelle swelling, and random catalytic processes *(1)*. The increase of plasma membrane permeability further leads to the release of the cell content into the extracellular milieu, which consequently evokes an inflammatory response. The induction of necrotic cell death during embryonal development or essential tissue cell turnover would have detrimental effects. Therefore, another kind of cell death was proposed to mediate these processes, which was initially termed "shrinkage necrosis" or "apoptosis" (Greek; *apo*:- apart; *-ptosis*:falling), referring to the cell death responsible for the falling of leaves in autumn *(2)*. Given its strictly regulated nature, this kind of cell death was also termed "programmed cell death." Apoptosis or programmed cell death refers to the morphological alterations exhibited by "actively" dying cells that include cell shrinkage, membrane blebbing, chromatin condensation, and DNA fragmentation *(3)*. Finally, apoptotic cells expose specific molecules on the surface to initiate phagocytosis either by resident cells or by specialized phagocytes, thus ensuring that no intracellular material is released into the tissue and, therefore, preventing an inflammatory reaction *(4)*. Thus, the apoptotic process is often referred to as "silent cell death."

The apoptotic process is regulated by a highly conserved signalling pathway, which has mainly been studied in *Caenorhabditis elegans*, with at least three families of genes being involved, termed *C. elegans* cell death gene 3 (ced-3), ced-4, and ced-9 *(5)*. The cysteine protease family of caspases, the mammalian homologs of ced-3, represents the main execution pathway, which ultimately leads to the activation of caspase-activated DNases *(6,7)*. The ced-9 homologs, the proteins of the Bcl-2 family, modulate cell death with either proapoptotic effectors such as Bax or Bad or antiapoptotic proteins like Bcl-2 or Bcl-X_L *(8,9)*.

Recent studies highlight the role of mitochondria in apoptotic signaling *(10,11)*. Cells undergoing apoptosis show an early reduction of the mitochondrial transmembrane potential with concomitant release of the mitochondrial protein cytochrome C *(12)*. In the cytosol, cytochrome C interacts with the mammalian homolog of ced-4, which has recently been identified as apoptosis-inducing factor 1 (Apaf-1), in a dATP/ATP-dependent (deoxyadenosine triphosphate) manner *(13)*. The Apaf-1/cytochrome C complex, in turn, activates caspase-9,

From: *Contemporary Cardiology, vol. 4: Nitric Oxide and the Cardiovascular System*
Edited by: J. Loscalzo and J. A. Vita © Humana Press Inc., Totowa, NJ

thereby amplifying the caspase cascade, which finally leads to the activation of caspase-3 and DNA-fragmentation *(12)*.

NO• AND CELL DEATH

The short-lived radical NO• exhibits various functions in the organism. NO• released by the constitutive endothelial NO•-synthase (eNOS) mediates vasodilation and inhibition of platelet aggregation, and prevents adhesion of leukocytes *(14)*. The synthesis of NO• in the neuronal system by the constitutive neuronal NOS (nNOS) is involved in neurotransmitter release and mediates signaling of nonadrenergic, noncholinergic nerves *(14)*. In contrast, generation of large amounts of NO• via the inducible NO•-synthase (iNOS) especially in macrophages, exerts cytotoxic effects thereby contributing to immune defense *(15)*. Thus, NO• not only mediates various physiological functions, but also induces cytotoxic effects, which are described in the following section. This chapter gives insights into the role of NO• in apoptosis and its potential physiological and pathophysiological sequelae.

Cytotoxic Effects of NO•

ROLE OF NO•-INDUCED CYTOTOXICITY

Inflammation or exposure of cells to inflammatory cytokines or toxins increases the synthesis of nitrite and nitrate *(16,17)* via activation of iNOS, which oxidizes L-arginine to L-citrulline and NO• *(18,19)*. Cytokine- or toxin-induced expression of iNOS occurs not only in macrophages, but also in various other cell types to produce large quantities of NO• *(15)*. The generation of high levels of NO• seems to contribute to the nonspecific immune defense by its potent cytotoxicity against bacteria and invading organisms *(20)*. The important role of NO•-induced cytotoxicity for mediating immune defense is supported by studies with iNOS-deficient mice, which are much more susceptible to specific pathogens such as *Mycobacterium tuberculosis* or *Leishmania major* (for review *see* ref. *[21]*). In addition, activated murine macrophages revealed cytotoxic and cytostatic effects on tumor cells suggesting a role for NO•-mediated cytotoxicity in tumor suppression *(19,22)*. However, the cytotoxic effects of NO• are also self-destructive, leading to the death of the stimulated macrophages and destruction of surrounding tissue *(23)*. For example, NO•-induced cytotoxicity has been proposed to be involved in the pathogenesis of autoimmune diabetes. Exogenous NO• as well as endogenous NO• generated by interleukin 1β-induced iNOS expression lead to the destruction of pancreatic β-cells *(24–26)*. Moreover, these in vitro studies were supported by animal experiments suggesting that the onset of diabetes is linked to NO•-generation *(27)*.

Taken together, at least in rodents, NO• cytotoxicity belongs to the weapons of the nonspecific immune defense system. The cytotoxic effects are mainly mediated via the expression of the iNOS, which generates high levels of NO•. However, as shown for other effector molecules of the immune system, this long-lasting, high-output NO• production may also have deleterious effects to the host leading to tissue destruction.

MECHANISMS OF NO•-MEDIATED CYTOTOXICITY

NO•-mediated cytotoxicity seems to be mainly caused by inhibition of energy metabolism by NO• via interaction with mitochondrial respiration, and further interference with glycolysis and the citric acid cycle *(19,28–30)*. NO• has been shown to inhibit mitochondrial respiration in bacteria and eukaryotic cells reversibly by binding to the oxygen-binding site of cytochrome oxidase in competition with oxygen *(30,31)*. In addition, Fe–S clusters of the respiratory chain, such as complex I/III and aconitase, also seem to be affected by NO• probably by *S*-nitros(yl)ation of the Fe–S clusters *(32,33)*. However, because of the reversibility of the *S*-nitros(ly)ation reaction by endogenous glutathione, it remains to be elucidated whether these effects take part in vivo or only occur when the level of the endogenous antioxidant capacity is reduced. Several studies suggest that the effects of NO• on energy metabolism are mainly due to the formation of peroxynitrite. Thus, the reaction of NO• with superoxide leading to the generation of peroxynitrite may enhance the cytotoxic potential of NO• *(34)*. Indeed, peroxynitrite has been shown to inhibit mitochondrial respiration irreversibly by interfering with complex I/III *(34)*. Furthermore, a recent study demonstrating that peroxynitrite induces the degradation of proteins such as aconitase suggests that further mechanisms might be involved in peroxynitrite cytotoxicity *(35)*.

Apoptosis and NO•

Having demonstrated that NO• induces cytotoxic effects on macrophages *(19)*, which was originally believed to be mediated by necrotic cell death, more detailed analysis revealed that NO• also triggers the apoptotic cell death pathway *(36,37)*. Induction of apoptosis by exogenous NO•-donors as well as endogenous synthesis of NO• mainly by iNOS has been demonstrated in various cell types including β-cells *(38,39)*, thymocytes *(40)*, neuronal cells *(41)*, and smooth muscle cells *(42)*. In contrast, other studies suggest an antiapoptotic effect of NO• *(43–45)*. Thus, NO• seems to play a complex role in modulating apoptosis. The following section of this chapter gives an overview of these contradictory effects of NO• on apoptosis with special focus on its potential role in physiology and pathophysiology.

IMMUNE SYSTEM

NO• and Apoptosis of Immune-Competent Cells. Activation of the immune system is important for defense against invading organisms as well as tumor cells, but also leads to damage of host tissue after prolonged stimulation. As outlined previously, NO• belongs to the nonspecific immune defense system, inducing the killing of the invading organisms (*see* "Cytotoxic Effects of NO•"). In addition, NO• also contributes to tumor cell destruction by inducing apoptotic cell death of tumor cells *(46)*. Moreover, transfection of cells with iNOS has been shown to be associated with apoptosis and suppression of tumorigenicity in vivo *(47)*. However, the immune competent cells themselves have also been shown to be rendered apoptotic by endogenously produced NO• *(36,37,40)*. One may speculate that production of high concentrations of NO• by macrophages leading to suicide of the cell may limit the inflammatory process. However, induction of iNOS during infection, which triggers excessive apoptosis of immune-competent cells, may also contribute to immune suppression or endotoxic shock *(40)*.

In contrast, other studies now demonstrated a potent inhibitory effect of NO• on apoptosis in lymphocytes. Thus, exogenous and endogenous NO• has been shown to inhibit soluble MHC- or Fas-induced apoptosis of B-cells *(43,44)*. Moreover, recent studies provide evidence that NO• protects T-lymphocytes against Fas–receptor-stimulated apoptotic cell death *(48–51)*. In addition, eosinophils were shown to be less susceptible to the induction of apoptosis after NO• treatment *(52,53)*.

Thus, both pro- as well as antiapoptotic effects of NO• have been demonstrated. It remains unclear whether the induction or inhibition of lymphocyte apoptosis is the major consequence of NO• production in vivo. These apparently opposing effects of NO• may be explained by a biphasic dose-dependent phenomenon. Under physiological conditions low levels of NO• may inhibit apoptosis of immune-competent cells and thereby support immune defense, whereas high levels may induce cell death, thus limiting the inflammatory process. However, as is typical for the immune defense system, the beneficial effects are overwhelmed when the mediator is released for prolonged time periods in high concentrations. Thus, excessive apoptosis induced by long-lasting, high-output NO• synthesis may also lead to tissue destruction. The cytotoxic effects of NO• toward specific pathogens clearly contribute to immune defense; however, further studies are necessary to determine the role and, more importantly, the functional consequences of NO•-modulated cell death of immune competent cells.

Role of NO•-Modulated Apoptosis in Inflammation. A number of studies suggested that NO•-induced apoptosis contributes to autoimmune disease and chronic inflammatory diseases. Indeed, destruction of pancreatic β-cells, which causes diabetes mellitus, has been shown to be mediated by NO•-triggered apoptosis. Thus, incubation with exogenous NO•-donors or induction of the iNOS by interleukin 1β induces apoptotic cell death of pancreatic β-cells in vitro *(38,39)*. Furthermore, NO•-induced stimulation of Fas-receptor expression in β-cells may enhance the pro-apoptotic effect of Fas-ligand-bearing lymphocytes infiltrating the islet *(54)*. Furthermore, IFNγ receptor knock out, which reduces the expression of the iNOS by IFNγ, leads to enhanced apoptosis of T-cells and increases the sensitivity to anti-CD-3-induced disease syndromes *(55)*. Proapoptotic effects of exogenous NO• donors were further described in mesangial cells, suggesting a possible role in glomerulonephritis *(56)*. However, as the endogenous production of NO• has also been shown to protect mesangial cells against apoptosis *(57)*, and as the iNOS knockout mouse is not resistant to autoimmune glomerulonephritis *(21)*, the contribution of NO•-induced apoptosis to the pathophysiology of glomerulonephritis remains controversial.

In contrast to these proapoptotic effects, various in vitro and in vivo studies suggest a cell-protective or antiapoptotic effect of NO• during inflammation. Thus, inhibition of NO• synthesis in endotoxic shock significantly enhanced DNA fragmentation in liver, lung, kidney, and intestine *(58)*, indicating an antiapoptotic effect of NO•. Moreover, tissue selective generation of NO• in the liver significantly suppresses apoptosis and protects hepatocytes in an animal model of liver failure *(59)*. In addition, ischemia/reperfusion injury-induced apoptotic cell death in the liver is prevented by infusion of the NO•-synthase substrate L-arginine *(60)*. The hepatoprotective effect of NO• is also supported by in vitro studies *(61,62)*. In summary, these studies suggest that the antiapoptotic effects of NO• may prevent tissue destruction and especially protect the liver against injurious insults.

CARDIOVASCULAR SYSTEM

Atherosclerosis. The pathophysiological events leading to the development of atherosclerotic lesions are initiated by endothelial cell injury followed by an inflammatory process with invasion of immune competent cells, smooth muscle cell proliferation, and development of the atherosclerotic plaque. Finally, the destabilization of the plaque characterized by degradation of matrix proteins and smooth muscle cell death leads to plaque rupture and induces the acute clinical manifestation of atherosclerosis, such as myocardial infarction or stroke. Apoptotic cells have been identified in human atherosclerotic lesions, atherectomy specimens, and saphenous vein grafts, suggesting a possible contribution of apoptosis to the pathophysiology of atherosclerosis *(63–65)*. Apoptotic cell death may play a role in at least three steps in the pathophysiology of atherosclerosis: (1) the initial endothelial cell injury, (2) apoptotic cell death of immune competent cells invading the plaque, and (3) smooth muscle cell death leading to plaque destabilization.

The nature of the initial endothelial cell injury preceding atherosclerotic lesion development is still unknown. Interestingly, lesion-prone regions, where atherosclerotic lesions preferentially develop, are characterized by enhanced endothelial cell turnover, which might be the consequence of underlying apoptotic cell death *(66)*. Indeed, proatherosclerotic factors, such as oxidized low-density lipoprotein (LDL), angiotensin II, or reactive oxygen species, induce apoptosis of endothelial cells in vitro *(67–69)*. NO• counteracts the proapoptotic effects of proatherosclerotic factors on endothelial cells. Thus, low doses of NO• donors potently inhibit endothelial cell apoptosis induced by classical apoptotic stimuli such as serum depletion or TNFα *(45,70)*. Moreover, apoptosis of endothelial cells induced by the proatherosclerotic factors angiotensin II, reactive oxygen species, oxidized LDL, and oxidized Lp(a) is completely prevented by exogenous NO• donors *(45,68,69,71)*. Most importantly, laminar flow-triggered release of endothelial NO• prevents apoptosis *(45,72,73)*. Increased concentrations of NO• donors also can induce endothelial cell apoptosis *(70)*; however, the concentrations required are beyond the levels produced by the endothelial cell itself. This view is supported by the finding that even overexpression of iNOS abolished lipopolysaccharide-induced apoptosis *(74)* and promotes endothelial cell proliferation *(75)*. Thus, the antiapoptotic effects of endothelial NO• contribute to the endothelial protective and antiatherosclerotic function of NO•.

In contrast, it has been suggested that NO• also function as a trigger of apoptosis in cells of the vascular wall (*see* Table 1). Indeed, expression of iNOS and nitrotyrosine, indicating significant NO• production, was demonstrated in atheroma *(76)*. Because the induction of iNOS in murine macrophages leads to apoptosis *(36)*, one may speculate about the contribution of NO• in triggering apoptotic cell death of macrophages, which has been demonstrated in the atheromatous plaque *(63,64)*. Moreover, apoptosis of smooth muscle cells in the atheromatous plaque *(64)* may be induced by NO•. Exogenous NO• donors, as well as endogenous generation of NO• via cytokine-induced iNOS expression, trigger apoptosis of smooth muscle cells *(42,77,78)*. In addition, NO•-induced upregulation of the Fas–receptor increases the susceptibility of smooth muscle cells toward Fas–receptor activation-triggered apoptosis *(79)*.

The consequences of apoptotic cell death in atherogenesis remain unclear. Recent studies provide evidence for an crucial role of NO• as a proapoptotic and antiproliferative factor for smooth muscle cells in the process of vascular remodeling *(80,81)*. In addition, one may speculate that apoptosis of inflammatory cells during the early pathogenesis of atherosclerosis may limit the inflammatory process. However, prolonged and enhanced apoptotic cell death, especially of the surrounding smooth muscle cells and endothelial cells, may promote atherosclerotic lesion development. The localization of apoptotic smooth muscle cells subendothelially within the fibrous cap and surrounding the necrotic core suggests a role for apoptosis in destabilization of the plaque *(64,82)*.

However, because human cells produce lower amounts of NO• compared to murine cells, it remains controversial whether the endogenous generation of NO• in humans is sufficient to induce apoptosis. Taken together, endothelial NO• clearly exhibits an antiatherosclerotic potential as demonstrated recently in eNOS knockout animals *(83)*. Moreover, the first and convincing evidence that iNOS also confers protection against atherosclerotic lesion development was recently provided by the finding that transplant atherosclerosis is exacerbated in iNOS-deficient mice *(84)*. Thus, generally NO• seems to exert a beneficial effect on atherosclerotic lesion development. The contribution of apoptosis—either inhibited or promoted by NO•—in atherogenesis, however, remains to be elucidated.

Myocardial Disease. Recent studies provide evidence that apoptotic cell death of cardiac myocytes is involved in the pathophysiology of heart failure and reperfusion injury (for review see *[85]*); however, the role of NO• is largely unknown. Some studies suggest that the induction of iNOS may play a role in myocardial cell apoptosis. Thus, in experimentally induced myocardial infarction, a colocalization of iNOS in infiltrating macrophages with apoptosis of macrophages and adjacent cardiomyocytes is observed *(86,87)*. A causal relationship was suggested by the finding that inhibition of NOS prevented myocardial infarction-induced cardiomyocyte apoptosis and further improved myocardial function *(87)*. In addition, adenovirus-mediated gene transfer of eNOS induced cardiomyocyte cell shrinkage, which was prevented by NOS inhibitors *(88)*. Further studies revealed that enhanced expression of iNOS may contribute to apoptosis of cardiac myocytes during cardiac allograft rejection *(89,90)*.

In contrast, other studies demonstrated a protective effect of NO• on cardiomyocyte cell death. Thus, inhibition of the endogenous NO• synthesis with N^G-monomethyl-L-arginine significantly enhanced reperfusion-induced apoptosis in isolated perfused hearts *(91)*. Moreover, stretch-induced cardiomyocyte cell death, an in vitro model of load-induced cardiac hypertrophy, was prevented by NO• donors *(92)*.

Table 1
Role of NO•-Modulated Apoptosis in Cardiovascular Disorders

Cardiovascular disorder	Cell type	Proposed effect of NO•	Suggested functional consequence		References
			Beneficial	Harmful	
Atherosclerosis	Endothelial cell	Antiapoptotic	Protection of the endothelium		45,68–74
	Smooth muscle cell	Proapoptotic	Reduction of neointima formation? Remodeling	Plaque destabilization	42,77–79 80,81
	Leukocytes/macrophages	Proapoptotic	Limitation of inflammation?	Atheroma formation?	36,37
Ischemia/reperfusion	Cardiomyocytes	Proapoptotic		Impairment of ventricular function	86–88
	Leukocytes/macrophages	Antiapoptotic	Improvement of ventricular function		89,90
Heart failure		Proapoptotic	Limitation of inflammation?		87,88
	Cardiomyocytes	Proapoptotic		Impairment of ventricular function Heart chamber enlargement Ventricular remodeling	
	Cardiomyocytes	Antiapoptotic	Improvement of ventricular function		92

Taken together, currently available data indicate that NO•-modulated apoptosis does play a role in myocardial disorders (*see* Table 1). However, it remains unclear whether NO• triggers or inhibits cardiomyocyte apoptosis and, thus, improves or impairs myocardial function.

NEURONAL SYSTEM

Besides the function of NO• as a neurotransmitter, NO• also has been proposed to be involved in the pathophysiology of neurodegenerative diseases. Indeed, apoptosis of neuronal as well as glial cells was demonstrated to occur after NO• addition in vitro (41,93,94). NO• further indirectly induced the release of glutamate, thereby stimulating the *N*-methyl-D-aspartate (NMDA) receptor and, thus, promoting apoptotic cell death (95,96).

The proapoptotic effects of NO• demonstrated in vitro were supported by animal experiments. Apoptotic cell death and iNOS colocalized in inflammatory lesions in mice with multiple sclerosis (97). Moreover, inhibition of neuronal NO• release prevented apoptotic cell death induced by hypothermic circulatory arrest (98) or dopaminergic neurotoxicity (99). Most importantly, striatal malonate lesion formation and apoptosis was attenuated in nNOS knockout mice (100). Interestingly, eNOS knockout mice were more susceptible to neuronal injury, thus indicating that NO• produced by eNOS might be protective against neuronal injury whereas NO• produced by the nNOS exerts cytotoxic effects.

Mechanisms of the Pro- and Antiapoptotic Effect of NO•

PROAPOPTOTIC EFFECTS

The precise mechanisms that determine cellular sensitivity to NO• mediated toxicity are not clear; however, the toxic and proapoptotic effects of NO• seem to be independent of the activation of guanylyl cyclase (101). The induction of apoptosis by NO• more likely is the result of direct DNA damage (102). It has been demonstrated that NO• incubation leads to direct deamination of cytosine to uracil and of 5-methylcytosine to thymidine, thereby promoting DNA strand breaks and apoptosis (102). Moreover, accumulation of the tumor suppressor protein p53, which is induced by DNA damage, has been described as an essential and early indicator of NO•-induced apoptosis (103). Subsequently, p53 elevation induces the expression of the proapoptotic protein Bax and the downregulation of the antiapoptotic protein Bcl-2 (103,104). However, NO• can also induce apoptosis in p53-depleted cells (105), which indicates that p53 elevation is not prerequisite for NO•-triggered apoptotic cell death. In addition, cleavage of the poly(ADP-ribose) polymerase (PARP) indicating the activation of caspases or related proteases may contribute to the induction of apoptosis (105). Subsequent studies, however, have not supported this assumption, as specific caspase inhibitors did not prevent apoptotic cell death (106), suggesting that the NO•-induced proapoptotic signal transduction may be more complex and questioning the assumption that there is really a causal relationship between activation of caspases and PARP cleavage and NO•-induced apoptotic cell death. Indeed, further studies suggest that NO• induces apoptosis by blocking the antiapoptotic effect of cyclooxygenase-2 (106).

Recent studies investigating the effects of NO• on mitochondria provide a novel and interesting mechanism by which to explain NO•-induced apoptosis and cytotoxicity. NO• has been shown to act as a regulator of mitochondrial permeability transition (107,108). Because opening of the mitochondrial transmembrane permeability pore seems to be involved in the release of mitochondrial cytochrome C into the cytosol, thereby promoting apoptotic cell death (10), it has been postulated that NO• may trigger apoptosis by this pathway. Indeed, pharmacological inhibition of the mitochondrial permeability pore prevented NO•-induced mitochondrial permeability and subsequent apoptosis (108).

The downregulation of protein kinase C (PKC) has also been proposed to mediate p53-independent NO•-induced apoptosis (109). In contrast, other studies demonstrated that

NO•-induced upregulation of PKC mediates the proapoptotic effect of NO• *(78,110)*. The explanation for these different outcomes may be the use of different cell systems and/or the involvement of different PKC isoforms.

In conclusion, several pathways have been shown to be affected by NO•, which might trigger the proapoptotic response in different cell lines as illustrated in Table 2. Although the sequential events are unclear, the induction of mitochondrial dysfunction or direct DNA damage by NO• are possible candidates for initiating the apoptotic pathway.

In the neuronal system, it has been suggested that the NMDA–receptor activation-triggered stimulation of the calcium-dependent nNOS induces neuronal cell death *(93)*. Neurotoxic effects were thereby proposed to be mainly caused by the reaction of NO• with superoxide radicals leading to peroxynitrite generation *(111)*. In addition, NO• also enhances the release of glutamate, which results in NMDA–receptor activation and calcium overload and, thereby, indirectly promotes neuronal cell death *(95,96)*.

ANTIAPOPTOTIC EFFECTS

The mechanisms by which NO• inhibits apoptosis may include several transcriptional and posttranscriptional events (*see* Table 2). Especially in hepatocytes, but also in other cell lines, NO• has been shown to stimulate the expression of antiapoptotic proteins. NO•-induced expression of the heat shock protein 70 (HSP70) inhibits apoptosis of hepatocytes induced by TNFα and actinomycin D *(62)*. Moreover, the upregulation of the antiapoptotic Bcl-2 protein by NO• has been suggested to prevent apoptosis in B cells *(44)*. NO• further increased the expression of the cytoprotective proteins heme oxygenase-1 and ferritin *(61,112,113)*, which have been proposed to inhibit endothelial cell and hepatocyte cytotoxicity *(61,112, 114)*. Other studies questioned a causal role for NO•-induced heme oxygenase upregulation in the antiapoptotic effects of NO• *(115)*. The antiapoptotic effect of NO•, however, does not only rely on the induction of antiapoptotic proteins, as NO• also inhibits apoptotic cell death when protein biosynthesis is inhibited *(49)*.

Initially, the well-known activation of the guanylyl cyclase by NO• leading to the formation of the second messenger cGMP was proposed to mediate the antiapoptotic effects of NO•. Membrane-permeable cGMP analogs reduced apoptosis in B-cells, eosinophils, and T-lymphocytes *(44,52)*. In contrast, other studies failed to demonstrate a protective effect for cGMP. Neither membrane-permeable cGMP analogs *(43,45,49,50)* nor pharmacological activation of the guanylyl cyclase *(68)* mimicked the NO• effect. Most importantly, protective effects of NO• were demonstrated in human umbilical vein endothelial cells, which lack cGMP-dependent protein kinase *(116)*.

The key mediators of apoptosis signaling are the caspases. The activation of these cysteine proteases by various stimuli, including TNFα, Fas–receptor activation, growth factor withdrawal, reactive oxygen species, as well as angiotensin II, has been shown to be inhibited by NO• *(45,48,68,70,73)*. The inhibition of caspase activation was not the result of downregulation of gene expression, but seems to be mediated by *S*-nitrosation of the essential cysteine residue located in the active site of the enzyme *(45)*. The *S*-nitrosation of the essential cysteine residue of the purified caspases (caspase-1 to capase-8) by NO• correlated with the inhibition of enzymatic activity *(45,49,70,117)*. A direct interference of NO• with the caspase cascade was further supported by the finding that apoptosis induced by overexpression of Fas-associated death domain protein (FADD), which directly activates the caspase cascade, or by the FADD-associated caspase-8 (FLICE) was prevented by NO•-donors *(49)*. Moreover, NO• donors stimulated the *S*-nitrosation of overexpressed caspase-3 in vivo, thereby preventing the induction of cell death and inhibited the enzyme activity of caspase-3 *(118)*.

A further potential mechanism by which NO• may interfere with apoptotic signaling is stabilization of the mitochondria. The disruption of mitochondrial membrane function induced by several proapoptotic stimuli by an undefined mechanism has been shown to evoke the

Table 2
Proposed Mechanisms Underlying the Pro- and Antiapoptotic Effects of NO•

	Proapoptotic effects	References	Antiapoptotic effects	References
Transcriptional effects	Inhibition of COX-2 expression	166	Upregulation of HSP70	62
	Upregulation of Bax	103,104	Upregulation of Bcl-2	44
	Downregulation of Bcl-2	103,104	Upregulation of heme oxygenase	112
			Upregulation of ferritin	61,113
Posttranscriptional effects	DNA damage	102	cGMP	44,52,53
	p53-accumulation	103,104	Inhibition of caspases by S-nitrosation	45,48,68, 70,73
	PKC modulation	78,109,110	Inhibition of ceramide-induced JNK-activation	53
	Activation of caspases	105,106		
	Increase of mitochondrial membrane permeability	107,108	Mitochondrial stabilization	119
			Scavenging of reactive oxygen species	57
	Enhanced glutamate release	95,96		

77

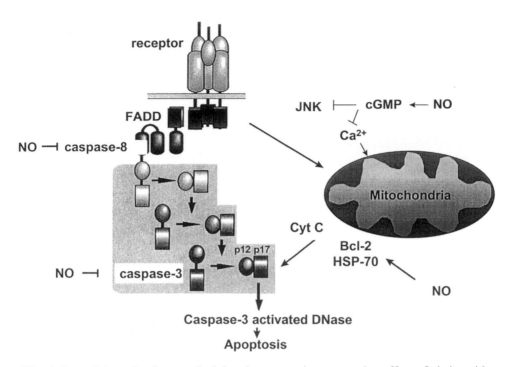

Fig. 1. Potential mechanisms underlying the apoptosis-suppressive effect of nitric oxide.

release of cytochrome C, which activates the caspase cascade by formation of the apoptosome complex with caspase-9 and Apaf-1 *(12)*. We recently demonstrated that NO• donors prevented the TNFα-induced release of cytochrome C into the cytosol in human umbilical endothelial cells (S. Dimmeler, personal communication). The potential mechanisms may include the stabilization or upregulation of the mitochondrial protective protein Bcl-2 by NO• *(44,119)* or the inhibition of upstream caspases such as caspase-8 or caspase-1, which may be involved in triggering mitochondrial membrane dysfunction *(10)*. Potentially, the upregulation of the HSP70 *(62)*, which also modulates mitochondrial function, may further contribute to mitochondrial stabilization in hepatocytes. NO• may also inhibit mitochondrial ATP-generation by blockade of complex I/III (*see* "Apoptosis and NO•"), thereby preventing the dATP/ATP-dependent activation of caspases by cytochrome C. However, if NO• reduced ATP levels but did not affect mitochondrial cytochrome C release, one would expect to induce necrotic instead of apoptotic cell death. A shift toward necrosis by incubation with NO•, however, has not been detected in endothelial cells (S. Dimmeler, personal communication).

Finally, NO• interferes with the activation of kinases involved in the apoptotic cascade. Thus, NO• blocked Fas- or ceramide-induced activation of the proapoptotic stress-activated jun-kinase (JNK), an effect that was mimicked by cGMP analogs *(53)*. The activation of the growth promoting mitogen-activated kinase cascade by NO• *(120)* may support cell survival, and, thereby inhibit the susceptibility of cells towards apoptotic cell death.

Taken together, NO• interacts with several components of the apoptotic signal transduction pathway as illustrated in Fig. 1. The importance of the specific NO•-effect in inhibiting apoptosis is difficult to interpret and may vary with the cell type investigated and the stimulus used. With regard to the various biochemical reactions by which NO• can interact with proteins (e.g., nitrotyrosine formation, *S*-nitrosation), and the interference with the oxidative flux in cells, it is not surprising that several steps in apoptotic signal transduction are inhibited by NO• and may underlie the important role of NO• in cell death signaling.

CONCLUSION

Having demonstrated that NO$^\bullet$ can induce or inhibit cell death, the question remains as to how to explain these different actions. Overall, it appears that the effects of NO$^\bullet$ formation by nNOS or iNOS are predominantly associated with cytotoxic and proapoptotic effects, whereas endothelial NO$^\bullet$ production protects against cytotoxicity and apoptosis. Most importantly, these in vitro observations have been supported by studies with gene knockout animals, which demonstrate an atheroprotective and antiinflammatory role of the eNOS *(83)* and a pro-inflammatory and cytotoxic effect of iNOS and nNOS *(21,100)*. Why does NO$^\bullet$ exert distinct effects when generated by the iNOS or nNOS compared to the eNOS ? The most plausible explanation might be a biphasic dose-dependent effect with low concentrations of NO$^\bullet$ generated by eNOS being antiapoptotic and antiinflammatory, whereas high concentrations generated by iNOS being proapoptotic. This conclusion is in accordance with in vitro studies clearly demonstrating a biphasic dose dependence of the effects of NO$^\bullet$ *(70)*. Other studies suggested that the different effects of NO$^\bullet$ are caused by different NO$^\bullet$ redox congeners being either cytotoxic or cytoprotective *(93)*. However, at least the exogenous addition of different redox species of NO$^\bullet$ produced similar effects in one study *(70)*. Another hypothesis might be that the biological action of NO$^\bullet$ depends on the redox state of the cell, which would implicate that endothelial cells are different compared to other cell types. All of these possible explanations, however, beg the question of differential molecular mechanism(s).

In conclusion, the challenge in investigating the effects of NO$^\bullet$ on cell death is to elucidate its contribution to physiology and pathophysiology. Because NO$^\bullet$ also exerts various other biological function, which might interfere with inflammatory processes, the specific contribution of NO$^\bullet$-modulated cell death remains to be clarified.

REFERENCES

1. Buja LM, Eigenbrodt ML, Eigenbrodt EH. Apoptosis and necrosis. Basic types and mechanisms of cell death. Arch Pathol Lab Med 1993;117:1208–1214.
2. Kerr JF, Wyllie AH, Currie AR. Apoptosis: a basic biological phenomenon with wide-ranging implications in tissue kinetics. Br J Cancer 1972;26:239–257.
3. Wyllie AH. Apoptosis: cell death in tissue regulation. J Pathol 1987;153:313–316.
4. Devitt A, Moffatt OD, Raykundalia C, Capra JD, Simmons DL, Gregory CD. Human CD14 mediates recognition and phagocytosis of apoptotic cells. Nature 1998;392:505–509.
5. White E. Life, death, and the pursuit of apoptosis. Genes Dev 1996;10:1–15.
6. Nagata S. Apoptosis by death factor. Cell 1997;88:355–365.
7. Enari M, Sakahira H, Yokoyama H, Okawa K, Iwamatsu A, Nagata S. A caspase-activated DNase that degrades DNA during apoptosis, and its inhibitor ICAD. Nature 1998;391:43–50.
8. Kroemer G. The proto-oncogene Bcl-2 and its role in regulating apoptosis. Nat Med 1997;3:614–620.
9. Reed JC. Double identity for proteins of the Bcl-2 family. Nature 1997;387:773–776.
10. Reed JC. Cytochrome c: can't live with it—can't live without it. Cell 1997;91:559–562.
11. Kroemer G, Zamzami N, Susin SA. Mitochondrial control of apoptosis. Immunol Today 1997;18:44–51.
12. Li P, Nijhawan D, Budihardjo I, Srinivasula SM, Ahmad M, Alnemri ES, et al. Cytochrome c and dATP-dependent formation of Apaf-1/Caspase-9 complex initiates an apoptotic protease cascade. Cell 1997;91:479–489.
13. Zou H, Henzel WJ, Liu X, Lutschg A, Wang X. Apaf-1, a human protein homologous to C. elegans CED-4, participates in cytochrome c-dependent activation of caspase-3. Cell 1997;90:405–413.
14. Moncada S, Higgs A. The L-arginine-nitric oxide pathway. N Engl J Med 1993;329:2002–2012.
15. Nathan C. Nitric oxide as a secretory product of mammalian cells. FASEB J 1992;6:3051–3064.
16. Ochoa JB, Udekwu AO, Billiar TR, Curran RD, Cerra FB, Simmons RL, et al. Nitrogen oxide levels in patients after trauma and during sepsis. Ann Surg 1991;214:621–626.
17. Stuehr DJ, Marletta MA. Mammalian nitrate biosynthesis: mouse macrophages produce nitrite and nitrate in response to Escherichia coli lipopolysaccharide. Proc Natl Acad Sci USA 1985; 82:7738–7742.
18. Stuehr DJ, Gross SS, Sakuma I, Levi R, Nathan CF. Activated murine macrophages secrete a metabolite of arginine with the bioactivity of endothelium-derived relaxing factor and chemical reactivity of nitric oxide. J Exp Med 1989;169:1011–1020.

19. Hibbs JB Jr, Taintor RR, Vavrin Z, Rachlin EM. Nitric oxide: a cytotoxic activated macrophage effector molecule. Biochem Biophys Res Commun 1988;157:87–94.

20. Granger DL, Hibbs JB Jr. High-output nitric oxide: weapon against infection? Trends Microbiol 1996; 4:46,47.

21. Nathan C. Inducible nitric oxide synthase: what difference does it make? J Clin Invest 1997;100: 2417–2423.

22. Dinapoli MR, Calderon CL, Lopez DM. The altered tumoricidal capacity of macrophages isolated from tumor-bearing mice is related to reduce expression of the inducible nitric oxide synthase gene. J Exp Med 1996;183:1323–1329.

23. Mulligan MS, Hevel JM, Marletta MA, Ward PA. Tissue injury caused by deposition of immune complexes is L-arginine dependent. Proc Natl Acad Sci USA 1991;88:6338–6342.

24. Appels B, Burkart V, Kantwerk-Funke G, Funda J, Kolb-Bachofen V, Kolb H. Spontaneous cytotoxicity of macrophages against pancreatic islet cells. J Immunol 1989;142:3803–3808.

25. Corbett JA, Wang JL, Sweetland MA, Lancaster JR Jr, McDaniel ML. Interleukin 1 beta induces the formation of nitric oxide by beta-cells purified from rodent islets of Langerhans. Evidence for the beta-cell as a source and site of action of nitric oxide. J Clin Invest 1992;90:2384–2391.

26. Dimmeler S, Ankarcrona M, Nicotera P, Brüne B. Exogenous nitric oxide (NO) generation or IL-1 beta-induced intracellular NO production stimulates inhibitory auto-ADP-ribosylation of glyceraldehyde-3-phosphate dehydrogenase in RINm5F cells. J Immunol 1993;150:2964–2971.

27. Corbett JA, McDaniel ML. Does nitric oxide mediate autoimmune destruction of beta-cells? Possible therapeutic interventions in IDDM. Diabetes 1992;41:897–903.

28. Stadler J, Billiar TR, Curran RD, Stuehr DJ, Ochoa JB, Simmons RL. Effect of exogenous and endogenous nitric oxide on mitochondrial respiration of rat hepatocytes. Am J Physiol 1991;260:C910–C916.

29. Dimmeler S, Lottspeich F, Brüne B. Nitric oxide causes ADP-ribosylation and inhibition of glyceraldehyde-3-phosphate dehydrogenase. J Biol Chem 1992;267:16,771–16,774.

30. Brown GC. Nitric oxide inhibition of cytochrome oxidase and mitochondrial respiration: implications for inflammatory, neurodegenerative and ischemic pathologies. Mol Cell Biochem 1997;174:189–192.

31. Lizasoain I, Moro MA, Knowles RG, Darley-Usmar V, Moncada S. Nitric oxide and peroxynitrite exert distinct effects on mitochondrial respiration which are differentially blocked by glutathione or glucose. Biochem J 1996;314:877–880.

32. Drapier JC. Interplay between NO and [Fe-S] clusters: relevance to biological systems. Methods 1997; 11:319–329.

33. Gardner PR, Costantino G, Szabo C, Salzman AL. Nitric oxide sensitivity of the aconitases. J Biol Chem 1997;272:25,071–25,076.

34. Hausladen A, Fridovich I. Superoxide and peroxynitrite inactivate aconitases, but nitric oxide does not. J Biol Chem 1994;269:29,405–29,408.

35. Grune T, Blasig IE, Sitte N, Roloff B, Haseloff R, Davies KJ. Peroxynitrite increases the degradation of aconitase and other cellular proteins by proteasome. J Biol Chem 1998;273:10,857–10,862.

36. Sarih M, Souvannavong V, Adam A. Nitric oxide synthase induces macrophage death by apoptosis. Biochem Biophys Res Commun 1993;191:503–508.

37. Albina J, Cui S, Mateo R, Reichner J. Nitric oxide-mediated apoptosis in murine peritoneal macrophages. J Immunol 1993;150:5080–5085.

38. Kaneto H, Fujii J, Seo HG, Suzuki K, Matsuoka T, Nakamura M, et al. Apoptotic cell death triggered by nitric oxide in pancreatic beta-cells. Diabetes 1995;44:733–738.

39. Ankarcrona M, Dypbukt JM, Brune B, Nicotera P. Interleukin-1 beta-induced nitric oxide production activates apoptosis in pancreatic RINm5F cells. Exp Cell Res 1994;213:172–177.

40. Fehsel K, Kröncke KD, Meyer KL, Huber H, Wahn V, Kolb-Bachofen V. Nitric oxide induces apoptosis in mouse thymocytes. J Immunol 1995;155:2858–2865.

41. Estevez AG, Spear N, Manuel SM, Radi R, Henderson CE, Barbeito L, et al. Nitric oxide and superoxide contribute to motor neuron apoptosis induced by trophic factor depriviation. J Neurosci 1998;18: 923–931.

42. Nishio E, Fukushima K, Shiozaki M, Watanabe Y. Nitric oxide donor SNAP induces apoptosis in smooth muscle cells through cGMP-independent mechanism. Biochem Biophys Res Commun 1996; 221:163–168.

43. Mannick JB, Asano K, Izumi K, Kieff E, Stamler JS. Nitric oxide produced by human B lymphocytes inhibits apoptosis and Epstein-Barr virus reactivation. Cell 1994;79:1137–1146.

44. Genaro AM, Hortelano S, Alvarez A, Martinez C, Bosca L. Splenic B lymphocyte programmed cell death is prevented by nitric oxide release through mechanisms involving sustained Bcl-2 levels. J Clin Invest 1995;95:1884–1890.

45. Dimmeler S, Haendeler J, Nehls M, Zeiher AM. Suppression of apoptosis by nitric oxide via inhibition of ICE-like and CPP32-like proteases. J Exp Med 1997;185:601–608.

46. Gal A, Tamir S, Kennedy LJ, Tannenbaum SR, Wogan GN. Nitrotyrosine formation, apoptosis and oxidative damage: relationships to nitric oxide production in SJL mice bearing the RcsX tumor. Cancer Res 1997;57:1823–1828.

47. Xie K, Huang S, Dong Z, Juang S.-H, Gutman M, Xie Q, et al. Transfection with the inducible nitric oxide synthase gene suppresses tumorgenicity and abrogates metastasis by K-1735 murine melanoma cells. J Exp Med 1995;181:1333–1343.

48. Melino G, Bernassola F, Knight RA, Corasaniti MT, Nistico G, Finazzi-Agro A. S-nitrosylation regulates apoptosis. Nature 1997;388:432,433.

49. Dimmeler S, Haendeler J, Sause A, Zeiher AM. Nitric oxide inhibits APO-1/Fas-mediated cell death. Cell Growth Differ 1998;9:415–422.

50. Mannick JB, Miao XQ, Stamler JS. Nitric oxide inhibits Fas-induced apoptosis. J Biol Chem 1997;272: 24,125–24,128.

51. Sciorati C, Rovere P, Ferrarini M, Heltai S, Manfredi AA, Clementi E. Autocrine nitric oxide modulates CD95-induced apoptosis in gamma delta T lymphocytes. J Biol Chem 1997;272:23,211–23,215.

52. Beauvais F, Michel L, Dubertret L. The nitric oxide donors, azide and hydroxylamine, inhibit the programmed cell death of cytokine-deprived human eosinophils. FEBS Lett 1995;361:229–232.

53. Hebestreit H, Dibbert B, Balatti I, Braun D, Schapowal A, Blaser K, et al. Disruption of Fas receptor signaling by nitric oxide in eosinophils. J Exp Med 1998;187:415–425.

54. Stassi G, Maria RD, Trucco G, Rudert W, Testi R, Galluzzo A, et al. Nitric oxide primes pancreatic beta-cells for Fas-mediated destruction in insulin-dependent diabetes mellitus. J Exp Med 1997;186: 1193–1200.

55. Matthys P, Froyen G, Verdot L, Huang S, Sobis H, Damme JV, et al. IFNgamma receptor-deficient mice are hypersensitive to the anti-CD3-induced cytokine release syndrome and thymocyte apoptosis. J Immunol 1995;155:3823–3829.

56. Muhl H, Sandau K, Brüne B, Briner VA, Pfeilschifter J. Nitric oxide donors induce apoptosis in glomerular mesangial cells, epithelial cells and endothelial cells. Eur J Pharmacol 1996;317:137–149.

57. Sandau K, Pfeilschifter J, Brüne B. The balance between nitric oxide and superoxide determines apoptotic and necrotic death of rat mesangial cells. J Immunol 1997;158:4938–4946.

58. Bohlinger I, Leist M, Gantner F, Angermüller S, Tiegs G, Wendel A. DNA fragmentation in mouse organs during endotoxic shock. Am J Pathol 1996;149:1381–1393.

59. Saavedra JE, Billiar TR, Williams DL, Kim YM, Watkins SC, Keefer LK. Targeting nitric oxide (NO) delivery in vivo. Design of a liver-selective NO donor prodrug that blocks tumor necrosis factor-alpha-induced apoptosis and toxicity in the liver. J Med Chem 1997;40:1947–1954.

60. Calabrese F, Valente M, Pettenazzo E, Ferraresso M, Burra P, Cadrobbi R. et al. The protective effects of L-arginine after liver ischemia/reperfusion injury in a pig model. J Pathol 1997;183:477–485.

61. Kim YM, Bergonia H, Lancaster JR Jr. Nitrogen oxide-induced autoprotection in isolated rat hepatocytes. FEBS Lett 1995;374:228–232.

62. Kim YM, de Vera ME, Watkins SC, Billiar TR. Nitric oxide protects cultured rat hepatocytes from tumor necrosis factor-alpha-induced apoptosis by inducting heat shock protein 70 expression. J Biol Chem 1997;272:1402–1411.

63. Geng YJ, Libby P. Evidence for apoptosis in advanced human atheroma. Colocalization with interleukin-1 beta-converting enzyme. Am J Pathol 1995;147:251–266.

64. Cai W, Devaux B, Schaper W, Schaper J. The role of Fas/APO 1 and apoptosis in the development of human atherosclerotic lesions. Atherosclerosis 1997;131:177–186.

65. Bjorkerud S, Bjorkerud B. Apoptosis is abundant in human atherosclerotic lesions, especially in inflammatory cells (macrophages and T cells), and may contribute to the accumulation of gruel and plaque instability. Am J Pathol 1996;149:367–380.

66. Caplan BA, Schwartz CJ. Increased endothelial cell turnover in areas of in vivo Evans Blue uptake in the pig aorta. Atherosclerosis 1973;17:401–417.

67. Dimmeler S, Haendeler J, Galle J, Zeiher AM. Oxidized low density lipoprotein induces apoptosis of human endothelial cells by activation of CPP32-like proteases: a mechanistic clue to the response to injury hypothesis. Circulation 1997;95:1760–1763.

68. Dimmeler S, Rippmann V, Weiland U, Haendeler J, Zeiher AM. Angiotensin II induces apoptosis of human endothelial cells. Protective effect of nitric oxide. Circ Res 1997;81:970–976.

69. Hermann C, Zeiher AM, Dimmeler S. Shear stress inhibits H2O2-induced apoptosis of human endothelial cells by modulation of the glutathione redox cycle and nitric oxide synthase. Arter Thromb Vasc Biol 1997;17:3588–3592.

70. Haendeler J, Weiland U, Zeiher AM, Dimmeler S. Effects of redox-related congeners on apoptosis and caspase-3 activity. Nitric Oxide 1997;1:282–293.

71. Haendeler J, Zeiher AM, Dimmeler S. Nitric oxide and Apoptosis. Vitamins Horm, 1998, in press.

72. Dimmeler S, Haendeler J, Rippmann V, Nehls M, Zeiher AM. Shear stress inhibits apoptosis of human endothelial cells. FEBS Lett 1996;399:71–74.

73. Hermann C, Zeiher AM, Dimmeler S. Shear stress-induced up-regulation of superoxide dismutase inhibits tumor necrosis factor alpha-mediated apoptosis of endothelial cells. Circulation 1997;96:2732.

74. Tzeng E, Kim YM, Pitt BR, Lizonova A, Kovesdi I, Billiar TR. Adenoviral transfer of the inducible nitric oxide synthase gene blocks endothelial cell apoptosis. Surgery 1997;122:255–263.

75. Fukuo K, Inoue T, Morimoto S, Nakahashi T, Yasuda O, Kitano S, et al. Nitric oxide mediates cytotoxicity and basic fibroblast growth release in cultured vascular smooth muscle cells. A possible mechanism of neovascularization in atherosclerotic plaques. J Clin Invest 1995;95:669–676.

76. Ravalli S, Albala A, Ming M, Szabolcz M, Barbone A, Michler RE, et al. Inducible nitric oxide synthase expression in smooth muscle cells and macrophages of human transplant coronary artery disease. Circulation 1998;97:2338–2345.

77. Pollman MJ, Yamada T, Horiuchi M, Gibbons GH. Vasoactive substances regulate vascular smooth muscle cell apoptosis. Countervailing influences of nitric oxide and angiotensin II. Circ Res 1996;79: 748–756.

78. Nishio E, Watanabe Y. Nitric oxide donor-induced apoptosis in smooth muscle cells is modulated by protein kinase C and protein kinase A. Eur J Pharmacol 1997;339:245–251.

79. Fukuo K, Hata S, Suhara T, Nakahashi T, Shinto Y, Tsujimoto Y, et al. Nitric oxide induces upregulation of Fas and apoptosis in vascular smooth muscle. Hypertension 1996;27:823–826.

80. Iwashina M, Shichiri M, Marumo F, Hirata Y. Transfection of inducible nitric oxide synthase gene causes apoptosis in vascular smooth muscle cells. Circulation 1988;98:1212–1218.

81. Rudic RD, Shesely EG, Maeda N, Smithies O, Segal SS, Sessa WC. Direct evidence for the importance of endothelium-derived nitric oxide in vascular remodeling. J Clin Invest 1998;101:731–736.

82. Kockx MM, De Meyer GR, Muhring J, Jacob W, Bult H, Herman AG. Apoptosis and related proteins in different stages of human atherosclerotic plaques. Circulation 1998;97:2307–2315.

83. Moroi M, Zhang L, Yasuda T, Virmani R, Gold HK, Fishman MC, et al. Interaction of genetic deficiency of endothelial nitric oxide, gender, pregnancy in vascular responses to injury in mice. J Clin Invest 1998;101:1225–1232.

84. Koglin J, Glysing-Jensen T, Mudgett JS, Russell ME. Exacerabated transplant arteriosclerosis in inducible nitric oxide-deficient mice. Circulation 1998;97:2059–2065.

85. MacLellan WR, Schneider MD. Death by design: programmed cell death in cardiovascular biology and disease. Circ Res 1997;81:137–144.

86. Suzuki H, Wildhirt SM, Dudek RR, Narayan KS, Bailey AH, Bing RJ. Induction of apoptosis in myocardial infarction and its possible relationship to nitric oxide synthase in macrophages. Tissue Cell 1996;28:89–97.

87. Wildhirt SM, Dudek RR, Suzuki H, Bing RH. Involvement of inducible nitric oxide synthase in the inflammatory process of myocardial infarction. Int J Cardiol 1995;50:253–261.

88. Kawaguchi H, Shin WS, Wang Y, Inukai M, Kato M, Matsuo-Okai Y, et al. In vivo gene transfection of human endothelial cell nitric oxide synthase in cardiomyocytes causes apoptosis-like cell death. Identification using Sendai virus-coated liposomes. Circulation 1997;95:2441–2447.

89. Szabolcs M, Michler RE, Yang X, Aji W, Roy D, Athan E, et al. Apoptosis of cardiac myocytes during cardiac allograft rejection. Relation to induction of nitric oxide synthase. Circulation 1996;94: 1665–1673.

90. Szabolcs MJ, Ravalli S, Minanov O, Sciacca RR, Michler RE, Cannon PJ. Apoptosis and increased expression of inducible nitric oxide synthase in human allograft rejection. Transplantation 1998;65: 804–812.

91. Weiland U, Haendeler J, Ihling C, Albus U, Scholz W, Dimmeler S. Inhibition of endogenous nitric oxide synthase potentiates ischemia/reperfusion-induced myocardial apoptosis via a caspase-3 dependent pathway. Circulation 1998;98(Suppl):3833.

92. Cheng W, Li B, Kajustra J, Li P, Wolin MS, Sonnenblick EH, et al. Stretch-induced programmed myocyte cell death. J Clin Invest 1995;96:2247–2259.

93. Lipton SA, Choi YB, Pan ZH, Lei SZ, Chen HS, Sucher NJ, et al. A redox-based mechanism for the neuroprotective and neurodestructive effects of nitric oxide and related nitroso-compounds. Nature 1993;364:626–632.

94. Lipton SA, Singel DJ, Stamler JS. Neuroprotective and neurodestructive effects of nitric oxide and redox congeners. Ann NY Acad Sci 1994;738:382–387.

95. Leist M, Fava E, Montecucco C, Nicotera P. Peroxynitrite and nitric oxide donors induce neuronal apoptosis by eliciting autocrine excitotoxicity. Eur J Neurosci 1997;9:1488–1498.

96. Bonfoco E, Leist M, Zhivotovsky B, Orrenius S, Lipton SA, Nicotera P. Cytoskeletal breakdown and apoptosis elicited by NO donors in cerebellar granule cells require NMDA receptor activation. J Neurochem 1996;67:2484–2493.

97. Okuda Y, Sakoda S, Fujimura H, Yanagihara T. Nitric oxide via an inducible isoform of nitric oxide synthase is a possible factor to eliminate inflammatory cells from the central nervous system of mice with experimental allergic encephalomyelitis. J Neuroimmunol 1997;73:107–116.

98. Tseng EE, Brock MV, Lange MS, Blue ME, Troncoso JC, Kwon CC, et al. Neuronal nitric oxide synthase inhibition reduces neuronal apoptosis after hypothermic circulatory arrest. Ann Thoracic Surg 1997;64:1639–1647.

99. Schulz JB, Matthews RT, Muqit MM, Browne SE, Beal MF. Inhibition of neuronal nitric oxide synthase by 7-nitroindazole protects against MPTP-induced neurotoxicity in mice. J Neurochem 1995;64:936–939.

100. Schulz JB, Huang PL, Matthews RT, Passov D, Fishman MC, Beal MF. Striatal malonate lesions are attenuated in neuronal nitric oxide synthase knockout mice. J Neurochem 1996;67:430–433.

101. Brüne B, Mohr S, Messmer UK. Protein thiol modification and apoptotic cell death as cGMP-independent nitric oxide (NO) signaling pathways. Rev Physiol Biochem Pharmacol 1996;127:1–30.

102. Nguyen T, Brunson D, Crespi CL, Penman BW, Wishnok JS, Tannenbaum SR. DNA damage and mutation in human cells exposed to nitric oxide in vitro. Proc Natl Acad Sci USA 1992;89:3030–3034.

103. Messmer UK, Reed JC, Brüne B. Bcl-2 protects macrophages from nitric oxide-induced apoptosis. J Biol Chem 1996;271:20,192–20,197.

104. Nishio E, Watanabe Y. NO induced apoptosis accompanying the change of oncoprotein expression and the activation of CPP32 protease. Life Sci 1998;62:239–245.

105. Messmer UK, Reimer DM, Reed JC, Brüne B. Nitric oxide induced poly(ADP-ribose) polymerase cleavage in RAW 264.7 macrophage apoptosis is blocked by Bcl-2. FEBS Lett 1996;384:162–166.

106. von Knethen A, Brune B. Cyclooxygenase-2: an essential regulator of NO-mediated apoptosis. FASEB J 1997;11:887–895.

107. Balakirev MY, Khramtsov VV, Zimmer G. Modulation of the mitochondrial permeability transition by nitric oxide. Eur J Biochem 1997;246:710–718.

108. Hortelano S, Dallaporta B, Zamzami N, Hirsch T, Susin SA, Marzo I, et al. Nitric oxide induces apoptosis via triggering mitochondrial permeability transition. FEBS Lett 1997;410:373–377.

109. Messmer U, Brüne B. Nitric oxide-induced apoptosis: p53-dependent and p53-independent signalling pathways. Biochem J 1996;319:299–305.

110. Jun CD, Park SJ, Choi BM, Kwak HJ, Park YC, Kim MS, et al. Potentiation of the activity of nitric oxide by the protein kinase C activator phorbol ester in human myeloid leukemic HL-60 cells; association with enhanced fragmentation of mature genomic DNA. Cell Immunol 1997;176:41–49.

111. Estevez AG, Radi R, Barbeito L, Shin JT, Thompson JA, Beckman JS. Peroxynitrite-induced cytotoxicity in PC12 cells: evidence for an apoptotic mechanism differentially modulated by neurotrophic factors. J Neurochem 1995;65(4):1543–1550.

112. Motterlini R, Foresti R, Intaglietta M, Winslow RM. NO-mediated activation of heme oxygenase: endogenous cytoprotection against oxidative stress to endothelium. Am J Physiol 1996;270:H107–H114.

113. Juckett MB, Balla J, Balla G, Jessurun J, Jacob HS, Vercellotti GM. Ferritin protects endothelial cells from oxidized low density lipoprotein in vitro. J Pathol 1995;147:782–789.

114. Polte T, Oberle S, Schröder H. The nitric oxide donor SIN-1 protects endothelial cells from tumor necrosis factor-alpha-mediated cytotoxicity: possible role for cyclic GMP and heme oxygenase. J Mol Cell Cardiol 1997;29:3305–3310.

115. Sandau K, Pfeilschifter J, Brüne B. Nitrosative and oxidative stress induced heme oxygenase-1 accumulation in rat mesangial cells. Eur J Pharmacol 1998;342:77–84.

116. Draijer R, Vaandrager AB, Nolte C, de Jonge HR, Walter U, van Hinsbergh VW. Expression of cGMP-dependent protein kinase I and phosphorylation of its substrate, vasodilator-stimulated phosphoprotein, in human endothelial cells of different origin. Circ Res 1995;77:897–905.

117. Li J, Billiar TR, Talanian RV, Kim YM. Nitric oxide reversibly inhibits seven members of the caspase family via S-nitrosylation. Biochem Biophys Res Commun 1997;240:419–424.

118. Rössig L, Fichtlscherer B, Breitschopf K, Haendeler J, Zeiher AM, Mülsch A, et al. Nitric oxide inhibits caspase-3 by S-nitrosation in vivo. J Biol Chem 1999, in press.

119. Dimmeler S, Haendeler J, Zeiher A.M. TNFα induces Bcl-2 degradation in endothelial cells: involvement of the MAP kinase pathway. Circulation 1998;98(Suppl):1145.

120. Lander HM, Jacovina AT, Davis RJ, Tauras JM. Differential activation of mitogen-activated protein kinases by nitric oxide-related species. J Biol Chem 1996;271:19,705–19,709.

6

Nitric Oxide and Ion Channels

Victoria M. Bolotina

INTRODUCTION

A variety of different ion channels are expressed in smooth muscle cells (SMC) and many of them are known to play an important role in the vascular regulation of vascular tone (Table 1 provides a list of all abbreviations used in this chapter). Ion channels regulate not only vessel contraction, but also relaxation to nitric oxide (NO$^\bullet$) and nitrovasodilators. This chapter summarizes the present knowledge of the mechanisms by which NO$^\bullet$ affects distinct ion channels to cause SMC relaxation. This is a first attempt to review the rapidly accumulating data in what is a very controversial area regarding the effects of NO$^\bullet$ on ion channels in SMC.

Ion Channels as Regulators of Intracellular Ca^{2+} and SMC Concentration

It is commonly accepted that intracellular free Ca^{2+} concentration ([Ca^{2+}]$_{in}$) is one of the major determinants of SMC tone *(1–3)*; increase in [Ca^{2+}]$_{in}$ causes SMC contraction, and decrease in [Ca^{2+}]$_{in}$ causes relaxation. A variety of different ion channels are thought to be involved in the regulation of [Ca^{2+}]$_{in}$. Figure 1 shows a simplified scheme of a SMC with the major ion channels that are discussed in this chapter. Voltage-gated Ca^{2+} channels of L- and T-type (Ca$^{2+}_{L,T}$), various kinds of nonselective cation channels (NSC), and store-operated channels (SOC) are located in the plasma membrane and directly allow extracellular Ca^{2+} to enter the cytoplasm. These channels are known to be responsible for Ca^{2+} influx into SMC. IP$_3$-sensitive (IP$_3$R) and ryanodine-sensitive (RyR) channels are located in the membrane of the endoplasmic reticulum, and allow Ca^{2+} to be released into the cytoplasm from intracellular Ca^{2+} stores. There are other ion channels located in the plasma membrane, which do not conduct Ca^{2+}, but can change the membrane potential, of SMC. A variety of K$^+$ channels like Ca^{2+}-activated (K$^+_{Ca}$), delayed rectifier (K$^+_{dr}$), ATP-sensitive (K$^+_{ATP}$) and inward-rectifier (K$^+_{ir}$) channels as well as Ca^{2+}-activated Cl$^-_{Ca}$ (Cl$^-_{Ca}$) channels, NSC and SOC channels are thought to produce positive or negative feedback by regulating membrane potential, which determines the activity of voltage-gated Ca^{2+}-conducting channels (such as Ca$^{2+}_L$ and Ca$^{2+}_T$) or other related processes (e.g., IP$_3$ production) , thus indirectly modulating [Ca^{2+}]$_{in}$ and SMC tone.

The literature regarding the fundamental properties of different ion channels and their physiological role in the regulation of [Ca^{2+}]$_{in}$ in SMC is rather extensive and is not reviewed in this chapter. For more details on the properties of each channel the reader is referred to the more specialized reviews.

Here, we intend to concentrate on the mechanism by which each kind of ion channel (shown in Fig. 1) is presently thought to participate in NO$^\bullet$-induced SMC relaxation. First, we review the main mechanisms by which NO$^\bullet$ is believed to affect ion channels, and then we will discuss the experimental data showing the effects of NO$^\bullet$ on each individual type of ion channels in SMC.

From: *Contemporary Cardiology, vol. 4: Nitric Oxide and the Cardiovascular System*
Edited by: J. Loscalzo and J. A. Vita © Humana Press Inc., Totowa, NJ

Table 1
Abbreviations Used in this Chapter

Abbreviation	Full name
$[Ca^{2+}]_{in}$	Intracellular Ca^{2+} concentration
Ca_L^{2+} channel	L-type Ca^{2+} channel
Ca_T^{2+} channel	T-type Ca^{2+} channel
cAMP	Adenosine 3',5'-cyclic monophosphate
cGMP	Guanosine 3',5'-cyclic monophosphate
Cl_{Ca}^- channel	Ca^{2+}-activated Cl^- channel
EDRF	Endothelium-derived relaxing factor
GSNO	S-nitrosoglutathione
IP_3	Inositol 1,4,5-triphosphate
IP_3R channel	IP_3-sensitive channel
K_{ATP}^+ channel	ATP-dependent K^+ channel
K_{Ca}^+ channel	Ca^{2+}-dependent K^+ channel
K_{dr}^+ channel	Delayed rectifier K^+ channel
K_{ir}^+ channel	Inward rectifier K^+ channel
NTG	Nitroglycerin
NO	Nitric oxide
NSC channel	Nonselective cation channel
ODQ	H-(1,2,4) oxadiazole (4,3-a) quinoxallinone
PKA	cAMP-dependent protein kinase
PKG	cGMP-dependent protein kinase
ROC	Receptor-operated channel
RSNOs	S-nitrosothiols
RyR channel	Ryanodine-sensitive channel
SERCA	Sarcoplasmic-endoplasmic reticulum Ca^{2+}-ATPase
SIN-1	3-Morpholino-sydnonimine
SMC	Smooth muscle cell
SNAP	S-nitroso-N-acetylpenicillamine
SNP	Sodium nitropruside
SNC	S-nitrosocysteine
SOC channel	store-operated channel

GENERAL MECHANISMS
OF DIRECT AND INDIRECT EFFECT
OF NO• ON ION CHANNELS

There are two major mechanisms by which NO• and other nitrovasodilators are thought to affect ion channels and cause SMC relaxation. The first is based on NO•-induced stimulation of guanylyl cyclase, accumulation of its product cyclic guanosine 3', 5'- monophosphate (cGMP), and indirect cGMP-dependent modulation of the activity of different ion channels. The second mechanism is based on the direct NO•-induced S-nitrosation of thiols on the channel protein or closely associated proteins that may serve as allosteric regulators of ion channel function.

The existence of these two mechanisms for NO•-induced modification of ion channel function is now well accepted, but there is still much controversy on the exact mechanisms and the relative role of indirect (cGMP-dependent) and direct (nitrosation) effects of NO• on individual ion channels that are discussed further for each individual channel.

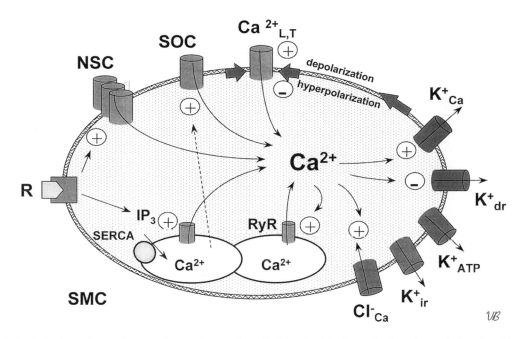

Fig. 1. A simplified scheme of smooth muscle cell (SMC) with the major ion channels involved in regulation of intracellular Ca^{2+}. *See text* for details.

The Indirect cGMP-Dependent Regulation of Ion Channels and Vascular Tone

Historically, NO•-induced activation of guanylyl cyclase leading to an increase in intracellular cGMP and relaxation of contracted arterial and bronchiolar smooth muscle strips was established *(4,5)* even before NO• was proposed to be an endothelium-derived relaxing factor (EDRF) *(6,7)*. Inhibition of guanylyl cyclase was shown to impair the NO•-induced relaxation, and for a long time nearly all the effects of NO• in SMC (including the effects on ion channels) were thought to be associated exclusively with the rise in cGMP. Cyclic GMP-dependent signaling actions of NO• are generally observed at relatively low (nanomolar) concentrations of NO• or NO• donors, and are thought to be mainly associated with activation of cGMP-dependent protein kinase (PKG) (for review *see* ref. *8*), although there is also a possibility of cGMP-dependent cross activation of cAMP-dependent protein kinase (PKA) *(9)*.

Several different types of ion channels are presently thought to be regulated by cGMP-dependent mechanisms, and we discuss the evidence that exists for indirect cGMP-dependent effects of NO• on Ca^{2+}_L, K^+_{Ca}, K^+_{ATP}, and IP_3R, channels. The conclusions about the indirect cGMP-dependent effects of NO• on ion channels are usually based on (1) the similarity of the effects of NO• or NO•-donors and membrane permeable analogs of cGMP and (2) the inhibition of the effects of NO• by inhibitors of guanylyl cyclase (ODQ, LY83583, methylene blue) or PKG (KT-5823 or Rp-8-bromo-cGMPS). Although in many studies such evidence appears convincing, it remains largely indirect and circumstantial. Only in one case (for K^+_{Ca} channels) has the direct cGMP-dependent phosphorylation of the channel by PKG been demonstrated.

The Direct, cGMP-Independent Effect of NO• on Ion Channels

The existence of cGMP-independent, ion channel-mediated pathways for NO•-induced SMC relaxation was proposed by different groups who found that inhibitors of guanylyl cyclase and PKG suppress, but not necessarily eliminate, the effects of NO$^\bullet$ and NO$^\bullet$ donors on single channels, whole-cell currents, $[Ca^{2+}]_{in}$, and vascular tone. Indeed, at the micromolar concentrations of NO$^\bullet$ released physiologically from endothelial cells *(10,11)*, cGMP-dependent pathways may not account for all the effects of NO$^\bullet$ in SMC.

As an alternative to indirect cGMP-dependent effects, it has been proposed that NO$^\bullet$ can directly affect different ion channels via interaction with their thiol groups *(12–16)*, similar to what was found for other proteins *(17,18)*. It is thought that sulfur-containing amino-acids (like cysteine) in the channel molecule contribute to protein stability by being donors or acceptors in intrachain hydrogen bonding with nitrogen, carbonyl oxygen, or hydroxyl oxygen. These bonds could add stability to preferred conformational states that are optimal for channel function. By interfering with these bonds, NO$^\bullet$ could change the conformational transitions in the channel molecule, and thus affect the channel function.

Stamler and coauthors *(19–22)* proposed that NO$^\bullet$ can modify thiol groups in ion channels in two ways. NO$^\bullet$ may undergo a transnitrosation reaction with thiols in the channel to form *S*-nitrosothiols, or, if two thiols are localized close to each other (i.e., are vicinal), NO$^\bullet$ can facilitate the formation of disulfide bonds. NO$^\bullet$ released by different *S*-nitrosothiols may modify channel thiols in a similar way, whereas some *S*-nitrosothiols themselves can also facilitate the formation of mixed disulfide bonds with cysteines. Recently, they also proposed *(16)* that poly-*S*-nitrosation of the channel can functionally cause an effect different from thiol oxidation. For more details on the chemistry of NO$^\bullet$-induced modification of ion channels and other proteins, *see* Chapters 1 and 4.

Presently, the possibility of the direct NO$^\bullet$-induced modification of ion channels is well accepted, but because of the complexity of the chemistry of NO$^\bullet$ and NO$^\bullet$ donors, experimental data obtained by different groups are still inconsistent.

EFFECTS OF NO$^\bullet$ ON INDIVIDUAL ION CHANNELS

The following is a review of the current experimental evidence for direct and indirect effects of NO$^\bullet$ and NO$^\bullet$ donors on each individual type of ion channel in SMC. It is important to emphasize that in many cases the results obtained by different groups vary, and often even contradict each other, so there is still no consensus on the exact mechanisms of the effect of NO$^\bullet$ on most ion channels. This field of research is quite new and quickly developing, so there are still more controversies and questions than definitive answers on how NO$^\bullet$ affects different ion channels. Figure 2 summarizes the current knowledge in this field.

Voltage-Gated Ca^{2+} Channels of the L- and T-Type

From all presently recognized subtypes of voltage-gated Ca^{2+} channels, only channels of the L- and T-types have been found in SMC. The properties, mechanisms of regulation, and physiological role of these channels in SMC have been extensively studied and reviewed elsewhere *(23,24)*.

L-TYPE CA^{2+} CHANNELS (CA$_L^{2+}$)

These channels are known to play a major role in regulation of $[Ca^{2+}]_{in}$ in SMC. Their activation by agonists and/or membrane depolarization causes substantial Ca^{2+} influx leading to an increase in $[Ca^{2+}]_{in}$ and SMC contraction. Inhibition or inactivation of Ca$_L^{2+}$ channels stops such influx and allows different pumps and exchangers to remove Ca^{2+} from the cytoplasm, decreasing $[Ca^{2+}]_{in}$ and relaxing SMC. Thus, one could expect inhibition of Ca$_L^{2+}$ channels to be one of the physiologically relevant mechanisms for NO$^\bullet$-induced SMC relaxation.

The effect of NO$^\bullet$ and NO$^\bullet$ donors on whole-cell Ca$_L^{2+}$ currents have been extensively studied in SMC and cardiomyocytes, although the results appear to be controversial. Indeed,

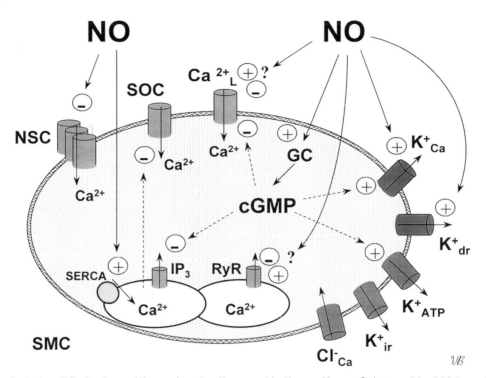

Fig. 2. A simplified scheme illustrating the direct and indirect effects of nitric oxide (NO˙) on the major ion channels in smooth muscle cell (SMC). *See text* for details.

inhibition of basal whole-cell Ca_L^{2+} current by NO˙ donors has been reported in SMC *(15, 25–27)*. In cardiomyocytes most groups found no effect of NO˙ on basal Ca_L^{2+} current *(28–31)*, whereas some investigators reported that NO˙ donors inhibit cardiac Ca_L^{2+} channels expressed in human embryonic kidney (HEK 293) cells *(15)*, or stimulate basal Ca_L^{2+} current in human atrial myocytes *(32)*, or dually modulate basal Ca_L^{2+} current in ferret ventricular myocytes *(14)* causing either inhibition or activation of the Ca_L^{2+} channels. When Ca_L^{2+} in cardiomyocytes was stimulated by cAMP, NO˙ donors either inhibited Ca_L^{2+} current *(29,31)*, or produced dual effects *(28,30)*. For example, Mery and coauthors *(28)* showed in frog ventricular myocytes that SIN-1 at low concentrations (0.1–10 nM) induced a pronounced stimulation of Ca_L^{2+} current, whereas when applied at high concentration (100 nM–1 mM) it reduced Ca_L^{2+} current. Several explanations have been proposed to account for major differences in the effects of NO˙ on Ca_L^{2+} in different preparations.

Most authors believe that NO˙ affects Ca_L^{2+} channels indirectly via different cGMP-dependent pathways, some of which can inhibit, whereas others can activate the channel. In SMC it is well established that cGMP-induced activation of PKG causes Ca_L^{2+} channel inhibition *(33–35)*. This indirect cGMP-dependent mechanism is thought to underlie the inhibitory effect of NO˙ on Ca_L^{2+} channels (and Ca^{2+} influx), which causes SMC relaxation *(25–27,36)*. Indeed, the membrane-permeable analog of cGMP (8-bromo-cGMP) mimicked the inhibition of whole-cell Ca_L^{2+} current by NO˙ donors, whereas inhibition of guanylyl cyclase and cGMP production with methylene blue inhibited the effects of NO˙ donors. Not only cGMP, but also NO˙-donor SNP have been shown to inhibit single Ca_L^{2+} channels in SMC from basilary artery *(36)* and in embryonic chick heart cells *(37)*.

The same mechanism of NO˙-induced cGMP-dependent activation of PKG is thought to account for NO˙-induced inhibition of Ca_L^{2+} channels in cardiomyocytes *(29,30,38,39)*. Ca_L^{2+}

channels in cardiomyocytes are known to be dually regulated by two opposing kinases: PKG, which inhibits, and PKA, which activates the channels (for review, *see* ref. *24*). Such dual regulation can account for different effects produced by the cGMP rise (stimulated by NO$^\bullet$). The NO$^\bullet$-induced stimulation of Ca_L^{2+} channels in cardiomyocytes could be explained by indirect cGMP-induced inhibition of phosphodiesterases, which can increase cAMP and stimulate Ca_L^{2+} current *(28,40)*. Activation of cGMP-dependent cAMP-phosphodiesterase was also proposed to account for NO$^\bullet$-induced inhibition of Ca_L^{2+} channels *(28)*. It is important to mention that in SMC the role of PKA in regulation of Ca_L^{2+} channels is still under debate. Xiong and Sperelakis *(34)* suggest that PKA in SMC inhibits Ca_L^{2+} channels similarly to PKG. In contrast, several other groups *(33,35,41,42)* showed that PKA activates Ca_L^{2+} channels in SMC, as it does in cardiomyocytes. To complicate the situation even more, it is important to mention that cGMP and cAMP, along with their primer action, can also have a secondary and opposite action mediated by the opposing kinases *(35)*. These findings can provide a possible explanation for the variable and controversial results on the effect of NO$^\bullet$ on Ca_L^{2+} channels in different preparations.

Another possible explanation for high variability and even dual effects of NO$^\bullet$ and NO$^\bullet$ donors on Ca_L^{2+} channels has been proposed by Campbell and coauthors *(14)*. They showed that 3-morpholino-sydnonimine (SIN-1), which is known to generate both NO$^\bullet$ and O_2^-, either inhibited or stimulated whole-cell Ca_L^{2+} current in ferret ventricular myocytes. When O_2^- was eliminated by superoxide dismutase (SOD), only inhibition of Ca_L^{2+} current was observed. The later effect could be also mimicked by 8-bromo-cGMP. On the other hand, *S*-nitrosothiols, that donate NO$^\bullet$, stimulated Ca_L^{2+} in a manner that did not depend on activation of kinases, inhibition of phosphatases, or alteration in cGMP levels. Similarity of the effects of *S*-nitrosothiols and thiol oxidants (effects of which were reversed by thiol reductants) brought this group to the conclusion that activation of Ca_L^{2+} channels by NO$^\bullet$ and NO$^\bullet$ donors results from the NO$^\bullet$-induced direct *S*-nitrosation of Ca_L^{2+} channel-forming proteins.

Direct effects of NO$^\bullet$ on the Ca_L^{2+} channel have been also proposed by Hu and coworkers *(15)*, but instead of activation they reported NO$^\bullet$-induced inhibition of Ca_L^{2+} channel activity. They showed that SNAP, SNC, and GSNO reduced the Ba^{2+} current through channels formed by different combinations of channel subunits ($\alpha_{1C} \pm \beta_{1a} \pm \alpha_2$ or $\alpha_{1C} \pm \beta_{2a} \pm \alpha_2$) expressed in HEK293 cells, and coexpressed β subunits intended to potentiate the inhibitory effects of *S*-nitrosothiols. This inhibition seems to be independent of cGMP pathways, as it was observed even in the presence of methylene blue, an inhibitor of guanylyl cyclase. Oxidizing agents (thimerosal and DTDP) similarly inhibit the α_{1C} channel subunit *(43)* with or without the β_{2a} subunit *(15)*. Interestingly, the effect of thimerosal and DTDP could be reversed by DDT, whereas the effects of *S*-nitrosothiols were not. These results imply that even if the targets for NO$^\bullet$ donors are the same as those for thiol-specific modifying agents (which are still unknown), the chemical reactions may be not the same.

Thus, in spite of many efforts of different groups, there are still unresolved questions about how NO$^\bullet$ and NO$^\bullet$ donors affect Ca_L^{2+} channels in different preparations. It is clear, though, that the effects of NO$^\bullet$ can be mediated by indirect cGMP-dependent pathways, or may result from the direct S-nitrosation and/or oxidation of some (still to be determined) thiol groups in the channel protein.

T-Type Ca^{2+} Channels

These are thought to be involved in the generation of pacemaker currents in phasically contracting SMC *(24)*, but it is presently absolutely unclear what role (if any) Ca_T^{2+} channels can play in NO$^\bullet$-induced relaxation of SMC. The only study that recently addressed this question *(27)* showed that Ca_T^{2+} channels (as opposed to Ca_L^{2+} channels) were unaffected by NO$^\bullet$ donors, or by permeable analogs of cGMP in cultured human coronary myocytes.

K⁺ Channels

Ca²⁺-Dependent K⁺ Channels (K⁺_Ca)

These have been extensively studied and characterized in variety of SMC (for review *see* ref. *44*). The molecular properties of K^+_{Ca} channels have been recently reviewed elsewhere *(45)*. K^+_{Ca} channels cannot alter $[Ca^{2+}]_{in}$ directly, but they may do so indirectly by modulating Ca^{2+} influx through voltage-gated Ca^{2+} channels. Indeed, activation of K^+_{Ca} channels (leading to K^+ efflux from SMC) produces membrane hyperpolarization, which can indirectly inhibit (deactivate) L-type Ca^{2+} channels, thus serving as a negative feedback mechanism to control vascular tone *(23,44,46)*.

The role of K^+_{Ca} channels in vascular relaxation induced by NO· and NO· donors has been extensively studied in a variety of different blood vessels. It was shown that charybdotoxin (CTX) or iberitoxin (IbTX), inhibitors of K^+_{Ca} channels, significantly reduce relaxation to NO·, NO· donors, or acetylcholine in rabbit mesenteric *(47)* and carotid artery *(48,49)*, in guinea-pig aorta, pulmonary artery, carotid artery, and trachea *(50,51)*, in rat aorta *(52)*, mesenteric *(53)*, pulmonary *(54–56)*, and basilar artery *(57)*. These data provide strong support to the idea that activation of K^+_{Ca} channels play an important role in mediating relaxation caused by NO· and related compounds.

Indeed, NO· and a variety of NO· donors increase the activity of single K^+_{Ca} channels in cell-attached membrane patches in SMC from different vessels. Two different pathways have been proposed for NO·-induced activation of K^+_{Ca} channels: indirect cGMP-dependent activation, which is thought to be mediated by PKG *(49,53,55,58–63)*, and direct cGMP-independent activation, which is thought to be a result of nitrosation of the channel or a closely associated protein *(13,49,64–66)*.

The cGMP-dependent activation of K^+_{Ca} channels in SMC is well established. Williams et al. *(67)* first demonstrated that in cultured bovine aortic SMC, single K^+_{Ca} channels can be activated in cell-attached membrane patches by the NO· donor SNP and other vasodilatory agents (adenosine and atrial natriuretic factor [ANF]) that increase intracellular cGMP levels. Dibutyryl cGMP (membrane permeable analog of cGMP) produced similar effects on K^+_{Ca} channels. Activation of single K^+_{Ca} channels and whole-cell currents by both NO· donors and by membrane-permeable analogs of cGMP has been subsequently confirmed by many other groups in SMC *(54,55,58,59,61–63,68)* and other cells *(69–71)*. Activation of single K^+_{Ca} channels (in cell-attached membrane patches) and whole-cell currents, as well as relaxation of blood vessels by NO· donors, was attenuated or completely inhibited by inhibition of guanylyl cyclase with ODQ *(49,68)* and LY83583 *(55)*, or by inhibition of PKG with KT-5823 *(63)* or Rp-8-bromo-cGMPS *(61)*.

The first evidence that cGMP-dependent activation of K^+_{Ca} channels is mediated by PKG was presented in 1993 by three independent groups *(59,60,69)*. They showed that PKG added to the cytoplasmic side of excised membrane patches activates single K^+_{Ca} channels, but only in the presence of cGMP and ATP. It is interesting to note that in some studies, cGMP and ATP alone (without PKG) were able to activate K^+_{Ca} channels *(58,67,69)*, whereas in others channel activation occurred only if PKG is also added to cGMP and ATP *(59,60,72)*. This discrepancy can be possibly explained by the presence of endogenous PKG in the vicinity of the K^+_{Ca} channel in some, but not all, membrane preparations.

Thus, all the authors agree on the crucial role of PKG in mediating cGMP-dependent activation of K^+_{Ca} channels. However, there is still no consensus on the substrate that is phosphorylated by PKG. Recent experiments on the reconstituted α-subunit of K^+_{Ca} channel from tracheal SMC suggested that the target may be the channel itself *(72)*, although other studies provide strong evidence that a protein phosphatase may be essential for K^+_{Ca} channel activation with PKG *(69–71)*. Either way, cGMP-dependent PKG-mediated activation of K^+_{Ca} channels is one of the mechanisms of NO·-induced relaxation of SMC.

The idea of a cGMP-independent K_{Ca}^+ channel-mediated pathway for NO$^{\bullet}$-induced SMC relaxation was triggered by the findings that NO$^{\bullet}$-induced relaxation does not always disappear when the increase in cGMP in SMC is prevented. It was shown, for instance, that in atherosclerotic vessels from cholesterol-fed rabbits, guanylyl cyclase activity and its sensitivity to nitrovasodilators is dramatically decreased (73), and there is no significant rise in cGMP in SMC in response to stimulation by nitrovasodilators or acetylcholine (48,74). Nevertheless, considerable relaxation of such blood vessels persists despite the impairment of the NO$^{\bullet}$-induced rise in cGMP. Moreover, cGMP-independent relaxation, which persists in atherosclerotic blood vessels, appeared to be highly sensitive to CTX, pointing to the direct involvement of K_{Ca}^+ channels (48). The existence of cGMP-independent, NO$^{\bullet}$-induced relaxation was also found in normal rabbit aorta (13), bronchial smooth muscle (75), rat mesenteric and rabbit carotid artery (49), and coronary arteries (68).

Recently, Plane and coworkers provided strong evidence for the existence of both cGMP-dependent and -independent pathways that are both mediated by K_{Ca}^+ channels in rabbit carotid artery (49). They showed that inhibition of guanylyl cyclase with ODQ (which prevented the rise in cGMP) only attenuated, but did not inhibit, relaxation induced by acetylcholine or exogenous NO$^{\bullet}$. The relaxation remaining in the presence of ODQ was effectively blocked by CTX. This observation is similar to that in rabbit aorta in which the relaxation caused by NO$^{\bullet}$ persisted even after NO$^{\bullet}$-induced cGMP rise was prevented by pretreatment with methylene blue (in the presence of SOD), a nonspecific inhibitor of guanylyl cyclase (13). Interestingly, Plane and coauthors showed that, contrary to relaxation caused by authentic NO$^{\bullet}$, relaxation caused by such NO$^{\bullet}$ donors as SIN-1 and SNAP was almost completely eliminated by ODQ. These data clearly point to the existence of a cGMP-independent mechanism of NO$^{\bullet}$-induced vessel relaxation mediated by K_{Ca}^+ channels. Also, they emphasize possible differences in the mechanisms of SMC relaxation caused by authentic NO$^{\bullet}$ and different donors.

The direct cGMP-independent effect of NO$^{\bullet}$ on single K_{Ca}^+ channels was first shown in SMC from rabbit aorta (13), and then in rat pulmonary artery (64). In some recent studies the same effect was also found on K_{Ca}^+ channels reconstituted in planar lipid bilayers (65,66). In all these studies, to exclude the possibility of indirect cGMP-mediated activation, the activity of single K_{Ca}^+ channels was recorded in excised membrane patches, or in planar lipid bilayers in the absence of cGMP, ATP, and PKG. Under such conditions, exogenous NO$^{\bullet}$ (13) and such NO$^{\bullet}$ donors as SNP (64,65), SNAP (65), PAPA NONOate (a diazeniumdiolate), and SIN-1 (66) significantly increased the activity of single K_{Ca}^+ channels in a dose-dependent manner. NO$^{\bullet}$ released upon illumination of streptozotocin, a light-sensitive NO$^{\bullet}$ donor, produced K_{Ca}^+ channel activation, which depended on the initial activity of the channel: the lower the basal activity, the greater the increase produced by NO$^{\bullet}$ release (65). It is important to mention that NO$^{\bullet}$ produced by a donor aorta following stimulation of its endothelial cells with acetylcholine also activated single K_{Ca}^+ channels in excised membrane patches in a manner similar to that of exogenously applied NO$^{\bullet}$ (13).

Similar to other ion channels, direct cGMP-independent activation of K_{Ca}^+ channels by NO$^{\bullet}$ was dependent on the redox state, and was prevented by prior modification of sulfhydryl groups with N-ethylmaleimide (NEM) (13,66). These results suggest that the direct effect of NO$^{\bullet}$ on K_{Ca}^+ channels most likely is caused by S-nitrosation of the critical sulfhydryl groups on the channel-forming protein, or a closely associated regulatory protein. Recent studies on the redox modulation of single K_{Ca}^+ channels in excised membrane patches (76) strongly support such a possibility.

It is important to mention that in some preparations of SMC, the direct cGMP-independent activation of K_{Ca}^+ channels by NO$^{\bullet}$ was not observed, and the entire effect of NO$^{\bullet}$ on K_{Ca}^+ channels was attributed solely to the cGMP-dependent pathway (62,63). The reason why NO$^{\bullet}$ and NO$^{\bullet}$ donors activate K_{Ca}^+ channels in some, but not all, preparations is presently unclear. A possible explanation may relate to the dependence of K_{Ca}^+ channel activity on the cytosolic

redox potential *(76)*, and the importance of a redox-sensitive thiol for the direct effect of NO•
on the channel *(13)*. Under these conditions, treatment of excised membrane patches with
reducing agents may recover the ability of the K_{Ca}^+ channel to be activated by NO•.

Thus, direct (cGMP-independent) and indirect (cGMP-dependent) activation of K_{Ca}^+
channels are both involved in blood vessel relaxation by NO• and nitrovasodilators. The relative physiological role of these two pathways can vary depending on the type of the vessel,
and presumably can also change during some pathological conditions.

DELAYED RECTIFIER K^+ CHANNELS (K_{DR}^+)

These are involved in regulation of resting membrane potential, and their inhibition can
produce membrane depolarization, which could be sufficient to activate Ca_L^{2+} channels and
Ca^{2+} influx in some SMC (for review *see* ref. *44*). In this way, K_{dr}^+ are believed to control the
contractile behavior of SMC.

The involvement of K_{dr}^+ channels in NO•-induced relaxation has been proposed by Yuan
and coworkers *(64)* who reported that exogenous NO• and SNP activate whole-cell K_{dr}^+
currents and cause hyperpolarization in cultured SMC from rat pulmonary artery. They also
found that SNP can activate single K_{dr}^+ channels in excised outside-out membrane patches,
and proposed that it is due to a direct effect of NO• on the K_{dr}^+ channel. Indeed, similar to
the studies on K_{Ca}^+ channels, Yuan and others found that the NO• donor SNP activates K_{dr}^+
channels in the absence of cGMP, ATP, and PKG, which excludes a cGMP-dependent
mechanism. Other authors, however, found no activation of K_{dr}^+ channels by authentic NO•
or SNP *(55,62)*. Thus, further studies are necessary to confirm a possible direct effect of NO•
on K_{dr}^+ channels. There are presently no reports of indirect cGMP-dependent modulation of
K_{dr}^+ channels in SMC.

ATP-SENSITIVE K^+ CHANNELS (K_{ATP}^+)

These are known to serve as a critical link between metabolism and electrical activity in
many cell types (for review *see* refs. *77,78*), including SMC (for a recent review *see* ref. *44*).
Activation of K_{ATP}^+ channels and resulting SMC hyperpolarization is thought to underlie
vasorelaxation induced by hypoxia *(79)* and by some endogenous vasodilators *(23,80)*.

A variety of physiological studies point to the possible involvement of K^+_{ATP} channels in
NO•-induced vascular relaxation. NO• and NO• donors were reported to inhibit glucose-
induced insulin secretion *(81,82)* in rat pancreatic β-cells, and this effect was sensitive to
glibenclamide, a commonly used specific inhibitor of K_{ATP}^+ channels. In rabbit mesenteric
arteries, SIN 1 caused concentration-dependent hyperpolarization, which was inhibited by
glibenclamide *(83)*. The important role of K_{ATP}^+ channels in cGMP-mediated pial artery
vasodilation has also been reported *(84)*. These experimental data clearly indicate that K_{ATP}^+
channels could be another physiological target for NO• in vascular SMC.

The exact mechanism by which NO• affects K_{ATP}^+ channels still remains unclear. There
are a few studies suggesting that NO• donors can activate K_{ATP}^+ channels indirectly via a
cGMP-dependent pathway. Tsuura and coworkers *(81)* showed that SNP and SNAP activated single K_{ATP}^+ channels in cell-attached, but not in inside-out, membrane patches in
pancreatic β-cells. Interestingly, the same authors found no activation of K_{ATP}^+ channels by
SNP in ventricular myocytes. In vasculature, activation of single K_{ATP}^+ channels by endogenous NO• (in cell-attached membrane patches) has been reported in cultured SMC from porcine
coronary artery *(85)*. This activation was blocked by methylene blue, pointing to the possible
involvement of cGMP. In another study, zaprinast, an inhibitor of cGMP-specific phosphodiesterases, shifted the concentration-dependent SIN-1 induced glibenclamide-sensitive
hyperpolarization to the left in rabbit mesenteric arteries *(83)*. Furthermore, an increase in
intracellular cGMP by ANF activates single K_{ATP}^+ channels in cultured aortic SMC *(86)*.

All these data are consistent with indirect cGMP-dependent activation of K^+_{ATP} channels by NO$^{\bullet}$. Further studies are needed to determine how cGMP affects K^+_{ATP} channels, and if PKG is involved. Also, it is important to test further the possibility of a direct effect of NO$^{\bullet}$ on K^+_{ATP}, as diverse effects of sulfhydryl (-SH)-group modifying agents have been recently demonstrated on cardiac K^+_{ATP} channels (87), pointing to the possibility of redox modulation of K^+_{ATP} channels.

OTHER K$^+$ CHANNELS

Inward Rectifier K$^+$ Channels (K$^+_{ir}$). These have been found in small coronary and cerebral arteries, and in cerebral and mesenteric arterioles (for review *see* ref. 44). The role of K^+_{ir} in SMC is not well established, but they are thought to be involved in regulation of resting membrane potential and may also participate in K$^+$-induced dilation. It is presently unknown if K^+_{ir} channels are involved in NO$^{\bullet}$-induced SMC hyperpolarization and relaxation.

Novel K$^+$ Channels of Intermediate and Low Conductance (80 and 4 pS, Respectively). These were recently reported by Sanders and coworkers (62) to be activated by authentic NO$^{\bullet}$ and NO$^{\bullet}$ donors (SNAP and SNP) in colonic SMC. They showed that NO$^{\bullet}$, SNP, and SNAP activated these channels in both cell-attached and inside-out membrane patches. These effects were prevented by pretreatment with oxidizing (NEM) or reducing (dithiothreitol [DTT]) agents, supporting the possibility of a direct NO$^{\bullet}$-induced modification of free sulfhydryl groups similar to what was found for K^+_{Ca} channels. On the other hand, they also found that the membrane-permeable analog of cGMP (dibutyryl-cGMP) activated these channels in cell-attached patches pointing to the possible involvement of an indirect cGMP-dependent process. The authors proposed that these new K$^+$ channels are activated by NO$^{\bullet}$ via both direct and indirect mechanisms, leading to SMC hyperpolarization and relaxation.

Ca^{2+}-Activated Cl$^-$ Channels (Cl$^-_{Ca}$)

Ca^{2+}-activated Cl$^-$ channels (Cl$^-_{Ca}$) have been described in a variety of SMC (for review *see* ref. 88). Their activation by the rise in $[Ca^{2+}]_{in}$ produces an inward current and membrane depolarization that can activate Ca^{2+}_{L} channels and cause SMC contraction (88–90).

Inhibition of Cl$^-_{Ca}$ channels was proposed as one of the possible mechanisms of endothelium-dependent SMC hyperpolarization and relaxation (91), although very little is known about whether NO$^{\bullet}$ really affects Cl$^-_{Ca}$, or not. In SMC of opossum esophagus, NO$^{\bullet}$ donor diethylenetriamine-NO (DETA-NO$^{\bullet}$) and 8-bromo-cGMP were shown to suppress some part of Ca^{2+}-dependent, whole-cell current that authors attributed to Cl$^-_{Ca}$ (92). These results have been interpreted in favor of cGMP-mediated NO$^{\bullet}$-induced inhibition of Cl$^-_{Ca}$ channels, although the Cl$^-_{Ca}$ nature of the whole-cell current in these studies was not established, leaving a possibility that nonselective cation channels, rather than Cl$^-_{Ca}$ channels, could be the ones affected by NO$^{\bullet}$ in reported experiments.

Recently, we found no direct effect of NO$^{\bullet}$ and its donor, SNAP, on single Cl$^-_{Ca}$ channels (2 pS conductance) and whole-cell currents activated by caffeine in SMC from rabbit and mouse aorta (93). We also demonstrated that caffeine-induced activation of Cl$^-_{Ca}$ channels by Ca^{2+} release from intracellular stores could be suppressed by high doses of SNAP indirectly, through its effect on ryanodine-sensitive stores and intracellular Ca^{2+}. Thus, NO$^{\bullet}$ does not affect Cl$^-_{Ca}$ channels directly, but their activity can be decreased by NO$^{\bullet}$ indirectly as a result of an NO$^{\bullet}$-induced decrease in $[Ca^{2+}]_{in}$ via other mechanisms.

It is important to mention that in epithelial cells, Ca^{2+}-independent Cl$^-$ channels were found to be activated by NO$^{\bullet}$, presumably indirectly by phosphorylation via PKG (94,95). It is presently unknown if Cl$^-_{Ca}$ channels in SMC can be stimulated in the same way, although activation of Cl$^-_{Ca}$ channels by cGMP would cause contraction rather than relaxation, which is counter to any known physiological effect of cGMP and NO$^{\bullet}$ in SMC.

Receptor-Operated Nonselective Cation Channels (NSC)

Along with voltage-activated Ca_L^{2+} channels, a variety of different nonselective cation (NSC) channels is thought to be responsible for agonist-induced Ca^{2+} influx and contraction of different SMC (for review *see* refs. *96–98*). These NSC channels have different characteristics and mechanisms of regulation, but most of them are activated by some stimuli originated from the binding of agonists to their receptors. For this reason, these channels are frequently called receptor-operated channels (ROC). NSC channels provide an alternative to the Ca_L^{2+}-channel pathway for Ca^{2+} influx and SMC contraction, and may also be an ideal target for NO˙. Indeed, receptor-dependent agonist-induced contractions are generally more sensitive to inhibition by NO˙ than are those caused by depolarization mediated by Ca_L^{2+}.

Although NSC channels are known to play a very important role in an agonist-induced $[Ca^{2+}]_{in}$ rise and contraction of SMC, very little is presently known about the effects of NO˙ and nitrovasodilators on these channels. Recently, Masaki and coauthors *(99)* found that SNP and SNAP, as well as 8-bromo-cGMP, inhibit the NSC current activated by low concentrations of endothelin-1, and they proposed that agonist-induced NSC current in rat aortic SMC is inhibited by NO˙ indirectly via the cGMP-dependent pathway.

There is presently no evidence for a direct effect of NO˙ on NSC channels in vascular SMC, although in brown fat cells Ca^{2+}-activated NSC channels were found to be directly inhibited by NO˙ donors. Koivisto and Nedergaard *(100,101)* first showed that these channels can be reversibly inhibited by sulfhydryl reagents (mercury and thimerosal), and they also found that *S*-nitrosocysteine, SNP, SNAP, and nitroglycerin inhibit single Ca^{2+}-activated NSC channels in inside out membrane patches in the absence of ATP and cGMP. This inhibition was reversed by DTT, but not oxidized DTT. These results are consistent with NO˙-induced nitrosation (or oxidation) of critical sulfhydryl groups within the channel.

Thus, it is still unclear which nonselective cation channels in SMC are physiologically regulated by NO˙, and by what mechanisms such regulation could occur. Further studies are necessary to answer these important questions.

Store-Operated Channels (SOC) and Capacitative Ca^{2+} Influx

Capacitative Ca^{2+} influx mediated by the store-operated Ca^{2+} channels (SOC) is well-described in a variety of nonexitable cells (for review *see* refs. *102–105*). These SOC channels are regulated by the state of filling of intracellular Ca^{2+} stores through a still-unknown mechanism that transmits the signal from the empty stores to the plasma membrane to open SOC channels and allow Ca^{2+} to enter the cell and refill the stores. The best-known and characterized SOC channel is highly Ca^{2+}-selective CRAC (calcium release activated current) channel first described by Hoth and Penner *(106)* in mast cells. CRAC channels have been found in a variety of nonexitable cells, but there is no evidence for their existence in SMC. Although the presence of capacitative Ca^{2+} influx in SMC have been proposed by several different groups *(107–110)* who found that depletion of the stores produced by the inhibitors of sarcoplasmic–endoplasmic reticulum Ca^{2+}-ATPase (SERCA) causes Ca^{2+} and Mn^{2+} influx. Recently, we proposed that small (3 pS) NSC channels which we found in SMC from rabbit and mouse aorta could be responsible for capacitative nonselective cation influx and agonist-induced contraction in a variety of SMC *(109,110)*. These channels can provide sufficient Ca^{2+} influx to increase $[Ca^{2+}]_{in}$ and refill the stores. Also, because of their poor cation selectivity, they can amplify the signal derived from the empty stores by producing an inward Na^+ current that will cause SMC depolarization, which in turn can trigger the opening of Ca_L^{2+} channels leading to additional Ca^{2+} influx. Inhibition of SOC channels can prevent agonist-induced Ca^{2+} influx, leading to a reduction in $[Ca^{2+}]_{in}$ and SMC relaxation.

We have proposed that inhibition of these SOC and corresponding capacitative Ca^{2+} influx is an important mechanism of NO˙-induced SMC relaxation *(109,110)*. We showed that authentic NO$^\bullet$ and SNAP inhibit agonist-induced capacitative Ca^{2+} and Mn^{2+} influx in SMC, but functional SERCA, is required to inhibit cation influx. Indeed, there was no effect of NO$^\bullet$ on capacitative cation influx in the presence of SERCA inhibitor thapsigargin (TG), or in the absence of extracellular Ca^{2+}, excluding the possibility of a direct effect of NO$^\bullet$ on SOC. We also found that NO$^\bullet$ promotes the refilling of intracellular stores, and that the decrease in Ca_i^{2+} precedes the inhibition of cation influx by NO$^\bullet$. Thus, NO$^\bullet$ does not affect SOC directly, but it can inhibit capacitative Ca^{2+} influx indirectly via SERCA-dependent refilling of the stores. It is still unclear, though, whether NO$^\bullet$ affects SERCA directly or indirectly via cGMP-dependent phosphorylation of phospholamban (*see* Chapter 7).

Little is known about the NO$^\bullet$ effect on capacitative Ca^{2+} influx in other cells. Recently, we showed that the same pathway for indirect NO$^\bullet$-induced inhibition of capacitative Ca^{2+} influx also exists in human platelets *(111)*. Okamoto et al. *(112)* previously reported the lack of an effect of SNP on capacitative cation influx evoked by inhibition of SERCA with TG in human platelets. Similarly, Bischof et al. *(113)* found no effect of the cGMP rise caused by overexpression of nitric oxide synthase (NOS) on capacitative Ca^{2+} influx evoked by inhibition of SERCA with cyclopiazonic acid (CPA) in HEK 293 cells. These negative results brought both groups to the conclusion that NO$^\bullet$ cannot regulate the capacitative Ca^{2+} influx. Our recent findings, however, provided another interpretation of their results. Indeed, by inhibiting SERCA (which seems to be the real target for NO$^\bullet$) they simply eliminated the possibility of an indirect inhibition of capacitative Ca^{2+} influx by NO$^\bullet$. Thus, we would conclude that SOC and capacitative Ca^{2+} influx in SMC can be inhibited by NO$^\bullet$, but only indirectly, through NO$^\bullet$-induced acceleration of SERCA-dependent Ca^{2+} back sequestration and refilling of the stores.

Ca^{2+} *Release Channels*

Intracellular Ca^{2+} release channels have been extensively studied in a variety of different cells, and are described in several recent reviews *(114–119)*.

IP$_3$-Sensitive Ca^{2+} Release Channels (IP$_3$R)

These mediate agonist-induced Ca^{2+} release from intracellular Ca^{2+} stores. These channels are physiologically activated by IP$_3$, which is produced from PIP$_2$ during agonist-induced activation of phospholipase C (for review *see* ref. *120*). The structure and mechanisms of regulation of the IP$_3$R channels in variety of cells, including SMC, have been recently reviewed *(120–122)*. Even in the absence of Ca^{2+} influx from the extracellular space, agonist-induced Ca^{2+} release from the stores through IP$_3$R channels is known to produce a transient rise in $[Ca^{2+}]_{in}$ and SMC contraction. In many studies NO$^\bullet$ and NO$^\bullet$ donors have been shown to reduce significantly agonist-induced Ca^{2+} release from the stores, which was interpreted as NO$^\bullet$-induced inhibition of IP$_3$R channels.

Nothing is presently known about the possibility of a direct effect of NO$^\bullet$ on single IP$_3$R channels, but there is some evidence pointing to an indirect cGMP-dependent inhibition of IP$_3$R channels. Indeed, Komalavilas and Lincoln *(123)* showed cGMP-dependent phosphorylation of IP$_3$R channel by PKG. This result provides one possible explanation for the inhibition of Ca^{2+} release from the stores by the NO$^\bullet$-induced cGMP rise in intact rabbit aorta *(124,125)* and in isolated gastric SMC *(126)*. Indeed, IP$_3$R channels might be a physiological target for NO$^\bullet$, but it is important to mention that there are also other ways in which NO$^\bullet$ can suppress agonist-induced Ca^{2+} release without affecting IP$_3$R channels. For example, recently we showed that the effect of NO$^\bullet$ on the agonist-induced transient rise in Ca^{2+} can arise from NO$^\bullet$-induced acceleration of Ca^{2+} back-sequestration into the stores *(109,110)*.

Ryanodine-Sensitive Ca^{2+} Release Channels (RyR)

These are responsible for Ca^{2+}-induced Ca^{2+} release (CICR *[127]*) which is a cornerstone of excitation-contraction coupling in cardiomyocytes and skeletal muscle. RyR channels have been extensively studied and characterized (for review *see* refs. *115,116,118,119,121*).

In cardiomyocytes local increases in $[Ca^{2+}]_{in}$ (Ca^{2+} sparks *(128,129)* caused by release of Ca^{2+} from the stores through RyR channels) are recruited throughout the whole cell. That could explain both the spontaneous and the triggered rise in $[Ca^{2+}]_{in}$ that causes cell contraction. RyR channels also have been found and described in SMC (for review see ref. *122*), but their functional role is not that clear. Massive Ca^{2+} release from intracellular stores and SMC contraction resulting from caffeine-induced opening of RyR channels have been described in a variety of SMC. On the other hand, Nelson and coworkers *(130)* recently described spontaneous Ca^{2+} sparks in SMC that cause arterial dilation instead of contraction. They showed that Ca^{2+} sparks in SMC are generated mainly beneath the plasma membrane, which can activate a cluster of K^+_{Ca} channels causing a spontaneous outward current (STOC) and leading to membrane hyperpolarization. Such negative feedback deactivates Ca^{2+}_L channels leading to the global reduction of $[Ca^{2+}]_{in}$ and SMC relaxation. Thus, RyR channel-mediated Ca^{2+} release from the stores can participate in both contraction and relaxation of SMC. Such a dual role of RyR channels in the regulation of SMC tone makes these channels an interesting and puzzling target for NO• in SMC, and controversial data have been obtained showing both activation and inhibition of RyR channels by NO• and related compounds.

Several recent studies clearly showed that the function of single RyR channels incorporated into planar lipid bilayers can be modulated directly (without the involvement of cGMP-dependent pathways) by NO• and related species, but the results of these studies are conflicting, and there is still no consensus on whether NO• inhibits or activates RyR channels. Zahradnikova and coworkers *(131,132)* found that activity of single RyR channels (from skeletal and cardiac muscle) was suppressed by 0.1 mM SNAP. They also showed that RyR channel-mediated Ca^{2+} release is reduced by presumably NO• generated *in situ* from L-arginine by endogenous NOS. Later, detailed studies by Stoyanovski and co-authors *(133)* obtained the opposite results. Exogenous NO•, as well as its donors (NONOates and RSNO), promoted Ca^{2+} release from skeletal and cardiac sarcoplasmic reticulum vesicles and inhibited ryanodine binding to RyR receptors. Moreover, single RyR channels incorporated into planar lipid bilayers were activated by 0.5–1 mM SNAP. A similar activation of single cardiac RyR channels was recently reported by Stamler and co-investigators *(16)* who experimentally linked the effect of NO• with direct poly S nitrosation of free thiols in RyR channel. By measuring and comparing S-nitrosation and oxidation of the RyR channels by different NO• donors, and linking it to the changes in channel activity, this group proposed that ion channels can functionally differentiate nitrosation from oxidation. Their results suggest that S-nitrosylation of 3 sites per RyR channel subunit (up to 12 sites total) leads to progressive channel activation that can be reversed by thiol reduction. In contrast, oxidation of 5–6 thiols per RyR subunit (presumably forming 2–3 disulfides) by GSNO occurs without affecting RyR channel function, whereas oxidation of 7 or more thiols per subunit by SIN-1 and CysNO (formation of more than 3 disulfides) is associated with irreversible activation of RyR channels. Activation of RyR channels and Ca^{2+} release by NO• and related compounds is in good agreement with earlier studies, which reported that sulfhydryl oxidation triggers Ca^{2+} release from the stores *(134–137)*.

These interesting findings, though, cannot be directly transferred to SMC without experimental confirmation. Indeed, three forms of RyR channels have been identified: RyR1, expressed predominantly in skeletal muscle; RyR2, expressed predominantly in cardiac muscle and in SMC; and RyR3, expressed in specialized muscle, including SMC (for review *see* ref. *118*). Thus, RyR2 and RyR3 channels are expressed in SMC, and it is presently unknown if they have the same or different structures and stoichiometries of thiol groups, which can be responsible for NO•-induced channel S-nitrosation or oxidation of RyR channels found in cardiac and skeletal muscle. Alternatively spliced RyR channel molecules in different tissues could be differentially phosphorylated by protein kinases, and this might explain the apparently conflicting results mentioned.

CONCLUSION:
THE COMPLEXITY OF ION CHANNEL REGULATION BY NO•

It is presently clear that NO• can affect ion channels in two major ways. First, NO• acts indirectly through NO•-induced activation of guanylyl cyclase, which increases intracellular cGMP level and affects different cGMP-dependent processes involved in the regulation of ion channel function. Second, NO• causes cGMP-independent direct modification of S-nitrosothiols in the channel or closely associated regulatory protein. The existence of these two pathways and the current controversies about the end results of each pathway (activation versus inhibition) make the regulation of some of the channels by NO• rather complicated (see Fig. 2). Indeed, it is still unclear if a rise in cGMP necessarily causes inhibition of Ca_L^{2+} channels (which one would expect from the physiological point of view), or if it can also activate them under some circumstances. It is also unclear if the direct effect of NO• on Ca_L^{2+} channels causes inhibition, or if activation is also possible. The effect of NO• on K_{Ca}^+ channels is more certain, as K_{Ca}^+ channels are activated by NO• both directly and indirectly. The result of a direct effect of NO• on RyR channels is still unclear, as both activation and inhibition has been observed by different groups. The information about the effects of NO• on other ion channels is still incomplete: most of them have shown them to be regulated by NO• through only one pathway, but, in most cases, there is not enough evidence to definitely exclude the possibility of their regulation through other mechanisms as well.

Tremendous progress have been achieved in enumerating the ways in which NO• can affect different ion channels in different blood vessels and under a variety of conditions to produce its major physiological function—SMC relaxation. Further studies are necessary to resolve the remaining controversies, and to define better the physiological and potential pathological effects of NO• on each type of ion channel.

REFERENCES

1. Van Breemen C. Calcium requirement for activation of intact aortic smooth muscle. J Physiol (Lond) 1997;272:317–329.
2. Fay FS. Isometric contractile properties of single isolated smooth muscle cells. Nature 1997;265:553–556.
3. Yagi S, Becker PL, Fay FS. Relationship between force and Ca^{2+} concentration in smooth muscle as revealed by measurements on single cell. Proc Natl Acad Sci USA 1988;85:4109–4113.
4. Gruetter CA, Gruetter DY, Lyon JE, Kadowitz PJ, Ignarro LJ. Relationship between cyclic guanosine 3':5'-monophosphate formation and relaxation of coronary arterial smooth muscle by glyceryl trinitrate, nitroprusside, nitrite and nitric oxide: effects of methylene blue and methemoglobin. J Pharm Exp Ther 1981;219:181–186.
5. Arnold WP, Mittal CK, Katsuki S, Murad F. Nitric oxide activates guanylate cyclase and increases guanosine 3',5'-cyclic monophosphate levels in various tissue preparations. Proc Natl Acad Sci USA 1997;74:3203–3207.
6. Ignarro LJ, Byrns RE, Buga GM, Wood KS. Endothelium-derived relaxing factor from pulmonary artery and vein possess pharmacologic and chemical properties identical to those of nitric oxide radical. Circ Res 1987;61:866–879.
7. Palmer RM, Ferrige AG, Moncada S. Nitric oxide release accounts for the biological activity of endothelium-derived relaxing ractor. Nature 1987;327:524–526.
8. Lincoln TM, Cornwell TL, Komalavilas P, Boerth N. Cyclic GMP-dependent protein kinase in nitric oxide signaling. Methods Enzymol 1996;269:149–166.
9. Cornwell TL, Arnold E, Boerth N, Lincoln TM. Inhibition of smooth muscle cell growth by nitric oxide and activation of cAMP-dependent protein kinase by cGMP. Am J Physiol 1994;429:C1405–C1413.
10. Malinski T, Taha Z, Grunfeld S, Patton S, Kapturczak M, Tomboulian P. Diffusion of nitric oxide in the aorta wall monitored in situ by porphyrinic microsensors. Biochem Biophys Res Commun 1993;193:1076–1082.
11. Cohen RA, Plane F, Najibi S, Huk I, Malinski T, Garland CJ. Nitric oxide is the mediator of both endothelium-dependent relaxation and hyperpolarization of the rabbit carotid artery. Proc Natl Acad Sci USA 1997;94:4193–4198.

12. Lei SZ, Pan ZH, Aggarwal SK, Chen HS, Hartman J, Sucher NJ, Lipton SA. Effect of nitric oxide production on the redox modulatory site of the NMDA receptor-channel complex. Neuron 1992;8: 1087–1099.
13. Bolotina VM, Najibi S, Palacino JJ, Pagano PJ, Cohen RA. Nitric oxide directly activates calcium-dependent potassium channels in vascular smooth muscle. Nature 1994;368:850–853.
14. Campbell DL, Stamler JS, Strauss HC. Redox modulation of L-type calcium channels in ferret ventricular myocytes. Dual mechanism of regulation by nitric oxide and S-nitrosothiols. J Gen Physiol 1996; 108:277–293.
15. Hu H, Chiamvimonvat N, Yamagishi T, Marban E. Direct inhibition of expressed cardiac L-type Ca^{2+} channels by S-nitrosothiol nitric oxide donors. Circ Res 1997;81:742–752.
16. Xu L, Eu JP, Meissner G, Stamler JS. Activation of the cardiac calcium release channel (ryanodine receptor) by poly-S-nitrosylation. Science 1998;279:234–237.
17. Stamler JS, Singel DJ, Loscalzo J. Biochemistry of nitric oxide and its redox-activated forms. Science 1992;258:1898–1902.
18. Stamler JS, Simon DI, Osborne JA, Mullins ME, Jaraki O, Michel T, Singel DJ, Loscalzo J. S-nitrosylation of proteins with nitric oxide: synthesis and characterization of biologically active compounds. Proc Natl Acad Sci USA 1992;89:444–448.
19. Lipton SA, Choi YB, Pan ZH, Lei SZ, Chen HS, Sucher NJ, Loscalzo J, Singel DJ, Stamler JS. A redox-based mechanism for the neuroprotective and neurodestructive effects of nitric oxide and related nitroso-compounds. Nature 1993;364:626–632.
20. Stamler JS. Redox signaling: nitrosylation and related target interactions of nitric oxide. Cell 1994;78: 931–936.
21. Stamler JS, Feelisch M. Biochemistry of nitric oxide and redox-related species. In: Feelisch M, Stamler JS, eds. Methods of Nitric Oxide Research. Wiley, Chichester, UK, 1996, pp. 20–27.
22. Stamler JS, Toone EJ, Lipton SA, Sucher NJ. (S)NO signals: translocation, regulation and a consensus motif. Neuron 1997;18:691–696.
23. Nelson MT, Patlak JB, Worley JF, Standen NB. Calcium channels, potassium channels, and voltage dependence of arterial smooth muscle tone. Am J Physiol 1990;259:C3–C18.
24. McDonald TF, Pelzer S, Trautwein W, Pelzer DJ. Regulation and modulation of calcium channels in cardiac, skeletal, and smooth muscle cells. Physiol Rev 1994;74:365–507.
25. Clapp LH, Gurney AM. Modulation of calcium movements by nitroprusside in isolated vascular smooth muscle cells. Pflugers Arch 1991;418:462–470.
26. Blatter LA, Wier WG. Nitric oxide decreases $[Ca^{2+}]_i$ in vascular smooth muscle by inhibition of the calcium current. Cell Calcium 1994;15:122–131.
27. Quignard JF, Frapier JM, Harricane MC, Albat B, Nargeot J, Richard S. Voltage-gated calcium channel currents in human coronary myocytes. Regulation by cyclic GMP and nitric oxide. J Clin Invest 1997; 99:185–193.
28. Mery PF, Pavoine C, Belhassen L, Pecker F, Fischmeister R. Nitric oxide regulates cardiac Ca^{2+} current: involvement of cGMP-inihibited and cGMP-stimulated phosphodiesterases through guanylyl cyclase activation. J Biol Chem 1993;268:26,286–26,295.
29. Levi RC, Alloatti G, Penna C, Gallo MP. Guanylate-cyclase-mediated inhibition of cardiac ICa by carbachol and sodium nitroprusside. Pflugers Arch 1994;426:419–426.
30. Wahler GM, Dollinger SJ. Nitric oxide donor SIN-1 inhibits mammalian cardiac calcium current through cGMP-dependent protein kinase. Am J Physiol 1995;268:C45–C54.
31. Han X, Kobzik L, Balligand J-L, Kelly RA, Smith TW. Nitric oxide synthase (NOS3)-mediated cholinergic modulation of Ca^{2+} current in adult rabbit atrioventricular nodal cells. Circ Res 1996;78: 998–1008.
32. Kirstein M, Rivet-bastide M, Hatem S, Benardeau A, Mercadier JJ, Fischmeister R. Nitric oxide regulates the calcium current in isolated human atrial myocytes. J Clin Invest 1995;95:794–802.
33. Ishikawa T, Hume JR, Keef KD. Regulation of Ca^{2+} channels by cAMP and cGMP in vascular smooth muscle cells. Circ Res 1993;73:1128–1137.
34. Xiong Z, Sperelakis N. Regulation of L-type calcium channels of vascular smooth muscle cells. J Mol Cell Cardiol 1995;27:75–91.
35. Ruiz-Velasco V, Zhong J, Hume JR, Keef KD. Modulation of Ca^{2+} channels by cyclic nucleotide cross activation of opposing protein kinases in rabbit portal vein. Circ Res 1998;82:557–565.
36. Tewari K, Simard JM. Sodium nitroprusside and cGMP decrease Ca^{2+} channel avaliability in basilar artery smooth muscle cells. Pflugers Arch 1997;433:304–311.
37. Tohse M, Sperelakis N. cGMP inhibits the activity of single calcium channels in embrionic chick heart cells. Circ Res 1991;69:325–331.

38. Mery PF, Lohmann SM, Walter U, Fischmeister R. Ca^{2+} current is regulated by cyclic GMP-dependent protein kinase in mammalian cardiac myocytes. Proc Natl Acad Sci USA 1991;88:1197–1201.
39. Sumii K, Sperelakis N. cGMP-dependent protein kinase regulation of the L-type Ca^{2+} current in rat ventricular myocytes. Circ Res 1995;77:803–812.
40. Ono K, Trautwein W. Potentiation by cyclic GMP β-adrenergic effect on Ca^{2+} current in guinea-pig ventricular cells. J Physiol (Lond) 1991;443:387–404.
41. Tewari K, Simard JM. Protein kinase A increases availability of calcium channels in smooth muscle cells from guinea pig basilar artery. Pflugers Arch 1994;428:9–16.
42. Koh SD, Sanders KM. Modulation of Ca^{2+} current in canine colonic myocytes by cyclic nucleotide-dependent mechanisms. Am J Physiol 1996;271:C794–C803.
43. Chiamvimonvat N, O'Rourke B, Kamp TJ, Kallen RG, Hofmann F, Flockerzi V, Marban E. Functional consequences of sulfhydryl modification in the pore-forming subunits of cardiovascular Ca^{2+} and Na^+ channels. Circ Res 1995;76:325–334.
44. Nelson MT, Quayle JM. Physiological roles and properties of potassium channels in arterial smooth muscle. Am J Physiol 1995;268:C799–C822.
45. Toro L, Meera MW, Tanaka Y. Maxi-K_{Ca}, a unique member of the voltage-gated K channel super-family. News Physiol Sci 1998;13:112–117.
46. Brayden JE, Nelson MT. Regulation of arterial tone by activation of calcium-dependent potassium channels. Science 1992;256:532–535.
47. Khan SA, Mathews WR, Meisheri KD. Role of calcium-activated K^+ channels in vascodilation induced by nitroglycerine, acetylcholine and nitric oxide. J Pharmacol 1993;267:1327–1335.
48. Najibi S, Cowan CL, Palacino JJ, Cohen RA. Enhanced role of potassium channels in relaxations to acetyecholine in hypercholesterolemic rabbit carotid artery. Am J Physiol 1994;266:H2061–H2067.
49. Plane F, Wiley KE, Jeremy JY, Cohen RA, Garland CJ. Evidence that different mechanisms underlie smooth muscle relaxation to nitric oxide and nitric oxide donors in the rabbit isolated carotid artery. Br J Pharmacol 1998;123:1351–1358.
50. Jones TR, Charette L, Garcia ML, Kaczorowski GJ. Selective inhibition of relaxation of guinea-pig trachea by charybdotoxin, a potent Ca^{++}-activated K^+ channel inhibitor. J Pharm Exp Ther 1990;255:697–706.
51. Bialecki RA, Stinson-Fisher C. K_{Ca} channel antagonists reduce No donor-mediated relaxation of vascular and tracheal smooth muscle. Am J Physiol 1995;268:L152–L159.
52. Magliola L, Jones AW. Sodium nitroprusside alters Ca^{2+} flux components and Ca^{2+}-dependent fluxes of K^+ and Cl^- in rat aorta. J Physiol (Lond) 1990;421:411–424.
53. Plane F, Hurrell A, Jeremy JY, Garland CJ. Evidence that potassium channels make a major contribution to SIN-1-evoked relaxation of rat isolated mesenteric artery. Br J Pharmacol 1996;119:1557–1562.
54. Archer SL, Huang JMC, Hampl V, Nelson DP, Shultz PJ, Weir EK. Nitric oxide and cGMP cause vasorelaxation by cGMP-kinase-dependent activation of a charybdotoxin-sensitive K channel. Proc Natl Acad Sci USA 1994;91:7583–7587.
55. Archer SL, Huang JM, Reeve HL, Hampl V, Tolarova S, Michelakis E, Weir EK. Differential distribution of electrophysiologically distinct myocytes in conduit and resistance arteries determines their response to nitric oxide and hypoxia. Circ Res 1996;78:431–442.
56. Zhao YJ, Wang J, Rubin LJ, Yuan XJ. Inhibition of K_v and K_{Ca} channels antagonizes NO-induced relaxation in pulmonary artery. Am J Physiol 1997;272:H904–H912.
57. Kitazono T, Ibayashi S, Nagao T, Fujii K, Fujishima M. Role of Ca^{2+}-activated K^+ channels in acetylcholine-induced dilatation of basilar artery in vivo. Br J Pharmacol 1997;120:102–106.
58. Fujino K, Nakaya S, Wakatsuki T, Miyoshi Y, Nakaya Y. Effects of nitroglycerin on ATP-induced Ca^{++} mobilization, Ca^{++}-activated K channels and contraction of cultured smooth muscle cells of porcine coronary artery. J Pharm Exp Ther 1991;256:371–377.
59. Robertson BE, Schubert R, Hescheler J, Nelson MT. cGMP-dependent protein kinase activates Ca-activated K channels in cerebral artery smooth muscle cells. Am J Physiol 1993;265:C299–C303.
60. Taniguchi J, Furukawa KI, Shigekawa M. Maxi K^+ channels are stimulated by cyclic guanosine monophosphate-dependent protein kinase in canine coronary artery smooth muscle cells. Pflugers Arch 1993;423:167–172.
61. Lander HM, Sehajpal PK, Novogrodsyk A. Nitric oxide signalling: a possible role for G-proteins. J Immunol 1993;151:7182–7187.
62. Koh SD, Campbell JD, Carl A, Sanders KM. Nitric oxide activates multiple potassium channels in canine colonic smooth muscle. J Physiol 1995;489:735–743.

63. Carrier GO, Fuchs LC, Winecoff AP, Giulumian AD, White RE. Nitrovasodilators relax mesenteric microvessels by cGMP-induced stimulation of Ca-activated K channels. Am J Physiol 1997;273: H76–H84.
64. Yuan XJ, Tod ML, Rubin LJ, Blaunstein MP. NO hyperpolarizes pulmonary artery smooth muscle cells and decreases the intracellular Ca2+ concentration by activating voltage-gated K+ channels. Proc Natl Acad Sci USA 1996;93:10,489–10,494.
65. Shin JH, Chung S, Park EJ, Uhm DY, Suh CK. Nitric oxide directly activates calcium-activated potassium channels from rat brain reconstituted into planar lipid bilayer. FEBS Lettt 1997;415:299–302.
66. Abderrahmane A, Salvail D, Mumoulin M, Garon J, Cadiuex A, Rousseau E. Direct activation of K_{Ca} channel in airway smooth muscle by nitric oxide: involvement of a nitrothiosylation mechansim. Am J Resp Cell Mol Biol 1998;18:1–13.
67. Williams DLJ, Katz GM, Roy-Contancin L, Reuben JP. Guanosine 5'-monophosphate modulates gating of high-conductance Ca^{2+}-activated K^+ channels in vascular smooth muscle cells. Proc Natl Acad Sci USA 1988;85:9360–9364.
68. Li PL, Jin MW, Campbell WB. Effect of selective inhibition of soluble guanylyl cyclase on the K_{Ca} channel activity in coronary artery smooth muscle. Hypertension 1998;31:303–308.
69. White RE, Lee AB, Scherbatko AD, Lincoln TM, Schonbrunn A, Armstrong DL. Potassium channel stimulation by natriuretic peptides through cGMP-dependent dephosphorylation. Nature 1993;361: 263–266.
70. Zhou XB, Ruth P, Schlossmann J, Hofmann F, Korth M. Protein phosphatase 2A is essential for the activation of Ca^{2+}-activated K^+ currents by cGMP-dependent protein kinase in tracheal smooth muscle and chinese hamster ovary cells. J Biol Chem 1996;271:19,760–19,767.
71. Sansom SC, Stockand JD, Hall D, Williams B. Regulation of large calcium-activated potassium channels by protein phosphatase 2A. J Biol Chem 1997;272:9902–9906.
72. Alioua A, Huggins JP, Rousseau E. PKG-Iα phosphorylates the α-subunit and upregulates reconstituted GK_{Ca} channels from tracheal smooth muscle. Am J Physiol 1995;268:L1057–L1063
73. Schmidt K, Klatt P, Mayer B. Hypercholesterolemia is associated with a reduced response of smooth muscle guanylyl cyclase to nitrovasodilators. Arterioscler Thromb 1993;13:1159–1163.
74. Simonet S, Porro de Bailliencourt J, Descombes JJ, Mennecier P, Laubie M, Verbeuren TJ. Hypoxia causes an abnormal contractile response in the atherosclerotic rabbit aorta. Implication of reduced nitric oxide and cGMP production. Circ Res 1993;72:616–630.
75. Wong WS, Roman CR, Fleisch JH. Differential relaxant responses of guinea-pig lung strips and bronchial rings to sodium nitroprusside: a mechanism independent of cGMP formation. J Pharm Pharmacol 1995;47:757 761.
76. Wang ZW, Nara M, Wang YX, Kotlikoff MI. Redox regulation of large conductance Ca^{2+}-activated K+ channels in smooth muscle cells. J Gen Physiol 1997;110:35–44.
77. Ashcroft FM. Adenosine 5-triphosphate-sensitive potassium channels. Annu Rev Neurosci 1988;11: 97–118.
78. Trapp S, Ashcroft FM. A metabolic sensor in action: news from the ATP-sensitive K^+-channel. News Physiol Sci 1997;12:255–263.
79. Daud J, Mayer-Rudolph W, von Beckerath N, Mehrke G, Gunther K, Goedel-Meinen L. Hypoxic dilation of coronary arteries is mediated by ATP-sensitive potassium channels. Science 1990;247.1341–1344.
80. Standen NB, Quayle JM, Davies NW, Brayden JE, Huang Y, Nelson MT. Hyperpolarizing vasodilators activate ATP-sensitive K^+ channels in arterial smooth muscle. Science 1989;245:177–180.
81. Tsuura Y, Ishida H, Hayashi S, Sakamoto K, Horie M, Seino Y. Nitric oxide opens ATP-sensitive K^+ channels through suppression of phosphofructokinase activity and inhibits glucose-induced insulin release in pancreatic β cells. J Gen Physiol 1994;104:1079–1098.
82. Antoine MH, Hermann M, Herchuelz A, Lebrun P. Sodium nitroprusside inhibits glucose-induced insulin release by activating ATP-sensitive K^+ channels. Biochem Biophys Acta 1993;1175:293–301.
83. Murphy ME, Brayden JE. Nitric oxide hyperpolarizes rabbit mesenteric arteries via ATP-sensitive potassium channels. J Physiol (Lond) 1995;486:47–58.
84. Armstead WM. Role of activation of calcium-sensitive K^+ channels in NO- and hypoxia-induced pial artery vasodilation. Am J Physiol 1997;272:H1785–H1790.
85. Miyoshi H, Nakaya Y, Moritoki H. Nonendothelial-derived nitric oxide activates the ATP-sensitive K^+ channel of vascular smooth muscle cells. FEBS Lett 1994;345:47–49.
86. Kubo M, Nakaya Y, Matsuoka S, Saito K, Kuroda Y. Atrial natriuretic factor and isosorbide dinitrate modulate the gating of ATP-sensitive K^+ channels in cultured vascular smooth muscle cells. Circ Res 1994;74:471–476.

87. Coetzee WA, Nakamura TY, Faivre J.-F. Effects of thiol-modifying agents on K_{ATP} channels in guinea pig ventricular cells. Am J Physiol 1998;269:H1625–H1633.

88. Large WA, Wang Q. Characteristics and physiological role of the Ca^{2+}-activated and Cl^- conductance in smooth muscle. Am J Physiol 1996;271:C435-C454.

89. Pacuad P, Loirand G, Baron A, Mironneau C, Mironneau J. Ca^{2+} channel activation and membrane depolarization mediated by Cl^- channels in response to noradrenaline in vascular myocytes. Br J Pharmacol 1991;104:1000–1006.

90. Nelson MT, Conway MA, Knot HJ, Brayden JE. Chloride channel blockers inhibit myogenic tone in rat cerebral arteries. J Physiol (Lond) 1997;502:259–264.

91. Droogmans G, Callewaert G, Declerck I, Casteels R. ATP-induced Ca^{2+} release and Cl^- current in cultured smooth muscle cells from pig aorta. J Physiol (Lond) 1991;440:623–634.

92. Zhang Y, Vogalis F, Goyal RK. Nitric oxide supresses a Ca^{2+}-stimulated Cl^- current in smooth muscle cells of opossum esophagus. Am J Physiol 1998;274:G886–G890.

93. Hirakawa Y, Gericke M, Cohen RA, Bolotina VM. Ca^{2+}-dependent Cl^- channels in mouse and rabbit aortic smooth muscle cells: regulation by intracellular Ca^{2+} and nitric oxide. Am J Physiol 1999;277: H1732–H1744.

94. Lin M, Nairn AC, Guggino SE. cGMP-dependent protein kinase regulation of a chloride channel in T84 cells. Am J Physiol 1992;262:C1304–C1312.

95. Kamosinska B, Radomski MW, Duszyk M, Radomski A, Man SF. Nitric oxide activates chloride currents in human lung epithelial cells. Am J Physiol 1997;272:L1098–L1104.

96. Swandulla D, Partridge LD. Non-specific cation channels. In: Cook NS, ed. Potassium Channels: Structure, Classification, Function and Therapeutic Potential. Sandoz Ltd., Basel, Switzerland, 1990, pp. 167–180.

97. Isenberg G. Nonselective cation channels in cardiac and smooth muscle cells. In: Siemen D, Hescheler J, eds. Nonselective Cation Channels: Pharmacology, Physiology and Biophysics. Burkhauser Verlag, Basel, Switzerland, 1993, pp. 247–260.

98. Fasolato C, Innocenti B, Pozzan T. Receptor-activated Ca2+ influx: how many mechanisms for how many channels? TIPS 1994;15:77–83.

99. Minowa T, Miwa S, Kobayashi S, Enoki T, Zhang XF, Komuro T, Iwamuro Y, Masaki T. Inhibitory effect of nitrovasodilators and cyclic GMP on ET-1-activated Ca^{2+}-permeable nonselective cation channel in rat aortic smooth muscle cells. Br J Pharmacol 1997;120:1536–1544.

100. Koivisto A, Siemen D, Nedergaard J. Reversible blockade of the calcium-activated nonselective cation channel in brown fat cells by the sulfhydryl reagents mercury and thimerosal. Pflugers Arch 1993;425: 549–551.

101. Koivisto A, Nedergaard J. Modulation of calcium-activated non-selective cation channel activity by nitric oxide in rat brown adipose tissue. J Physiol (Lond) 1995;486:59–65.

102. Clapham DE. Calcium signaling. Cell 1995;80:259–268.

103. Berridge MJ. Capacitative calcium entry. Biochem J 1995;312:1–11.

104. Berridge MJ. Elementary and global aspects of calcium signaling. J Physiol (Lond) 1997;499:291–306.

105. Parekh AB, Penner R. Store depletion and calcium influx. Physiol Rev 1997;77:901–930.

106. Hoth M, Penner R. Depletion of intracellular calcium stores activates a calcium current in mast cells. Nature 1992;355:353–356.

107. Xuan Y-T, Wang O-L, Whorton AR. Thapsigargin stimulates Ca^{2+} entry in vascular smooth muscle cells: nicardipine-sensitive and -insensitive pathways. Am J Physiol 1992;262:C1258–C1265.

108. Byron KL, Taylor CW. Vasopressin stimulation of Ca^{2+} mobilization, two bivalent cation entry pathways and Ca^{2+} efflux in A7r5 rat smooth muscle cells. J Physiol (Lond) 1995;485:455–468.

109. Bolotina VM, Weisbrod RM, Gericke M, Cohen RA. Novel mechanism of nitric oxide-induced relaxation: accelerated refilling of intracellular calcium stores and inhibition of store-operated calcium influx. Circulation 1997;96:I–448.

110. Cohen RA, Weisbrod RM, Gericke M, Yaghoubi M, Bierl C, Bolotina VM. Mechanism of nitric oxide-induced vasodialtion. Refilling of intracellular stores by sarcoplasmic reticulum Ca^{2+} ATPase and inhibition of store-operated Ca^{2+} influx. Circ Res 1999;84:210–219.

111. Trepakova ES, Cohen RA, Bolotina VM. Nitric oxide inhibits capacitative cation influx in human platelets by promoting sarcoplasmic/endoplasmic reticulum Ca^{2+}-ATPase-dependent refilling of Ca^{2+} stores. Circ Res 1999;84:201–209.

112. Okamoto Y, Ninomiya H, Miwa S, Masaki T. Capacitative Ca^{2+} entry in human platelets is resistant to nitric oxide. Biochem Biophys Res Commun 1995;212:90–96.

113. Bischof G, Brenman J, Bredt DS, Machen TE. Possible regulation of capacitative Ca^{2+} entry into colonic epithelial cells by NO and cGMP. Cell Calcium 1995;17:250–262.

114. Pozzan T, Rizzuto R, Volpe P, Meldolesi J. Molecular and cellular physiology of intracellular calcium stores. Physiol Rev 1994;74:595–636.

115. Meissner G. Ryanodine receptor/Ca^{2+} release channels and their regulation by endogenous effectors. Annu Rev Physiol 1994;56:485–508.

116. Sutko JL, Airey JA. Ryanodine receptor Ca^{2+} release channels: does diversity in form equal diversity in function? Physiol Rev 1996;76:1027–1071.

117. Katz AM. Calcium channel diversity in the cardiovascular system. JACC 1996;28:522–529.

118. Marks AR. Intracellular calcium-release channels: regulators of cell life and death. Am J Physiol 1997; 272:H597–H605.

119. Zucchi R, Ronca-Testoni S. The sarcoplasmic reticulum Ca^2 channel/rianodine receptor: modulation by endogenous effectors, drugs, and disease states. Pharmacol Rev 1997;49:1–51.

120. Berridge MJ. Inositol trisphosphate and calcium signalling. Nature 1993;361:315–325.

121. Ehrlich BE, Kaftan E, Bezprozvannaya S, Bezprozvanny I. The pharmacology of intracellular Ca^{2+}-release channels. TIPS 1994;15:145–149.

122. Himpens B, Missiaen L, Casteels R. Ca^{2+} homeostasis in vascular smooth muscle. J Vasc Res 1995;32: 207–219.

123. Komalavilas P, Lincoln TM. Phosphorylation of the inositol 1,4,5-trisphosphate receptor by cyclic GMP-dependent protein kinase. J Biol Chem 1994;269:8701–8707.

124. Meisheri KD, Taylor CJ, Saneii H. Synthetic atrial peptide inhibits intracellular calcium release in smooth muscle. Am J Physiol 1986;250:C171–C174.

125. Collins P, Griffith TM, Henderson AH, Lewis MJ. Endothelium-derived relaxation factor alters calcium fluxes in rabbit aorta: a cyclic guanosine monophosphate-mediated effect. J Physiol (Lond) 1986; 381:427–437.

126. Jin JG, Murthy KS, Grider JR, Makhlouf GM. Activation of distinct cAMP- and cGMP-dependent pathways by relaxant agents in isolated gastric muscle cells. Am J Physiol 1993;264:G470–G477.

127. Fabiato A. Time and calcium dependence of activation and inactivation of calcium-induced release of calcium from the sarcoplasmic reticulum of a skinned canine cardiac Purkinje cell. J Gen Physiol 1985; 85:247–289.

128. Cheng H, Lederer WJ, Cannell MB. Calcium sparks: elementary events underlying excitation-contraction coupling in heart muscle. Science 1993;262:740–744.

129. Cannell MB, Cheng H, Lederer WJ. The control of calcium release in heart muscle. Science 1995;268: 1045–1049.

130. Nelson MT, Cheng H, Rubart M, Santana LF, Bonev AD, Knot HJ, Lederer WJ. Relaxation of arterial smooth muscle by calcium sparks. Science 1995;270:633–637.

131. Meszaros LG, Minarovic I, Zahradnikova A. Inhibition of the skeletal muscle ryanodine receptor calcium release channel by nitric oxide. FEBS Lett 1996;380:49–52.

132. Zahradnikova A, Minarovic I, Venema RC, Meszaros LG. Inactivation of the cardiac ryanodine receptor calcium release channel by nitric oxide. Cell Calcium 1997;22:447–454.

133. Stoyanovsky D, Murphy T, Anno PR, Kim YM, Salama G. Nitric oxide activates skeletal and cardiac ryanodine receptors. Cell Calcium 1997;21:19–29.

134. Trimm JL, Salama G, Abramson JJ. Sulfhydryl oxidation induces rapid calcium release from sarcoplasmic reticulum vesicles. J Biol Chem 1986;261:16,092–16,098.

135. Zaidi NF, Lagenaur CF, Abramson JJ, Pessah I, Salama G. Reactive disulfides trigger Ca^{2+} release from sarcoplasmic reticulum via an oxidation reaction. J Biol Chem 1989;264:21,725–21,736.

136. Prabhu SD, Salama G. Reactive disulfide compounds induce Ca^{2+} release from cardiac sarcoplasmic reticulum. Arch Biochem Biophys 1990;282:275–283.

137. Salama G, Abramson JJ, Pike GK. Sulphydryl reagents trigger Ca^{2+} release from the sarcoplasmic reticulum of skinned rabbit psoas fibres. J Physiol (Lond) 1992;454:389–420.

7

Role of Nitric Oxide in Vasomotor Regulation

Richard A. Cohen

INTRODUCTION

The contractile tone of the smooth muscle of blood vessels is regulated through neural, humoral, and local control mechanisms. The discovery of nitric oxide (NO•) as a biological mediator occurred coincidentally with the realization that it played a major role in the local control of vasomotor tone as a result of its release from endothelial cells and diffusion to smooth muscle cells in the arterial media *(1)*. It is also likely that NO• participates in neural control of the vasculature because it participates in regulating both sympathetic and parasympathetic reflex control mechanisms, and is now a recognized neurotransmitter that influences vascular as well as other cells. This chapter reviews the many aspects of the control of vasomotor tone in which NO• participates.

ENDOTHELIUM-DERIVED NO• AND VASOMOTOR REGULATION

Before the discovery of NO•, the endothelium was thought to behave as a passive lining to the vasculature. Even so the endothelium was recognized in the 1970s to regulate vascular tone, albeit indirectly, as a result of the fact that the endothelium was shown to prevent platelet aggregation *(2)*. Damage to the endothelium was shown to result in platelet aggregation on the exposed underlying matrix and to result in the release of vasoconstrictor agents including thromboxane A_2 and 5-hydroxytryptamine. In this respect, the endothelium plays a vital hemostatic role.

In 1979 and 1980 Robert Furchgott was responsible for showing that the endothelium plays an active role in vasomotor regulation *(1,3)*. He found that mechanical denudation of the endothelium from isolated arteries eliminated the relaxation to agents such as bradykinin and acetylcholine (*see* Fig. 1). In so doing, he resolved a long-standing debate over the relevance of isolated blood vessel studies. It was well known that acetylcholine was a potent vasodilator when administered in vivo. Furchgott found that isolated artery studies failed to demonstrate such a response because the common technique of studying spiral strips of smooth muscle inadvertently removed the endothelial cells. Furchgott also demonstrated that a diffusible substance mediated the vasodilation of an artery with intact endothelial cells by showing that an artery without endothelium apposed to that with endothelium, or superfused with the perfusate of an intact artery, also relaxed *(1)*. Furchgott *(3)*, Ignarro et al. *(4,5)*, and Palmer et al. *(6)* studied the physical and chemical properties of the diffusible "endothelium-derived relaxing factor" and found them to be identical to NO•. This included the demonstration that the relaxing factor like NO• stimulated soluble guanylyl cyclase, had a half-life in

From: *Contemporary Cardiology, vol. 4: Nitric Oxide and the Cardiovascular System*
Edited by: J. Loscalzo and J. A. Vita © Humana Press Inc., Totowa, NJ

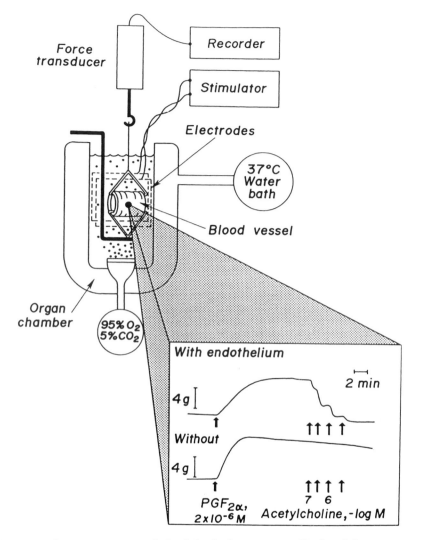

Fig, 1. Apparatus for measurement of physiological responses of isolated ring segments of blood vessels. The recording shows an experiment like that of Furchgott and Zawadzki *(1)* in which it is demonstrated in a ring of dog coronary artery contracted with prostaglandin $F_{2\alpha}$ ($PGF_{2\alpha}$) that the concentration-dependent relaxation caused by acetylcholine depends on an intact endothelial cell layer. The lower ring, which was denuded of endothelium prior to mounting in the organ chamber, does not relax. From Vanhoutte and Cohen *(170)* by permission of the Federation of American Societies of Experimental Biology.

physiological solutions of approx 5 s, and was scavenged by oxyhemoglobin. The identity of the relaxing factor as NO˙ was further established by showing that, like NO˙, the diffusible factor was inactivated by superoxide anion *(7,8)*. Following the demonstration that NO˙ was synthesized from arginine in macrophages, Palmer et al. showed that the relaxing factor was derived from this amino acid, and that arginine analogs prevented the formation of the factor *(9)*. These studies established that the enzymatic synthesis of NO˙ from arginine in endothelial cells accounted for the vasodilator discovered by Furchgott. There have been suggestions that NO˙ might be released from the endothelium as a S-nitrosothiol *(10)* or chemically complexed with nonheme iron *(11)*, but NO˙ would be the active species released rapidly from these alternative species. Despite studies suggesting the importance of vasodilator factors other than NO˙, notably a putative distinct endothelium-derived hyperpolarizing factor *(12)*, several studies have confirmed that NO˙ released from the endothelium is the major vasomotor regulator *(13,14)*.

Taking advantage of the ability of the arginine analogs, N^G-monomethyls-L-arginine and L-N^G-arginine methyl ester, to inhibit NO˙ release, Moncada's group quickly established the widespread role of NO˙ in vasomotor regulation. Not only was it shown that endothelium-dependent relaxation of isolated arteries was inhibited by these analogs *(15)*, but it was also shown that NO˙ could be implicated as a vasodilator of the microcirculation in the coronary *(16)*, pulmonary *(17)*, skeletal muscle *(18)*, and renal *(19)* circulation in experimental animals, as a well as in the human forearm circulation *(20)*. In each of these vascular beds the arginine analogs caused vasoconstriction, which was reversible by exogenous L-arginine, implying that the tonic production of NO˙ maintained a vasodilator influence on the circulation. Of particular importance, N^G-monomethyl-L-arginine was found to increase blood pressure, establishing a role for NO˙ in blood pressure regulation *(21)*.

REGULATION OF ENDOTHELIAL NO˙ RELEASE

Basal Release of NO˙

Vasoconstrictor responses of isolated blood vessels are larger when either the endothelium is removed or NOS inhibitors are present, suggesting that NO˙ is released under resting conditions from intact endothelial cells and inhibits contraction of neighboring smooth muscle cells *(22–25)*. The basal release of NO˙ is thought to occur as a result of the fact that basal endothelial cell intracellular calcium levels are sufficient to activate calmodulin, which binds to and stimulates NOS in endothelial cells (eNOS) *(26)*. Basal levels of intracellular calcium are maintained by a balance between the influx of calcium through ion channels and the removal of calcium from the cytoplasm by transport pumps either out of the cell or into intracellular storage compartments. Calcium-conducting ion channels in endothelium are nonselective ion channels. Unlike L-type calcium channels, which are absent from endothelium, the nonselective cation channels in endothelial cells do not increase conductance with depolarization. Rather, influx through theses channels, and therefore greater activation of NOS, occurs at more negative membrane potentials and is enhanced by endothelial cell hyperpolarization (*see* Fig. 2) *(27)*.

Shear Stress Stimulation of NO˙ Release

By as yet poorly understood mechanisms, increased blood flow stimulates the release of NO˙ by increasing shear forces on endothelial cells. Mechanical deformation by pulsatile pressure and flow variations probably also contributes to the stimulation of cells *(28,29)*. The proteins that sense shear forces are unknown, but probably consist of cytoskeletal proteins *(29)*. A recent study implicated the structural protein vimentin by showing that flow-mediated vasodilation was greatly suppressed in knockout mice lacking the protein *(30)*. The cellular response to shear stress may be mediated by activation of potassium channels in the cell membrane *(31–34)*. The resulting hyperpolarization causes greater calcium influx *(34,35)*, and therefore the production of NO˙ by eNOS *(32)*. Interestingly, shear stress on an arterial segment increases NO˙ release by a calcium-dependent mechanism only transiently. This is then followed by a calcium-independent phase, which persists as long as the mechanical stimulation, and which may be mediated by tyrosine phosphorylation-signaling cascades *(36–38)*. Shear stress-induced tyrosine phosphorylation of eNOS may lead to translocation between the cytosol and plasma membrane, and changes in function *(38)*. Endothelium is very sensitive to shear forces and can respond to very small changes in shear stress associated with small increases in viscosity *(39)*. Shear stress induced increase in NO˙ explains the

Table 1
Humoral Stimuli of Endothelial Cell Vasoactive Factors

Stimulus	Endothelial cell receptor	References
Acetylcholine	M_2	155,156
Histamine	$H_{1,2}$	157–159
Arginine vasopressin	VP_1	61
Norepinephrine/epinephrine	$Alpha_2$	160
Bradykinin	B_2	161,162
Adenosine di-, triphosphate	P_{2y}	163,164
5-Hydroxytryptamine	$5\text{-}HT_1$	165,166
Thrombin	T	63
Endothelin	ET_B	167
Insulin	I	68,169

arterial dilation observed in vivo caused by increased blood flow or pulsations (39–44). In some blood vessels, prostacylcin release is provoked by shear stress and contributes to the vasodilation. The vasomotor response to shear stress is complex and may be partially attributable to a decrease in endothelin release (45), and an increase in platelet-derived growth factor (PDGF) release from the endothelium (46).

Shear stress, or "flow-mediated," vasodilation is thought to be important for the physiological regulation of blood flow in exercising muscle in which blood flow may vary by more than 100-fold between the resting and exercising state. Resistance arteries dilate in response to metabolism of the ischemic muscle. This causes an increase in flow in the upstream arteries that dilate as a result of the shear-induced NO• release. This positive feedback mechanism can maximally dilate the arteries feeding ischemic or exercising muscle (47,48). For instance, blood flow in exercising forearm muscle is decreased and oxygen extraction augmented by 15–20% by inhibitors of NOS (49). Also, the hyperemia that immediately follows ischemia is decreased by 25% by NOS inhibitors (50). This contribution to total muscle blood flow by shear stress thus contributes importantly to exercise capacity.

It is likely that shear stress mediated tonic regulation of NO• release as mentioned above also regulates blood pressure. This suggestion is based on the hypertensive response to infused NOS inhibitors (21) and the fact that knockout mice lacking eNOS are hypertensive (51,52).

Humoral Stimulation of NO• Release

In addition to those originally reported by Furchgott (1), multiple other substances have been reported to increase the release of NO• from endothelial cells and to therefore mediate vasodilation (see Table 1). Many humoral substances stimulate specific receptors that are present on the endothelial cell surface and that consequently mediate an increase in endothelial cell calcium and NOS. The rise in intracellular calcium results from receptor-dependent activation of G-proteins and phospholipase C, production of inositol trisphosphate, and release of calcium from intracellular stores (53). In addition, the emptying of intracellular stores causes calcium influx into the cytosol (54). The rise in intracellular free calcium also activates calcium-dependent potassium channels, which promote hyperpolarization and greater calcium influx (see Fig. 2).

It is currently uncertain whether or not acetylcholine or bradykinin, which were the first substances noted to stimulate endothelial cell release of NO•, actually do so under in vivo physiological conditions. It has been reported that acetylcholine, when it is released from the motor endplates in skeletal muscle, diffuses to the endothelium of feeder arteries and increases

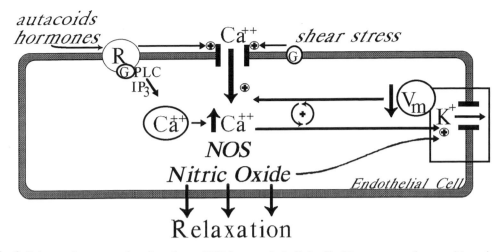

Fig. 2. Scheme demonstrating the release NO˙ from endothelial cells. Hormones and autacoids acting at endothelial membrane receptors (R), or shear stress cause G-protein (G) mediated increases in calcium (Ca^{2+}) influx and phospholipase C (PLC)-mediated hydrolysis of phosphatidyl inositol bisphosphate yielding inositol trisphosphate (IP_3), which releases calcium from intracellular stores. The resulting increase in calcium activates NOS to produce NO˙. The endothelial cell membrane potential (V_m) is hyperpolarized, possibly due to activation of calcium-dependent potassium channels, either by the rise in calcium or by NO˙ acting in an autocrine manner. The resulting hyperpolarization accentuates calcium influx due to the increased electrochemical gradient for calcium, and thereby through positive feedback potentiates the release of NO˙. Revised from Cohen and Vanhoutte (*12*); reproduced by permission of the American Heart Association.

blood flow to help meet metabolic requirements (*55,56*). Although bradykinin is synthesized by endothelial cells, it may not stimulate endothelial cells normally. However, by preventing its degradation, angiotensin-converting enzyme (ACE) inhibitors may increase the levels of bradykinin sufficiently for it to stimulate the release of NO˙ (*57*). Adenosine diphosphate, 5-hydroxytryptamine, and epinephrine, which are released from aggregating platelets stimulate endothelial cells (*58–60*). Vasopressin (*61*) and PDGF (*62*), which are also released from human platelets, may contribute to the NO˙ release that occurs. By virtue of its proteolytic activity, which activates a specific endothelial cell receptor—thrombin—formed during intravascular coagulation may also stimulate NO˙ release (*63,64*). Because many of these substances released by aggregating platelets cause smooth muscle contraction when the endothelium is absent, the normal release of NO˙ is important in determining the vascular response during intravascular hemostasis and thrombosis. Activated leukocytes also release adenosine diphosphate and 5-hydroxytryptamine, as well as leukotrienes and prostaglandin E_2, which can stimulate endothelial cells to release NO˙ (*65,66*).

RELEASE OF NO˙ FROM NITRERGIC VASCULAR NERVES AND PREJUNCTIONAL VASCULAR NEURONAL EFFECTS OF NO˙

Many blood vessels that receive parasympathetic neurogenic input demonstrate nonadrenergic, noncholinergic vasodilation. This includes blood vessels supplying the brain (*67,68*), and internal organs including the heart (*69*), lungs (*70*), and gastrointestinal (*71,72*) and urogenitary systems (*73–76*). Nerves supplying the blood vessels in these regions contain nNOS, the neuronal NOS isoform, and are denoted "nitrergic nerves." These nerves are believed to serve such diverse physiological functions as cerebral vasodilation, facial flushing, and penile erection. Rather than exocytotic release as for other neurotransmitters, it is thought that an increase in neuronal cell calcium on stimulation leads to activation of nNOS, which like eNOS, is calcium-dependent. In tissues supplied by parasympathetic vasodilator nerves, NO• may serve as a primary neurotransmitter, or as one which supplements the actions of vasodilator cotransmitters including acetylcholine or vasoactive intestinal polypeptide. In the microvasculature of the human penis and in the horse penile artery, NO• functions as the principal vasodilator neurotransmitter, with only a supplemental role played by acetylcholine *(73,77)*. Impaired NO• vasodilation in these tissues may contribute to impotence *(78)*. In cerebral arteries, nitrergic nerves mediate vasodilation. Interestingly, this vasodilation is enhanced by acetylcholine which is also released by the nerves and may stimulate the endothelium to release more NO• *(68)*.

In pial cerebral arterioles nNOS plays a compensatory role following chronic eNOS disruption. The pial vasodilation to acetylcholine in eNOS knockout mice is blocked by a selective nNOS inhibitor *(79)*. As in wild-type mice, a soluble guanylyl cyclase inhibitor also blocks the response indicating that NO• produced by nNOS stimulates the same enzyme as in wild-type mice *(79)*. The response to acetylcholine is also prevented by blocking electrical conduction in the nerves, indicating the neuronal origin of the stimulated nNOS *(80)*. The absence of these nNOS characteristics in the acetylcholine response of wild-type mice indicates that its involvement is truly compensatory following targeted disruption of the eNOS gene *(79)*.

In addition to its role as a neurotransmitter in blood vessels, NO• may be a prejunctional regulator of the sympathetic neurotransmitter, norepinephrine. The source of the NO• may be from vascular nerves or the endothelium. An intact endothelium inhibits the release of norepinephrine in blood vessels, an action that may be mediated by NO• and cyclic guanosine 5' monophosphate (cGMP) *(75,81,82)*. As a result of the inhibition exerted by the endothelium on the release of neuronal norepinephrine, the neurogenic vasoconstriction mediated by norepinephrine is attenuated in the isolated rabbit carotid *(81)* and renal *(75)* arteries much more than that to exogenous norepinephrine. This suggests that an important component of the vasodilation mediated by the endothelium is via prejunctional inhibition of peripheral sympathetic vasoconstrictor nerves *(83)*. This effect has been demonstrated in the cutaneous circulation of the rabbit ear where an NOS inhibitor increases neurogenic vasoconstriction *(84)*. There may well be a central neural role for NO•. In the conscious rabbit, an NOS inhibitor augments the increase in renal sympathetic nerve activity caused by angiotensin II *(85)*, suggesting a central or ganglionic neural regulatory role for NO•.

RELEASE OF NO• FROM OTHER CELLS AND INOS

If one records the tone of the isolated rat aorta continuously over several hours, the tone gradually decreases. This effect is greater if the blood vessel is treated with the cytokine interleukin-1 (IL-1) or endotoxin. The decrease in tone can be prevented by inhibiting new mRNA or protein synthesis *(86–88)*, or by glucocorticoids *(89–93)*. The response is explained by the fact that the cytokines or endotoxin rapidly induce iNOS, the inducible NOS, in vascular smooth muscle cells and fibroblasts *(94)*. The iNOS becomes a source of large amounts of NO• derived from L-arginine. Consequently, NOS inhibitors prevent the decrease in tone *(94–99)*. This mechanism may, in large part, explain the hypotension associated with bacterial endotoxin release during sepsis, as the hypotension may be reversed by NOS inhibitors *(100)*.

Release of cytokines by leukocytes in a variety of inflammatory conditions, including arthritis *(101,102)*, may induce iNOS. The high amounts of NO• that iNOS is capable of producing may by itself, or together with the formation of peroxynitrite, contribute to the local inflammatory response *(102)*. The anti-inflammatory properties of glucocorticoids and salicylates *(103)* may be the result of their ability to limit the induction iNOS. The expression of iNOS caused by leukocyte-derived cytokines may also affect vascular reactivity in athero-

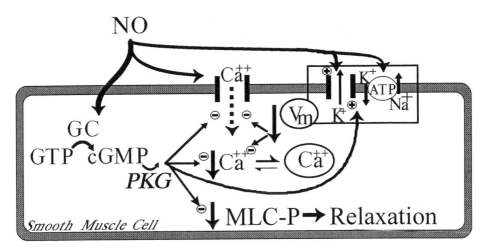

Fig. 3. Scheme showing mechanisms by which vascular smooth muscle cells respond to NO˙. NO˙ stimulates guanylyl cyclase (GC), which converts guanosine triphosphate (GTP) to cyclic guanosine monophosphate (cGMP). The cyclic nucleotide through protein kinase G (PKG) phosphorylates proteins, which favor reuptake of calcium, increase calcium extrusion from the cell, and inhibit calcium influx, all leading to a decrease in intracellular free calcium and relaxation. Cyclic GMP may also hyperpolarize the smooth muscle cell by activating potassium channels. NO˙ may also have direct calcium inhibitory effects, as well as direct hyperpolarizing actions via activation of potassium channels or the Na^+/K^+ ATPase. The resulting hyperpolarization decreases smooth cell calcium levels by inhibiting influx through voltage-dependent calcium channels and favoring the reuptake of calcium into intracellular stores and extrusion of calcium from the cell, resulting in a decrease in intracellular free calcium levels. The decrease in myosin light-chain phosphorylation (MLC-P) by the calcium-dependent myosin light chain kinase relaxes the smooth muscle cell. Revised from Cohen and Vanhoutte *(12)*; reproduced by permission of the American Heart Association.

sclerotic blood vessels. In hypercholesterolemic atherosclerotic rabbits, contractile tone is reduced by arginine, and an NOS inhibitor increases the tone. The removal of the endothelium has no effect on the reduced tone, suggesting that it is NO˙ production by iNOS, which has been demonstrated by immunohistochemistry in atherosclerotic lesions *(104–106)*, that mediates the reduction in tone *(107)*.

MECHANISMS BY WHICH NO˙ REGULATES VASCULAR TONE

In resting smooth muscle there is little or no effect of NO˙ on contractile tone. It follows that vasodilation caused by NO˙ depends on the contractile state of the vascular smooth muscle cell (SMC) (*see* Fig. 3). Because the contractile tone is dictated primarily by the intracellular calcium concentration which, in turn, regulates contractile protein activity, the mechanism of action of NO˙ also involves the regulation of intracellular calcium. The principal action of NO˙ is to prevent a rise in intracellular calcium concentration or to decrease an already elevated level caused by contractile agents or myogenic mechanisms *(108)*. The decrease in intracellular calcium concentration may occur through several processes, including decreasing the influx of extracellular calcium, accelerating the reuptake of calcium into stores within the muscle or increasing extrusion of calcium from the cell. An additional mechanism of NO˙-induced relaxation is the reduction of calcium sensitivity of smooth muscle contractile proteins *(108,109)*. NO˙ relaxes smooth muscle whether it is contracted by depolarization-induced activation of L-type calcium channels or by contractile agonists such as norepinephrine, angiotensin II, or endothelin (cf. Chapter 6). The later mediators contract the smooth muscle by G-protein-mediated phospholipase C stimulation, inositol trisphosphate formation, release of intracellular calcium, and influx of extracellular calcium. As indicated as follows, NO• may inhibit contraction through diverse and redundant mechanisms. The early phylogenetic appearance of endothelium-dependent vasodilation *(110)* suggests the primordial importance of this mechanism, and may help to explain the complexity of the evolved mechanisms.

The Role of cGMP

Before NO• was identified as the mediator of endothelium-dependent relaxation, cGMP was suggested to play a key role. The observations that endothelium-dependent relaxations are associated with a rise in smooth muscle content of cGMP, and that inhibitors of soluble guanylyl cyclase such as methylene blue and LY83583 decrease endothelium-dependent relaxations were important pieces of evidence that the endogenous endothelial mediator was similar to NO• released from nitrovasodilators such as sodium nitroprusside and nitroglycerin *(111)*.

Guanylyl Cyclase

Soluble guanylyl cyclase is a heme-containing enzyme present in all cells. Activation of the enzyme, which has a high affinity for NO•, depends only on the concentration of NO• and the diffusion distance. In fact, guanylyl cyclase stimulation occurs in the endothelial cell when NO• is synthesized *(112)*. When NO• reacts with the iron-containing heme moiety of the enzyme, the enzymatic guanosine conversion of GTP to cGMP increases greatly.

Cyclic GMP-Dependent Protein Kinase (Protein Kinase G)

The most important target of cGMP is cGMP-dependent protein kinase. This kinase is responsible for phosphorylating multiple intracellular targets, which are ultimately responsible for regulating intracellular calcium levels. The sequence of guanylyl cyclase stimulation by NO•, followed by protein kinase G (PKG) activation, and its phosphorylation of calcium regulatory proteins provides for an amplifying signaling mechanism that is very sensitive to very low concentrations of NO•. The multiple protein targets of PKG coordinately decrease vascular tone by differing mechanisms, providing for a mechanism that is not only sensitive but also redundant.

PKG is present in mammalian cells in two isoforms: type I is the form present in smooth muscle and endothelium, and type II is expressed in brain and intestinal epithelium *(113)*. The smooth muscle isoform is a cytosolic enzyme, although it may be associated with intracellular membranes *(113)*. The specificity for activation of the protein kinase by cGMP is sufficiently low that cyclic adenosine monophosphate (cAMP), which is present in cells at levels significantly higher than cGMP, also activates the enzyme. Activation of PKG, in fact, may be more important for cAMP-induced smooth muscle relaxation than is activation of protein kinase A (PKA) *(113)*.

The multiple targets of PKG include calcium ion transporters, which decrease cytosolic calcium by either pumping calcium from the cell or mediating the reuptake of calcium into intracellular stores. This includes the plasma membrane calcium adenosine triphosphate (ATPase), the sodium-calcium exchanger, and the sarcoplasmic reticulum calcium ATPase. The activation of the sarcoplasmic membrane calcium ATPase pump may occur indirectly following phosphorylation of phospholamban by PKG. Phospholamban, when unphosphorylated, is electrostatically bound to the calcium ATPase and inhibits the sequestration of calcium into the intracellular storage pool by the enzyme *(114)*. Phospholamban dissociates from the ATPase when it becomes phosphorylated, and ATPase activity increases. PKG may also interfere with agonist-induced calcium store emptying by limiting the generation of inositol trisphosphate by phospholipase C, or by decreasing the sensitivity of its receptor on the sarcoplasmic reticulum membrane. PKG also apparently inhibits the activity of L-type calcium channels (cf. Chapter 6). This could be by directly inhibiting the calcium channels or may be by activating calcium-dependent potassium channels, which mediate membrane hyperpolarization and thereby inhibit voltage-dependent calcium channels. Although its major effects are those related to a decrease in intracellular calcium, PKG can also directly inhibit the activity of myosin light-chain kinase, which catalyzes the phosphorylation of the light chain of myosin leading to contraction *(115)*. In addition, an increase in myosin light-chain phosphatase activity has been attributed to PKG *(116)*. These latter effects decrease the sensitivity of the contractile apparatus to calcium, and, thus, mediate relaxation. This redundancy of mechanisms ensures that NO• reduces intracellular calcium and relaxes vascular smooth muscle.

The intracellular level of cGMP is regulated by a variety of phosphodiesterases that breakdown the cyclic nucleotide *(117)*. In smooth muscle, a calcium–calmodulin-dependent phosphodiesterase is activated by agonists that elevate intracellular calcium and powerfully decrease NO•-stimulated cGMP levels *(118)*. A cGMP-binding phosphodiesterase is expressed in smooth muscle and may also breakdown the cyclic nucleotide and, therefore, contributes to the regulation of the response to NO• *(117)*.

Cyclic GMP-Independent Mechanisms of NO• Action

The amplifying nature of signaling by NO• through cGMP likely allows for responses to concentrations of NO• below the nanomolar level. Cyclic GMP-independent mechanisms exist, however, that may be responsible for actions of NO• in concentrations in the micromolar range. Because the concentration of NO• released after stimulating endothelial cell receptors reaches this concentration range *(14,119)*, cGMP may not account for all the actions of NO• *(120)*. For instance, blocking the generation of cGMP with the guanylyl cyclase inhibitors, methylene blue, or 1H-[1,2,4]oxadiazolo[4,3-a]quinoxaline-1-one] (ODQ), only partially inhibits relaxation and hyperpolarization of the rabbit carotid artery to acetylcholine *(121)* or NO• *(120–122)*. In addition, in an experimental model of atherosclerosis, endothelium-dependent, NO•-mediated relaxation may be mediated without a measurable rise in cGMP level *(123,124)*. These cGMP-independent responses may be caused by direct activation by NO• of calcium-dependent potassium channels *(122)* or other ion channels and transporters responsible for intracellular calcium homeostasis (cf. Chapter 6). Indeed, in the case of the arteries in which guanylyl cyclase is inhibited, or in that of the atherosclerotic arteries mentioned, the residual relaxations were significantly inhibited by blockers of calcium-dependent potassium channels *(122–124)*. The effect of NO• on these potassium channels has been attributed to nitrosation of redox-sensitive protein thiol groups that regulate the function of the ion channel *(122)*. Another ion transport mechanism that could contribute to hyperpolarization and vascular relaxation, the sodium–potassium ATPase, which also contains redox-sensitive thiol groups, may also be stimulated by NO• without the involvement of cGMP *(125)*.

INTERACTION OF NO• WITH OTHER ENDOTHELIUM-DERIVED VASODILATORS

Eicosanoids

Although NO• is the primary vasodilator released from endothelial cells, it is not the only endogenous substance that may serve this purpose. Prostacyclin was discovered long before NO• as an endothelium-derived vasodilator substance *(2,126)*. The endothelial cell stimulation caused by shear stress and agonists also increases the activity of calcium-dependent phospholipase A_2, which releases arachidonic acid from phospholipids, and via the action of various cyclooxygenases, prostaglandin synthases, lipoxygenases, and epoxygenases produces eicosanoids of the prostaglandin, hydroxyeicosatatraenoic acid (HETE), and epoxyeicostrienoic acid (EET) groups, all of which are vasoactive to some extent. Although any of these endogenous substances potentially may alter, supplement, or supplant the role of NO•, the evidence for a major role of any is not as well established as that of NO•. For instance, the lack of any consistent increase in blood pressure caused by cyclooxygenase inhibitors, like that caused by NOS inhibitors, indicates no prominent role in systemic blood pressure regulation of vasodilatory prostaglandins. Nevertheless, evidence does exist both in vivo and in vitro that eicosanoids, particularly prostacyclin, play a physiological modulatory role in endothelial vasomotor regulation by NO•. For instance, flow-mediated coronary and renal artery vasodilation *(127)*, as well as that caused by endothelium-dependent vasodilators such as acetylcholine, bradykinin, and endothelin *(128–131)*, are, in part, inhibited by cyclooxygenase blockers indicating a role for prostacyclin, the major vasodilatory prostaglandin. In the eNOS knockout mouse, the role of vasodilatory prostaglandins is increased apparently in a compensatory role *(52)*. Thus, in the heart and kidney, released prostacylin supplements the action of NO•. This supplemental role is in part because prostacyclin mediates vasodilation by stimulating cAMP which is a distinct second messenger system to that mediated by NO•. The part played by prostacyclin in endothelium-dependent vasodilation is more heterogeneous across different vascular beds and blood vessels than is that of NO•. This is due to the fact that in some blood vessels prostacylcin is only a weak vasodilator, or as in the rabbit aorta, causes paradoxical vasoconstriction *(132)*.

Endothelium-Derived Hyperpolarizing Factor

In some blood vessels endothelium-dependent vasodilation is thought to be mediated in part by endothelium-dependent hyperpolarization of the smooth muscle *(12)*. The hyperpolarization is thought to limit the activation of L-type, voltage-dependent calcium channels, thus limiting calcium entry and favoring relaxation of the smooth muscle. The importance of hyperpolarization to the overall relaxation therefore depends on the membrane potential and the activity of L-type channels (cf. Chapter 6). The existence of an endothelium-derived vasodilator distinct from NO•, termed endothelium-derived hyperpolarizing factor (EDHF), was suggested in early studies by the fact that inhibitors of NOS and guanylyl cyclase were ineffective in blocking the relaxation or hyperpolarization of endothelium-intact isolated blood vessels to endothelium-dependent vasodilators. Many studies also have attributed the vasodilation which persists in many vascular beds after the administration of NOS inhibitors to a part played by this putative factor *(12)*. The identity of such a distinct factor has been difficult to demonstrate because of the difficulty in measuring a transferable substance *(133)*. One potential candidate is prostacyclin, which does hyperpolarize smooth muscle *(134)*. In the guinea pig coronary artery, part of the endothelium-dependent hyperpolarization is blocked, unlike in most blood vessels, by cyclooxygenase inhibitors, suggesting that prostacyclin could play a role. EETs have also been implicated as EDHF because EET's activate potassium channels, hyperpolarize smooth muscle, and inhibitors of their synthesis do block endothelium-dependent hyperpolarization in some arteries *(135,136)*. Identification of EETs as distinct EDHFs awaits chemical measurements demonstrating that they are released in high enough concentrations by the endothelium to mediate the response. The nonspecific nature of the inhibitors of EET synthesis *(137,138)*, and the fact that endothelium-derived EET's may subserve an autocrine function by regulating the synthesis of NO• *(139)*, makes the direct measurement of alternative endothelium-derived mediators essential to proving this thesis.

The latter point is important given the fact that NOS inhibitors block only a portion of the release of NO• caused by agonists such as acetylcholine *(14,140)*. It has been proposed that the persistent release of NO• after treatment with NOS inhibitors can adequately explain endothelium-dependent hyperpolarization due to the fact that measurement of NO• release from the endothelium closely correlated with both relaxation and hyperpolarization, and that NO• itself has been demonstrated to activate potassium channels *(122)* and to hyperpolarize smooth muscle *(121,141)*. This membrane-hyperpolarizing mechanism may occur through both cyclic GMP-dependent and -independent pathways and be mediated by activation of potassium channels or other electrogenic membrane ion transport (cf. Chapter 6).

REGULATION OF VASCULAR TONE
VIA THE BREAKDOWN OF NO·

NO· was identified as the endothelium-derived vasodilator in part because of its susceptibility to oxidation by superoxide anion *(7,8)*. Although this was first demonstrated by showing that NO· released from endothelium was inactivated by chemicals which generate superoxide anion, it soon became apparent that superoxide anion is constitutively generated by blood vessels, and that the integrity and activity of NO· depends on adequate scavenging of superoxide anion. This is demonstrable in normal blood vessels by inhibiting superoxide dismutase, the superoxide anion-scavenging enzyme. In many vascular disease states, levels of superoxide anion increase and exceed the capacity of superoxide dismutase, and the bioactivity of NO· is thereby decreased *(142,143)* (cf. Chapter 13).

In the normal rabbit aorta, inhibition of superoxide dismutase with diethyldithiocarbamate increases measurable levels of superoxide anion produced by the artery by more than 10-fold *(144)* and inhibits NO·-mediated relaxations *(142,145)*. This indicates that normal arteries produce large amounts of superoxide anion, and that the normal activity of NO· depends on the activity of endogenous superoxide dismutase. Without superoxide dismutase, NO· is inactivated by reaction with superoxide anion to form peroxynitrite, a less active relaxant and highly reactive oxidizing agent *(146–149)*.

Superoxide anion is produced in the rabbit *(150,151)* and rat *(152,153)* aorta and the bovine coronary artery *(154)* by an enzyme(s) that resembles the neutrophil nicotinamide adenine dinucleotide phosphate (NAD(P)H) oxidase, but unlike the neutriphil enzyme is apparently constitutively active. In both the rat *(153)* and rabbit aorta *(150,151)*, the enzyme is localized to the adventitia where its production of superoxide anion has been shown to attenuate NO·-induced relaxation *(153)*. Although little is known about the regulation of this enzyme, its activity is increased by angiotensin II and in hypertension *(152)*.

CONCLUSIONS

NO· was discovered as a biological-signaling molecule by virtue of its fundamental role as a regulator of vascular function. Although diversity exists across species and different vascular beds, NO· is the primary local mediator produced by endothelial cells. Although its release may be stimulated by humoral substances, its primary role as a physiological regulator stems from its constitutive production under the influence of shear forces on the endothelium. Following its diffusion to smooth muscle cells, NO· stimulates diverse mechanisms which effect relaxation by decreasing intracellular free calcium concentration and sensitivity to calcium of contractile proteins. The effect of low concentrations of NO· mediate their effect primarily through amplifying and redundant mechanisms involving cGMP and PKG, whereas higher concentrations mediate other effects through ion channels and transporters. The activity of NO· depends on effective scavenging of tissue superoxide anion, which arises from enzymatic sources within cells and otherwise reacts with and inactivates the vasodilator action of NO·.

REFERENCES

1. Furchgott RF, Zawadzki JV. The obligatory role of the endothelial cells in the relaxation of arterial smooth muscle by acetylcholine. Nature 1980;288:373–376.
2. Moncada S, Vane JR. Pharmacology and endogenous roles of prostaglandin endoperoxides, thromboxane A_2, and prostacyclin. Pharmacol Rev 1979;30:293–331.

3. Furchgott RF. Studies on relaxation of rabbit aorta by sodium nitrate: basis for the proposal that the acid-activatable component of the inhibitory factor from retractor penis is inorganic nitrate and the endothelium-derived relaxing factor is nitric oxide. In: Vanhoutte PM, ed. Vasodilation: Vascular Smooth Muscle, Peptides, Autonomic Nerves, and Endothelium. Raven, New York, 1988, pp. 401–414.

4. Ignarro LJ, Byrns RE, Wood KS. Biochemical and pharmacological properties of endothelium-derived relaxing factor and its similarity to nitric oxide radical. In: Vanhoutte PM, ed. Mechanisms of Vasodilatation. Raven, New York, 1988, pp. 427–435.

5. Ignarro LJ, Buga GM, Wood KS, Byrns RE, Chaudhuri G. Endothelium-derived relaxing factor produced and released from artery and vein is nitric oxide. Proc Natl Acad Sci USA 1987;84:9265–9269.

6. Palmer RM, Ferrigo AG, Moncada S. Nitric oxide release accounts for the biological activity of endothelium-derived relaxing factor. Nature 1987;327:524,525.

7. Rubanyi GM, Vanhoutte PM. Superoxide anions and hyperoxia inactivate endothelium-derived relaxing factor. Am J Physiol 1986;250:H822–H827.

8. Gryglewski RJ, Palmer RM, Moncada S. Superoxide anion is involved in the breakdown of endothelium-derived vascular relaxing factor. Nature 1986;320:454–456.

9. Palmer RM, Ashton DS, Moncada S. Vascular endothelial cells synthesize nitric oxide from L-arginine. Nature 1988;333:664–666.

10. Myers PR, Minor RL Jr, Guerra R Jr, Bates JN, Harrison DG. Vasorelaxant properties of the endothelium-derived relaxing factor more closely resemble S-nitrosocysteine than nitric oxide. Nature 1990; 345:161–163.

11. Mulsch A, Mordvintcev P, Vanin AF, Busse R. The potent vasodilating and guanylyl cyclase activating dinitrosyl-iron(II) complex is stored in a protein-bound form is vascular tissue and is released by thiols. FEBS Lett 1991;294(3):252–256.

12. Cohen RA, Vanhoutte PM. Endothelium-dependent hyperpolarization—beyond nitric oxide and cyclic GMP. Circulation 1995;92:3337–3349.

13. Feelisch M, te Poel M, Zamora R, Deussen A, Moncada S. Understanding the controversy over the identity of EDRF. Nature 1994;368:62–65.

14. Cohen RA, Plane F, Najibi S, Huk I, Malinski T, Garland CJ. Nitric oxide is the mediator of both endothelium-dependent relaxation and hyperpolarization of the rabbit carotid artery. Proc Natl Acad Sci USA 1997;94:4193–4198.

15. Rees DD, Palmer RM, Hodson HF, Moncada S. A specific inhibitor of nitric oxide formation from L-arginine attenuates endothelium-dependent relaxation. Br J Pharmacol 1989;96:418–424.

16. Amezcua JL, Palmer RM, de Souza BM, Moncada S. Nitric oxide synthesized from L-arginine regulates vascular tone in the coronary circulation of the rabbit. Br J Pharmacol 1989;97:1119–1124.

17. Wiklund NP, Persson MG, Gustafsson LE, Moncada S, Hedqvist P. Modulatory role of endogenous nitric oxide in pulmonary circulation in vivo. Eur J Pharmacol 1990;185:123,124.

18. Persson MG, Gustafsson LE, Wiklund NP, Hedqvist P, Moncada S. Endogenous nitric oxide as a modulator of rabbit skeletal muscle microcirculation in vivo. Br J Pharmacol 1990;100:436–466.

19. Lahera V, Salom MG, Miranda-Guardiola F, Moncada S, Romero JC. Effects of N^G-nitro-L-arginine methyl ester on renal function and blood pressure. Am J Physiol 1991;261:F1033–F1037.

20. Vallance P, Collier JG, Moncada S. Effect of endothelium-derived nitric oxide on peripheral arteriolar tone in man. Lancet 1989;28:997–1000.

21. Rees DD, Palmer RM, Moncada S. Role of endothelium-derived nitric oxide in the regulation of blood pressure. Proc Natl Acad Sci USA 1989;86:3375–3378.

22. Martin W, Villani GM, Jothianandan D, Furchgott RF. Selective blockade of endothelium-dependent and glyceryl trinitrate-induced relaxation by hemoglobin and by methylene blue in rabbit aorta. J Pharmacol Exp Ther 1985;232:708–716.

23. Martin W, Furchgott RF, Villani GM, Jothianandan D. Depression of contractile responses in rat aorta by spontaneously released endothelium-derived relaxing factor. J Pharmacol Exp Ther 1986;237: 529–538.

24. Cohen RA, Zitnay KM, Weisbrod RM, Tesfamariam B. Influence of the endothelium on tone and the response of islated pig coronary artery to norepinephrine. J Pharmacol Exp Ther 1988;244:550–555.

25. Tesfamariam B, Weisbrod RM, Cohen RA. Endothelium inhibits responses of rabbit carotid artery to adrenergic nerve stimulation. Am J Physiol 1987;22:H792–H798.

26. Schmidt HH, Pollock JS, Nakane M, Forstermann U, Murad F. Ca^{2+}/calmodulin-regulated nitric oxide synthases. Cell Calcium 1992;13:427–434.

27. Nilius B, Droogmans G, Gericke M, Schwarz G. Nonselective ion pathways in human endothelial cells. In: Siemen D, Hescheler J, eds. Nonselective Cation Channels: Pharmacology, Physiology and Biophysics. Birkhauser Verlag, Basel/Switzerland, 1993, pp. 269–280.

28. Lamontagne D, Pohl U, Busse R. Mechanical deformation of vessel wall and shear stress determine the basal release of endothelium-derived relaxing factor in the intact rabbit coronary vascular bed. Circ Res 1992;70:123–130.

29. Davies PF, Barbee KA. Endothelial cell surface imaging: insights into hemodynamic force transduction. NIPS 1994;9:153–158.

30. Henrion D, Terzi F, Matrougui K, Duriez M, Boulanger CM, Colucci-Guyon E, et al. Impaired flow-induced dilation in mesenteric resistance arteries from mice lacking vimentin. J Clin Invest 1997;100: 2909–2914.

31. Olesen SP, Clapham DE, Davies PF. Haemodynamic shear stress activates a K+ current in vascular endothelial cells. Nature 1988;331:168–170.

32. Jacobs ER, Cheliakine C, Gebremedhin D, Birks EK, Davies PF, Harder DR. Shear activated channels in cell-attached patches of cultured bovine aortic endothelial cells. Pflugers Arch 1995;431:129–131.

33. DePaola N, Gimbrone MA Jr, Davies PF, Dewey CF Jr. Vascular endothelium responds to fluid shear stress gradients. Arterioscler Thromb 1992;12:1254–1257.

34. Cooke JP, Rossitch E Jr, Andon NA, Loscalzo J, Dzau VJ. Flow activates an endothelial potassium channel to release an endogenous nitrovasodilator. J Clin Invest 1991;88·1663–1671.

35. Luckhoff A, Busse R. Calcium influx into endothelial cells and formation of endothelium-derived relaxing factor is controlled by the membrane potential. Pflugers Arch 1990;416:305–311.

36. Fleming I, Bauersachs J, Busse R. Calcium-dependent and calcium-independent activation of the endothelial NO synthase. J Vasc Res 1997;34:165–174. [Abstract]

37. Ayajiki K, Kindermann M, Hecker M, Fleming I, Busse R. Intracellular pH and tyrosine phosphorylation but not calcium determine shear stress-induced nitric oxide production in native endothelial cells. Circ Res 1996;78:750–758. [Abstract]

38. Fleming I, Bauersachs J, Fisslthaler B, Busse R. Ca^{2+}-independent activation of the endothelial nitric oxide synthase in response to tyrosine phosphatase inhibitors and fluid shear stress. Circ Res 1998;82: 686–695.

39. Tesfamariam B, Cohen RA. Inhibition of adrenergic vasoconstriction by endothelial cell shear stress. Circ Res 1988;63:720–725.

40. Tesfamariam B, Halpern W. Modulation of adrenergic responses in pressurized resistance arteries by flow. Am J Physiol 1987;253:H1112–H1119.

41. Kaiser L, Sparks HV Jr. Mediation of flow-dependent arterial dilation by endothelial cells. Circ Shock 1986;18:109–114.

42. Lansman JB. Going with the flow. Nature 1988;331:481,482.

43. Rubanyi GM, Lorenz RR, Vanhoutte PM. Bioassay of endothelium-derived relaxing factor(s): inactivation by catecholamines. Am J Physiol 1985;249:H95–H101.

44. Laurent S, Brunel P, Lacolley P, Billaud E, Pannier B, Safar ME. Flow-dependent vasodilation of the brachial artery in essential hypertension: preliminary report. J Hypertens 1988;6:S182–S184.

45. Malek A, Izumo S. Physiological fluid shear stress causes downregulation of endothelin-1 mRNA in bovine aortic endothelium. Am J Physiol 1992;263:C389–C396.

46. Hsieh H, Li N, Frangos JA. Shear-induced platelet-derived growth factor gene expression in human endothelial cells is mediated by protein kinase C. J Cell Physiol 1992;150:552–558.

47. Meredith IT, Currie KE, Anderson TJ, Roddy MA, Ganz P, Creager MA. Postischemic vasodilation in human forearm is dependent on endothelium-derived nitric oxide. Am J Physiol 1996;270: H1435–H1440.

48. Yamabe H, Okumura K, Ishizaka H, Tsuchiya T, Yasue H. Role of endothelium-derived nitric oxide in myocardial reactive hyperemia. Am J Physiol 1992;263:H8–H14.

49. Gilligan DM, Panza JA, Kicoyne CM, Waclawiw MA, Casino Quyyumi AA. Contribution of endothelium-derived nitric oxide to exercise-induced vasodilation. Circulation 1994;90:2853–2858.

50. Tagawa T, Imaizumi T, Endo T, Shiramoto M, Harasawa Y, Takeshita A. Role of nitric oxide in reactive hyperemia in human forearm vessels. Circulation 1994;90:2285–2290.

51. Huang PL, Huang Z, Mashimo H, Bioch KD, Moskowitz MA, Bevan JA, Fishman MC. Hypertension in mice lacking the gene for endothelial nitric oxide synthase. Nature 1995;377(239), 239–242.

52. Godecke A, Decking UK, Ding Z, Hirchenhain J, Bidmon H-J, Godecke S, Schrader J. Coronary hemodynamics in endothelial NO synthase knockout mice. Circ Res 1998;82:186–194.

53. Freay AD, Johns A, Adams DJ, Ryan US, van Breemen C. Bradykinin and inositol 1,4,5-triphosphate-stimulated calcium release from intracellular stores in cultured bovine endothelial cells. Pflugers Arch 1989;414:377–384.

54. Gericke M, Droogmans G, Nilius B. Thapsigargin discharges intracellular calcium stores and induces transmembrane currents in human endothelial cells. Eur J Physiol 1993;422:552–557.

55. Gath I, Closs EI, Godtel-Ambrust U, Schmitt S, Nakane M, Wessler I, et al. Inducible NO synthase II and neuronal NO synthase I are constitutively expressed in different structures of guinea pig skeletal muscle: implications for contractile function. FASEB J 1996;10:1614–1620.

56. Welsh DG, Segal SS. Acetylcholine release from motor nerves triggers vasodilation. FASEB J 1996; 10:A55

57. Mombouli JV, Vanhoutte PM. Heterogeneity of endothelium-dependent vasodilator effects of angiotensin-converting enzyme inhibitors: role of bradykinin generation during ACE inhibition. J Cardiovasc Pharmacol 1992;20:S74–S83.

58. Cohen RA, Shepherd JT, Vanhoutte PM. Inhibitory role of the endothelium in the response of isolated coronary arteries to platelets. Science 1983;221:273,274.

59. Lopez JA, Armstrong ML, Piegors DJ, Heistad DD. Effect of early and advanced atherosclerosis on vascular responses to serotonin, thromboxane A_2, and ADP. Circulation 1989;79:698–705.

60. Cohen RA, Vanhoutte PM. Platelets, serotonin, and endothelial cells. In: Vanhoutte PM, ed. Serotonin and the Cardiovascular System. Raven, New York, 1985, pp. 105–112.

61. Katusic ZS, Shepherd JT, Vanhoutte PM. Vasopressin causes endothelium-dependent relaxations of the canine basilar artery. Circ Res 1984;55:575–579.

62. Cunningham LD, Brecher P, Cohen RA. PDGF receptors on macrovascular endothelial cells mediate relaxation via nitric oxide in rat aorta. J Clin Invest 1992;89:878–882.

63. Hollenberg MD, Laniyonu AA, Saifeddine M, Moore GJ. Role of the amino- and carboxyl-terminal domains of thrombin receptor-derived polypeptides in biological activity in vascular endothelium and gastric smooth muscle: evidence for receptor subtypes. Mol Pharmacol 1993;43:921–930.

64. Ku DD. Mechanism of thrombin-induced endothelium-dependent coronary vasodilation in dogs: role of its proteolytic enzymatic activity. J Cardiovasc Pharmacol 1986;8:29–36.

65. Mugge A, Lopez JA, Heistad DD, Lichtlen PR. Vasoconstriction in response to activated leukocytes: implications for vasospasm. Eur Heart J 1993;14:87–92.

66. Kaul S, Padgett RC, Heistad DD. Role of platelets and leukocytes in modulation of vascular tone. Ann NY Acad Sci 1994;714:122–135.

67. Gonzalez C, Barroso C, Martin C, Gulbenkian S, Estrada C. Neuronal nitric oxide synthase activation by vasoactive intestinal peptide in bovine cerebral arteries. J Cereb Flow Metab 1997;17:977–984.

68. Jiang F, Li CG, Rand MJ. Mechanisms of electrical field stimulation-induced vasodilation in the guinea-pig basilar artery: the role of endothelium. J Auton Pharmacol 1997;17:71–76.

69. Klimaschewski L, Kummer W, Mayer B, Couraud JY, Preissler U, Philippin B, et al. Nitric oxide synthase in cardiac nerve fibers and neurons of rat and guinea pig heart. Circ Res 1992;71:1533–1537.

70. Haberberger R, Schemann M, Sann H, Kummer W. Innervation pattern of guinea pig pulmonary vasculature depends on vascular diameter. J Appl Physiol 1997;82:426–434.

71. De Man JG, Boeckxstaens GE, Pelckmans PP, De Winter BY, Herman AG, Van Maercke YM. Prejunctional modulation of the nitrergic innervation of the canine ileocolonic junction via potassium channels. Br J Pharmacol 1993;110:559–564.

72. Yamamoto R, Wada A, Asada Y, Niina H, Sumiyoshi A. N-nitro-l-arginine an inhibitor of nitric oxide synthesis, decreases noradrenaline outflow in rat isolated perfused mesenteric vasculature. Naunyn–Schmiedeberg's Arch Pharmacol 1993;347:238–240.

73. Kim N, Azadzoi KM, Goldstein I, Saenz de Tejada I. A nitric oxide-like factor mediates nonadrenergic-noncholinergic neurogenic relaxation of penile corpus cavernosum smooth muscle. J Clin Invest 1991; 88:112–118.

74. Cellek S, Kasakov L, Moncada S. Inhibition of nitrergic relaxations by a selective inhibitor of the soluble guanylate cyclase. Br J Pharmacol 1996;118:137–140.

75. Vials AJ, Crowe R, Burnstock G. A neuromodulatory role for neuronal nitric oxide in the rabbit renal artery. Br J Pharmacol 1997;121:213–220.

76. Cellek S, Moncada S. Nitrergic control of peripheral sympathetic responses in the human corpus cavernosum: a comparison with other species. Proc Natl Acad Sci USA 1997;94:8226–8231.

77. Simonsen U, Prieto D, Sanez de Tejada I, Garcia-Sacristan A. Involvement of nitric oxide in the non-adrenergic non-cholinergic neurotransmission of horse deep penile arteries: role of charybdotoxin-sensitive K(+)-channels. Br J Pharmacol 1995;116:2582–2590.

78. Saenz de Tejada I, Goldstein I, Azadzoi K, Krane RJ, Cohen RA. Impaired neurogenic and endothelium-dependent relaxation of human penile smooth muscle: the pathophysiological basis for impotence in diabetes mellitus. N Engl J Med 1989;320:1025–1030.

79. Meng W, Ayata C, Waeber C, Huang PL, Moskowitz MA. Neuronal NOS-cGMP-dependent ACh-induced relaxation in pial arterioles of endothelial NOS knockout mice. Am J Physiol 1998;274: H411–H415.

80. Meng W, Ma J, Ayata C, Hara H, Huang PL, Fishman MC, Moskowitz MA. Ach dilates pial arterioles in endothelial and neuronal NOS knockout mice by NO-dependent mechanisms. Am J Physiol 1996; 271:H1145–H1150.

81. Cohen RA, Weisbrod RM. Endothelium inhibits norepinephrine release from adrenergic nerves of the rabbit carotid artery. Am J Physiol 1988;254:H871–H878.

82. Greenberg SS, Diecke FP, Peevy K, Tanaka TP. Release of norepinephrine from adrenergic nerve endings of blood vessels is modulated by endothelium-derived relaxing factor. Am. J Hypertens 1990; 3:211–218.

83. Cohen RA, Tesfamariam B, Weisbrod RM. Endothelium inhibits adrenergic neurotransmission. In: Rubanyi GM, Vanhoutte PM. eds. Endothelium–Derived Vasoactive Factors. Karger Publications, New York, 1990, pp. 206–212.

84. Khan F, Palacino JJ, Coffman JD, Cohen RA. Chronic inhibition of nitric oxide production augments skin vasoconstriction in the rabbit ear. J Cardiovasc Pharmacol 1993;22:280–286.

85. Liu J-L, Murakami H, Zucker IH. Angiotensin II-nitric oxide interaction on sympathetic outflow in conscious rabbits. Circ Res 1998;82:496–502.

86. Beasley D, Cohen RA, Levinsky NG. Endotoxin inhibits contraction of vascular smooth muscle in vitro. Am J Physiol 1990;27:H1187–H1192.

87. Beasley D, Cohen RA, Levinsky NG. Interleukin 1 inhibits contraction of vascular smooth muscle. J Clin Invest 1989;83:331–335.

88. Beasley D, Schwartz JH, Brenner BM. Interleukin 1 induces prolonged L-arginine-dependent cyclic guanosine monophosphate and nitrite production in rat vascular smooth muscle cells. J Clin Invest 1991;87:602–608.

89. Szabo C, Thiemermann C, Wu C-C, Perretti M, Vane JR. Attenuation of the induction of nitric oxide synthase by endogenous glucocorticoids accounts for endotoxin tolerance in vivo. Proc Natl Acad Sci USA 1994;91:271–275.

90. Knowles RG, Salter M, Brooks SL, Moncada S. Anti-inflammatory glucocorticoids inhibit the induction by endotoxin of nitric oxide synthase in the lung, liver and aorta of the rat. Biochem Biophys Res Commun 1990;172:1042–1048.

91. Palmer RMJ, Bridge L, Foxwell NA, Moncada S. The role of nitric oxide in endothelial cell damage and its inhibition by glucocorticoids. Br J Pharmacol 1992;105(1):11,12.

92. Wright CE, Rees DD, Moncada S. Protective and pathological roles of nitric oxide in endotoxin shock. Cardiovasc Res 1992;26:48–57.

93. Geller DA, Nussler AK, DiSilvio M, Lowenstein CJ, Sharpiro RA, Wang SC, et al. Cytokines, endotoxin, and glucocorticoids regulate the expression of inducible nitric oxide synthase in hepatocytes. Proc Natl Acad Sci USA 1993;90:522–526.

94. Zhang H, Chobanian AV, Brecher P. Aortic adventitia is a source of nitric oxide: a possible paracrine role. Hypertension 1995;26:569

95. Marsden PA, Ballermann BJ. Tumor necrosis factor a activates soluble guanylate cyclase in bovine glomerular mesangial cells via an L-arginine-dependent mechanism. J Exp Med 1990;172:1843–1852.

96. Werner-Felmayer G, Werner ER, Fuchs D, Hausen A, Reibnegger G, Wachter H. Tetrahydrobiopterin-dependent formation of nitrite and nitrate in murine fibroblasts. J Exp Med 1990;172:1599–1607.

97. Kilbourn RG, Belloni P. Endothelial cell production of nitrogen oxides in response to interferon gamma in combination with tumor necrosis factor, interleukin-1:or endotoxin. J Natl Cancer Inst 1990; 82:772–776.

98. Busse R, Mulsch A. Induction of nitric oxide synthase by cytokines in vascular smooth muscle cells. FEBS Lett 1990;275:87–90.

99. Schini VB, Junquero DC, Scott-Burden T, Vanhoutte PM. Interleukin-1β induces the production of an L-arginine-derived relaxing factor from cultured smooth muscle cells from rat aorta. Biochem Biophys Res Commun 1991;176:114–121.

100. Nava E, Palmer RM, Moncada S. Inhibition of nitric oxide synthesis in septic shock: how much is beneficial? Lancet 1991;338:1555–1557.

101. Sakurai H, Kohsaka H, Liu MF, Higashiyama H, Hirata Y, Kanno K, et al. Nitric oxide production and inducible nitric oxide synthase expression in inflammatory arthritides. J Clin Invest 1995;96:2357–2363.

102. Ialenti A, Moncada S, DiRosa M. Modulation of adjuvant arthritis by endogenous nitric oxide. Br J Pharmacol 1993;110:701–706.

103. Farivar RS, Brecher P. Salicylate is a transcripitional inhibitor of the inducible nitric oxide synthase in cultured cardiac fibroblasts. J Biol Chem 1996;271:31,585–31,592.

104. Sobey CG, Brooks RM II, Heistad DD. Evidence that expression of inducible nitric oxide synthase in response to endotoxin is augmented in atherosclerotic rabbits. Circ Res 1995;77:536–543.

105. Buttery LDK, Springall DR, Chester AH, Evans TJ, Standfield N, Parums DV, et al. Inducible nitric oxide synthase is present within human atherosclerotic lesions and promotes the formation and activity of peroxynitrite. Lab Invest 1996;75:77–85.

106. Luoma JS, Stralin P, Marklund SL, Hiltunen TP, Sarkioja T, Yla-Herttuala S. Expression of extracellular SOD and iNOS in macrophages and smooth muscle cells in human and rabbit atheroclerotic lesions: colocalization with epitopes characteristic of oxidized LDL and peroxynitrite modified proteins. Arterioscler Thromb Vasc Biol 1998;18:157–167.

107. Verbeuren TJ, Bonhomme E, Laubie M, Simonet S. Evidence for induction of non-endothelial NO synthase in aortas of cholesterol-fed rabbits. J Cardiovasc Pharmacol 1993;21:841–845.

108. McDaniel NL, Chen XL, Singer HA, Murphy RA, Rembold CM. Nitrovasodilators relax arterial smooth muscle by decreasing $[Ca^{2+}]_i$ and uncoupling stress from myosin phosphorylation. Am J Physiol 1992;263:C461–C467.

109. Chen XL, Rembold CM. Nitroglycerin relaxes rat tail artery primarily by lowering Ca^{2+} sensitivity and partially by repolarization. Am J Physiol 1996;271:H962–H968.

110. Miller VM, Vanhoutte PM. Endothelium-dependent responses in isolated blood vessels of lower vertebrates. Blood Vessels 1986;23:225–235.

111. Ignarro LJ, Byrns RE, Buga GM, Wood KS. Endothelium-derived relaxing factor from pulmonary artery and vein possesses pharmacologic and chemical properties identical to those of nitric oxide radical. Circ Res 1987;61:866–879.

112. Schini V, Grant NJ, Miller RC, Takeda K. Morphological characterization of cultured bovine aortic endothelial cells and the effects of atriopeptin II and sodium nitroprusside on cellular and extracellular accumulation of cyclic GMP. Eur J Cell Biol 1988;47:53–61.

113. Lincoln TM, Cornwell TL, Komalavilas P, MacMillan-Crow LA, Boerth N. The nitric oxide-cyclic GMP signaling system. In: Barany M. ed. Biochemistry of Smooth Muscle Contraction. Academic, San Diego, CA, 1996, pp. 257–268.

114. Karczewski P, Kelm M, Hartmann M, Schrader J. Role of phospholamban in NO/EDRF-induced relaxation in rat aorta. Life Sci 1992;51:1205–1210.

115. Taylor DA, Bowman BF, Stull JT. Cytoplasmic Ca^{2+} is a primary determinant for myosin phosphorylation in smooth muscle cells. J Biol Chem 1989;264;6207–6213.

116. Wu X, Somlyo AV, Somlyo AP. Cyclic GMP-dependent stimulation reverses G-protein-coupled inhibition of smooth muscle myosin light chain phosphate. Biochem Biophys Res Commun 1996; 220:658–663.

117. Beltman J, Sonnenburg WK, Beavo JA. The role of protein phosphorylation in the regulation of cyclic nucleotide phosphodiesterases. Mol Cell Biochem 1993;127/128:239–253.

118. Smith JB, Lincoln TM. Angiotensin decreases cyclic GMP accumulation produced by atrial natriuretic factor. Am J Physiol 1987;253:C147–C150.

119. Malinski T, Taha Z, Grunfeld S, Patton S, Kapturczak M, Tomboulian P. Diffusion of nitric oxide in the aorta wall monitored in situ by porphyrinic microsensors. Biochem Biophys Res Commun 1993; 193:1076–1082.

120. Weisbrod RM, Griswold MC, Yaghoubi M, Komalavilas P, Lincoln TM, Cohen RA. Evidence that additional mechanisms to cyclic GMP mediate the decrease in intracellular calcium and relaxation of rabbit aortic smooth muscle to nitric oxide. Br J Pharmacol 1998;125:1695–1707.

121. Plane F, Wiley KE, Jeremy JY, Cohen RA, Garland CJ. Evidence that different mechanisms underlie smooth muscle relaxation to nitric oxide and nitric oxide donors in the rabbit isolated carotid artery. Br J Pharmacol 1998;123:1351–1358.

122. Bolotina VM, Najibi S, Palacino JJ, Pagano PJ, Cohen RA. Nitric oxide directly activates calcium-dependent potassium channels in vascular smooth muscle cells. Nature 1994;368:850–853.

123. Najibi S, Cowan CL, Palacino JJ, Cohen RA. Enhanced role of potassium channels in relaxations to acetylcholine in hypercholesterolemic rabbit carotid arteries. Am J Physiol 1994;266:H2061–H2067.

124. Najibi S, Cohen RA. Enhanced role of potassium channels in relaxation of hypercholesterolemic rabbit carotid artery to nitric oxide and sodium nitroprusside. Am J Physiol 1995;269:H805–H811.

125. Gupta S, McArthur C, Grady C, Ruderman NB. Stimulation of vascular Na^+-K^+-ATPase activity by nitric oxide: a cGMP-independent effect. Am J Physiol 1994;266:H2146–H2151.

126. Moncada S, Vane JR, Higgs EA. Human arterial and venous tissues generate prostacyclin (prostaglandin X), a potent inhibitor of platelet aggregation. Lancet 1977;1:18–20.

127. Holtz J, Forstermann U, Pohl U, Giesler M, Bassenge E. Flow-dependent, endothelium-mediated dilation of epicardial coronary arteries in conscious dogs: effects of cyclooxygenase inhibition. J Cardiovasc Pharmacol 1984;6:1161–1169.

128. Lamontagne D, Konig A, Bassenge E, Busse R. Prostacyclin and nitric oxide contribute to the vasodilator action of acetylcholine and bradykinin in the intact rabbit coronary bed. J Cardiovasc Pharmacol 1992;20:652–657.

129. Forstermann U, Hertting G, Neufang B. The importance of endogenous prostaglandins other than prostacyclin, for the modulation of contractility of some rabbit blood vessels. Br J Pharmacol 1984; 81:623–630.

130. Cairns HS, Rogerson ME, Westwick J, Neild GH. Regional heterogeneity of endothelium-dependent vasodilation in the rabbit kidney. J Physiol 1994;436:421–429.

131. Herman F, Magyar K, Chabrier PE, Braquet P, Filep J. Prostacyclin mediates antiaggregatory and hypotensive actions of endothelin in anesthetized beagle dogs. Br J Pharmacol 1989;98:38–40.

132. Vegesna RVK, Diamond J. Elevation of cyclic AMP by prostacyclin is accompanied by relaxation of bovine coronary arteries and contraction of rabbit aortic rings. Eur J Pharmacol 1986;128:25–31.

133. Kauser K, Rubanyi GM. Bradykinin-induced N-nitro-l-arginine-insensitive endothelium-dependent relaxation of porcine coronary arteries is not mediated by bioassayable relaxing substances. J Cardiovasc Pharmacol 1992;20:S101–S104.

134. Parkington HC, Tare M, Tonta MA, Coleman HA. Stretch revealed three components in the hyperpolarization of guinea-pig coronary artery in response to acetylcholine. J Physiol 1993;465:459–476.

135. Campbell WB, Gebremedhin G, Pratt PF, Harder DR. Identification of epoxyeicosatrienoic acids as endothelium-derived hyperpolarizing factors. Circ Res 1996;78:415–423.

136. Hecker M, Bara AT, Bauersachs J, Busse R. Characterization of endothelium-derived hyperpolarizing factor as a cytochrome P_{450}-derived arachidonic acid metabolite in mammals. J Physiol 1994;481: 407–414.

137. Corriu C, Feletou M, Canet E, Vanhoutte PM. Inhibitors of the cytochrome P450-mono-oxygenase and endothelium-dependent hyperpolarizations in the guinea-pig isolated carotid artery. Br J Pharmacol 1996;117:607–610.

138. Biel M, Altenhofen W, Hullin R, Ludwig J, Freichel M, Flockerzi V, et al. Primary structure and functional expression of a cyclic nucleotide-gated channel from rabbit aorta. FEBS Lett 1993;329(1,2):134–138.

139. Graier WF, Simecek S, Sturek M. Cytochrome P_{450} mono-oxygenase-regulated signalling of Ca^{2+} entry in human and bovine endothelial cells. J Physiol 1995;482:259–274.

140. Myers PR, Guerra Jr, Harrison DG. Release of multiple endothelium-derived relaxing factors from porcine coronary arteries. J Cardiovasc Pharmacol 1992;20:392–400.

141. Tare M, Parkington HC, Coleman HA, Neild TO, Dusting GJ. Hyperpolarization and relaxation of arterial smooth muscle caused by nitric oxide derived from the endothelium. Nature 1990;346:69–71.

142. Cohen RA, Pagano PJ. Other factors in endothelial cell dysfunction in hypertension and diabetes. In: Vallance P, Webb D, eds. Endothelial Function in Hypertension. Springer Verlag Berlin, 1997, pp. 39–51.

143. Cohen RA. The role of nitric oxide and other endothelium-derived vasoactive substances in vascular disease. Prog Cardiovasc Dis 1995;38:105–128.

144. Pagano PJ, Tornheim K, Cohen RA. Superoxide anion production by the rabbit thoracic aorta: effect of endothelium-derived nitric oxide. Am J Physiol 1993;265:H707–H712.

145. Omar HA, Cherry PD, Mortelliti MP, Burke-Wolin T, Wolin MS. Inhibition of coronary artery superoxide dismutase attenuates endothelium-dependent and -independent nitrovasodilator relaxation. Circ Res 1991;69(3):601–608.

146. Beckman JS, Beckman TW, Chen JC, Marshall PA, Freeman BA. Apparent hydroxyl radical production by peroxynitrite: Implications of endothelial injury from nitric oxide and superoxide. Proc Natl Acad Sci USA 1990;87:1620–1624.

147. Radi R, Beckman JS, Bush KM, Freeman BA. Peroxynitrite-induced membrane lipid peroxidation: the cytotoxic potential of superoxide and nitric oxide. Arch Biochem Biophys 1991;288:481–487.

148. Hogg N, Darley-Usmar VM, Wilson MT, Moncada S. Production of hydroxyl radicals from the simultaneous generation of superoxide and nitric oxide. Biochemistry J 1992;281:419–424.

149. Darley-Usmar VM, Gogg N, O'Leary VJ, Wilson MT, Moncada S. The simultaneous generation of superoxide and nitric oxide can initiate lipid peroxidation in human low density lipoprotein. Free Radic Res Commun 1992;17:9–20.

150. Pagano PJ, Ito Y, Tornheim K, Gallop P, Cohen RA. An NADPH oxidase superoxide generating system in the rabbit aorta. Am J Physiol 1995;268:H2274–H2280.

151. Pagano PJ, Clark JK, Cifuentes-Pagano ME, Clark SM, Callis GM, Quinn MT. Localization of a constitutively active, phagocyte-like NADPH oxidase in rabbit aortic adventitia: enhancement by angiotensin II. Proc Natl Acad Sci USA 1997;94:14,483–14,488.

152. Fukui T, Ishizaka N, Rajagopalan S, Laursen JB, Capers G 4th, Taylor WR, et al. p22phox mRNA expression and NADPH oxidase activity are increased in aortas from hypertensive rats. Circ Res 1997; 80:45–51.

153. Wang HD, Pagano PJ, Du Y, Cayatte AJ, Quinn MT, Brecher P, et al. Superoxide anion from the adventitia of the rat thoracic aorta inactivates nitric oxide. Circ Res 1998;82:810–818.

154. Mohazzab KM, Kaminski PM, Wolin MS. NADH oxidoreductase is a major source of superoxide anion in bovine coronary artery endothelium. Am J Physiol 1994;266:H2568–H2572.

155. Tsukahara T, Hongo K, Kassell NF, Ogawa H. Characterization of muscarinic cholinergic receptors on the endothelium and the smooth muscle of the rabbit thoracic aorta. J Cardiovasc Pharmacol 1989; 13:870–878.

156. Hynes MR, Banner W Jr, Yamamura HI, Duckles SP. Characterization of muscarinic receptors of the rabbit ear artery smooth muscle and endothelium. J Pharmacol Exp Ther 1986;238:100–105.

157. Niimi N, Noso N, Yamamoto S. The effect of histamine on cultured endothelial cells. A study of the mechanism of increased vascular permeability. Eur J Pharmacol 1992;221:325–331.

158. Hide M, Fukui H, Watanabe TX, Wada H, Yamamoto S. Histamine H^1-receptor in endothelial and smooth muscle cells of guinea-pig aorta. Eur J Pharmacol 1988;148:161–170.

159. Van de Voorde J, Leusen I. Influence of prostaglandin-synthesis inhibitors on carbachol-and histamine-induced vasodilatation in perfused rat hindquarters. Pflugers Arch 1983;397:290–294.

160. Miller VM, Vanhoutte PM. Endothelial alpha–2-adrenoceptors in canine pulmonary and systemic blood vessels. Eur J Pharmacol 1985;118:123–129.

161. Keravis TM, Nehlig H, Delacroix M-F, Regoli D, Hilley CR, Stoclet JC. High-affinity bradykinin B_2 binding sites sensitive to nucleotides in bovine aortic endothelial cells. Eur J Pharmacol 1991;207: 149–155.

162. Sung C-P, Arleth AJ, Shikano K, Berkowitz BA. Characterization and function of bradykinin receptors in vascular endothelial cells. J Pharmacol Exp Ther 1988;247:8–13.

163. Boeynaems JM, Pearson JD. P_2 purinoceptors on vascular endothelial cells: physiological significance and transduction mechanisms. TIPS 1990;11:34–37.

164. Houston DA, Burnstock G, Vanhoutte PM. Different P_2-purinergic receptor subtypes of endothelium and smooth muscle in canine blood vessels. J Pharmacol Exp Ther 1987;241:501–506.

165. Houston DS, Vanhoutte PM. Comparison of serotonergic receptor subtypes on the smooth muscle and endothelium of the canine coronary artery. J Pharmacol Exp Ther 1988;244:1–10.

166. Schoeffter P, Hoyer D. 5-Hydroxytryptamine (5-HT)-induced endothelium-dependent relaxation of pig coronary arteries is mediated by 5-HT receptors similar to the 5-HT_{1D} receptor subtype. J Pharmacol Exp Ther 1990;252:387–395.

167. Karaki H, Sudjarwo SA, Hori M, Sakata K, Urade Y, Takai M, et al. ET_B receptor antagonist, IRL 1038, selectively inhibits the endothelin-induced endothelium-dependent vascular relaxation. Eur J Pharmacol 1993;231:371–374.

168. Zeng G, Quon MJ. Insulin-stimulated production of nitric oxide is inhibited by wortmannin. J Clin Invest 1996;98:894–898.

169. Hu RM, Levin ER, Pedram A, Frank HJ. Insulin stimulates production and secretion of endothelin from bovine endothelial cells. Diabetes 1993;42:351–358.

170. Vanhoutte PM, Cohen RA. Effects of acetylcholine on the coronary artery. Fed Proc 1984;43:2878–2880.

8

Nitric Oxide and Platelet-Mediated Hemostasis

Elisabeth M. Battinelli and Joseph Loscalzo

Nitric oxide (NO•) inhibits platelet function by limiting platelet adhesion and aggregation, as well as disaggregating previously aggregated platelets *(1–5)*. Under resting conditions, blood flow stimulates the endothelium to produce NO•, which regulates platelet activity *(6–8)*. NO• activates soluble guanylyl cyclase leading to a concomitant increase in the production of cyclic guanosine monophosphate (cGMP), the principal mediator of NO•'s effects. As a consequence of disease states, the amount of NO• being produced by the endothelium and the platelet itself may be adversely altered, resulting in impairment in platelet aggregation and function. In this chapter we provide evidence for the importance of NO• in regulating platelet function and hemostasis, and we also illustrate the role of NO• deficiency in thrombotic disease.

AN INTRODUCTION TO PLATELET BIOLOGY

Platelets were first recognized in 1881 by Bizzozero, who is credited with describing their adhesive characteristics and their involvement in thrombosis and blood coagulation *(9)*. Morphologically, the platelet appears as a colorless, anucleate cell that is discoid in shape in the resting state. In response to blood vessel injury or exposure to a foreign surface, platelets rapidly undergo activation, adhesion, and aggregation reactions, thereby promoting hemostasis *(see* Fig. 1). These reactions are modulated by a myriad of excitatory and inhibitory effectors that initiate intracellular signal casades within the platelet.

Platelet Formation

The progenitor cell of the platelet is the megakaryocyte. Like all hematopoietic cells, it is produced from a pluripotent stem cell that gives rise to progenitors that are committed to the megakaryocytic cell lineage. As these early megakaryocytic cells mature, they cease cell division, yet continue to replicate their DNA by a process that is termed endomitosis *(10)*. Endomitotic replication produces mature megakaryocytes with polyploid nuclei (ranging from 4–64 *N*) *(11)*. As the megakaryocyte matures, it produces platelet-specific products that are packaged into granules. The α-granule is the most abundant granule and contains many proteins that are essential for platelet function, including fibrinogen, von Willebrand Factor (vWF), platelet factor 4, β-thromboglobulin, platelet-derived growth factor (PDGF), and P-selectin *(12)*. The dense granules are storage sites for serotonin (5-HT), adenosine diphosphate (ADP), adenosine triphosphate (ATP), and Ca^{2+}. As the mature megakaryocyte moves through the sinusoids in the bone marrow, the cytoplasm fragments along the platelet fields,

From: *Contemporary Cardiology, vol. 4: Nitric Oxide and the Cardiovascular System*
Edited by: J. Loscalzo and J. A. Vita © Humana Press Inc., Totowa, NJ

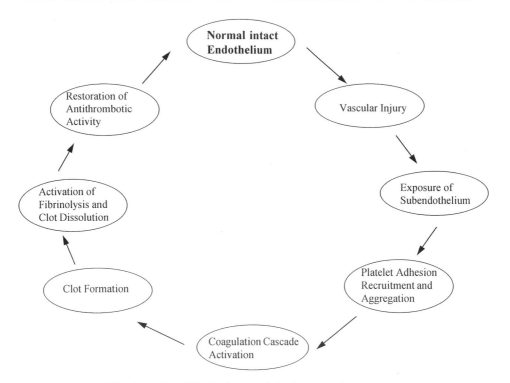

Fig. 1. A simplified scheme of the hemostatic response.

formed by the demarcation membrane system, which results in platelet production by cytoplasmic budding *(13)*. Controversy has arisen as to the actual site of platelet formation, however, as megakaryocytes have also been observed in the pulmonary circulation *(14)*. An alternative theory of platelet production suggests that the megakaryocytic cytoplasm may break off as the megakaryocytes travel through the rapidly flowing pulmonary circulation *(11)*. Regardless of the site, production of platelets is a regulated process in which the hematopoietic growth factor, thrombopoietin (TPO), is believed to be the main mediator *(15)*. Upon exposure to TPO, megakaryocyte size and number greatly increase, thereby producing many more mature megakaryocytes that are available for platelet production *(15)*.

Mechanism of Platelet Activation

Platelet activation occurs in three stages: exposure to a platelet agonist, generation of second messengers, and initiation of a response cascade that includes cytoskeletal rearrangement, shape change, storage granule release, and, ultimately, platelet aggregation.

Many factors can initiate platelet activation including collagen, a constituent of the subendothelium matrix; vWF, a plasma protein; thrombin, a plasma protease; hormones like epinephrine or vasopressin; and products of the platelet's own metabolism, such as ADP and thromboxane A_2 (TXA_2) *(16)*. Agonists can initiate platelet activation by binding to receptors present on the surface of the platelet initiating biochemical cascades (*see* Fig. 2). The structures of many of the agonist receptors have been characterized, and structural analysis has classified many of them as GTP-binding proteins (G proteins) *(17)*. There are as many as nine different types of G proteins associated with the surface of a platelet, and these are grouped into three functionally distinct types: G_p, which couples activating ligand–receptor interations to stimulation of phosphoinositide-specific phospholipase C (PLC); G_s, which couples inhibitory ligand–receptor interactions to activation of adenylyl cyclase; and G_i, which couples platelet agonist–receptor interactions to inhibition of adenylyl cyclase *(18)*. Presumably, the difference between strong and weak agonists is due to the second messenger

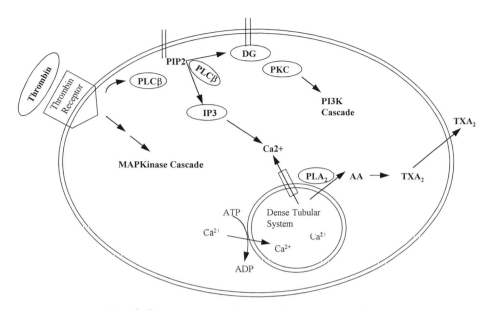

Fig. 2. Biochemical pathways of platelet activation.

systems they recruit within the platelet. Strong agonists, such as thrombin and collagen, are known to stimulate phosphoinositide hydrolysis and eicosanoid formation with direct increases in cytosolic free Ca^{2+}. These processes are mediated through PLC and phospholipase A_2 (PLA$_2$). The weak agonists, including ADP and epinephrine, by contrast, do not initiate phosphoinositide hydrolysis and are mainly regulated through PLA$_2$-mediated signal cascades (18).

Phosphoinositide-specific PLC hydrolyzes phosphotidylinositol 4,5-bisphosphate (PIP$_2$) to form two second messengers, inositol 1,4,5-triphosphate (IP$_3$) and sn-1,2-diacylglycerol (DAG). These molecules then diverge to modulate different biochemical pathways within the platelet. IP$_3$ binds to receptors on the dense tubular system resulting in release of Ca^{2+}, thereby increasing the level of free cytosolic Ca^{2+}. DAG leads to initiation of another biochemical cascade within the platelet through the activation of protein kinase C (PKC). Both Ca^{2+} release and PKC activation can independently result in platelet activation, but together they act synergistically to stimulate platelet secretion and release of arachidonic acid from membrane phospholipids via PLA$_2$ (19).

Calcium functions as a second messenger within the platelet. In the resting state the platelet concentration of Ca^{2+} is 50–100 nM, but on activation the level rises, depending on the strength of the agonist used, to as high as 1 mM (19). Normally, platelet Ca^{2+} concentration is kept low due to the limited permeability of the platelet plasma membrane to Ca^{2+} and the action of Ca^{2+}–Mg^{2+} ATPase pumps within the dense tubular system (18). As the calcium level rises in the activated platelet, many Ca^{2+}-dependent enzymes are activated, including PLA$_2$, PLC, calpain, phosphorylase kinase, and myosin light-chain kinase.

Protein kinase C is a Ca^{2+}-dependent, serine–threonine-specific protein kinase that functions in signal transduction cascades within the platelet. In a stimulated platelet, DAG triggers the translocation of inactive PKC to the plasma membrane where it becomes activated in the presence of Ca^{2+} and phosphatidylserine. DAG functions principally by increasing the affinity of PKC for Ca^{2+}. Stimulation of PKC leads to activation of the fibrinogen receptor glycoprotein (GP)IIb/IIIa, which binds fibrinogen. Owing to its bivalent structure, fibrinogen can form crossbridges between two activated platelets to support aggregation. Perhaps most importantly, PKC mediates platelet activation through its role in activating PLA$_2$ (19).

PLA$_2$ is responsible for the release of arachidonic acid (AA) from the plasma membrane. The role of PKC in this activation process may be to phosphorylate and inactivate platelet lipocortin, which normally inhibits PLA_2, thus enhancing PLA_2-mediated AA release *(17)*. It has also been postulated that a second level of control exists to modulate PLA_2 activity through a Na^+/H^+ exchanger. This antiporter is important in regulating the pH of the platelet, and it has been shown that platelet cytosolic alkalinization can lead to activation of PLA_2 *(19)*. Upon release from phospholipids by PLA_2, AA is rapidly converted into many eicosanoids through the actions of the cyclooxygenase and lipooxygenase pathways. In the platelet, cyclooxygenase oxygenates AA to the prostaglandin endoperoxides, PGG_2 and PGH_2, which are then converted to TXA_2, a potent agonist of platelet function.

As the process of platelet activation begins, the platelet changes from its normal discoid shape to a more spherical configuration, after which multiple pseudopodial projections form. As this shape change occurs, the platelet granules migrate toward the center of the cell and contraction of the cellular cytoskeleton ensues, resulting in the granule release reaction *(17)*. Secretion of granular contents from the platelet appears to occur through a unique form of exocytosis in which granules, instead of moving towards the periphery of the cell and fusing with the plasma memebrane, move to the center of the cell and fuse with the open canalicular system to form a route by which the constituents of the granules are delivered extracellularly *(12,20)*. Granule release occurs when the cytoskeletal microtubule coil contracts. Ca^{2+}-dependent phosphorylation cascades prepare actin and myosin filaments for contractile interactions. Activation of Ca^{2+}-dependent calpains results in proteolytic cleavage of actin binding proteins making actin filaments available to crosslink myosin that simultaneously has been activated by Ca^{2+}-dependent myosin light-chain kinase *(17)*. The actin–myosin filaments are linked to the platelet surface receptor, GPIb/IX, whose ligand, vWF, is found in exposed subendothelial matrix, is localized to Weibel–Palade bodies of endothelial cells, and is released by activated platelets themselves.

The molecules secreted during the release reaction are able to regulate the platelet response. The contents of the dense granules and the molecules that are synthesized from platelet membrane phospholipids via PLA_2 are short-acting, rapidly secreted mediators *(18)*. Their effects, therefore, are locally active, with a tendency to modulate the actions of surrounding platelets as well as the tone of the vascular smooth muscle in its vicinity. The most rapidly released molecule is ADP, which is a potent agonist for the recruitment of additional platelets to the primary hemostatic plug. Hydrolysis of plasma membrane phospholipids and concomitant formation of the arachidonate-derived mediator TXA_2 results in further platelet recruitment. Slower-acting mediators are released from the α-granules, including PDGF, which is essential for modulating growth and gene expression of cells in the blood vessel wall; factors V and VIII, which are important in the coagulation cascade; and P-selectin *(12)*.

Mechanisms of Platelet Adhesion, Aggregation, and Recruitment

Platelets adhere to the subendothelial matrix by the binding of integrin glycoproteins, found on the platelet surface, to the connective tissue components of the matrix. These glycoproteins include GPIb/IX/V, GPIa/IIa, and GPIIb/GPIIIa. GPIb complexes noncovalently with GPIX and GPV to form a surface receptor for the adhesion of platelets to the subendothelium via vWF, linking the platelet integrin to collagen in the subendothelium *(21)*. Von Willebrand factor undergoes a conformational change that is essential for maintaining the contact between the platelet and subendothelium. The platelet is also able to bind directly to collagen via the GPIa/IIa receptor.

After adhering to the subendothelial matrix, the platelet initiates the release reaction, secreting the contents of its granules as discussed before. Through the release of ADP, 5-HT, and the formation of TXA_2, more platelets are recruited to the platelet plug. Platelet recruitment occurs through the GPIIb/GPIIIa complex, also known as the fibrinogen receptor, which is activated by a calcium-dependent conformational change *(22,23)*. Two RGD sequences in the fibrinogen molecule's A α-chain and a dodecapeptide sequence near the carboxytermi-

Table 1
Characterization of Inducible and Constitutive Nitric Oxide Synthases

NOS isoform	iNOS	eNOS
Calcium dependence	No	Yes
Calmodulin dependence	Yes	Yes
Cell prototype	Macrophage	Endothelial cells
Subcellular localization	Cytosolic	Membrane associated
Expression	17q11.2–1.12	7q35–q36

nus of the γ-chain directly interact with platelets via the GPIIb/IIIa receptor *(24)*. Simultaneously, the platelet aggregate activates the coagulation cascade via the assembly of prothrombinase on the platelet surface. Subsequently, further platelet aggregation is initiated by this series of reactions through the production of yet another platelet agonist, thrombin *(25)*. Thrombin, a serine protease, cleaves the Aα and Bβ chains of fibrinogen to form fibrin. Fibrin is stabilized through transamidination reactions by factor XIIIa, which itself is generated by the action of thrombin on factor XIII *(25)*. The production of a fibrin meshwork is essential for the stability of the newly formed platelet aggregate.

Endothelial Antithrombotic Mechanisms

Under normal circumstances, platelet activation and aggregation are suppressed by endothelial products that inhibit the platelet response, including cyclooxygenase, and lipooxygenase pathway products, such as prostacyclin and 13-hydroxyoctadecadienoic acid (13-HODE); ectonucleotidase ADP diphosphohydrolase (ecto-ADPase); and NO· *(4,26,27)*. Prostacyclin has been shown to inhibit platelet aggregation *(3)*, whereas 13-HODE regulates platelet adhesion to the vessel wall, modulating integrin receptor expression *(27)*. The ectonucleotidases(s) metabolize ADP to AMP and adenosine, resulting in a decrease in platelet recruitment and activity by the dinucleotide agonist *(28)*; this molecule has recently been identified as CD39 *(29)*. The role of NO· as an inhibitor of platelet aggregation is discussed below.

The endothelium further limits thrombus formation by degrading prothrombotic vasoactive amines present in the blood, by inactivating thrombin, and by inducing expression of thrombomodulin. Thrombomodulin acts as a thrombin-binding surface protein that facilitates thrombin-dependent activation of protein C, a naturally occurring anticoagulant that degrades factors Va and VIIIa *(30)*. Endothelial surface glycosaminoglycans that catalyze the binding of the anticoagulant serine protease inhibitors (serpins) antithrombin III and heparin cofactor II to specific coagulation proteins, such as thrombin, attenuate coagulation *(31)*. Plasmin, the fibrinolytic counterpart to thrombin, is produced when it is converted from its plasma zymogen plasminogen by plasminogen activators, including tissue-type plasminogen activator (t-PA) and the urokinase-type plasminogen activators, both of which are serine proteases that are produced by the endothelium. Plasmin, once formed, cleaves fibrin leading to the dissolution of the fibrin clot or the thrombus.

PLATELETS AND NO·

NO· synthesis occurs in both the vascular endothelium and the platelet. NO· is produced when the terminal guanidino nitrogen of L-arginine undergoes a five-electron oxidation to form L-citrulline and NO· *(32,33)*. This reaction is catalyzed by the NO· synthase (NOS) family of enzymes of which there are two isoform classes, constitutive NOS (cNOS) and inducible NOS (iNOS, *NOS*2 gene product). The differences between these isoforms are shown in Table 1. Constitutive NOS is found in vascular endothelial cells (eNOS, *NOS*3 gene product) as well as in neuronal cells (nNOS, *NOS*1 gene product), and is regulated by Ca^{2+}

and calmodulin. Ca^{2+} is released from intracellular stores via binding of inositol 1,4,5-tri-phosphate (IP_3) to receptors on the endoplasmic reticulum. Released Ca^{2+} is then free to interact with calmodulin, and the Ca^{2+}-calmodulin complex activates cNOS *(34–37)*. The production of NO• by cNOS is, therefore, rapid, transient, and continuous until the Ca^{2+} level returns to baseline. Inducible NOS is expressed in many cell types including the macrophage and the neutrophil *(38,39)*. Inducible NOS is stimulated by exposure to bacterial endotoxin or cytokines *(40–42)*, and its activity is regulated at the transcriptional level and, therefore, not dependent on Ca^{2+} concentration *(43)*. The production of NO• by iNOS is delayed in comparison to production by cNOS, but the amounts of NO• generated by this isoform far exceed that of cNOS.

NO• binds to the heme moiety of guanylyl cyclase and induces a conformational change that displaces the iron out of the plane of the porphyrin ring *(44)*. This effect results in the enzymatic conversion of guanosine 5'-triphosphate (GTP) to guanosine 3',5'-monophos-phate (cGMP) with concomitant stimulation of cGMP-dependent protein kinase. Cyclic GMP-dependent protein kinase phosphorylates intracellular enzyme targets resulting in activation of intracellular signaling molecule cascades.

NO• and Platelet Aggregation

NO• suppresses platelet adhesion to the endothelium thereby preventing platelet recruit-ment and aggregation, as well. When stimulated with bradykinin, endothelial cells release NO• in amounts sufficient to inhibit platelet adhesion *(6,45)*. Immediately downstream from where NO• is released, platelet aggregation is diminished, suggesting that the endothelium is responsible for regulating platelets in its vicinity as opposed to platelets at a distance from the endothelial source of NO• *(8)*. Cholinergic stimulation and substance P can also stimulate the release of NO• from endothelial cells, which is then available to inhibit platelet aggregation induced by collagen or ADP *(46)*. NO• can also disaggregate preformed platelet aggregates that come in contact with the endothelial surface *(3)*. Freedman and colleagues have demonstrated that platelet-derived NO• inhibits platelet recruitment to a growing platelet thrombus *(47)*.

Once NO• is released from the endothelium or the platelet, it can react with thiols in the presence of oxygen to produce *S*-nitrosothiols. In plasma, *S*-nitrosothiols are a principal redox state of NO_x *(48)*. In contrast to free NO•, *S*-nitrosothiols appear to be a more stable source of bioactive NO_x and, therefore, *S*-nitrosothiols have been postulated to be a storage form of bioactive NO_x. *S*-Nitrosothiols activate platelet soluble guanylyl cyclase and elevate cGMP levels, leading to inhibition of platelet aggregation *(49)*. Mendelsohn and colleagues showed that *S*-nitroso-N-acetylcysteine, an *S*-nitrosothiol compound, decreases the intracellular cal-cium flux in response to ADP stimulation leading to inhibition of fibrinogen binding in activated platelets *(50)*. Keaney and colleagues demonstrated that endogenous NO• can react with serum albumin to form *S*-nitroso-serum albumin, which has antiplatelet properties *(51)*. Simon and colleagues established that the platelet surface is able to facilitate the release of NO• from *S*-nitrosothiols by transnitrosation reactions *(52)*. Recently, it has been shown that the ability of *S*-nitrosothiols to limit platelet responses is dependent on the presence of copper. Gordge and colleagues showed that inhibition of platelet aggregation by *S*-nitroso-glutathione (GSNO) is diminished by incubation with the copper(I)-specific chelator batho-cuproine disulfonic acid (BCS) *(53)*.

Other molecules present within the vicinity of NO• can attenuate NO•'s ability to limit the platelet response. Superoxide anions produced by activated or dysfunctional endothelial cells, leukocytes, activated platelets, and smooth muscle cells can inactivate NO• through the formation of peroxynitrite, which is further metabolized to nitrate. The highly reactive peroxynitrite causes cellular toxicity through lipid peroxidation and nitrosation of protein tyrosyl residues. Unlike NO•, peroxynitrite does not have antiplatelet properties *(54)*. Super-oxide dismutase (SOD) is an enzyme that catalyzes the dismutation of superoxide into water and hydrogen peroxide, thereby limiting the amount of superoxide available to react with NO*. SOD, therefore, potentiates the antiplatelet activity of NO* to prevent adhesion and aggregation of platelets induced by thrombin in vivo, as demonstrated by Meng and colleagues who showed that administration of SOD to damaged and stenotic carotid arteries led to a decrease in thrombus formation at the site of vascular injury (55).

Other molecules produced by the endothelial cell and the platelet work in concert with NO* to potentiate inhibition of platelet activation and aggregation, including PGI_2, PGD_2, and t-PA (1,2,56). No factor alone, however, is able to limit fully the activated-platelet response. Instead, synergistic interactions of several factors optimally limit platelet aggregation. Prostacyclin, whose synthesis is stimulated by mechanical injury, PDGF, and bradykinin, is a potent inhibitor of aggregation and a very weak inhibitor of platelet adhesion (57). It has limited or no antiadhesive properties, which do not potentiate those of NO* (3). Prostacyclin's ability to limit platelet activation is dependent on cGMP in contrast to its usual mechanism of action through cAMP-dependent responses. NO* and prostacyclin do appear, however, to act synergistically to limit platet aggregation and disaggregation (58,59).

Because both the platelet and the endothelium produce factors that are necessary for hemostasis, our group recently investigated the importance of platelet-derived NO*, in contrast to endothelial-derived NO*, in the hemostatic response. We have characterized platelet function in knockout mice lacking eNOS, the NOS3 gene product. Using a NO*-selective microelectrode, we showed that ADP-stimulated platelets from NOS3-deficient (NOS3–/–) mice were unable to release NO*, in contrast to platelets from wild-type mice. Bleeding times in the NOS3 knockout mice were significantly decreased compared with those in wild-type mice. To determine the contribution of endothelial vs. platelet-derived NO* to the bleeding time, isolated platelets from either NOS3-deficient or wild-type mice were transfused into thrombocytopenic NOS3-deficient mice and the bleeding times were measured. Transfusion with platelets from NOS3 knockout mice significantly decreased the bleeding times in these animals compared to transfusion with platelets from wild-type mice, suggesting that platelet-derived NO* is essential for maintenance of the normal hemostatic response (60).

Platelet Isoforms of NOS

Isoforms of NO* synthase have been characterized in platelets. Controversy, however, exists as to which isoforms are, indeed, present, and as to the biochemical characteristics of these isoforms. An eNOS-like isoform has been isolated from platelets and appears to require similar cofactors as eNOS itself. Muruganandam and colleagues (61) suggested that the molecular size of this constitutively expressed NOS is 80 kDa, in contrast to the 130-kDa protein found in endothelial cells, attributable either to differential splicing or posttranslational modifications. Others, however, have not found this size differential and believe that platelet eNOS is similar in size to endothelial eNOS.

An isoform of NOS2 has also been characterized in platelets. Because the platelet is anucleate with a minimal pool of mRNA, and thus able to synthesize only modest amounts of protein, most platelet proteins represent residual megakaryocyte protein pools (62). Megakaryocytes express both constitutive and inducible NOSs (63). Wallerath and colleagues, however, have shown that platelets are heterogeneous with respect to iNOS protein expression, which is substantiated by their finding that megakaryocytes are also variable in their expression with only 30% of bone marrow megakaryocytes characterized as containing iNOS (64). Because iNOS induction is dependent on cytokine exposure, the population differences observed are dependent on the immediate environment of the megakaryocyte. The molecular mass of platelet iNOS was determined by Chen and Mehta to be 200 kDa (65). These authors believe that in unstimulated platelets iNOS exists in an inactivated form complexed with an unknown protein to form the 200-kDa unit. Wallerath and colleagues, however, have characterized platelet iNOS as a 130-kDa protein (64).

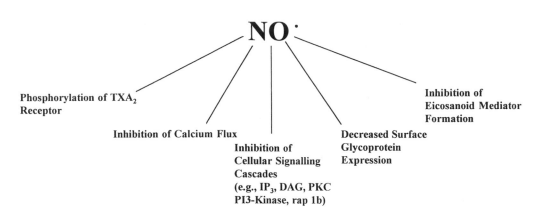

Fig. 3. NO•'s mechanisms of platelet inhibition.

Although there is much controversy as to the isoforms of NOS present in platelets, it is clear that platelets synthesize and release NO• *(66)*. Stimulation of platelet NO• synthase leads to activation of soluble guanylyl cyclase and, ultimately, to inhibition of platelet aggregation *(67)*.

NO•'s Mechanism of Action in Platelets

Production of NO• via L-arginine has been shown to inhibit the platelet aggregation response in vivo and in vitro (Fig. 3). A single, saturable, sodium-independent transporter system for movement of L-arginine into human platelets has been postulated *(68)*. Radomski *(67)* showed that L-arginine inhibited platelet aggregation induced by ADP and arachidonic acid. Inhibition of thrombin-induced aggregation, however, occurred only when prostacyclin and cGMP phosphodiesterase inhibitors were also present.

NO•'s ability to regulate cGMP and cGMP-dependent protein kinase has been postulated as its principal mechanism of inhibition of platelet activity (Fig. 3). An inhibitor of guanylyl cyclase, 1H-(1,2,4) oxadiazolo (4,3-a) quinoxalin-1-one, blocks these cGMP-dependent effects, resulting in an increase in platelet aggregation *(69)*. Inhibition of cGMP-mediated platelet responses can also occur through cyclic nucleotide phosphodiesterases, which can degrade cGMP. Radomski and colleagues showed that M + B 22984, a cGMP phosphodiesterase inhibitor, can potentiate L-arginine-mediated antiplatelet effects *(67)*.

One mechanism by which cGMP may regulate aggregation is through inhibition of receptor-mediated calcium influx in platelets. An increase in soluble guanylyl cyclase leads to a reduction of intracellular Ca^{2+} in platelets through cGMP-mediated inhibition of Ca^{2+} release from intracellular stores, an increased rate of Ca^{2+} extrusion, and decreased Ca^{2+} entry from extracellular stores *(70–74)*. Trepakova and colleagues have established that NO• accelerates sarcoplasmic/endoplasmic reticulum Ca^{2+}-ATPase-dependent refilling of the Ca^{2+} store *(75)*. As a result of this effect, less Ca^{2+} is available for the platelet response, thereby limiting aggregation. Pernollet and colleagues have shown that NO• slows down the initial rate of ATP-dependent Ca^{2+} uptake by as much as 80% *(76)*. The authors also demonstrated that NO• can induce an increase in the basal concentrations of Ca^{2+} in unstimulated platelets through a decrease in Ca^{2+} uptake by intracellular storage granules *(76)*. Their work is supported by Sang and colleagues who showed that addition of NO• to unstimulated platelets can lead to an increase in the cytosolic Ca^{2+} level by as much as 48% because of a decrease in Ca^{2+} uptake *(77)*.

Recently, an alternative mechanism by which NO• may modulate platelet aggregability via cGMP has been proposed. Reep and Lapetina have suggested that phosphorylation of the signaling molecule rap 1b in platelets is induced by NO• activation of guanylyl cyclase and cGMP-dependent protein kinase *(78)*. They showed that incubation with *S*-nitroso-serum albumin leads to inhibition of collagen-stimulated platelet aggregation that correlated with phosphorylation of rap 1b in a dose-dependent manner.

Yet another mechanism of how NO˙ may limit the platelet response is also related to the activation of cGMP-dependent protein kinase. Wang and colleagues, using immunoaffinity techniques, have shown that the TXA_2 receptor is a substrate for cGMP-dependent protein kinase (79). In support of this theory, the authors have established that the carboxyterminus of the TXA_2 receptor can be phosphorylated by cGMP and its related kinase. These data identify a novel mechanism by which NO˙ is able to inhibit platelet activity by blocking signaling mechanisms of the TXA_2 receptor through catalyzing its phosphorylation via cGMP-dependent protein kinase (79).

Platelet adhesion can also be regulated by NO˙. P selectin, a mediator of platelet adhesion, is found in the Weibel–Palade bodies of endothelial cells and also in the α-granules of platelets. NO˙ synthase inhibitors, such as L-nitroarginine methyl ester (L-NAME), have been shown to induce P-selectin expression on the endothelial cell surface in the rat mesenteric circulation in vivo. This observation suggests that NO˙ may regulate platelet adhesion by decreasing the expression of P-selectin, which is needed for the initial attachment of the platelet to the (activated) endothelium (80). In support of this theory, the endothelium of patients with acute respiratory distress syndrome who were treated with inhaled NO˙ exhibited diminished P-selectin expression (81). Michelson and colleagues have shown that S-nitroso-N-acetyl-L-cysteine can also markedly inhibit the upregulation of P-selectin on the platelet surface (82). Because NO˙ and cGMP inhibit PKC activity, Murohara and colleagues have suggested that NO˙, via cGMP-dependent kinase, may regulate PKC activity and thereby downregulate P-selectin expression on the surface of both platelets and endothelial cells (80).

Recently, cGMP has also been shown to regulate the surface expression of not only P-selectin but also CD63 and the GPIIb/IIIa complex. NO˙ regulates fibrinogen binding to the GPIIb/IIIa receptor by increasing the dissociation constant of the receptor for fibrinogen and decreasing the total number of available fibrinogen molecules bound to the platelet (50) through inhibiting the activation-induced exposure of the fibrinogen binding site on the platelet GPIIb/IIIa complex (82).

Yet another factor in the mechanism by which endothelial NO˙ regulates platelet aggregation is by modulating the activity of the hemoprotein isomerase enzymes that transform prostaglandin I_2 into prostaglandin I_2 and TXA_2 via catalytic inactivation (83). Using various NO˙ donors, Wade and colleagues have established that NO˙ regulates prostaglandin I_2 synthase activity in a biphasic manner, with moderate concentrations increasing enzyme activity and higher concentrations inhibiting enzyme activity (83). In the case of TXA_2, NO˙ donors irreversibly inhibited TXA_2 synthase at all concentrations tested. They conclude that by inhibiting prostanoid enzyme catalysis, NO˙ attenuates the formation of eicosanoid mediators of hemostasis.

NO˙ may also exert its antiplatelet effects by modulating the p85/PI3K pathway (84). Pigazzi and colleagues have shown that the NO˙ donor, S-nitroso-glutathione, and wortmannin synergistically inhibit the effects of thrombin receptor-activating peptide (TRAP)-induced platelet aggregation and also inhibit the expression of GPIIb/IIIa on the platelet surface (84). Both wortmannin and GSNO inhibit PI3-kinase's lipid and protein kinase activities in phosphotyrosine and lyn immunoprecipitates of platelet proteins. This observation suggests yet another signaling mechanism by which NO˙ regulates function.

NO˙ AND HEMOSTATIC DISORDERS

Clinical evidence substantiates the antiplatelet role of NO˙. Thrombotic complications associated with atherosclerosis, hypertension, and diabetes mellitus have been shown to involve an impairment in NO˙ synthesis and mechanism of action (85,86). In contrast, excessive NO˙ production has been associated with increased bleeding times and frank hemorrhage.

NO• and Thrombosis

NO• regulates the platelet response to injury, thereby limiting thrombosis formation. Nishimura and colleagues showed that NO• synthase blockade in brain pial arteries enhanced the accumulation of activated platelets in areas of endothelial damage *(87)*. L-NAME potentiates pulmonary accumulation and prolongs the rate of disaggregation of [^{111}In]-labeled platelets in an in vivo model of platelet aggregation *(1,2)*. In an experimental model of coronary stenosis in rabbits, massive platelet adhesion and aggregation in areas of damaged endothelium was observed in those animals treated with N^G-monomethyl-L-arginine (L-NMMA), another inhibitor of NO• synthesis *(88)*. Folts and colleagues used a canine model of coronary artery stenosis to demonstrate that intravenous nitroglycerin, an organic nitrate metabolized to NO•, can improve coronary flow at sites of stenosis and endothelial injury by inhibiting platelet thrombus formation *(89)*.

In addition, studies with inhibitors of NOS have shown that decreased generation of NO• in vivo can lead to platelet and polymorphonuclear leukocyte activation and thrombosis *(88,90–92)*. When L-NMMA was given to healthy subjects and platelet function monitored in vivo, hemostasis was disturbed and platelets became activated as measured by the increase in plasma levels of markers of platelet activation, including β-thromboglobulin and platelet factor-4 *(93)*. Recently, other investigators have shown that inhibition of NOS activity in areas of endothelial damage can result in enhanced platelet adhesion to the injured arterial surface *(94)*. Using a model of the vascular endothelium, Watanabe and colleagues *(95)* demonstrated that exposure of the intact endothelium to a preformed platelet aggregate transiently stimulated the production of basal NO• release, whereas prolonged exposure to this aggregate resulted in dose-dependent inhibition of NO• release at both basal levels and in response to ATP or serotonin, with NO• activity being attenuated in these cells. Thus, prolonged exposure to aggregated platelets may affect the antiplatelet properties of the endothelium by directly inhibiting NO• elaboration or activity and platelet function *(95)*.

Two brothers with a cerebral thrombotic disorder have provided further information regarding NO•'s ability to regulate platelet function. We originally observed that platelets from these individuals could not be inhibited by NO•. Plasma glutathione peroxidase, an antioxidant enzyme, was found to be decreased in these patients, who had half the normal complement of activity and protein. Addition of exogenous glutathione peroxidase led to restoration of platelet inhibition by NO•. The mechanism of action of glutathione peroxidase involves reduction of lipid hydroperoxides to their corresponding alcohols *(96)*. Impaired metabolism of eicosanoids, such as lipid hydroperoxides, as occurs when glutathione peroxidase activity is decreased, can lead to an increase in hydroperoxyl radical concentration, which itself can react with and decrease bioactive NO•. These reactions, thus, impair the ability of NO• to inhibit platelet activation. Previously, Freedman and colleagues had shown that glutathione peroxidase can potentiate the ability of the naturally occurring *S*-nitrosothiol *S*-nitroso-glutathione to inhibit platelets, an in vitro observation consistent with these observations in patients *(97)*.

Balloon angioplasty, a technique used to treat occlusive arterial lesions, can ultimately lead to enhanced thrombus formation owing to vascular injury resulting from endothelial denudation and impaired NO• synthesis. Marks and colleagues found that local administration of a relatively stable *S*-nitrosothiol, poly-*S*-nitroso-bovine serum albumin, can inhibit thrombosis formation and platelet deposition after arterial balloon injury *(98)*. In a model of vascular injury in which the endothelium was denuded by balloon angioplasty, NO• production could be restored by using gene transfer techniques to deliver the *NOS3* gene to the site of vascular injury, leading to inhibition of neointima formation and preventing platelet aggregation *(99)*. Using a balloon-injury model, Chen and colleagues have demonstrated that retroviral-mediated overexpression of eNOS in smooth muscle cells can limit neointimal formation by inhibiting cell proliferation and increasing the production of NO˙ *(100)*. In addition, *NOS2* gene transfer using an adhesive vector has been shown to inhibit neointimal hyperplasia following balloon injury in rats and pigs *(101)*. NO˙ inhalation significantly decreases platelet-mediated coronary artery thrombotic occlusion in dogs. After inhalation of NO˙, cGMP levels in blood were increased significantly and platelet aggregation was inhibited *(102)*. Nong and colleagues have suggested that inhaled NO˙ may be a method by which to commpensate for the reduced platelet or endothelial NO˙ production that occurs in patients with coronary atherosclerosis and is associated with increased platelet aggregation, especially in acute coronary syndromes *(103)*. Inhaled NO˙ inhibits platelet aggregation, P-selectin expression, and fibrinogen binding to the GPIIb/IIIa receptor of human platelets in vitro in a dose-dependent manner. A depression in NO˙ synthase actvity has also been observed in atrial fibrillation, a disease that is associated with thromboembolism. Patients with this disease had decreased plasma levels of nitrate and lower platelet cGMP levels in comparison to subjects with normal sinus rhythm *(104)*.

NO˙ and Decreased Hemostasis

In contrast to the conditions just discussed in which diminished NO˙ production leads to an increase in the platelet aggregatory response, excessive NO˙ bioactivity can lead to hemorrhagic states. Severe hypotension and disturbances in the hemostatic balance are among the major clinical signs of septicemic reactions. The bleeding diathesis of sepsis is believed to be caused by disseminated intravascular coagulation with consumption coagulopathy, fibrinolysis, and thrombocytopenia from bacterial lipopolysaccharide (LPS) production and its subsequent induction of iNOS activity *(1,2)*. Stimulation of endothelial cells with LPS and interferon-γ, a cytokine produced during inflammatory reactions, results in expression of iNOS, which can lead to the production of large amounts of NO˙ for a prolonged period of time. Thus, bleeding complications that accompany endotoxemia may result, in part, from upregulated expression of iNOS in vascular cells and leukocytes.

Uremia can result in hemostatic defects, including prolonged bleeding times and decreased platelet adhesion and aggregation. Metabolites of the urea cycle accumulate, including L-arginine, which can lead to increased NO˙ production *(105)*. Bode-Boger and colleagues showed that L-arginine increases the excretion of NO˙ byproducts, including nitrate *(106)*. It has been shown that the prolonged bleeding times in uremic rats can be normalized by systemic administration of L-NMMA *(107)*. Simon and colleagues have supported this finding by demonstrating that inhibition of NO˙ production by L-NMMA shortens the bleeding time modestly *(108)*.

NO˙ may also affect bleeding times by interfering with the fibrinolytic system. In patients with peripheral vascular disease, NO˙ donors activate the plasma fibrinolytic system by inhibiting the release of PAI-1 *(109)*. Gryglewski *(109)* reported that prostaglandin synergizes with the NO˙ donor molsidomine to increase the activity of the fibrinolytic system in patients with peripheral vascular disease by both increasing the release of t-PA from cells and inhibiting the release of the antifibrinolytic molecule PAI-1, as has also been demonstrated by Korbut and colleagues *(110)*.

CONCLUSION

In this chapter, we have provided an overview of the importance of NO˙ in regulating hemostasis through its effects on platelet function. Clearly, much has been achieved in this field in recent years, and the observations reviewed here suggest that the role of NO˙ in modulating platelet function is, indeed, complex. An ongoing challenge is to develop unique and potentially useful therapeutic strategies to treat patients with hemostatic diseases that are a consequence of abnormalities in NO˙ synthesis or metabolism.

REFERENCES

1. Radomski MW, Moncada, S. Role of nitric oxide in endothelial cell-platelet interactions. In: Herman AG, ed. Antithrombotics, Pathophysiological Rationale for Pharmacological Interventions. Kluwer Academic Publishers, Dordrecht, The Netherlands, 1991, pp. 27–48.
2. Stamler J, Mendelsohn ME, Amarante P, Smick D, Andon N, Davies PF, Cooke JP, Loscalzo S. N-acetylcysteine potentiates platelet inhibition by endothelium-derived relaxing factor. Circ Res 1989;65: 789–795.
3. Radomski MW, Palmer RM, Moncada S. The anti-aggregating properties of vascular endothelium: interactions between prostacyclin and nitric oxide. Br J Pharmacol 1987;92:639–646.
4. Radomski MW, Palmer RM, Moncada S. Endogenous nitric oxide inhibits human platelet adhesion to vascular endothelium. Lancet 1987; 2:1057,1058.
5. Radomski MW, Palmer RM, Moncada S. The role of nitric oxide and cGMP in platelet adhesion to vascular endothelium. Biochem Biophys Res Commun 1987;148:1482–1489.
6. Pohl U, Busse R. EDRF increases cyclic GMP in platelets during passage through the coronary vascular bed. Circ Res 1989;65:1798–1803.
7. Cooke JP, Tsao P. Cellular mechanisms of atherogenesis and the effects of nitric oxide. Curr Opin Cardiol 1992;7:799–804.
8. de Graaf JC, Banga JD, Moncada S, Palmer RM, de Groot PG, Sixma JJ. Nitric oxide functions as an inhibitor of platelet adhesion under flow conditions. Circulation 1992;85:2284–2290.
9. Bizzozero G. Su di un nuovo elemento morfologico del sangue dei mammiferi e della sua importanza nella trombosi e nella coagulazione. L'Osservatore Gazetta delle Cliniche 1881;XVII: 785–787.
10. Long MW, Hoffman R. Thrombocytopoiesis. In: Hoffman R, Benz EJ Jr, Shattil ST, Furie B, Cohen HJ, Silberstein LE, eds. Hematology: Basic Principles and Practice, 2nd ed. Churchill Livingstone, New York, 1995, pp 274–286.
11. Burstein SA, Breton-Gorius J, Megakaryopoiesis and platelet formation. In: Butler E, Lichtman MA, Coller BS, Kipps TJ, eds. Williams' Hematology, 5th ed. McGraw-Hill, New York, 1995, pp. 1149–1161.
12. Lind SE, Platelet morphology. In: Loscalzo J, Schafer A, eds. Thrombosis and Hemorrhage. Blackwell Scientific, Boston. 1994, pp. 201–212.
13. Isenberg WM, Bainton DF, Megakaryocyte and platelet structure. In: Hoffman R, Benz EJ, Shattil ST, Furie B, Cohen HJ, Silberstein LE, eds. Hematology: Basic Principles and Practice, 2nd ed. Churchill Livingstone, New York, 1995, pp 1516–1524.
14. Trowbridge EA, Martin JF, Slater DN. Evidence for a theory of physical fragmentation of megakaryocytes, implying that all platelets are produced in the pulmonary circulation. Thromb Res 1982;28: 461–475.
15. Kuter KJ, Hemorrhagic Disorders II. Platelets. In: Beck WS, ed. Hematology, 5th ed. The MIT Press, Cambridge, 1994, pp. 543–575.
16. Brass LF, Molecular basis for platelet activation. In: Hoffman R, Benz EJ, Shattil ST, Furie B, Cohen HJ, Silberstein LE, eds. Hematology: Basic Principles and Practice, 2nd ed. Churchill Livingstone, New York, 1995, pp 1536–1552.
17. Kroll MH, Mechanisms of platelet activation. In Loscalzo J, Schafer A, eds. Thrombosis and Hemorrhage, Blackwell Scientific Publications, Boston, 1994, pp. 247–266.
18. Plow FE, Ginsberg MH, Molecular basis of platelet function. In: Hoffman R, Benz EJ, Shattil ST, Furie B, Cohen HJ, Silberstein LE, eds. Hematology: Basic Principles and Practice, 2nd ed. Churchill Livingstone, New York, 1995, pp 1524–1535.
19. Kroll MH, Schafer AI. Biochemical mechanisms of platelet activation. Blood 1984;74:1181–1195.
20. Droller MJ. Ultrastructure of the platelet release reaction in response to various aggregating agents and their inhibitors. Lab Invest 1973;29:595–606.
21. Vaughan D, Schafer A, Loscalzo J. Normal mechanisms of hemostasis and fibrinolysis. In: Loscalzo J, Creager M, Dzau VJ, ed. Vascular Medicine, A Textbook of Vascular Biology and Diseases, 2nd ed. Little Brown, Boston, 1996, pp. 207–216.
22. George JN, Nurden AT, Phillips DR. Molecular defects in interactions of platelets with the vessel wall. N Engl J Med 1984;311:1084–1098.
23. Ginsberg MH, Loftus JC, Plow EF. Cytoadhesions, integrins, and platelets. Thromb Haemost 1988; 59:1–6.
24. Hawiger J, Timmons S, Kloczewiak M, Strong DD, Doolittle RF. Gamma and alpha chains of fibrinogen possess sites reactive with human receptors. Proc Natl Acad Sci USA 1982;79:2068–2071.

25. Loscalzo J. Pathogenesis of thrombosis. In; Beutler MA, Lichtman BL, Coller BS, Kipps TJ, eds. Williams' Hematology, 5th ed. Saunders, Philadelphia, 1994, pp. 4485–4508.
26. Moncada S. Eighth Gaddum Memorial Lecture—University of London Institute of Education. Biological importance of prostacyclin. Br J Pharmacol 1982;76:3–31.
27. Buchanan MR, Brister SJ. Antithrombotics and the lipoxygenase pathway. In: Herman AG, ed. Antithrombotics. Kluwer Academic Publishers, Dordrecht, The Netherlands, 1991, pp. 159–180.
28. Marcus AJ, Safier LB. Thromboregulation: multicellular modulation of platelet reactivity in hemostasis and thrombosis. FASEB J 1993;7:516–522.
29. Marcus AJ, Broekman MJ, Drosopoulos JH, Islam N, Alyonycheva TN, Safier LB, et al. The endothelial cell ecto-ADPase responsible for inhibition of platelet function is CD39. J Clin Invest 1997;99: 1351–1360.
30. Esmon CT. Molecular events that control the protein C anticoagulant pathway. Thromb Haemost 1993; 70:29–35.
31. Rosenberg RD, Bauer KA. The heparin-antithrombin system: a natural anticoagulant mechanism. In: Coleman RW, Hirsch J, Marder VJ, Salmon EW, eds. Hemostasis and Thrombosis. Lippincott, Philadelphia, 1994, pp. 837–860.
32. Palmer RM, Ashton DS, Moncada S. Vascular endothelial cells synthesize nitric oxide from L-arginine. Nature (Lond) 1988;333:664–666.
33. Nathan C. Nitric oxide is a secretory product of mammalian cells. FASEB J 1992;6:3051–3064.
34. Dinerman JL, Lowenstein CJ, Snyder SH. Molecular mechanisms of nitric oxide regulation. Potential relevance to cardiovascular disease. Circ Res 1993;73:217–222.
35. Bredt DS, Snyder SH. Isolation of nitric oxide synthase, a calmodulin-requiring enzyme. Proc Natl Acad Sci USA 1990;87:682–685.
36. Busse R, Mulsch A. Calcium-dependent nitric oxide synthesis in endothelial cytosol is mediated by calmodulin. FEBS Lett 1990;265:133–136.
37. Mayer B, Schmidt K, Humbert P, Bohme E. Biosynthesis of endothelium-derived relaxing factor: a cytosolic enzyme in porcine endothelial cells Ca^{2+}-dependently converts L-arginine into an activator of soluble guanylyl cyclase. Biochem Biophys Res Commun 1989;164:678–685.
38. Marletta MA, Yoon PS, Iyengar R, Leaf CD, Wishnok JS. Macrophage oxidation of L-arginine to nitrite and nitrate: nitric oxide is an intermediate. Biochemistry 1988;27:8706–8711.
39. Yui Y, Hattori R, Kosuga K, Eizawa H, Hiki K, Ohkawa S, et al. Calmodulin-independent nitric oxide synthase from rat polymorphonuclear neutrophils. J Biol Chem 1991;266:3369–3371.
40. Drapier JC, Hibbs JB Jr. Differentiation of murine macrophages to express nonspecific cytotoxicity for tumor cells results in L-arginine-dependent inhibition of mitochondrial iron-sulfur enzymes in the macrophage effector cells. J Immunol 1988;140:2829–2838.
41. Steuhr DJ, Marletta MA. Induction of nitrite/nitrate synthesis in murine macrophages by BCG infection, lymphokines or interferon-gamma. J Immunol 1987;139:518–525.
42. Ding AH, Nathan CF, Steuhr DJ. Release of reactive nitrogen intermediates and reactive oxygen intermediates from mouse peritoneal macrophages. Comparison of activating cytokines and evidence for independent production. J Immunol 1988;141:2407–2412.
43. Xie QW, Cho XJ, Calaycay J, Mumford RA, Swiderek KM, Lee TD, et al. Cloning and characterization of inducible nitric oxide synthase from mouse macrophages. Science 1992;256:225–228.
44. Ignarro LJ, Adams JB, Horowitz PM, Wood KS. Activation of soluble guanylyl cyclase by NO-hemoproteins involves NO-heme exchange. Comparison of heme-containing and heme-deficient enzyme forms. J Biol Chem 1986;261:4997–5002.
45. Venturini CM, Del Vecchio PJ, Kaplan JE. Thrombin induced platelet adhesion to endothelium is modified by endothelial derived relaxing factor (EDRF). Biochem Biophys Res Commun 1989;159:349–354.
46. Humphries RG, Tomlinson W, O'Connor SE, Leff P. Inhibition of collagen- and ADP-induced platelet aggregation by substance P in vivo: involvement of endothelium-derived relaxing factor; involvement of endothelium-derived relaxing factor. J Cardiovasc Pharmacol 1990;16:292–297.
47. Freedman JE, Loscalzo J, Barnard MR, Alpert C, Keaney JF Jr, Michelson AD. Nitric oxide released from activated platelets inhibits platelet recruitment. J Clin Invest 1997;100:350–356.
48. Stamler JS, Jaraki O, Osborne J, Simon DI, Keaney JF Jr, Vita JA, et al. Nitric oxide circulates in mammalian plasma primarily as an S-nitroso adduct of serum albumin. Proc Natl Acad Sci USA 1992; 89:7674–7677.
49. Mellion BT, Ignarro LJ, Ohlstein EH, Pontecorvo EG, Hyman AL, Kadowitz PJ. Evidence for the inhibitory role for guanosine 3'-5'-monophosphate in ADP-induced human platelet aggregation in the presence of nitric oxide and related vasodilators. Blood 1981;57:946–955.

50. Mendelsohn ME, O'Neill S, George D, Loscalzo J. Inhibition of fibrinogen binding to human platelets by S-nitroso-N-acetylcycsteine. J Biol Chem 1990;265:19,028–19,034.

51. Keaney JF Jr, Simon DI, Stamler JS, Jaraki O, Scharfstein J, Vita JA, et al. NO forms an adduct with serum albumin that has endothelium-derived relaxing factor-like properties. J Clin Invest 1993;91: 1582–1589.

52. Simon DI, Stamler JS, Jaraki O, Keaney JF Jr, Osborne JA, Francis SA, et al. Antiplatelet properties of protein S-nitrosothiols dervied from nitric oxide and endothelium-derived relaxing factor. Arterioscler Thromb 1993;13:791–799.

53. Gordge MP, Hothersall JS, Neild GH, Dutra AA. Role of a copper (I)-dependent enzyme in the antiplatelet action of S-nitrosoglutathione. Br J Pharmacol 1996;119:533–538.

54. Moro MA, Darley-Usmar VM, Goodwin DA, Read NG, Zamora-Pino R, Feelisch M, et al. Paradoxical fate and biological action of peroxynitrite on human platelets. Proc Natl Acad Sci USA 1994;91: 6702–6706.

55. Meng Y, Trachtenburg J, Ryan US, Abendschein D. Potentiation of endogenous nitric oxide with superoxide dismutase inhibits platelet-mediated thrombosis in injured and stenotic arteries. J Am Coll Cardiol 1995;25:269–275.

56. Loscalzo J, Vaughan DE. Tissue plasminogen activator promotes platelet disaggregation in plasma. J Clin Invest 1987;79:1749–1755.

57. Gerrard JM, White JG. Prostaglandins and thromboxanes: "middlemen" in modulating platelet function in hemostasis and thrombosis. In: Spaet TH, ed. Progress in Hemostasis and Thrombosis, Vol. 4. Grunne & Stratton, New York, 1992, pp. 87–126.

58. Maurice DH, Haslam RJ, Molecular basis of the synergistic inhibition of platelet function by nitrovasodilators and activators of adenylate cyclase: inhibition of cyclic AMP breakdown by cyclic GMP. Mol Pharmacol 1990;37:671–681.

59. Stamler JS, Vaughan DE, Loscalzo J. Synergistic dissagregation of platelets by tissue-type plasminogen activator, prostaglandin E1, and nitroglycerin. Circ Res 1989;65:796–804.

60. Freedman JE, Sauter R, Battinelli EM, Ault K, Knowles C, Huang PL, et al. Deficient platelet-derived nitric oxide and enhanced hemostasis in mice lacking the NOS3 gene. Circulation 1998;1(Suppl):18.

61. Muruganandam A, Mutus B. Isolation of nitric oxide synthase from human platelets. Biochim Biophys Acta 1994;1200:1–6.

62. Djaffar I, Vilette D, Bray PF, Rosa JP. Quantitative isolation of RNA from human platelets. Thromb Res 1991;62:127–135.

63. Lelchuk R, Radomski MW, Martin JF, Moncada S. Constitutive and inducible nitric oxide synthases in human megakaryoblastic cells. J Pharmacol Exp Ther 1992;262:1220–1224.

64. Wallerath T, Gath I, Aulitzky WE, Pollock JS, Kleinert H, Forstermann U. Identification of the NO synthase isoforms expressed in human neutrophil granulocytes, megakaryocytes and platelets. Thromb Haemost 1997;77:163–167.

65. Chen LY, Mehta JL. Further evidence of the presence of constitutive and inducible nitric oxide synthase isoforms in human platelets. J Cardiovasc Pharmacol 1996;27:154–158.

66. Zhou Q, Hellermann GR, Solomonson LP. Nitric oxide release from resting platelets. Thromb Res 1995;77:87–96.

67. Radomski MW, Palmer RM, Moncada S. An L-arginine/nitric oxide pathway present in human platelets regulates aggregation. Proc Natl Acad Sci USA 1990;87:5193–5197.

68. Vasta V, Meacci E, Farnararo M, Bruni P. Identification of a specific transport system for L-arginine in human platelets. Biochem Biophys Res Commun 1995;206:878–884.

69. Moro MA, Russell RJ, Cellek S, Lizasoain I, Su Y, Darley-Usmar VM, et al. cGMP mediates the vascular and platelet actions of nitric oxide: confirmation using an inhibitor of the soluble guanylyl cyclase. Proc Natl Acad Sci USA 1996;93:1480–1485.

70. Nakashima S, Tohmatsu T, Hattori H, Okano Y, Nozawa Y. Inhibitory action of cyclic GMP on secretion, polyphosphoinositide hydrolysis and calcium mobilization in thrombin-stimulated human platelets. Biochem Biophys Res Commun 1986;135:1099–1104.

71. Matsuoka I, Nakahata N, Nakanishi H. Inhibitory effect of 8-bromo cyclic GMP on an extracellular Ca^{2+}-dependent arachidonic acid liberation in collagen-stimulated rabbit platelets. Biochem Pharmacol 1989;38:1841–1847.

72. Morgan RO, Newby AC. Nitroprusside differentially inhibits ADP-stimulated calcium influx and mobilization in human platelets. Biochem J 1989;258:447–454.

73. Geiger J, Nolte C, Butt E, Sage SO, Walter U. Role of cGMP and cGMP-dependent protein kinase in nitrovasodilator inhibition of agonist-evoked calcium-elevation in human platelets. Proc Natl Acad Sci USA 1992;89:1031–1035.

74. Johansson JS, Hayness DH. Cyclic GMP increases the rate of the calcium reflux extrusion pump in intact human platelets but has no direct effect on the dense tubular calcium accumulation system. Biochim Biophys Acta 1992;1105:40–50.

75. Trepakova ES, Cohen RA, Bolotina VM. Nitric oxide inhibits store-operated nonselective cation influx in platelets and smooth muscle cells via Ca^{2+}-ATPase dependent refilling of Ca^{2+} stores. Circulation 1998;1(Suppl):4316.

76. Pernollet MG, Lantoine F, Devynck MA. Nitric oxide inhibits ATP-dependent Ca^{2+} uptake into platelet membrane vesicles. Biochem Biophys Res Commun 1996;222:780–785.

77. Le Quan Sang KH, Lantoine F, Devynck MA. Influence of authentic nitric oxide on basal cytosolic $[Ca^{2+}]$ and Ca^{2+} release from internal stores in human platelets. Br J Pharmacol 1996;119:1361–1366.

78. Reep B, Lapetina EG. Nitric oxide stimulates the phosphorylation of rap1b in human platelets and acts synergistically with iloprost. Biochem Biophys Res Commun 1996;219:1–5.

79. Wang GR, Zhu Y, Halushka PV, Lincoln TM, Mendelsohn ME. Mechanism of platelet inhibition by nitric oxide: *in vivo* phosphorylation of thromboxane receptor by cyclic GMP-dependent protein kinase. Proc Natl Acad Sci USA 1998;95:4888–4893.

80. Murohara T, Parkinson SJ, Waldman SA, Lefer AM. Inhibition of nitric oxide biosynthesis promotes P-selectin expression in platelets. Role of protein kinase C. Arterioscler Thromb Vasc Biol 1995;15: 2068–2075.

81. Gries A, Bode C, Peter K, Herr A, Bohrer H, Motsch J, et al. Inhaled nitric oxide inhibits human platelet aggregation, P-selectin expression, and fibrinogen binding in vitro, and in vivo. Circulation 1998;97: 1481–1487.

82. Michelson AD, Benoit SE, Furman MI, Breckwoldt WL, Rohrer MJ, Barnard MR, et al. Effects of nitric oxide/EDRF on platelet surface glycoproteins. Am J Phys 1996;270:H1640–H1648.

83. Wade ML, Fitzpatrick FA. Nitric oxide modulates the activity of the hemoproteins prostaglandin I_2 synthase and thromboxane A_2 synthase. Arch Biochem Biophys 1997;347:174–180.

84. Pigazzi A, Heydrick SJ, Folli F, Benoit SE, Michelson AD, Loscalzo J. Nitric oxide inhibits thrombin receptor activating peptide-induced phosphoinositdie 3-kinase activity in human platelets. J Biol Chem 274:14,368–14,375.

85. Cadwgan T, Benjamin N. Reduced platelet nitric oxide synthesis in essential hypertension. J Vasc Biol 1991;3:455A.

86. Calver A, Collier J, Vallance P. Inhibition and stimulation of nitric oxide synthesis in the human forearm arterial bed of patients with insulin-dependent diabetes. J Clin Invest 1992;90:2548–2554.

87. Nishimura H, Rosenblum WI, Nelson GH, Boynton S. Agents that modify EDRF formation alter antiplatelet properties of brain arteriolar endothelium *in vivo*. Am J Physiol 1991;261:H15–H21.

88. Herbaczynska-Cedro K, Lembowicz K, Pytel B. N_G-monomethyl-L-arginine increases platelet deposition on damaged endothelium in vivo. A scanning electron microscopic study. Thromb Res 1991;64: 1–9.

89. Folts JS, Stamler JS, Loscalzo J. Intravenous nitroglycerin infusion inhibits cyclic blood flow responses caused by periodic platelet thrombus formation in stenosed dog coronary arteries. Circulation 1991;83: 2122–2127.

90. May GR, Crook P, Moore PK, Page CP. The role of nitric oxide as an endogenous regulator of platelet and neutrophil activation within the pulmonary circulation of the rabbit. Br J Pharmacol 1991;102: 759–763.

91. Golino P, Capelli-Bigazzi M, Ambrosio G, Ragni M, Russolillo E, Condorelli M, et al. Endothelium-derived relaxing factor modulates platelet aggregation in an in vivo model of recurrent platelet activation. Circ Res 1992;71:1447–1456.

92. Yao SK, Ober JC, Krishnaswami A, Ferguson JJ, Anderson HV, Golino P, et al. Endogenous nitric oxide protects against platelet aggregation and cyclic flow variations in stenosed and endothelium-injured arteries. Circulation 1992;86:1302–1309.

93. Bodzenta-Lukaszyk A, Gabryelewicz A, Lukaszyk A, Bielawiec M, Konturek JW, Domschke W. Nitric oxide synthase inhibition and platelet function. Thromb Res 1994;75:667–672.

94. Yan ZQ, Yokota T, Zhang W, Hansson GK. Expression of inducible nitric oxide synthase inhibits platelet adhesion and restores blood flow in the injured artery. Circ Res 1996;79:38–44.

95. Watanabe R, Kishi Y, Sakita S, Numano F. Impaired NO release from bovine aortic endothelial cells exposed to activated platelets. Atherosclerosis 1997;128:19–26.

96. Freedman JE, Frei B, Welch GN, Loscalzo J. Glutathione peroxidase potentiates the inhibition of platelet function by S-nitrosothiols. J Clin Invest 1995;96:394–400.

97. Freedman JE, Loscalzo J, Benoit SE, Valeri CR, Barnard MR, Michelson AD. Decreased platelet inhibition by nitric oxide in two brothers with a history of arterial thrombosis. J Clin Invest 1996;97:979–987.

98. Marks DS, Vita JA, Folts JS, Keaney JF Jr, Welch GN, Loscalzo J. Inhibition of neointimal prolifera-
    tion in rabbits after vascular injury by a single treatment with a protein adduct of nitric oxide. J Clin
    Invest 1995;96:2630–2638.

99. von der Leyen HE, Gibbons GH, Morishita R, Lewis NP, Zhang L, Nakajima M, et al. Gene therapy
    inhibiting neointimal vascular lesion: *in vivo* transfer of endothelial cell nitric oxide synthase gene.
    Proc Natl Acad Sci USA 1995;92:1137–1141.

100. Chen L, Daum G, Forough R, Clowes M, Walter U, Clowes AW. Overexpression of human endothelial
     nitric oxide synthase in rat vascular smooth muscle cells and in balloon-injured carotid artery. Circ Res
     1998;82:862–870.

101. Miyagoshima M, Tzeng E, Shears LJ, Kawaharada N, Watkins Billiar TR. Perivascular iNOS gene
     transfer using a novel non-occlusive gene delivery device inhibits intimal hyperplasia. Circulation
     1997;96:I–13.

102. Andrie C, Bloch KD, Moreno PR, Hurford WE, Guerrero JL, Holt R. Inhaled nitric oxide increases
     coronary artery patency after thrombolysis. Circulation 1996;94:1919–1926.

103. Nong Z, Hoylaerts M, Van Pelt N, Collen D, Janssens S. Nitric oxide inhalation inhibits platelet
     aggregation and platelet-mediated pulmonary thrombosis in rats. Circ Res 1997;81:865–869.

104. Minamino T, Kitakaze M, Sato H, Asanuma H, Funaya H, Koretsune Y, Hori M. Plasma levels of
     nitrite/nitrate and platelet cGMP levels are decreased in patients with atrial fibrillation. Arterioscl
     Thromb Vasc Biol 1997;17:3191–3195.

105. Radomski MW, Salas E. Biological significance of nitric oxide in platelet function. In: Kubes P,
     ed. Nitric Oxide: A Modulator of Cell-Cell Interactions in the Microcirculation. R.G. Landes, 1995,
     pp. 43–75.

106. Bode-Boger SM, Boger RH, Kienke S, Junker W, Frolich JC. Elevated L-arginine/dimethylarginine
     ratio contributes to enhanced NO production by dietary L-arginine in hypercholesterolemic rabbits.
     Biochem Biophys Res Commun 1996;219:598–603.

107. Remuzzi G, Perico N, Zoja C, Corna D, Macconi D, Vigano G. Role of endothelium-derived nitric
     oxide in the bleeding tendency of uremia. J Clin Invest 1990;86:1768–1771.

108. Simon DI, Stamler JS, Loh E, Loscalzo J, Francis SA, Creager MA. Effect of nitric oxide synthase
     inhibition on bleeding time in humans. J Cardiovasc Pharmacol 1995;26:339–342.

109. Gryglewski RJ. Interactions between nitric oxide and prostacyclin. Sem Thromb Hemost 1993;19:
     158–166.

110. Korbut R, Ocetkiewicz A, Gryglewski RJ. Nitric oxide complements prostacyclin in the regulation of
     endothelial thromboresistance under flow conditions. Methods Find Exp Clin Pharmacol 1993;15:
     179–181.

9 Nitric Oxide Modulates Leukocyte–Endothelial Cell Adhesion

Wolfgang Cerwinka and D. Neil Granger

INTRODUCTION

Although the role of leukocytes in certain inflammatory diseases (e.g., arthritis, inflammatory bowel diseases) has long been appreciated, there is a large body of recent evidence that implicates leukocytes in a number of other pathological conditions, including atherosclerosis, hypertension, ischemia–reperfusion injury, venous thrombosis, and gastric ulceration. The recognition that a leukocyte must first adhere to vascular endothelium before it can exert its deleterious effects on blood vessels and neighboring parenchymal cells has led to an intensive effort to define the factors that influence the ability of leukocytes to adhere to endothelial cells. Data derived from both in vitro and in vivo models of leukocyte–endothelial cell adhesion invoke a role for several factors in the modulation of this cell-adhesion process. These factors include adhesion glycoproteins that are expressed on the surface of activated leukocytes and endothelial cells, hydrodynamic dispersal forces (e.g., shear rate) that are generated by the movement of blood through the circulation, and some products of leukocyte and endothelial cell activation.

Inflamed tissues produce and liberate a variety of chemical substances that can determine the intensity and duration of the inflammatory response by modulating the adhesion and emigration of leukocytes in postcapillary venules. Cytokines (such as tumor necrosis factor and interleukins), platelet-activating factor, and leukotrienes represent some of the factors that can promote and perpetuate an inflammatory reaction by enhancing leukocyte–endothelial cell adhesion. The enhanced leukocyte adhesion that is mediated by these proinflammatory agents can be explained by their ability to increase the expression of leukocyte and endothelial cell adhesion glycoproteins, and, in some instances, by reducing the shear forces in blood vessels that tend to oppose leukocyte adhesion. The reduction in venular shear rate is a consequence of the constrictor action of some mediators (e.g., serotonin, thromboxane A_2) on upstream arterioles.

There are several substances produced by endothelial cells in inflamed tissue that are known to exert anti-inflammatory actions, including inhibition of leukocyte–endothelial cell adhesion. Prostacyclin, adenosine, and nitric oxide (NO•) have all been shown to exert potent anti-inflammatory actions that are independent of their potent vasodilator effects. Of these three endogenous inhibitors of leukocyte–endothelial cell adhesion, NO• has recently received the greatest attention. This focus on NO• largely results from the fact that an alteration in NO• production or bioavailability (because of superoxide-mediated inactivation) has been invoked as a key initiating factor in the pathogenesis of a number of systemic cardiovascular diseases

From: *Contemporary Cardiology, vol. 4: Nitric Oxide and the Cardiovascular System*
Edited by: J. Loscalzo and J. A. Vita © Humana Press Inc., Totowa, NJ

(e.g., atherosclerosis, diabetes, sepsis) and regional circulatory disorders (ischemia–reperfusion) in which there is evidence of an inflammatory component.

This chapter summarizes the available information that implicates NO$^\bullet$ as a modulator of the adhesion of different populations of leukocytes (neutrophils, monocytes, and lymphocytes) to endothelial cells and to discuss the mechanisms that may underlie this important biological property. In addition, evidence that implicates NO$^\bullet$ as a mediator of the adhesive interactions between adjacent endothelial cells and the relevance of this action to vascular permeability changes in inflamed tissue is discussed.

LEUKOCYTE–ENDOTHELIAL CELL ADHESION

Molecular Determinants of Leukocyte–Endothelial Cell Adhesion

A number of different adhesion molecules have been identified that mediate the recruitment of leukocytes to sites of inflammation. Table 1 summarizes the different adhesion glycoproteins that are expressed on the surface of leukocytes and endothelial cells after stimulation *(1,2)*. The selectins comprise a family of lectin-like adhesion molecules that mediate the low-affinity adhesive interaction manifested as leukocyte rolling. L-selectin, which is constitutively expressed on neutrophils, can bind to P- or E-selectin found on the surface of activated endothelial cells. P-selectin is normally stored in granular structures (Weibel–Palade bodies) within endothelial cells but can be mobilized to the cell surface after stimulation with thrombin, histamine, oxygen radicals, or other mediators. This rapid upregulation of P-selectin allows for the recruitment of rolling leukocytes within 5–10 min after an inflammatory stimulus. The expression of P-selectin can also occur via transcription-dependent processes after cytokine stimulation, requiring approx 4 h for peak expression on activated endothelial cells. E-selectin expression on activated endothelial cells is entirely dependent on a transcription-dependent mechanism, requiring approx 3 h for peak expression.

The firm adhesion of leukocytes to endothelial cells is mediated by different families of adhesion molecules *(1,2)*. Neutrophils activated by stimuli such as platelet activating factor (PAF), leukotriene B$_4$ (LTB$_4$), and C5a exhibit rapid (<5 min) expression of the β_2-integrin CD11/CD18. This leukocyte adhesion glycoprotein exists as three heterodimers, each of which consists of a functionally and structurally distinct α-subunit (designated as CD11a, CD11b, and CD11c) noncovalently associated with a common β-subunit (designated as CD18). The major counterreceptor for CD11/CD18 on endothelial cells belongs to the immunoglobulin superfamily of adhesion glycoproteins, i.e., intercellular adhesion molecule-1 (ICAM-1). ICAM-1 is constitutively expressed on endothelial cells in all vascular beds and its expression can increase substantially after activation of endothelial cells with cytokines or endotoxin. A related endothelial cell adhesion molecule VCAM-1 (vascular cell adhesion molecule-1) mediates the firm adhesion of monocytes and lymphocytes by binding to its counterreceptor (VLA$_4$) on the leukocyte. VCAM-1, like ICAM-1, expression on endothelial cells is entirely under transcriptional regulation, with profound increases noted after cytokine challenge. Another member of this family of endothelial cell adhesion molecules, PECAM-1 (platelet-endothelial cell adhesion molecule-1), has been implicated as a key mediator of transendothelial migration of neutrophils (diapedesis). However, this adhesion molecule is largely unresponsive to the stimulating effects of cytokines; hence, its density of expression on endothelial cells remains fairly constant during inflammatory reactions *(1,2)*.

A multistep model has been proposed to explain how the different leukocyte and endothelial cell adhesion molecules interact in a sequential and coordinated fashion to recruit leukocytes to sites of inflammation (Fig. 1). As blood exits capillaries to enter postcapillary venules, lateral displacement forces generated by the faster-moving red blood cells push leukocytes toward the vessel wall. If selectins are expressed on venular endothelial cells, the leukocytes will roll along the vessel wall with a progressive decline in leukocyte rolling

Table 1
Adhesion Molecules That Mediate Leukocyte–Endothelial Adhesion

Adhesion molecule	Distribution of molecule	Ligand	Distribution of ligand	Basal surface expression	Stimuli for expression	Function
Endothelial						
P-Selectin	Activated endothelial cells and platelets	Sialyl-Lewis X, Sialyl-Lewis A, PGSL-1, L-selectin	Platelets, leukocytes	Yes	Histamine, thrombin, cytokines, LPS	Leukocyte and platelet rolling
E-Selectin	Activated endothelial cells	PGSL-1, Sialyl-Lewis X, Sialyl-Lewis A, ESL-1, L-selectin	Leukocytes	No	Cytokines, LPS	Leukocyte rolling
ICAM-1	Endothelial cells, monocytes	CD11a/CD18, CD11b/CD18, CD11c/CD18	Leukocytes	Yes	Cytokines, LPS	Leukocyte adhesion and emigration
ICAM-2	Endothelial cells	CD11a/CD18	Leukocytes	Yes	?	Leukocyte adhesion and emigration
VCAM-1	Endothelial cells	VLA-4	Leukocytes	Yes	Cytokines, LPS	Leukocyte adhesion and emigration
PECAM-1	Endothelial cells, leukocytes, platelets	PECAM-1 (homophilic)	Endothelial cells, leukocytes, platelets	Yes	?	Leukocyte adhesion and emigration
MAdCAM-1	Endothelial cells, lymphoid tissue	L-Selectin, CD49d?	Leukocytes	Yes	Cytokines, LPS	Leukocyte adhesion and emigration

(continued)

Table 1 (Continued)

Adhesion molecule	Distribution of molecule	Ligand	Distribution of ligand	Basal surface expression	Stimuli for expression	Function
Leukocyte L-Selectin	Leukocytes	Sialyl-Lewis X, Sialyl-Lewis A, CD34, GlyCAM-1, P-, E-selectin	Endothelial cells and high endothelial venules	Yes	Down-regulated by FMLP, LTB$_4$, PAF	Leukocyte rolling
CD11a/CD18 (LFA-1)	T and B lymphocytes, monocytes	ICAM-1, ICAM-2	Endothelial cells	Yes	C5a, FMLP, LTB$_4$, PAF	Leukocyte adhesion and emigration
CD11b/CD18 (MAC-1)	All leukocytes	ICAM-1	Endothelial cells	Yes	FMLP, LTB$_4$, PAF	Leukocyte adhesion and emigration
CD11c/CD18 (p150,95)	Neutrophils, monocytes	Fb, iC3b		Yes	?	?
CD49d/CD29 (VLA-4)	Lymphocytes, monocytes, eosinophils, basophils	VCAM-1	Endothelial cells	Yes	FMLP, LTB$_4$, PAF	Leukocyte adhesion and emigration
CD49d/7	Lymphocytes	MAdCAM-1 VCAM-1		Yes	No	Leukocyte adhesion and emigration

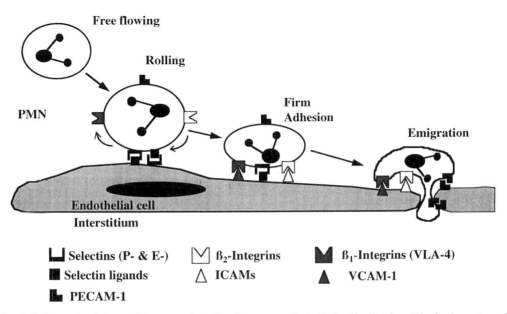

Fig. 1. Schematic of the multistep model of leukocyte–endothelial cell adhesion. The leukocyte and endothelial cell receptors that contribute to the different steps (rolling, firm adhesion, emigration) in the recruitment cascade are also illustrated.

velocity. This slow rolling exposes leukocytes to inflammatory stimuli generated in proximity to venules (e.g., mast cells) or by endothelial cells (e.g., PAF). Endothelial cells exposed to cytokines released from adjacent cells begin the transcription-dependent production and expression of ICAM-1 and VCAM-1. Slow-rolling leukocytes exposed to inflammatory agents (e.g., PAF) rapidly express CD11b/CD18, which allow the leukocyte to bind to ICAM-1 on endothelial cells. Both ICAM-1 and PECAM-1 are utilized by the leukocyte to traverse the vessel wall and enter the adjacent interstitial compartment. The process of leukocyte rolling, adherence, and emigration can be sustained over several hours to days, provided the stimuli (e.g., cytokines) for transcription-dependent expression of E-selectin, ICAM-1, and VCAM-1 are generated by the inflamed tissue *(1,2)*. It must be emphasized that adhesion molecules that mediate a specific step (e.g., rolling) in this cascade can exert effects on a subsequent step (e.g., transmigration) in the recruitment of leukocytes.

NO• and Neutrophil Adhesion

The possibility that NO• may contribute to the regulation of neutrophil–endothelial cell adhesion was initially considered as a result of published reports that described a role for NO• in the inhibition of homotypic aggregation of platelets *(3–8)* and studies that invoked a role for superoxide as a mediator of leukocyte–endothelial cell adhesion. The latter observation led to the proposal that the ability of superoxide dismutase (SOD) to inhibit ischemia–reperfusion-induced neutrophil adhesion in mesenteric venules may be related to superoxide-mediated inactivation of an endogenous antiadhesion molecule *(9–11)*. Because NO• is known to react with superoxide at a rate that is three times faster than the reaction between superoxide and SOD *(12)*, it was proposed that pathologic conditions associated with an excess production of superoxide would diminish the bioavailability of NO• and consequently limit the accumulation and actions of this putative antiadhesion molecule.

Inhibitors of nitric oxide synthase (NOS) like L-NMMA (N^G-monomethyl-L-arginine) or L-NAME (N^G-nitro-L-arginine methylester) have been shown to elicit increased leukocyte

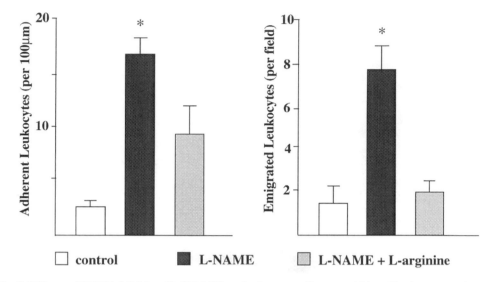

□ control   ■ L-NAME   ▨ L-NAME + L-arginine

Fig. 2. Effects of NOS inhibition (L-NAME) on leukocyte adherence (**A**) and leukocyte emigration (**B**) in rat mesentery. Data are presented for 30 min after starting each superfusion. Data from ref. *14.* * indicates $p < 0.05$ relative to control.

adherence in postcapillary venules (*13,14*; Fig. 2A,B). Aminoguanidine, a putative selective inhibitor of the inducible form of NOS (iNOS), has also been shown to promote leukocyte adhesion in mesenteric venules (*15*). However, it remains unclear whether this action of aminoguandine relates to an overlapping ability to inhibit the constitutive form of NOS that is found in endothelial cells (eNOS). The specificity of action of the L-arginine derivatives (L-NMMA and L-NAME) as inhibitors of NOS is supported by a reversal of their proadhesive actions with supplemental (fivefold excess) L-arginine, but not D-arginine (*14*; Figs. 2–4A).

L-NMMA, but not L-NAME, was shown to elicit directly increased surface expression of CD11/CD18 on isolated neutrophils (*13*). Furthermore, neither NOS inhibitor was able to promote neutrophil adhesion to inert surfaces, suggesting that endothelial cells must be present for the NOS inhibitors to exert their antiadhesive effects. Monoclonal antibodies (MAbs) directed against either the common β-subunit of the leukocyte adhesion glycoprotein CD11/CD18, ICAM-1, or P-selectin significantly blunt the increased leukocyte adherence and emigration elicited by L-NAME in mesenteric venules (*16*). These observations indicate that inhibition of NO• synthesis leads to adhesive interactions between neutrophils and venular endothelial cells that are mediated by CD11/CD18 on leukocytes and ICAM-1 on endothelial cells. The observation that L-NAME also elicits PAF and LTB_4 production (*16,17*) is consistent with L-NAME-induced CD11/CD18-ICAM-1 adhesive interactions because it has been shown that LTB_4 as well as PAF increase the surface expression of CD11/CD18 on leukocytes, which can bind to constitutively expressed ICAM-1 on venular endothelial cells (*1*).

P-selectin appears to modulate the leukocyte rolling elicited by L-NAME. The recruitment of rolling leukocytes caused by L-NAME can be inhibited by a P-selectin MAb, and immunohistochemical techniques have been used to show that L-NAME increases the expression of P-selectin in mesenteric venules (*18*). A role for NO• in modulating P-selectin expression is also supported by reports showing diminished ischemia–reperfusion-induced upregulation of P-selectin in vascular beds treated with NO• donors (*19,20*). A similar downregulation of endothelial cell adhesion molecule expression by NO• has been observed in studies assessing VCAM-1 expression on cytokine-stimulated monolayers of human umbilical vein endothelial cells (*21,22*). The latter studies also suggest that NO• may blunt

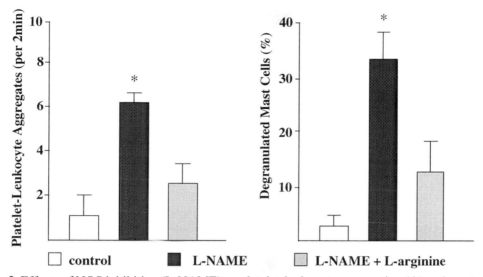

Fig. 3. Effects of NOS inhibition (L-NAME) on platelet-leukocyte aggregation (**A**) and mast cell degranulation (**B**) in rat mesentery. Data are presented for 30 min after starting each superfusion. Data from ref. *14*. *indicates $p < 0.05$ relative to control.

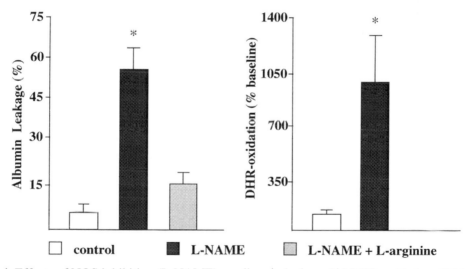

Fig. 4. Effects of NOS inhibition (L-NAME) on albumin leakage (**A**) DHR-oxidation, (**B**) in rat mesentery. Data are presented for 30 min after starting each superfusion. Data from refs. *14* and *27*. *indicates $p < 0.05$ relative to control.

transcription-dependent expression of endothelial cell adhesion molecules via an inhibitory action on the nuclear transcription factor, NFκB.

A major line of evidence that supports a role for NO• in mediating leukocyte–endothelial cell adhesion are reports showing a potent inhibitory action of NO•-donating agents on the leukocyte adhesion elicited by either ischemia–reperfusion *(19)*, NOS inhibition *(14)*, oxygen radical generating system *(11)*, or oxidized low-density lipoproteins *(23,24)*. These findings indicate that replenishment of NO• in tissues subjected to reduced bioavailability of NO• restores leukocyte–endothelial cell adhesion to its normal low level.

Reactive Oxygen Metabolite–NO• Interactions

The ability of NO• to inhibit leukocyte–endothelial adhesion may be related to its ability to interact with superoxide. NO• may exert its antiadhesive action by preventing the accumulation of superoxide (which promotes leukocyte adhesion) or by reacting with superoxide to form the peroxynitrite ($ONOO^-$) anion. The results of a recent report (25) indicates that nanomolar levels of peroxinitrite can inhibit leukocyte–endothelial cell adhesion. The possibility that NO• acts to inhibit leukocyte adhesion in much the same manner as SOD is also plausible. SOD completely blocks the leukocyte–endothelial cell adhesion induced by NOS inhibitors (10) as well as the adhesion elicited by superfusion of mesenteric venules with the oxygen radical generating system, hypoxanthine–xanthine oxidase (11).

The possibility that NO• serves as an important scavenger of superoxide generated by endothelial cells and other cells (e.g., mast cells) is supported by intravital microscopic studies employing oxidant-sensitive fluorochromes (26,27). Inhibitors of NOS (e.g., L-NAME, L-NMMA) have been shown to promote the oxidation of dihydrorhodamine-123, an oxidant-sensitive fluorochrome, by endothelial cells lining postcapillary venules (27; Fig. 4B). Administration of catalase or dimethylthiourea (DMTU) significantly attenuates, whereas inhibition of endogenous catalase by aminotriazole or depletion of intracellular glutathione by dimethylmaleate enhances the L-NAME-induced oxidation of DHR. These observations indicate that NOS inhibition and the consequent elimination of NO• results in an enhanced production of hydrogen peroxide that is likely generated from the spontaneous dismutation of superoxide, which accumulates in the absence of NO•. The resulting accumulation of superoxide and hydrogen peroxide may initiate a variety of biochemical and molecular changes that ultimately lead to neutrophil–endothelial cell adhesion.

Hydrogen peroxide (28) and NOS inhibitors (17) appear to activate phospholipase A_2, which generates lipid mediators of leukocyte–endothelial cell adhesion, i.e., PAF and LTB_4 (17). It has been shown that 8-bromo-cyclic GMP is as effective as a PAF-receptor antagonist in blunting the enhanced leukocyte adherence/emigration elicited by L-NAME (16). This observation suggests that the loss of cyclic guanosine monophosphate (cGMP) that normally accompanies inhibition of NO• synthesis contributes to leukocyte–endothelial adhesion, since restoring cellular cGMP levels with 8-bromo-cGMP greatly attenuates the adhesive response.

Mast Cell–NO• Interactions

There is a significant body of evidence that implicates mast cells in the leukocyte–endothelial cell adhesion mediated by NO•. For example, it has been shown that sodium nitroprusside decreases the amount of histamine released from mast cells (29), and that NO• inhibits PAF production by mast cells (30). Administration of L-NAME elicits the degranulation of mast cells that surround postcapillary venules (14; Fig. 3B). Ketotifen (mast cell stabilizer) and SOD are effective in abolishing this response. Because both agents were also effective in blunting the recruitment of adherent leukocytes normally elicited by L-NAME, it was proposed that mast cell degranulation contributes to the leukocyte–endothelial cell adhesion. The fact that SOD can attenuate L-NAME-induced mast cell degranulation implicates superoxide in this process. Using dihydrorhodamine to detect oxidant production, it has been demonstrated that a significant fraction of the mast cells surrounding mesenteric postcapillary venules undergo an oxidant stress after NOS inhibition with L-NAME (10). This suggests that inhibition of NO• synthesis leads to an accumulation of superoxide in mast cells, which may trigger the release of a variety of inflammatory mediators, such as PAF, tumor necrosis factor (TNF), and LTB_4. These mediators may then contribute to NO•/superoxide-dependent leukocyte–endothelial cell adhesion via activation of CD11/CD18 on leukocytes as well as selectins and ICAM-1 on endothelial cells.

NO• Mediates Leukocyte–Platelet Aggregation

NOS inhibitors have also been shown to promote the formation of platelet–leukocyte aggregates within postcapillary venules (14,16; Fig. 3A). The formation of these aggregates can be inhibited by mAbs directed against P-selectin but not CD11/CD18 or ICAM-1. These findings are consistent with reports showing that stimulated platelets rapidly mobilize P-selectin from α-granules to the cell surface. Circulating leukocytes can bind with platelets via an interaction between P-selectin and oligosaccharide ligands that are constitutively expressed on the leukocyte surface. Although the physiological relevance of the platelet–leukocyte aggregation associated with NOS inhibition remains unclear, it may explain the presence of such aggregates in the blood after administration of oxidized LDL (31), which is known to lower endothelial production of NO• (32,33).

Role of Shear Rate in NO•-Mediated Modulation of Leukocyte Adhesion

The shear rate generated by the movement of blood in postcapillary venules (estimated from red blood cell velocity divided by vessel diameter) can exert a profound influence on leukocyte–endothelial cell adhesion. Reductions in shear stress tend to promote leukocyte adherence, whereas elevations in shear rate oppose leukocyte adhesion (34). Three mechanisms may explain this negative correlation between shear rate and leukocyte adhesion. As shear rates are reduced, the hydrodynamic dispersal forces acting on the leukocyte (which tends to sweep the leukocyte away from the vessel wall) are reduced such that the ratio of adhesive forces to dispersive forces increases, thereby promoting the rolling and subsequent adherence of leukocytes. Another possibility is that when venular wall shear rate is reduced, the washout of inflammatory mediators basally generated by tissues is also reduced, thus resulting in an increased expression of adhesion molecules on both leukocytes and endothelial cells (35). A final mechanism that may explain the inverse relationship between leukocyte adherence and venular shear rate relates to the influence of shear rate on endothelial production of NO•. An elevated shear rate is a potent stimulus for increased production of NO• (36–38) and diminished generation of endothelins (which can promote leukocyte adhesion via upregulation of adhesion molecules) (39–41). Hence, it is conceivable that low shear rates favor leukocyte adhesion because NO• levels are diminished, whereas endothelin levels are elevated above control values.

The contribution of shear rate to the recruitment of adherent leukocytes in postcapillary venules treated with NOS inhibitors has been addressed. The increased number of adherent leukocytes after L-NAME treatment cannot be explained by the corresponding (approx 30%) reduction in venular blood flow and shear rate (13). Comparable reductions in venular shear rate induced by mechanical constriction of the arterial inflow elicited an increased leukocyte adhesion, which was only a small fraction of the value observed by NOS inhibition.

NO• and Monocyte Recruitment

Monocytes and macrophages are able to generate NO• from both constitutive and inducible isoforms of NOS. Unstimulated monocytes/macrophages express only cNOS, but after cytokine stimulation iNOS becomes the predominant isoform (42). Macrophages/monocytes appear capable of modulating their adhesion to endothelial cells by generating NO• in an autocrine process (43–45). In vitro studies indicate that NO• donors inhibit monocyte–endothelial cell adhesion (46) and inhibit monocyte chemotaxis (47–49). Shear stress reduces (38), whereas hypercholesterolemia enhances (23,50), the adhesiveness of endothelial cells for monocytes via the activation and inhibition of eNOS, respectively.

NO• and Lymphocyte Recruitment

The adhesion of lymphocytes to endothelial cells is not as profoundly affected by NO• as noted for neutrophils and monocytes. Quiescent and cytokine-stimulated lymphocytes exhibit no change in adhesive behavior when L-NMMA or NO• donors like sodium nitroprusside or spermine–NO• are administered *(51)*. This may be related to the relative inability of lymphocytes to produce superoxide, or it may reflect a lesser dependence of homing lymphocytes on those endothelial–cell adhesion molecules (e.g., P-selectin) that are regulated by NO• *(52)*.

NO• AND THE ENDOTHELIAL BARRIER

The leukocyte–endothelial cell adhesion that is associated with diminished NO• production is often accompanied by an increased microvascular permeability *(14,53;* Fig. 4A). Because preventing leukocyte adhesion with mAbs directed against CD11/CD18 also blunts the protein extravasation that results from NOS inhibition *(54)*, it has been proposed that factors released from activated, adherent leukocytes mediate the endothelial barrier dysfunction. There is also evidence, however, that invokes a direct action of NO• to diminish the restrictive properties of the endothelial barrier and consequently increase vascular permeability. Studies on isolated buffer-perfused postcapillary venules have revealed that increases in shear rate result in an enhanced albumin extravasation that can be prevented by an NOS inhibitor *(55)*. Other studies have implicated NO• as the mediator of bradykinin- *(56–58)* and histamine- *(57)* induced increases in vascular permeability. Because these agents are known to affect barrier function by eliciting the contraction (and retraction) of adjacent endothelial cells, the foregoing findings suggest that NO• can alter the adhesion of adjacent endothelial cells. There is some controversy, however, regarding the role of NO• as a direct inducer of albumin extravasation in vivo. Some investigators have obtained data that suggest that NO• mediates bradykinin-induced vascular protein leakage by virtue of its ability to elicit arteriolar vasodilation and consequently increase the pressure within postcapillary venules *(58)*. Others have proposed that ablation of basal NO• release (using a NOS inhibitor) by postcapillary venules elicits a transient increase in water permeability of the endothelial barrier, which is related to the antioxidant role of NO• *(59)*. The contradictory evidence concerning the role of NO• in modulating endothelial barrier function is difficult to explain. However, it appears likely that the direct actions of endothelial cell-derived NO• on junctional integrity differ from the responses noted when NO•-responsive intravascular (e.g., leukocytes and platelets) and perivascular (mast cells, macrophages) cells participate in the vascular permeability responses. The relative rates of NO• and superoxide production are also likely to be important determinants of the net effect of NO• depletion or overproduction on endothelial barrier function.

CONCLUSIONS

A role for NO• in the modulation of leukocyte–endothelial cell adhesion is now well established. Although the molecular basis for this NO•-mediated, heterotypic cell adhesion response has not been clearly defined, it appears to contribute to the inflammatory responses noted in different experimental models of cardiovascular disease, including atherosclerosis, ischemia–reperfusion, and circulatory shock. Because leukocyte–endothelial cell adhesion has been invoked as an important component of these and other pathological processes, the use of drugs that either replenish tissue NO• levels or prevent superoxide-mediated NO• metabolism to limit the inflammatory response appears to be worthy of further consideration.

ACKNOWLEDGMENT

D.N.G. was supported by grants from the National Heart Lung and Blood Institute (HL26441) and National Institute of Diabetes, Digestive and Kidney Diseases (P01 DK43786).

REFERENCES

1. Granger DN, Kubes P. The microcirculation and inflammation: modulation of leukocyte-endothelial cell adhesion. J Leukoc Biol 1994;55:662–675.
2. Panes J, Granger DN. Leukocyte-endothelial cell interactions: molecular mechanisms and implications in gastrointestinal disease. Gastroenterology 1998;114:1066–1090.
3. Stamler J, Mendelsohn ME, Amarante P, Smick D, Andon N, Davies PF, et al. N-acetylcysteine potentiates platelet inhibition by endothelium-derived relaxing factor. Circ Res 1989;65:789–795.
4. Yao SK, Ober JC, Krishnaswami A, Ferguson JJ, Anderson HV, Golino P, et al. Endogenous nitric oxide protects against platelet aggregation and cyclic flow variations in stenosed and endothelium-injured arteries. Circulation 1992;86:1302–1309.
5. Michelson AD, Benoit SE, Furman MI, Breckwoldt WL, Rohrer MJ, Barnard MR, et al. Effects of nitric oxide/EDRF on platelet surface glycoproteins. Am J Physiol 1996;270:H1640–H1648
6. Hogan JC, Lewis MJ, Henderson AH. In vivo EDRF activity influences platelet function. Br J Pharmacol 1988;94:1020–1022.
7. Mendelsohn ME, O'Neill S, George D, Loscalzo J. Inhibition of fibrinogen binding to human platelets by S-nitroso-N-acetylcysteine. J Biol Chem 1990;265:19,028–19,034.
8. Houston DS, Buchanan MR. Influence of endothelium-derived relaxing factor on platelet function and hemostasis in vivo. Thromb Res 1994;74:25–37.
9. Suzuki M, Inauen W, Kvietys PR, Grisham MB, Meininger C, Schelling ME, et al. Superoxide mediates reperfusion-induced leukocyte-endothelial cell interactions. Am J Physiol 1989;257:H1740–H1745.
10. Kubes P, Kanwar S, Niu XF, Gaboury JP. Nitric oxide synthesis inhibition induces leukocyte adhesion via superoxide and mast cells. FASEB J 1993;7:1293–1299.
11. Gaboury J, Woodman RC, Granger DN, Reinhardt P, Kubes P. Nitric oxide prevents leukocyte adherence: role of superoxide. Am J Physiol 1993;265:H862–H867.
12. Beckman JS, Koppenol WH. Nitric oxide, superoxide, and peroxynitrite: the good, the bad, and ugly. Am J Physiol 1996;271:C1424–C1437.
13. Kubes P, Suzuki M, Granger DN. Nitric oxide: an endogenous modulator of leukocyte adhesion. Proc Natl Acad Sci USA 1991;88:4651–4655.
14. Kurose I, Wolf R, Grisham MB, Granger DN. Effects of an endogenous inhibitor of nitric oxide synthesis on postcapillary venules. Am J Physiol 1995;268:H2224–H2231.
15. Lopez-Belmonte J, Whittle BJ. Aminoguanidine-provoked leukocyte adherence to rat mesenteric venules: role of constitutive nitric oxide synthase inhibition. Br J Pharmacol 1995;116:2710–2714.
16. Kurose I, Kubes P, Wolf R, Anderson DC, Paulson J, Miyasaka M, et al. Inhibition of nitric oxide production. Mechanisms of vascular albumin leakage. Circ Res 1993;73:164–171.
17. Arndt H, Russell JB, Kurose I, Kubes P, Granger DN. Mediators of leukocyte adhesion in rat mesenteric venules elicited by inhibition of nitric oxide synthesis. Gastroenterology 1993;105:675–680.
18. Davenpeck KL, Gauthier TW, Lefer AM. Inhibition of endothelial-derived nitric oxide promotes P-selectin expression and actions in the rat microcirculation. Gastroenterology 1994;107:1050–1058.
19. Gauthier TW, Davenpeck KL, Lefer AM. Nitric oxide attenuates leukocyte-endothelial interaction via P-selectin in splanchnic ischemia-reperfusion. Am J Physiol 1994;267:G562–G568.
20. Eppihimer MJ, Russell J, Anderson DC, Epstein CJ, Laroux S, Granger DN. Modulation of P-selectin expression in the postischemic intestinal vasculature. Am J Physiol 1997;273:G1326–G1332.
21. Takahashi M, Ikeda U, Masuyama J, Funayama H, Kano S, Shimada K. Nitric oxide attenuates adhesion molecule expression in human endothelial cells. Cytokine 1996;8:817–821.
22. Khan BV, Harrison DG, Olbrych MT, Alexander RW, Medford RM. Nitric oxide regulates vascular cell adhesion molecule 1 gene expression and redox-sensitive transcriptional events in human vascular endothelial cells. Proc Natl Acad Sci USA 1996;93:9114–9119.
23. Tsao PS, McEvoy LM, Drexler H, Butcher EC, Cooke JP. Enhanced endothelial adhesiveness in hypercholesterolemia is attenuated by L-arginine. Circulation 1994;89:2176–2182.
24. Liao L, Granger DG. Modulation of oxidized low-density lipoprotein-induced microvascular dysfunction by nitric oxide. Am J Physiol 1995;268:H1643–H1650.
25. Lefer DJ, Scalia R, Campbell B, Nossuli T, Hayward R, Salamon M, et al. Peroxynitrite inhibits leukocyte-endothelial cell interactions and protects against ischemia-reperfusion injury in rats. J Clin Invest 1997;99:684–691.
26. Suematsu M, Tamatani T, Delano FA, Miyasaka M, Forrest M, Suzuki H, et al. Microvascular oxidative stress preceding leukocyte activation elicited by in vivo nitric oxide suppression. Am J Physiol 1994;266:H2410–H2415.
27. Kurose I, Wolf R, Grisham MB, Aw TY, Specian RD, Granger DN. Microvascular responses to inhibition of nitric oxide production. Role of active oxidants. Circ Res 1995;76:30–39.

28. Otamiri T, Lindahl M, Tagesson C. Phospholipase A2 inhibition prevents mucosal damage associated with small intestinal ischemia in rats. Gut 1988;29:489–494.
29. Mannaioni PF, Masini E, Pistelli A, Salvemini D, Vane JR. Mast cells as a source of superoxide anions ans nitric oxide-like factor: relevance to histamine release. Int J Tissue React 1991;13:271–278.
30. Hogaboam CM, Befus AD, Wallace JL. Modulation of rat mast cell reactivity by IL-1 beta. Divergent effects on nitric oxide and platelet-activating factor release. J Immunol 1993;151:3767–3774.
31. Lehr HA, Olofsson AM, Carew TE, Vajkoczy P, von Andrian UH, Hubner C, et al. P-selectin mediates the interaction of circulating leukocytes with platelets and microvascular endothelium in response to oxidized lipoprotein in vivo. Lab Invest 1994;71:380–386.
32. Tanner FC, Boulanger CM, Luscher TF. Endothelium-derived nitric oxide, endothelin, and platelet vessel wall interaction: alterations in hypercholesterolemia and atherosclerosis. Semin Thromb Hemost 1993;19:167–175.
33. Liao JK, Shin WS, Lee WY, Clark SL. Oxidized low-density lipoprotein decreases the expression of endothelial nitric oxide synthase. J Biol Chem 1995;270:319–324.
34. Perry MA, Granger DN. Role of CD11/CD18 in shear rate-dependent leukocyte-endothelial cell interactions in cat mesenteric venules. J Clin Invest 1991;87:1798–1804.
35. Bienvenu K, Russell J, Granger DN. Leukotriene B$_4$ mediates shear rate-dependent leukocyte adhesion in mesenteric venules. Circ Res 1992;71:906–911.
36. Pohl U, Holtz J, Busse R, Bassenge E. Crucial role of endothelium in the vasodilator response to increase flow in vivo. Hypertension 1986;8:37–44.
37. Cooke JP, Rossitch E Jr, Andon NA, Loscalzo J, Dzau VJ. Flow activates an endothelial potassium channel to release an endogenous nitrovasodilator. J Clin Invest 1991;88:1663–1671.
38. Tsao PS, Lewis NP, Alpert S, Cooke JP. Exposure to shear stress alters endothelial adhesiveness. Role of nitric oxide. Circulation 1995;92:3513–3519.
39. Kuchan MJ, Frangos JA. Shear stress regulates endothelin-1 release via protein kinase C and cGMP in cultured endothelial cells. Am J Physiol 1993;264:H150–H156.
40. McCarron RM, Wang L, Stanimirovic DB, Spatz M. Endothelin induction of adhesion molecule expression on human brain microvascular endothelial cells. Neurosci Lett 1993;156:31–34.
41. Lopez Farre A, Riesco A, Espinosa G, Digiuni E, Cernadas MR, Alvarez V, et al. Effect of endothelin-1 on neutrophil adhesion to endothelial cells and perfused heart. Circulation 1993;88:1166–1171.
42. Reiling N, Ulmer AJ, Duchrow M, Ernst M, Flad HD, Hauschildt S. Nitric oxide synthase: mRNA expression of different isoforms in human monocytes/macrophages. Eur J Immunol 1994;24:1941–1944.
43. Cartwright JE, Johnstone AP, Whitley GS. Inhibition of nitric oxide synthase by antisense techniques: investigations of the roles of NO produced by murine macrophages. Br J Pharmacol 1997;120:146–152.
44. Magazine HI, Liu Y, Bilfinger TV, Fricchione GL, Stefano GB. Morphine-induced conformational changes in human monocytes, granulocytes, and endothelial cells and in invertebrate immunocytes and microglia are mediated by nitric oxide. J Immunol 1996;156:4845–4850.
45. King JM, Srivastava KD, Stefano GB, Bilfinger TV, Bahou WF, Magazine HI. Human monocyte adhesion is modulated by endothelin B receptor-coupled nitric oxide release. J Immunol 1997;158:880–886.
46. De Caterina R, Libby P, Peng HB, Thannickal VJ, Rajavashisth TB, Gimbrone MA Jr, et al. Nitric oxide decreases cytokine-induced endothelial activation. Nitric oxide selectively reduces endothelial expression of adhesion molecules and proinflammatory cytokines. J Clin Invest 1995;96:60–68.
47. Bath PM, Hassal DG, Gladwin AM, Palmer RM, Martin JF. Nitric oxide and prostacyclin. Divergence of inhibitory effects on monocyte chemotaxis and adhesion to endothelium in vitro. Arterioscler Thromb 1991;11:254–260.
48. Belenky SN, Robbins RA, Rubinstein I. Nitric oxide synthase inhibitors attenuate human monocyte chemotaxis in vitro. J Leukoc Biol 1993;53:498–503.
49. Zeiher AM, Fisslthaler B, Schray-Utz B, Busse R. Nitric oxide modulates the expression of monocyte chemoattractant protein 1 in cultured human endothelial cells. Circ Res 1995;76:980–986.
50. Theilmeier G, Chan JR, Zalpour C, Anderson B, Wang BY, Wolf A, et al. Adhesiveness of mononuclear cells in hypercholesterolemic humans is normalized by dietary L-arginine. Arterioscler Thromb Vasc Biol 1997;17:3557–3564.
51. Cartwright JE, Whitley GS, Johnstone AP. Endothelial cell adhesion molecule expression and lymphocyte adhesion to endothelial cells: effect of nitric oxide. Exp Cell Res 1997;235:431–434.
52. Westphal JR, de Waal RM. The role of adhesion molecules in endothelial cell accessory function. Mol Biol Rep 1992;17:47–59.
53. Gaboury JP, Kubes P. Endogenous antiadhesive molecules. In: Granger DN, Schmid-Schönbein GW, eds. Physiology and Pathophysiology of Leukocyte Adhesion. Oxford University Press, New York, 1995, pp. 241–260.

54. Kubes P, Granger DN. Nitric oxide modulates microvascular permeability. Am J Physiol 1992;262: H611–H615.
55. Yuan Y, Granger HJ, Zawieja DC, Chilian WM. Flow modulates venular permeability by a nitric oxide-related mechanism. Am J Physiol 1992;263:H641–H646.
56. Mayhan WG. Role of nitric oxide in modulating permeability of hamster cheek pouch in response to adenosine 5'-diphosphate and bradykinin. Inflammation 1992; 16:295–305.
57. Paul W, Douglas GJ, Lawrence L, Khawaja AM, Perez AC, Schachter M, et al. Cutaneous permeability responses to bradykinin and histamine in the guinea-pig: possible differences in their mechanism of action. Br J Pharmacol 1994;111:159–164.
58. Feletou M, Bonnardel E, Canet E. Bradykinin and changes in microvascular permeability in the hamster cheek pouch: role of nitric oxide. Br J Pharmacol 1996;118:1371–1376.
59. He P, Zeng M, Curry FE. Effect of nitric oxide synthase inhibitors on basal microvessel permeability and endothelial cell [Ca2+]i. Am J Physiol 1997;273:H747–H755.

10

Nitric Oxide and Cardiomyocyte Function

Jean-Luc Balligand and Paul J. Cannon

CELL BIOLOGY OF CARDIAC NO•

Myocardial NO• Synthases

There is ample evidence that all three isoforms of nitric oxide synthase (NOS) are expressed within the various cell types in the myocardium (*see* Table 1). The coordinate physiological regulation of cardiac muscle contraction by the NO• (*see* Table 2) produced by each of these isoforms mandates a tight regulation of both the expression and the activity of each NOS isoform within a specific cell type. Therefore, despite the apparent promiscuity of having all three NOS isoforms within cardiac muscle, the predominant cellular source of the NO• that is produced in the heart may vary according to specific transcriptional and posttranscriptional stimuli differentially affecting each cell type and/or isoform (as will subsequently be illustrated for eNOS).

NOS 1 protein has been identified in both cholinergic and nonadrenergic, noncholinergic nerve terminals, in specialized conduction tissue and in sympathetic nerve terminals of the guinea pig heart *(1,2)*. Immunohistochemical colocalization of NOS 1 with tyrosine hydroxylase in cardiac neurons definitively demonstrated that orthosympathetic nerve terminals express NOS1 in the rodent heart *(3)*. NO• produced endogenously by nerve terminals was also shown to play a role in the control of catecholamine release during electrical sympathetic nerve stimulation in isolated perfused hearts *(3)*, a finding also confirmed in PC-12 cells in vitro *(4)*. Cardiac myocytes, however, do not seem to express the canonical NOS 1, at least in the rat *(5,6)*. Nor was the muscle-specific isoform of n-NOS (n-NOS-mu) *(7)* detectable in extracts of purified rat ventricular myocytes *(8)*. Recently, a NOS isoform with nNOS immunoreactivity, but slightly slower electrophoretic mobility (160 vs 155 kDa), was identified in SR vesicles from rabbit hearts, where it was shown to inhibit calcium uptake by the sarcoplasmic reticulum (SR) *(9)*.

The expression of NOS 3 (eNOS) has been demonstrated in endothelial cells from the endocardium and from arterial capillaries and veins in rodents and a variety of mammalian species *(5,10,11)* including humans *(12,13)*. The abundance of the immunostained proteins seems to be heterogenous along the coronary vascular bed *(11)*. In addition to endothelial cells, there is unequivocal evidence that eNOS is expressed in cardiomyocytes from atria and atrioventricular nodal and ventricular tissue in several species *(5,14,15)*, including in humans *(12,13,16)*. This conclusion is based on several complementary experimental approaches including single-cell contractility or ionic current measurements, *in situ* hybridization, and immunohistochemistry. In addition, Feron and colleagues showed that, as in endothelial cells, palmitoylated and miristoylated eNOS in cardiac myocytes is localized to caveolae which are

From: *Contemporary Cardiology, vol. 4: Nitric Oxide and the Cardiovascular System*
Edited by: J. Loscalzo and J. A. Vita © Humana Press Inc., Totowa, NJ

Table 1
Cell Source and Isoforms of NOS in the Myocardium

Cell type	Isoform	Physiol./pathol. condition	Reference
Endocardial endothelium	eNOS	Constitutive	11
	iNOS	Sepsis, transplant rejection	10,25
Endothelium,	eNOS	Constitutive	11
Macro/microvascular	iNOS	Sepsis, transplant rejection	10,25
Intracardial neurons	nNOS	Constitutive	3,10
Vascular smooth muscle cells, fibroblasts	iNOS	Sepsis, transplant rejection	10,25
Cardiomyocytes			
Atrial	eNOS	Constitutive	16
AV node	eNOS	Constitutive	14
Ventricular	eNOS	Constitutive	5
	nNOS[a]	Constitutive	9
	iNOS	Sepsis, infarction, transplant rejection, heart failure	10,25,55
Infiltrating inflammatory cells	iNOS	Sepsis, transplant rejection, infarction	10,25

Because of space constraints, only a limited number of original references are cited. Many other original references may be found in the bibliography of refs. *10* and *25*; note also that NOS expression in each type may vary from one species to another.

[a] May be an isoform different from canonical nNOS.

detergent-insoluble glycosphingolipid-rich microdomains in the plasmalemma *(17)*. These authors demonstrated, using extracts of rat cardiac myocytes, that eNOS is coimmunoprecipitated with the isoform of caveolin (caveolin 3), that is specifically expressed in myocytes but not endothelial cells, consistent with myocyte-specific expression of eNOS *(17)*. The identification of caveolin-binding domains within the eNOS protein is consistent with a direct protein–protein interaction between eNOS and caveolin-3 in cardiomyocytes, such as had been previously demonstrated between eNOS and caveolin-1 *(18–21)* *(see* Chapter 2). This molecular interaction alone, however, is insufficient for correct targeting of eNOS to caveolae, which may be facilitated by posttranslational lipidation (e.g., palmitoylation) *(22)*. Of additional interest, Parton and colleagues *(23)* recently showed that caveolin-3 is also expressed in the T-tubular system in skeletal and cardiac muscle. It had been suggested for years that the T-tubular system developed from the coalescence of clusters of caveolae at the sarcolemmal membrane *(24)*. Together, these separate pieces of evidence may be relevant to the potential role of eNOS in the regulation of excitation–contraction coupling in the heart, as discussed as follows.

Virtually all cell types within heart muscle are now known to express iNOS after appropriate stimulation with specific combinations of inflammatory cytokines, e.g., cardiac microvascular endothelial cells and cardiac myocytes (for a review, *see* refs. *10* and *25*). The relative abundance of iNOS expression within the different cell types in pathophysiological situations in vivo may be substantially different from the results observed after exposure of the cells to recombinant cytokines in vitro. In human allograft rejection, e.g., there is a clear expression of iNOS within macrophages and myocytes that (along with endothelial cells) account for most of the iNOS immunoreactivity *(26)*. In other circumstances, such as the rabbit model of acute myocardial infarction, however, iNOS staining seems to be restricted to infiltrating macrophages with little or no staining of adjacent cardiomyocytes *(27)*. The amount of iNOS expression, as detected by immunostaining appears to be more heterogenous in the myocardium of patients with heart failure *(28–30)*. In a recent study *(31)*, iNOS

Table 2
Functional Effects of NO• in Normal and Diseased Heart

	Healthy hearts/myocytes	Diseased hearts/myocytes
Inotropic state (systolic contraction)	"Baseline" contraction (i.e., in the absence of an agonist) Positive inotropic effect (low doses of exogenous NO• donors) Negative inotropic effect (high doses of exogenous NO• donors)	Myocardial depression[b] (sepsis, transplant rejection, heart failure)
	"Stimulated" contraction (i.e., β-adrenergic response) Negative inotropic effect[a] Positive inotropic effect	Attenuation of β-adrenergic responsiveness[b]
Lusitropic state (diastolic relaxation)	Hastening of relaxation, shortening of contraction Improvement of diastolic filling (paracrine effect[a])	Loss of NO•[a]: diastolic dysfunction
Chronotropic state	Mediation of muscarinic cholinergic effects on heart rate and conduction in S.A., A.V. nodal, and ventricular tissue[a]	Loss of NO•[a]: decreased threshold for arrhythmias
Force–frequency relationship	Attenuation of positive rate-staircase[a]	—
Myocardial oxygen consumption	Decrease in O_2 consumption (paracrine effect[a])	Loss of NO•[a]: increase in O_2 consumption
Ischemia/reperfusion	—	Trigger for preconditioning stimulus[a] Mediator for late preconditioning effect[b]
Growth/remodeling	—	Control of hypertrophic response[a]
Others	Control of substrate (glucose) utilization[a]	Induction of apoptosis[b] Immune response against bacteria and viruses[b]

[a] eNOS-mediated.
[b] iNOS-mediated.

immunostaining in patients with end-stage heart failure due to ischemic cardiomyopathy and myocarditis was present in cardiac myocytes within infarcted and noninfarcted regions and was present in infiltrating macrophages; iNOS activity was variable and correlated significantly with the density of infiltrating macrophages. From these studies, it seems that the positivity of iNOS immunostaining varies according to the etiology of the cardiomyopathy with some studies reporting increase in iNOS expression restricted to idiopathic cardiomyopathy (30) in myocardial dysfunction associated with sepsis (32), or ischemic myocardium (31). Even though most of these diseases are likely to be associated with increased expression and production of inflammatory cytokines, which are known to increase iNOS gene transcription in vitro (as directly demonstrated for tumor necrosis factor-α [TNF-α]) (30,33), one should keep in mind that iNOS protein expression is discontinuous over time. Temporal variations in iNOS expression in different cells in the myocardium may explain some of the discrepancy among different reports depending on the time interval of sampling and the progression of the disease in the tissue samples that have been examined.

eNOS Activation by Cytokines

Aside from the well-known effect of inflammatory cytokines on increasing iNOS expression and NO• production, cytokines may also increase NO• production in cardiac muscle through direct activation of the constitutively expressed eNOS. The first hint of such an acute effect that is independent of increased gene transcription or protein expression was the study of Finkel and colleagues, who demonstrated that exposure of hamster papillary muscles to TNF-α, IL-2 (interleukin), or IL-6 decreased the amplitude of the muscles' contraction within minutes *(34)*. The inhibition of this negative inotropic effect by NOS inhibitors such as ^GN-mono-methyl-L-arginine (L-NMMA) strongly suggested that a constitutively expressed isoform of NOS within cardiac muscle was involved in the effect. More recently, Goldhaber and colleagues showed that recombinant TNF-α decreased the contractile amplitude of shortening of isolated rabbit ventricular myocytes through L-NMMA-sensitive mechanisms, a finding consistent with the aforementioned reported results *(35)*. These data are also consistent with earlier observations of the acute release of a NO•-like factor from aortic endothelial cells induced by endotoxin within a time course that would exclude de novo gene expression *(36)*.

eNOS Activation by Mechanical Activity

In endothelial cells, mechanical forces like flow-dependent shear stress are known to be important stimuli regulating basal (i.e., in the absence of agonists) release of NO• in the vasculature (for a review, *see* ref. *37*). This receptor-independent activation of eNOS is thought to be mediated by calcium-independent mechanisms, possibly involving changes in the phosphorylation state of eNOS-associated cytoskeletal proteins *(38)*. Even though this has been demonstrated mainly in endothelial cells from the macrovasculature, there is also initial evidence that similar mechanical forces may be acting on endothelial or endocardial cells within cardiac muscle. Using a NO•-specific porphyrinic electrode implanted within different layers of beating ventricular myocardium, Pinsky and colleagues demonstrated that the NO• signals were modulated by changes in preload and afterload *(39)*. In addition, mechanical deformation of ventricular muscle ex vivo was accompanied by parallel changes in NO• production, suggesting that cyclic variations in mechanical constraints such as those experienced by ventricular muscle during the cardiac cycle, may exert autoregulatory effects on coronary flow and ventricular relaxation mediated through changes in endogenous NO• production. Because deendothelization of these preparations abrogated the NO• signals, the authors concluded that endothelial cells were the predominant source of NO• production under their experimental conditions *(39)*.

eNOS Activation by Beating and Beta-Adrenergic Agonists

The constitutive NOS isozymes (nNOS, eNOS) are classically activated by calcium–calmodulin binding to its specific target sequence on each NOS monomer, which enables electrons to flow from the reductase to the oxygenase domains *(40)*. For both neuronal and endothelial NOS, the EC 50 for calcium activation of enzyme activity is about 200–400 μ*M*, i.e., within the range of intracellular calcium concentrations observed after the binding of agonists known to elevate intracellular calcium concentrations. It is also close to intracellular calcium levels measured during systole in cardiac myocytes. Using electrically stimulated cultures of adult rat ventricular myocytes, Kaye and colleagues showed that myocyte NO• production is activated by increasing the frequency of contraction and can be inhibited by NOS inhibitors *(41)*. Similarly, the force–frequency relationship was shown to be modulated by endogenously produced NO• in guinea-pig papillary muscle through an L-NMMA-sensitive mechanism *(42)*.

It is well known that beta-adrenergic agonists increase intracellular calcium concentration in cardiac myocytes through cyclic adenosine monophosphate (cAMP) and protein kinase A (PKA)-dependent upregulation of calcium current through voltage-sensitive calcium channels. Accordingly, exposure of cultured neonatal or adult rat ventricular myocytes to beta 1 or beta 2 (but not alpha) adrenergic agonists evoked L-NMMA-inhibitable increases in NO• release, as measured with a porphyrinic microelectrode *(43)*. These findings are consistent with the previous demonstration of eNOS expression within cardiac myocytes as mentioned earlier. The subsequent observation that the NO• signal was similarly enhanced by cAMP analogs, GTPγs, and the calcium channel-activating dihydropyridine (BAYK 8644) all suggested that the classical beta 1 or beta 2 adrenergic pathway stimulated eNOS enzyme activity by G-protein mediated activation of adenylyl cyclase and subsequent calcium influx. More recently, however, Gauthier and colleagues observed that exposure of human ventricular biopsies to norepinephrine in the presence of full alpha- and beta 1 and beta 2-adrenoceptor blockade induced an increase in the intracellular concentration of cGMP associated with a strikingly negative inotropic effect *(13)*. Gauthier et al. noted that these observations were reproduced upon exposure of ventricular tissue to specific agonists of the beta 3–adrenoceptor subtype and that both the increases in cGMP and the negative inotropic effect were fully inhibited upon incubation with either pertussis toxin or L-NMMA. These results strongly suggest that beta 3–adrenoceptors in the human heart are coupled to NOS activation through $G\alpha_i$ proteins *(13)*. The additional direct measurements of increases in NO° production with a porphyrinic electrode in the solution bathing human ventricular tissue specimens in these experiments demonstrated that the aforementioned effects are specifically the result of beta 3–adrenoceptor mediated activation of NOS.

eNOS Activation by Muscarinic Cholinergic Agonist

Muscarinic receptors that are predominantly expressed on cardiomyocytes are mainly of the M2 subtype. M2 receptors mediate acetylcholine's negative actions on heart rate and force of contraction through $G\alpha_i$-mediated inhibition of adenylyl cyclase or $G\alpha_q$-coupling to specific potassium currents (I_{KAch}). The specific coupling of any muscarinic receptor subtype to eNOS activation is poorly characterized. According to the classical paradigm of Ca–calmodulin-dependent NOS activation, such coupling could involve muscarinic receptor-mediated release of intracellular calcium. This has been shown to occur following agonist binding to M1, M3, and M5 receptors in other cell types; it may also occur following M2 receptor stimulation in heart cells *(44)*. In isolated ventricular myocytes from rat hearts, Feron et al. demonstrated that muscarinic receptor stimulation promotes the translocation of the receptors to caveolae *(45)* where components of the phosphoinositide pathway (including phospholipase C), sarcoplasmic reticulum calcium release channels and eNOS are colocalized, thus rendering their functional interaction likely. Reports from several laboratories have shown that in endothelial cells, the formation of a heteroduplex between eNOS and caveolin inhibits the enzyme activity, and that this protein–protein interaction is in equilibrium with the calcium-dependent binding of calmodulin to eNOS (for a review, *see* ref. *46*). According to this scheme, agonist-dependent increases in intracellular calcium would promote eNOS activation in two ways: by displacing caveolin, thereby relieving its tonic inhibition of eNOS and by enabling the conformational change within eNOS protein that allows the electron flow for the oxidation of L-arginine in its oxygenase domain. As a corollary, the efficient coupling of muscarinic receptors to eNOS activation could theoretically be hampered by the competitive displacement of eNOS binding toward its inhibitory heteroduplex formation with caveolin, if, e.g., the abundance of the latter was increased. Indeed, this was directly demonstrated in experiments in which the muscarinic cholinergic-induced increase in intracellular cGMP and decrease in beating rate (which were previously shown to be eNOS-dependent) *(47)*, were abolished on overexpression of caveolin 3 in transfected neonatal rat myocytes *(48)*. A similar uncoupling of the muscarinic receptor was reproduced on reversible permeabilisation of the myocytes with peptides containing the caveolin scaffolding sequence (thereby mimicking formation of the inhibitory heteroduplex), whereas control peptides with a scrambled sequence were inactive *(48)*.

Another corollary to these observations is that the physical colocalization of all the necessary signalling proteins within the same subcellular compartment may be required for the efficient coupling of any membrane receptor to eNOS activation. This assumption is supported by the observations that the cholinergic muscarinic-dependent increase in cyclic

GMP and decrease in beating rate, which are lost in cultured neonatal myocytes from mice deficient in the eNOS gene (eNOS–/–, *see* next section), can be restored on transfection of the myocytes with wild-type eNOS. These responses cannot be restored by transfection with the eNOS mutant (G2AeNOS) deficient for the miristoylation site, which cannot be targeted to the plasma membrane *(48)*. In addition to facilitating receptor-dependent activation of the enzyme, targeting eNOS to the plasma membrane may also promote its interaction with other proteins, (e.g., from the cytoskeleton), which could participate in mechanical (i.e., through increases in stretch, shear) or other potentially calcium-independent mechanisms of eNOS activation *(49)*.

REGULATION OF NOS EXPRESSION AND ACTIVITY IN CARDIOMYOCYTES

eNOS

In addition to the molecular mechanisms that govern acute increases in eNOS activity, as outlined earlier, the abundance of eNOS mRNA and protein is also regulated in the long term by several other factors. In cultured ventricular cardiac myocytes, as in macrovascular endothelial cells *(50)*, the abundance of eNOS mRNA is downregulated by inflammatory cytokines, such as TNF-α, IL-1β, and IFN-γ *(5)*. In animal models of heart failure, such as the chronically paced dog, the expression of eNOS is similarly downregulated, at least in the vasculature *(51)*. Studies of NO•- and endothelium-dependent relaxation in the vasculature of patients with heart failure have led to similar observations of eNOS downregulation, which may explain in part the increased vascular resistance in heart failure. Few studies, however, have addressed the question of whether eNOS is similarly downregulated in cardiac myocytes. In fact, a recent report supports the opposite *(52)*. This question is of special relevance given the previous demonstration of a differential regulation of eNOS expressed in cardiac myocytes versus microvascular endothelial cells in rat ventricular muscle. Increases in cAMP following treatment of cultured cells with beta adrenergic agonists in vitro or treatment of rats with milrinone in vivo were associated with selective downregulation of both eNOS mRNA and protein in cardiac myocytes but not in microvascular endothelial cells. Such treatment in vitro was also associated with the appearance of a higher molecular weight form of eNOS (150 kDa) and its translocation to cytosolic fractions *(6,8)*. A similar upregulation of a 150-kDa protein with immunoaffinity characteristics of eNOS was shown in left atria of dogs with long-term (21 d), pacing-induced heart failure, which exhibited enhanced Ca-dependent NOS activity *(53)*. Similarly, we observed a transient upregulation of Ca-dependent NOS activity in both atrial and ventricular tissue in a dog model of hypertensive cardiomyopathy (A. Piech and J.L. Balligand, unpublished observations). This increased NOS activity may represent a compensatory mechanism against the development of cardiac hypertrophy in the prefailing heart. Finally, Hare and colleagues reported observations suggesting that eNOS activity and protein levels are influenced by pertussis toxin in the rat heart, through mechanisms that are presently uncharacterized *(54)*.

iNOS

Many inflammatory cytokines, including IL-1β, TNF-α, IFN-γ (interferon), and TGF-β (transforming growth factor), have been shown to exert transcriptional and posttranscriptional regulation of iNOS gene expression. These data include specific studies of cytokines with cardiac myocytes *(55–59)*. Recent experiments using neonatal rat ventricular myocytes transfected with the iNOS promoter allowed the identification of key transcriptional regulators of iNOS gene expression in this specific cellular context; these include NF-κB, interferon regulatory factor (IRF)-1, and cAMP responsive element binding protein (CREB) *(60)*. Interactions with CREB may explain previous observations of the potentiation of iNOS induction following angiotensin II or phenylephrine stimulation by increases in intracellular cAMP *(61,62)*. Additional experiments, however, suggested that the effect of cAMP was mediated through enhanced iNOS–mRNA stability *(63)*. Other experiments have identified intracellular mitogen-activated protein (MAP) kinase and protein kinase C (PKC) phosphorylation pathways as critical regulators of iNOS expression *(57,64*; for a review, *see* refs. *10* and *25*). Of interest, the same pathways were found to be activated when mechanical strain was applied to cardiac myocytes and shown to decrease iNOS expression *(65)*. The activity of iNOS is also regulated posttranslationally by increases in the availability of its substrate L-arginine following cytokine induction of L-arginine transporters *(66)*. The same cytokines also induce the expression of guanosine triphosphate (GTP) cyclohydrolase, the rate-limiting enzyme for *de novo* synthesis of tetrahydrobiopterin, a key cofactor for NOS activity *(55,67)*.

MECHANISMS OF ACTION OF NO• IN CARDIAC TISSUE

NO• has effects in cardiomyocytes, which are cyclic GMP-dependent and other effects that are cyclic GMP-independent (*see* Fig. 1). Heart muscle cells express the soluble isoform of guanylyl cyclase that catalytically increases intracellular levels of cyclic GMP in reponse to stimulation by NO• or by thionitrite derivatives of NO•, such as *S*-nitrosoglutathione, which was recently identified as an intermediate for NO• signaling following bradykinin stimulation in rat hearts *(68)*. Cardiomyocytes from most mammalian species also express isoforms of phosphodiesterases such as PDE_2, which is activited by intracellular cyclic GMP, or PDE_3, which is inhibited by it. PDE_3 was suggested to mediate NO•-induced increases in cAMP with subsequent activation of L-type calcium current and inotropy in isolated cardiac myocytes from rodents and also human atria *(69,70)*. The same pathway may mediate the rebound increase in L-type calcium current, calcium transient, and contraction after the acute removal of acetylcholine in feline cardiac myocytes *(71)*. On the other hand, activation of PDE_2 by cGMP produces opposite effects, with decreases in intracellular cAMP and its downstream effectors, including L-type calcium current, thereby decreasing myocyte contraction. This pathway involving PDE_2 was shown to be operative in the muscarinic cholinergic-dependent "accentuated antagonism" involving eNOS activation in sinoatrial, atrioventricular, and ventricular myocytes from rabbits and rats *(5,14,72)*, with resultant decreases in adrenergically-stimulated L type calcium current and myocyte contraction. Of note, these dual actions of cGMP probably explain the bimodal effect of exogenous NO• donors on both calcium current and contraction of cardiomyocytes in vitro and in vivo. Because the relative abundance of each isoform of phosphodiesterase in heart cells may vary from one species to another, these variations may explain some of the discrepancies in earlier reports of the effects of NO• on cardiac contraction. However, bimodal effects of cGMP have also been observed previously within the same cell *(73,74)*, suggesting that other factors, (e.g., the concentrations of exogenous NO• donors used and the resultant intracellular concentrations of cGMP generated) may influence the final functional response. Even though it has been suggested that low concentrations of exogenous NO• potentiate inotropic parameters, whereas higher concentrations do the opposite, one should bear in mind that concentrations generated locally from exogenous NO• donors may only approximate the concentrations and effects of NO• produced endogenously within specific subcellular compartments. In cardiac myocytes in which endogenous NO• is produced following iNOS induction with cytokines, the resultant increases in intracellular cGMP were shown to be associated with an attenuation of isoproterenol-stimulated increases in cyclic AMP paralleling the attenuation of the shortening of adult rat cardiac myocytes in culture *(75)*. The fact that the attenuation in cAMP generation was partly abrogated on treatment of the cells with isobutyl-methylxanthine (IBMX) clearly implicated PDE stimulation as one mechanism of the attenuation of cardiac myocyte contraction by endogenously produced NO•.

In addition to activating PDE_2, cGMP can attenuate cardiomyocyte contraction by activating cGMP-dependent protein kinase G (PKG). PKG may in turn downregulate the L-type

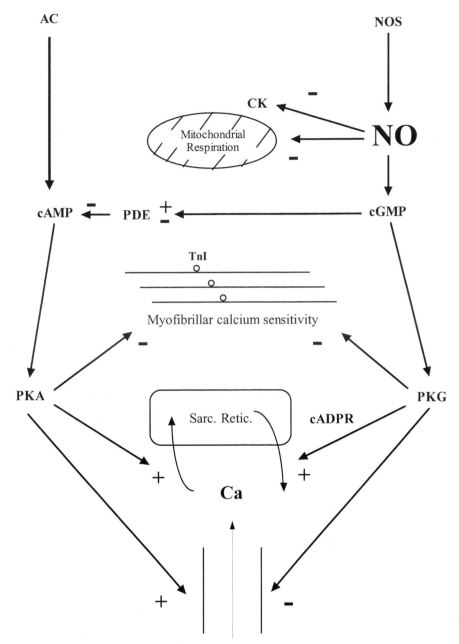

Fig. 1. Multiple targets for the effect of NO· on cardiomyocyte contraction. Left side: Cyclic AMP, produced by the membrane-bound enzyme, adenylyl cyclase (AC), activates protein kinase A (PKA) that mediates most of the classic inotropic effects of adrenergic stimulation of heart muscle; i) positive inotropic effect through increase in L-type calcium current; ii) positive lusitropic effect through increase in sarcoplasmic reticulum (SR) calcium uptake, and phosphorylation of troponin I to decrease myofilament calcium sensitivity. Right side: Nitric oxide (NO·), produced by eNOS or iNOS in cardiac myocytes (or neighbouring cells), may oppose or potentiate the above-mentioned effects through mechanisms that are dependent or independent of cGMP, formed by NO·'s activation of guanylyl cyclase (GC). Cyclic GMP-dependent effects: through allosteric interactions, cGMP stimulates or inhibits specific isoforms of phosphodiesterases (PDE) that hydrolyze cAMP.

calcium current stimulated by PKA *(76,77)*, or downregulate the contractile responses of cardiac myofilaments independently of changes in calcium transients *(35,78)*. The latter mechanism could operate through the previously described phosphorylation of troponin I, which desensitized cardiac myofilaments to calcium *(79,80)*. However, the demonstration that such mechanism contributes to the contractile response to endogenously produced NO• is still lacking.

Other mechanisms involving intracellular calcium channels in cardiac myocytes may also participate in the contractile responses to NO•. In the early 1990s, Galione and colleagues provided evidence that intracellular cGMP could activate intracellular calcium release from the ryanodine channel in sea urchin eggs through activation of adenosine diphosphate (ADP) ribosyl cyclase and subsequent increases in cADP ribose *(81)*. The same group subsequently demonstrated that the ryanodine calcium channel could be activated by exogenous NO• not only in reconstituted lipid bilayers but also in intact sea urchin eggs, which prompted the search for a putative similar action of NO• to regulate calcium-induced calcium release in intact cardiac myocytes. Despite early negative data (apparently ruling out such a pathway in intact guinea pig cardiac myocytes *(82)*, Galione and colleagues more recently demonstrated that, at physiological temperatures, exogenous NO• was able to increase calcium release from the sarcoplasmic reticulum in intact guinea-pig myocytes *(83)*. However, other experiments from Meszaros and colleagues recently demonstrated in membrane preparations that the cardiac-specific ryanodine receptor channel was inhibited by NO• produced endogenously by the eNOS protein *(84)*. Although the latter effect probably occurred independently of increases in cGMP, these observations emphasize the need to integrate the various often antagonistic effects of NO• on excitation–contraction coupling and the need to systematically verify that any effect produced with pharmacological concentrations of NO• donors is representative of the action of NO• following NOS activation.

Accumulating evidence indicates that the oxidation of critical thiol residues on regulatory proteins by NO• or peroxynitrite may account for effects of NO• on various parameters of cardiac contraction. Again, much of the evidence was provided by experiments using exogenous NO• donors. This includes the demonstration of direct inhibition of heterologously expressed cardiac L-type calcium channels by *S*-nitrothiols *(85)* and the redox-dependent bimodal effect of NO• donors on L-type calcium currents in intact ferret ventricular myocytes, where thiol oxydants were shown to stimulate calcium currents *(86)*. Xu and coworkers recently reported that poly-*S*-nitrosylation of the calcium release channel (ryanodine receptor) resulted in activation of cardiac calcium release channels in lipid bilayers and that this effect was reversed by denitrosylation. The channel reacted differently to nitrosation or more profound oxidative signals (which produced loss of control) *(87)*.

In addition to the effects on excitation–contraction coupling and calcium transients discussed previously, NO• may also potentially regulate key glycolytic enzymes and mitochondrial respiration thereby affecting oxygen consumption and ATP generation within heart muscle *(88,89*; for reviews, *see* refs. *10* and *25)*. NO• has also been shown to *S*-nitrosate the glycolytic enzyme glyceraldehyde-3-phosphate-dehydrogenase (GAPDH), which increases its

---

cGMP activates protein kinase G (PKG) that phosphorylates troponin I to decrease myofilament calcium sensitivity, or the L-type calcium channel (or an intermediate protein) to decrease calcium current. Cyclic GMP also stimulates the formation of cyclic ADP ribose (cADPR) which activates the release of calcium through the ryanodine-sensitive channel. Cyclic GMP-independent effects: NO• binds non-heme iron and inactivates enzymes (complex I, II, IV) in the mitochondrial chain to decrease mitochondrial respiration and oxygen consumption. Through *S*-nitrosylation of critical thiol residues, NO• inhibits creatine kinase (CK). It can also reversibly activate the ryanodine channel (or irreversibly upon further oxidation); alternatively, NO• produced by eNOS may downregulate the ryanodine receptor and decrease calcium-induced calcium release (not shown).

auto-ADP-ribosylation and reduces its activity, impeding glycolysis *(90,91)*. *S*-nitrosation of creatinine kinase was shown to decrease its activity in intact isolated guinea-pig hearts and isolated rat ventricular myocytes in vitro *(92,93)*. This effect was reproduced by endogenously produced NO[.] following iNOS induction in endothelial cells cocultured with cardiomyocytes *(93)*. In studies using slices of canine myocardium, it has been reported that NO[.] reduced myocardial oxygen consumption presumably by inhibiting mitochondrial electron transport, an effect that was reproduced in experiments using neonatal myocytes treated with IL-1β *(88,94,95)*

Peroxynitrite, the product of the interaction of NO[.] and superoxide is a strong oxidant that can cause autoperoxidation of lipids and proteins and decomposes to form toxic hydroxyl radicals *(96)*. Peroxynitrite can also produce nitrate tyrosines of myocardial proteins, altering their function *(96)*. Peroxynitrite has been demonstrated to inhibit enzymes of the citric acid cycle such as *cis*-aconitase *(97)*. DNA damage induced by peroxynitrite is associated with poly-ADP-ribose-synthase, resulting in mitochondrial inhibition and depletion of cellular energy stores in cultures of cardiac myoblasts *(98)*. These effects of peroxynitrite probably account for some of the myocardial dysfunction in conditions such as septic shock, where high amounts of NO[.] and superoxide anions are likely to be produced by the high-output iNOS under cytokine stimulation. As has been recently demonstrated, similarly high levels of oxidative stress may result from inhibition of glutathione peroxidase following iNOS induction in cultured cardiac myocytes, which increases the susceptibility of the cells to oxidant-mediated injury *(99)*.

EFFECTS OF eNOS ON BASAL SYSTOLIC-DIASTOLIC FUNCTION

In Vivo Whole Organ

In patients with normal cardiac function, and in transplant recipients free of rejection or vasculopathy, intracoronary infusion of substance P, which is known to increase the release of NO[.] from the vasculature, produced a fall in peak left ventricular systolic pressure and an earlier onset of left ventricular relaxation in the absence of any change in left ventricular *dp/dt* or left ventricular end-diastolic volume. The earlier onset of relaxation in the absence of changes in end-diastolic volume or pressure was consistent with an increase in distensibility induced by NO[.] *(100)*. In other experiments, inhibition of endogenous eNOS with NOS inhibitors inhibits myocardial oxygen consumption; this effect possibly results from the abolition of the small positive inotropic effect of low concentration of endogenous NO[.] *(101)*. Conversely increases in NO[.] production with angiotensin-converting enzyme (ACE) inhibitors were shown to depress basal myocardial oxygen consumption *(102,103)*, a finding consistent with a modulatory effect of NO[.] on mitochondrial respiration.

Isolated Hearts

Stimulation of endothelial NOS with bradykinin or substance P in isolated ejecting guinea-pig hearts induced an earlier onset and accelaration of the diastolic left ventricular pressure fall, with no significant alteration of systolic parameters *(104)*. These data are consistent with the positive lusitropic effects of NO[.] as described earlier. More recently, the same group reported that inhibition of eNOS decreased the Frank–Starling responses of isolated, perfused hearts by a mechanism that was apparently independent of changes in coronary vasomotor tone; these data were interpreted to be consistent with a role for constitutively expressed eNOS in modulating appropriate diastolic relaxation in response to increases in preload *(105)*.

Isolated Cardiac Muscle or Cardiomyocytes

A positive lusitropic effect of NO[.], produced endogenously by an endocardial NOS, was shown in ferret papillary muscle, in which application of substance P shortened the duration of contraction by inducing earlier onset of relaxation, with little effect on peak force of contraction *(106)*. Because the effect was abrogated on damaging the endocardial layer, the authors attributed most of the NO• produced to endothelial cells within the endocardium. Using cocultures of isolated guinea-pig cardiomyocytes and endothelial cells from macrovessels, Brady and colleagues have shown that paracrinally produced NO• following stimulation of endothelial cells with bradykinin reduced the amplitude of shortening of the cocultured myocytes *(107)*. In contrast to these results, inhibition of eNOS expressed in human endomyocardial biopsy specimens (which contain a mixture of endocardial, microvascular endothelial cells, and myocytes) did not change any parameter of systolic contraction or diastolic relaxation on electrical stimulation in vitro in the absence of any agonist *(13)*. Similarly, inhibition of eNOS that was shown to be expressed in isolated rat cardiomyocytes did not affect the rate of systolic shortening or diastolic relaxation measured by videomicroscopy in electrically stimulated cardiomyocytes in the absence of adrenergic agonists (i.e., under baseline conditions) *(47)*. Qualitatively and quantitatively similar results were also recently obtained in isolated ventricular myocytes from homozygous mice in which the eNOS gene had been disrupted; the myocytes from the eNOS-deficient mice exhibited baseline contractility parameters that were not significnatly different from those of the wild-type animals *(108)*.

eNOS REGULATION OF BETA-ADRENERGIC RESPONSE

In Vivo Whole Organ

To examine the potential modulation of the positive inotropic effect of beta-adrenergic stimulation by endogenously expressed eNOS, Hare and colleagues administered an intracoronary infusion of L-NMMA in patients and examined the inotropic response following intravenous infusion of dobutamine (a peripheral infusion to avoid confounding effects of a higher amine concentration in a vasoconstricted coronary vascular bed). In patients with heart failure, they observed a significant potentiation of the positive inotropic effect of dobutamine that was not observed in patients with normal heart function *(109,110)*. One possible explanation for this discrepancy is a difference in the sensitivity to the regulatory influence of endogenously produced NO• between these two groups of patients. A higher sensitivity to NO• of the failing hearts compared to normal controls would more consistently result in a potentiation of the beta-adrenergic response to dobutamine infusion when NOS is inhibited. Consistent with this interpretation, the peak LV pressure response to dobutamine was markedly blunted when cardiac eNOS was activated by intracoronary substance P infusion in transplanted patients and patients with dilated nonischemic cardiomyopathy *(111)*. Altogether, these results point to a role of endogenously produced NO• to attenuate the inotropic responsiveness to beta-adrenergic stimulation. Such a role has been clearly demonstrated for the contractile response to isoproterenol in anesthetized dogs *(112)*, and in preliminary experiments in transgenic mice deficient for eNOS, which exhibited an enhanced contractile responsiveness to positive inotropic agents in comparison to wild-type controls *(113,114)*. In addition to modulation of the inotropic state, endogenous production of NO• in the myocardium may also elevate the threshold for adrenergically induced ventricular arrythmias in animals with acute coronary artery occlusion; this was recently shown in experiments in open-chest dogs in which intrapericardial perfusion with L-arginine to increase NOS activity, as reflected by an increased NO• effluent in the coronary sinus *(115)*, prevented the occurrence of ventricular arrythmias.

Isolated Cardiac Muscle or Cardiomyocytes

Consistent with the results we mentioned above, inhibition of NOS in human atrial strips in vitro enhanced the arrhythmogenic effects of submaximal concentrations of isoproterenol *(116)*. In the same preparations, NOS inhibitors also potentiated the inotropic responsiveness to isoproterenol *(116)*, as had been shown initially in isolated rat ventricular myocytes *(47)* and later in isolated rat atria *(117)*. Such potentiation of the inotropic responsiveness to isoproterenol, however, was not observed in isolated ventricular myocytes from eNOS-deficient transgenic mice. In the latter experiments, however, the use of maximally stimulating concentrations of isoproterenol ($1\ \mu M$) may explain the lack of an identifiable difference in responses between myocytes from eNOS-deficient and wild-type animals *(108)*.

eNOS REGULATION OF MUSCARINIC CHOLINERGIC RESPONSE

In Vivo, Whole Organ

As a corollary to the demonstration that eNOS activity is stimulated by muscarinic cholinergic agonists, it was important to demonstrate that NO• mediates some of the effects of vagal stimulation on the heart in vivo. Using a model of open-chest, anesthetized dogs, Hare and colleagues observed that inhibition of myocardial NOS after intracoronary infusion of L-NMMA attenuated the effect of vagal stimulation on the contractile response to beta-adrenergic agonists *(118)*. Blunting the positive inotropic effect of dobutamine on stimulation of the vagus nerve in these dogs (thereby reproducing the classical accentuated antagonism) was significantly attenuated after NOS inhibition *(118)*. In a different set of experiments, Zipes and colleagues found that NOS inhibition abolished the protective effect of vagal stimulation against ventricular arrhythmias in dogs *(119)*. Moreover, on selective infusion of the NOS inhibitor L-NMMA into the sinoatrial nodal artery in the same animals, they found that endogenous NO• production within the sinoatrial node cells modulated sinus discharge rate and atrioventricular conduction *(119)*.

Isolated Cardiac Muscle or Cardiomyocytes

The aforementioned experiments nicely extend to an in vivo whole-organ setting the paradigm first demonstrated in cultures of rat neonatal ventricular myocytes, which illustrates the obligatory role of endogenously expressed eNOS in mediating the negative chronotropic effect of muscarinic cholinergic stimulation *(47)*. This paradigm was later verified in isolated rabbit sinoatrial node cells *(71,120)*, rabbit atrioventricular cells *(14)*, and rat ventricular myocytes *(5)*, where eNOS was shown to mediate the accentuated parasympathetic antagonism. Despite earlier negative data *(121)*, the same paradigm was also verified in atrial strips from human hearts, in which the muscarinic cholinergic attenuation of isoproterenol-stimulated contraction was also found to be significantly blunted on NOS inhibition with L-NMMA *(116)*. Earlier data obtained in frog atrial myocytes *(122)*, and even some rodent myocytes *(123)*, had apparently disputed the involvement of eNOS in parasympathetic signaling in cardiomyocytes, but as with most of these negative studies, there was no confirmation with an independent technique that NOS was active under the particular experimental conditions used. This and other limitations also appear to invalidate the negative conclusions from a recent study by Vandecasteele and colleagues in transgenic mice deficient for eNOS *(124)*. Foremost is the fact that their eNOS–/– mice are not matched with the appropriate controls, i.e., aside from incomplete back-crossing into the appropriate strains to obtain homogenous genetic background, their knockout animals were studied at 3 mo of age and over, at a time when chronic hypertension had resulted in a significant myocardial hypertrophy, a phenotype not independently accounted for in their comparison with normal controls. In their multicellular (papillary muscle or atrial) preparations, the expression of $I_{K\text{-}Ach}$ may have accounted for the persistence of the responsiveness to muscarinic cholinergic stimulation despite eNOS genetic deficiency. Finally, in their single myocyte experiments, the authors again provide no independent evidence that NOS is active under the experimental conditions used, e.g., measuring currents at room temperature may well have dampened any enzymatic activity of NOS expressed in control myocytes, thereby preventing any NOS-dependent difference from appearing between wild-type and eNOS–/– myocytes. By contrast, when matched with the appropriate genetic controls in another study *(108)*, eNOS–/– mice allowed to confirm the role of eNOS in mediating the parasympathetic-accentuated antagonism, i.e., the muscarinic cholinergic attenuation of isoproterenol-stimulated L-type calcium current was lost in ventricular myocytes from eNOS–/– mice. Importantly, the NOS-dependent increase in cGMP, which was inhibited by L-NMMA in myocytes from control animals, was also abolished in those from eNOS–/– mice, showing that NOS was activatable under the experimental conditions used. Of note, the eNOS–/– mice used in this study were younger than 3 mo and exempt from significant hypertrophy. Others have since demonstrated a similar involvement of a constitutive NOS pathway in modulating the L-type calcium current in guinea-pig cardiomyocytes *(125)* and also in the purinergic attenuation of L-type calcium current in rabbit pacemaker and atrioventricular nodal cells *(126–128)*.

A critical reading of earlier and recent reports on this subject emphasizes the importance of the experimental protocol, in addition to species variation, on the functional effects observed with eNOS inhibition. For example, when the role of endogenous NO· is examined in the absence of prestimulation with beta-adrenergic agonists in cat cardiomyocytes, it is found that eNOS inhibition does not affect the attenuating effect of acetylcholine on L-type calcium current and contractile shortening, but clearly blunts the rebound increase in these parameters following abrupt removal of the muscarinic cholinergic agonist *(71,129)*. The latter effect was proposed to involve NO· and cGMP-dependent inhibition of PDE3, resulting in increases in intracellular cAMP. Similarly, inhibition of cNOS slowed the heart rate recovery following vagal stimulation of isolated guinea-pig atria in the absence of prestimulation with beta-adrenergic agonists *(130)*. Finally, electrophysiological experiments in single isolated cardiomyocytes in transgenic eNOS-deficient mice, as mentioned previously, apparently exclude any modulating effect of eNOS on other ionic currents, such as chloride currents *(131)* or muscarinic cholinergic-activated potassium currents ($I_{K\text{-Ach}}$) *(108)*.

eNOS AND CARDIAC HYPERTROPHY

Earlier findings that NO· attenuates the release or the action of several growth factors in the vasculature *(132)* prompted a search for qualitatively similar effects of NO· produced by eNOS in modulating the phenotype of cardiomyocytes, especially following hypertrophic stimuli. Calderone and colleagues using cultured neonatal cardiac myocytes and fibroblasts exposed to several growth factors, including endothelin and alpha-adrenergic agonists, provided direct evidence that NO·, atrial natriuretic peptide (ANP), and cGMP inhibit the growth-promoting effects of the agonists on cardiac cells *(133)*. Such findings would appear to be corroborated by the observation that chronic NOS inhibition in vivo is accompanied with the development of cardiac hypertrophy *(134)*, even though the experiments did not distinguish between direct effects of NOS inhibition on cardiomyocytes from indirect effects secondary to increases in blood pressure in the animals. There is, however, some evidence supporting a protective effect of bradykinin activation of eNOS against hypertrophy in cultures of cardiomyocytes *(135,136)*.

iNOS AND BASAL CONTRACTILE FUNCTION

In Vivo, Whole Organ

In cardiac transplant recipients, the expression of iNOS mRNA in endomyocardial biopsies was reported to be inversely related to left ventricular performance, i.e., ejection fraction *(28)*. In patients with idiopathic dilated cardiomyopathy, iNOS enzyme activity and iNOS protein measured by immunohistochemistry in cardiac muscle were increased and correlated with impaired contractile performance *(28,29,137)*. In the study of Fukuchi and coworkers, iNOS immunostaining was increased in macrophages and cardiomyocytes in cardiac tissue from patients with heart failure caused by ischemic and nonischemic cardiomyopathy and myocarditis *(31)*. Even though increases in iNOS activity or protein have been found in many disease states with cardiac dysfunction, such as myocardial infarction, immune cardiomyopathy, postpartum myopathy, and idiopathic dilated cardiomyopathy, this circumstantial evidence is insufficient to demonstrate a direct causal role of NO• in the pathogenesis of these diseases. Such demonstration would be clearer if there were unequivocal evidence for a beneficial role of iNOS inhibition in reversing some or all of the myocardial dysfunction. However, results using NOS inhibitors in vivo are discordant at best, if not entirely negative. In endotoxemic rats, e.g., inhibition of iNOS with a nonselective inhibitor resulted in myocardial ischemia with a subsequent deleterious functional effect *(138)*. Myocardial ischemia following nonselective NOS inhibition could be caused by direct vasoconstriction or an increase in the adhesion of platelets or neutrophils through the inhibition of NOS in endothelial cells *(139,140)*. NOS inhibition may also reverse the NO•-mediated downregulation of nicotinamide adenine dinucleotide phosphate (NADPH) oxidase activity in neutrophils that control oxygen radical formation *(141)*, thereby enhancing oxidative damage and the permeability of the endothelium to macromolecules *(142,143)*.

The functional role of iNOS in septic shock in vivo has been investigated in three studies using mice deficient in the iNOS gene (iNOS−/−). One group reported that there was no mortality in iNOS−/− mice treated with 12.5 mg/kg of lipopolysaccharide (LPS) *(144)*. Another group reported that the iNOS−/− mice exibited significantly less mortality after LPS injection at 30 mg/kg in comparison with wild-type controls *(145)*. The benefit in, terms of mortality, however, was lost when mice were coinjected with *Propionibacterium acnes*, a model of infection that may mimic the clinical situation more closely. A third group found that F2 iNOS−/− mice did not show a significant survival advantage over F2 iNOS+/+ mice treated with LPS at either 12.5 or 25 mg/kg *(146)*. In these experiments using three different iNOS−/− transgenic lines, the potential participation of myocardial dysfunction in shock was not specifically studied.

TNF-α, an inflammatory cytokine involved in iNOS induction, is known to be elevated in sepsis and in heart failure *(147)*. TNF-α has recently received much attention in light of the report of beneficial effects of soluble TNF receptors in heart failure patients *(148)*. Despite the clear demonstration of coexpression and localization of both TNF protein and iNOS in myocardium from failing hearts *(30,137)*, a specific role for iNOS in the beneficial effect of TNF-α suppression is only speculative. TNF-α at pathophysiologically relevant concentrations has been shown to induce cardiomyocyte dysfunction through alternative mechanisms *(149)*, including activation of the sphingomyelinase pathway *(150)* and induction of myocyte apoptosis *(151,152)*. In this regard, however, it is interesting to note that iNOS inhibition with a partially selective iNOS inhibitor, aminoguanidine (which also has antioxidant and other properties), was shown to improve allografted rat survival and developed tension in papillary muscles from the cardiac allografts *(153)*.

In Vitro Whole Hearts or Cardiomyocytes

In support of the previously mentioned hypothesis, the use of NOS inhibitors has been shown to ameliorate the contractile dysfunction of isolated perfused hearts treated with IL-1β and TNF-α *(154)*, or of isolated cardiomyocytes from LPS-treated guinea pigs *(155)*. Similarly, the relatively selective iNOS inhibitor, aminoguanidine, was shown to reverse the decrease in basal shortening of cardiomyocytes taken from heterotransplanted rat hearts *(156)*. In some experiments, the depressing effect of inflammatory cytokines or LPS was apparent when the contractile shortening of isolated myocytes was studied under baseline (i.e., in absence of agonists) conditions *(64,78)*, although in other cases, the contractile deficit was only apparent on stimulation of the myocytes with adrenergic agonists *(157)*. Even though the evidence mentioned earlier favors a pathogenetic role for iNOS in mediating contractile dysfunction, especially after endotoxin infusion, other cardiodepressant factors are probably involved in the complete septic shock syndrome *(139)*. For example, infusion of LPS was reported to be followed by myocardial depression in the absence of measurable increases in NOS activity in one study *(158)*.

iNOS AND THE BETA-ADRENERGIC RESPONSE

In the early 1990s, experiments in neonatal cardiac myocytes had shown that cytokine treatment resulted in decreased contractile responsiveness to adrenergic agonists that was associated with an attenuation of the normal increase in intracellular cAMP *(159,160)*. A similar decreased responsiveness to beta-adrenergic agonists was later observed in ventricular myocytes isolated from rejecting cardiac allografts, although the specific involvement of the NO• pathway was not determined in these experiments *(161)*. Using specific combinations of recombinant cytokines or a mixture of inflammatory cytokines obtained from the culture supernatants of rat macrophages stimulated with LPS, Balligand and colleagues found that the reduced contractile response of isolated myocytes exposed to submaximal concentrations of isoproterenol was fully reversed upon cotreatment of the cells with NOS inhibitors, thereby clearly implicating NO• production in the contractile dysfunction, at least under these experimental conditions *(157)*. Similar findings were subsequently observed by the same investigators using cultures of rat ventricular myocytes in coculture with iNOS-expressing endothelial cells *(56)* as well as by many other groups using either isolated contracting cardiomyocytes or papillary muscles exposed to LPS alone or in combination with other cytokines *(78,162;* for a review *see* ref. *10)*.

iNOS AND CARDIOMYOCYTE BIOLOGY

The effects of NO• on cardiac myocyte biology are not restricted to alterations in contractile function. Consistent with the role of the inducible isoform of NOS as part of the early, innate immune response, iNOS expression in the myocardium was shown to modulate the degree of myocardial injury subsequent to viral infection. Experiments in a murine model of viral myocarditis induced by coxackie B-3 virus have suggested a deleterious role for the NO• produced, as low doses of the NOS inhibitor nitro-L-arginine methyl ester (L-NAME) decreased myocardial injury and mortality *(163)*. High doses of the NOS inhibitor were associated with increased mortality, however. A protective role for iNOS was reported by others using a similar model. In these experiments, iNOS induction in macrophages within the myocardium was demonstrated along with increased mortality and higher viral titers in mice fed NOS inhibitors *(164)*. Discordant results have also been found regarding the role of iNOS in modulating the oxidative stress in several models. In a rat transplantation model of ischemia–reperfusion, studies with a porphyrinic electrode indicated that low levels of NO• quenched oxygen-derived radicals *(165)*. On the other hand, inducing of iNOS with recombinant cytokines in cultured myocytes was shown to increase oxidative damage through inhibition of glutathione synthesis *(99)*. The latter finding would be consistent with prior observations that iNOS expression is associated with myocardial damage and cell death in models of cardiac allograft rejection *(153,166)*. In different cells and in different settings it has been demonstrated that NO• and its reaction products such as peroxinitrite can promote apoptosis or inhibit it *(167)*. Induction of apoptosis by NO• and/or peroxinitrite derived from iNOS expressed in macrophages and cardiac myocytes is one of the potential pathways by which iNOS may promote the death of heart cells. This has been suggested by the observations of the parallel occurrence of iNOS mRNA, protein expression, and enzyme activity together with several markers of apoptosis of macrophages and cardiomyocytes in a model of rat cardiac allograft rejection (168). It is of interest to note that the expression of immuno-detected iNOS protein also accompanied apoptosis of cardiac myocytes in endomyocardial biopsies from patients with cardiac allograft rejection (169). In these studies, cardiomyocytes also showed positive immunostaining for nitrotyrosine, which is a marker for the formation of peroxinitrite (168,169). Both NO· and peroxinitrite have also been shown to produce DNA damage and DNA strand breaks, which can trigger the apoptotic response in appropriate cells (170–172). In a preliminary report, a group studying cardiac allograft rejection in transgenic mice found that apoptosis during rejection was less in iNOS-knockout mice than in wild-type control mice (173). In addition to its effects on cardiomyocyte viability, NO· produced in response to exposure to LPS has also been shown to induce cell shrinkage of cultured rabbit ventricular myocytes through a mechanism involving increases in cGMP and inhibition of Na+/K+/2Cl-cotransport (174).

EFFECTS OF EXOGENOUS NO· DONORS

Not all of the effects of endogenously produced NO· can be reproduced by drugs that release NO· in solution. Some of the discrepancies may be explained by concentration differences and biochemical differences between the NO· (or any derivative thereof) produced by the NOS enzymes targeted to specific intracellular compartments and the NO· provided by NO· donors delivered to the extracellular space. The availability of endogenous thiol-containing molecules, and/or the accessibility of endogenous versus exogenous NO· to these molecules to form thionitrite intermediates, may affect the biological fate and functional effect on any cellular target. In addition, the redox state in the microenvironment in which NO· is synthesized may significantly alter its biological effects. Low levels of NO· quench oxygen-derived radicals, whereas high concentrations of NO· (such as those produced by iNOS) in the presence of superoxide form peroxynitrite, which is a powerful oxidant.

In addition to these potential biochemical differences, experiments using NO· donor drugs have shown that the functional results vary with many other parameters, such as the concentrations of the donor drugs used, the species (i.e., amphibians versus mammalians), or the region of the heart (i.e., atria versus ventricle) studied. The effect of NO· on parameters such as L-type calcium current or contraction may also be dependent on prestimulation of the preparation with an adrenergic agonist and/or with the endogenous baseline level of cAMP. Despite these limitations, NO· donor drugs have proven to be useful tools for characterizing the various intracellular signaling pathways activated by NO· in cardiomyocytes. In frog and human atrial myocytes, low concentrations of NO· donors were shown to potentiate L-type calcium current (69,70). Similar doses induced a moderate, positively inotropic effect in adult rat ventricular myocytes (74) and in open-chest dog hearts (175). When higher concentrations of the NO· donors were used in rat and guinea-pig ventricular myocytes, however, an inhibition of both L-type calcium current and contractility were observed, mostly after prestimulation of the preparations with an adrenergic agonist or following increases in intracellular cAMP with analogs of the cyclic nucleotide or inhibition of phosphodiesterases with isobutylmethyl-xanthine (76,77). These negatively inotropic effects may have been secondary to greater increases in intracellular cGMP levels. Consistent with this hypothesis, incubation of cat papillary muscle with the PDE V inhibitor, zaprinast, to increase intracellular cGMP concentrations was shown to decrease the force of contraction after pretreatment with the beta-adrenergic agonist, isoproterenol (176). The downstream signaling events leading to either of these two opposing contractile responses were also shown to involve either cGMP-mediated activation or inhibition of specific isoforms of PDEs to hydrolyze intracellular cAMP, as well as PKG-dependent pathways. Finally, high concentrations of the exogenous NO· donor S-nitroso-N-acetylpenicillamine (SNAP) were shown to trigger apoptosis of adult rat cardiomyocytes in culture. Increased apoptosis was not observed when the cardiomyocytes were incubated with the same concentrations of *N*-acetyllpenicillamine (NAP) or SNAP along with reduced hemoglobin to scavenge NO• released from the drug *(177)*. Similarly, effects from inducing apoptosis of neonatal cardiac myocytes were observed with the NO• donor *S*-nitrosoglutathione *(178)*. In both studies, iNOS induction by cytokines in the cardiomyocytes was also associated with NO•-dependent apoptosis of these cells *(177,178)*.

CONCLUSION

It is apparent that all three isoforms of NOS are present in the cells constituting the myocardium, and that the local intramyocardial concentration of NO• is the summation of that produced by different isoforms in different cell types, including endocardial and endothelial cells, vascular smooth muscle cells, cardiac myocytes, and, in disease states, infiltrating inflammatory cells. The biological effects of NO• are related to its diffusion, to the number and affinity of multiple competing target molecules and to the ambient redox state, which can influence the formation of derivative compounds such as peroxynitrite. Important roles for eNOS and iNOS in cardiomyocytes have been demonstrated, which include the muscarinic–cholinergic modulation of heart rate and of the inotropic response to beta adrenergic agonists. The expression of iNOS in the heart has been demonstrated in a variety of cardiac diseases including myocardial infarction, transplant allograft rejection, and ischemic and idiopathic dilated cardiomyopathies. It is likely that in the near future the role of eNOS in excitation–contraction coupling, the significance of the localization of eNOS in caveolae, and the local determinants of whether the NO• produced by iNOS in cardiac diseases is helpful or harmful will be clarified. Despite rapid advances in research in this area, much remains to be learned.

REFERENCES

1. Schmidt HH, Gagne GD, Nakane M, Pollock JS, Miller MF, Murad F. Mapping of neural nitric oxide synthase in the rat suggests frequent co-localization with NADPH diaphorase but not with soluble guanylyl cyclase and novel paraneural functions for nitrinergic signal transduction. J Histochem Cytochem 1992;40:1439–1456.
2. Tanaka K, Hassall CJ, Burnstock G. Distribution of intracardiac neurons and nerve terminals that contain a marker for nitric oxide, NADPH-diaphorase, in the guinea-pig heart. Cell Tissue Res 1993; 273:293–300.
3. Schwarz P, Diem R, Dun NJ, Förstermann U. Endogenous and exogenous nitric oxide inhibits norepinephrine release from rat heart sympathetic nerves. Circ Res 1995;77:841–848.
4. Kaye DM, Wiviott D, Kobzik L, Kelly RA, Smith TW. S-nitrisothiols inhibit neuronal norepinephrine transport. Am J Physiol 1997;272:H875–H883.
5. Balligand JL, Kobzik L, Han X, Kaye DM, Belhassen L, O'Hara DS, et al. Nitric oxide-dependent parasympathetic signaling is due to activation of constitutive endothelial (type III) nitric oxide synthase in cardiac myocytes. J Biol Chem 1995;270:14,582–14,586.
6. Belhassen L, Kelly RA, Smith TW, Balligand JL. Nitric oxide synthase (NOS3) and contractile responsiveness to adrenergic and cholinergic agonists in the heart. Regulation of NOS3 transcription in vitro and in vivo by cAMP in rat cardiac myocytes. J Clin Invest 1996;97:1908–1915.
7. Silvagno F, Xia H, Bredt DS. Neuronal nitric oxide synthase mu, an alternatively spliced isoform expressed in differentiated skeletal muscle. J Biol Chem 1996;271:11,204–11,208.
8. Belhassen L, Feron O, Kaye DM, Michel T, Kelly RA. Regulation by cAMP of post-translational processing and subcellular targeting of endothelial nitric-oxide synthase (type 3) in cardiac myocytes. J Biol Chem 1997;272:11,198–11,204.
9. Xu KY, Huso DL, Dawson TH, Bredt DS, Becker LC. Nitric oxide synthase in cardiac sarcoplasmic reticulum. Proc Natl Acad Sci USA 1999;96:657–662.
10. Balligand JL, Cannon PJ. Nitric oxide synthases and cardiac muscle. Autocrine and paracrine influences. Arterioscler Thromb Vasc Biol 1997;17:1846–1858.
11. Andries LJ, Brutsaert DL, Sys SU. Nonuniformity of endothelial constitutive nitric oxide synthase distribution in cardiac endothelium. Circ Res 1998;82:195–203.

12. Balligand JL, Smith TW. Molecular regulation of NO synthase in the heart. In: Shah AM, Lewis MJ, eds. Endothelial Modulation of Cardiac Contraction. Harwood Academic Publishers, Amsterdam, The Netherlands, 1997, pp. 53–71.

13. Gauthier C, Leblais V, Kobzik L, Trochu JN, Khandoudi N, Bril A, Balligand JL, Le Marec H. The negative inotropic effect of beta-3-adrenoceptor stimulation is mediated by activation of a nitric oxide synthase pathway in human ventricle. J Clin Invest 1998;102:1377–1384.

14. Han X, Kobzik L, Balligand JL, Kelly RA, Smith TW. Nitric oxide synthase (NOS3)-mediated cholinergic modulation of Ca2+ current in adult rabbit atrioventricular nodal cells. Circ Res 1996;78:998–1008.

15. Seki T, Hagiwara H, Naruse K, Kadowaki M, Kashiwagi M, Demura H, et al. In situ identification of messenger RNA of endothelial type nitric oxide synthase in rat cardiac myocytes. Biochem Biophys Res Commun 1996;218:601–605.

16. Wei CM, Jiang SW, Lust JA, Daly RC, MacGregor CG. Genetic expression of endothelial nitric oxide synthase in human atrial myocardium. Mayo Clin Proc 1996;71:346–350.

17. Feron O, Belhassen L, Kobzik L, Smith TW, Kelly RA, Michel T. Endothelial nitric oxide synthase targeting to caveolae. Specific interaction with caveolin isoforms in cardiac myocytes and endothelial cells. J Biol Chem 1996;271:22,810–22,814.

18. Michel JB, Feron O, Sase K, Prabhakar P, Michel T. Caveolin versus calmodulin. Counterbalancing allosteric modulators of nitric oxide synthase. J Biol Chem 1997;272: 25,907–25,912.

19. Garcia-Cardena G, Martasek P, Masters BS, Skidd PM, Couet J, Li S, et al. Dissecting the interaction between nitric oxide synthase (NOS) and caveolin. Functional significance of the NOS caveolin binding domain in vivo. J Biol Chem 1997;272:25,437–25,440.

20. Ghosh S, Gachhui R, Crooks C, Wu C, Lisanti MP, Stuehr DJ. Interaction beween caveolin-1 and the reductase domain of endothelial nitric oxide synthase. J Biol Chem 1998;273:22,267–22,271.

21. Ju H, Zou R, Venema VJ, Venema RC. Direct interaction of endothelial nitric-oxide synthase and caveolin-1 inhibits synthase activity. J Biol Chem 1997;272:18,522–18,525.

22. Feron O, Saldana JB, Michel JB, Michel T. The eNOS-caveolin regulatory cycle. J Biol Chem 1998; 273:3125–3128.

23. Parton RG, Way M, Zorzi N, Stang E. Caveolin-3 associates with developing T-tubules during muscle differentiation. J Cell Biol 1997;136:137–154.

24. Ishikawa H. Formation of elaborate networks of T-system tubules in cultured skeletal muscle with special reference to the T-system formation. J Cell Biol 1968;38:51–66.

25. Kelly RA, Balligand JL, Smith T. Nitric oxide and cardiac function. Circ Res 1996;79:363–380.

26. Szabolcs MJ, Ravalli S, Minanov O, Sciacca RR, Michler RE, Cannon PJ. Apoptosis and increased expression of inducible nitric oxide synthase in human allograft rejection. Transplantation 1998;65: 804–812.

27. Wildhirt SM, Dudek RR, Suzuki H, Bing RJ. Involvement of inducible nitric oxide synthase in the inflammatory process of myocardial infarction. Int J Cardiol 1995;50:253–261.

28. Lewis NP, Tsao PS, Rickenbacher PR, Xue C, Johns RA, Haywood GA, et al. Induction of nitric oxide synthase in the human cardiac allograft is associated with contractile dysfunction of the left ventricle. Circulation 1996;93:720–729.

29. Haywood GA, Tsao PS, von der Leyen HE, Mann MJ, et al. Expression of inducible nitric oxide synthase in human heart failure. Circulation 1996;93:1087–1094.

30. Habib FM, Springall DR, Davies GJ, Oakley CM, Yacoub MH, Polak JM. Tumor necrosis factor and inducible nitric oxide synthase in dilated cardiomyopathy. Lancet 1996;347:1151–1155.

31. Fukuchi M, Hussain SNA, Giaiad A. Heterogeneous expression and activity of endothelial and inducible nitric oxide synthases in end-stage human heart failure: their relation to lesion site and β-adrenergic receptor therapy. Circulation 1998;98:132–139.

32. Thoenes M, Forstermann U, Tracey WR, Bleese NM, Nussler AK, Scholz H, et al. Expression of inducible nitric oxide synthase in failing and non-failing human heart. J Mol Cell Cardiol 1996;28:165–169.

33. Torre-Amione G, Kapadia S, Benedict C, Oral H, Young JB, Mann DL. Proinflammatory cytokine levels in patients with depressed left ventricular ejection fraction: a report from the Studies of Left Ventricular Dysfunction (SOLVD). J Am Coll Cardiol 1996;27:1201–1206.

34. Finkel MS, Oddis CV, Jacob TD, Watkin SC, Hattler BG, Simmons RL. Negative inotropic effects of cytokines on the heart mediated by nitric oxide. Science 1992;257:387–389.

35. Goldhaber JI, Kim KH, Natterson PD, Lawrence T, Yang P, Weiss JN. Effects of TNF-alpha on [Ca2+]$_i$ and contractility in isolated adult rabbit ventricular myocytes. Am J Physiol 1996;271:H1449–H1455.

36. Salvemini D, Korbut R, Anggard E, Vane J. Immediate release of a nitric oxide-like factor from bovine aortic endothelial cells by Escherichia coli lipopolysaccharide. Proc Natl Acad Sci USA 1990; 87:2593–2597.

37. Harrison DG. Cellular and molecular mechanisms of endothelial cell dysfunction. J Clin Invest 1997; 100:2153–2157.

38. Fleming I, Bauersachs J, Fisslthaler B, Busse R. Ca^{2+}-independent activation of the endothelial nitric oxide synthase in response to tyrosine phosphatase inhibitors and fluid shear stress. Circ Res 1998;82: 686–695.

39. Pinsky DJ, Patton S, Mesaros S, Brovkovych V, Kubaszewski E, Grunfeld S, et al. Mechanical transduction of nitric oxide synthesis in the beating heart. Circ Res 1997;81:372–379.

40. Nathan C, Xie QW. Regulation of biosynthesis of nitric oxide. J Biol Chem 1994;269:13725–13728.

41. Kaye DM, Wiviott SD, Balligand JL, Simmons WW, Smith TW, Kelly RA. Frequency-dependent activation of a constitutive nitric oxide synthase and regulation of contractile function in adult rat ventricular myocytes. Circ Res 1996;78:217–224.

42. Finkel MS, Oddis CV, Mayer OH, Hattler BG, Simmons RL. Nitric oxide synthase inhibitor alters papillary muscle force-frequency relationship. J Pharmacol Exp Ther 1995;272:945–952.

43. Kanai AJ, Mesaros S, Finkel MS, Oddis CV, Birder LA, Malinski T. Beta-adrenergic regulation of constitutive nitric oxide synthase in cardiac myocytes. Am J Physiol 1997;273:C1371–C1377.

44. Felder CC. Muscarinic acetylcholine receptors: signal transduction through mutiple effectors. FASEB J 1995;9:619–625.

45. Feron O, Smith TW, Michel T, Kelly RA. Dynamic targeting of the agonist-stimulated m2 muscarinic acetylcholine receptor to caveolae in cardiac myocytes. J Biol Chem 1997;272:17,744–17,748.

46. Michel T, Feron O. Nitric oxide synthases: which, where, how and why? J Clin Invest 1997;100: 2146–2152.

47. Balligand JL, Kelly RA, Marsden PA, Smith TW, Michel T. Control of cardiac muscle cell function by an endogenous nitric oxide signaling system. Proc Natl Acad Sci USA 1993;90:347–351.

48. Feron O, Dessy C, Opel DJ, Arstall MA, Kelly RA, Michel T. Modulation of the eNOS-caveolin interactions in cardiac myocytes: implications for the autonomic regulation of heart rate. J Biol Chem 1998;273:30,249–30,354.

49. Fleming I, Bauersachs J, Busse R. Calcium-dependent and calcium-independent activation of the endothelial NO synthase. J Vasc Res 1997;34:165–174.

50. Yoshizumi M, Perrella MA, Burnett JC Jr, Lee HE. Tumor necrosis factor downregulates an endothelial nitric oxide synthase mRNA by shortening its half-life. Circ Res 1993;73:205–209.

51. Smith CJ, Sun D, Hoegler C, Roth BS, Zhang X, Zhao G, et al. Reduced gene expression of vascular endothelial NO synthase and cyclooxygenase-1 in heart failure. Circ Res 1996;78:58–64.

52. Stein B, Eschenhagen T, Rudiger J, Scholz H, Forstermann U, Gath I. Increased expression of constitutive nitric oxide synthase III, but not inducible nitric oxide synthase II in human heart failure. J Am Coll Cardiol 1998;32:1179–1186.

53. Khadour FH, O'Brien DW, Fu Y, Armstrong PW, Schulz R. Endothelial nitric oxide synthase increases in left atria of dogs with pacing-induced heart failure. Am J Physiol 1998;275:H1971–H1978.

54. Hare JM, Kim B, Flavahan NA, Ricker KM, Peng X, Colman L, et al. Persussis-toxin-sensitive G proteins influence nitric oxide synthase III activity and protein levels in rat heart. J Clin Invest 1998;101: 1424–1431.

55. Balligand JL, Ungureanu-Longrois D, Simmons WW, Pimental D, Malinski TA, Kapturczak M, et al. Cytokine-inducible nitric oxide synthase (iNOS) expression in cardiac myocytes. Characterization and regulation of iNOS expression and detection of iNOS activity in single cardiac myocytes in vitro. J Biol Chem 1994;269:27,580–27,588.

56. Ungureanu-Longrois D, Balligand JL, Okada I, Simmons WW, Kobzik L, Lowenstein CJ, et al. Contractile responsiveness of ventricular myocytes to isoproterenol is regulated by induction of nitric oxide synthase activity in cardiac microvascular endothelial cells in heterotypic primary culture. Circ Res 1995;77:486–493.

57. Singh K, Balligand JL, Fischer TA, Smith TW, Kelly RA. Regulation of cytokine-inducible nitric oxide synthase in cardiac myocytes and microvascular endothelial cells. Role of extracellular signal-regulated kinases 1 and 2 (ERK1/ERK2) and STAT1 alpha. J Biol Chem 1996;271:1111–1117.

58. Pinsky DJ, Cai B, Yang X, Rodriguez C, Sciacca RR, Cannon PJ. The lethal effects of cytokine-induced nitric oxide on cardiac myocytes are blocked by nitric oxide synthase antagonism or transforming growth factor β. J Clin Invest 1995;95:677–685.

59. Roberts AB, Vodovotz Y, Roche NS, Sporn MB, Nathan CF. Role of nitric oxide in antagonistic effects of transforming growth factor-beta and interleukin-1 beta on the beating rate of cultured cardiac myocytes. Mol Endocrinol 1992;6:1921–1930.

60. Kinugawa K, Schimizu T, Yao A, Kohmoto O, Serizawa T, Takahashi T. Transcriptional regulation of inducible nitric oxide synthase in cultured neonatal rat cardiac myocytes. Circ Res 1997;81:911–921.

61. Ikeda U, Maeda Y, Kawahara Y, Yokoyama M, Shimada K. Angiotensin II augments cytokine-stimulated nitric oxide synthesis in rat cardiac myocytes. Circulation 1995;92:2683–2689.

62. Ikeda U, Murakami Y, Kanbe T, Shimada K. Alpha-adrenergic stimulation enhances inducible nitric oxide synthase expression in rat cardiac myocytes. J Mol Cell Cardiol 1996;28:1539–1545.

63. Oddis CV, Simmons RL, Hattler BG, Finkel MS. cAMP enhances inducible nitric oxide synthase mRNA stability in cardiac myocytes. Am J Physiol 1995;269:H2044–H2050.

64. McKenna TM, Li S, Tao S. PKC mediates LPS- and phorbol-induced cardiac cell nitric oxide synthase activity and hypocontractility. Am J Physiol 1995;269:H1891–H1898.

65. Yamamoto K, Dang QN, Kelly RA, Lee RT. Mechanical strain suppresses inducible nitric oxide synthase in cardiac myocytes. J Biol Chem 1998;273:11,862–11,866.

66. Simmons WW, Closs EI, Cunningham JM, Smith TW, Kelly RA. Cytokines and insulin induce cationic amino acid transporter (CAT) expression in cardiac myocytes. Regulation of L-arginine transport and NO production by CAT-1, CAT-2A, and CAT-2B. J Biol Chem 1996;271:11,694–11,702.

67. Simmons WW, Ungureanu-Longrois D, Smith GK, Smith TW, Kelly RA. Glucocorticoïds regulate inducible nitric oxide synthase by inhibiting tetrahydrobiopterin synthesis and L-arginine transport. J Biol Chem 1996;271:23,928–23,937.

68. Mayer B, Pfeiffer S, Schrammel A, Koesling D, Schmidt K, Brunner F. A new pathway of nitric oxide/cyclic GMP signaling involving S-nitrosoglutathione. J Biol Chem 1998;273:3264–3270.

69. Méry PF, Pavoine C, Belhassen L, Pecker F, Fischmeister R. Nitric oxide regulates cardiac Ca2+ current. Involvement of cGMP-inhibited and cGMP-stimulated phosphodiesterases through guanylyl cyclase activation. J Biol Chem 1993;268:26,286–26,295.

70. Kirstein M, Rivet-Bastide M, Hatem S, Benardeau A, Mercadier JJ, Fischmeister R. Nitric oxide regulates the calcium current in isolated human atrial myocytes. J Clin Invest 1995;95:794–802.

71. Wang YG, Rechenmacher CE, Lipsius SL. Nitric oxide signaling mediates stimulation of L-Type Ca2+ current elicited by withdrawal of acetylcholine in cat atrial myocytes. J Gen Physiol 1998;111:113–125.

72. Han X, Shimoni Y, Giles WR. A cellular mechanism for nitric oxide-mediated cholinergic control of mammalian heart rate. J Gen Physiol 1995;106:45–65.

73. Ono K, Trautwein W. Potentiation by cyclic GMP of beta-adrenergic effect on Ca2+ current in guinea-pig ventricular cells. J Physiol 1991;443:387–404.

74. Kojda G, Kottenberg K, Nix P, Schluter KD, Piper HM, Noack E. Low increase of cGMP induced by organic nitrates and nitrovasodilators improves contractile response of rat ventricular myocytes. Circ Res 1996;78:91–101.

75. Joe EK, Schussheim AE, Longrois D, Mäki T, Kelly RA, Smith TW, et al. Regulation of cardiac myocyte contractile function by inducible nitric oxide synthase (iNOS): mechanisms of contractile depression by nitric oxide. J Mol Cell Cardiol 1998;30:303–315.

76. Méry PF, Lohmann SM, Walter U, Fischmeister R. Ca2+ current is regulated by cyclic GMP-dependent protein kinase in mammalian cardiac myocytes. Proc Natl Acad Sci USA 1991;88:1197–1201.

77. Wahler GM, Dollinger SJ. Nitric oxide donor SIN-1 inhibits mammalian cardiac calcium current through cGMP-dependent protein kinase. Am J Physiol 1995;268:C45–C54.

78. Yasuda S, Lew WY. Lipopolysaccharide depresses cardiac contractility and beta-adrenergic contractile response by decreasing myofilament response to Ca2+ in cardiac myocytes. Circ Res 1997;81:1011–1020.

79. Robertson SP, Johnson JD, Holroyde MJ, Kranias EG, Potter JD, Solaro RJ. The effect of troponin I phosphorylation on the Ca2+-binding properties of the Ca2+-regulatory site of bovine cardiac troponin. J Biol Chem 1982;257:260–263.

80. Pfitzer G, Ruegg JC, Flockerzi V, Hofmann F. cGMP-dependent protein kinase decreases calcium sensitivity of skinned cardiac fibers. FEBS Lett 1982;149:171–175.

81. Galione A, Lee HC, Busa WB. Ca(2+)-induced Ca2+ release in sea urchin egg homogenates: modulation by cyclic ADP-ribose. Science 1991;253:1143–1146.

82. Guo X, Laflamme MA, Becker PL. Cyclic ADP-ribose does not regulate sarcoplasmic reticulum Ca2+ release in intact cardiac myocytes. Circ Res 1996;79:147–151.

83. Iino S, Cui Y, Galione A, Terrar DA. Actions of cADP-ribose and its antagonists on contraction in guinea pig isolated ventricular myocytes. Influence of temperature. Circ Res 1997;81:879–884.

84. Zahradnikova A, Minarovic I, Venema RC, Meszaros LG. Inactivation of the cardiac ryanodine receptor calcium release channel by nitric oxide. Cell Calcium 1997;22:447–454.

85. Hu H, Chiamvimonvat N, Yamaghishi T, Marban E. Direct inhibition of expressed cardiac L-type Ca2+ channels by S-nitrosothiol nitric oxide donors. Circ Res 1997;81:742–752.

86. Campbell DL, Stamler JS, Strauss HC. Redox modulation of L-type calcium channel in ferret ventricular myocytes. Dual mechanism regulation by nitric oxide and S-nitrosothiols. J Gen Physiol 1996;108:277–293.

 87. Xu L, Eu JP, Meissner G, Stamler JS. Activation of the cardiac calcium release channel (ryanodine receptor) by poly-S-nitrosylation. Science 1998;279:234–237.
 88. Shen W, Hintze TH, Wolin MS. Nitric oxide. An important signaling mechanism between vascular endothelium and parenchymal cells in the regulation of oxygen consumption. Circulation 1995;92: 3505–3512.
 89. Kelm M, Schafer S, Dahmann R, Dolu B, Perings S, Decking UK, et al. Nitric oxide induced contractile dysfunction is related to a reduction in myocardial energy generation. Cardiovasc Res 1997;36: 185–194.
 90. Molina y Vedia L, Mc Donald B, Reep B, Brune B, Di Silvio M, et al. Nitric oxide-induced S-nitrosylation of glyceraldehyde-3 phosphate dihydrogenase inhibits enzymatic activity and increases endogenous ADP-ribosylation. J Biol Chem 1992;267:24,929–24,932.
 91. Mohr S, Stamler JS, Brune B. Post-tranlational modification of glyceraldehyde-3 phosphate dehydrogenase by S-nitrosylation and subsequent NADH attachment. J Biol Chem 1996;271:4209–4214.
 92. Gross WL, Bak MI, Ingwall JS, Arstall MA, Smith TW, Balligand JL, et al. Nitric oxide inhibits creatine kinase and regulates rat heart contractile reserve. Proc Natl Acad Sci USA 1996;93:5604–5609.
 93. Arstall MA, Bailey C, Gross WL, Bak M, Balligand JL, Kelly RA. Reversible S-nitrosation of creatinine kinase by nitric oxide in adult rat ventricular myocytes. J Mol Cell Cardiol 1998;30:979–988.
 94. Shen W, Xu X, Ochoa M, Zhao G, Wolin MS, Hintze TH. Role of nitric oxide in the regulation of oxygen consumption in conscious dogs. Circ Res 1994;75:1086–1095.
 95. Oddis CV, Finkel MS. Cytokine-stimulated nitric oxide production inhibits mitochondrial activity in cardiac myocytes. Biochem Biophys Res Commun 1995;213:1002–1009.
 96. Beckman JS, Koppenol WH. Nitric oxide, superoxide and peroxynitrite: the good, the bad and ugly. Am J Physiol 1996;271:1424–1437.
 97. Hausladen A, Fridovich K. Superoxide and peroxinitrite inactivate aconitases, but nitric oxide does not. J Biol Chem 1994;269: 29,405–29,408.
 98. Gilad E, Zingarelli B, Salzman AL, Szabo C. Protection by inhibition of poly (ADP-ribose) synthetase against oxidant injury in cardiac myoblasts in vitro. J Mol Cell Cardiol 1997;29:2585–2597.
 99. Igarashi J, Nishida M, Hoshida S, Yamashita N, Kosaka H, Hori M, et al. Inducible nitric oxide synthase augments injury elicited by oxidative stress in rat cardiac myocytes. Am J Physiol 1998;274: C245–C252.
100. Paulus WJ, Vantrimpont PJ, Shah AM. Paracine coronary endothelial control of left ventricular function in humans. Circulation 1995;92:2119–2126.
101. Sherman AJ, Davis CA 3rd, Klocke FJ, Harris KR, Srinivasan G, Yaacoub AS, et al. Blockade of nitric oxide synthesis reduces myocardial oxygen consumption in vivo. Circulation 1997;95:1328–1334.
102. Zhang X, Xie YW, Nasjletti A, Xu X, Wolin MS, Hintze TH. ACE inhibitors promote nitric oxide accumulation to modulate myocardial oxygen consumption. Circulation 1997;95:176–182.
103. Laursen JB, Harrisson DG. Modulation of myocardial oxygen consumption through ACE inhibitors. No effect? Circulation 1997;95:14–16.
104. Grocott-Mason R, Fort S, Lewis MJ, Shah AM. Myocardial relaxant effect of exogenous nitric oxide in isolated ejecting hearts. Am J Physiol 1994;266:H1699–H1705.
105. Prendergast BD, Sagach VF, Shah AM. Basal release of nitric oxide augments the Frank-Starling response in the isolated heart. Circulation 1997;96:1320–1329.
106. Smith JA, Shah AM, Lewis MJ. Factors released from endocardium of the ferret and pig modulate myocardial contraction. J Physiol 1991;439:1–14.
107. Brady AJ, Warren JB, Poole-Wilson PA, Williams TJ, Harding SE. Nitric oxide attenuates cardiac myocyte contraction. Am J Physiol 1993;265:H176–H182.
108. Han X, Kubota I, Feron O, Opel DJ, Arstall MA, Zhao YY, et al. Muscarinic cholinergic regulation of cardiac myocyte ICa-L is absent in mice with targeted disruption of endothelial nitric oxide synthase. Proc Natl Acad Sci USA 1998;95:6510–6515.
109. Hare JM, Loh E, Creager MA, Colucci WS. Nitric oxide inhibits the positive inotropic response to beta-adrenergic stimulation in humans with left ventricular dysfunction. Circulation 1995;92:2198–2203.
110. Hare JM, Givertz MM, Creager MA, Colucci WS. Increased sensitivity to nitric oxide synthase inhibition in patients with heart failure: potentiation of beta-adrenergic inotropic responsiveness. Circulation 1998;97:161–166.
111. Bartunek J, Shah AM, Vanderheyden M, Paulus WJ. Dobutamine enhances cardiodepressant effects of receptor-mediated coronary endothelial stimulation. Circulation 1997;95:90–96.
112. Keaney JF Jr, Hare JM, Balligand JL, Loscalzo J, Smith TW, Colucci WS. Inhibition of nitric oxide synthase augments myocardial contractile responses to beta-adrenergic stimulation. Am J Physiol 1996;271:H2646–H2652.

113. Gyurko R, Fishman MC, Huang PL. Enhanced systolic contractility and preserved diastolic relaxation in mice deficient in endothelial nitric oxide synthase. Presented at the 4th International Meeting on the Biology of Nitric Oxide, Kyoto, Japan, September 1997.

114. Godecke A, Heinicke T, Decking UKM, Stumpe T, Schrader J. B-adrenergic stimulation of eNOS-deficient mice hearts. Circulation 1998;98:I–70 (abstract).

115. Fei L, Baron AD, Henry DP, Zipes DP. Intrapericardial delivery of L-arginine reduces the increased severity of ventricular arrhythmias during sympathetic stimulation in dogs with acute coronary occlusion: nitric oxide modulates sympathetic effects on ventricular electrophysiological properties. Circulation 1997;96:4044–4049.

116. Gauthier C, Erfanian M, Baron O, Balligand JL. Control of contractile and rhythmic properties of human atrial tissue by a NO pathway. Circulation 1998;98:I–732 (abstract).

117. Sterin-Borda L, Genaro A, Perez Leiros C, Cremaschi G, Echague AV, Borda E. Role of nitric oxide in cardiac beta-adrenoceptor-inotropic response. Cell Signal 1998;10:253–257.

118. Hare JM, Keaney JF Jr, Balligand JL, Loscalzo J, Smith TW, Colucci WS. Role of nitric oxide in parasympathetic modulation of β-adrenergic myocardial contractility in normal dogs. J Clin Invest 1995;95:360–366.

119. Elvan A, Rubart M, Zipes DP. NO modulates autonomic effects on sinus discharge rate and AV nodal conduction in open-chest dogs. Am J Physiol 1997;272:H263–H271.

120. Han X, Shimoni Y, Giles WR. An obligatory role of nitric oxide in autonomic control of mammalian heart rate. J Physiol 1994;476:309–314.

121. Kilter H , Lenz O, La Rosée K, Flesch M, Schwinger RH, Mädge M, et al. Evidence against a role of nitric oxide in the indirect negative inotropic effect of M-cholinoreceptor stimulation in human ventricular myocardium. Naunyn-Schmiedeberg's Arch Pharmacol 1995;352:308–312.

122. Méry-PF, Hove-Madsen L, Chesnais JM, Hartzell HC, Fischmeister R. Nitric oxide synthase does not participate in negative inotropic effect of acetylcholine in frog heart. Am J Physiol 1996;270: H1178–H1188.

123. Stein B, Droemuller A, Mulsch A, Schmitz W, Scholz H. Ca (++)-dependent constitutive nitric oxide synthase is not involved in the cyclic GMP-increasing effects of carbachol in ventricular cardiomyocytes. J Pharmacol Exp Ther 1993;266:919–925.

124. Vandecasteele G, Eschenhagen T, Scholz H, Stein B, Verde I, Fischmeister R. Muscarinic and beta-adrenergic regulation of heart rate, force of contraction and calcium current is preserved in mice lacking endothelial nitric oxide synthase. Nat Med 1999;5:331–334.

125. Gallo MP, Ghigo D, Bosia A, Allaotti G, Costamagna C, Penna C, et al. Modulation of guinea-pig cardiac L-type calcium current by nitric oxide synthase inhibitors. J Physiol (Lond) 1998;506:639–651.

126. Shimoni Y, Han X, Severson D, Giles WR. Mediation by nitric oxide of the indirect effects of adenosine on calcium current in rabbit heart pacemaker cells. Br J Pharm 1996;119:1463–1469.

127. Martynyuk AE, Kane KA, Cobbe SM, Rankin AC. Nitric oxide mediates the anti-adrenergic effect of adenosine on calcium current in isolated rabbit atrioventricular nodal cells. Pflugers Arch 1996;431: 452–457.

128. Martynyuk AE, Kane KA, Cobbe SM, Rankin AC. Role of nitric oxide, cGMP and superoxide in inhibition by adenosine of calcium current in rabbit atrioventricular nodal cells. Cardiovasc Res 1997; 34:360–367.

129. Wang YG, Lipsius SL. Acetylcholine elicits a rebound stimulation of Ca2+ current mediated by pertussis toxin-sensitive G protein and cAMP-dependent protein kinase A in atrial myocytes. Circ Res 1995;76:634–644.

130. Sears CE, Choate JK, Paterson DJ. Inhibition of nitric oxide synthase slows heart rate recovery from cholinergic activation. J Appl Physiol 1998;84:1596–1603.

131. Zakharov SI, Pieramici S, Kumar GK, Prabhakar NR, Harvey RD. Nitric oxide synthase activity in guinea-pig ventricular myocytes is not involved in muscarinic inhibition of cAMP-regulated ion channels. Circ Res 1996;78:925–935.

132. Ruschittzka FT, Noll G, Luscher TF. The endothelium in coronary artery disease. Cardiology 1997; 3:3–19.

133. Calderone A, Thaik CM, Takahashi N, Chang DLF, Colucci WS. NO, ANP, cGMP, inhibit the growth-promoting effects of norephephrine in cardiac myocytes and fibroblasts. J Clin Invest 1998;101:812–818.

134. Devlin AM, Brosnan MJ, Graham D, Morton JJ, McPhaden AR, Mcintyre M, et al. Vascular smooth muscle cell polyploidy and cardiomyocyte hypertrophy due to chronic NOS inhibition in vivo. Am J Physiol 1998;274:H52–H59.

135. Ishigai Y, Mori T, Ikeda T, Fukuzawa A, Shibano T. Role of bradykinin-NO pathway in prevention of cardiac hypertrophy by ACE inhibitor in rat cardiomyocytes. Am J Physiol 1997;273:H2659–H2663.

136. Takaori K, Kim S, Ohta K, Hamaguchi A, Yagi K, Iwao H. Inhibition of nitric oxide synthase causes cardiac phenotypic modulation in rat. Eur J Pharmacol 1997;322:59–62.
137. de Belder A, Robinson N, Richardson P, Martin J, Moncada S. Expression of inducible nitric oxide synthase in human heart failure. Circulation 1997;95:1672,1673.
138. Avontuur JA, Bruining HA, Ince C. Inhibition of nitric oxide synthesis causes myocardial ischemia in endotoxemic rats. Circ Res 1995;76:418–425.
139. Ungureanu-Longrois D, Balligand JL, Kelly RA, Smith TWJ. Myocardial contractile dysfuncion in the systemic inflammatory response syndrome: role of a cytokine-inducible nitric oxide synthase in cardiac myocytes. J Mol Cell Cardiol 1995;27:155–167.
140. Balligand JL, Ungureanu-Longrois D, Simmons WW, Kobzik L, Lowenstein CJ, Lamas S, et al. Induction of NO synthase in rat cardiac microvascular endothelial cells by IL-1β and IFN-γ. Am J Physiol 1995;268:H1293–H1303.
141. Fujii H, Ichimori K, Hoshiai K, Nakazawa H. Nitric oxide inactivates NADPH oxidase in pig neutrophils by inhibiting its assembling process. J Biol Chem 1997;272:32,773–32,778.
142. Kubes P, Grisham MB, Barrowman JA, Gaginella T, Granger DN. Leukocyte-induced vascular protein leakage in cat mesentery. Am J Physiol 1991;261:H1872–H1879,
143. Kubes P. Nitric oxide affects microvascular permeability in the intact and inflamed vasculature. Microcirculation 1995;2:235–244.
144. Wei XQ, Charles IG, Smith A, Ure J, Feng GJ, Huang FP, et al. Altered immune responses in mice lacking inducible nitric oxide synthase. Nature (Lond) 1995;375:408–411.
145. MacMicking JD, Nathan C, Hom G, Chartrain N, Fletcher DS, Trumbauer M, et al. Altered responses to bacterial infection and endotoxic shock in mice lacking inducible nitric oxide synthase. Cell 1995; 81:641–650.
146. Laubach VE, Sheseley EG, Smithies O, Sherman PA. Mice lacking inducible nitric oxide synthase are not resistant to lipopolysaccharide-induced death. Proc Natl Acad Sci USA 1995;92:10,688–10,692.
147. Levine B, Kalman J, Mayer L, Fillit HM, Packer M. Elevated levels of tumor necrosis factor in severe chronic heart failure. N Engl J Med 1990;323: 236–241.
148. Deswal A, Bozkurt B, Seta Y, Parilti-Eiswirth S, Hayes FA, Blosch C, Mann DL. Safety and efficacy of a soluble P75 tumor necrosis factor receptor (Enbrel, etanercept) in patients with advanced heart failure. Circulation 1999;99:3224–3226.
149. Muller-Werdan U, Schumann H, Fuchs R, Reithmann C, Loppnow H, Koch S, et al. TNF alpha is cardiodepressant in pathophysiologically relevant concentrations without inducing iNOS or triggering cytotoxicity. J Mol Cell Cardiol 1997;29:2915–2923.
150. Oral H, Dorn GW, Mann DL. Sphingosine mediates the immediate negative inotropic effects of tumor necrosis factor-alpha in the adult mammalian cardiac myocyte. J Biol Chem 1997;272:4836–4842.
151. Anversa P, Myocyte apoptosis and heart failure. Eur Heart J 1998;19:359,360.
152. Anversa P, Kajstura J. Myocyte cell death in the diseased heart. Circ Res 1998;82:1231–1233.
153. Worrall NK, Lazenby WD, Misko TP, Lin TS, Rodi CP, Manning PT, et al. Modulation of in vivo alloreactivity by inhibition of inducible nitric oxide synthase. J Exp Med 1995;181:63–70.
154. Schulz R, Panas DL, Catena R, Moncada S, Olley PM, Lopaschuk GD. The role of nitric oxide in cardiac depression induced by interleukin 1 and tumor necrosis factor-α. Br J Pharmacol 1995;114:27–34.
155. Brady AJ, Poole-Wilson PA, Harding SE, Warren JB. Nitric oxide production within cardiac myocytes reduces their contractility in endotoxemia. Am J Physiol 1992;263:H1963–H1966.
156. Ziolo MT, Dollinger SJ, Wahler GM. Myocytes isolated from rejecting transplanted rat hearts exhibit reduced basal shortening which is reversible by aminoguanidine. J Mol Cell Cardiol 1998;30: 1009–1017.
157. Balligand JL, Ungureanu D, Kelly KA, Kobzik L, Pimental D, Michel T, et al. Abnormal contractile function due to induction of nitric oxide synthesis in rat cardiac myocytes follows exposure to activated macrophage-conditioned medium. J Clin Invest 1993;91:2314–2319.
158. Decking UK, Flesche CW, Godecke A, Schrader J. Endotoxin-induced contractile dysfunction in guinea pig hearts is not mediated by nitric oxide. Am J Physiol 1995;268:H2460–H2465.
159. Gulick T, Chung MK, Pieper SJ, Lange LG, Schreiner GF. Interleukin 1 and tumor necrosis factor inhibit cardiac myocyte beta-adrenergic responsiveness. Proc Natl Acad Sci USA 1989;86: 6753–6757.
160. Chung MK, Gulick TS, Rotondo RE, Schreiner GF, Lange LG. Mechanism of cytokine inhibition of beta-adrenergic agonist stimulation of cyclic AMP in rat cardiac myocytes. Impairment of signal transduction. Circ Res 1990;67:753–763.
161. Pyo RT, Wahler GM. Ventricular myocytes isolated from rejecting cardiac allografts exhibit a reduced beta-adrenergic contractile response. J Mol Cell Cardiol 1995;27:773–776.

162. Sun X, Delbridge LMD, Dusting GY. Cardiodepressant effects of interferon-gamma and endotoxin reversed by inhibition of NO synthase 2 in rat myocardium. J Mol Cell Cardiol 1998;30:989–997.

163. Mikami S, Kawashima S, Kanazawa K, Hirata K, Hotta H, Hayashi Y, et al. Low-dose N omega-nitro-L-arginine methyl ester treatment improves survival rate and decreases myocardial injury in a murine model of viral myocarditis induced by coxackie virus B3. Circ Res 1997;81:504–511.

164. Lowenstein CJ, Hill SL, Lafond-Walker A, Wu J, Allen G, Landavere M, et al. Nitric oxide inhibits viral replication in murine myocarditis. J Clin Invest 1996;97:1837–1843.

165. Pinsky DJ, Oz MC, Koga S, Taha Z, Broekman MJ, Marcus AJ, et al. Cardiac preservation is enhanced in a heterotopic rat transplant model by supplementing the nitric oxide pathway. J Clin Invest 1994;93:2291–2297.

166. Yang X, Chowdhury N, Cai B, Brett J, Marboe C, Sciacca RR, et al. Induction of myocardial nitric oxide synthase by cardiac allograft rejection. J Clin Invest 1994;94:714–721.

167. Kim Y-M, Bombeck CA, Billiar TR. Nitric oxide as a bifunctional regulator of apoptosis. Circ Res 1999;84:253–256.

168. Szabolcs M, Michler RE, Yang X, Aji W, Royd Athan E, et al. Apoptosis of cardiac myocytes during cardiac allograft rejection. Relation to induction of nitric oxide synthase. Circulation 1996;94:1665–1673.

169. Szabolcs MJ, Ravalli S, Minanov O, Sciacca RR, Michler RE, Cannon PJ. Apoptosis and increased expression of inducible nitric oxide synthase in human allograft rejection. Transplantation 1998;65:804–812.

170. Nguyen T, Brunson D, Crespi CL, Penamn BW, Wishnok JS, Tannenbaum SR. DNA damage and mutation in human cells exposed to nitric oxide in vitro. Proc Natl Acad Sci USA 1992;89:3033,3034.

171. Burney S, Tamir S, Gal S, Tannenbaum SR. A mechanistic analysis of nitric oxide-induced cellular toxicity. Nitric Oxide Biol Chem 1997;1:130–144.

172. Hounstetter A, Izumo S. Apoptosis: basic mechanisms and implication for cardiovascular disease. Circ Res 1998;82:1111–1129.

173. Koglin J, Granville DJ, Glysing-Jensen T, Mudgalt JS, Carthy CM, McManus BM, Russell ME. Attenuated acute cardiac rejection in NOS2–/– recipients correlates with reduced apoptosis. Circulation 1999;99:836–842.

174. Lew WYW. LPS induces cell shrinkage in rabbit ventricular cardiac myocytes. Am J Physiol 1997;272:H2989–H2993.

175. Preckel B, Kojda G, Schlack W, Ebel D, Kottenberg K, Noack E, et al. Inotropic effects of glyceryl trinitrate and spontaneous NO donors in the dog heart. Circulation 1997;96:2675–2682.

176. Mohan P, Brutsaert DL, Paulus WS, Sys V. Myocardial contractile response to nitric oxide and cGMP. Circulation 1996;93:1223–1229.

177. Pinsky DJ, Aji W, Szabolcs M, Athan ES, Liu Y, Yang YM, et al. Nitric oxide triggers programmed cell death (apoptosis) of adult rat cardiac myocytes in culture. Am J Physiol 1999;277:H1189–H1199.

178. Ing DJ, Zang J, Dzau VJ, Webster KA, Bishopric NH. Modulation of cytokine-induced cardiac myocyte apoptosis by nitric oxide, Bak and Bcl-x. Circ Res 1999;84:21–33.

11   The Fibroblast and Nitric Oxide

Peter Brecher

The fibroblast typically is found in loose connective tissue where it is considered to be the principal cell type. Fibroblasts are responsible for the synthesis of the extracellular matrix proteins including collagen, elastin, and reticular fibers, as well as the complex carbohydrates of the ground substance. In addition, during pathophysiological processes such as wound healing, the fibroblast can change phenotype, differentiate into a myofibroblast, and exhibit properties characteristic of both smooth muscle and conventional fibroblast cells. The role of fibroblasts during wound repair was reviewed recently, and the diverse functions for fibroblasts and their interaction with other cell types during wound healing was discussed [1,2]. In addition to matrix production, those functions include growth factor production, proliferation and migration, protease release, formation and contraction of granulation tissue, and phenotypic changes to a myofibroblast or to apoptosis.

Although usually identified morphologically by an elongated and spindly shape and by its presence within connective tissue, there is no distinct biochemical marker for the fibroblast; thus positive identification can be difficult, particularly when inflammation is present and the shape and staining characteristics of the cell may change. The problems associated with identifying fibroblasts are even greater when they are studied in cell culture. Hynes [3], in an incisive monograph on the properties of fibronectins, discusses this problem and suggests that a fibroblast "is a term now used to refer to a class of cells that adheres, migrates, and grows readily in tissue culture, adopting a flattened and/or elongated morphology." Although morphology may be adequate to distinguish cultured fibroblasts from cells such as epithelial cells, it is more difficult when mixed with endothelial cells, smooth muscle cells, or chondrocytes, where additional biochemical criteria or growth characteristics must be used.

Functionally, fibroblasts are most frequently associated with the deposition of extracellular matrix during nonpathological processes and for diverse roles in wound healing. Nitric oxide (NO·) has often been associated with inflammatory and wound-repair sites, but the specific cell types responsible for NO· production are not always well defined. There is a paucity of information on the role of NO· in the regulation of extracellular matrix production by fibroblasts or any other cell type, whereas a role for NO· in inflammation has been studied more extensively. In this chapter, emphasis is placed on the ability of the fibroblast to produce NO· during inflammation, and the possible functional role of fibroblast-derived NO· in pathological events. Initial consideration will be given to the different organ systems where fibroblasts have been studied with respect to NO·, and then to the cardiovascular system, emphasizing studies with cardiac fibroblasts as well as the possible role of the adventitia in vascular disease.

From: *Contemporary Cardiology, vol. 4: Nitric Oxide and the Cardiovascular System*
Edited by: J. Loscalzo and J. A. Vita © Humana Press Inc., Totowa, NJ

PRODUCTION OF NO•
BY FIBROBLASTS FROM DIFFERENT ORGAN SYSTEMS

Skin

A recent overview of NO• in human skin provides an excellent summary of available data in this field *(4)*. Skin contains varied cell types, and all isoforms of NO• synthase have been described in the different cell types. The functional role of NO•, although not clearly established, appears to be diverse both in physiological and pathophysiological situations. A role for NO• is under investigation for psoriasis, skin cancer, and other cutaneous diseases, but no definitive studies are yet available. In human skin, fibroblasts obtained in culture spontaneously produce NO•, and this production was enhanced by stimulation with a combination of interferon-gamma (IFN-γ) and lipopolysaccharide (LPS) *(5)*. Enzymatic studies, polymerase chain reaction (PCR) techniques, and immunohistochemistry indicated that both the constitutive and inducible isoforms of NO synthase (NOS) are present in these cells, although at levels somewhat lower than in other fibroblasts cell types. The suggestion was made that NO• production by dermal fibroblasts could be important during the inflammatory stages of wound healing, and subsequently in tissue remodeling after skin injury in humans. In a subsequent study *(6)*, dermal fibroblasts from hypertrophic scar tissue and site-matched normal dermis were compared. Both NO• production and levels of the constitutive eNOS were reduced in the cells derived from scar tissue using enzymatic techniques as well as flow cytometry. Because NO• inhibits cell proliferation, it was speculated that the low levels of endogenous NO• might be responsible for the cellularity of postburn hypertrophic scar tissue, which is a characteristic feature of this fibrotic condition.

Fibroblasts obtained from wounds produced by inserting sponges subcutaneously in rats for 10 d were studied *(7)*, and it was shown that cells in the first in vitro passage produced NO• spontaneously, but this capacity was markedly diminished in subsequent passages. Normal dermal fibroblasts did not produce nitrite, and it required about 7 d of in vivo implantation of the sponge to obtain the phenotype of wound fibroblasts that did produce nitrite. *In situ* hybridization studies demonstrated iNOS mRNA both in fibroblasts and macrophages from the wound area, and immunohistochemical studies confirmed the *in situ* hybridization findings. Of interest in this study was the additional observation that NO• appeared to regulate fibroblast collagen synthesis. Inhibition of NO• synthesis by competitive inhibitors of the synthase resulted in decreased collagen synthesis, whereas collagen synthesis was enhanced when NO• release was increased following stimulation with LPS and IFN-γ. Inhibition of NO• synthesis also enhanced fibroblast-mediated collagen contraction, but did not influence proliferation. The data indicated that during wound healing, the phenotypic changes in fibroblasts lead to altered NO• production, which in turn regulates collagen synthesis and contractile activity.

Further evidence for the role of NO• in wound healing, and more specifically for the role of iNOS in the process, was recently reported *(8)*. These investigators used a model for wound closure in mice and compared the process using iNOS knockout mice with wild-type animals. Delayed wound healing in inducible NOS (iNOS)-deficient mice was completely reversed by application of an adenoviral vector containing human iNOS cDNA at the time of wounding. The results established a key role for iNOS in wound closure, and suggested that gene therapy could improve wound healing in other iNOS-deficient states such as diabetes or during steroid treatment.

Gastrointestinal Tract

A study on the effects of LPS and interferon-γ (IFN-γ) on fibroblasts from the human small intestinal lamina propria, undertaken because of a presumed role for fibroblast participation in inflammatory disorders of the intestine, indicated that LPS addition alone induce increased cell proliferation and collagen synthesis concomitant with a suppression of basal levels of NO• *(9)*. If IFN-γ was also added with LPS, there was an increase in NO• production and concurrently a decrease in cell proliferation and collagen production. Inhibitors of NO• production partially restored cell proliferation and collagen synthesis in cells treated with both LPS and IFN-γ, implicating NO• as a negative effector of both proliferation and connective tissue production. Thus, completely opposing results of NO• on collagen production were found when LPS and IFN-γ were added to either human fibroblasts from skin *(7)* or lamina propria *(9)*. A regulatory role for NO• in gastrointestinal healing using an in vivo model *(10)* showed that LPS administration to animals given a left colonic anastomosis led to iNOS expression; and enhanced NO• production in systemic sepsis led to impaired collagen synthesis, dysregulation of collagen gene expression, and decreased anastomotic strength.

Lung

Other than the studies mentioned using human dermal fibroblasts, there is relatively little evidence for either of the constitutive forms of NOS in fibroblasts. However, the addition of cytokines to cultured fibroblasts from several cell types leads to the expression of iNOS and the subsequent production of NO•. As might be expected, the pattern of expression of iNOS in response to various cytokines differs considerably among fibroblasts from different sources. In a study *(11)* on the induction of iNOS in mouse and rat fibroblasts from embryonic tissue and adult lung, it was reported that nitrite production was induced by cytokines, particularly when IFN-γ was present with either tumor necrosis factor-α (TNF-α) or interleukin 1β (IL 1β). LPS also was studied and found to be synergistic with either TNF-α or IL-1β. These responses with fibroblast cell populations contrasted with previous studies from the same laboratory using cultured macrophages where synergy with LPS was not found. The comparisons suggested that fibroblasts were activated more readily to produce NO• than interstitial macrophages, and the authors speculated that fibroblasts could be the major source of NO• in tissues. In a subsequent study *(12)*, it was found that when macrophages that lacked the ability to make NO• were cocultured with transformed fibroblasts with this capability, macrophages could induce NO• production in the fibroblasts by releasing TNF-α and IL-1β, and subsequently suppress cell proliferation.

In rat lung fibroblasts, Zhang et al. *(13)* found that IL-1b added alone could decrease expression of a-smooth muscle actin, inhibit contractility of collagen gels, reduce cell number, and increase apoptosis. All these changes were associated with increased NO• production, and when NO• production was inhibited by N^G-monomethyl-L-arginine (L-NMMA), the other changes were also reversed. These studies, addressing a role for NO• in pulmonary fibrosis, suggested that NO• may be an important regulator of the contractile phenotype for lung fibroblasts. A rat-lung cell line was used to examine a potential mechanism by which NO• could play a protective role in cell injury *(14)*. It was found that NO• increased cellular glutathione levels several fold in these fibroblasts, most likely by increasing glutathione biosynthesis, and the increased glutathione could have a protective role through its ability to modulate oxidative stress during inflammation.

Heart

In a study on NO• synthesis in cardiac myocytes and fibroblasts by inflammatory cytokines, Shindo et al. *(15)* found that such substances as IL-1β or LPS could induce nitrite or cGMP levels in myocytes, but not in cardiac fibroblasts obtained from the neonatal cardiac tissue from the same species. These findings are representative of other studies with cultured fibroblasts indicating a need for more than one cytokine to induce iNOS in fibroblast cell populations. A related study *(16)* showed that IL-1β induced cardiac myocyte hypertrophy but when incubated with cardiac fibroblasts, IL-1β had an antiproliferative effect. Unfortunately, NO• was not measured in those studies, but would be a likely mediator of the antiproliferative effect if the cells could increase iNOS expression solely in response to IL-1β.

The need for more than one cytokine to induce iNOS expression in some, but not all, cultured fibroblasts is most likely due to the requirement for several transcription factors to be induced simultaneously in order to activate gene expression. The transcription factors most studied to date with respect to iNOS are NF-κB, induced by cytokines such as IL-1β or TNF-α, and members of the Stat family, most frequently induced by IFN-γ. A mechanistic study on the relationship between transcription factors and iNOS induction was performed in murine 3T3 fibroblasts (17). In that study, it was shown that agents other than cytokines, such as protein kinase C-stimulating agents or cyclic adenosine monophosphate (cAMP)-elevating agents, were efficacious inducers of iNOS expression. Using electrophoresis mobility shift assays, NF-κB was shown to be activated in all cases regardless of the signaling pathway. Agents that inhibited iNOS expression, such as dexamethasone, pyrrolidine dithiocarbamate, and 3,4-dichloroisocoumarin (all inhibitors of NF-κB activation), suppressed iNOS mRNA induction. These studies clearly indicated a key regulatory role of NF-κB in fibroblast iNOS expression. Although it was not addressed directly in the study, the data suggested that alterations in oxidative stress could activate iNOS via a mechanism involving NF-κB.

Studies from the author's laboratory (18,19) have examined in detail the induction of iNOS in cardiac fibroblasts using combinations of cytokines, and explored indirectly the possibility that the anti-inflammatory effects of salicylates are caused by their ability to inhibit iNOS in fibroblasts. In primary cultures, IFN-γ, IL-1β, or TNF-α separately did not stimulate nitrite production, whereas IFN-γ combined with IL-1β or TNF-α synergistically induced iNOS, both at the level of steady-state mRNA and nitrite accumulation. Steady-state mRNA levels for iNOS were obvious as early as 3 h after addition of IFN-γ plus TNF-α and remained elevated for at least 72 h. Sodium salicylate, at anti-inflammatory doses, inhibited cytokine-induced nitrite accumulation. The inhibition was reversible and occurred when salicylate was added either before or after cytokine induction. Aspirin also inhibited nitrite production, whereas indomethacin and acetaminophen did not. TNF-α, either alone or combined with IFN-γ, significantly stimulated prostaglandin E_2, which was inhibited by either salicylate or indomethacin. Salicylate, when given either before or after IFN-γ plus TNF-α, reduced mRNA levels of iNOS induced by cytokines. These studies (18) implicated cardiac fibroblasts as a source of NO• in inflammatory cardiac diseases, and suggest a possible therapeutic role for salicylate and aspirin in diminishing the steady-state levels of iNOS mRNA.

To define further the mechanism of inhibition of iNOS by salicylate in cardiac fibroblasts, iNOS mRNA induction by cytokines was investigated with regard to the kinetics of inhibition by salicylate, as compared to dexamethasone (19). IFN-γ plus TNF-α induced iNOS mRNA synergistically. Both dexamethasone and salicylate equally inhibited the induction of iNOS mRNA, both before and after cytokine induction. Salicylate also inhibited IFN-γ plus IL-1β-induced iNOS mRNA. After 24 h of cytokine stimulation, salicylate stopped the induction of iNOS mRNA, whereas dexamethasone delayed the accumulation of transcript. In half-life experiments of iNOS mRNA, dexamethasone reduced the half-life of iNOS mRNA, whereas salicylate had no effect on mRNA stability. TNF-α and IFN-γ induced NF-κB and Stat-1, respectively, as assessed by gel-shift assays. Salicylate did not inhibit the cytokine induction of NF-κB or Stat-1. This study suggested that the anti-inflammatory mechanism of salicylate involved inhibition of iNOS transcription and showed that the effect was independent of NF-κB activation.

Studies summarized earlier on the production of NO• in a variety of fibroblast types from different sources have in common a requirement for two cytokines acting synergistically to activate iNOS. There have been reports showing that a single cytokine can induce iNOS in myocytes (16) or vascular smooth muscle (20), e.g., but not in fibroblasts. Perhaps the need for multiple cytokines, and presumably the requirement for a combination of requisite transcription factors, ensures that iNOS will not be induced physiologically unless there is an appropriate inflammatory environment. Most studies to date involving fibroblasts and NO˙ have emphasized the pathophysiological role of the fibroblast in fibrosis, be it dermal, pulmonary, or cardiac. In most cases of fibrosis, there exists a situation where fibroblasts are located adjacent to inflammatory cells, and can serve either as the source or target of secreted cytokines. It remains to be shown in a pathophysiological setting whether the fibroblast actually produces NO˙ or releases cytokines that influence other fibroblasts or other cell types to produce NO˙ in an autocrine or paracrine manner, respectively.

EFFECTS OF NO˙ ON FIBROBLAST CELL GROWTH

There now exists a fairly extensive literature on the effects of NO˙ on cell proliferation, but the results are inconsistent, both among cell types and in a given cell type. Fibroblasts from various sources have been used to examine the mechanisms underlying the effects of NO˙ on the cell cycle. The antiproliferative effect of NO˙ was initially described in cultured vascular smooth muscle cells *(21)*, where its antiproliferative effects were mimicked by cyclic guanosine monophosphate (cGMP), and subsequently in many other cell types including fibroblasts. Using BALB/c3T3 fibroblasts, which lack soluble guanylyl cyclase, addition of NO˙ donors nevertheless inhibited mitogenesis and proliferation, suggesting a mechanism that did not require cGMP in these fibroblasts *(22)*. In another study *(23)*, also using BALB/C3T3 cells, a low concentration of NO˙ donors was shown to enhance proliferation as measured by increased labeled thymidine incorporation in stationary cells and increased thymidine kinase activity in exponentially growing cells. To complicate the issue further, the same investigators who first described the inhibitory effects of NO˙ on DNA synthesis in cultured vascular smooth muscle cells later showed that in primary cultures of smooth muscle cells, NO˙ enhanced fibroblast growth factor-induced mitogenesis, whereas in subsequent passages in vitro, NO˙ inhibited mitogenesis *(24)*.

The complexity of the response to NO˙ was recently explored *(25)* using NIH-3T3 fibroblasts overexpressing epidermal growth factor (EGF) receptors as a model for cell proliferative mechanisms. A cGMP-dependent stimulation of growth was demonstrated early in the cell cycle and involved the formation of the AP-1 transcription complex, whereas a cGMP-independent inhibition of cell growth was found to be mediated by a slowing of the cell cycle occurring in the G_1 and S phase, and partly mediated by negative regulation of ribonucleotide reductase. The multiple and conflicting effects of NO˙, even in a single cell type, were suggested to act in a coordinated program of cell growth regulation, although the mechanistic details remain to be studied. In another study *(26)* relating NO˙, EGF, and proliferation, NO˙ was shown to stimulate tyrosine phosphorylation of a relatively small population of proteins with molecular masses of 126, 56, and 43 kDa in murine fibroblasts exposed to different NO˙ donors. This effect was shown to be independent of the presence of EGF. This effect was mimicked by 8-bromo-cGMP and blocked by oxyhemoglobin. The authors suggested that the antiproliferative effects of NO˙ could be due to its ability to subvert the normal growth factor-associated signaling pathways of the cell by influencing tyrosine kinase activity.

The effects of both exogenously added and endogenously produced NO˙ on cell proliferation were recently studied in WI38 cells, which are human embryonal cells that were used in later passages to mimic a senescent cell population *(27)*. It was found that induction of iNOS by a combination of cytokines led to arrest in the G_1 phase of the cell cycle and to inhibition of proliferation. However, addition of the NO˙ donors sodium nitroprusside or *S*-nitroso-*N*-acetyl-penicillamine increased cell proliferation rates and the population of cells in the S/G_2 fraction. The data suggested a functional role for NO˙ in cell cycle regulation and cell proliferation, which depended both on the mode of NO˙ generation and the culture conditions used.

It is well known that NO˙ can induce apoptosis in various cell types, and this event may occur in vivo during the progression of fibrosis. With respect to the fibroblast, there are as yet few studies documenting NO˙-induced apoptosis. Shin et al. *(28)* showed that acidic fibroblast growth factor (FGF-1) enhanced apoptosis in primary murine fibroblasts, presumably because of peroxynitrite formation resulting from the reaction between NO˙ and superoxide anion. It was speculated that FGF-1 made fibroblasts more sensitive to peroxynitrite-induced apoptosis, and this effect may have a pivotal role during inflammation and repair processes in vivo.

Studies performed in vivo in the author's laboratory *(29)* showed that chronic inhibition of NOS led to an exaggerated response to relatively low doses of angiotensin II, resulting in a rapid and marked cardiac fibrosis. This in vivo effect, which resulted in cardiac fibroblast proliferation and matrix deposition, was blocked both by agents that antagonized angiotensin II or enhanced NO˙ production. To examine further the importance of angiotensin II in inducing cardiac fibrosis and the possibility that NO˙ serves as a modulator of the proliferative effects of angiotensin II, cultured rat cardiac fibroblasts were used to study the interrelationships between these substances *(30)*. Angiotensin II induced a delayed DNA synthetic response in quiescent cells that occurred 30 h after exposure to the hormone. This response was inhibited in a dose-dependent manner by the addition of either *S*-nitroso-*N*-acetylpenicillamine (SNAP) or sodium nitroprusside, each a source of NO˙. The NO˙ donor was most effective in reducing thymidine incorporation when added 12 h after angiotensin II, whereas the metabolite *N*-acetylpenicillamine (NAP) had no effect at any time. The inhibitory effect of SNAP was mimicked by 8-bromoguanosine 3':5'-cyclic monophosphate but not by 8-bromoadenosine 3':5'-cyclic monophosphate. NO˙ donors did not appear to inhibit the induction of *c-fos*, *Egr-1*, or other immediate early genes in response to angiotensin II. The results suggested that NO˙ affects the cell cycle following the transition into G_1 and modulates the proliferation of fibroblasts during cardiac fibrosis induced by angiotensin II.

Although a molecular explanation for how NO˙ exerts an antiproliferative or apoptotic effect on fibroblasts, or other cell types, is not yet forthcoming, there is new information relating the effects of NO˙ signaling pathways that could affect the cell cycle. NO˙ is known to induce DNA damage in several cell types, and it was shown *(31)* that the expression of p53, a transcriptional activator of several growth regulatory genes, is induced concomitant with NO˙-induced DNA damage. Using fibroblasts, it was shown in the same study that overexpression of p53 led to a downregulation of iNOS expression through inhibition of the iNOS promoter, implicating a negative feedback loop where DNA damage and p53 expression prevent additional NO˙ production. One important growth regulatory gene that is induced by p53 is the cyclin-dependent kinase inhibitor p21. Of particular interest is a study *(32)* showing that NO˙ induces p21, which can arrest the cell cycle in G_1, preventing the cell from entering S phase and subsequently replicating. These studies were conducted using cultured vascular smooth muscle cells, but studies have recently confirmed the basic observation in rat aortic adventitial fibroblasts *(33)*. This induction of p21 provides an explanation for the antiproliferative effects of NO˙, and leads to further mechanistic questions regarding how NO˙ influences gene expression. A summary of the proliferative and antiproliferative effects of NO˙ on fibroblasts is shown in Table 1.

ADVENTITIAL FIBROBLASTS IN THE VASCULATURE

Localization of iNOS

Most studies in vascular biology have focused on the interrelationships between endothelial cells and vascular smooth muscle, localized within the intima and media respectively, with emphasis on the paracrine relationships that modulate vascular growth and tone. Less attention has been given to the role of the adventitia in normal vascular function and in diseases such as atherosclerosis, hypertension, and restenosis. The major cell type within the

Table 1
Effects of NO• on Fibroblasts

Antiproliferative effects of NO•
    Most common in cultured cells
    Requires high concentrations of NO• donors
    Slows cell cycle in G_1–S phase
    Induces p53, p21, and apoptosis
Proliferative effects of NO•
    Observed in primary cell culture
    Low concentrations of NO• more effective
    Influences early cell cycle changes
    cGMP-dependent

adventitia is the fibroblast, and the adventitia has been recognized as a site for inflammatory cells to enter and influence the resident fibroblasts as well as other portions of the vessel wall. Previous studies have shown that when LPS was given to rats in vivo, there was a rapid and transient increase in NO• production due to the induction of iNOS. In vivo studies have documented increased NOS activity in rat aortic tissue following administration of endotoxin (34). In those studies, endothelial removal eliminated completely the Ca^{2+}-dependent activity, but had only a minor effect on the substantial amount of Ca^{2+}-independent activity induced by endotoxin in aortic tissue, suggesting that medial smooth muscle was the source of iNOS. The adventitia was not specifically examined as a potential source of the activity in the vascular segments tested.

Using a monoclonal antibody against iNOS in adult rats in which septic shock was induced by intravenous LPS injection, iNOS-positive cells were identified in the aorta and other organs (35,36). Aortic endothelial cells showed a strong reaction 4–6 h after LPS administration, whereas iNOS appeared only weakly in medial smooth muscle cells. In other studies where aortic rings were incubated in vitro using organ chamber techniques (37–39), iNOS induction was demonstrated both in intact and denuded rat aortic rings after LPS or cytokine treatment, and smooth muscle cells were implicated as a site of iNOS induction. Again, the adventitia was not examined directly. A comparison between cultured vascular smooth muscle cells and aortic strips showed distinctions between mechanisms involved in the induction of iNOS in those preparations (40). That study showed that aortic rings produced increased mRNA for iNOS following either addition of LPS alone or in combination with IFN-γ, whereas cultured cells required a synergy between these agents to promote expression. In that study, the authors suggested that phenotypic differences in smooth muscle cells in culture and in the intact aorta could account for the different responses, but the possible contribution of the adventitia was not considered.

Recent studies from the author's laboratory (41) have utilized in situ hybridization techniques to show that iNOS induction in response to LPS occurred primarily in the adventitia and intima. These studies showed that fibroblasts, localized in the aortic adventitia, express iNOS following administration of LPS, and suggest that the adventitia may be an important source of NO• within the aorta during the inflammatory response. In addition to adventitial fibroblasts, in situ hybridization indicated that endothelial cells also express iNOS following LPS treatment. Interestingly, we found little or no induction of iNOS in medial smooth muscle cells following this in vivo treatment.

Role of the Adventitia in Vascular Disease

Wilcox and Scott (42) reviewed the literature relating the potential role of the adventitia in the development of both arteritis and atherosclerosis. In that review it was noted that inflammatory cells have been observed in the adventitia of atherosclerotic vessels for over

100 yr, yet most of the available data show a correlation between inflammatory cells in the adventitia and vascular injury, but do not indicate a causal relationship. With regard to a specific role for adventitial fibroblasts in vascular disease, a porcine model of restenosis was used where young pigs underwent balloon overinflation injury to the coronary arteries, and the study showed that adventitial myofibroblasts contributed to the process of vascular lesion formation by proliferation, growth factor production, and possibly migration *(43)*. A similar study *(44)* also used balloon injury of a pig coronary artery to show that adventitial myofibroblasts translocate from the adventitia to the neointima of the progressing lesion. These two independent studies provide strong evidence for a role of the adventitial fibroblast in neointimal formation in an injured large blood vessel. Subsequent studies have indicated that transforming growth factor-β (TGF-β), made by the porcine coronary adventitial fibroblasts, may have a role in regulating the phenotype of these cells during injury *(45)*, and the possibility that differentiated fibroblasts (myofibroblasts) from the vascular adventitia may have a role in other vascular diseases has been reviewed and discussed *(46)*.

There have been relatively few studies relating adventitial changes to the pathogenesis of vascular injury in experimental hypertension. In a model of aortic ligation between renal arteries to produce hypertension in rats, it was shown that adventitial fibroblasts respond with increased DNA synthesis and matrix production *(47)*. The authors suggested that the adventitia might participate in the development of vascular hypertrophy and arterial disease. Studies by Kato et al. *(48)* have utilized a model of angiotensin II infusion and chronic treatment with an inhibitor of NOS in rats to show that adventitial fibroblasts responded specifically to angiotensin II by increased DNA synthesis, even when the drug was given at subpressor doses. During remodeling processes that occur in pulmonary hypertension, changes in adventitial connective tissue metabolism were induced by a factor derived from vascular smooth muscle *(49)*. Interestingly, a recent report indicated that the adventitia is a diffusion barrier to NO• in the pulmonary artery *(50)*. A few studies have utilized aortic adventitial fibroblasts in tissue culture and shown that when taken from spontaneously hypertensive rats, proliferative activity *(51)* and expression of cyclins *(52)* differ from comparable cells obtained from Wistar-Kyoto controls. Although there are many studies implicating paracrine relationships between endothelial and vascular smooth muscle cells, both in normal and pathophysiological situations, the role of the adventitial cell population in modulating smooth muscle cell function has not been examined intensively and is a research area that should be given greater attention.

NO• and Atherosclerosis

There has been considerable efforts to determine the role of NO• in atherosclerotic lesions (also see Chapter 16). Suprisingly, there have been relatively few studies identifying cell types where iNOS might be present in the vessel wall. Using the Watanabe heritable hyperlipidemic rabbit as a model for atherosclerosis, Sobey et al. *(53)* showed that LPS administration to atherosclerotic rabbits resulted in an augmented production of NO• using contractile responsiveness, enzymatic assays, and immunodetection as criteria. The authors used nicotinamide adenine dinucleotide phosphate (NADPH) diaphorase antibodies to detect iNOS, as specific antibodies to iNOS did not indicate the presence of enzyme that was there by other criteria. Localization was thought to be in smooth muscle cells and not macrophages of the atherosclerotic animals, although adventitia was not examined specifically. No iNOS was found in the intima or media of normal rabbit aortic tissue. Another study *(54)* used cholesterol-fed rabbits to produce atherosclerosis and found that iNOS was present in T lymphocytes and macrophages of atherosclerotic vessels, but not in smooth muscle cells. Again, nothing was found in normal rabbit aorta. In human atherosclerotic lesions, iNOS was detected by immunocytochemistry, Western blotting, and *in situ* hybridization and shown to be localized to macrophages (CD68-positive), foam cells, and the vascular smooth muscle *(55)*. A recent study *(56)* using both human and rabbit atherosclerotic lesions employed immunocytochemistry and *in situ* hybridization. They found that iNOS (and superoxide dismutase) were highly expressed in lesion macrophages with lesser amounts present in vascular smooth muscle. Finally, a study in human aortic tissue using lesions of varying severity showed that there was a loss of eNOS expression by endothelial cells as the lesions progressed and a significant increase in overall NOS synthesis by other cell types in advanced lesions, including eNOS, iNOS, and nNOS *(57)*. Thus, the studies so far agree that little or no iNOS is present in normal vessels, but there is no clear consensus as to the localization of iNOS in lesions or media from atherosclerotic tissue. Although most investigators agree that atherosclerosis has an inflammatory component to its pathogenesis, and the adventitia certainly can be a site for infiltration of inflammatory cells, there has not yet been a systematic and prospective study on the adventitia as a potential site for iNOS expression in atherosclerosis.

A novel approach to understanding the functional role of the adventitial fibroblast with respect to NO˙ production involved the use of adenoviral vectors to deliver endothelial NOS (eNOS) in vivo to the adventitia of cerebral arteries *(58)*. Using the canine model, gene transfer of eNOS was accomplished via the cerebrospinal fluid, and functional studies were documented by showing increased NOS activity in the adventitia of major cerebral arteries. The increased local NO˙ production led to augmentation of cGMP production and enhanced bradykinin-induced relaxations. Morphological examination indicated the adventitial fibroblast as the cell site for gene transfer. Another study involving gene therapy *(59)* showed that recombinant eNOS could be transduced into human saphenous veins. The vein segments were subsequently analyzed for eNOS expression and activity and these were shown to be present in both endothelial and adventitial cells. Furthermore, the generation of nitrite after stimulation with a calcium ionophore correlated with augmented maximal relaxation. These studies indicate that if NO˙ is generated in the adventitia, then functional changes in vascular tone might result.

Adventitial Fibroblasts and Superoxide Anion

A series of studies by Pagano and Cohen *(60–62)* have implicated the adventitia as a source of superoxide anion. Since superoxide reacts rapidly with NO˙ and can markedly influence the biological effects of NO˙, the colocalization of either NO˙ or superoxide anion could have pathophysiological significance. Pagano et al. *(60)* first showed that an NADPH oxidase was present in aortic tissue that generated superoxide anion based on chemiluminescent measurements with lucigenin. These studies further indicated that the adventitia was the major site for superoxide production in the vessel wall. A subsequent study *(61)* showed that a constitutively active NADPH oxidase, resembling the enzyme that has been well characterized in phagocytic cells, was present in relatively large amounts in the rabbit aortic adventitia, and that addition of angiotensin II increased superoxide generating activity in aortic rings from these rabbits. Constitutive superoxide generating activity was localized to aortic adventitial fibroblasts, and immunohistochemical studies showed the presence of subunits of the NADPH oxidase localized primarily in the adventitia. In a more recent study, Wang et al. *(62)* found that superoxide anion was produced endogenously in the rat aorta, and in sufficient quantities so that there was interference with the response of the rat aorta to NO˙. These experiments showed that nitroblue tetrazolium staining, indicative of superoxide anion, was present primarily in the adventitia of rat aortic rings and that when rings were oriented so the adventitial or luminal surface was preferentially exposed to NO˙, the response to NO˙ was attenuated more strongly with adventitial exposure. These data suggested that extracellular superoxide anion can inactivate and decrease the effect of NO˙ on adjacent smooth muscle cells.

Figure 1 illustrates schematically several possible roles for the fibroblast in a pathophysiological condition associated with inflammation, injury, and wound repair in a vascular environment. Initially, leukocytes infiltrate the adventitia and, during inflammation, release cytokines.

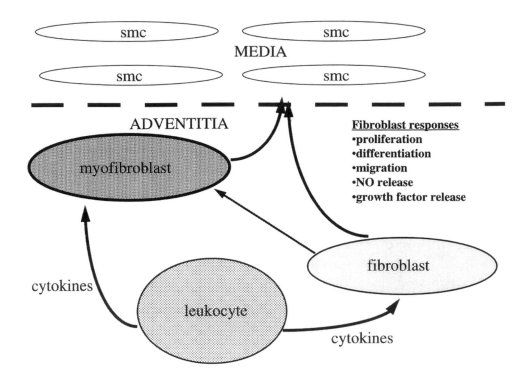

Fig. 1. Possible roles for the adventitial fibroblast during vascular injury.

Paracrine effects of those cytokines on fibroblasts could influence iNOS induction and NO•
production leading to a possible relaxation or antiproliferative effect on medial cells. Differentiation of resident fibroblasts into myofibroblasts, proliferation of either fibroblast phenotype, and perhaps migration into either the media or neointima of lesioned regions has been suggested. The possibility that growth factors or cytokines released by fibroblasts could influence medial smooth muscle cells to hypertrophy, migrate, or proliferate remains to be studied. The general concept of fibroblasts in any organ responding to inflammatory signals and releasing substances, such as NO•, with concomitant paracrine effects should be considered in any type of inflammatory or fibrotic process.

REFERENCES

1. Clark RA. Wound repair: overview and general considerations. In: Clark RA, ed. The Molecular and Cellular Biology of Wound Repair, 2nd ed. Plenum, New York, 1996, pp. 3–50.
2. Desmouliere A, Gabbiani G. The role of the myofibroblast in wound healing and fibrocontractive diseases. In: Clark RA, ed. The Molecular and Cellular Biology of Wound Repair, 2nd ed. Plenum, New York, 1996, pp. 391–423.
3. Hynes RO. Expression of fibronectin by cells in culture. In: Fibronectins. Springer Verlag, New York, 1990, p. 51.
4. Bruch-Gerharz C, Ruzicka T, Kolb-Bachofen V. Nitric oxide in human skin: current status and future prospects. J Invest Dermatol 1998;110:1–7.
5. Wang R, Ghahary A, Shen YJ, Scott PG, Tredget EE. Human dermal fibroblasts produce nitric oxide and express both constitutive and inducible nitric oxide synthase isoforms. J Invest Dermatol 1996;106: 419–427.
6. Wang R, Ghahary A, Shen YJ, Scott PG, Tredget EE. Nitric oxide synthase expression and nitric oxide production are reduced in hypertrophic scar tissue and fibroblasts. J Invest Dermatol 1997;108:438–444.
7. Schaffer MR, Efron PA, Thornton FJ, Klingel K, Gross SS, Barbul A. Nitric oxide, an autocrine regulator of wound fibroblast synthetic function. J Immunol 1997;158:2375–2381.

8. Yamasaki K, Edington HD, McClosky C, Tzeng E, Lisonova A, Kovesdi I, et al. Reversal of impaired wound repair in iNOS-deficient mice by topical adenoviral-mediated iNOS gene transfer. J Clin Invest 1998;101:967–971

9. Chakravortty D, Kumar KS. Induction of cell proliferation and collagen synthesis in human small intestinal lamina propria fibroblasts by lipopolysaccharide: possible involvement of nitric oxide. Biochem Biophys Res Commun 1997;240:458–463.

10. Thornton FJ, Ahrendt GM, Schaffer MR, Tantry US, Barbul A. Sepsis impairs anastomotic collagen gene expression and synthesis: a possible role for nitric oxide. J Surg Res 1997;69:81–86.

11. Lavnikova N, Laskin DL. Unique patterns of regulation of nitric oxide production in fibroblasts. J Leukoc Biol 1995;58:451–458.

12. Lavnikova N, Prokhorova S, Burdelia L, Lakhotia A, Laskin DL. Mechanisms regulating macrophage-induced nitric oxide production by spontaneously transformed hamster fibroblasts. J Leukoc Biol 1996; 60:473–479.

13. Zhang H, Gharaee-Kermani M, Phan SH. Regulation of lung fibroblast α-smooth muscle actin expression, contractile phenotype, and apoptosis by IL-1β. J Immunol 1997;158:1392–1399.

14. White AC, Maloney EK, Boustani MR, Hassoun PM, Fanburg BL. Nitric oxide increases cellular glutathione levels in rat lung fibroblasts. Am J Respir Cell Mol Biol 1995;13:442–448.

15. Shindo T, Ikeda U, Ohkawa F, Kawahara Y, Yokoyama M, Shimada K. Nitric oxide synthesis in cardiac myocytes and fibroblasts by inflammatory cytokines. Cardiovasc Res 1995;29:813–819.

16. Palmer JN, Hartogensis WE, Patten M, Fortuin FD, Long CS. Interleukin-1β induces cardiac myocyte growth but inhibits cardiac fibroblast proliferation in culture. J Clin Invest 1995;95:2555–2564.

17. Kleinert H, Euchenhofer C, Ihrig-Biedert I, Forstermann U. In murine 3T3 fibroblasts, different second messenger pathways resulting in the induction of NO synthase II (iNOS) converge in the activation of transcription factor NF-κB. J Biol Chem 1996;271:6039–6044.

18. Farivar RS, Chobanian AV, Brecher P. Salicylate or aspirin inhibits the induction of the inducible nitric oxide synthase in rat cardiac fibroblasts. Circ Res 1996;78:759–768.

19. Farivar RS, Brecher P. Salicylate is a transcriptional inhibitor of the inducible nitric oxide synthase in cultured cardiac fibroblasts. J Biol Chem 1996;271:31,585–31,592.

20. Koide M, Kawahara Y, Nakayama I, Tsuda T, Yokoyama M. Cyclic AMP-elevating agents induce an inducible type of nitric oxide synthase in cultured vascular smooth muscle cells. Synergism with the induction elicited by inflammatory cytokines. J Biol Chem 1993;268:24,959–24,966.

21. Garg UC, Hassid A. Nitric oxide-generating vasodilators and 8-bromo-cyclic guanosine monophosphate inhibit mitogenesis and proliferation of cultured rat vascular smooth muscle cells. J Clin Invest 1989;83:1774–1777.

22. Garg UC, Hassid A. Nitric oxide-generating vasodilators inhibit mitogenesis and proliferation of BALB/ C 3T3 fibroblasts by a cyclic GMP-independent mechanism. Biochem Biophys Res Commun 1990;171: 474–479.

23. Du M, Islam M, Lin L, Ohmura Y, Moriyama Y, Fujimura S. Promotion of proliferation of murine BALB/C3T3 fibroblasts mediated by nitric oxide at lower concentrations. Biochem Mol Biol Int 1997; 41:625–631.

24. Hassid A, Arabshahi H, Bourcier T, Dhaunsi GS, Matthews C. Nitric oxide selectively amplifies FGF-2-induced mitogenesis in primary rat aortic smooth muscle cells. Am J Physiol 1994;267:H1040–H1048.

25. Sciorati C, Nistico G, Meldolesi J, Clementi E. Nitric oxide effects on cell growth: GMP-dependent stimulation of the AP-1 transcription complex and cyclic GMP-independent slowing of cell cycling. Br J Pharmacol 1997;122:687–697.

26. Peranovich TM, daSilva AM, Fries DM, Stern A, Monteiro HP. Nitric oxide stimulates tyrosine phosphorylation in murine fibroblasts in the absence and presence of epidermal growth factor. Biochem J 1995;305:613–619.

27. Gansuage S, Gansauge F, Nussler AK, Rau B, Poch B, Schoenberg MH, et al. Exogenous, but not endogenous, nitric oxide increases proliferation rates in senescent human fibroblasts. FEBS Lett 1997; 410:160–164.

28. Shin JT, Barbeito L, MacMillan-Crow LA, Beckman JS, Thompson JA. Acidic fibroblast growth factor enhances peroxynitrite-induced apoptosis in primary murine fibroblasts. Arch Biochem Biophys 1996; 335:32–41.

29. Hou J, Kato H, Cohen RA, Chobanian AV, Brecher P. Angiotensin II-induced cardiac fibrosis in the rat is increased by chronic inhibition of nitric oxide synthase. J Clin Invest 1995;96:2469–2477.

30. Takizawa T, Gu M, Chobanian AV, Brecher P. The effect of nitric oxide on DNA replication induced by angiotensin II in rat cardiac fibroblasts. Hypertension 1997;30:1035–1040.

31. Forrester K, Ambs S, Lupold SE, Kapust RB, Spillare EA, Weinberg WC, et al. Nitric oxide-induced p53 accumulation and regulation of inducible nitric oxide synthase expression by wild-type p53. Proc Natl Acad Sci USA 1996;93:2442–2447.

32. Ishida A, Sasaguri T, Kosaka C, Nojima H, Ogata J. Induction of the cyclin-dependent kinase inhibitor p21Sdi1/Cip1/Waf1 by nitric oxide-generating vasodilator in vascular smooth muscle cells. J Biol Chem 1997;272:10,050–10,057.

33. Gu M, Brecher P. Nitric oxide increased the expression of p21 in proliferating fibroblasts from the aortic adventitia. FASEB J 1998;12:A79.

34. Knowles RG, Salter M, Brooks SL, Moncada S. Anti-inflammatory glucocorticoids inhibit the induction by endotoxin of nitric oxide synthase in the lung, liver, and aorta of the rat. Biochem Biophys Res Commun 1990;172:1042–1048.

35. Cook HT, Bune AJ, Jansen AS, Taylor GM, Loi RK, Cattell V. Cellular localization of inducible nitric oxide synthase in experimental endotoxic shock in the rat. Clin Sci 1994;87:179–186.

36. Sato K, Miyakawa K, Takeya M, Hattori R, Yui Y, Sunamoto M, et al. Immunohistochemical expression of inducible nitric oxide synthase (iNOS) in reversible endotoxic shock studied by a novel monoclonal antibody against rat iNOS. J Leukoc Biol 1995;57:36–44.

37. Fleming I, Gray AG, Stoclet J. Influence of endothelium on induction of the L-arginine-nitric oxide pathway in rat aortas. Am J Physiol 1993;264:H1200–H1207.

38. Fleming I, Gray AG, Julou-Schaeffer G, Parratt J, Stoclet J. Incubation with endotoxin activates the L-arginine pathway in vascular tissue. Biochem Biophys Res Commun 1990;172:562–568.

39. Schini-Kerth V, Bara A, Mylsch A, Busse R. Pyrrolidine dithiocarbamate selectively prevents the expression of the inducible nitric oxide synthase in the rat aorta. Eur J Pharmacol 1994;265:83–87.

40. Sirsjo A, Soderkvist P, Sundqvist T, Carlsson M, Ost M, Gidlof A. Different induction mechanisms of mRNA for inducible nitric oxide synthase in rat smooth muscle cells in culture and in aortic strips. FEBS Lett 1994;338:191–196.

41. Zhang H, Du Y, Chobanian AV, Brecher P. Adventitia as a source of inducible nitric oxide synthase in the rat aorta. Am J Hyper 1999;12:467–475.

42. Wilcox JN, Scott NA. Potential role of the adventitia in arteritis and atherosclerosis. Int J Cardiol 1996; 54(Suppl):S21–S35.

43. Scott NA, Cipolia GD, Ross CE, Dunn B, Martin FH, Simonet L, et al. Identification of a potential role for the adventitia in vascular lesion formation after balloon overstretch injury of porcine coronary arteries. Circulation 1996;93:2178–2187.

44. Shi Y, Pienick M, Fard A, O'Brien J, Mannion JD, Zalewski A. Adventitial remodeling after coronary arterial injury. Circulation 1996;93:340–348.

45. Shi Y, O'Brien JE, Fard A, Zalewski A. Transforming growth factor-β1 expression and myofibroblast formation during arterial repair. Arterioscler Thromb Vasc Biol 1996;16:1298–1305.

46. Zalewski A, Shi Y. Vascular myofibroblast lessons from coronary repair and remodeling. Arterioscler Thromb Vasc Biol 1997;17:417–422.

47. Chatelain RE, Dardik BN. Increased DNA replication in the arterial adventitia after aortic ligation. Hypertension 1988;11:I130–I134.

48. Kato H, Hou J, Chobanian AV, Brecher P. Effects of angiotensin II infusion and inhibition of nitric oxide synthase on the rat aorta. Hypertension 1996;28:153–158.

49. Mecham RP, Whitehouse LA, Wrenn DS, Parks WC, Griffen GL, Senior RM, et al. Smooth muscle-mediated connective tissue remodeling in pulmonary hypertension. Science 1987;237:423–426.

50. Steinhorn RH, Morin FC, Russell JA. The adentitia may be a barrier specific to nitric oxide in rabbit pulmonary artery. J Clin Invest 1994;94:1883–1888.

51. Zhu DL, Herembert T, Marche P. Increased proliferation of adventitial fibroblasts from spontaneously hypertensive rat aorta. J Hypertens 1991;9:1161–1168.

52. Venance SL, Watson MH, Wigle DA, Mak AS, Pang SC. Differential expression and activity of p34cdc2 in cultured aotic adventitial fibroblasts derived from spontaneously hypertensive and Wistar-Kyoto rats. J Hypertens 1993;11:483–489.

53. Sobey CG, Brooks RM, Heistead DD. Evidence that expression of inducible nitric oxide synthase in response to endotoxin is augmented in atherosclerotic rabbits. Circ Res 1995;77:536–543.

54. Esaki T, Hayashi T, Asai Y, Kumar TN, Kano H, Muto E, et al. Expression of inducible nitric oxide synthase in T lymphocytes and macrophages in vessels with advanced atherosclerosis. Blood Vessels 1997;12(Suppl):89–92.

55. Buttery LD, Springall DR, Chester AH, Evans TJ, Standfield EN, Parums DV, et al. Inducible nitric oxide sytnhase is present within human atherosclerotic lesions and promotes the formation and activity of peroxynitrite. Lab Invest 1996;75:77–85.

56. Luoma JS, Stralin P, Marklund SL, Hiltunen TP, Sarkioja T, Yla-Herttuala S. Expression of extracellular SOD and iNOS in macrophages and smooth muscle cells in human and rabbit atheroscerotic lesions: colocalization with epitopes characteristic of oxidized LDL and peroxynitrite-modified proteins. Arterioscler Thromb Vasc Biol 1998;18:157–167.
57. Wilcox JN, Subramanian RR, Sundell CL, Tracey WR, Pollock JS, Harrison DG, et al. Expression of multiple isoforms of nitric oxide sythase in normal and atherosclerotic vessels. Arterioscler Thromb Vasc Biol 1997;17:2479–2488.
58. Chien AF, Jiang S-W, Crotty TB, Tsutsui M, Smith LA, O'Brian T, et al. Effects of in vivo adventitial expression of recombinant endothelial nitric oxide synthase gene in cerebral arteries. Proc Natl Acad Sci USA 1997;94:12,568–12,573.
59. Cable DG, O'Brian T, Schaff HV, Pompili VJ. Recombinant endothelial nitric oxide synthase-transduced human saphenous veins: gene therapy to augment nitric oxide production in bypass conduits. Circulation 1997;96:II-173–II-178.
60. Pagano PJ, Ito H, Tornheim K, Gallop PM, Tauber AI, Cohen RA. An NADPH oxidase superoxide-generating system in the rabbit aorta. Am J Physiol 1995;268:H2274–H2280.
61. Pagano PJ, Clark JK, Cifuentes-Pagano ME, Clark SM, Callis GM, Quinn MT. Localization of a constitutively active, phagocyte-like NADPH oxidase in rabbit aortic adventitia: enhancement by angiotensin II. Proc Natl Acad Sci USA 1997;94:14,483 14,488.
62. Wang HD, Pagano PJ, Du Y, Cayatte AJ, Quinn MT, Brecher P, et al. Superoxide anion from the adventitia of the rat throacic aorta inactivates nitric oxide. Circ Res 1998;82:810–818.

12

Nitric Oxide
in Cardiac Electrophysiology

Lü Fei and Douglas P. Zipes

INTRODUCTION

Nitric oxide (NO•) has become one of the most important molecular determinants of cardiovascular physiological responses. Although its vital role in preserving vascular function is well established, the impact of NO• on cardiac electrophysiology is less widely appreciated. This chapter summarizes current knowledge in this area.

EFFECTS OF NO• ON CELLULAR
ELECTROPHYSIOLOGICAL RESPONSES

Several studies have evaluated the role of NO• in modulating β-adrenergic effects on calcium currents in isolated cardiac cells (1–5). Although it had no significant effects on basal calcium currents in frog and guinea-pig ventricular myocytes (1,4), NO• manifests biphasic effects on the enhanced calcium currents stimulated by isoproterenol and other agents (such as cyclic adenosine monophosphate [cAMP] or forskolin) (1). At high concentrations (100 nM– 1 mM), the NO• donor 3-morpholino-syndnonimine (SIN-1) significantly reduced the isoproterenol-induced increase in calcium currents (by up to 85%) (Fig. 1). In contrast, at lower concentrations (0.1–10 nM) SIN-1 enhanced (by approx 40%) the isoproterenol-induced increase in calcium currents. These actions of SIN-1 on calcium currents seem to result from an inhibition of cGMP-dependent protein kinase via the NO•-guanylyl cyclase pathway (1,4). Because SIN-1 generates NO• and O^{2-}, both indirect (cGMP-dependent) and direct (oxidation) effects of SIN-1 play an important role in the regulation of ventricular calcium currents (6). There is evidence that cardiac ion channels can differentiate nitrosative from oxidative signals (7). NO• and related molecules can inhibit the L-type calcium channel via cyclic guanosine monophosphate (cGMP); on the other hand, they sensitize the muscle to Ca^{2+}-induced Ca^{2+} release by chemical modifications of thiols (7). Pacing-induced changes in electrophysiological responses may partially be produced through the regulation of a constitutive nitric oxide synthase (NOS) in rat ventricular myocytes (8).

In guinea-pig ventricular myocytes, interleukin-1β significantly decreased the β-adrenergic response of calcium currents to isoproterenol (3). The role of NO• in the modulation of the chronotropic effects of cytokines has been questioned (9). NO• significantly inhibited calcium currents in a manner similar to intracellular cGMP analogs in human coronary myocytes (10), which may relate to the therapeutic effects of nitrovasodilators. There is evidence that NO• directly activates calcium-dependent potassium channels in rabbit aortic smooth muscle

From: *Contemporary Cardiology, vol. 4: Nitric Oxide and the Cardiovascular System*
Edited by: J. Loscalzo and J. A. Vita © Humana Press Inc., Totowa, NJ

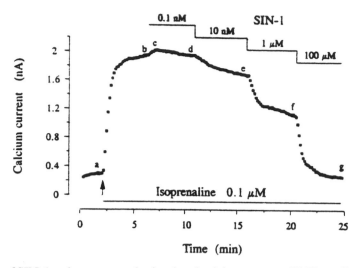

Fig, 1. Effects of SIN-1 on isoproterenol-stimulated calcium current *(1)*. The cell was successively exposed to 0.1 μM isoproterenol, and to successively increasing concentrations of SIN-1 (0.1 n*M*, 10 n*M*, 1 μ*M*, and 100 μ*M*). Reproduced with permission from the American Society for Biochemistry and Molecular Biology.

(11), independent of guanylyl cyclase activity. The inhomogeneity in the distribution of potassium channels in pulmonary arterial smooth muscle cells might account for their differential reactions to NO•. However, little is known about the effects of NO• on cardiac potassium currents in myocardial and nodal cells, and on the specific conduction system in the heart.

Chen and colleagues *(12)* have demonstrated that NO• plays an important role in modulating calcium-dependent neurotransmission in sympathetic neurons. Intracellular application of NO• donors such as sodium nitroprusside increased calcium currents and reduced norepinephrine-induced inhibition of calcium currents in rat superior cervical ganglionic neurons. This mechanism may be operative in NO•-induced autonomic actions that regulate its cardiac electrophysiological effects *(13)*.

EFFECTS OF NO• ON SINUS NODE FUNCTION

NO• plays an important role in the cholinergic inhibition of L-type calcium currents in rabbit sinus nodal cells. Carbamoylcholine significantly inhibited calcium currents enhanced by isoproterenol, and activated outward potassium currents *(2)*. Inhibition of NOS abolished the inhibitory effects of carbamoylcholine on calcium currents but had no significant effect on the activation by carbamoylcholine of potassium currents. L-arginine reversed these effects induced by the NOS inhibitor. The NO• donor SIN-1 inhibited the augmented calcium currents by isoproterenol, which was prevented by maximal carbamoylcholine. There is also evidence that NO• may not be important in the negative chronotropic effects of endothelin in the presence of isoproterenol *(14)*.

Recently, we demonstrated that NO• plays an important role in the autonomic modulation of the sinus rate in α-chloralose-anesthesized, autonomically denervated, open-chest dogs *(15)*. Injection of L-arginine or a NOS inhibitor, N^G-monomethyl-L-arginine (L-NMMA), into the sinus nodal artery caused no significant effects on sinus cycle length. However, L-NMMA significantly attenuated the lengthening of sinus cycle length induced by vagal stimulation, which was reversed toward baseline after administration of L-arginine. The effects of L-NMMA increased with greater vagal effects on sinus cycle length. L-NMMA also augmented isoproterenol- or sympathetic stimulation-induced sinus cycle length shortening, which was abolished by L-arginine (Fig. 2), but not by D-arginine. Similar results were observed during

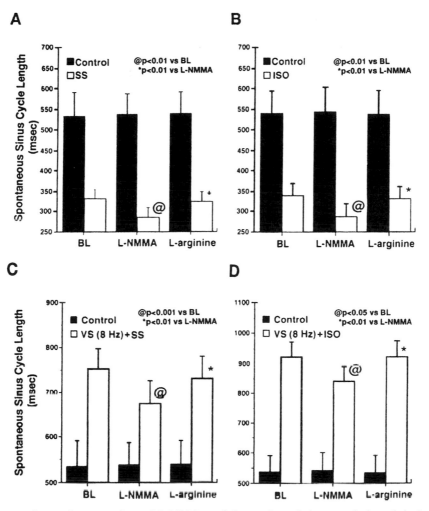

Fig. 2. Comparison of extent of vagal inhibition of shortening of sinus cycle length induced by sympathetic stimulation (**A**) or isoproterenol (Iso) infusion (**B**) during baseline (BL), L-NMMA infusion into sinus node artery, and after injection of L-arginine. Comparison of extent of vagal modulation of sympathetic shortening of sinus cycle length induced by sympathetic (VS + SS; C) or isoproterenol infusion (VS + Iso; D) during saline baseline, L-NMMA infusion into sinus node artery, and after intravenous administration of L-arginine *(13)*. Reproduced with permission from the American Physiological Society.

simultaneous sympathetic and vagal stimulation. NO• had no significant effect on acetylcholine-induced lengthening in sinus cycle length, suggesting that NO• may not have significant direct postjunctional vagal actions. Neither L-NMMA nor L-arginine altered sinus cycle length at baseline or during vagal stimulation at a high stimulation frequency (8 Hz). Data from this study suggested that NO• plays a stimulatory role in mediating vagal neurotransmission and vagal modulation of sympathetic effects and an inhibitory role in mediating sympathetic neurotransmission *(15)*.

There is evidence that nitrinergic neural function plays an important role in reflex regulation of the heart rate and blood pressure *(16)*. Several studies *(17–20)* have demonstrated that NO• may affect autonomic control of the heart rate through the baroreflex, although this hypothesis has been questioned *(21)* and other mechanisms may be more important *(22–24)*. Inhibition of NOS by L-NAME did not impair the function of either the afferent or efferent limbs of the baroreflex in rats *(25)*, whereas blockade of neural nitric oxide synthase signifi-cantly altered the baroreflex control of heart rate in rabbits *(20)*. In conscious rats, oral N^G-nitro-L-arginine methyl ester (L-NAME, 50 mg/kg/d) administered for 4 wk significantly decreased the gain of the baroreflex *(17)*. In contrast, Minami and colleagues *(18)* demon-strated that intravenous injection of L-NAME (10 mg/kg) enhanced the gain of the baroreflex in conscious rats. Interestingly, although L-NMMA, but not L-arginine, infusion increased mean blood pressure and decreased heart rate, neither of them significantly changed the relationship between heart rate response and mean blood pressure in rabbits *(26)*. Widdop and colleagues *(27)* reported that L-NAME (10 mg/kg, iv) caused a significant increase in mean blood pressure and a decrease in heart rate in conscious rats, which was reversed by atropine. At a higher dose (50–100 mg, iv), L-NAME significantly reduced the bradycardia induced by vagal stimulation after β-blockade by propranolol in the anesthetized ferret *(28)*.

Scrogin and colleagues *(29)* reported that 1-wk treatment with L-NAME significantly depressed the baroreflex (–3.5 vs control –5.7 beats/min/mmHg) without significant changes in resting plasma catecholamine concentrations in rats. This resulted in a significant decrease in heart rate (16% reduction) and an increase in blood pressure. In contrast, Cunha and colleagues *(30)* have shown that L-NAME significantly increased both blood pressure and heart rate (28% increase). This difference in the response of heart rate to L-NAME may be explained by different doses used and biphasic responses *(29)*. On the other hand, Kennedy and colleagues *(31)* reported that NO• did not have a significant chronotropic action in isolated rat atrial preparation. In their study, NOS inhibitors did not alter the chronotropic effects of acetylcholine or norepinephrine. Methylene blue, which inhibits NO• activation of guanylyl cyclase, did not antagonize the SIN-1 (>300 µmol)-induced negative chronotropic action. Further studies are warranted to define the role of NO• in the modulation of the heart rate.

It is well known that sodium nitroprusside-induced hypotension may be responsible for the drug-related tachycardia mediated by the baroreflex. However, sodium nitroprusside can also increase heart rate in patients following heart transplantation *(32)*. Therefore, mecha-nisms other than the baroreflex may contribute to this effect. For example, intracoronary injection of a low dose of sodium nitroprusside, which has been reported to generate NO• intracellularly *(33)*, has been shown to increase the heart rate without significant changes in blood pressure *(34)*. In a similar study, 50-fold higher doses of sodium nitroprusside caused a slight reduction in heart rate *(35)*. In isolated perfused hearts, a low concentration of sodium nitroprusside (10 µmol/L) caused a 20% increase in beating rate *(36)*. Pharmacological blockade of NOS reduced beating rate by 15% *(36)*. In isolated sinus nodal–atrial preparations, Musialek and colleagues *(37)* demonstrated a biphasic response of the beating rate to NO• donors (sodium nitroprusside or SIN-1). A low concentration of NO• donors gradually increased the beating rate, whereas high concentrations decreased it. Calcium blockade using nifedipine had no significant effect on NO• donor-induced changes in beating rate, whereas blockade of the hyperpolarization-activated inward current (I_f) using CsCl abolished this effect of NO•. These authors have also shown that superoxide dismutase, guanylyl cyclase, and cGMP were involved in these NO•-mediated actions. They concluded that tachycardia associated with myocardial production of NO• was caused by stimulation of I_f via a NO•–cGMP pathway. However, this hypothesis has recently been questioned *(19)*.

In addition to alteration in the baroreflex, L-NAME also causes a marked enhancement of the Bezold-Jarish reflex (a decrease in heart rate accompanied by a decrease in diastolic arterial pressure) because of the hyperresponsiveness of the cardiac pacemaker to cholin-ergic stimulation *(38)*.

Human studies on NO•-mediated effects on heart rate are scarce and less conclusive. Intravenous L-NMMA-induced changes in heart rate were associated with changes in blood pressure in humans *(39)*, which was similar to that induced by phenylephrine. Intravenous infusion of L-arginine caused a significant tachycardia associated with decreased blood pressure and increased cardiac output in healthy volunteers *(40,41)*. This effect was accompanied by increased urinary output of nitrite/nitrate *(40)*.

There have been no reports on the actions of NO˙ on atrial arrhythmias. A decreased plasma NO˙ level may contribute to the hemostatic abnormalities in patients with atrial fibrillation *(42)*, thus implicating the therapeutic value of NO˙ in atrial fibrillation *(43)*.

EFFECTS OF NO˙ ON ATRIOVENTRICULAR NODE FUNCTION

Using immunohistochemical staining, Han and colleagues *(5)* identified the presence of the endothelial constitutive NOS in both single-rabbit atrioventricular nodal cells and in cryostat sections of atrioventricular nodal tissue. In isolated atrioventricular nodal cells, their investigation demonstrated that the NO˙ donor SIN-1 significantly suppressed isoproterenol-induced increases in calcium currents and decreased the frequency and amplitude of spontaneous action potentials in single atrioventricular nodal cells *(5)*. SIN-1 had no additional effects on calcium currents when currents were attenuated by carbamoylcholine. Han et al. showed that changes in calcium currents resulted from effects of the NO˙–cGMP pathway. From the same study *(5)*, they also showed that blockade of the NO˙ pathway had no effects on carbamoylcholine-activated potassium currents. These NO˙-induced changes on cellular electrophysiology may be responsible for the observations that NO˙ is involved in the autonomic modulation of atrioventricular nodal conduction in intact animals *(15)*.

In autonomically denervated dogs, we *(15)* demonstrated that infusion of L-NMMA into the coronary artery supplying the atrioventricular nodal region reduced vagal stimulation-induced atrial-His (A-H) interval prolongation. L-arginine reduced this effect of L-NMMA toward baseline. Neither L-NMMA nor L-arginine had significant effect on the A-H interval at baseline without vagal stimulation. Shortening of the A-H interval produced by isoproterenol or by sympathetic stimulation was enhanced by L-NMMA; again, L-arginine blunted the effects of L-NMMA. L-NMMA significantly decreased the vagal modulation of sympathetic effects on the atrioventricular (AV) interval and L-arginine reversed this effect toward baseline. Similar to results on sinus cycle length, neither L-NMMA nor L-arginine had significant effects on acetylcholine-induced prolongation in the AV interval. A significant effect of NO˙ on vagal modulation of sympathetic effects on the AV interval was noted. These observations suggest that NO˙ is involved in the autonomic regulation of AV nodal conduction by decreasing the positive dromotropic effects of sympathetic stimulation and increasing vagal modulation of these sympathetic actions *(15)*.

EFFECTS OF NO˙ ON VENTRICULAR ELECTROPHYSIOLOGY

The biphasic effects of NO˙ on β-adrenergic enhancement of calcium currents was discussed at the beginning of this chapter. In rat ventricular myocytes, Balligand and colleagues *(44)* reported that NO˙ plays an important role in the carbachol-induced inhibition of spontaneous beating rate. Inhibition of the NO˙ pathway using a NO˙/guanylyl cyclase inhibitor, methylene blue, or a NOS inhibitor, N^G-monomethyl-L-arginine, blocked the negative chronotropic effects of carbachol. Adding excessive L-arginine reversed the inhibition of the N^G-monomethyl-L-arginine-induced reduction of the negative chronotropic effects of carbachol. Similar to its action on calcium currents, NO˙ had no significant effects on basal beating rate. In the same study *(44)*, NO˙ was shown to be in involved in the modulation of isoproterenol-induced change in contractility. No data were presented on the effects of NO˙ on isoproterenol-induced chronotropic actions.

NO˙ has also been shown to modulate autonomic effects on cardiac contractility *(45)* and sinus and AV nodal electrophysiology in vivo *(15)*. Data on the role of NO˙ in the modulation of ventricular electrophysiology in intact animals are scarce. Because NOS is present in cardiac nerve fibers and neurons and in the ventricular myocardium *(46,47)*, it is quite

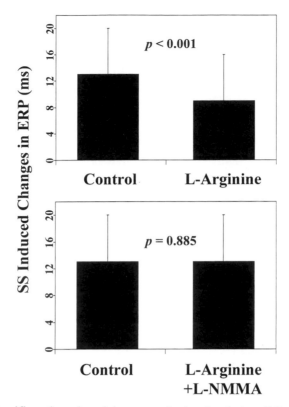

Fig. 3. L-Arginine significantly reduced the sympathetic stimulation (SS)-induced shortening in ventricular effective refractory periods (ERP) (**top**), but simultaneous superfusion of both L-arginine and L-NMMA revealed no significant difference in sympathetic stimulation induced shortening in ventricular ERPs compared with control (**bottom**) *(11)*. Reproduced with permission from the American Heart Association.

possible that NO˙ is also involved in the autonomic modulation of ventricular electrophysiology. This hypothesis, if true, will be clinically important because substantial evidence indicates that heightened sympathetic activity can increase the prevalence and severity of life-threatening ventricular arrhythmias both in animals and in humans. We conducted a study in autonomically denervated dogs to test this hypothesis and to determine a potential mechanism by investigating the impact of NO˙ on norepinephrine release from cardiac sympathetic nerves *(13)*. Cardiac sympathetic nerves were superfused *(48–50)* by introducing normal Tyrode's solution (approx 40–80 mL) containing either L-arginine or L-arginine and L-NMMA. Ventricular effective refractory periods were measured in the presence of pericardial superfusion with L-arginine or L-arginine and L-NMMA before and during sympathetic stimulation. In the baseline state without sympathetic stimulation, pericardial superfusion with L-arginine had no significant effect on ventricular effective refractory period; however, it significantly decreased sympathetic stimulation-induced shortening of ventricular effective refractory periods by 31% ($p < 0.001$), an effect abolished by L-NMMA (Fig. 3).

In another group of animals, ischemic ventricular arrhythmias were induced by repeated 7-min occlusions of the left anterior descending coronary artery between the first and second diagonal branches during constant atrial pacing at a rate of 150 beats/min. The first coronary artery occlusion was performed 30 min after normal Tyrode's solution was infused into the pericardial sac. Because intramyocardial conduction delay and ventricular arrhythmias were usually more exaggerated during the first occlusion than subsequent ones *(49)*, possibly owing to preconditioning mechanisms *(51)*, results from this first occlusion were discarded

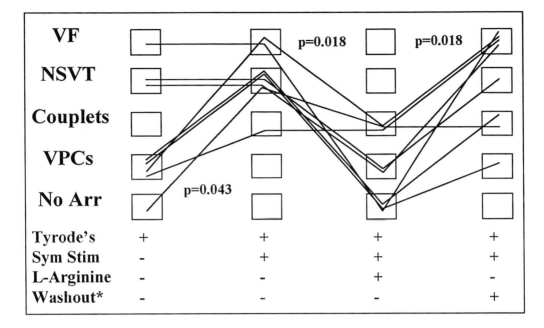

Fig. 4. In this study *(11)*, ventricular arrhythmias were classified into five categories of increasing severity: (1) no ventricular arrhythmias, (2) isolated ventricular ectopic beats, (3) couplets, (4) nonsustained ventricular tachycardia (≥3 consecutive beats but <15 s), and (5) ventricular fibrillation. The highest category of ventricular arrhythmias was scored for each occlusion. The severity of ventricular arrhythmia significantly increased during sympathetic stimulation. L-Arginine significantly reduced this increase caused by sympathetic stimulation (*p* = 0.018). There was no significant difference in the severity of ventricular arrhythmia after washout of L-arginine using normal Tyrode's solution compared to that before pericardial superfusion with L-arginine. Reproduced with permission from the American Heart Association.

and the second occlusion was used as a control. The second coronary occlusion was performed 15 min after the first occlusion. The third occlusion was performed 15 min later in the presence of sympathetic stimulation. Thereafter, the Tyrode's solution containing L-arginine was infused into the pericardial sac to replace the normal Tyrode's solution and the fourth coronary artery occlusion was performed. The fifth coronary artery occlusion was performed after superfusion with normal Tyrode's solution for 30 min (washout). Both the fourth and the fifth coronary occlusions were performed in the presence of sympathetic stimulation. Consistent with previous observations, we found that sympathetic stimulation significantly increased the severity of ventricular arrhythmias during coronary artery occlusion. L-arginine significantly reduced this increase caused by sympathetic stimulation (Fig. 4).

In this study *(13)*, we also measured NO• production and norepinephrine release in the heart. Five-milliliter samples of coronary sinus blood were obtained during pericardial superfusion with (1) Tyrode's solution, (2) Tyrode's solution and L-arginine, and (3) washout with Tyrode's solution after atrial pacing at 150 beats/min for 3 min. These samples were again obtained during sympathetic stimulation for 3 min. The concentration of norepinephrine in coronary sinus blood reached a steady state within 1 min of sympathetic stimulation in normal dog hearts *(52)*. Norepinephrine or NO• spillover (overflow) was defined as the product of norepinephrine or NO• concentration, respectively, and blood flow from the coronary sinus. We found that pericardial superfusion of the heart with L-arginine significantly increased NO• production in the heart in this experimental preparation. We also demonstrated that L-arginine significantly decreased norepinephrine release from sympathetic nerves in the heart, which is consistent with the findings in the study by Schwarz and colleagues *(53)*. This reduction in norepinephrine release in the heart may be at least in part responsible for the effects of NO• on cardiac electrophysiology observed in this study.

In isolated perfused heart preparations, Pabla and Curtis *(54)* showed a role of NO• in protection against reperfusion-induced ventricular fibrillation in rats and rabbits. They found that a neuronal nitric oxide synthase (nNOS) inhibitor 7-nitro-indazole increased the incidence of ventricular fibrillation from 0–60% ($p < 0.05$). Simultaneous perfusion of L-arginine reduced the incidence of ventricular fibrillation to 20%. The nonselective NOS inhibitor L-NMMA increased ventricular fibrillation incidence from 0–50% ($p < 0.05$). These authors proposed that enhanced production of NO• was cardioprotective in this animal model by virtue of its ability to scavenge free radicals.

Thus, current data *(13,54)* indicate that NO• is involved in the modulation of autonomic action on cardiac electrophysiology and may protect against both ischemic and reperfusion arrhythmias.

EFFECTS OF NO• ON AUTONOMIC
NERVOUS SYSTEM ACTIVITY IN CONGESTIVE HEART FAILURE

NO• production has been shown to be altered in congestive heart failure (CHF) *(55)*. It has been shown that increased NO• production in CHF did not alter basal sarcomere mechanics, but did attenuate the positive inotropic response to isoproterenol *(55)*. This type of effect may also be manifest in the regulation of autonomic effects on cardiac electrophysiology in the presence of CHF.

There is a significant autonomic disturbance with a sympathetic predominance in patients with CHF. Modification of this sympathovagal imbalance may be beneficial. NO•-induced vasodilation and modulation of autonomic action of cardiac mechanical and electrophysiological activities may have important therapeutic potential. Intravenous infusion of L-arginine in patients with moderate CHF resulted in an increase in NO• production and in cardiac output without a significant change in heart rate *(56)*. Rector and colleagues *(57)* reported that supplemental oral L-arginine had a significant beneficial effect in these patients. Compared with placebo, L-arginine significantly improved functional status as indicated by increased walking distance during a 6-min walk test in addition to a significant increase in forearm blood flow during forearm exercise.

We have conducted a preliminary randomized, double-blind, placebo-controlled, cross-over study to investigate whether supplemental oral L-arginine has beneficial effects on autonomic imbalance and impaired left ventricular function in patients with CHF. Preliminary results (unpublished data) indicate that L-arginine (4 g three times per day for 4 wk) did not cause significant changes in left ventricular ejection fraction, the scores on a CHF questionnaire *(58)*, or short- (10 min during supine position) and long-term (24 h) heart rate variability. These findings are consistent with the observation that intracoronary injection of L-NMMA had no significant effect on heart rate in patients with left ventricular dysfunction (left ventricular ejection fraction 21 ± 3%) *(59)*. In a study in conscious rats, blood pressure variability has been shown to be significantly increased following intravenous injection of L-NAME *(60)*. Thus, the therapeutic value of NO• remains to be determined in the presence of CHF.

POTENTIAL MECHANISMS UNDERLYING
THE EFFECTS OF NO• ON CARDIAC ELECTROPHYSIOLOGY

The exact mechanisms responsible for the foregoing effects of NO• are unclear. NO• can modulate autonomic actions on cardiac electrophysiology either centrally or peripherally *(22–25)*. It has been reported that NO• plays an important role in the modulation of autonomic actions in the nucleus tractus solitarius *(61)*, in the rostral and caudal ventrolateral medulla *(62)*, in the hypothalamus *(63)*, and in the paraventricular nucleus *(64)*. NOS has been shown to be present extensively in the medullary neurons including the nucleus tractus solitarius *(65)*. Intravenous infusion of L-NAME has been shown to decrease the activity of baroreceptor-sensitive neurons in the nucleus of the solitary tract, whereas L-arginine infusion reversed this effect *(66)*. Microinjection of NO° donor or inhibitors into the paraventricular nucleus in rats caused a significant decrease or increase, respectively, in heart rate *(64)*. Similarly, the sympathoexcitatory effects of glutamate (such as an increase in heart rate) were potentiated by inhibition of nNOS in the brain *(67)*. However, intravenous L-NMMA had no significant effect on sympathetic activity in humans *(39)*. A redox-based mechanism involving NMDA (*N*-methyl-D-aspartate) receptor has been proposed for the neuroprotective and neurodestructive effects of NO° in the central nervous system *(68)*. However, the importance of the NMDA receptor in the regulation of the autonomic effects of NO° on cardiac electrophysiological responses is not known.

The potential peripheral sites of NO°-mediated actions may be ventricular myocytes, cardiac neurons, or both. Horackova and colleagues *(69)* reported that NO° did not affect cultured adult guinea-pig myocytes directly. The beating rate of such myocytes could be indirectly affected when they were cultured with intrinsic or stellate ganglia neurons. Considering that there was a significant L-arginine-mediated effect on ventricular effective refractory periods during sympathetic stimulation, whereas there was no significant change without sympathetic stimulation in totally denervated hearts *(13)*, a likely locus of the effects of NO° is the signaling between cardiac neurons and ventricular myocardium. This is consistent with the finding in the study of Horackova and colleagues *(69)* that the effect of NO° on the beating rates of ventricular myocytes depended on neuronal activation. Several investigators *(70–73)* reported that nonadrenergic and noncholinergic actions may be involved in certain physiological responses to NO°. The findings *(13,53)* that NO° reduced cardiac norepinephrine release in response to sympathetic stimulation makes nonadrenergic and noncholinergic actions of NO° less important in the NO°-mediated autonomic modulation of ventricular electrophysiology. There is also evidence that alkyl esters of L-arginine can function as muscarinic antagonists *(74)*. Thus, the modulation of autonomic action on cardiac electrophysiology by NO° is multifactorial.

SUMMARY

NOS has been shown to exist in the central cardiovascular regulatory centers; cardiac ganglion cells, and nerve fibers innervating the sinus and atrioventricular nodes, the myocardium, local neurons, and coronary arteries *(46)*, implicating their potential importance in the modulation of cardiovascular electrophysiology. However, data on NO°-mediated effects on cardiac electrophysiology are scarce and inconclusive. It is our current understanding that NO° has minimal actions on cardiac electrophysiological responses in a basal state without distinct autonomic stimulation. However, NO° has significant effects on chronotropic and dromotropic responses to autonomic stimulation. Several studies have shown that NO° is involved in the baroreflex control of heart rate. NO° seems to reduce norepinephrine release in the heart during sympathetic stimulation and may have significant protective effects against the development of ventricular arrhythmias during ischemia and reperfusion. Whether NO° has therapeutic action in CHF is uncertain. NO° exerts its effects by modulating autonomic effects on cardiac electrophysiology either centrally or peripherally. Its effects are generally thought to be associated with activation of guanylyl cyclase and subsequent formation of guanosine 3', 5'-cyclic monophosphate, at least at the cellular level, however, other mechanisms may also be involved and include direct effects on specific ion channels and neuronal receptors that modulate ion channel activity.

ACKNOWLEDGMENT

This work is supported by the Herman C. Krannert Fund and by grant HL-52323 from the National Heart, Lung and Blood Institute of Health.

REFERENCES

1. Méry PF, Pavoine C, Belhassen L, Pecker F, Fischmeister R. Nitric oxide regulates cardiac Ca^{2+} current. Involvement of cGMP-inhibited and cGMP-stimulated phosphodiesterases through guanylyl cyclase activation. J Biol Chem 1993;268:26,286–26,295.
2. Han X, Shimoni Y, Giles WR. An obligatory role for nitric oxide in autonomic control of mammalian heart rate. J Physiol 1994;476:309–314.
3. Rozanski GJ, Witt RC. IL-1 inhibits beta-adrenergic control of cardiac calcium current: role of L-arginine/nitric oxide pathway. Am J Physiol 1994;267:H1753–H1758.
4. Wahler GM, Dollinger SJ. Nitric oxide donor SIN-1 inhibits mammalian cardiac calcium current through cGMP-dependent protein kinase. Am J Physiol 1995;268:C45–C54.
5. Han X, Kobzik L, Zhao YY, Opel DJ, Liu WD, Kelly RA, et al. Nitric oxide regulation of atrioventricular node excitability. Can J Cardiol 1997;13:1191–1201.
6. Campbell DL, Stamler JS, Strauss HC. Redox modulation of L-type calcium channels in ferret ventricular myocytes. Dual mechanism regulation by nitric oxide and S-nitrosothiols. J Gen Physiol 1996;108: 277–293.
7. Xu L, Eu JP, Meissner G, Stamler JS. Activation of the cardiac calcium release channel (ryanodine receptor) by poly-S-nitrosylation. Science 1998;279:234–237.
8. Kaye DM, Wiviott SD, Balligand JL, Simmons WW, Smith TW, Kelly RA. Frequency-dependent activation of a constitutive nitric oxide synthase and regulation of contractile function in adult rat ventricular myocytes. Circ Res 1996;78:217–224.
9. Oddis CV, Simmons RL, Hattler BG, Finkel MS. Chronotropic effects of cytokines and the nitric oxide synthase inhibitor, L-NMMA, on cardiac myocytes. Biochem Biophys Res Commun 1994;205:992–997.
10. Quignard JF, Frapier JM, Harricane MC, Albat B, Nargeot J, Richard S. Voltage-gated calcium channel currents in human coronary myocytes. Regulation by cyclic GMP and nitric oxide. J Clin Invest 1997;99: 185–193.
11. Bolotina VM, Najibi S, Palacino JJ, Pagano PJ, Cohen RA. Nitric oxide directly activates calcium-dependent potassium channels in vascular smooth muscle. Nature 1994;368:850–853.
12. Chen C, Schofield GG. Nitric oxide modulates Ca^{2+} channel currents in rat sympathetic neurons. Eur J Pharmacol 1993;243:83–86.
13. Fei L, Baron AD, Henry DP, Zipes DP. Intrapericardial delivery of L-arginine reduces the increased severity of ventricular arrhythmias during sympathetic stimulation in dogs with acute coronary occlusion: nitric oxide modulates sympathetic effects on ventricular electrophysiological properties. Circulation 1997;96:4044–4049.
14. Zhu Y, Yang HT, Endoh M. Does nitric oxide contribute to the negative chronotropic and inotropic effects of endothelin-1 in the heart? Eur J Pharmacol 1997;332:195–199.
15. Elvan A, Rubart M, Zipes DP. Nitric oxide modulates autonomic effects on sinus discharge rate and AV nodal conduction in open chest dogs. Am J Physiol 1997;272:H263–H271.
16. Toda N, Kitamura Y, Okamura T. Neural mechanism of hypertension by nitric oxide synthase inhibitor in dogs. Hypertension 1993;21:3–8.
17. Lantelme P, Lo M, Sassard J. Decreased cardiac baroreflex sensitivity is not due to cardiac hypertrophy in N^G-nitro-L-arginine methyl ester-induced hypertension. J Hypertens 1994;12:791–795.
18. Minami N, Imai Y, Hashimoto J, Abe K. The role of nitric oxide in the baroreceptor-cardiac reflex in conscious Wistar rats. Am J Physiol 1995;269:H851–H855.
19. Matsuda T, Bates JN, Lewis SJ, Abboud FM, Chapleau MW. Modulation of baroreceptor activity by nitric oxide and S-nitrosocysteine. Circ Res 1995;76:426–433.
20. Murakami H, Liu JL, Yoneyama H, Nishida Y, Okada K, Kosaka H, et al. Blockade of neuronal nitric oxide synthase alters the baroreflex control of heart rate in the rabbit. Am J Physiol 1998;274:R181–R186.
21. Miyano H, Kawada T, Sugimachi M, Shishido T, Sato T, Alexander J Jr, et al. Inhibition of NO synthesis does not potentiate dynamic cardiovascular response to sympathetic nerve activity. Am J Physiol 1997; 273:H38–H43.
22. Sakuma I, Togashi H, Yoshioka M, Saito H, Yanagida M, Tamura M, et al. NG-methyl-L-arginine, an inhibitor of L-arginine-derived nitric oxide synthesis, stimulates renal sympathetic nerve activity

in vivo. A role for nitric oxide in the central regulation of sympathetic tone? Circ Res 1992;70: 607–611.

23. Togashi H, Sakuma I, Yoshioka M, Kobayashi T, Yasuda H, Kitabatake A, et al. A central nervous system action of nitric oxide in blood pressure regulation. J Pharmacol Exp Ther 1992;262:343–347.

24. Lo WC, Lin HC, Ger LP, Tung CS, Tseng CJ. Cardiovascular effects of nitric oxide and N-methyl-D-aspartate receptors in the nucleus tractus solitarii of rats. Hypertension 1997;30:1499–1503.

25. Habler HJ, Wasner G, Bartsch T, Janig W. Responses of rat postganglionic sympathetic vasoconstrictor neurons following blockade of nitric oxide synthesis in vivo. Neuroscience 1997;77:899–909.

26. Jimbo M, Suzuki H, Ichikawa M, Kumagai K, Nishizawa M, Saruta T. Role of nitric oxide in regulation of baroreceptor reflex. J Auton Nerv Syst 1994;50:209–219.

27. Widdop RE, Gardiner SM, Kemp PA, Bennett T. The influence of atropine and atenolol on the cardiac haemodynamic effects of N^G-nitro-L-arginine methyl ester in conscious, Long Evans rats. Br J Pharmacol 1992;105:653–656.

28. Conlon K, Collins T, Kidd C. Modulation of vagal actions on heart rate produced by inhibition of nitric oxide synthase in the anaesthetized ferret. Exp Physiol 1996;81:547–550.

29. Scrogin KE, Hatton DC, Chi Y, Lutt FC. Chronic nitric oxide inhibition with L NAME: effects on autonomic control of the cardiovascular system. Am J Physiol 1998;274:R367–R374.

30. Cunha RS, Cabral AM, Vasquez, EC. Evidence that the autonomic nervous system plays a major role in the L-NAME-induced hypertension in conscious rats. Am J Hypertens 1993;6:806–809.

31. Kennedy RH, Hicks KK, Brian JE Jr, Seifen E. Nitric oxide has no chronotropic effect in right atria isolated from rat heart. Eur J Pharmacol 1994;255:149–156.

32. Levine TB, Olivari MT, Cohen JN. Effects of orthotopic heart transplantation on sympathetic control mechanisms in congestive heart failure. Am J Cardiol 1986;58:1035–1040.

33. Fung HL, Kowaluk EA, Chung SJ, Jhun BH, Seth P. Nitric oxide generation from nitrovasodilators in coronary artery smooth muscle cells is mediated by multiple enzymes. In: Moncada S, Marletta MA, Hibbs JB Jr, Higgs EA, eds. The Biology of Nitric Oxide: Physiological and Clinical Aspects. Portland Press, London, UK, 1992, pp. 139–141.

34. Crystal GJ, Gurevicius J. Nitric oxide does not modulate myocardial contractility acutely in in situ canine hearts. Am J Physiol 1996;270:H1568–H1576.

35. Paulus WJ, Vantrimpont PJ, Shah AM. Acute effects of nitric oxide on left ventricular relaxation and diastolic distensibility in humans. Assessment by bicoronary sodium nitroprusside infusion. Circulation 1994;89:2070–2078.

36. Pabla R, Curtis MJ. Effects of NO modulation on cardiac arrhythmias in the rat isolated heart. Circ Res 1995;77:984 992.

37. Musialek P, Lei M, Brown HF, Paterson DJ, Casadei B. Nitric oxide can increase heart rate by stimulating the hyperpolarization-activated inward current, I(f). Circ Res 1997;81:60–68.

38. Araujo MT, Barker LA, Cabral AM, Vasquez, EC. Inhibition of nitric oxide synthase causes profound enhancement of the Bezold-Jarisch reflex. Am J Hypertens 1998;11:66–72.

39. Hansen J, Jacobsen TN, Victor RG. Is nitric oxide involved in the tonic inhibition of central sympathetic outflow in humans? Hypertension 1994;24:439–444.

40. Hishikawa K, Nakaki T, Tsuda M, Esumi H, Ohshima H, Suzuki H, et al. Effect of systemic L-arginine administration on hemodynamics and nitric oxide release in man. Jpn Heart J 1992;33:41–48.

41. Nakaki T, Hishikawa K, Suzuki H, Saruta T, Kato R. L-arginine-induced hypotension. Lancet 1990; 336:696.

42. Minamino T, Kitakaze M, Sato H, Asanuma H, Funaya H, Koretsune Y, et al. Plasma levels of nitrite/nitrate and platelet cGMP levels are decreased in patients with atrial fibrillation. Arterioscler Thromb Vasc Biol 1997;17:3191–3195.

43. Loscalzo J, Welch G. Nitric oxide and its role in the cardiovascular system. Prog Cardiovasc Dis 1995; 38:87–104.

44. Balligand JL, Kelly RA, Marsden PA, Smith TW, Michel T. Control of cardiac muscle cell function by an endogenous nitric oxide signaling system. Proc Natl Acad Sci USA 1993;90:347–351.

45. Hare JM, Keaney JF Jr, Balligand JL, Loscalzo J, Smith TW, Colucci WS. Role of nitric oxide in parasympathetic modulation of beta-adrenergic myocardial contractility in normal dogs. J Clin Invest 1995;95:360–366.

46. Klimaschewski L, Kummer W, Mayer B, Couraud JY, Preissler U, Philippin B, et al. Nitric oxide synthase in cardiac nerve fibers and neurons of rat and guinea pig heart. Circ Res 1992;71:1533–1537.

47. Schulz, R, Nava E, Moncada S. Induction and potential biological relevance of a Ca^{2+}-independent nitric oxide synthase in the myocardium. Br J Pharmacol 1992;105:575–580.

48. Miyazaki T, Pride HP, Zipes DP. Modulation of cardiac autonomic neurotransmission by epicardial superfusion. Effects of hexamethonium and tetrodotoxin. Circ Res 1989;65:1212–1219.

49. Miyazaki T, Zipes DP. Pericardial prostaglandin biosynthesis prevents the increased incidence of reperfusion-induced ventricular fibrillation produced by efferent sympathetic stimulation in dogs. Circulation 1990;82:1008–1019.

50. Miyazaki T, Pride HP, Zipes DP. Prostaglandins in the pericardial fluid modulate neural regulation of cardiac electrophysiological properties. Circ Res 1990;66:163–175.

51. Miyazaki T, Zipes DP. Protection against autonomic denervation following acute myocardial infarction by preconditioning ischemia. Circ Res 1989;64:437–448.

52. Masuda Y, Levy MN. Heart rate modulates the disposition of neurally released norepinephrine in cardiac tissues. Circ Res 1985;57:19–27.

53. Schwarz, P, Diem R, Dun NJ, Forstermann U. Endogenous and exogenous nitric oxide inhibits norepinephrine release from rat heart sympathetic nerves. Circ Res 1995;77:841–848.

54. Pabla R, Curtis MJ. Endogenous protection against reperfusion-induced ventricular fibrillation: role of neuronal versus non-neuronal sources of nitric oxide and species dependence in the rat versus rabbit isolated heart. J Mol Cell Cardiol 1996;28:2097–2110.

55. Yamamoto S, Tsutsui H, Tagawa H, Saito K, Takahashi M, Tada H, et al. Role of myocyte nitric oxide in beta-adrenergic hyporesponsiveness in heart failure. Circulation 1997;95:1111–1114.

56. Koifman B, Wollman Y, Bogomolny N, Chernichowsky T, Finkelstein A, Peer G, et al. Improvement of caridac performance by intravenous infusion of L-arginine in patients with moderate congestive heart failure. Am J Coll Cardiol 1995;26:1251–1256.

57. Rector TS, Bank AJ, Mullen KA, Tschumperlin LK, Sih R, Pillai K, et al. Randomized, double-blind, placebo-controlled study of supplemental oral L-arginine in patients with heart failure. Circulation 1996;93:2135–2141.

58. Rector TS, Cohn JN. Assessment of patient outcome with the Minnesota Living with Heart Failure questioinaire: reliability and validity during a randomized, double-blind, placebo-controlled trial of pimobendan (Pimobendan Multicenter Research Group). Am Heart J 1992;124:1017–1025.

59. Hare JM, Loh E, Creager MA, Colucci WS. Nitric oxide inhibits the positive inotropic response to beta-adrenergic stimulation in humans with left ventricular dysfunction. Circulation 1995;92:2198–2203.

60. Nafz, B, Wagner CD, Persson PB. Endogenous nitric oxide buffers blood pressure variability between 0.2 and 0.6 Hz in the conscious rat. Am J Physiol 1997;272:H632–H637.

61. Harada S, Tokunaga S, Momohara M, Masaki H, Tagawa T, Imaizumi T, et al. Inhibition of nitric oxide formation in the nucleus tractus solitarius increases renal sympathetic nerve activity in rabbits. Circ Res 1993;72:511–516.

62. Shapoval LN, Sagach VF, Pobegailo LS. Nitric oxide influences ventrolateral medullary mechanisms of vasomotor control in the cat. Neurosci Lett 1991;132:47–50.

63. Hashiguchi H, Ye SH, Ross-Cisneros F, Alexander N. Central nitric oxide donors attenuate cardiovascular and central norepinephrine responses to stress. Am J Physiol 1997;272:R1447–R1453.

64. Zhang K, Mayhan WG, Patel KP. Nitric oxide within the paraventricular nucleus mediates changes in renal sympathetic nerve activity. Am J Physiol 1997;273:R864–R872.

65. Lawrence AJ. Nitric oxide as a modulator of medullary pathways. Clin Exp Pharmacol Physiol 1997;24: 760–763.

66. Ma S, Abboud FM, Felder RB. Effects of L-arginine-derived nitric oxide synthesis on neuronal activity in nucleus tractus solitarius. Am J Physiol 1995;268:R487–R491.

67. Zanzinger J, Czachurski J, Seller H. Neuronal nitric oxide reduces sympathetic excitability by modulation of central glutamate effects in pigs. Circ Res 1997;80:565–571.

68. Lipton SA, Choi YB, Pan ZH, Lei SZ, Chen HS, Sucher NJ, et al. A redox-based mechanism for the neuroprotective and neurodestructive effects of nitric oxide and related nitroso-compounds. Nature 1993;364:626–632.

69. Horackova M, Armour JA, Hopkins DA, Huang MH. Nitric oxide modulates signaling between cultured adult peripheral cardiac neurons and cardiomyocytes. Am J Physiol 1995;269:C504–C510.

70. Li CG, Rand MJ. Nitric oxide and vasoactive intestinal polypetide mediate non-adrenergic, non-cholinergic inhibitory transmission to smooth muscle of the rat gastric fundus. Eur J Pharmacol 1990;191: 303–309.

71. Gibson A, Mirzazadeh S, Hobbs AJ, Moore PK. L-N^G-monomethyl arginine and L-N^G-nitro arginine inhibit non-adrenergic, non-cholinergic relaxation of the mouse anococcygeus muscle. Br J Pharmacol 1990;99:602–606.

72. McKirdy HC, McKirdy ML, Lewis MJ, Marshall RW. Evidence for involvement of nitric oxide in the non-adrenergic non-cholinergic (NANC) relaxation of human lower oesophageal sphincter muscle strips. Exp Physiol 1992;77:509–511.
73. Rajfer J, Aronson WJ, Bush PA, Dorey FJ, Ignarro LJ. Nitric oxide as a mediator of relaxation of the corpus cavernosum in response to nonadrenergic, noncholinergic neurotransmission. N Engl J Med 1992;326:90–94.
74. Buxton IL, Cheek DJ, Eckman D, Westfall DP, Sanders KM, Keef KD. N^G-nitro L-arginine methyl ester and other alkyl esters of arginine are muscarinic receptor antagonists. Circ Res 1993;72:387–395.

II

CARDIOVASCULAR PATHOPHYSIOLOGY OF NITRIC OXIDE

13

Nitric Oxide and Endothelial Dysfunction

Gerard A. Dillon and Joseph A. Vita

INTRODUCTION

In the past, the vascular endothelium was viewed largely as a passive, semipermeable barrier between blood and tissues for the exchange of substrates and products of metabolism. More recently, it has become clear that the endothelium plays an active role in the regulation of vascular homeostasis. A turning point in this altered perception of the endothelium occurred in 1980 with the seminal observation by Furchgott and Zawadzki that an intact endothelium is required for acetylcholine-induced vasodilation *(1)*. Subsequent studies identified "endothelium-derived relaxing factor" (EDRF) as nitric oxide (NO•) *(2,3)*. Since then, studies have shown that in addition to controlling vascular tone, endothelium-derived NO• (EDNO) also regulates platelet function, vascular growth and remodeling, and adhesion of inflammatory cells to the endothelial surface.

The importance of the endothelium in cardiovascular disease states has also been recently recognized. Previously, the endothelium was viewed as a passive target for injury. However, this concept began to change with the observation that endothelial vasodilator function is abnormal in the setting of atherosclerosis *(4,5)*. Subsequent studies have shown that endothelial dysfunction is present prior to the development of atherosclerosis in a variety of associated disease states including hypercholesterolemia *(6,7)*, hypertension *(8)*, and diabetes mellitus *(9)*. There now is convincing evidence that loss of EDNO action contributes to the development of atherosclerotic lesions and to the clinical expression of coronary artery disease (CAD). Furthermore, recent studies suggest that restoration of EDNO action may explain, in part, the reduction in cardiovascular risk associated with interventions such as cholesterol-lowering therapy.

In addition to releasing NO•, it is clear that the endothelium regulates vascular homeostasis through the expression and/or release of a large number of other factors that influence vasomotor tone, fibrinolysis, thrombosis, vascular growth, and vascular inflammation (Table 1). The term "endothelial dysfunction" or "endothelial activation" usually indicates a generalized alteration in endothelial cell phenotype that influences many of these functions *(10)*. Importantly, loss of EDNO action is a central feature of endothelial dysfunction that has been extensively studied and is clinically relevant. This chapter briefly reviews the general regulatory functions of the endothelium and then focuses on EDNO and its role in endothelial function and dysfunction. Specific mechanisms of impaired EDNO action will be considered and related to relevant disease states and potential interventions for improvement. This chapter serves as an introduction for subsequent chapters in this section that discuss in greater detail the importance of EDNO in specific disease states and potential therapies to restore its bioactivity.

From: *Contemporary Cardiology, vol. 4: Nitric Oxide and the Cardiovascular System*
Edited by: J. Loscalzo and J. A. Vita © Humana Press Inc., Totowa, NJ

Table 1
Opposing Regulatory Functions of the Vascular Endothelium

Vasomotor tone	
Vasodilators	Vasoconstrictors
Nitric oxide	Endothelin
Prostacyclin	Angiotensin II
Endothelial-derived hyperpolarizing	Endothelium-derived constricting factor
factor	Platelet-derived growth factor (PDGF)
Adenosine	Prostaglandin H_2
	Thromboxane A_2
Fibrinolysis	
Profibrinolytic factors	Antifibrinolytic factors
Tissue plasminogen activator (t-PA)	Plasminogen activator inhibitor-1
Urokinase-type plasminogen activator	
Thrombosis	
Platelet inhibitors	Platelet activators
Nitric oxide	von Willebrand factor
Prostacyclin	Platelet-activating factor
Ecto-ADPase[a]	
Anticoagulants	Procoagulants
Thrombomodulin	Tissue factor
Heparan sulfate	von Willebrand factor
Dermatan sulfate	
Cell growth	
Growth inhibition	Growth promotion
Nitric oxide	Angiotensin II
Heparan sulfate	Platelet-derived growth factor
Prostacyclin	Endothelin
Inflammation	
Anti-inflammatory factors	Proinflammatory factors
Nitric oxide	E-selectin
	Intracellular adhesion molecule-1 (ICAM-1)
	Vascular cell adhesion molecule-1 (VCAM-1)
	Monocyte chemotactic protein-1 (MCP-1)
	Interleukin-8

[a]ADP = adenosine diphosphate.

NO• AND NORMAL ENDOTHELIAL FUNCTION

As detailed in prior chapters, NO• is produced in endothelial cells from L-arginine and oxygen by the endothelial isoform of nitric oxide synthase (eNOS). In endothelial cells, eNOS is constitutively expressed and is localized to caveolae (11). In the presence of calcium, eNOS interacts with calmodulin and is activated to synthesize NO•. Production of NO• by endothelial cells is stimulated by mechanical forces including shear stress (12) and following exposure to receptor-dependent agonists such as acetylcholine, adenosine diphosphate (ADP), bradykinin, thrombin, and serotonin (5-HT) (13). EDNO diffuses locally within the blood vessel wall and produces vasodilation primarily by activating soluble guanylyl cyclase and increasing intracellular cyclic guanosine monophosphate (cGMP) in vascular smooth muscle cells. As detailed in Chapter 7, NO• also induces vasorelaxation by non-cGMP-dependent mechanisms, including activation of calcium-dependent potassium channels in vascular smooth muscle cells (15). When the endothelium is mechanically removed and EDNO is no longer available, acetylcholine and other agonists have unopposed direct vasoconstrictor effects *(1)*. In general, EDNO acts to limit arterial shear stress and oppose vasoconstrictor stimuli within the vasculature.

There is convincing evidence that EDNO is involved in the normal regulation of vaso-motor tone in humans. An intracoronary infusion of acetylcholine produces epicardial vaso-dilation in young subjects with angiographically normal coronary arteries *(4)*. Increased shear stress also stimulates epicardial coronary dilation in angiographically normal vessels *(16)*. In addition to its effects on conduit vessels, infusion of acetylcholine also increases coronary blood flow, reflecting vasodilation of coronary resistance vessels *(17)*. The epicar-dial and resistance vessel vasodilator responses to acetylcholine *(18)* and other EDNO ago-nists such as substance P *(19)* and bradykinin *(20)* are inhibited by concomitant infusion of the NOS inhibitor N^G-monomethyl-L-arginine (L-NMMA), confirming their dependence on NO• synthesis. In addition to these effects in the coronary circulation, these agonists and shear stress also produce NO•-dependent vasodilation of conduit and resistance vessels in the brachial circulation of normal subjects *(7,21)*. Furthermore, exercise-induced vasodilation and postischemic dilation of forearm resistance vessels also depend in part on NO• synthesis in humans *(22–24)*.

In addition to releasing NO•, the endothelium regulates vasomotor tone through the release of other vasodilator substances including prostacyclin *(25)*, adenosine *(26)*, and endothe-lium-derived hyperpolarizing factor (EDHF) *(27)*. The identity of EDHF remains unknown, and it likely plays a secondary role in controlling vasomotor tone under normal conditions. However, EDHF may play a more important compensatory role when EDNO release is impaired in certain disease states *(28)*. In addition to releasing vasodilators, the endothelium also produces vasoconstrictor substances including endothelin *(29)*, angiotensin II *(30)*, thromboxane A_2 *(31)*, and other prostanoid vasoconstrictors *(32)*. Thus, the endothelium participates in the regulation of vasomotor tone via a balanced release of vasodilator and vaso-constrictor substances. Under normal conditions, this balance favors vasodilation; however, vasoconstriction may predominant under pathological conditions, as is discussed shortly.

In addition to its role in modulating tone, EDNO has other important effects in the vascu-lature, which are reviewed in detail in previous chapters. For example, NO• inhibits platelet adhesion and activation by a cGMP-dependent mechanism *(33)*, and, thus, has important antithrombotic effects. EDNO and exogenous NO• donors also inhibit proliferation of smooth muscle cells *(34,35)*, and by these mechanisms influence the response to arterial injury. Further-more, EDNO modulates leukocyte adhesion to the endothelial surface *(36)* and expression of monocyte chemotactic factor-1 (MCP-1) *(37)*. The effect of NO• on leukocyte adhesion appears to be mediated in part by a reduction in the expression of endothelial–leukocyte adhesion molecules, including vascular cell adhesion molecule-1 (VCAM-1) *(38,39)*.

A large number of other endothelial products also are important for the maintenance of vascular homeostasis *(40)*. For example, the endothelium participates in the control of fibrin-olysis through the production of tissue-type plasminogen activator (t-PA) and its primary inhibitor in plasma, plasminogen activator inhibitor-1 (PAI-1) *(41)*. In addition to inhibiting platelets through the effects of NO• and prostacyclin, the endothelium also inhibits thrombo-sis by producing heparan sulfate proteoglycans *(42)* and through the action of thrombomod-ulin, which reduces thrombin activity at the endothelial surface *(43)*. Like NO•, prostacyclin and heparan sulfates also inhibit the growth of vascular smooth muscle cells *(40)*.

Finally, the vascular endothelium plays a critical role in the regulation of the inflammatory response, which is also relevant to the process of atherogenesis. The normal endothelium provides a barrier to attachment and infiltration by leukocytes. However, following exposure to cytokines such as interleukin 1-β (IL-1β) or tumor necrosis factor alpha (TNF-α), endo-thelial cells are activated to produce endothelial–leukocyte adhesion molecules including VCAM-1, intercellular adhesion molecule (ICAM-1), and E-selectin, all of which promote leukocyte binding *(44)*. Furthermore, the endothelium also produces chemoattractants such

Table 2
Disease States Associated with Endothelial Dysfunction

Atherosclerosis
Hypercholesterolemia
Diabetes mellitus
Hypertension
Cigarette smoking
Congestive heart failure
Hyperhomocysteinemia
Ischemia/reperfusion
Posttransplantation
Pulmonary hypertension
Vascular injury/regenerated endothelium

as interleukin 8 (IL-8) and monoctye chemotactic protein (MCP-1), further accelerating the inflammatory process. As discussed earlier, NO• inhibits adhesion molecule expression, in part by preventing activation of nuclear factor-κB (NF-κB) *(39)*.

NO• AND ENDOTHELIAL DYSFUNCTION

Endothelial dysfunction is present in atherosclerosis, risk factors for atherosclerosis, and a large number of other vascular disease states (Table 2). Although impaired endothelial control of fibrinolysis and inflammation have also been documented in a number of these disease states, this chapter focuses on impaired bioactivity of EDNO and its clinical relevance. For broader discussions of endothelial dysfunction in vascular disease, the reader is referred to several reviews of this subject *(40,45,46)*.

The first evidence that atherosclerosis is associated with impaired EDNO activity was provided by Ludmer and colleagues with the demonstration that an intracoronary infusion of acetylcholine produces vasoconstriction of epicardial coronary arteries in patients with angiographic evidence of atherosclerosis *(4)*. In these patients, intracoronary nitroglycerin infusion produces normal coronary dilation. Thus, the ability of vascular smooth muscle to respond to a direct NO• donor appears to be preserved suggesting that the constrictor response to acetylcholine reflects a loss of EDNO. Using coronary arteries isolated from the explanted hearts of patients undergoing cardiac transplantation, Bossaller and colleagues demonstrated that coronary atherosclerosis is associated with impaired relaxation and decreased accumulation of tissue cGMP in response to acetylcholine and other EDNO agonists, but intact responses to nitroglycerin *(5)*. Subsequent in vivo studies in patients with coronary artery disease also demonstrated impaired vasodilator responses to other stimuli for EDNO release including shear stress *(16)*, serotonin *(47)*, and substance P *(48)*.

Impaired EDNO action is present very early in the atherosclerotic process. For example, the coronary vasodilator response to acetylcholine is impaired prior to the development of angiographic evidence of atherosclerosis in patients with hypercholesterolemia *(6)*, hypertension *(49)*, cigarette smoking *(50)*, and diabetes mellitus *(9)*. Endothelial vasomotor dysfunction may also be present prior to the development of intimal thickening as assessed by intracoronary ultrasound, which provides a more sensitive method for detecting early atherosclerosis *(51)*. Flow-mediated dilation of the brachial artery is impaired in young children with familial hypercholesterolemia *(52)* and in the otherwise healthy offspring of patients with coronary artery disease *(53)*. Interestingly, impaired flow-mediated dilation of the brachial artery correlates with impaired endothelial vasomotor function in the coronary circulation *(54)*, suggesting that noninvasive studies in the arm may have clinical relevance to CAD. Forearm blood flow responses to acetylcholine or methacholine are impaired in patients with hypercholesterolemia *(7)*, hypertension *(8)*, and diabetes *(55)*, reflecting impaired EDNO action in resistance vessels, which do not develop atherosclerotic lesions. Thus, impaired EDNO action precedes atherosclerosis and is associated with a broad array of coronary risk factors. These observations are consistent with the idea that loss of EDNO action is more than a consequence of atherosclerosis and plays a causative role in atherogenesis *(see* Chapter 16).

In addition to effects on the early stages of atherosclerosis, a number of studies suggest that loss of EDNO action in the coronary circulation also contributes to the pathogenesis of myocardial ischemia in patients with advanced coronary artery disease and chronic angina. For example, Yeung and colleagues reported that atherosclerotic coronary segments with a constrictor response to acetylcholine tend to constrict in response to mental stress, whereas segments with intact endothelial function demonstrate a vasodilator response *(56)*. Similar observations were made for exercise *(57)* and the cold pressor test *(58)*. These clinically relevant stimuli have complex effects on the cardiovascular system, including increases in coronary blood flow, activity of the sympathetic nervous system, and circulating catecholamines. In atherosclerotic vessels, impaired EDNO release in response to flow *(16)* or α_2-adrenergic agonists *(59)* could contribute to unopposed vasoconstriction and/or impaired conduit and resistance vessel vasodilator responses. Thus, under conditions of increased myocardial oxygen demand, loss of EDNO action may limit coronary blood supply and contribute to myocardial ischemia.

In addition to this role in stable coronary disease, loss of EDNO action may also contribute to the pathogenesis of acute coronary syndromes. It is now understood that plaque rupture and intracoronary thrombosis play causative roles in unstable angina and acute myocardial infarction *(60)*. Because EDNO blunts platelet aggregation and the constrictor responses to serotonin, thrombin, and other products of aggregating platelets *(47,61)*, loss of EDNO may contribute to the severity of thrombosis and vasoconstriction under these circumstances. Consistent with this possibility are the observations that patients with a recent myocardial infarction *(62)* or unstable angina *(63)* have more severe endothelial dysfunction than patients with stable symptoms. Loss of NO'-dependent vasodilation may also lead to local increases in shear stress *(64)*, which could increase the risk for plaque rupture. Because accumulation of inflammatory cells in plaque is believed to contribute to plaque vulnerability, loss of the anti-inflammatory effects of EDNO could also contribute to this process *(65)*.

The studies reviewed previously make it clear that impaired bioactivity of EDNO is both an early feature of the atherogenic process and a contributor to the clinical expression of disease in its advanced stages. Given its importance in atherosclerosis, one might predict that an intervention that improves EDNO action would reduce cardiovascular risk. Although there currently is no direct evidence for such an effect, circumstantial evidence is accumulating. For example, cholesterol-lowering therapy improves endothelium-dependent vasodilation in patients with hypercholesterolemia and has proven to be effective for the primary and secondary prevention of cardiovascular disease. Other interventions that improve EDNO action may also reduce cardiovascular risk, including antioxidants and estrogen replacement therapy.

MECHANISMS OF IMPAIRED EDNO ACTION

Given the importance of endothelial dysfunction and impaired EDNO bioactivity in vascular disease, there currently is great interest in elucidating the mechanisms of this impairment. As outlined in Fig. 1, investigators have considered a number of potential defects in the pathway leading from *NOS3* gene expression to the biological effects of EDNO. This section considers these potential defects in different vascular disease states and, when relevant, discusses potential interventions.

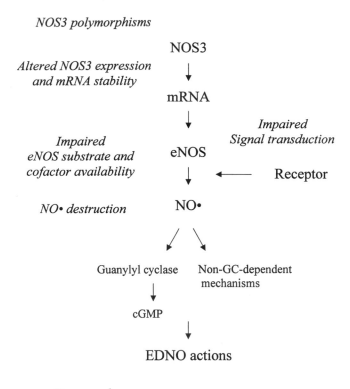

NOS3 polymorphisms

NOS3

Altered NOS3 expression
and mRNA stability

mRNA

Impaired
Signal transduction

Impaired
eNOS substrate and
cofactor availability

eNOS

Receptor

NO• destruction

NO•

Guanylyl cyclase   Non-GC-dependent
mechanisms

cGMP

EDNO actions

Decreased
responsiveness to NO•

Fig. 1. The pathway from eNOS gene expression to endothelium-derived NO• action is presented schematically. Potential mechanisms of impaired EDNO action discussed in the text are indicated in italics. Abbreviations: NOS3 = *NOS3* gene, mRNA = messenger ribonucleic acid, eNOS = endothelial nitric oxide synthase protein, GC = guanylyl cyclase, cGMP = 3',5'-cyclic guanosine monophosphate, NO• = nitric oxide.

NOS3 Polymorphisms

eNOS is the product of the *NOS3* gene, which is located on chromosome 7 *(66)*. A number of *NOS3* polymorphisms have been described that could cause variation in EDNO bioactivity and contribute to cardiovascular disease. Given that the eNOS knockout mouse is hypertensive *(67)*, investigators have proposed that polymorphisms of the *NOS3* gene might be a genetic cause of human hypertension. Studies of this issue have provided conflicting results. For example, several studies have failed to show linkage between polymorphisms of the intron regions of *NOS3* and hypertension *(68,69)*. However, there is evidence for linkage between the missense variant Glu298Asp in exon 7 of the *NOS3* gene and hypertension *(69)*. The Glu298Asp variant has also been linked to vasospastic angina *(70)* and acute myocardial infarction *(71,72)*. These observations were made in Japanese populations, and it is notable that investigators have been unable to demonstrate linkage between this polymorphism and ischemic stroke in a Caucasian population *(73)*.

The significance of Glu298Asp and other polymorphisms for the enzymatic activity of eNOS remains unclear. A preliminary study does suggest that a $T^{-786} \rightarrow C$ mutation in the 5'-flanking region of the *NOS3* gene, is associated with more severe acetylcholine-induced coronary artery constriction and a reduction in serum nitrite/nitrate concentrations *(74)*. The 27-bp repeat intron 4 polymorphism has also been associated with decreased plasma nitrite/nitrate concentrations *(75)*. Thus, in certain situations, a genetically based decrease in eNOS activity could explain impaired EDNO action and contribute to the development of vascular disease.

Altered NOS3 Gene Expression and mRNA Stability

Altered regulation of *NOS3* gene expression and posttranscriptional mRNA processing may be relevant to endothelial dysfunction in cardiovascular disease. The *NOS3* gene is expressed constitutively in endothelial cells, but a number of factors may influence the level of expression *(76)*. For example, the 5'-flanking region contains a number of shear stress-responsive elements *(77)*. eNOS expression and NO' production are increased by shear stress *(78)* and exercise-induced increases in coronary blood flow *(79)*. Endothelium-dependent vasodilation is enhanced under conditions of high flow/shear stress *(80)* and impaired in low flow states *(81)*. Investigators have postulated that the reduction in cardiovascular risk associated with exercise may relate, in part, to improved EDNO action *(82)*.

The *NOS3* promoter region contains a number of other regulatory sites that may be clinically relevant, including cytokine responsive elements *(66,83)*. For example, transforming growth factor β-1 (TGFβ-1) has been shown to increase *NOS3* gene transcription *(84)*. Estrogen-responsive elements are also present in the *NOS3* promoter region, but there are conflicting reports regarding the effect of estrogens on *NOS3* expression *(85–87)*. Although the specific regulatory mechanisms remain unclear, endothelial cell proliferation is associated with an increase in eNOS expression *(88)*, whereas oxidized low-density lipoprotein (LDL) and hypoxia *(90)* have the opposite effect.

Posttranscription regulation of eNOS mRNA also appears to influence the bioavailability of EDNO. In addition to their effects on *NOS3* transcription, oxidized low-density lipoprotein (ox-LDL) *(89)* and hypoxia *(90)* have been shown to decrease the stability of eNOS mRNA and to decrease NO' production. Other factors that destabilize eNOS mRNA include tumor necrosis factor-α (TNF-α) *(91)* and lipopolysaccharide (LPS) *(92)*. Because inflammation and ox-LDL play important roles in the atherogenic process *(93)*, these effects are likely to be clinical relevant. Furthermore, hydroxymethylglutaryl coenzyme A (HMG CoA) reductase inhibitors, which are known to reduce cardiovascular risk, may act, in part, by improving eNOS mRNA stability *(94)* in addition to their effects on lipid levels.

Decreased Substrate/Cofactor Availability

As discussed in Chapter 30, there is convincing evidence that administration of L-arginine, the substrate for NO' synthesis, enhances EDNO action in a variety of disease states in humans including hypercholesterolemia *(95,96)*, variant angina *(97)*, and coronary atherosclerosis *(98)*. These findings suggest that deficiency or decreased bioavailablity of L-arginine may contribute to abnormal endothelial function. However, investigators have argued on a kinetic basis that it is doubtful that L-arginine availability is rate limiting under physiological conditions *(76)*. The K_m of L-arginine for NOS is approx 2.9 μM *(99)*, whereas plasma and intracellular L-arginine concentrations greatly exceed this level *(76)*. In addition, endothelial cells are able to synthesize L-arginine from L-citrulline *(100)*, making an intracellular deficiency unlikely, even when exogenous sources are restricted. However, it is possible that L-arginine improves endothelial function by some other mechanism other than simply repleting the eNOS substrate. For example, L-arginine stimulates insulin release, which is known to increase NO' production *(101)*. L-arginine also stimulates release of other potentially vasoactive hormones including atrial natriuretic peptide, glucagon, and growth hormone *(102)*. Finally, L-arginine is also a potential reducing agent that may act nonspecifically to improve EDNO action. Investigators have also speculated that altered transport may affect local availability of L-arginine in endothelial cells in certain disease states *(103)*.

Another mechanism of endothelial dysfunction that relates to eNOS substrate availability is the presence of NOS inhibitors in vivo. One such inhibitor is asymmetrical dimethyl arginine (ADMA), a naturally occurring analog of L-arginine *(104)*. Plasma levels of ADMA are approximately twofold higher in hypercholesterolemic subjects compared to control subjects, and correlate inversely with brachial artery flow-mediated dilation *(105)*. ADMA levels are elevated in hypertension *(106)* and in patients with renal failure *(107)*, a condition that is also associated with impaired endothelium-dependent vasodilation *(108)*. In patients with peripheral vascular disease, ADMA levels are also elevated and have been shown to correlate with the extent of disease *(109)*. L-Arginine supplementation increases the L-arginine:ADMA ratio and improves endothelial function in patients with hypercholesterolemia *(105)*, and in experimental hypercholesterolemia *(110)*. Investigators have speculated that this improvement in L-arginine:ADMA ratio may explain the paradoxical benefits of L-arginine in the face of apparently adequate plasma and/or intracellular levels *(105)*.

Tetrahydrobiopterin (BH_4) is required for NO• synthesis by eNOS, and there is evidence that impaired availability of this cofactor may contribute to endothelial dysfunction in vascular disease. Inhibition of BH_4 synthesis induces endothelial vasomotor dysfunction in canine coronary arteries *(111)*. Conversely, BH_4 administration improves abnormal endothelium-dependent vasodilation in the forearm of hypercholesterolemic patients *(112)*, in isolated saphenous vein harvested from cigarette smokers *(113)*, and in experimental models of diabetes *(114)* and reperfusion injury *(115)*. Although chronic parenteral BH_4 administration is not practical, a recent study demonstrated that oral administration of 5-methyltetrahydrofolate, which increases intracellular BH_4, improved EDNO action in patients with familial hypercholesterolemia *(116)*.

There are several possible explanations for the observed beneficial effects of BH_4. Although intracellular levels of BH_4 have not been examined, an absolute or relative deficiency of BH_4 and decreased enzyme activity could be present in certain disease states. In addition, BH_4 deficiency has been associated with the uncoupling of electron transfer to L-arginine by eNOS with decreased NO• production and increased production of reactive oxygen species including superoxide anion that can "inactivate" NO• *(111,117)*. There is evidence that BH_4 prevents eNOS-mediated superoxide production by coupling L-arginine oxidation to nicotinamide adenine dinucleotide phosphate (NADPH) consumption and preventing dissociation of the ferrous–dioxygen complex *(118)*. A recent study demonstrated that BH_4 decreased superoxide anion and hydrogen peroxide production and increased NO• release in vascular tissue from spontaneously hypertensive rats *(117)*.

Altered Signal Transduction

Several lines of evidence suggest that abnormalities of endothelial receptor signal transduction may contribute to impaired EDNO action in vascular disease. In humans, vasodilation following exposure to receptor-dependent agonists, such as acetylcholine, are impaired early in the course of atherosclerosis, whereas dilation to nonreceptor-dependent stimuli are preserved until more advanced stages of the disease *(119)*. Similarly, in isolated coronary arteries from patients with atherosclerosis, relaxation to receptor-dependent EDNO agonists, such as acetylcholine and substance P, is impaired, whereas relaxation to the nonreceptor-dependent calcium ionophore A23187 is largely preserved *(5)*. A similar pattern is observed when normal arterial segments are exposed to ox-LDL *(120)*.

Further insight into altered signal transduction as a cause of endothelial dysfunction is provided by the observation that NO•-dependent dilation by agonists coupled to a pertussis toxin-sensitive G_{i-2} protein (serotonin, thrombin, $alpha_2$-adrenergic agonists) is impaired in hypercholesterolemic swine. In contrast, vasodilation to agonists dependent on other signal transduction mechanisms (adenosine diphosphate, bradykinin, A23187) is relatively preserved *(121)*. Products of ox-LDL have a similar effect on G_i-dependent relaxation *(122)*. A number of mechanisms for this effect have been proposed, including altered membrane fluidity, decreased receptor density, and altered expression of G proteins *(123,124)*.

In human hypertension, resistance vessel dilation to acetylcholine and bradykinin are impaired *(125)*, whereas dilation to isoproterenol is preserved *(126)*. Both the muscarinic and bradykinin receptors act via G proteins with activation of phospholipase C (PLC), generation of inositol-1,4,5-triphosphate (IP3), and increases in intracellular calcium. In contrast, beta-adrenergic receptor activation leads to increased intracellular cyclic adenosine monophosphate (cAMP). On the basis of these observations, this group has proposed that human hypertension is associated with a defect in the PLC/IP3 pathway (126). A similar defect has been observed under hyperglycemic conditions (127).

Destruction of NO•

The mechanisms of impaired EDNO action discussed earlier all relate to decreased production of NO• by endothelial cells either due to a reduction in eNOS level or eNOS activity or to impaired signaling between endothelial receptor and the enzyme. However, there is evidence that production of NO• may be intact or increased in certain vascular disease states, and that the defect in EDNO action relates to NO• destruction by reactive oxygen species (see Chapter 26). Superoxide anion and NO• react rapidly to form peroxynitrite eliminating the biological activity of NO• (128). Superoxide production by vascular tissue is increased in hypercholesterolemia (129), and under these conditions, release of NO• oxidation products (nitrite/nitrate) is increased despite markedly impaired endothelium-dependent vasodilation (130). Furthermore, superoxide dismutase (SOD) restores endothelial function in this setting (129,131). Increased production of superoxide anion and destruction of NO• appear to contribute to endothelial dysfunction in other disease states, including diabetes mellitus (132) and hypertension (133). Ascorbic acid is capable of scavenging superoxide anion and preserving EDNO action when administered in sufficiently high concentration (134). Thus, support for the clinical importance of increased superoxide production is provided by the observation that acute administration of high-dose ascorbic acid improves endothelium-dependent dilation in patients with diabetes mellitus (135), hypercholesterolemia (136), and hypertension (137).

A number of studies have provided insight into the enzymatic sources of superoxide anion in vascular disease states. In hypercholesterolemia, xanthine oxidase inhibitors decrease superoxide production and improve endothelium-dependent vasodilation (129). Furthermore, a recent study suggests that hypercholesterolemia is associated with increased plasma levels of xanthine oxidase and binding of the enzyme to heparin-binding sites on the endothelial surface with increased local production of superoxide anion and inactivation of EDNO (138). In patients with hypercholesterolemia, an intra-arterial infusion of oxypurinol improves endothelium-dependent dilation in the forearm circulation, although this intervention had no effect in patients with hypertension (139).

NADH/NADPH oxidase is also a source of superoxide production in vascular tissue and its level of expression in vascular smooth muscle cells is enhanced following exposure to angiotensin-II (140). In a rat model of angiotensin-II-induced hypertension, increased NADH/NADPH oxidase activity is associated with an increase in vascular superoxide production and impaired endothelium-dependent relaxation (133). Under these conditions, treatment with SOD improves endothelium-dependent vasodilation. These findings are specific for angiotensin-II-induced hypertension, as these findings were absent in a control animals with norepinephrine-induced hypertension. There is evidence that NADPH oxidase in adventitial fibroblasts also is an important source of vascular superoxide anion production and that this activity is increased by angiotensin II (141). Investigators (142) have proposed that NADH/NADPH-mediated superoxide production and endothelial dysfunction may explain the increased risk for cardiovascular events in hypertensive patients with increased plasma renin levels (143).

Finally, recent studies suggest that eNOS itself may be a source of superoxide anion production and that, under pathological conditions, such as hypercholesterolemia, the relative production of NO• and superoxide anion may be altered and contribute to endothelial dysfunction. As noted before, deficiency of BH_4 is associated with increased superoxide production by eNOS. In cultured endothelial cells, exposure to native LDL is associated with an increase in the production of NO•, superoxide anion, and nitrotyrosine suggesting peroxynitrite formation (144). These findings were not attributable to iNOS or formation of ox-LDL, but appeared to reflect an as yet undefined effect of native LDL on eNOS.

Other reactive oxygen species can inactive EDNO and impair endothelium-dependent vasodilation. For example, in addition to interrupting signal transduction (120), there is evidence that ox-LDL can react directly with NO• and eliminate its bioactivity (145). Lipid peroxyl radicals are capable of reacting with NO• to form organic peroxynitrite (146), and it is known that organic hydroperoxides induce contraction and decrease cGMP in isolated arteries, suggesting loss of EDNO action (147). In contrast to superoxide anion, NO• does not react directly with hydrogen peroxide. However, there is evidence that hydrogen peroxide impairs EDNO action (148), possibly by oxidizing thiols required for EDNO generation or stabilization. In rabbits, chronic administration of advanced glycosylation end products (AGES), which have been implicated in the complications of diabetes mellitus, impairs acetylcholine- and nitroglycerin-mediated vascular relaxation (149). These results suggest that AGES inactivate NO•; however, the precise chemical mechanism for this interaction remains unknown.

One problem with the paradigm that destruction of NO• accounts for impaired EDNO action in vascular disease states is the observation that vasodilation to exogenous sources of NO• is largely intact. For example, vasodilation to nitroglycerin and nitroprusside is largely preserved in atherosclerosis (4), diabetes mellitus (9), and hypertension (8). It is possible that preserved responses to nitrovasodilators may reflect the relatively high doses used in many of these studies.

Compartmentalization of the sources of superoxide and NO• could also reconcile these observations; however, further investigation in this area is required. It is notable that Creager and colleagues reported a significant impairment of the vasodilator responses of forearm microvessels to nitroprusside in patients with hypercholesterolemia (7). This finding could reflect destruction of nitroprusside-derived NO•.

Decreased Responsiveness to NO•

In addition to decreased production and increased destruction of NO•, there is evidence that in certain situations, impaired target cell responsiveness may account for impaired EDNO action in vascular disease. In addition to reflecting destruction of nitroprusside-released NO•, the finding that nitroprusside-mediated dilation is impaired in hypercholesterolemia (7) is also consistent with an impairment of the ability of vascular smooth muscle to respond to NO•. In a study of 800 subjects, the vasodilator response to nitroglycerin was shown to be significantly reduced in patients with coronary risk factors (150). Consistent with these observations, Weisbrod and colleagues observed decreased relaxation to authentic NO• in arterial tissue isolated from hypercholesterolemic rabbits (151). This impairment was attributable to a decrease in cGMP-mediated inhibition of calcium entry to vascular smooth muscle cells. The impairment was not reversed by SOD, suggesting that superoxide-mediated inactivation of NO• did not account for the impairment. An earlier study suggested an impairment of NO•-stimulated guanylate cyclase activity in the setting of atherosclerosis (152).

In summary, there are multiple potential mechanisms for impaired EDNO action in vascular disease states. It is likely that multiple mechanisms are operative, and that different mechanisms are involved at different stages of disease. It also appears likely that different coronary risk factors impair endothelium-dependent vasodilation by different mechanisms (153), possibly contributing to the additive effects of these risk factors on endothelial function (6) and cardiovascular risk (154).

Table 3
Human Studies of Cholesterol-Lowering Therapy and Endothelial Vasomotor Function

Study first author	Baseline total cholesterol (mg/dL)	Intervention	Treatment duration (mo)	Improvement demonstrated
Coronary circulation				
Leung (173)	275 ± 31	Cholestyramine	6	+
Egashira (174)	272 ± 8	Pravastatin	6	+
Treasure (159)	230 ± 33	Lovastatin	5.5	+
Anderson (164)	209 ± 33	Lovastatin plus cholestyramine	12	±
Yeung (160)	204 ± 32	Simvastatin	6	–
Forearm circulation				
O'Driscoll (175)	255 ± 33	Simvastatin	1	+
Drury (176)	209 ± 17	Pravastatin	5 yr	+
Vogel (177)	200 ± 12	Simvastatin	3	+
Tamai (178)	195 ± 34	LDL apheresis	Immediate	+

TREATMENT OF ENDOTHELIAL DYSFUNCTION

Many of the studies that provide insight into the pathophysiological mechanisms of endo-thelial dysfunction also suggest potential therapies. As discussed before, L-arginine and BH_4 have been shown to improve NO˙-dependent vasodilation in patients with vascular disease, although the clinical significance of these treatments remain to be determined. Importantly, several other interventions that reverse endothelial dysfunction also have been shown to reduce cardiovascular risk. For example, lipid-lowering therapy has been shown to be effec-tive for primary and secondary prevention of CAD events (155–158) and overall mortality (155). A number of studies have convincingly shown that lipid-lowering therapy improves EDNO action in the coronary and peripheral circulations of patients with coronary artery disease and hypercholesterolemia (Table 3). Although improved endothelial vasomotor func-tion has been demonstrated with short-term treatment of patients with elevated cholesterol levels (159), a large, well-controlled study demonstrated that 6 mo of lipid-lowering therapy failed to improve the endotheial function in patients with relatively low baseline LDL choles-terol levels (130 mg/dL) (160). These findings suggest that more prolonged therapy may be necessary to impact endothelial function. The findings are also consistent with the observa-tion that 2–3 yr of treatment are required to impact cardiovascular events in patients with similar baseline lipid levels (156,161).

As discussed in Chapter 26, antioxidant treatment has been shown to improve EDNO action, and recent studies support the clinical importance of antioxidant treatment in CAD. A large, well-controlled randomized trial demonstrated that vitamin E treatment is associated with a reduction in nonfatal myocardial infarction in patients with CAD (162). A recent study demonstrated improved endothelial function with vitamin E treatment (163) and with pro-bucol (164), another lipid-soluble antioxidant. Decreased dietary intake of ascorbic acid is associated with increased risk of cardiovascular events (165). As already noted, ascorbic acid treatment improves EDNO action in patients with CAD (166), diabetes mellitus (135), hyper-cholesterolemia (136), and hypertension (137).

A number of other interventions associated with reduced cardiovascular risk have also been shown to improve endothelial function. For example, premenopausal women and women receiving estrogen replacement therapy have a reduced risk of cardiovascular disease *(167)*. Although estrogens favorably impact lipid profile and have other beneficial effects, estrogen replacement therapy has also been shown to improve endothelium-dependent vasodilation in postmenopausal women *(168)*. However, a recent, well-controlled study failed to demonstrate a reduction in CAD events in women receiving estrogen replacement therapy in combination with progesterone *(169)*. Thus, important questions remain about the clinical importance of improved EDNO action with estrogen replacement therapy. Angiotensin converting enzyme inhibitors are known to reduce CAD events in patients with a previous myocardial infarction *(170)*. Treatment of patients with CAD with quinapril for 6 mo improves coronary artery endothelial function *(171)*. As noted earlier, exercise is associated with reduced cardiovascular risk and chronic exercise has been shown to improve EDNO action *(82)*. Cessation of cigarette smoking also is associated with improved endothelium-dependent vasodilation *(172)*.

CONCLUSIONS

This chapter has reviewed the importance of NO• in the normal and abnormal functions of the vascular endothelium. Impaired EDNO action is a consistent feature in patients with coronary risk factors and more advanced atherosclerosis, and likely contributes to the pathogenesis of CAD. Conisistent with this possibility is the observation that interventions that improve EDNO action also reduce cardiovascular risk. New approaches for therapy will likely arise from ongoing studies of the mechanisms of impaired EDNO action in atherosclerosis. Large-scale trials are currently in progress that will further examine the clinical relevance and predictive value of endothelial vasomotor dysfunction for CAD events. Examination of EDNO action may prove to be a useful surrogate marker of cardiovascular risk and a useful guide to therapy.

ACKNOWLEDGMENTS

Dr. Vita is the recipient of an Established Investigator Award from the American Heart Association. Portions of the work cited in this chapter were supported by grants from the National Institutes of Health (HL53398 and HL55993).

REFERENCES

1. Furchgott RF, Zawadzki JV. The obligatory role of endothelial cells in the relaxation of arterial smooth muscle by acetylcholine. Nature 1980;288:373–376.
2. Ignarro LJ, Buga GM, Wood KS, Byrns RE, Chaudhuri G. Endothelium-derived relaxing factor produced and released from artery and vein is nitric oxide. Proc Natl Acad Sci USA 1987;84:9265–9269.
3. Palmer RM, Ferrige AG, Moncada S. Nitric oxide release accounts for the biological activity of endothelium-derived relaxing factor. Nature 1987;327:524–526.
4. Ludmer PL, Selwyn AP, Shook TL, Wayne RR, Mudge GH, Alexander RW, et al. Paradoxical vasoconstriction induced by acetylcholine in atherosclerotic coronary arteries. N Engl J Med 1986;315: 1046–1051.
5. Bossaller C, Habib GB, Yamamoto H, Williams C, Wells S, Henry PD. Impaired muscarinic endothelium-dependent relaxation and cyclic guanosine 5'-monophosphate formation in atherosclerotic human coronary artery and rabbit aorta. J Clin Invest 1987;79:170–174.
6. Vita JA, Treasure CB, Nabel EG, McLenachan JM, Fish RD, Yeung AC, et al. Coronary vasomotor response to acetylcholine relates to risk factors for coronary artery disease. Circulation 1990;81:491–497.
7. Creager MA, Cooke JP, Mendelsohn ME, Gallagher SJ, Coleman SM, Loscalzo J, et al. Impaired vasodilation of forearm resistance vessels in hypercholesterolemic humans. J Clin Invest 1990;86: 228–234.
8. Panza JA, Quyyumi AA, Brush JE, Epstein SE. Abnormal endothelium-dependent vascular relaxation in patients with essential hypertension. N Engl J Med 1990;323:22–27.

9. Nitenberg A, Valersi P, Sachs R, Dali M, Aptecar E, Attali JR. Impairment of coronary vascular reserve in and ACH-induced coronary vasodilation in diabetic patients with angiographically normal coronary arteries and normal left ventricular systolic function. Diabetes 1993;42:1017–1025.

10. Levine GN, Keaney JF Jr, Vita JA. Cholesterol reduction in cardiovascular disease: Clinical benefits and possible mechanisms. N Engl J Med 1995;332:512–521.

11. Michel T, Feron O. Nitric oxide synthases: which, where, how, and why? J Clin Invest 1997;100: 2146–2152.

12. Olesen SP, Clapham DE, Davies PF. Haemodynamic shear stress activates a K+ current in vascular endothelial cells. Nature 1988;331:168–170.

13. Moncada S, Higgs A. The L-arginine nitric oxide pathway. N Engl J Med 1993;329:2002–2012.

14. Arnold WP, Mittal CK, Katsuki S, Murad F. Nitric oxide activates guanylate cyclase and increases guanosine 3',5'-cyclic monophosphate levels in various tissue preparations. Proc Natl Acad Sci USA 1977;74:3203–3207.

15. Bolotina VM, Najibi S, Palacino JJ, Pagano PJ, Cohen RA. Nitric oxide directly activates calcium-dependent potassium channels in vascular smooth muscle. Nature 1994;368:850–853.

16. Cox DA, Vita JA, Treasure CB, Fish RD, Alexander RW, Ganz P, et al. Atherosclerosis impairs flow-mediated dilation of coronary arteries in humans. Circulation 1989;80:458–465.

17. Treasure CB, Vita JA, Cox DA, Fish RD, Gordon JB, Mudge GH, et al. Endothelium-dependent dilation of the coronary microvasculature is impaired in dilated cardiomyopathy. Circulation 1990;81: 772–779.

18. Quyyumi AA, Dakak N, Andrews NP, Husain S, Arora S, Gilligan DM, et al. Nitric oxide activity in the human coronary circulation. Impact of risk factors for atherosclerosis. J Clin Invest 1995;95:1747–1755.

19. Quyyumi AA, Mulcahy D, Andrews NP, Husain S, Panza JA, Cannon RO III. Coronary nitric oxide activity in hypertension and hypercholesterolemia: comparison of acetylcholine and substance P. Circulation 1997;95:104–110.

20. Kato M, Shiode N, Yamagata T, Matsuura H, Kajiyama G. Bradykinin induced dilatation of human epicardial and resistance coronary arteries in vivo: effect of inhibition of nitric oxide synthesis. Heart 1997;78:493–498.

21. Lieberman EH, Gerhard MD, Uehata A, Selwyn AP, Ganz P, Yeung AC, et al. Flow-induced vasodilation of the human brachial artery is impaired in patients <40 years of age with coronary artery disease. Am J Cardiol 1996;78:1210–1214.

22. Meredith IT, Currie KE, Anderson TJ, Roddy MA, Ganz P, Creager MA. Postischemic vasodilation in human forearm is dependent on endothelium-derived nitric oxide. Am J Physiol 1996;270: H1435–H1440.

23. Gilligan DM, Panza JA, Kilcoyne CM, Waclawiw MA, Casino PR, Quyyumi AA. Contribution of endothelium-derived nitric oxide to exercise-induced vasodilation. Circulation 1994;90:2853–2858.

24. Quyyumi AA, Dakak N, Andrews NP, Gilligan DM, Panza JA, Cannon RO. Contribution of nitric oxide to metabolic coronary vasodilation in the human heart. Circulation 1995;92:320–326.

25. Oates JA, Fitzgerald GA, Branch RA, Jackson EK, Knapp HR, Roberts LJ. Clinical implications of prostaglandin and thromboxane A2 formation. N Engl J Med 1988;319:689–698.

26. Pearson JD, Gordon JL. Vascular endothelial and smooth muscle cells in culture selectively release adenine nucleotides. Nature 1979;281:384–386.

27. Chen G, Suzuki H, Weston AH. Acetylcholine releases endothelium-derived hyperpolarizing factor and EDRF from rat blood vessels. Br J Pharmacol 1988;95:1165–1174.

28. Cohen RA, Vanhoutte PM. Endothelium-dependent hyperpolarization: beyond nitric oxide and cyclic GMP. Circulation 1995;92:3337–3349.

29. Yanagisawa M, Kurihara H, Kimura S, Tomobe Y, Kobayashi M, Mitsui Y, et al. A novel potent vasoconstrictor peptide produced by vascular endothelial cells. Nature 1988;332:411–415.

30. Dzau VJ. Circulating versus local renin-angiotensin system in cardiovascular homeostasis. Circulation 1988;77(6 pt 2), I4–I13.

31. Tesfamariam B, Brown ML, Deykin D, Cohen RA. Elevated glucose promotes generation of endo-0thelium-derived vasoconstrictor prostanoids in rabbit aorta. J Clin Invest 1990;85:929–932.

32. Luscher TF, Vanhoutte PM. Endothelium-dependent contractions to acetylcholine in the aorta of the spontaneously hypertensive rat. Hypertension 1986;8:344–348.

33. Radomski MW, Palmer RMJ, Moncada S. The role of nitric oxide and cGMP in platelet adhesion to the vascular endothelium. Biochem Biophys Res Commun 1987;148:1482–1489.

34. Garg UC, Hassid A. Nitric oxide-generating vasodilators and 8-bromo-cyclic guanosine monophosphate inhibit mitogenesis and proliferation of cultured rat vascular smooth muscle cells. J Clin Invest 1989;83:1774–1777.

35. Scott-Burden T, Vanhoutte PM. Regulation of smooth muscle cell growth by endothelium-derived factors. Tex Heart Inst J 1994;21:91–97.
36. Kubes P, Suzuki M, Granger DN. Nitric oxide: an endogenous modulator of leukocyte adhesion. Proc Natl Acad Sci USA 1991;88:4651–4655.
37. Zeiher AM, Fisslthaler B, Schray-Utz B, Busse R. Nitric oxide modulates the expression of monocyte chemoattractant protein 1 in cultured human endothelial cells. Circ Res 1995;76(6):980–986.
38. Tsao PS, Buitrago R, Chan JR, Cooke JP. Fluid flow inhibits endothelial adhesiveness: nitric oxide and transcriptional regulation of VCAM-1. Circulation 1996;94:1682–1689.
39. De Caterina R, Libby P, Peng HB, Thannickal VJ, Rajavashisth TB, Gimbrone MA, et al. Nitric oxide decreases cytokine-induced endothelial activation. Nitric oxide selectively reduces endothelial expression of adhesion molecules and proinflammatory cytokines. J Clin Invest 1995;96:60–68.
40. Gokce N, Keaney JF Jr, Vita JA. Endotheliopathies: clinical manifestations of endothelial dysfunction. In: Loscalzo J, Shafer AI, eds. Thrombosis and Hemorrhage. Williams and Wilkins, Philadelphia, 1998, pp. 901–924.
41. Loskutoff D, Edgington T. Synthesis of a fibrinolytic activator and inhibitor by endothelial cells. Proc Natl Acad Sci USA 1977;74:3903–3907.
42. Marcum JA, Rosenberg RD. Heparin-like molecules with anticoagulant activity are synthesized by cultured endothelial cells. Biochem Biophys Res Commun 1985;126:365–372.
43. Esmon NL, Owen WG, Esmon CT. Isolation of a membrane bound cofactor for thrombin-catalyzed activation of protein C. J Biol Chem 1982;257:859–864.
44. Collins T. Endothelial nuclear factor-κB and the initiation of the atherosclerotic lesion. Lab Invest 1993;68:499–508.
45. Cohen RA. The role of nitric oxide and other endothelium-derived vasoactive substances in vascular disease. [Review]. Prog Cardiovasc Dis 1995;38:105–128.
46. Gimbrone MAJ. Vascular endothelium: an integrator of pathophysiologic stimuli in atherosclerosis. Am J Cardiol 1995;75:67B–70B.
47. Golino P, Piscione F, Willerson JT, Capelli-Bigazzi M, Focaccio A, Villari B, et al. Divergent effects of serotonin on coronary artery dimensions and blood flow in patients with coronary atherosclerosis and control patients. N Engl J Med 1991;324:641–648.
48. Crossman DC, Larkin SW, Dashwood MR, Davies GJ, Yacoub M, Maseri A. Responses of atherosclerotic human coronary arteries in vivo to substance P. Circulation 1991;84:2001–2010.
49. Treasure CB, Manoukian SV, Klein JL, Vita JA, Nabel EG, Renwick GH, et al. Epicardial coronary artery responses to acetylcholine are impaired in hypertensive patients. Circ Res 1992;71:776–781.
50. Nitenberg A, Antony I, Foult JM. Acetylcholine-induced coronary vasoconstriction in young, heavy smokers with normal coronary arteriographic findings. Am J Med 1993;95:71–77.
51. Nishimura RA, Lerman A, Chesebro JH, Ilstrup DM, Hodge DO, Higano ST, et al. Epicardial vasomotor responses to acetylcholine are not predicted by coronary atherosclerosis as assessed by intracoronary ultrasound. J Am Coll Cardiol 1995;26:41–49.
52. Sorensen KE, Celermajer DS, Georgakopoulos D, Hatcher G, Betteridge DJ, Deanfield JE. Impairment of endothelium-dependent dilation is an early event in children with familial hypercholesterolemia and is related to the lipoprotein (a) level. J Clin Invest 1994;93:50–55.
53. Clarkson P, Celermajer DS, Powe AJ, Donald AE, Henry RM, Deanfield JE. Endothelium-dependent dilatation is impaired in young healthy subjects with a family history of premature coronary disease. Circulation 1997;96:3378–3383.
54. Anderson TJ, Uehata A, Gerhard MD, Meredith IT, Knab S, Delagrange D, et al. Close relation of endothelial function in the human coronary and peripheral circulations. J Am Coll Cardiol 1995;26: 1235–1241.
55. Johnstone MT, Creager SJ, Scales KM, Cusco JA, Lee BK, Creager MA. Impaired endothelium-dependent vasodilation in patients with insulin-dependent diabetes mellitus. Circulation 1993;88: 2510–2516.
56. Yeung AC, Vekshtein VI, Krantz DS, Vita JA, Ryan TJ Jr, Ganz P, et al. The effect of atherosclerosis on the vasomotor response of coronary arteries to mental stress. N Engl J Med 1991;325:1551–1556.
57. Gordon JB, Ganz P, Nabel EG, Fish RD, Zebede J, Mudge GH, et al. Atherosclerosis influences the vasomotor response of epicardial coronary arteries to exercise. J Clin Invest 1989;83:1946–1952.
58. Nabel EG, Ganz P, Gordon JB, Alexander RW, Selwyn AP. Dilation of normal and constriction of atherosclerotic coronary arteries caused by the cold pressor test. Circulation 1988;77:43–52.
59. Vita JA, Treasure CB, Yeung AC, Vekshtein VI, Fantasia GM, Fish RD, et al. Patients with evidence of coronary endothelial dysfunction as assessed by acetylcholine infusion demonstrate marked increase in sensitivity to constrictor effects of catecholamines. Circulation 1992;85:1390–1397.

60. Fuster V, Badimon L, Badimon JJ, Chesebro JH. The pathogenesis of coronary artery disease and the acute coronary syndromes (Part 1). N Engl J Med 1992;326:242–250.
61. Shimokawa H, Vanhoutte PM. Impaired endothelium-dependent relaxation to aggregating platelets and related vasoactive substances in porcine coronary arteries in hypercholesterolemia and atherosclerosis. Circ Res 1989;64:900–914.
62. Okumura K, Yasue H, Matsuyama K, Ogawa H, Morikami Y, Obata K, et al. Effect of acetylcholine on the highly stenotic coronary artery: difference between the constrictor response of the infarct-related coronary artery and that of the noninfarct-related artery. J Am Coll Cardiol 1992;19:752–758.
63. Bogaty P, Hackett D, Davies G, Maseri A. Vasoreactivity of the culprit lesion in unstable angina. Circulation 1994;90:5–11.
64. Vita JA, Treasure CB, Ganz P, Cox DA, Fish RD, Selwyn AP. Control of shear stress in the epicardial coronary arteries of humans: impairment by atherosclerosis. J Am Coll Cardiol 1989;14:1193–1199.
65. Libby P. Molecular basis of the acute coronary syndromes. Circulation 1995;91:2844–2850.
66. Marsden PA, Heng HQ, Scherer SW, Stewart RJ, Hall AV, Shi XM, et al. Structure and chromosomal localization of the human constitutive endothelial nitric oxide synthase gene. J Biol Chem 1993;268: 17,478–17,488.
67. Shesely EG, Maeda N, Kim HS, Desai KM, Krege JH, Laubach VE, et al. Elevated blood pressure in mice lacking endothelial nitric oxide synthase. Proc Natl Acad Sci USA 1996;93:13,176–13,181.
68. Bonnardeaux A, Nadaud S, Charru A, Jeunemaitre X, Corvol P, Soubrier F. Lack of evidence for linkage of the endothelial cell nitric oxide synthase gene to essential hypertension. Circulation 1995; 91:96–102.
69. Miyamoto Y, Saito Y, Kajiyama N, Yoshimura M, Shimasaki Y, Nakayama M, et al. Endothelial nitric oxide synthase gene is positively associated with essential hypertension. Hypertension 1998;32:3–8.
70. Yoshimura M, Yasue H, Nakayama M, Shimasaki Y, Sumida H, Sugiyama S, et al. A missense Glu298Asp variant in the endothelial nitric oxide synthase gene is associated with coronary spasm in the Japanese. Hum Genet 1998;103:65–69.
71. Shimasaki Y, Yasue H, Yoshimura M, Nakayama M, Kugiyama K, Ogawa H, et al. Association of the missense Glu298Asp variant of the endothelial nitric oxide synthase gene with myocardial infarction. J Am Coll Cardiol 1998;31:1506–1510.
72. Hibi K, Ishigami T, Tamura K, Mizushima S, Nyui N, Fujita T, et al. Endothelial nitric oxide synthase gene polymorphism and acute myocardial infarction. Hypertension 1998;32:521–526.
73. Markus HS, Ruigrok Y, Ali N, Powell JF. Endothelial nitric oxide synthase exon 7 polymorphism, ischemic cerebrovascular disease, and carotid atheroma. Stroke 1998;29:1908–1911.
74. Yoshimura M, Yasue H, Nakayama M, Shimasaki Y, Kugiyama K, Harada E, Hirashima O, Miyamoto Y, Kamitani S, Saito Y, Nakao K. A T⁻⁷⁸⁶-C mutation in the endothelial nitric oxide synthase gene affects coronary vasomotor responses and serum nitrite/nitrate levels. Circulation 1998;98:I–673(Abstr).
75. Tsukada T, Yokoyama K, Arai T, Takemoto F, Hara S, Yamada A, et al. Evidence of association of the ecNOS gene polymorphism with plasma NO metabolite levels in humans. Biochem Biophys Res Commun 1998;245:190–193.
76. Harrison DG. Cellular and molecular mechanisms of endothelial cell dysfunction. J Clin Invest 1997; 100:2153–2155.
77. Venema RC, Nishida K, Alexander RW, Harrison DG, Murphy TJ. Organization of the bovine gene encoding the endothelial nitric oxide synthase. Biochim Biophys Acta 1994;1218:413–420.
78. Uematsu M, Ohara Y, Navas JP. Regulation of endothelial cell nitric oxide synthase mRNA expression by shear stress. Am J Physiol 1995;269:C1371–C1378.
79. Sessa WC, Pritchard K, Seyedi N, Wang J, Hintze TH. Chronic exercise in dogs increases coronary vascular nitric oxide production and endothelial cell nitric oxide synthase gene expression. Circ Res 1994;74:349–353.
80. Miller VM, Vanhoutte PM. Enhanced release of endothelium-derived relaxing factor by chronic increases in blood flow. Am J Physiol 1988;255:H446–H451.
81. Sellke FW, Quillen JE, Brooks LA, Harrison DG. Endothelial modulation of the coronary vasculature in vessels perfused via mature collaterals. Circulation 1990;81:1938–1947.
82. Niebauer J, Cooke JP. Cardiovascular effects of exercise: role of endothelial shear stress. J Am Coll Cardiol 1996;28:1652–1660.
83. Robinson LJ, Weremowicz S, Morton CC, Michel T. Isolation and chromosomal localization of the human endothelial nitric oxide synthase (NOS3) gene. Genomics 1994;19:350–357.
84. Inoue N, Venema RC, Sayegh HS, Ohara Y, Murphy TJ, Harrison DG. Molecular regulation of the bovine endothelial cell nitric oxide synthase by transforming growth factor-beta 1. Arterioscler Thromb Vasc Biol 1995;15:1255–1261.

85. Hishikawa K, Nakaki T, Marumo T, Suzuki H, Kato R, Saruta T. Up-regulation of nitric oxide synthase by estradiol in human aortic endothelial cells. FEBS Lett 1995;360:291–293.

86. Weiner CP, Lizasoain I, Baylis SA, Knowles RG, Charles IG, Moncada S. Induction of calcium-dependent nitric oxide synthases by sex hormones. Proc Natl Acad Sci USA 1994;91:5212–5216.

87. Arnal JF, Clamens S, Pechet C, Negre-Salvayre A, Allera C, Girolami JP, et al. Ethinylestradiol does not enhance the expression of nitric oxide synthase in bovine endothelial cells but increases the release of bio-active nitric oxide by inhibiting superoxide anion production. Proc Natl Acad Sci USA 1996; 93:4108–4113.

88. Arnal JF, Yamin J, Dockery S, Harrison DG. Regulation of endothelial nitric oxide synthase mRNA, protein, and activity during cell growth. Am J Physiol 1994;267:C1381–C1388.

89. Liao JK, Shin WS, Lee WY, Clark SL. Oxidized low-density lipoprotein decreases the expression of endothelial nitric oxide synthase. J Biol Chem 1994;270:319–324.

90. McQuillan LP, Leung GK, Marsden PA, Kostyk SK, Kourembanas S. Hypoxia inhibits expression of eNOS via transcriptional and posttranscriptional mechanisms. Am J Physiol 1994;267:H1921–H1927.

91. Yoshizumi M, Perrella MA, Burnett JC Jr, Lee ME. Tumor necrosis factor downregulates an endothelial nitric oxide synthase mRNA by shortening its half-life. Circ Res 1993;73:205–209.

92. Lu JL, Schmiege LM, Kuo L, Liao JC. Downregulation of endothelial constitutive nitric oxide synthase expression by lipopolysaccharide. Biochem Biophys Res Commun 1996;225:1–5.

93. Diaz MN, Frei B, Vita JA, Keaney JF Jr. Antioxidants and atherosclerotic heart disease. N Engl J Med 1997;337:408–417.

94. Laufs U, La Fata V, Plutzky J, Liao JK. Upregulation of endothelial nitric oxide synthase by HMG CoA reductase inhibitors. Circulation 1998;97:1129–1135.

95. Drexler H, Zeiher AM, Meinzer K, Just H. Correction of endothelial dysfunction in coronary microcirculation of hypercholesterolemic patients by L-arginine. Lancet 1991;338:1546–1550.

96. Creager MA, Gallagher SJ, Girerd XJ, Coleman SM, Dzau VJ, Cooke JP. L-Arginine improves endothelium-dependent vasodilation in hypercholesterolemic humans. J Clin Invest 1992;90:1248–1253.

97. Egashira K, Katsuda Y, Mohri M, Kuga T, Tagawa T, Shimokawa H, et al. Basal release of endothelium-derived nitric oxide at site of spasm in patients with variant angina. J Am Coll Cardiol 1996;27: 1444–1449.

98. Quyyumi AA, Dakak N, Diodati JG, Gilligan DM, Panza JA, Cannon RO. Effect of L-arginine on human coronary endothelium-dependent and physiologic vasodilation. J Am Coll Cardiol 1997;30:1220–1227.

99. Pollock JS, Forstermann U, Mitchell JA, Warner TD, Schmidt HH, Nakane M, et al. Purification and characterization of particulate endothelium-derived relaxing factor synthase from cultured and native bovine aortic endothelial cells. Proc Natl Acad Sci USA 1991;88:10,480–10,484.

100. Hecker M, Sessa WC, Harris HJ, Anggard EE, Vane JR. The metabolism of L-arginine and its significance for the biosynthesis of endothelium-derived relaxing factor: cultured endothelial cells recycle L-citrulline to L-arginine. Proc Natl Acad Sci USA 1990;87:8612–8616.

101. Giugliano D, Marfella R, Verrazzo G, Acampora R, Coppola L, Cozzolino D, et al. The vascular effects of L-arginine in humans: the role of endogenous insulin. J Clin Invest 1997;99(3):433–438.

102. Pedrinelli R, Ebel M, Catapano G, Dell'Omo G, Ducci M, Del Chicca M, et al. Pressor, renal and endocrine effects of L-arginine in essential hypertensives. Eur J Clin Pharmacol 1995;48:195–201.

103. McDonald KK, Zharikov S, Block ER, Kilberg MS, Durante W, Liao L, et al. A caveolar complex between the cationic amino acid transporter 1 and endothelial nitric-oxide synthase may explain the "arginine paradox." J Biol Chem 1997;272:31,213–31,216.

104. Vallance P, Leone A, Calver A, Collier J, Moncada S. Endogenous dimethylarginine as an inhibitor of nitric oxide synthesis. J Cardiovasc Pharmacol 1992;20(Suppl 12):S60–S62.

105. Boger RH, Bode-Boger SM, Szuber A, Tsao PS, Chan JR. Asymmetric dimethylarginine (ADMA): a novel risk factor for endothelium dysfunction. Circulation 1998;98:1842–1847.

106. Goonasekera CD, Rees DD, Woolard P, Frend A, Shah V, Dillon MJ. Nitric oxide synthase inhibitors and hypertension in children and adolescents. J Hypertens 1997;15:901–909.

107. Vallance P, Leone A, Calver A, Collier J, Moncada S. Accumulation of an endogenous inhibitor of nitric oxide synthesis in chronic renal failure. Lancet 1992;339:572–575.

108. Kari JA, Donald AE, Vallance DT, Bruckdorfer KR, Leone A, Mullen MJ, et al. Physiology and biochemistry of endothelial function in children with chronic renal failure. Kidney Int 1997;52:468–472.

109. Boger RH, Bode-Boger SM, Thiele W, Junker W, Alexander K, Frolich JC. Biochemical evidence for impaired nitric oxide synthesis in patients with peripheral arterial occlusive disease. Circulation 1997; 95:2068–2074.

110. Bode-Boger SM, Boger RH, Kienke S, Junker W, Frolich JC. Elevated L-arginine/dimethylarginine ratio contributes to enhanced systemic NO production by dietary L-arginine in hypercholesterolemic rabbits. Biochem Biophys Res Commun 1996;219:598–603.

111. Cosentino F, Katusic ZS. Tetrahydrobiopterin and dysfunction of endothelial nitric oxide synthase in coronary arteries. Circulation 1995;91:139–144.
112. Stroes E, Kastelein J, Cosentino F, Erkelens W, Wever R, Koomans H, et al. Tetrahydrobiopterin restores endothelial function in hypercholesterolemia. J Clin Invest 1997;99:41–46.
113. Higman DJ, Strachan AM, Buttery L, Hicks RC, Springall DR, Greenhalgh RM, et al. Smoking impairs the activity of endothelial nitric oxide synthase in saphenous vein. Arterioscler Thromb Vasc Biol 1996;16:546–552.
114. Pieper GM. Acute amelioration of diabetic endothelial dysfunction with a derivative of the nitric oxide synthase cofactor, tetrahydrobiopterin. J Cardiovasc Pharmacol 1997;29:8–15.
115. Tiefenbacher CP, Chilian WM, Mitchell M, Defily DV. Restoration of endothelium-dependent vasodilation after reperfusion injury by tetrahydrobiopterin. Circulation 1996;94:1423–1429.
116. Verhaar MC, Wever RMF, Kastelein JJP, van Dam T, Koomans HA, Rabelink TJ. 5-Methyltetrahydrofolate, the active form of folic acid, restores endothelial function in familial hypercholesterolemia. Circulation 1998;97:237–241.
117. Cosentino F, Patton S, d'Uscio LV, Werner ER, Werner-Felmayer G. Tetrahydrobioprotein alters superoxide and nitric oxide release in prehypertensive rats. J Clin Invest 1998;101:1530–1537.
118. Vasquez-Vivar J, Kalyanaraman B, Martasek P, Hogg N, Masters BS, Karoui H, et al. Superoxide generation by endothelial nitric oxide synthase: the influence of cofactors. Proc Natl Acad Sci USA 1998;95:9220–9225.
119. Zeiher AM, Drexler H, Wollschlager H, Just H. Modulation of coronary vasomotor tone in humans. Progressive endothelial dysfunction with different early stages of coronary atherosclerosis. Circulation 1991;83:391–401.
120. Kugiyama K, Kerns SA, Morrisett JD, Roberts R, Henry PD. Impairment of endothelium-dependent arterial relaxation by lysolecithin in modified low-density lipoproteins. Nature 1990;344:160–162.
121. Shimokawa H, Flavahan NA, Vanhoutte PM. Loss of endothelial pertussis toxin-sensitive G-protein function in atherosclerotic porcine coronary arteries. Circulation 1991;83:652–660.
122. Freeman JE, Kuo WY, Drenger B, Barnett TN, Levine MA, Flavahan NA. Analysis of lysophosphatidylcholine-induced endothelial dysfunction. J Cardiovasc Pharmacol 1996;28:345–352.
123. Van DV, Bast A. Effect of oxidative stress on receptors and signal transmission. Chem Biol Interact 1992;85:95–116.
124. Liao JK, Clark SL. Regulation of G-protein alpha(i2) subunit expression by oxidized low-density lipoprotein. J Clin Invest 1995;95:1457–1463.
125. Panza JA, Garcia CE, Kilcoyne CM, Quyyumi AA, Cannon RO. Impaired endothelium-dependent vasodilation in patients with essential hypertension: evidence that nitric oxide abnormality is not localized to a single signal transduction pathway. Circulation 1995;91:1732–1738.
126. Cardillo C, Kilcoyne CM, Quyyumi AA, Cannon RO, Panza JA. Selective defect in nitric oxide synthesis may explain the impaired endothelium-dependent vasodilation in patients with essential hypertension. Circulation 1998;97:851–856.
127. Pieper GM, Dondlinger L. Glucose elevations alter bradykinin-stimulated intracellular calcium accumulation in cultured endothelial cells. Cardiovasc Res 1997;34:169–178.
128. Gryglewski RJ, Palmer RM, Moncada S. Superoxide anion is involved in the breakdown of endothelium-derived vascular relaxing factor. Nature 1986;320:454–456.
129. Ohara Y, Peterson TE, Harrison DG. Hypercholesterolemia increases endothelial superoxide anion production. J Clin Invest 1993;91:2546–2551.
130. Minor RL Jr, Myers PR, Guerra R Jr, Bates JN, Harrison DG. Diet-induced atherosclerosis increases the release of nitrogen oxides from rabbit aorta. J Clin Invest 1990;86:2109–2116.
131. Mugge A, Elwell JH, Peterson TE, Hofmeyer TG, Heistad DD, Harrison DG. Chronic treatment with polyethylene-glycolated superoxide dismutase partially restores endothelium-dependent vascular relaxations in cholesterol-fed rabbits. Circ Res 1991;69:1293–1300.
132. Hattori Y, Kawasaki H, Abe K, Kanno M. Superoxide dismutase recovers altered endothelium-dependent relaxation in diabetic rat aorta. Am J Physiol 1991;261:H1086–H1094.
133. Rajagopalan S, Kurz S, Munzel T, Tarpey M, Freeman BA, Griendling KK, et al. Angiotensin II-mediated hypertension in the rat increases vascular superoxide production via membrane NADH/NADPH oxidase activation. J Clin Invest 1996;97:1916–1923.
134. Jackson TS, Xu A, Vita JA, Keaney JF Jr. Ascorbate prevents the interaction of superoxide and nitric oxide only at high physiologic concentrations. Circ Res 1998;83:916–922.
135. Ting HH, Timimi FK, Boles KS, Creager SJ, Ganz P, Creager MA. Vitamin C improves endothelium-dependent vasodilation in patients with non-insulin-dependent diabetes mellitus. J Clin Invest 1996;97:22–28.

136. Ting HH, Timimi FK, Haley EA, Roddy MA, Ganz P, Creager MA. Vitamin C improves endothelium-dependent vasodilation in forearm resistance vessels of humans with hypercholesterolemia. Circulation 1997;95:2617–2622.
137. Taddei S, Virdis A, Ghiadoni L, Magagna A, Salvetti A. Vitamin C improves endothelium-dependent vasodilation by restoring nitric oxide activity in essential hypertension. Circulation 1997;97:2222–2229.
138. White CR, Darley-Usmar V, Berrington WR, McAdams M, Gore JZ, Thompson JA, et al. Circulating plasma xanthine oxidase contributes to vascular dysfunction in hypercholesterolemic rabbits. Proc Natl Acad Sci USA 1996;93:8745–8749.
139. Cardillo C, Kilcoyne CM, Cannon RO, Quyyumi AA, Panza JA. Xanthine oxidase inhibition with oxypurinol improves endothelial vasodilator function in hypercholesterolemic but not in hypertensive patients. Hypertension 1997;30:57–63.
140. Griendling KK, Minieri CA, Ollerenshaw JD, Alexander RW. Angiotensin II stimulates NADH and NADPH oxidase activity in cultured vascular smooth muscle cells. Circ Res 1994;74:1141–1148.
141. Pagano PJ, Clark JK, Cifuentes-Pagano ME, Clark SM, Callis GM, Quinn MT. Localization of a constitutively active, phagocyte-like NADPH oxidase in rabbit aortic adventitia: enhancement by angiotensin II. Proc Natl Acad Sci USA 1997;94:14,483–14,488.
142. Laursen JB, Rajagopalan S, Galis Z, Tarpey M, Freemam BA, Harrison DG. Role of superoxide in angiotensin II-induced but not catecholamine-induced hypertension. Circulation 1997;95:588–593.
143. Alderman MH, Madhavan S, Ooi WL. Association of the renin-sodium profile with the risk of myocardial infarction in patients with hypertension. N Engl J Med 1991;324:1098–1104.
144. Pritchard KA Jr, Groszek L, Smalley DM, Sessa WC, Wu M, Villalon P, et al. Native low-density lipoprotein increases endothelial cell nitric oxide synthase generation of superoxide anion. Circ Res 1995;77:510–518.
145. Chin JH, Azhar S, Hoffman BB. Inactivation of endothelium-derived relaxing factor by oxidized lipoproteins. J Clin Invest 1992;89:10–18.
146. Padmaja S, Huie RE. The reaction of nitric oxide with organic peroxyl radicals. Biochem Biophys Res Commun 1993;195:539–544.
147. Zembowicz A, Hatchett RJ, Jakubowski AM, Gryglewski RJ. Involvement of nitric oxide in the endothelium-dependent relaxation induced by hydrogen peroxide in rabbit aorta. Br J Pharmacol 1993; 110:151–158.
148. Wei EP, Kantos HE. H₂O₂ and endothelium-dependent cerebral arteriolar dilation. Implications for the identity of endothelium-derived relaxing factor generated by acetylcholine. Hypertension 1990;16: 162–169.
149. Vlassara H, Fuh H, Makita Z, Krungkrai S, Cerami A, Bucala R. Exogenous advanced glycosylation end products induce complex vascular dysfunction in normal animals: a model of diabetic and aging complications. Proc Natl Acad Sci USA 1992;89:12,043–12,047.
150. Adams MR, Robinson J, McCredie R, Seale JP, Sorensen KE, Deanfield JE, et al. Smooth muscle dysfunction occurs independently of impaired endothelium-dependent dilation in adults at risk of atherosclerosis. J Am Coll Cardiol 1998;32:123–127.
151. Weisbrod RM, Griswold MC, Du Y, Bolotina VM, Cohen RA. Reduced responsiveness of hypercholesterolemic rabbit aortic smooth muscle cells to nitric oxide. Arterioscler Thromb Vasc Biol 1997; 17:394–402.
152. Schmidt K, Klatt P, Mayer B. Hypercholesterolemia is associated with a reduced response of smooth muscle guanylyl cyclase to nitrovasodilators. Arterioscler Thromb 1993;13:1159–1163.
153. Thorne S, Mullen MJ, Clarkson P, Donald AE, Deanfield JE. Early endothelial dysfunction in adults at risk from atherosclerosis: different responses to L-arginine. J Am Coll Cardiol 1998;32:110–116.
154. Wilson PWF, D'Agostino RB, Levy D, Belanger AM, Silbershatz H, Kannel WB. Prediction of coronary heart disease using risk factor categories. Circulation 1998;97:1837–1847.
155. Scandinavian Simvastatin Survival Study Group. Randomized trial of cholesterol lowering in 4444 patients with coronary heart disease: The Scandinavian Simvastatin Survival Study (4S). Lancet 1994; 344:1383–1389.
156. Sacks FM, Pfeffer MA, Moye LA, Rouleau JL, Rutherford JD, Cole TG, et al. The effect of pravastatin on coronary events after myocardial infarction in patients with average cholesterol levels. N Engl J Med 1996;335:1001–1009.
157. Influence of pravastatin and plasma lipids on clinical events in the West of Scotland Coronary Prevention Study (WOSCOPS). Circulation 1998;97:1440–1445.
158. Downs JR, Clearfield M, Weis S, Whitney E, Shapiro DR, Beere PA, et al. Primary prevention of acute coronary events with lovastatin in men and women with average cholesterol levels. Results of AFCAPS/TexCAPS. JAMA 1998;279:1615–1622.

159. Treasure CB, Klein JL, Weintraub WS, Talley JD, Stillabower ME, Kosinski AS, et al. Beneficial effects of cholesterol-lowering therapy on the coronary endothelium in patients with coronary artery disease. N Engl J Med 1995;332:481–487.

160. Yeung A, Hodgson JM, Winniford M, Vita J, Klein L, Treasure C, Kern M, Plotkin D, Shih WC, Mitchel YB, Charbonneau F, Ganz P. Assessment of coronary vascular reactivity after cholesterol lowering. Circulation 1996;94:I–402 (Abstr).

161. The Long-Term Intervention with Pravastatin in Ischaemic Disease (LIPID) Study Group. Prevention of cardiovascular events and death with pravastatin in patients with coronary heart disease and a broad range of initial cholesterol levels. N Engl J Med 1998;339:1349–1357.

162. Stephens NG, Parsons A, Schofield PM, Kelly F, Cheeseman K, Mitchinson MJ. Randomised controlled trial of vitamin E in patients with coronary disease: Cambridge Heart Antioxidant Study (CHAOS). Lancet 1996;347:781–786.

163. Heitzer T, Yla HS, Wild E, Luoma J, Drexler H. Effect of vitamin E on endothelial vasodilator function in patients with hypercholesterolemia, chronic smoking or both. J Am Coll Cardiol 1999;33:499–505.

164. Anderson TJ, Meredith IT, Yeung AC, Frei B, Selwyn A, Ganz P. The effect of cholesterol lowering and antioxidant therapy on endothelium-dependent coronary vasomotion. N Engl J Med 1995;332: 488–493.

165. Enstrom JE, Kanim LE, Klein MA. Vitamin C intake and mortality among a sample of the United States population. Epidemiology 1992;3:194–202.

166. Levine GN, Frei B, Koulouris SN, Gerhard MD, Keaney JF Jr, Vita JA. Ascorbic acid reverses endothelial vasomotor dysfunction in patients with coronary artery disease. Circulation 1996;96:1107–1113.

167. Barrett-Connor E, Bush TL. Estrogen and coronary heart disease in women. JAMA 1991;265: 1861–1867.

168. Lieberman EH, Gerhard MD, Uehata A, Walsh BW, Selwyn AP, Ganz P, et al. Estrogen improves endothelium-dependent, flow mediated vasodilation in post menopausal women. Ann Intern Med 1994;121:936–941.

169. Hulley S, Grady D, Bush T, Furberg C. , Herrington D, Riggs B, et al. Randomized trial of estrogen plus progestin for secondary prevention of coronary heart disease in postmenopausal women. Heart and Estrogen/progestin Replacement Study (HERS) Research Group. JAMA 1998;280:605–613.

170. Pfeffer MA, Braunwald E, Moye LA, Basta L, Brown EJ Jr, Cuddy TE, et al. Effect of captopril on mortality and morbidity in patients with left ventricular dysfunction after myocardial infarction. N Engl J Med 1992;327:669–677.

171. Mancini GB, Henry GC, Macaya C, O'Neill BJ, Pucillo AL, Carere RG, et al. Angiotensin-converting enzyme inhibition with quinapril improves endothelial vasomotor dysfunction in patients with coronary artery disease. The TREND (Trial on Reversing Endothelial Dysfunction) Study. Circulation 1996;94:258–265.

172. Celermajer DS, Sorensen KE, Georgakopoulos D, Bull C, Thomas O, Robinson J, et al. Cigarette smoking is associated with dose-related and potentially reversible impairment of endothelium-dependent dilation in healthy young adults. Circulation 1993;88:2149–2155.

173. Leung WH, Lau CP, Wong CK. Beneficial effect of cholesterol-lowering therapy on coronary endothelium-dependent relaxation in hypercholesterolemic patients. Lancet 1993;341:1496–1500.

174. Egashira K, Hirooka Y, Kai H, Sugimachi M, Suzuki S, Inou T, et al. Reduction in serum cholesterol with pravastatin improves endothelium-dependent coronary vasomotion in patients with hypercholesterolemia. Circulation 1994;89:2519–2524.

175. O'Driscoll G, Green D, Taylor RR. Simvastatin, a HMG-coenzyme A reductase inhibitor, improves endothelium function within 1 month. Circulation 1997;95:1126–1131.

176. Drury J, Cohen JD, Veerendrababu B, Flaker G, Donohue TJ, Labovitz AJ. Brachial artery endothelium-dependent vasodilation in patients enrolled in the Cholesterol and Recurrent Events (CARE) Study. Circulation 1996;94:I–402.

177. Vogel RA, Corretti M, Plotnick GD. Changes in flow-mediated brachial artery vasoactivity with lowering of desirable cholesterol levels in healthy, middle-aged men. Am J Cardiol 1995;77:37–40.

178. Tamai O, Matsuoka H, Itabe H, Wada Y, Kohno K, Iamaizumi T. Single LDL apheresis improves endothelium-dependent vasodilation in hypercholesterolemic humans. Circulation 1997;95:76–82.

14

Nitric Oxide and Hypertension

M. Audrey Rudd,
María R. Trolliet, and Joseph Loscalzo

INTRODUCTION

Although hypertension has been studied extensively for decades, its etiology remains an enigma. An increase in systemic intravascular pressure or systemic hypertension can result from changes in two basic hemodynamic parameters: (1) a decrease in intravascular size as occurs during vasoconstriction, or (2) an increase in intravascular volume. The latter may occur as a result of either increased salt and water retention or cardiac output. Nitric oxide (NO•) has emerged as a critically important agent in the regulation of vascular tone, renal fluid and volume regulation, and cardiac function. Consequently, an alteration in NO• action on vessel tone, volume regulation, or heart function can lead to hypertension (Fig. 1).

There are at least five potential sites in the L-arginine/NO• pathway that, when deranged, can result in an apparent decrease in NO• bioactivity. These include (1) an alteration in intracellular substrate availability because of either a decrease in L-arginine transport or extracellular concentrations; (2) impaired NO• synthase (NOS) activity from mutations in the NOS genes, alterations in gene regulation, inhibition by endogenous or exogenous inhibitors, product feedback inhibition, or cofactor(s) deficiency; (3) increased metabolism of NO• to products with either no effect or detrimental actions that ultimately lead to potentiation of the pathogenesis and development of hypertension; (4) uncoupling of NO• and guanylyl cyclase (GC) as a result of enzyme dysfunction; and (5) alterations at any one of a number of signaling sites downstream from or independent of GC. This chapter reviews the literature on models of hypertension, as well as human essential hypertension, and presents evidence that implicates a role for the L-arginine/NO• pathway in either the etiology or maintenance of hypertension.

VESSEL TONE

Vessel tone is modulated by both vasoconstrictor as well as vasorelaxant substances released from the endothelium, as well as the neurohumoral system. Nitric oxide (NO•), a potent vasorelaxant and a modulator of endothelial vasoconstrictors and growth factors, has been shown to be one of the major contributors to basal vessel diameter or tone (1–7). Consequently, an impairment in NO• vascular action may be a significant contributing factor in the pathogenesis of hypertension. Vascular NO• that controls vessel diameter is synthesized principally by endothelial NO• synthase (eNOS). This enzyme can be stimulated to release NO• by increasing blood flow and consequently shear stress; receptor agonists such as bradykinin, serotonin, adenosine-5'-diphosphate, acetylcholine, thrombin, and substance P;

From: *Contemporary Cardiology, vol. 4: Nitric Oxide and the Cardiovascular System*
Edited by: J. Loscalzo and J. A. Vita © Humana Press Inc., Totowa, NJ

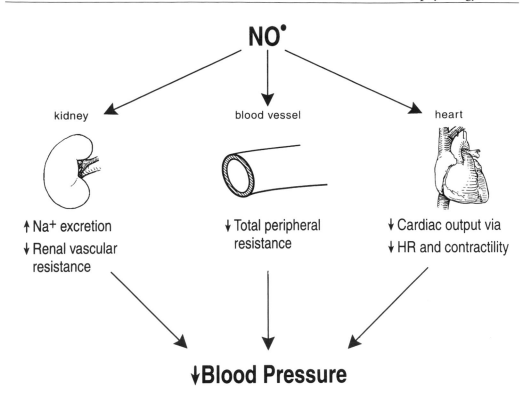

Fig. 1. The role of NO• in blood pressure regulation.

or calcium agonists *(8)*. NO• is also produced in vascular smooth muscle cells by inducible NOS (iNOS). However, iNOS is not present under normal conditions in the vasculature, but is expressed in states of inflammation. Additionally, iNOS has been reported to be present in fibroblasts located within the arterial adventitia, as well as microvascular endothelial cells *(9,10)*.

Because NO• appears to play a critical role in the normal maintenance of blood pressure (Fig. 1), many investigators in the area of hypertension have attempted to determine whether or not there is an abnormality in vascular NO• in animal models of hypertension as well as in humans with essential hypertension. Some of these data are reviewed next (*see* Table 1).

Endothelial Function

Over the years several animal models have been developed to mimic human essential hypertension. These models have been studied extensively to assess the role of NO• in the etiology of the development and maintenance of hypertension. One of the most widely studied models is the Okamoto and Aoki spontaneously hypertensive rat (SHR). This model is characterized by an early rise in blood pressure, perhaps even *in utero*, as compared with the normotensive control strain, the Wistar Kyoto rat (WKY) *(11)*. Using chronically instrumented rats, Smith and Hutchins demonstrated an increase in cardiac output in the early phase of hypertension (5–6 wk of age), followed by an increase in total peripheral resistance in later stages of hypertension (10–12 wk of age) *(12)*. There is modest but significant cardiac hypertrophy associated with the hypertension in this model *(13)*, and renal damage is often absent even in much older rats *(14)*. Vascular endothelial function has been examined almost exclusively in SHR in the established phase of the disease, i.e., older than 8 wk of age.

In vivo studies in SHR using NO• inhibitors, such as L-nitro-arginine methylester (L-NAME) and N^G-monomethyl-L-arginine (L-NMMA), reveal that NO• contributes to basal blood pressure similarly as in WKY *(15–18)*. Indeed, SHR excrete greater NO_X than WKY but less

Table 1
Vascular Actions of Nitric Oxide in Hypertension

Model	NO· bioactivity	Mechanism	Reference
Animals			
SHR	Decreased	Decreased NOS activity and increased NO· degradation	20–32 33,34
Goldblatt			
A-II dependent			
during clipping	Normal or elevated	Unknown	43–46
during unclipping	Normal or elevated	Unknown	47
A-II independent			
during clipping	Normal (increased early but returns to normal)	Unknown	52
during unclipping	Normal or elevated	Unknown	53–55
DOCA-salt			
Normal rats	Decreased	Increased NO· and cGMP, therefore decreased response due to uncoupling of NO·/GC and cellular response	59–61
Sabra	Decreased	Decreased NOS activity	4,63
Dahl salt-sensitive	Decreased	Decreased NO· and GC response to NO·	67–73
Humans	Decreased	Unknown	78–85

N^G,N^G-dimethyl-L-arginine (ADMA), an endogenous NOS inhibitor [19]. However, stroke-prone SHR cerebral vessels were unresponsive to superfusion with acetylcholine (ACh), whereas WKY vessels vasodilated [20]. These same authors reported similar findings in SHR basilar vessels [21]. A diminished L-arginine depressor response has also been observed in SHR relative to WKY [22]. Additionally, Chou and colleagues detected reduced eNOS activity as well as protein levels in aortic tissue of SHR compared to their normotensive counterparts [23].

In vitro studies show a consistent decrease or impairment in vascular responsiveness to stimulated NO· release using ACh. Decreased NO·-dependent relaxation has been noted in skeletal muscle arteries [24], coronary vessels [25,26], mesenteric arteries [27–29], and aortae [13,30,31]. Other investigators have shown increased contraction in response to vaso-constrictors, suggesting a decrease in endothelium-dependent relaxation [31,32]. In addition to measuring NO· release in endothelial cells from isolated vessels, investigators have also measured eNOS expression in the coronary arteries of isolated, perfused hearts from SHR and WKY. Crabos and associates found a decrease in eNOS expression in SHR, and the level of expression correlated inversely with the extent of NO·-dependent relaxation or L-NAME-induced vasoconstriction [25]. Other investigators have focused on NO· inactivation by super-oxide. Specifically, Tschudi and colleagues found increased superoxide production and subsequent NO· oxidation in aortae of older SHR compared with younger animals and with age-matched WKY [33].

Furthermore, Nakazono and colleagues observed a significant decrease in the blood pressure of SHR with superoxide dismutase treatment. There was a similar effect of oxypurinol, a potent inhibitor of xanthine oxidase and no effect of either agent, on the blood pressure of WKY rats [34]. Since xanthine oxidase may be a source of superoxide anion, this model of hypertension may involve increased oxidative stress.

Interestingly, endothelial function in 4-wk-old SHR is not impaired as compared to normotensive controls *(23)*. The level of eNOS protein and activity were not different from that
of WKY at this age, unlike what was observed in 14- and 64-wk-old animals when eNOS
activity and protein are decreased.

The majority of the studies, both in vivo and in vitro, overwhelmingly suggest that there
is an impairment in NO• activity in the established phase of hypertension in the SHR model.
The reduced NO• activity appears to be caused by both a reduction in enzymatic activity and
increased NO• oxidative inactivation by superoxide. Endothelial function appears to be normal
during the early phase of hypertension in this model.

Other models of spontaneous hypertension have not been studied as extensively as the SHR.
New Zealand spontaneously hypertensive rats appear to be more sensitive to NO• inhibition
as compared to their normotensive counterparts. Specifically, NO• inhibition causes a greater
rise in blood pressure as well as left ventricular hypertrophy in the hypertensive group
whereas controls exhibited neither hypertension nor hypertrophy *(34)*.

The role of NO• in animal models of renovascular hypertension has also been examined.
Both two-kidney, one-clip (2K–1C) and one-kidney, one-clip (1K–1C) Goldblatt hypertensive models have been studied. The 2K–1C model is characterized as an angiotensin II-
dependent model of hypertension *(36,37)*. Angiotensin II rises early in the development of
hypertension and remains elevated throughout the duration of the clip phase. Cardiac hypertrophy and renal damage are also observed in this model of hypertension *(38–41)*. Blood
pressure rapidly returns to baseline once the clip is removed *(42)*. Investigators have assessed
the role of NO• in both the hypertensive phase and during blood pressure normalization after
removal of the clip. NO• does not appear to be impaired during the hypertension; in fact, NO•
production is enhanced during the developmental phase *(43–45)*. Consequently, L-NAME
causes a similar increase in blood pressure in 2K–1C as in the sham controls. However,
Ortenberg and colleagues, using videomicroscopy, found a rightward shift in the ACh dose-
response curve in 2K–1C renal afferent arterioles *(46)*. Following removal of the clip, blood
pressure returns to control levels usually within hours, and L-NAME prevents the fall in blood
pressure following unclipping *(47)* suggesting a role for NO• in the renal response to restoration of perfusion in this model.

Unlike the 2K–1C model, 1K–1C is not angiotensin II-dependent. Angiotensin II is elevated during the early clip phase, but returns to baseline once hypertension is established. As
in the 2K–1C model, left ventricular hypertrophy occurs over time but without glomerular
damage *(39,48–50)*. The initial rise in blood pressure is attributed to an increase in cardiac
output, whereas the more established phase of hypertension is caused by an increase in total
peripheral vascular resistance *(48)*. Unclipping returns blood pressure to normal within 24 h
(51). Dubey and colleagues monitored urinary nitrite/nitrate as well as cyclic guanosine monophosphate (cGMP) levels during 5 wk of clipping *(52)*. They observed an increase in nitrite/
nitrate and cGMP during the first 2 wk, but the levels returned to baseline by wk 5. Additionally, other investigators found decreased aortic cGMP content and ACh-dependent relaxation after 4 wk of clipping *(53)*. As in the 2K–1C model, NO• may also play a role in the fall
in blood pressure following clip removal. Gerkens and associates observed an endothelium-
dependent inhibition of vasoconstriction by sympathetic stimulation following unclipping
(54). Otsuka and associates measured elevated cGMP levels in the aorta 2 wk after clip
removal *(53)*. L-NAME significantly reduced the fall in blood pressure, whereas *N*-acetyl-
L-cysteine (NAC) caused an earlier return of blood pressure to baseline compared to clip
removal alone *(55)*.

Whereas NO• is decreased in the 1K–1C angiotensin II-independent Goldblatt model of
hypertension, NO• appears to act compensatorily in the 2K–1C model of hypertension. In both
models NO• is involved in the return of blood pressure to control levels after removal of the
clip. However, the degree to which NO• is involved in the normalization of blood pressure

following the removal of the clip may differ between the two models. It appears that NO• is pivotal in this response in the 2K–1C model but is only partially involved in the 1K–1C model.

The DOCA salt model is another frequently used animal model of hypertension. Hypertension is produced in this model by removing one kidney and administering deoxycorticosterone acetate (DOCA) and salt. The Sabra rat is a genetically selected DOCA salt model. Sabra hypertensive rats were selectively bred for their sensitivity to DOCA salt, whereas their normotensive counterparts are resistant to this treatment (56,57).

As in the previous models, there is significant left ventricular hypertrophy (LVH) and renal hypertrophy and damage in DOCA salt rats (58,59). Isolated aortic rings from DOCA salt rats show no change in tension in the presence of L-NAME (60) and have a decreased relaxation response to ACh. However, Van de Voode and Leusen found that impaired aortic ACh responsiveness was not due to a decrease in NO• release but, possibly, the result of decreased sensitivity of the smooth muscle cell to NO• (61). Interestingly, Xu and colleagues detected increased cGMP levels in the aorta of DOCA salt hypertensives compared to normotensive controls (59). This observation suggests that the impaired relaxation to ACh is a consequence of abnormal responses downstream from guanylyl cyclase. In contrast, Hagen and associates found no difference in the coronary vessel response to ACh, prostaglandin, or sodium nitroprusside (62).

In the Sabra–DOCA salt model, investigators have observed a decrease in NO•-dependent regulation of basal blood pressure as assessed with L-NMMA administration (4). Rees and associates (4) measured decreased plasma nitrite/nitrate and eNOS protein in cultured aortic endothelial cells from Sabra hypertensive rats compared to normotensive Sabra controls. WKY rats had levels that were in between those of these two strains. Lippoldt and coworkers measured all three isoform gene expression in both Sabra normotensive and hypertensive strains (63). Although eNOS gene expression was different between the two groups, iNOS and nNOS gene expression values were lower in the hypertensive group.

Another frequently used animal model of hypertension is the Dahl salt-sensitive (DS) strain developed by Lewis K. Dahl in the early 1960s (64). The Dahl salt-sensitive rat is characterized by increased blood pressure in response to increased dietary salt, an impaired pressure natriuresis response, cardiac hypertrophy, and renal lesions (65,66); its inbred control is the Dahl salt-resistant (DR) model. Chen and Sanders found no change in arterial pressure in DS rats given L-NMMA, but an increase in blood pressure in DR rats (67). Thus, NO• does not appear to contribute to basal blood pressure regulation in the DS hypertensive rat. Additionally, Boegehold showed a decrease in the contribution of NO• to skeletal arteriolar tone in DS as compared to DR controls (67a). The aortic ring response to ACh is also reduced in the DS rat compared to the DR (68,69). Although urinary excretion of NO_x increases in Sprague–Dawley and DR rats during a high salt diet, it remains unchanged in the DS rat (70–72). Simchon and Manger also measured reduced levels of urinary cGMP in DS rats during a high-salt diet (73). Additionally, L-arginine significantly reduced the hypertension normally seen in DS animals when given with the high-salt diet (70). Clearly, the DS rat has an impairment in the L-arginine/NO• pathway; however, it is not clear whether or not this impairment pre-exists or occurs only in response to the initiation of a high-salt diet. Deng and Rapp found that the region of chromosome 10 containing iNOS cosegregated with hypertension when the DS rat is crossed with Milan and WKY rats (74). This was not the case for the eNOS or nNOS genes. There was no correlation of phenotype and genotype when DS and DR rats were compared; however, it should be noted that the authors used very few polymorphic allelic markers for their linkage analysis. Owing to the high common genetic background of the DS and DR rats, many more markers are required in order to detect differences between the two strains. Therefore, it is distinctly possible that the impaired NO• response may preexist rather than be induced during salt feeding; this conclusion, however, remains to be proved.

Very little evidence is available that addresses the involvement of NO• in other forms of experimental hypertension, such as aortic banding, angiotensin II infusion, and transgenic models of hypertension. Aortic banding studies reveal that 2 wk after banding, endothelium-dependent relaxations were unchanged in vessel segments above the coarctation *(60,75)*; eNOS expression as well as NO• release are also normal *(60)*. However, prolonged exposure to banding leads to reduced eNOS expression in both aortic and coronary vessels *(75)*, with a corresponding decrease in endothelium-dependent relaxation *(53,75)*. Otsuka also found lower cGMP levels as compared to sham-operated rats *(53)*. Other hypertensive models produced by catecholamine and angiotensin II infusion or transgenic animals that overexpress components of the renin–angiotensin system have been less well studied *(76,77)*. Limited available data suggest that NO• is involved as a compensatory mechanism to return blood pressure to control levels in these models.

Human essential hypertension clearly is a multifactorial disease. Despite its complexity, investigators have been able to identify some of the factors that appear to play pivotal roles in the pathogenesis of essential hypertension. In recent years the role of NO• has been given considerable attention. Some of the earliest studies examined the effect of NO• inhibition on blood pressure in hypertensives as well as normotensive controls; hypertensive patients had a smaller rise in blood pressure as compared with normotensives *(78)*. Subsequent studies have supported these findings. Specifically, ACh-induced vasorelaxation is diminished in the forearm as well as coronary vessels in hypertensives *(79–81)*. Moreover, Panza and coauthors reported a significant inverse correlation between blood pressure and basal NO•/EDRF release showing an attenuated response to L-NMMA administration among hypertensives *(80)*. Additionally, hypertensive patients have lower plasma nitrite\nitrate levels when compared to normotensive controls *(82–84)*. Specifically, Node and associates observed a correlation between plasma nitrite/nitrate levels and systolic blood pressure *(84)*. Furthermore, L-arginine infusions appear to normalize the impaired ACh response in hypertensive individuals *(85)*. In contrast, Panza and associates *(79)* noted that L-arginine failed to augment the acetylcholine response of hypertensives. Despite these consistent findings of impaired endothelial function from several laboratories, Cockcroft and colleagues found preserved endothelial function in hypertensive patients independent of their treatment status *(86)*. The reasons for these discrepant results remain unclear.

Because dietary salt has been shown to be an important factor in the expression of high blood pressure, Campese and colleagues compared the plasma excretion of NO_X in black salt-sensitive and salt-resistant patients *(87)*. Interestingly, plasma NO_X decreased during the high-salt diet and increased during the low-salt diet in both salt-sensitive and salt-resistant hypertensive blacks as compared to normotensive blacks. Plasma NO_X was not measured in salt-sensitive and salt-resistant white hypertensives. In a separate study Campese and associates observed a greater fall in blood pressure in the salt-sensitive group as compared to salt-resistant and normal subjects during L-arginine infusion *(88)*. However, the salt-sensitive group had less of an increase in renal plasma flow than in either the salt-resistant or control groups. More recently, one group in Japan found a missense variant in exon 7 of the eNOS gene in a Japanese population *(89)*; this polymorphism was significantly linked to essential hypertension in this population. In contrast, it appears that hypertensive patients with coronary heart disease (CHD) have higher plasma nitrite levels compared to nonhypertensive CHD patients *(90)*.

Clearly more studies are required before the nature of the role of NO• in human essential hypertension is understood. Perhaps in some populations and/or conditions, NO• from eNOS is compensatorily increased, whereas in others it is impaired. Additionally, there may be variations in iNOS function and activity that may account for differences in populations. Few studies have attempted to examine the separate roles of each NOS isoform in hypertension.

Smooth Muscle Cell

Attempts have been made to evaluate vascular smooth muscle cell (VSMC) function in the SHR in order to determine whether or not a decrease in VSMC responsiveness to NO• may also contribute to hypertension. However, studies that have used stimuli to increase NO• release from vessels show normal smooth muscle responses *(20)*. Cultured VSMC from 4–8 wk-old SHR show enhanced NO• production as demonstrated by measuring cGMP levels in VSMC *(91)*. Chou detected iNOS protein in 14- and 64-wk-old SHR VSMC, but not in young (4-wk-old) SHR VSMC; WKY VSMC did not appear to express iNOS at any time over the range of ages studied *(23)*.

The role of VSMC iNOS in this model of hypertension remains unclear. If there is enhanced iNOS expression and NO• release, then one would expect greater relaxation in SHR. However, this does not appear to be the case. Perhaps there is an imbalance in the determinants of vasoconstriction and vasorelaxation. In support of this view, Kung and colleagues found that SHR had elevated levels of vasoconstrictor prostanoids *(91a)*, and Hayakawa and Raij showed that the reduced endothelium-dependent aortic ring relaxation could be normalized with indomethacin pretreatment in these animals *(13)*.

Thickening of the vascular media often accompanies hypertension; however, the mechanism of the VSMC proliferation in the media is unclear. Hayakawa and associates measured eNOS activity and aortic hypertrophy in both SHR and DS models of hypertension, and they found that eNOS activity was enhanced in SHR relative to WKY, DS, or DR rats. DS rats had normal eNOS activity compared to DR rats *(13)*. Interestingly, SHR had significantly less aortic hypertrophy than DS rats despite a similar degree of hypertension. Although the authors did not separate the endothelial layer from the rest of the aorta prior to homogenization for NOS activity, they termed the activity as eNOS activity owing to its calcium dependence. Taken together, these data suggest that the increased iNOS in SHR VSMC may be a compensatory mechanism to prevent vascular hypertrophy and a counterbalance to the increased production of vascular (prostanoid) vasoconstrictors.

Vascular hypertrophy may be due to an imbalance between endothelin (ET) and NO•. DOCA–salt hypertensive rats that have a decrease in vascular NO• bioactivity overexpress ET-1 and have severe vascular hypertrophy. SHR rats that have increased aortic NOS activity have decreased ET-1 expression and, consequently, have far less hypertrophy than that seen in DOCA salt or DS hypertensive rats. In fact ET-1 B type receptors appear to lead to an increase in NO• release in SHR *(13,92–94)*.

VASCULAR VOLUME REGULATION

The kidney is a regulatory organ that plays a crucial role in the maintenance of a balanced internal environment, mainly water volume and solute composition. This organ achieves this goal by ultrafiltration of plasma at the glomerular level and selective tubular reabsorption of water and solutes. Thus, through its ability to regulate the amount of water and salt output, the kidney plays a pivotal role in the long-term control of arterial pressure. The basis for this homeostatic function, termed pressure-natriuresis, has been described by Guyton and collaborators *(95)*. According to this theory, if the blood pressure becomes too high, the renal excretion of water and sodium will increase, even surpassing net intake, so that blood volume will decrease to bring arterial pressure down to normal levels. Many factors, including neurotransmitters and hormones, may mediate and influence the renal pressure–natriuresis response. If any of these factors resets the relationship between arterial pressure and renal hemodynamics and excretory function to higher levels of blood pressure, hypertension may result. In this section, evidence that NO• plays an essential role in the maintenance of renal glomerular, vascular, and tubular function is presented.

Table 2
Localization of Different NOS Isoforms in the Kidney

NOS	Location	Method	Reference
nNOS	Macula densa	Immunohistochemistry,	95–98
		in situ hybridization	99
	Inner medullary collecting duct	RT-PCR	100
iNOS	Preglomerular afferent arteriole, postglomerular efferent arteriole	vsm-iNOS immunostaining	97–104
	Interlobular and arcuate arteries	RT-PCR + restriction mapping for vsm-iNOS	102
	Intercalated cells of collecting duct	Mac-iNOS immunostaining	105
	Mesangial cells, glomeruli, proximal tubules, medullary thick ascending limb, cortical and inner medullary collecting ducts	RT-PCR + restriction mapping for mac-iNOS	102
	Thick ascending limb, medullary collecting duct	Southern blot of cDNA	106
eNOS	Glomerulus, preglomerular vasculature	RT-PCR	108

NORMAL PHYSIOLOGY

Localization of NO• in the Kidney

Immunohistochemistry and *in situ* hybridization as well as reverse-transcriptase polymerase chain reaction (RT-PCR) have been used to detect NOS protein and mRNA, respectively in various regions of the kidney (Table 2). All three NOS isoforms are found in various renal structures (96). In the rat kidney, immunohistochemical and *in situ* hybridization techniques have demonstrated that nNOS is present in the macula densa (97–100). Bachmann and coworkers also found nNOS mRNA almost exclusively localized to the macula densa of rat and mouse kidney as shown by *in situ* hybridization (101). However, Terada and colleagues (102) demonstrated the presence of nNOS mRNA mainly in the inner medullary collecting duct using semiquantitative RT-PCR on mRNA from microdissected renal tubule segments. Weaker signals for this constitutive isoform of NOS were also detected in the cortical collecting duct, outer medullary collecting duct, glomerulus, vasa recta, and arcuate artery.

In addition, two distinct isoforms of the inducible NOS (iNOS) have been found in rat kidney (103,104). These isoforms appear to have distinct expression patterns along the nephron, and even though they are highly homologous, their expression is differentially regulated by cytokine stimulation (105) and dietary salt (106). These isoforms, vsmiNOS and maciNOS, were found to be closely related to the rat vascular smooth muscle iNOS isoform and to the cultured murine macrophages iNOS, respectively. Although these isoforms share 93% amino-acid sequence identity, they appear to represent proteins encoded by different genes (96). Only a single iNOS isozyme, however, has been identified in mouse and human kidney. Conflicting immunohistochemical localization of iNOS has been reported, and may be a consequence of the different molecular variants of iNOS. Immunostaining for vsmiNOS was observed in the preglomerular portion of the afferent arteriole, and, less consistently, in the initial efferent arteriole of unstimulated rat kidneys (99,106). Additionally, faint signals were present in the thick ascending limb, macula densa, and distal convoluted tubule. The use of macrophage-type iNOS polyclonal antibody found positive staining in intercalated cells of collecting ducts (107). Basal expression of mRNA for iNOS was found in rat kidney.

Southern blot analysis of iNOS cDNA from microdissected renal structures detected positive signals in the outer medulla, primarily in the thick ascending limb, with minor amounts in the medullary collecting ducts *(108)*. Additionally, abundant iNOS mRNA was also found in the glomerulus; lesser amounts were found in the cortical tubules and inner medulla.

To characterize the expression of both vsm- and mac-iNOS genes topographically and quantitatively, Mohaupt and collaborators *(104)* used quantitative PCR followed by restriction mapping of total RNA isolated from microdissected rat kidneys. The authors found that maciNOS mRNA was preferentially expressed in cultured mesangial cells, microdissected glomeruli, proximal tubules, medullary thick ascending limbs, and cortical and inner medulla collecting ducts. The vsmiNOS mRNA, however, was mainly found in the interlobular and arcuate arteries. Normal, unstimulated rat kidney was used for the localization of both vsm-, and maciNOS, as well as their respective mRNAs, suggesting that tonic influences along the rat nephron result in the constitutive expression of iNOS.

eNOS has also been detected in the kidney. It is found primarily within the endothelial cells of the vasculature *(109,110)*. Consequently, it is most abundant in the cortical region and less so in the outer and inner medullary regions. Using RT-PCR on microdissected renal structures, eNOS mRNA was detected at high levels in the glomerulus and preglomerular vasculature, and less consistently in preglomerular tubules, thick ascending limb, and cortical and inner medullary collecting ducts *(110)*.

NOS Activity and NO• Synthesis in the Kidney

Direct in vivo determinations of NO• are limited owing to its short half life (5–8 s). Since NO• is a potent stimulator of soluble GC, the presence of cGMP and/or NOS activity is considered indicative of NO• production in tissues. Biondi and collaborators *(111)* showed that incubation of canine renal cortex and renal medullary slices with endothelium-dependent vasodilators increased the production of cGMP. This effect was prevented by preincubating the tissue with the NOS inhibitor L-NMMA and was restored by preincubation with L-arginine. These results indicate that renal tissue is able to induce cGMP formation through NO• synthesis. Furthermore, the authors *(112)* demonstrated that the renal medulla, more specifically the inner and middle portions of the inner medulla, has a greater capacity for NO•-induced cGMP formation than the renal cortex. This result is consistent with the presence of the iNOS isoform in this same area. This isoform is a high-capacity enzymatic form of NOS and, thus, can produce high fluxes of NO•. Using NADPH-dependent diaphorase activity, two independent groups located a strong NOS signal in the rat macula densa segment *(100,101,113)*. This area corresponds to the localization of high levels of nNOS mRNA and protein *(101)*. Both, NADPH–diaphorase staining *(109)*, and immunohistochemical detection *(101)* confirm the presence of eNOS in the endothelium of the renal vasculature.

NO• and Renal Function

The importance of NO• in the regulation of peripheral vascular tone under physiological and pathophysiological conditions has been described in the first part of this chapter. In this section we focus on the role of NO• in the regulation of renal hemodynamics as well as salt and water homeostasis.

NO• AND RENAL HEMODYNAMICS

Renal blood flow (RBF) usually comprises 20% of cardiac output. Sufficient glomerular capillary hydrostatic pressure is needed to achieve an adequate single nephron glomerular filtration rate (SNGFR) and sodium excretion. This pressure level, which favors ultrafiltration, is dependent on RBF and on the tone of preglomerular (afferent) and postglomerular (efferent) arteriolar resistance vessels. In response to changes in systemic arterial pressure, renal autoregulation attempts to maintain constant glomerular capillary pressure by altering the relative tone of the afferent and efferent arterioles. Vasoactive agents, including NO˙, have profound effects on the regulation of these parameters.

The renal circulation appears to be especially sensitive to NO˙ blockade, as administration of NOS inhibitors at low doses that produce no change in systemic blood pressure significantly increase renal vascular resistance *(114)*. In several species, including humans, local intrarenal and low-dose systemic NO˙ blockade cause renal vasoconstriction without changes in arterial blood pressure *(114–119)*. This increase in renal vascular resistance (RVR) is usually accompanied by a reduction in RBF.

The effects of NO˙ blockade on GFR are, however, still controversial. Some investigators observed no change in GFR, whereas others found a reduction *(116,118,120–125)*. These differences may be a consequence of the dose and type of NOS inhibitor used, the use of anesthetics, the vagaries of experimental protocols used, or species differences *(126)*.

In vivo micropuncture studies *(114)*, as well as in vitro experiments on isolated microperfused afferent and efferent arterioles *(127,128)*, have shown that inhibition of renal NO˙ synthesis decreases afferent, but not efferent, arteriolar diameter. It appears that locally synthesized NO˙ exerts tonic control of the cortical afferent, but not the efferent, arteriole, and thus is capable of regulating glomerular capillary pressure *(129)*. Systemic pressor doses of NO˙ synthesis blockers, however, increase the resistance of both the afferent (R_A) and efferent (R_E) arterioles *(115)*, suggesting that changes in R_E in this situation appear to be the result of secondary phenomena dependent on systemic blood pressure changes and not directly on local NO˙ influences. It is not yet clear whether the vasoconstriction produced by NOS inhibition is due to the blockade of an active vasodilatory stimulus or to an amplification of vasoconstrictor responses *(96)*.

NO˙ AND NA+ HOMEOSTASIS

Although renal hemodialysis appear to be exquisitely sensitive to NO˙ inhibition, several studies demonstrated that renal excretory function is even more sensitive to NO˙ blockade *(130,131)*. The tubuloglomerular feedback (TGF) system is an important regulator of GFR and water and NaCl excretion in response to perturbations in total Na+ balance. The TGF response acts as a negative feedback loop wherein the macula densa senses both the composition and flow rate of the thick ascending limb fluid and sends a signal to modify the afferent arteriole tone and SNGFR accordingly *(132)*. Thus, when NaCl delivery to the macula densa increases, R_A decreases, and, consequently, GFR increases. In addition macula densa-dependent renin release decreases. During high-salt intake, a blunted TGF would thereby maintain SNGFR and NaCl excretion, preventing the development of a positive Na+ balance.

The predominant location of nNOS activity in the macula densa suggests that NO˙ is involved in TGF and modulation of renin release. There is general consensus that inhibition of intratubular NO˙ synthesis results in an enhanced vasoconstrictor response during high-salt intake, whereas with low-salt intake, TGF is minimally affected *(100,132–135)*. These results imply that juxtaglomerular NO˙ decreases the sensitivity of the TGF response in conditions of salt overload, thus providing the means to restore salt and water homeostasis.

The pressure–natriuresis response is a phenomenon by which increases in renal arterial pressure cause proportional increases in medullary blood flow and interstitial pressure, resulting in increased urinary Na+ excretion. A decrease in NO˙ production induced by the administration of NOS inhibitors reduces the kidney's ability to excrete Na+, so that higher levels of arterial blood pressure are required to restore natriuresis *(114,136,137)*. However, when NO˙ blockade leads to hypertension, the initial antinatriuretic effect is replaced by a marked natriuresis *(114,138)*. The data presented in this review suggest that impaired NO˙ production could increase the resistance in the renal vasculature, shift rightward the pressure–natriuresis relationship, and result in an exaggerated TGF response. These altered parameters result in a condition known as salt sensitivity, and, ultimately, hypertension. In salt sensitivity, the pressure–natriuresis curve is not only shifted toward higher perfusion pressures, but the slope is altered so that urinary Na^+ excretion becomes proportional to renal perfusion pressure *(139)*.

HYPERTENSION

NO• Localization and Activity

Very few studies have been performed to address localization of NOS protein or activity in the various models of hypertension. A recent study by Ikeda and colleagues measured all three isoforms within the kidney of the Dahl strain *(140)*. These authors found no difference in the eNOS and iNOS isoforms between DS and DR rats, but noted reduced nNOS in DS rats maintained on a 4% salt diet. Contrary to these results suggesting nNOS as the critical isoform involved in salt sensitivity, Deng and Rapp showed that blood pressure cosegregates with the iNOS gene and not the nNOS or eNOS gene *(74)*. Rudd and associates observed a rise in systolic blood pressure of DR rats during an 8% salt diet when given a selective iNOS inhibitor *(141)*. These data are consistent with earlier work of Mattson and Higgins *(125)* and Shultz and Tolins *(72)*, which indicate a positive correlation between salt intake and urinary nitrite/nitrate excretion in normal rats and diminished nitrite/nitrate excretion in DS rats on high salt. Urinary cGMP also is diminished in the DS strain during high-salt administration compared to their normotensive counterparts *(73)*. L-Arginine not only normalized the blood pressure in DS following a high increased salt intake, but also urinary cGMP excretion *(67)*. Additionally, lower urinary cGMP has been detected in response to atrial natriuretic peptide as well as sodium nitroprusside, suggesting that there may be a primary defect in the ability to generate cGMP in this salt-sensitive model.

NO• and Renal Function

Even fewer studies have been done to address the role of NO• in the regulation of renal function in hypertension. Simchon et al. *(142)* observed a profound increase in renal vascular resistance (RVR) long before total peripheral resistance is elevated in the DS rat model; thus, it appears that the kidney is exquisitely sensitive to decreases in NO• *(2,124)*. Inhibition of NO• production results in alterations in urinary salt and water excretion, renal vascular resistance, and peripheral resistance in this order of sensitivity *(2)*. Thus, if high salt leads to a decrease in renal NO• in a salt-sensitive model, this could lead to a significant increase in RVR before any change in total peripheral resistance. Interestingly, black hypertensive patients are often characterized by an increase in RVR and subsequent decreases in RBF as compared to whites or normotensives *(143,144)*. Approximately 75% of black hypertensives are salt sensitive as compared to only 50% of whites *(145,146)*. The elevated RVR may be the result of a reduction in NO• production in these individuals *(88)*. Furthermore, hypertensive blacks also have a decreased vasodilatory response to isoproterenol relative to white hypertensive patients *(147)*.

Lahera and coauthors reported that NO• deficiency can lead to volume-dependent hypertension, suggesting that NO• inhibition increases salt and water retention and subsequent volume expansion *(130,148)*. Animal models of hypertension with accompanying volume expansion may have deficient medullary NO• production. It remains controversial whether hypertensive patients, particularly black salt-sensitive patients, are volume expanded *(149–151)*. There is no definitive evidence for decreased renal NO• production as a contributing factor in the development of hypertension.

CARDIAC FUNCTION

Increased cardiac output (CO) can also lead to elevated blood pressure. CO may rise following increases in either heart rate, stroke volume, or both. Recent studies have localized

NOS in both endocardial as well as myocardial cell types *(152)*. eNOS is found in endothelial and endocardial cells, whereas both eNOS and iNOS isoforms have been found in myocytes *(153–155)*. Using the SHR model, Hayakawa and colleagues observed an increase in left ventricular eNOS activity compared to WKY *(13)*. However, in the same study, DS rats had normal eNOS activity relative to DR rats. It is interesting to note that the DS rat had a greater hypertrophic response than the SHR despite similar blood pressure levels. Kelm and coauthors measured NO• release from isolated perfused hearts from SHR and WKY rats *(156)*. There was a greater release of NO• from SHR relative to WKY and a decrease in NO• with L-NAME in SHR, suggesting a greater basal NO• synthesis in the hearts of SHR. These findings suggest that compensatory increases in NO•, primarily from eNOS, limit the degree of cardiac hypertrophy during hypertension.

NO• has been reported to have both inotropic and chronotropic actions (Table 3). Ballingand and colleagues, using isolated cardiac myocytes, demonstrated an inhibitory effect of NO• on the frequency of spontaneous contractions *(157,158)*. Analogs of cGMP also decreased contraction rate *(157)*. Furthermore, NO• reduced the effects of isoproterenol in the contraction frequency. However, contrary to these results, Musialek and associates reported that high NO• levels cause an increase in heart rate using a sinoatrial node/atrial preparation, an effect that can be mimicked by cGMP analogs and blocked by cGMP inhibitors *(160)*.

The ionotropic actions of NO• are also controversial. Ballingand and colleagues observed no basal effects of NO• on isolated rat cardiac myocyte contractility *(157)*. However, these authors found that NO• decreases the β-adrenergic-stimulated increase in contractility. Others have also reported decreased contractility with high doses of NO• donors and cGMP in papillary muscle *(153,159)*. On the other hand, Klabunde and associates found a reduction in left ventricular developed pressure in isolated perfused rat hearts with either NO• or cGMP inhibition *(161,162)*, whereas Kirstein and associates reported an increase in calcium current in human atrial myocytes with 3-morpholino-sydnonimine (SIN-1) treatment *(164)*.

The apparent discrepancy in NO• action in the heart may involve the relative levels of cAMP and cGMP. It is postulated that low levels of NO• reduce cAMP via the cGMP-inhibited isoform of cAMP-dependent phosphodiesterase *(161–164)*, whereas high levels may be cardiodepressant through the cGMP-protein kinase pathway. Exogenously administered NO• may produce levels that exceed normal ambient levels and evoke these effects through the cGMP-protein kinase pathway, whereas NOS and guanylyl cyclase inhibitors decrease endogenous NO• and cGMP levels, respectively, below normal with the effect of the cAMP pathway predominating *(159,165,166)*.

Cardiac hypertrophy is also observed in other models of hypertension, including hypertension caused by inhibition of endogenous NO• production *(13,39,50,59,167,168)*. In WKY treated with L-NAME, antihypertensive treatment prevented the increase in blood pressure but not the hypertrophy normally observed with L-NAME administration *(169)*. Similarly, Moreno and associates found that enalapril prevents the hypertension as well as the hypertrophy, but not the fibrosis, following L-NAME treatment in rats *(170)*. Hou and associates demonstrated profound angiotensin II-induced fibrosis in rats pretreated with L-NAME *(171)*. Thus, cardiac hypertrophy and fibrosis may result when there is a relative decrease in NO• or an imbalance in the relative levels of NO• and angiotensin II independent of arterial blood pressure.

There are few studies that have focused on the role of NO• on in vivo cardiac function in hypertensive animal models or in humans. L-NAME administration, which leads to hypertension, produces a decrease in heart rate (HR) and CO (probably secondary to the fall in HR) in rats *(172,173)*; however, other investigators found an increase in HR with L-NAME treatment in rats *(174–176)*. These differences appear to be caused by the duration of L-NAME exposure. Acutely, L-NAME causes bradycardia, whereas longer treatment (3–12 d) produces tachycardia *(173,175–177)*. Chronically, L-NAME appears to decrease cardiac vagal tone with a compensatory increase in cardiac muscarinic receptors *(175,176)*. However, the increased

Table 3
Effect of NO• on Cardiac Function

Cardiac function	NO• action	Agents used	Preparation	Reference
Inotropy	Increase	cGMP inhibitor	Isolated rat hearts	162
		NOS inhibitor	Isolated rat hearts	161
		NO• donor (low concentrations)	Cat papillary muscle	159
	Decrease	NO• donor (high concentrations)	Cat papillary muscle	159
		NOS inhibitor	Dogs Humans	152,153
Chronotropy	Increase	NO• donor (low concentrations)	Sinoatrial preparation	160
	Decrease	NO• donor (high concentrations)	Sinoatrial preparation	160
		Carbachol or cGMP analogs	Cardiac myocytes	157,158
		L-NAME	Cardiac myocytes	157
Morphology				
Hypertrophy	Decrease	L-NAME	1K–1C Goldblatt	52
		L-NAME	New Zealand rats	35
		L-NAME	Wistar,WKY	167, 169–171,174
		cNOS activity	DS	13
		None	DOCA salt	59
		cNOS activity	SHR	13
Fibrosis	Decrease	L-NAME + A-II	Wistar	171
		L-NAME	Wistar	170

ACh responsiveness is not adequate to overcome the tachycardic response to L-NAME. The bradycardia associated with acute L-NAME administration may be the result of the baroreceptor reflex response evoked by the rise in blood pressure. Perhaps ganglionic blockade would eliminate these differences in heart rate response to L-NAME treatment and, thus, allow for direct effects of L-NAME to be manifested. To date are there are no studies that have addressed directly the role of NO• in regulating blood pressure through its effects on cardiac function. However, one can postulate that if endogenous NO• levels have both negative inotropic and chronotropic actions, then impairment in NOS activity or increased NO• degradation could potentially lead to increased inotropy and chronotropy. Both of these effects would increase CO and subsequently blood pressure. Relevant to this point, increased CO has been measured in patients with borderline and essential hypertension (178–180) as well as in SHR and the models of angiotensin hypertension (12,48). Interestingly, the CO in the animal models is short-lived and hypertension is maintained through increased total peripheral resistance. These various cardiac effects of NO• are summarized in Table 3.

SUMMARY

The evidence from both animal models and humans suggests that NO• contributes significantly to the regulation of blood pressure in hypertension. The effect of NO• on vascular function in hypertension has been studied extensively. In some models of hypertension, vascular NO• is upregulated compensatorily in an attempt to return blood pressure to normal, and in other cases it is depressed and, thereby, may directly account for the rise in systolic blood pressure. The mechanisms by which NO• bioactivity is reduced vary depending upon the model and include (1) decreased NOS levels, 2) decreased GC activity, and (3) increased NO• degradation. The effect of NO• on vascular volume and CO is less well studied. The data suggest that NO• plays a critical role in the regulation of sodium excretion and that the renal L-arginine/NO• pathway may be impaired in hypertension. The nature and extent of the impairment is unclear at this time, as is the role of NO• in cardiac function in hypertension.

REFERENCES

1. Baylis C, Mitruka B, Deng A. Chronic blockade of nitric oxide synthesis in the rat produces systemic hypertension and glomerular damage. J Clin Invest 1992;90:278–281.
2. Lahera V, Khraibi AA. Nitric oxide inhibition in hypertension. NIPS 1994;9:268–274.
3. Moreno H Jr, Metze K, Bento AC, Antunes E, Zatz R, de Nucci G. Chronic nitric oxide inhibition as a model of hypertensive heart muscle disease. Basic Res Cardiol 1996;91:248–255.
4. Rees DD, Palmer RMJ, Moncado S. Role of endothelium-derived nitric oxide in the regulation of blood pressure. Proc Natl Acad Sci USA 1989;86:3375–3378.
5. Shesely EG, Maeda M, Kim HS, Desai KM, Krege JH, Laubach VE, Sherman PA, Sessa WC, Smithies O. Elevated blood pressures in mice lacking endothelial nitric oxide synthase. Proc Natl Acad Sci USA 1996;93:13,176–13,181.
6. Tolins JP, Palmer RMJ, Moncada S, Raij L. Role of endothelium-derived relaxing factor in regulation of renal hemodynamic responses. Am J Physiol 1990;258:H655–H662.
7. Kourembanas S, McQuillan LP, Leung GK, Faller DV. Nitric oxide regulates the expression of vaso-constrictors and growth factors by vascular endothelium under both normoxia and hypoxia. J Clin Invest 1993;92:99–104.
8. Busse R, Müisch A, Fleming I, Hecker M. Mechanisms of nitric oxide release from the vascular endothelium. Circulation 1993;87(Suppl):V18–V25.
9. Zhang H, Chobanian AV, Brecher P. Aortic adventitia is a source of nitric oxide: a possible paracrine role. Hypertension 1995;25:33.
10. Yang X, Chowdhury N, Cai B, Brett J, Marboe C, Sciacca RR, Michler RE, Cannon PJ. Induction of myocardial nitric oxide synthase by cardiac allograft rejection. J Clin Invest 1994;94:714–721.
11. Bruno L, Azar S, Weller D. Abscence of a pre-hypertensive stage in post-natal Kyoto hypertensive rats. Jpn Heart J 1979;20(Suppl):90–92.
12. Smith TL, Hutchins PM. Central hemodynamics in the developmental stage of spontaneous hypertension in the unanesthetized rat. Hypertension 1979;1:508–517.
13. Hayakawa H, Raij L. The link among nitric oxide synthase activity, endothelial function, and aortic and ventricular hypertrophy in hypertension. Hypertension 1997;29:235–241.
14. Dworkin LD, Feiner HD. Glomerular injury in uninephrectomized spontaneously hypertensive rats. A consequence of glomerular capillary hypertension. J Clin Invest 1986;77:797–809.
15. Arnal JF, Battle T, Ménard J, Michel JB. The vasodilatory effect of endogenous nitric oxide is a major counter-regulatory mechanism in the spontaneously hypertensive rat. J Hypertens 1993;11:945–950.
16. Chen HI, Hu CT. Endogenous nitric oxide on arterial hemodynamics: a comparison between normotensive and hypertensive rats. Am J Physiol 1997;273:H1816–H1823.
17. Fozard JR, Part M-L. Hemodynamic responses to N^G-monomethyl-L-arginine in spontaneously hypertensive and normotensive Wistar-Kyoto rats. Br J Pharmacol 1991;102:823–826.
18. Minami N, Imai Y, Hasimoto J, Abe K. Contribution of vascular nitric oxide to basal blood pressure in conscious spontaneously hypertensive rats and normotensive Wistar Kyoto rats. Clin Sci 1995;89:177–182.
19. Matsuoka H, Itoh S, Kimoto M, Kohno K, Tamai O, Wada Y, et al. Asymmetrical dimethylarginine, an endogenous nitric oxide synthase inhibitor, in experimental hypertension. Hypertension 29:1997;242–247.
20. Mayhan WG, Faraci FM, Heistad DD. Impairment of endothelium-dependent responses of cerebral arterioles in chronic hypertension. Am J Physiol 1987;253:H1435–H1440.
21. Mayhan WG. Impairment of endothelium-dependent dilation of basilar artery during chronic hypertension. Am J Physiol 1990;259:H1455–H1462.
22. Lin K-F, Chao L, Chao J. Prolonged reduction of high blood pressure with human nitric oxide synthase gene delivery. Hypertension 1997;30:307–313.
23. Chou T-C, Yen M–H, Li C-Y, Ding Y-A. Alterations of nitric oxide synthase expression with aging and hypertension in rats. Hypertension 1998;31:643–648.

24. Huang A, Koller A. Both nitric oxide and prostaglandin-mediated responses are impaired in skeletal muscle arterioles of hypertensive rats. J Hypertens 1996;14:887–895.

25. Crabos M, Coste P, Paccalin M, Tariosse L, Daret D, Besse P, Bonoron-Adèle S. Reduced basal NO-mediated dilation and decreased endothelial NO-synthase expression in coronary vessels of spontaneously hypertensive rats. J Mol Cell Cardiol 1997;29:55–65.

26. Fujita H, Takeda K, Nakamura K, Uchida A, Takenaka K, Itoh H, Nakata T, Sasaki S, Nakagawa M. Role of nitric oxide in impaired coronary circulation and improvement by angiotensin II receptor antagonist in spontaneously hypertensive rats. Clin Exp Pharm Physiol 1995;(Suppl 1):S148–S150.

27. Dohi Y, Thiel MA, Bühler FR, Lüscher TF. Activation of endothelial L-arginine pathway in resistance arteries. Effect of age and hypertension. Hypertension 1990;16:170–179.

28. Li J-S, Deng LY, Grove K, Deschepper CF, Schiffrin EL. Comparison of effect of endothelin antagonism and angiotensin-converting enzyme inhibition on blood pressure and vascular structure in spontaneously hypertensive rats treated with N^G-nitro-L-arginine methyl ester. Correlation with topography of vascular endothelin-1 gene expression. Hypertension 1996;28:188–195.

29. Matrougui K, Maclouf J, Lévy BI, Henrion D. Impaired nitric oxide- and prostaglandin-mediated responses to flow in resistance arteries of hypertensive rats. Hypertension 1997;30:942–947.

30. Gil-Longo J, Fernandez-Grandal D, Àlvarez M, Sieira M, Orallo F. Study of in vivo and in vitro resting vasodilator nitric oxide tone in normotensive and genetically hypertensive rats. Eur J Pharmacol 1996; 310:175–183.

31. Konishi M, Su C. Role of endothelium in dilator responses of spontaneously hypertensive rat arteries. Hypertension 1983;5:881–886.

32. Dohi Y, Kojima M, Sato K. Endothelial modulation of contractile responses in arteries from hypertensive rats. Hypertension 1996;28:732–737.

33. Tschudi MR, Mesaros S, Luscher T, and Malinski T. Direct in situ measurement of nitric oxide in mesenteric resistance arteries: increased decomposition by superoxide in hypertension. Hypertension 1996;27:32–35.

34. Nakazono K, Watanabe N, Matsuno K, Sasaki J, Sato T, Inoue M. Does superoxide underlie the pathogenesis of hypertension? Proc Natl Acad Sci USA 1991;88:10,045–10,048.

35. Ledingham JM, Laverty R. Nitric oxide synthase inhibition with omega-nitro-L-arginine methyl ester affects blood pressure and cardiovascular structure in the genetically hypertensive rat strain. Clin Exp Pharmacol Physiol 1997;24:433–435.

36. Carretero OA, Gulati OP. Effects of angiotensin antagonist in rats with acute, subacute, and chronic two-kidney renal hypertension. J Lab Clin Med 1978;91:264–271.

37. Martinez-Maldonado M. Pathophysiology of renovascular hypertension. Hypertension 1991;17: 707–719.

38. Averill DB, Ferrario CM, Tarazi RC, Sen S, Bajibus R. Cardiac performance in rats with renal hypertension. Circ Res 1976;38:280–288.

39. Cabral AM, Antonio A, Moyses MR, Vasquez EC. Left ventricular hypertrophy differences between male and female renovascular hypertensive rats. Braz J Med Biol Res 1988;21:633–635.

40. Delacrétaz E, Zanchi A, Nussberger J, Hayoz D, Aubert J-F, Brunner HR, Waeber B. Chronic nitric oxide synthase inhibition and carotid artery distensibility in renal hypertensive rats. Hypertension 1995;26:332–336.

41. Wilson C, Byrom FB. The vicious cycle in chronic Bright's disease. Experimental evidence from the hypertensive rat. Q J Med 1941;34:65–93.

42. Thurston H, Bing RF, Swales JD. Reversal of two-kidney one clip renovascular hypertension in the rat. Hypertension 1980;2:256–265.

43. Nakamoto H, Ferrario CM, Fuller SB, Robaczewski DL, Winicov E, Dean RH. Angiotensin-(1–7) and nitric oxide interaction in renovascular hypertension. Hypertension 1995;25:796–802.

44. Sigmon DH, Beierwaltes WH. Influence of nitric oxide in the chronic phase of two-kidney, one clip renovascular hypertension. Hypertension 1998;31:649–656.

45. Sigmon DH, Beierwaltes WH. Renal nitric oxide and angiotensin II interaction in renovascular hypertension. Hypertension 1993;22:237–242.

46. Ortenberg JM, Cook AK, Inscho EW, Carmines PK. Attenuated afferent arteriolar response to acetylcholine in Goldblatt hypertension. Hypertension 1992;19:785–789.

47. Bierwaltes WH, Potter DL, Carretero OA, Sigmon DH. Nitric oxide synthesis inhibition blocks reversal of two-kidney, one clip renovascular hypertension after unclipping. Hypertension 1995;25: 174–179.

48. Hall JE. Renal function in one-kidney, one-clip hypertension and low renin essential hypertension. Am J Hypertens 1991;4:523S–533S.

49. Ledingham JM, Cohen RD. Circulatory changes during reversal of experimental hypertension. Clin Sci 1962;22:69–77.

50. O'Sullivan JB, Black MJ, Bertram JF, Bobik A. Cardiovascular hypertrophy in one-kidney, one clip renal hypertensive rats: a role for angiotensin II? J Hypertens 1994;12:1163–1170.

51. Vandongen R, O'Dwyer J, Barden A. Release of prostaglandins during reversal of one-kidney, but not two-kidney, one clip hypertension in the rat. J Hypertens 1983;1:177–182.

52. Dubey RK, Boegehold MA, Gillespie DG, Rosselli M. Increased nitric oxide activity in early renovascular hypertension. Am J Physiol 1996;270:R118–R124.

53. Otsuka Y, DiPiero A, Hirt E, Brennaman B, Lockette W. Vascular relaxation and cGMP in hypertension. Am J Physiol 1988;254:H163–H169.

54. Gerkens JF. Unclipping of two-kidney, one clip hypertensive rats produces endothelium-dependent inhibition of sympathetic vasoconstriction. J Hypertens 1989;7:961–966.

55. Fenoy FJ, Tornel J, Madrid MI, López E, García-Salom M. Effects of N^G-nitro-L-arginine and N-acetyl-L-cysteine on the reversal of one-kidney, one clip hypertension. Am J Hypertens 1997;10:1208–1215.

56. Ben-Ishay D, Saliternik R, Welner A. Separation of two strains of rats with inbred dissimilar sensitivity to DOCA-salt hypertension. Experientia 1972;28:1321,1322.

57. Yagil C, Katni G, Rubattu S, Stolpe C, Kreutz R, Lindpaintner K, Ganten D, Ben-Ishay DY, Yagil D. Development, genotype and phenotype of a new colony of the Sabra hypertension prone (SBH/y) and resistant (SBN/y) rat model of salt sensitivity and resistance. J Hypertens 1996;14:1175–1182.

58. Dworkin LD, Feiner HD, Randazzo J. Glomerular hypertension and injury in desoxycorticosterone-salt rats on antihypertensive therapy. Kidney Int 1987;31:718–724.

59. Xu Y, Arnal JF, Hinglais N, Appay MD, Laboulandine I, Bariety J, Michel J-B. Renal hypertensive angiopathy: comparison between chronic nitric oxide suppression and DOCA-salt intoxication. Am J Hypertens 1995;8:167–176.

60. Pucci ML, Miller KB, Dick LB, Guan H, Lin L, Nasjletti A. Vascular responsiveness to nitric oxide synthesis inhibition in hypertensive rats. Hypertension 1994;23(Pt 1):744–751.

61. Van de Voorde J, Leusen I. Endothelium-dependent and independent relaxation of aortic rings from hypertensive rats. Am J Physiol 1986;250:H711–H717.

62. Hagen EC, Webb RC. Coronary artery reactivity in deoxycorticosterone acetate hypertensive rats. Am J Physiol 1984;247:H409–H414.

62a. Rees D, Ben-Ishay D, Moncada S. Nitric oxide and the regulation of blood pressure in the hypertension-resistant Sabra rat. Hypertension 1996;28:367–371.

63. Lippoldt A, Gross V, Schneider K, Hansson A, Nadaud S, Schneider W, Bader M, Yagil C, Yagil Y, Luft FC. Nitric oxide synthase and renin-angiotensin system gene expression in salt-sensitive and salt-resistant Sabra rats. Hypertension 1997;30:409–415.

64. Dahl LK, Heine M, Tassinari L. Effects of chronic salt ingestion: evidence that genetic factors play an important role in susceptibility to experimental hypertension. J Exp Medicine 1962;115:1173–1190.

65. Giardin E, Caverzasio J, Iwai J, Bonjour JP, Muller AF, Grandchamp A. Pressure natriuresis in isolated kidneys from hypertension-prone and hypertension-resistant rats (Dahl rats). Kidney Int 1980;18:10–19.

66. Rapp JP, Dene H. Development and characteristics of inbred strains of Dahl salt-sensitive and salt-resistant rats. Hypertension 1985;7:340–349.

67. Chen PY, Sanders PW. L-arginine abrogates salt-sensitive hypertension in Dahl/Rapp rats. J Clin Invest 1991;88:1559–1567.

67a. Boegehold MA. Enhanced arteriolar vasomotion in rats with chronic salt-induced hypertension. Microvasc Res 1993;45:83–94.

68. Lüscher TF, Raij L, Vanhoutte PM. Endothelium-dependent vascular responses in normotensive and hypertensive Dahl rats. Hypertension 1987;9:157–163.

69. Lüscher TF, Vanhoutte PM, Raij L. Antihypertensive treatment normalizes decreased endothelium-dependent relaxations in rats with salt-induced hypertension. Hypertension 1987;9:III193–III197.

70. Chen PY, Sanders PW. Role of nitric oxide synthesis in salt-sensitive hypertension in Dahl/Rapp rats. Hypertension 1993;22:812–818.

71. Hu L, Manning RD Jr. Role of nitric oxide in regulation of long-term pressure-natriuresis relationship in Dahl rats. Am J Physiol 1995;268:H2375–H2383.

72. Shultz PJ, Tolins JP. Adaptation to increase dietary salt intake in the rat. Role of endogenous nitric oxide. J Clin Invest 1993;91:642–650.

73. Simchon S, Manger W, Blumberg G, Brensilver J, Cortell S. Impaired renal vasodilation and urinary cGMP excretion in Dahl salt-sensitive rats. Hypertension 1996;27:653–657.

74. Deng AY, Rapp JP. Locus for the inducible, but not a constitutive, nitric oxide synthase cosegregates with blood pressure in the Dahl salt-sensitive rat. J Clin Invest 1995;95:2170–2177.

75. Bouloumie A, Bauersacks J, Linz W, Schölkens BA, Wiemer G, Fleming I, Busse R. Endothelial dysfunction coincides with and enhanced nitric oxide synthase expression and superoxide anion production. Hypertension 1997;30:934–941.

76. Deng X, Welch WJ, Wilcox CS. Role of nitric oxide in short-term and prolonged effects of angiotensin II on renal hemodynamics. Hypertension 1996;27:1173–1179.

77. Granger J, Schnackenberg C, Novak J, Tucker B, Miller T, Morgan S, Kassab S. Role of nitric oxide in modulating the long-term renal and hypertesive actions of norepinephrine. Hypertension 1997; 29:205–209.

78. Calver A, Collier J, Moncada S, Vallance P. Effect of local intra-arterial N^G-monomethyl-L-arginine in patients with hypertension: nitric oxide dilator mechanism appears abnormal. J Hypertens 1992; 10:1025–1031.

79. Panza JA, Casino PR, Badar DM, Quyyumi AA. Effect of increased availability of endothelium-derived nitric oxide precursor on endothelium-dependent vascular relaxation in normal subjects and in patients with essential hypertension. Circulation 1993;87:1475–1481.

80. Panza JA, Casino PR, Kilcoyne CM, Quyyumi AA. Role of endothelium-derived nitric oxide in the abnormal endothelium-dependent vascular relaxation of patients with essential hypertension. Circulation 1993;87:1468–1474.

81. Taddei S, Virdis A, Mattei P, Salvetti A. Vasodilation to acetylcholine in primary and secondary forms of human hypertension. Hypertension 1993;21:929–933.

82. Forte P, Copland M, Smith LM, Milne E, Sutherland J, Benjamin N. Basal nitric oxide synthesis in essential hypertension. Lancet 1997;349:837–842.

83. Nobunaga T, Tokugawa Y, Hashimoto K, Matsuzaki N, Nitta Y, Kimura T, et al. Plasma nitric oxide levels in pregnant patients with preeclampsia and essential hypertension. Gynecol Obstet Invest 1996; 41:189–193.

84. Node K, Kitakaze M, Yoshikawa H, Kosaka H, Hori M. Reduced plasma concentrations of nitrogen oxide in individuals with essential hypertension. Hypertension 1997;30:405–408.

85. Hishikawa K, Nakaki T, Suzuki H, Kato R, Saruta T. Role of L-arginine-nitric oxide pathway in hypertension. J Hypertens 1993;11:639–645.

86. Cockcroft JR, Chowienczyk PJ, Benjamin N, Ritter JM. Preserved endothelium-dependent vasodilation in patients with essential hypertension. N Engl J Med 1994;330:1036–1040.

87. Campese VM, Tawadrous M, Bigazzi R, Bianchi S, Mann AS, Oparil S, Raij L. Salt intake and plasma atrial natriuretic peptide and nitric oxide in hypertension. Hypertension 1996;28:335–340.

88. Campese VM, Amar M, Anjali CTM, Wurgaft A. Effect of L-arginine on systemic and renal hemodynamics in salt-sensitive patients with essential hypertension. J Hum Hypertens 1997;11:527–532.

89. Miyamoto Y, Saito Y, Kajiyama N, Yoshimura M, Shimasaki Y, Nakayama M, et al. Endothelial nitric oxide synthase gene is positively associated with essential hypertension. Hypertension 1998;32:3–8.

90. Ferlito S, Gallina M. Nitrite plasma levels in acute and chronic coronary heart disease. Minerva Cardioangiol 1997;45:553–558.

91. Xiao J, Pang PKT. Activation of nitric oxide synthesis in vascular smooth muscle cells and macrophages during development in spontaneously hypertensive rats. Am J Hypertens 1996;9:377–384.

91a. Küng CF, Lüscher TF. Different mechanisms of endothelial dysfunction with aging and hypertension in rat aorta. Hypertension 1995;25:194–200.

92. Clozel M, Breu V. The role of ETB receptors in normotensive and hypertensive rats as revealed by the non-peptide selective ETB receptor antagonist Ro 46–8443. FEBS Lett 1996;383:42–45.

93. Noll G, Wenzel RR, Luscher TF. Endothelin and endothelin antagonists: potential role in cardiovascular and renal disease. Mol Cell Biochem 1996;157:259–267.

94. Sventek P, Li JS, Grove K, Deschepper CF, Schiffrin EL. Vascular structure and expression of endothelin-1 gene in L-NAME-treated spontaneously hypertensive rats. Hypertension 1996;27:49–55.

95. Guyton AC, Coleman TG, Cowley AW Jr, Scheel KW, Manning RD Jr, Norman RA Jr. Arterial pressure regulation overiding dominance of the kidneys in long term regulation and in hypertension. Am J Med 1972;52:584–594.

96. Kone BC, Baylis C. Biosynthesis and homeostatic roles of nitric oxide in the normal kidney. Am J Physiol 1997;272:F561–F578.

97. Mundel P, Bachmann S, Bader M, Fischer A, Kummer W, Mayer B, et al. Expression of nitric oxide synthase in kidney macula densa cells. Kidney Int 1992;42:1017–1019.

98. Scmidt HHHW, Gagne GD, Nakane M, Pollcok JS, Miller MF, Murad F. Mapping of neuronal nitric oxide synthase in the rat suggests frequent co-localization with NADPH-diaphorase but not with soluble guanylyl cyclase, and novel paraneural function for nitrinergic signal transduction. J Histochem Cytochem 1992;40:1439–1456.

99. Tojo A, Gross SS, Zhang L, Tisher CC, Schmidt HHHW, Wilcox CS, Madsen KM. Immunocyto-chemical localization of distinct isoforms of nitric oxide synthase in the juxtaglomerular apparatus of normal rat kidney. J Am Soc Nephol 1994;4:1438–1447.

100. Wilcox CS, Welch WJ, Murad F, Gross SS, Taylor G, Levi R, et al. Nitric oxide synthase in macula densa regulates glomerular capillary pressure. Proc Natl Acad Sci USA 1992;89:11,993–11,997.

101. Bachmann S, Bosse HM, Mundel P. Topography of nitric oxide synthesis by localizing constitutive NO synthases in mammalian kidney. Am J Physiol 1995;268:F885–F898.

102. Terada Y, Tomita K, Nonoguchi H, Marumo F. Polymerase chain reaction localization of constitutive nitric oxide synthase and soluble guanylate cyclase messenger RNAs in microdissected rat nephron segments. J Clin Invest 1992;90:659–665.

103. Ito S. Nitric oxide in the kidney. Curr Opin Nephrol Hypertens 1995;4:23–30.

104. Mohaupt MG, Elzie JL, Ahn KY, Clapp WL, Wilcox CS, Kone BC. Differential expression and induction of mRNAs encoding two inducible nitric oxide synthases in rat kidney. Kidney Int 1994; 46:653–665.

105. Lau, KS, Nakashima O, Aalund GR, Hogarth L, Ujie K, Yuen J, Star RA. TNF-alpha and IFN-gamma induce expression of nitric oxide synthase in cultured rat medullary interstitial cells. Am J Physiol 1995;269:F212–F217.

106. Tojo A, Madsen KM, Wilcox CS. Expression of immunoreactive nitric oxide synthase isoforms in rat kidney. Effects of dietary salt and losartan. Jpn Heart J 1995;36:389–398.

107. Tojo A, Garg LC, Guzman NJ, Tisher CC, Madsen KM. Nitric oxide inhibits bafilomycin-sensitive H^+-ATPase activity in rat cortical collecting duct. Am J Physiol 1994;267:F509–F515.

108. Morrissey JJ, McCracken R, Kaneto H, Vehaskari M, Montani D, Klahr S. Location of an inducible nitric oxide synthase mRNA in the normal kidney. Kidney Int 1994;45:998–1005.

109. Bachmann S, Mundel P. Nitric oxide in the kidney: synthesis, localization, and function. Am J Kidney Dis 1994;24(1):112–129.

110. Ujiie K, Yuen J, Hogarth L, Danziger R, Star RA. Localization and regualtion of endothelial NO synthase mRNA expression in rat kidney. Am J Physiol 1994;267:F296–F302.

111. Biondi ML, Dousa TP, Vanhoutte PM, Romero JC. Evidences for the existence of endothelium-derived relaxing factor in the renal medulla. Am J Hypertens 1990;3:876–878.

112. Biondi ML, Bolterman RJ, Romero JC. Zonal changes of cGMP related to EDRF in dog kidney. Renal Physiol Biochem 1992;15:16–22.

113. McKee M, Scavone C, Nathanson JA. Nitric oxide, cGMP, and hormone regulation of active sodium transport. Proc Natl Acad Sci USA 1994;91:12,056–12,060.

114. Lahera V, Salom MG, Miranda-Guardiola F, Moncada S, Romero JC. Effects of N^G-nitro-L-arginine methyl ester on renal function and blood pressure. Am J Physiol 1991;261:F1033–F1037.

115. Deng A, Baylis C. Locally produced EDRF controls preglomerular resistance and ultrafiltration coefficient. Am J Physiol 1993;264:F212–F215.

116. Granger JP, Alberola AM, Salazar FJ, Nakamura T. Control of renal hemodynamics during intrarenal and systemic blockade of nitric oxide synthesis in conscious dogs. J Cardiovasc Pharmacol 1992;20: S160–S162.

117. Slangen B, Weaver C, Baylis C. Renal effects of low dose nitric oxide (NO) inhibition in the rat. J Am Soc Nephrol 1993;4(Abstr):569A.

118. Walder CE, Thiemermann C, Vane JR. The involvement of endothelium-derived relaxing factor in the regulation of renal cortical blood flow in the rat. Br J Pharmacol 1991;102:967–973.

119. Woltz M, Schmetterer L, Ferber W, Artner E, Mensik C, Eichler H-G, Krejcy K. Effect of nitric oxide synthase inhibition on renal hemodynamics in humans: reversal by L-arginine. Am J Physiol 1997;272: F178–F182.

120. Bech JN, Nielsen CB, Pedersen EB. Effects of systemic NO synthesis inhibition on RPF, GFR, U_{Na}, and vasoactive hormones in healthy humans. Am J Physiol 1996;270:F845–F851.

121. Haynes WG, Hand MF, Dockrell MEC, Eadington DW, Lee MR, Hussein Z, Benjamin N, Webb DJ. Physiological role of nitric oxide in regulation of renal function. Am J Physiol 1997;272:F364–F371.

122. Lahera V, Navarro-Cid J, Cachofiero V, García-Estañ, J, Ruilope LM. Nitric oxide, the kidney, and hypertension. Am J Hypertens 1997;10:129–140.

123. Manning RD Jr, Hu L. Nitric oxide regulates renal hemodynamics and urinary sodium excretion in dogs. Hypertension 1994;22:619–625.

124. Mattson DL, Roman RJ, Cowley AW Jr. Role of nitric oxide in renal papillary blood flow and sodium excretion. Hypertension 1992;19:766–769.

125. Mattson DL, Higgins DJ. Influence of dietary sodium intake on renal medullary nitric oxide synthase. Hypertension 1996;27:688–692.

126. Just A. Nitric oxide and renal autoregulation. Kidney Blood Press Res 1997;20:201–204.
127. Ito S, Arima S, Ren Y, Juncos LA, Carretero OA. Endothelium-derived relaxing factor/nitric oxide modulates angiotensin II action in the isolated microperfused rabbit afferent but not efferent arteriole. J Clin Invest 1993;91:2012–2019.
128. Ito S, Johnson CS, Carretero OA. Modulation of angiotensin II-induced vasoconstriction by endothelium-derived relaxing factor in the isolated microperfused rabbit afferent but not efferent arteriole. J Clin Invest 1991;87:1656–1663.
129. Raij L, Baylis C. Glomerular actions of nitric oxide. Kidney Int 1995;48:20–32.
130. Romero JC, Lahera V, Salom MG, Biondi ML. Role of endothelium-dependent relaxing factor nitric oxide on renal function. J Am Soc Nephrol 1992;2:1371–1387.
131. Salazar FJ, Alberola A, Pinilla JM, Romero JC, Quesada T. Salt-induced increase in arterial pressure during nitric oxide synthesis inhibition. Hypertension 1993;22:49–55.
132. Thorup C, Persson AEG. Inhibition of locally produced nitric oxide resets tubuloglomerular feedback mechanism. Am J Physiol 1994;267:F606–F611.
133. Ito S, Ren Y. Evidence for the role of nitric oxide in macula densa control of glomerular hemodynamics. J Clin Invest 1993;92:1093–1098.
134. Vallon V, Thomson S. Inhibition of local nitric oxide synthase increases homeostatic efficiency of tubuloglomerular feedback. Am J Physiol 1995;269:F892–F899.
135. Wilcox CS, Welch WJ. TGF and nitric oxide: effects of salt-intake and salt-sensitive hypertension. Kidney Int 1996;49(Suppl 55):S-9–S-13.
136. Guarasci GR, Kline RL. Pressure natriuresis following acute and chronic inhibition of nitric oxide synthase in rats. Am J Physiol 1996;270:R469–R478.
137. Krier JD, Romero JC. Systemic inhibition of nitric oxide and prostaglandins in volume-induced natriuresis and hypertension. Am J Physiol 1998;274:R175–R180.
138. Haas JA, Khraibi AA, Perella MA, Knox FG. Role of renal interstitial hydrostatic pressure in natriuresis of systemic nitric oxide inhibition. Am J Physiol 1993;264:F411–F414.
139. Romero JC, Strick DM. Nitric oxide and renal function. Curr Opin Nephrol Hypertens 1993;2: 114–121.
140. Ikeda Y, Saito K, Kim JI, Yokoyama M. Nitric oxide synthase isoform activities in kidney of Dahl salt-sensitive rats. Hypertension 1995;26:1030–1034.
141. Rudd MA, Trolliet M, Hope S, Loscalzo J. Dahl salt-resistant rat becomes salt-sensitive with inducible nitric oxide synthase inhibition. Am J Hypertens 1997;10:20A.
142. Simchon S, Manger WM, Brown TW. Dual hemodynamic mechanisms for salt-induced hypertension in Dahl salt-sensitive rats. Hypertension 1991;17:1063–1071.
143. Campese VM, Parise M, Karubian F, Bigazzi R. Abnormal renal hemodynamics in black salt-sensitive patients with hypertension. Hypertension 1991;18:805–812.
144. Frohlich ED, Messerli FH, Dunn FG, Oigman W, Ventura HO, Sundgaard-Riise K. Greater renal vascular involvement in the black patient with essential hypertension. A comparison of systemic and renal hemodynamics in black and white patients. Mineral Electrolyte Metab 1984;10:173–177.
145. Svetkey LP, McKeown SP, Wilson AF. Heritability of salt sensitivity on black Americans. Hypertension 1996;28:854–858.
146. Weinberger MH, Miller JZ, Luft FC, Grim CE, Fineberg NS. Definitions and characteristics of sodium sensitivity and blood pressure resistance. Hypertension 1986;8:II127–II134.
147. Lang CC, Stein CM, Brown RM, Deegan R, Nelson R, He HB, Wood M, Wood AJ. Attenuation of isoproterenol-mediated vasodilation in blacks. New Engl J Med 1995;332:155–160.
148. Lahera V, Salazar J, Salom MG, Romero JC. Deficient production of nitric oxide induces volume-dependent hypertension. J Hypertens 1992;10(Suppl):S173–S177.
149. Chobanian AV, Gqavras H, Melby JC, Gavras I, Jick H. Relationship of basal plasma noradrenaline to blood pressure, age, sex, plasma renin activity and plasma volume in essential hypertension. Clin Sci Mol Med 1978;4(Suppl):939–969.
150. Julius S, Esler M. Increased central blood volume: a possible pathophysiological factor in mild low-renin essential hypertension. Clin Sci Mol Med 1976;3(Suppl):2079–2109.
151. Safar ME, Chau, NP, Weiss YA, London GM, Simon AC, Milliez PP. The pressure-volume relationship in normotensive and permanent essential hypertensive patients. Clin Sci Mol Med 1976;50:207–212.
152. Brady AJB, Warren JB, Poole-Wilson PA, Williams TJ, Harding SE. Nitric oxide attenuates cardiac myocyte contraction. Am J Physiol 1993;265:H176–H182.
153. Brady AJB, Poole-Wilson PA, Harding SE, Warren JB. Nitric oxide production within cardiac myocytes reduces their contractility in endotoxemia. Am J Physiol 1992;262:H1963–H1966.
154. Kelly RA, Ballingand JL, Smith TW. Nitric oxide and cardiac function. Circ Res 1996;79:363–380.

155. Shultz R, Nava E, Moncado S. Induction and potential biological relevance of a calcium-independent nitric oxide synthase in the myocardium. Br J Pharmacol 1992;105:575–580.

156. Kelm M, Feelisch M, Krebber T, Deussen A, Motz W, Strauer BE. Role of nitric oxide in the regulation of coronary vascular tone in hearts from hypertensive rats. Maintenance of nitric oxide-forming capacity and increased basal production of nitric oxide. Hypertension 1995;25:186–193.

157. Ballingand JL, Kelly RA, Marsden PA, Smith TW, Michel T. Control of cardiac muscle cell function by an endogenous nitric oxide signalling system. Proc Natl Acad Sci USA 1992;90:347–351.

158. Joe EK, Schussheim AE, Longrois D, Mäki T, Kelly RA, Smith TW, Balligand JL. Regulation of cardiac myocyte contractile function by inducible nitric oxide synthase (iNOS): mechanisms of contractile depression by nitric oxide. J Mol Cell Cardiol 1998;30:303–315.

159. Mohan P, Brutsaert DL, Paulus WJ, Sys SU. Myocardial contractile responce to nitric oxide and cGMP. Circulation 1996;92:1223–1229.

160. Musialek P, Lei M, Brown HF, Paterson DJ, Casadei B. Nitric oxide can increase heart rate by stimulating the hyperpolarization-activated inward current, I(f). Circ Res 1997;81:60–68.

161. Klabunde RE, Kimber ND, Kuk JE, Helgren MC, Forstermann U. N^G-methyl-L-arginine decreases contractility, cGMP and cAMP in isoproterenol-stimulated rat hearts in vitro. Eur J Pharmacol 1992; 222:1–7.

162. Klabunde RE, Tse J, Weiss HR. Guanylyl cyclase inhibition reduces contractility and decreases cGMP and cAMP in isolated rat hearts. Cardiovasc Res 1998;37:676–683.

163. Kojda G, Kottenberg K, Nix P, Schulter KD, Piper HM, Noack E. Low increase in cGMP induced by organic nitrates and nitrovasolidators improves contractile response of rat ventricular myocytes. Circ Res 1996;78:91–101.

164. Kirstein M, Rivet-Bastide M, Hatem S, Agnès B, Mercadier JJ, Fischmeister R. Nitric oxide regulates the calcium current in isolated human atrial myocytes. J Clin Invest 1995;95:794–802.

165. Beckman JS, Koppenol WH. Nitric oxide, superoxide, and peroxynitrite: the good, the bad, and the ugly. Am J Physiol 1996;271:C1424–C1437.

166. Wahler GM, Dollinger SJ. Nitric oxide donor SIN-1 inhibits mammalian cardiac calcium current through cGMP-dependent protein kinase. Am J Physiol 1995;268:C45–C54.

167. Arnal JF, el Amrani AI, Chatellier G, Ménard J, Michel J-B. Cardiac weight in hypertension induced by nitric oxide synthase blockade. Hypertension 1993;22:380–387.

168. de Simone G, Devereux RB, Volpe M, Camargo MJ, Wallerson DC, Laragh JH. Relation of left ventricular hypertrophy, afterload, and contractility to left ventricular performance in Goldblatt hypertension. Am J Hypertens 1992;5:292–301.

169. Numaguchi K, Egashira K, Takemoto M, Kadokami T, Shimokawa H, Sueishi K, Takeshita A. Chronic inhibition of nitric oxide synthesis causes coronary microvascular remodeling in rats. Hypertension 1995;26:957–962.

170. Moreno H Jr, Nathan LP, Costa SKP, Metze K, Antunes E, Zatz R, de Nucci G. Enalapril does not prevent the myocardial ischemia caused by the chronic inhibition of nitric oxide synthesis. Eur J Pharmacol 1995;287:93–96.

171. Hou J, Kato H, Cohen RA, Chobanian AV, Brecher P. Angiotensin II-induced cardiac fibrosis in the rat is increased by chronic inhibition of nitric oxide synthase. J Clin Invest 1995;96:2469–2477.

172. Hu CT, Chang K-C, Wu CY, Chen HI. Acute effects of nitric oxide blockade with L-NAME on arterial haemodynamics in the rats. Br J Pharmacol 1997;122:1237–1243.

173. Gardiner SM, Compton AM, Bennett T, Palmer RM, Moncada SM. Control of regional blood flow by endothelium-derived nitric oxide. Hypertension 1990;15:486–492.

174. Araujo MT, Barker LA, Cabral AM, Vasquez EC. Inhibition of nitric oxide synthase causes profound enhancement of the Bezold-Jarisch reflex. Am J Hypertens 1998;11:66–72.

175. Cunha RS, Cabral AM, Vasquez EC. Evidence that the autonomic nervous system plays a major role in the L-NAME-induced hypertension in conscious rats. Am J Hypertens 1993;6:806–809.

176. Vasquez EC, Cunha RS, Cabral AM. Baroreceptor reflex function in rats submitted to chronic inhibition of nitric oxide. Braz J Med Biol Res 1994;27:767–774.

177. Gardiner SM, Compton AM, Bennett T, Palmer RM, and Moncada S. Regional haemodynamic changes during oral ingestion of N^G-monomethyl-L-arginine or N^G-nitrol-l-arginine methyl ester in conscious Brattleboro rats. Br J Pharmacol 1990;101:10–12.

178. Frohlich ED, Kozul VJ, Tarazi RC, Dustan HP. Physiological comparison of labile and essential hypertension. Circ Res 1970;27(Suppl1):55–69.

179. Julius S, Pascual AV, London R. Role of parasympathetic inhibition in the hyperkinetic type of borderline hypertension. Circulation 1971;44:413–418.

180. Messerli FH, de Carvalho JGR, Christie B, Frohlich ED. Systemic and regional hemodynamics in low, normal, and high cardiac output in borderline hypertension. Circulation 1978;58:441–448.

15 Nitric Oxide and Pulmonary Hypertension

John J. Lepore and Kenneth D. Bloch

INTRODUCTION

The pulmonary arterial vasculature, like the systemic arterial vasculature, is a dynamic system in which the resistance to blood flow is tightly regulated. Pathophysiologic states that perturb the normal control of pulmonary artery blood pressure result in significant clinical manifestations. The discovery of the central role of the nitric oxide (NO·) signal transduction system in the regulation of pulmonary arterial tone in health and disease has increased our understanding of the pathophysiology of pulmonary hypertension. In this chapter, we review (1) the causes, clinical manifestations, and epidemiology of pulmonary hypertension; (2) the biology of the NO·/cyclic guanosine monophosphate (cGMP) signal transduction system; (3) the production of NO· by NO synthase (NOS) isoforms in the lung and upper respiratory system and its regulation in fetal development; (4) the role of NO· in maintaining basal pulmonary vascular tone; (5) the role of NO· in modulating acute hypoxic pulmonary vasoconstriction; (6) the role of NO· in chronic pulmonary hypertension; (7) abnormalities of NO· production in human disease; and (8) the use of NO· and NO·-donor compounds for the diagnosis and treatment of pulmonary hypertension.

PULMONARY HYPERTENSION: CAUSES, CLINICAL MANIFESTATIONS, AND EPIDEMIOLOGY

In the normal adult, the total blood flow through the pulmonary circulation and the systemic circulation is similar. Because the resistance to blood flow in the pulmonary circulation is much lower than the resistance in the systemic circulation, a proportionally lower pressure gradient is necessary to pump blood through the pulmonary circulation than through the systemic circulation. Therefore, in the adult, the pulmonary artery pressure (normally 18–25 mmHg systolic, 6–10 mmHg diastolic, 12–16 mmHg mean) is considerably lower than the systemic blood pressure.

The pulmonary artery pressure is abnormally elevated in disease states that increase the resistance to pulmonary blood flow. Pathophysiologic mechanisms leading to the increased pulmonary vascular resistance include hypoxia, toxic effects of drugs (e.g., anorexogens and cocaine), infection (including human immunodeficiency virus [HIV]), increased pulmonary venous pressure secondary to left-sided heart disease (left ventricular systolic or diastolic dysfunction, mitral valve disease, aortic valve disease, systemic hypertension), obstruction to pulmonary flow (pulmonary emboli, congenital pulmonary arterial or venous strictures), increased

From: *Contemporary Cardiology, vol. 4: Nitric Oxide and the Cardiovascular System*
Edited by: J. Loscalzo and J. A. Vita © Humana Press Inc., Totowa, NJ

pulmonary blood flow secondary to congenital heart disease with left to right shunting (atrial septal defect, ventricular septal defect, patent ductus arteriosus), and narrowing of the pulmonary arterioles secondary to pulmonary vascular diseases (arteritis or collagen vascular diseases with pulmonary involvement, cirrhosis). Conditions in which the cause of pulmonary hypertension can be identified are referred to as secondary pulmonary hypertension.

Primary pulmonary hypertension, on the other hand, is a disease in which the specific etiology of pulmonary hypertension is not identified. This disease has an incidence of approx 2 per million per year, has a female-to-male predominance (approx 1.7:1), and typically presents between the ages of 20 and 50 *(1)*. The clinical course is characterized by progressive elevation of the pulmonary artery pressure associated with the development of dyspnea, fatigue, syncope, cor pulmonale, and death. The mean survival after diagnosis in untreated patients is approx 2.5 yr *(2)*, but survival can be significantly prolonged by treatment with anticoagulants and vasodilators.

There are a number of pathologic features in the lung that are shared by patients with chronic pulmonary hypertension from all causes, although all of the characteristic features are not present in every patient. In contrast to the endothelial monolayer that exists in normal pulmonary arteries, focal proliferations of endothelial cells, known as "plexiform" lesions, can impinge on the arterial lumen in patients with chronic pulmonary hypertension. In addition, the arterial lumen can also be narrowed by focal concentric lamellar formations of endothelial cells and extracellular matrix components, known as "onionskin" lesions. There is frequently subintimal proliferation and thickening caused by migration of smooth muscle cells (SMC) and deposition of extracellular matrix components. The media is often extensively thickened by hyperplasia of vascular SMC. In some cases, there is *in situ* thrombosis within abnormal pulmonary artery segments. Collectively, these pathologic changes in the pulmonary vasculature in chronic pulmonary hypertension are referred to as remodeling *(3,4)*.

The initial goal of treatment of chronic pulmonary hypertension (CPH) is to eliminate reversible causes by correcting hypoxia, discontinuing toxic agents, preventing *in situ* thrombosis and pulmonary thromboembolism with anticoagulation, treating systemic inflammatory conditions, eliminating congestive heart failure (CHF), and correcting valvular, coronary, or congenital heart disease (CHD). Patients in whom pulmonary hypertension persists are candidates for therapy with vasodilator medications. Effective oral vasodilators include nitrate preparations, such as isosorbide dinitrate, and calcium channel blockers, such as nifedipine. In patients with primary pulmonary hypertension, prolonged therapy with oral nifedipine can reduce symptoms, produce sustained reduction of pulmonary artery pressure and pulmonary vascular resistance (PVR), allow regression of right ventricular hypertrophy (RVH), improve exercise tolerance, and increase survival *(5–7)*. Unfortunately, patients with advanced pulmonary hypertension often have little or no response to vasodilators or cannot tolerate these agents because of systemic hypotension, because of RV dysfunction associated with the negative inotropic effects of calcium channel blockers *(8)*, or because of hypoxemia due to exacerbation of ventilation–perfusion mismatching. Patients with severe pulmonary hypertension who do not respond to or cannot tolerate oral vasodilators can be treated with continuous intravenous infusion of epoprostenol (prostaglandin I2, prostacyclin). Epoprostenol improves symptoms and prolongs survival, but is limited by high cost, systemic vasodilatation, catheter-related complications, and side effects including jaw pain and diarrhea *(9)*. Lung transplantation is an option for only a small number of patients with primary pulmonary hypertension because of the shortage of donor organs *(10)*.

Pulmonary hypertension can also afflict newborn babies. This unusual form of pulmonary hypertension is referred to as persistent pulmonary hypertension of the newborn (PPHN). In this condition, the physiologic pulmonary hypertension that exists in the fetal circulation fails to progress to the lower pulmonary pressure of the postnatal circulation. Many disorders have been associated with PPHN, including meconium or amniotic fluid aspiration, congenital diaphragmatic hernia, neonatal infection, and metabolic abnormalities. Pathologic changes in the lung include smooth muscle hypertrophy and adventitial thickening of the small pulmonary arteries (11). The clinical syndrome is characterized by labile pulmonary artery pressure, right-to-left intracardiac shunting, severe hypoxemia, and high morbidity and mortality (12). Standard therapy includes administration of oxygen and oral vasodilators, which have the same limitations in this condition as are encountered in adults with pulmonary hypertension. Infants with PPHN who do not respond to standard therapy frequently require extracorporeal membrane oxygenation.

Pulmonary hypertension of any etiology features, at least in part, a relative excess of vasoconstrictors (e.g., endothelins, angiotensin II) relative to vasodilators (e.g., prostacyclin, NO•). The remainder of this chapter is focused on the role of NO•, one of the vasodilators, in the pathogenesis of pulmonary hypertension.

THE NO•/CGMP SIGNAL TRANSDUCTION SYSTEM

NO• is a free radical molecule that is produced throughout the body and has diverse physiologic functions. For example, in the nervous system, NO• is an important neurotransmitter, and, in macrophages, NO• is a mediator of cell-mediated cytotoxicity (13). In blood vessels, the role of NO• as the principal mediator of endothelium-dependent vasodilatation has been elucidated over the past two decades. In 1980, Furchgott and Zawadzki (14) demonstrated that an intact endothelium and a labile endothelium-derived relaxing factor (EDRF) are necessary for the vasodilator effects of acetylcholine. In 1987, two groups (15,16) demonstrated that NO• accounts for the biologic activity of EDRF. The vasodilator action of many of the drugs prescribed for patients with pulmonary hypertension, including nitroglycerin and nitroprusside, depends on the release of NO• (17).

NO• is synthesized from L-arginine by three NOS isoforms in a cell-type and isoform-specific fashion. As reviewed in Chapter 2, NOSs are divided into two classes, constitutive and inducible. Constitutive NOSs were first isolated from neuronal cells (NOS1) and endothelial cells (NOS3) and are regulated by calcium and calmodulin. In contrast, the inducible isoform (NOS2) is typically present in cells only after exposure to bacterial endotoxin or cytokines and does not require increased intracellular calcium levels for activation

In normal blood vessels, the signal transduction system that leads to the release of NO• and ultimately to vasodilatation begins when a stimulus, such as acetylcholine, bradykinin, or shear stress, causes increased calcium levels in vascular endothelial cells. Calcium stimulates calmodulin to bind to and activate NOS3. NO• diffuses into the subadjacent vascular smooth muscle cells (VSMC) where it interacts with multiple intracellular targets, one of which is soluble guanylate cyclase (sGC) (Fig. 1). Binding of NO• to the heme group in sGC stimulates the conversion of guanosine triphosphate (GTP) to cGMP (reviewed in ref. 18). sGC is a heterodimer composed of α and β subunits linked by disulfide bonds, and at least four sGC subunits have been identified in the mammalian genome: $\alpha1$, $\alpha2$, $\beta1$, and $\beta2$. Although α and β subunits each have catalytic domains, both subunits are required for enzyme activity (19). cGMP exerts its effects on vascular cells, in part, through its action on cGMP-dependent protein kinase (cGDPK). The two isoforms of cGDPK detected in vascular smooth muscle, Ia and Ib, share the same substrate-binding/catalytic domain, but differ in cGMP affinity. Additional cGMP targets include cGMP-gated ion channels and cGMP-regulated cyclic nucleotide phosphodiesterases (20). Phosphodiesterases (PDEs) inactivate cGMP by converting it to GMP. At least five types of PDEs appear to participate in the metabolism of cGMP in pulmonary tissues, including Types 1, 2, 3, 5, and 9, two of which are cGMP-specific, Types 5 and 9 (21,22).

The effects of NO• on vascular cells may also be mediated by cGMP-independent mechanisms. NO• can serve as an antioxidant, opposing the effect of superoxides. The antioxidant

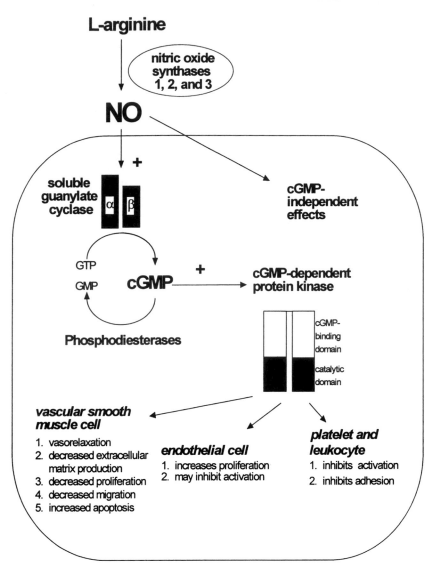

Fig. 1. The NO•/cGMP signal transduction system, In the lung, NO• is produced from L-arginine by three NOS isoforms (NOS1, NOS2, NOS3) in a variety of cell types including VSMCs, endothelial cells, bronchial epithelial cells, and macrophages. NO• diffuses into the cytoplasm of target cells and activates one of its receptors, soluble guanylate cyclase (sGC), which is a heterodimer composed of α and β subunits. sGC catalyzes the formation of cGMP from GTP. cGMP functions as a second messenger by activating cGMP-dependent protein kinase, which mediates the cell-specific effects of NO•. In VSMCs, NO• mediates VSMC relaxation and vasodilatation, decreased extracellular matrix production, decreased SMC proliferation and migration, and increased SMC apoptosis. Acting via cGMP-dependent protein kinase, NO• also inhibits activation and adhesion of platelets and leukocytes, prevents the activation of endothelial cells, and increases endothelial cell proliferation. An important regulatory step is the inactivation of cGMP by a family of PDEs. NO• also has cGMP-independent effects including changes in the intracellular redox state, and reaction with superoxides to form peroxynitrite.

properties of NO• appear to account for its ability to inhibit proinflammatory activation of endothelial cells *(23,24)*. In contrast, NO• may also react with superoxide to form peroxynitrite, which may be responsible for the cellular toxicity associated with high levels of NO• production *(25)*.

It is important to emphasize that increased pulmonary vascular tone is only one component of the pathophysiology of pulmonary hypertension. Additional processes that may be important in the development and maintenance of pulmonary hypertension include pulmonary vascular remodeling, platelet activation and *in situ* thrombosis, and apoptosis of pulmonary VSMC. There is abundant evidence demonstrating that NO• can modulate vascular endothelial and SMC proliferation, migration, apoptosis, and extracellular matrix synthesis *(26–29)*. In addition, NO• prevents adherence and activation of both platelets and leukocytes *(30,31)*.

PRODUCTION OF NO• IN THE LUNG

All three NOS isoforms contribute to pulmonary NO• production. Although NOS1 is predominantly localized to the central and peripheral nervous system, it has also been detected by immunohistochemistry in rats in the epithelium of terminal and respiratory bronchioli, but not in that of larger bronchi or in alveolar epithelial cells *(32)*. These observations were supported by Asano et al. *(33)*, who used the reverse-transcription polymerase chain reaction (RT-PCR) to detect NOS1 mRNA in cultured human bronchial epithelial cells. In normal human lung, Giaid *(34)* reported that NOS1 immunoreactivity was present in airway epithelium and SMCs, as well as in nerves and scattered macrophages. Of note, weak staining for NOS1 immunoreactivity was also detected in microvascular endothelium and the endothelium of larger pulmonary vessels.

High levels of NOS2 mRNA and protein have been consistently detected in pulmonary epithelial cells after exposure to inflammatory cytokines and bacterial lipopolysaccharide *(33)*. Compared with patients without airway inflammation, patients with asthma have increased NOS2 immunostaining in lung biopsy specimens *(35)* and increased concentrations of expired NO• *(36)*. Inflammatory cytokines also induce NOS2 expression in pulmonary alveolar macrophages *(37)*, VSMCs *(38)* and bronchial SMCs *(39)*. It remains controversial whether NOS2 is present in the normal lung in the absence of inflammatory conditions. Using immunohistochemical methods, Tracey et al. *(37)* found that NOS2 protein was not detectable in normal human lung tissue. Meng et al. *(40)* recently reported that, in normal human lungs, NOS2 immunoreactivity was detected only in macrophages and in occasional airway epithelial cells. In contrast, Guo et al. *(41)* detected both NOS2 mRNA and protein in airway epithelial cells from normal human lung tissue. This apparent discrepancy may reflect differences in the sensitivities of the techniques used to detect NOS2 expression.

In addition to NOS1 and NOS2, NOS3 has been detected in cultured human bronchial epithelial cells *(42)*. The role of NO• production by the three NOS isoforms in bronchial epithelium is incompletely defined. NOS3 is also present in pulmonary vascular endothelial cells *(43,44)*. Because of its location at the interface between VSMCs and intraluminal blood components, endothelial NOS3 is ideally situated to play an important role in the regulation of pulmonary vascular tone, pulmonary vascular remodeling, and *in situ* thrombosis. It is likely that, in noninflamed lung, NOS3 contributes most of the NO• that regulates pulmonary vascular tone. NO• production by NOS3 is regulated at the level of enzyme activation by intracellular calcium levels, enzyme intracellular localization and posttranslational modifications, substrate availability, and presence of cofactors such as nicotinamide adenine dinucleotide phosphate (NADPH), flavin adenine dinucleotide (FAD), and tetrahydrobiopterin (BH$_4$) *(45–47)*. Endothelial NOS3 expression is also spatially regulated with higher levels of expression in the endothelium of proximal pulmonary arteries compared with the pulmonary microvasculature *(48)*.

NO• released into the airways can be measured in the expired gas by chemiluminescence. In rabbits and guinea pigs, inhibition of NOS with the competitive inhibitors, N^G-nitro-L-arginine methylester (L-NAME) or N^G-monomethyl-L-arginine (L-NMMA), inhibits the release of NO•; and this inhibition can be overcome by administration of L-arginine *(49)*. In one study, mice with targeted deletion of the *NOS1* gene exhaled 60% less NO• than wild-type mice *(50)*, suggesting that *NOS1* makes an important contribution to total pulmonary NO• production. It is important to point out that the NO• measured in exhaled gas consists of NO• produced in both the lung and the upper respiratory tract. High levels of NO• are produced in the human paranasal sinuses *(51)*, and NOS2 and NOS3 mRNA and protein are present in human nasal mucosa *(52)*. In fact, nasopharyngeal NO• production may contribute importantly to pulmonary NO• levels. Settergren et al. *(53)* observed, in patients recovering from cardiac surgery, that nasal breathing (inspiration through the nose, expiration through the mouth) was associated with lower PVR than was associated with mouth breathing (inspiration thought the mouth, expiration through the nose). Exhaled NO• appears to be produced predominantly in the airways and not in the pulmonary vasculature because of the very low concentration of NO• in expired gas at end-expiration *(54,55)*.

Because of the dramatic changes in pulmonary vascular resistance that occur at birth, and because of the important contribution of NO• to perinatal pulmonary vasodilatation, the developmental regulation of pulmonary NOS expression has been extensively investigated. In the fetus, gas exchange takes place in the placenta, pulmonary blood flow is low, and high pulmonary artery pressures shunt right-sided blood flow into the systemic circulation through the foramen ovale and ductus arteriosus. At birth, with the initiation of ventilation, pulmonary vascular resistance (PVR) falls rapidly and pulmonary blood flow increases. A role for NO• in perinatal pulmonary vasodilatation is supported by observations, in fetal lambs, that administration of NOS inhibitors immediately prior to birth attenuated the increase in pulmonary blood flow associated with the onset of neonatal ventilation *(56–58)*. Moreover, longer-term antenatal NOS inhibition (10 d in the fetal lamb model) results in persistence of fetal pulmonary hypertension, which is reminiscent of the findings in persistent pulmonary hypertension of the newborn *(59)*. On the other hand, the pulmonary vascular transition from fetus to neonate does not appear to be impaired in mice deficient in any one of the NOS isoforms *(60)*. It is possible that other NOS isoforms or other vasodilators can compensate for the deficiency of a single NOS isoform during the perinatal pulmonary period.

All three NOS isoforms have been detected in the lungs of neonatal animals. North et al. *(61)* detected high levels of NOS1 and NOS3 mRNA and protein in lungs of fetal rats late in gestation. Kawai et al. *(62)* found that pulmonary *NOS3* gene expression in rats was highest just after birth and that NOS3 mRNA and protein levels declined during the postnatal period. Using *in situ* hybridization, these investigators also observed that the distribution of NOS3 mRNA in the lungs was developmentally regulated: in the neonate, abundant NOS3 mRNA was detected in the alveolar and serosal epithelial cells, as well as the vascular endothelium, whereas in the adult, *NOS3* gene expression was largely confined to the vascular endothelium. Rairigh et al. *(63)* identified NOS2 mRNA in the ovine fetal lung and demonstrated that administration of NOS2-selective inhibitors attenuated the pulmonary vasodilatation induced by ventilation suggesting that NOS2, probably in addition to NOS1 and NOS3, participates in the perinatal decrease in PVR.

It is important to note that the mechanisms responsible for pulmonary responsiveness to NO•, as well as NO• production, are developmentally regulated. For example, sGC, a NO• receptor *(64)*, and PDE 5, a cGMP-specific PDE *(65,66)*, are abundant in lungs of rats during the perinatal period. Interestingly, like NOS3, the distribution of mRNAs encoding sGC subunits and PDE5 is developmentally regulated in the lungs of rats. In the lungs of neonatal rats, sGC and PDE5 appear to be localized in the alveolar epithelium, as well as the vascular and bronchial smooth muscle, suggesting an important nonvascular role for pulmonary NO•/cGMP signal transduction during the perinatal period.

In summary, NO• is produced by three different NOS isoforms in many pulmonary cell types including bronchial and alveolar epithelium, bronchial and VSMCs, vascular endothelium, and alveolar macrophages. NO• production is spatially and developmentally regulated at the level of NOS isoform gene expression and enzyme activity, as well as at the level of NO$^\bullet$ responsiveness.

ROLE OF NO$^\bullet$ IN MAINTAINING BASAL PULMONARY VASCULAR TONE

Although the initial experiments leading to the identification of NO$^\bullet$ as EDRF were conducted in preparations of aortic endothelial cells, the potential role of NO$^\bullet$ in mediating pulmonary vascular tone was immediately appreciated. It was quickly demonstrated that EDRF produced in pulmonary arteries is also identical to NO$^\bullet$ *(67,68)*, that pulmonary artery endothelial cells produce NO$^\bullet$ in response to the vasodilator stimuli including acetylcholine or bradykinin *(67,69,70)*, and that NOS inhibitors block the pulmonary vascular response to these endothelium-dependent vasodilators *(71)*.

It was not immediately clear from animal models whether basal NO$^\bullet$ release is required to maintain normally low basal pulmonary tone. Several studies *(72–74)* demonstrated that inhibition of NO$^\bullet$ synthesis by exposure to L-NMMA or L-NAME did not change the baseline PVR, whereas other studies *(75–78)* indicated that administration of NOS inhibitors caused pulmonary vasoconstriction (reviewed in ref. 79). It is likely that some of the differences in the reported observations can be attributed to species differences. The notion that NO$^\bullet$ production by NOS3 can contribute to low basal PVR is supported by the observation that mice with targeted deletion of the *NOS3* gene have mild pulmonary hypertension relative to wild-type mice *(80)*.

Evidence that NO$^\bullet$ participates in the maintenance of normal basal pulmonary arterial tone in humans comes from a study in which L-NMMA was administered intravenously to healthy volunteers under normoxic conditions during right heart catheterization *(81)*. Administration of this NOS inhibitor resulted in an increase in systemic blood pressure (by 16%), an increase in systemic and PVR (by 63 and 40%, respectively), and a decrease in CO (by 28%). Similarly, Cooper et al. *(82)* observed, in normal human volunteers, that administration of L-NMMA selectively into a segmental lower lobe pulmonary artery decreased pulmonary arterial blood flow. These studies indicate that, in humans, basal production of NO$^\bullet$ is important for maintaining normal basal tone in both the systemic and the pulmonary arterial beds.

THE ROLE OF NO$^\bullet$ IN ACUTE HYPOXIC PULMONARY VASOCONSTRICTION

More than a century ago *(83)*, it was observed that acute alveolar hypoxia produces diffuse pulmonary vasoconstriction in humans that is readily reversible when the inspired oxygen tension is returned to normal. The anatomic site of most pronounced vasoconstriction is the small, muscular pulmonary artery *(84,85)*. Recent investigations have sought to define the cellular and molecular mechanisms responsible for the vasoconstrictor response to hypoxia. In pulmonary VSMCs, pathophysiologic processes associated with the development of hypoxic pulmonary vasoconstriction include shifts in the redox state *(86)*, inhibition of plasma membrane potassium channels *(87,88)*, activation of voltage-gated calcium channels *(89)*, and increases in intracellular calcium *(90)*. Exactly how these cellular and molecular events interact to produce hypoxic vasoconstriction is incompletely understood (reviewed in ref. *91*), but it does appear that NO$^\bullet$ is capable of modulating the process.

Experiments investigating the role of NO$^\bullet$ in modulating hypoxic pulmonary vasoconstriction have yielded conflicting results. Several experiments on pulmonary vascular rings from animals exposed to acute hypoxia have indicated that endothelial denudation abolishes hypoxic pulmonary vasoconstriction *(92,93)*, raising the possibility that NO$^\bullet$ or another endothelium-dependent factor contributes to hypoxic vasoconstriction. In contrast, other findings have suggested that hypoxic pulmonary vasoconstriction can occur in the absence of endo-thelium *(94,95)* and even in isolated pulmonary VSMCs *(96)*. These conflicting findings may be explained by differences in the species and vessel type (conduit vs resistance) studied, as well as the duration of hypoxia. For example, Leach et al. *(97)* found that endothelial denuda-tion of rat pulmonary vascular rings limited hypoxic vasoconstriction in small, but not large pulmonary artery segments.

The regulation of NO• production during acute hypoxia is highly complex. Although studies on pulmonary vascular rings from rats *(92)* and rabbits *(98)* have demonstrated that acute hypoxia is associated with decreased endothelium-dependent vasodilatation, it remained unclear whether NO• production is increased or decreased. In one study of isolated rat pulmonary artery segments, NO• production was decreased during acute hypoxia *(99)*. In contrast, studies in pulmonary vascular endothelial cells in culture have indicated that NO• production is increased during acute hypoxia *(100)*. Studies evaluating the regulation by oxygen of NOS3 expression have also yielded conflicting results. In most studies of cultured endothelial cells, NOS3 mRNA and protein levels were decreased during acute hypoxia *(101–104)*, whereas NOS3 mRNA was increased in the lungs of rats exposed to acute hypoxia *(105)*. Dweik et al. *(54)* suggested that an oxygen-sensitive mechanism participates in the regulation of pulmonary NO• production. They showed that the amount of NO• expired into the bronchi of human subjects was directly proportional to the inspired oxygen concen-tration. Because the in vivo K_mO_2 for NO• production was similar to the in vitro K_mO_2 for NO• production by purified NOS2, these authors proposed that the oxygen-sensitive source of NO• production in the bronchial epithelium is NOS2.

Evidence in favor of a role for NO• in limiting hypoxic vasoconstriction has come from experiments in isolated perfused rat lungs in which inhibitors of NO• activity *(106)* or NO• synthesis *(72)* augmented hypoxic vasoconstriction. Similarly, Blitzer and colleagues *(107)* observed, in normal human volunteers, that intravenous administration of L-NMMA increased PVR both under normoxic and hypoxic conditions. These studies suggested that NO• production serves as a counterregulatory mechanism to hypoxic pulmonary vasocon-striction. This hypothesis was supported by the findings of Frostell et al. *(108)*, using an awake lamb model, that inhaling low concentrations of NO• gas rapidly and completely reversed the pulmonary vasoconstriction associated with hypoxia (FiO$_2$ 0.06–0.08). Simi-larly, in human subjects breathing 12% oxygen, NO• inhalation reversed pulmonary vaso-constriction *(109)* (Fig. 2). Importantly, the pulmonary vasodilator effect of inhaled NO• was not accompanied by systemic hypotension. This demonstration of the selective pulmonary vasodilator effect of inhaled NO• had important implications for developing therapeutic applications of inhaled NO•, as described later in this chapter.

ROLE OF NO• IN CHRONIC PULMONARY HYPERTENSION

Whereas acute hypoxia causes rapidly reversible pulmonary vasoconstriction, chronic hypoxia is associated with remodeling of the small muscular pulmonary arteries, the devel-opment of CPH, and the eventual development of RVH *(110,111)*. The pulmonary vascular changes of chronic hypoxia have therefore been used in animal models to investigate the role of NO• in the pulmonary vascular changes of CPH. Despite extensive study of NO• signaling in lungs of animals breathing low concentrations of oxygen, the roles of NO• in the pulmo-nary vascular response to hypoxia remain controversial, as discussed as follows.

The first controversy is whether NO• production is increased or decreased during chronic hypoxia. Adnot et al. *(112)* studied isolated–perfused rat lungs and observed that chronic hypoxia diminished endothelium-dependent vasodilatation and NO• release, but that endo-thelium-independent vasodilatation (in response to nitroprusside) was preserved. These findings suggested that the production of NO• was diminished in chronic hypoxia, but that

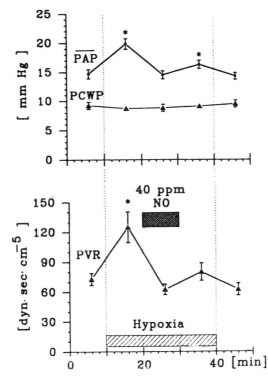

Fig. 2. Effect of NO$^{\bullet}$ inhalation on mean pulmonary artery pressure (PAP) and pulmonary vascular resistance (PVR) during hypoxia in normal subjects. PAP and PVR were measured at baseline, during hypoxia (PO$_2$ approx 50 mmHg), and during hypoxia plus administration of inhaled NO$^{\bullet}$ (40 ppm). During hypoxia, there was an increase in PAP and PVR (by 35 and 71%, respectively) compared with the PA and PVR in room air. With the addition of inhaled NO$^{\bullet}$, PA and PVR returned to the room air baseline. When inhaled NO$^{\bullet}$ was discontinued, PA was again increased (by 11%) compared with PA at baseline; PVR was not significantly increased compared with PVR at baseline. Pulmonary capillary wedge pressure (PCWP) did not change during hypoxia or during inhalation of NO$^{\bullet}$. (Adapted from ref. *109* with permission.)

the responsiveness to NO$^{\bullet}$ was intact. However, other studies demonstrated that expression of NOS1, NOS2, and NOS3 is increased during chronic hypoxia in rat bronchial epithelium, VSMCs, and vascular endothelial cells, respectively *(113–115)*. In addition, in one study, there was *de novo* expression of NOS3 in the small pulmonary resistance vessels of chronically hypoxic rats that was not present in normoxic rats *(43)*. LeCras et al. *(116)* used a model of surgical unilateral pulmonary artery constriction to demonstrate that hypoxia-induced upregulation of NOS3 expression was independent of the effects of hypoxia on pulmonary blood flow. Taken together, these studies demonstrate that although chronic hypoxia increases pulmonary NOS levels, NO$^{\bullet}$ production in response to endothelium-dependent vasodilators is impaired. To explain this apparent discrepancy, Shaul et al. *(115)* suggested that variability in the availability of NOS enzyme cofactors (such as NADPH, FAD, FMN [flavin mononucleotide], BH$_4$) may account for diminished NO$^{\bullet}$ synthesis despite increased pulmonary NOS levels in response to hypoxia. Alternatively, chronic hypoxia may disrupt the signaling pathways leading to the activation of constitutive NOS isoforms.

A second controversy is whether or not pulmonary vascular responsiveness to NO$^{\bullet}$ is changed during chronic hypoxia. Adnot et al. observed that pulmonary vasodilatation in response to nitroprusside was preserved in isolated lungs (as noted previously), as well as in pulmonary artery rings *(117)*, from rats exposed to 10–11% oxygen for 3 wk under normobaric conditions. In contrast, Maruyama and Maruyama *(118)* observed that pulmonary vascular relaxation in response to nitroprusside was impaired in pulmonary artery rings from rats exposed to hypobaric hypoxia for 10 d. Similarly, Crawley et al. *(119)* found that nitroprusside-induced vasodilatation was impaired in pulmonary arteries from rats exposed to 10% oxygen for 2 and 7 d. The explanation for these differing results remains uncertain.

The third controversy is whether NO• attenuates the pulmonary vascular remodeling that is associated with chronic hypoxia. The observations from studies of cultured cells that NO• can inhibit VSMC proliferation *(120)* led to the expectation that NO• would inhibit pulmonary vascular remodeling. Indeed, administration of inhaled NO• to chronically hypoxic newborn *(121)* or adult rats *(122,123)* prevented the development of RVH and pulmonary vascular remodeling. On the other hand, Hassid et al. *(124)* have reported that NO•-donor compounds augmented the mitogenic effect of fibroblast growth factor-2 on VSMCs in culture, and Xue and Johns *(43)* have proposed that NO• can promote pulmonary vascular remodeling because the hypoxia-induced increase in small pulmonary artery thickness and muscularity is temporally correlated with increased expression of NOS isoforms. It thus remained possible that NO• or non-NO• products of NOS, such as superoxide *(125)* could contribute to the development of pulmonary remodeling in chronic hypoxia. To test this hypothesis, Steudel et al. *(126)* studied mice with a targeted deletion of the *NOS3* gene exposed to 10% oxygen for 3–6 wk using open- and closed-chest hemodynamics, transesophageal echocardiography, and pulmonary morphometry. They found that the hypoxia-induced increases in RV pressure, pulmonary artery pressure, PVR, number of muscularized small pulmonary vessels, and RVH were greater in NOS3-deficient mice than in wild-type mice.

In summary, the available experimental evidence indicates that NO• plays an important protective role in modulating the pulmonary vasoconstriction, pulmonary vascular remodeling, and RVH associated with chronic hypoxia. It appears that increased production of NO• by the lung is a compensatory response to chronic hypoxia, but that the level of NO• produced, or perhaps the ability of the lung to respond to it, is inadequate to prevent the net vasoconstrictor and vascular remodeling effects of chronic hypoxia.

There are several other animal models of CPH in which abnormalities of NO• production or endothelium-dependent relaxation have been reported. As in the case of chronic hypoxia, studies in these models have yielded conflicting information about the role of NO• in the development of pulmonary hypertension. Monocrotaline-induced pulmonary hypertension, like the pulmonary hypertension of chronic hypoxia, is characterized by endothelial injury, VSMC hypertrophy and hyperplasia, and abnormal extracellular matrix deposition *(127)*. In this model, one group has reported that the development of pulmonary hypertension in rats is associated with decreased availability of bioactive NO• and impairment of endothelium-dependent, NO•-mediated vasodilatation *(128,129)*, whereas others have reported that monocrotaline administration results in increased NO• production, increased NOS3 protein, and improved agonist-induced endothelium-dependent vasodilatation *(130–131)*.

Apparently conflicting information has also been reported in models of fetal pulmonary hypertension induced by increasing pulmonary blood flow. In experiments in which pulmonary hypertension is produced in fetal lambs by closure of the ductus arteriosus, *NOS3* gene expression and endothelium-dependent vasodilatation to acetylcholine were decreased, suggesting that this form of CPH is associated with decreased NO• production *(132,133)*. In contrast, when pulmonary hypertension was produced in fetal lambs via an aortopulmonary vascular graft, endothelium-dependent vasodilatation was also impaired *(134)*, but NOS3 expression was increased *(135)* and pulmonary vasoconstriction was produced by treatment with an NOS inhibitor *(134)*, suggesting that NO• production is increased in this model. The differences observed in these studies may be attributable to the anatomic model used to increase pulmonary blood flow. These results suggest that different etiologies of pulmonary hypertension may differentially effect pulmonary NO• synthesis and NOS expression.

ABNORMALITIES OF NO• PRODUCTION
IN HUMAN PULMONARY HYPERTENSION

The ultimate goal of the studies in the animal models just described has been to elucidate the role of NO• in human pulmonary diseases. Indeed, the explosion of interest in the roles of NO• in human pulmonary diseases has brought much anticipation that these studies will lead both to new insights into the pathogenesis of common pulmonary diseases and to novel therapeutic applications of NO• and NO• donors. The role of NO• in human pulmonary hypertension has been studied at the levels of NOS expression and NO• production, as well as at the level of vascular responsiveness to endothelium-dependent and endothelium-independent vasodilating substances.

The expression of NOS1 and NOS3 isoforms has been investigated in tissue specimens from patients with primary pulmonary hypertension. Using RNA blot hybridization, *in situ* hybridization, and immunohistochemistry, Giaid and Saleh *(136)* reported that levels of NOS3 mRNA and protein were less in the pulmonary arteries of patients with both primary and secondary pulmonary hypertension than in those of patients with normal pulmonary artery pressure. They observed that the intensity of NOS3 immunoreactivity was inversely correlated with both PVR and the severity of the histologic changes. They suggested that reduced expression of NOS3 leading to reduced production of NO• could contribute to the development of primary pulmonary hypertension or other forms of chronic pulmonary hypertension by facilitating vasoconstriction, smooth muscle proliferation, and platelet activation. Alternatively, decreased NOS3 expression may be a secondary effect of established pulmonary hypertension but nonetheless may serve to promote disease progression *(137)*. In contrast, Xue and Johns *(138)* reported that NOS3-immunoreactivity was increased in pulmonary arteries from two patients with secondary pulmonary hypertension compared to specimens from individuals without pulmonary hypertension. Recently Mason et al. *(139)* reported a study of NOS3 expression in the lungs from 44 patients with pulmonary hypertension (22 primary and 22 secondary) and 12 patients without pulmonary hypertension. They found that NOS3 expression was decreased in the pulmonary arterioles of patients with both primary and secondary hypertension. However, in contrast to the observations of Giaid and Saleh, these investigators found consistently high levels of NOS3 expression in plexiform lesions. Taken together, these studies suggest that some patients have forms of pulmonary hypertension similar to chronically hypoxic rats (abundant NOS3), whereas other patients may have forms of pulmonary hypertension similar to chronically hypoxic NOS3(−/−) mice or neonatal sheep after ductus arteriosus occlusion *in utero* (deficient NOS3). Additionally, the natural history of pulmonary hypertension in some patients may be characterized by temporal and anatomic variations of NOS3 expression. Recently, Giaid *(34)* reported that NOS1 immunoreactivity was not altered in the lungs of patients with pulmonary hypertension. Studies describing pulmonary NOS2 levels in patients with pulmonary hypertension have not yet been published.

Dinh-Xuan et al. *(140)* compared endothelium-dependent vasodilatation in pulmonary vascular rings isolated from patients undergoing heart–lung transplantation for severe chronic obstructive lung disease (COLD) with that in vascular rings from normal portions of lungs of patients undergoing tumor resection. They found that the degree of acetylcholine (ACh)-induced vasodilatation was significantly reduced in the pulmonary vascular rings from patients with COLD compared with control subjects, but that nitroprusside-induced relaxation did differ in the two groups. Additionally, the degree of impairment of endothelium-dependent relaxation correlated directly with the degree of intimal thickening, implying that the histologic severity of pulmonary hypertension and the level of endothelial NO• production were inversely correlated. The same group also found impairment of endothelium-dependent pulmonary vascular relaxation in specimens from patients with Eisenmenger's syndrome

(141). Other investigators have used endothelium-dependent vasodilators to assess pulmonary vasoreactivity in patients with pulmonary hypertension. Palevsky and colleagues *(142)* observed that administration of ACh-induced pulmonary vasodilatation in only 4 of 23 patients with primary pulmonary hypertension. In contrast, Uren et al. *(143)* reported that endothelium-dependent vasodilators (ACh, calcitonin gene-related peptide, and substance P) failed to decrease PVR in five patients with primary pulmonary hypertension. In fact, Conraads et al. *(144)* reported two patients with pulmonary hypertension in whom ACh-induced paradoxic pulmonary vasoconstriction. This ACh-induced vasoconstrictor response may reflect the sum of impaired release of NO• by a dysfunctional endothelium and the direct constrictor action of ACh on vascular smooth muscle. These results suggest that only a minority of patients with pulmonary hypertension will have a vasodilator response to endothelium-dependent agonists.

Kaneko et al. *(145)* measured NO• production during bronchoscopy in patients with primary pulmonary hypertension. They found that NO• in airway gases and NO• biochemical reaction products in bronchoalveolar lavage were decreased in patients with primary pulmonary hypertension relative to normal controls. Moreover, the quantity of reaction products of NO• in the lavage fluid inversely correlated directly with the degree of pulmonary hypertension. In another study by Riley et al. *(146)*, the rate of NO• production measured in expired air at rest was similar in patients with primary pulmonary hypertension compared with that in normal control subjects. However, during exercise, the rate of NO• production doubled in normal control subjects, but did not change in patients with primary pulmonary hypertension. The ability to identify patients with pulmonary hypertension characterized by deficient NO• production may permit selection of appropriate replacement therapy, as outlined in the following section.

NO• AND THE TREATMENT OF PULMONARY HYPERTENSION

Because (1) pulmonary NO• production appears to be reduced in at least some patients with pulmonary hypertension; (2) NO• has an important role in maintaining basal pulmonary vasodilatation and attenuating hypoxic pulmonary vasoconstriction; and (3) NO• attenuates pulmonary vascular remodeling in animal models, therapies aimed at increasing the availability of NO• in the lung are attractive approaches to the treatment of pulmonary hypertension. Potential therapeutic approaches to augmenting NO• availability in the lung in patients with pulmonary hypertension include supplementation of NOS substrate and cofactors; administration of endothelium-dependent vasodilators, NO•-donor compounds, or inhaled NO•; and augmentation of pulmonary NOS levels using gene transfer (Table 1).

Because L-arginine is a critical substrate for NO• synthesis, Mehta et al. *(147)* sought to overcome the reduced production of NO• in patients with pulmonary hypertension by administering L-arginine intravenously. They found that acute administration of L-arginine to patients with pulmonary hypertension of various causes reduced mean PA pressure (by 16%) and PVR (by 28%). There is also evidence from animal studies that chronic administration of L-arginine can limit the adverse pulmonary vascular sequelae of chronic hypoxia. Mitani et al. *(148)* administered daily intraperitoneal L-arginine to rats exposed to chronic hypoxia (10 d). They found that rats who were treated with L-arginine had significantly lower PA pressure, reduced right ventricular hypertrophy, and less marked pulmonary vascular remodeling than rats exposed to hypoxia without treatment with L-arginine. These results suggest that supplementation with NOS substrate, and potentially NOS cofactors such as tetrahydrobiopterin (BH_4) *(149)*, may by useful for the treatment of patients with pulmonary hypertension.

As noted earlier, endothelium-dependent vasodilators reduce PVR in a subgroup of patients with primary *(142,143)* and secondary *(140,141)* pulmonary hypertension. However, administration of ACh to patients with pulmonary hypertension has been limited largely to the acute setting because of the possibility of producing systemic hypotension or worsening oxygenation by increasing perfusion in lung segments that are poorly ventilated *(150)*.

Table 1
Potential Therapeutic Approaches
to Increase Pulmonary NO˙ Concentrations in Patients with Pulmonary Hypertension

Therapeutic approach	Reference
Administration of NOS substrate (L-arginine)	147,148
Administration of NOS cofacator (BH_4)	149
Administration of endothelium-dependent vasodilators	140–143,150
Systemic administration of NO˙ -donor compounds	152,153
Selective delivery of NO˙ to the pulmonary vasculature	
Intravenous ultrashort half-life NO˙ donors	154–156
Inhaled NO˙ (see Table 2)	109,158–169,172–175
Inhaled NO˙ in combination with PDE inhibitor	185–190
NOS gene transfer to the pulmonary vasculature	101

Organic nitrates, such as isosorbide dinitrate, are effective pulmonary vasodilators because metabolism of these agents releases NO˙ *(17,151)*. In patients with pulmonary hypertension, organic nitrates lower PVR, increase CO, decrease symptoms, and increase exercise capacity *(152,153)*. Similarly, intravenous administration of sodium nitroprusside and nitroglycerin acutely lower PA pressure and PVR and increase CO. The principal limitation of oral and intravenous NO˙-donor compounds is that these agents do not act selectively in the lung, and concentrations of these drugs necessary to dilate the pulmonary vasculature typically produce symptomatic hypotension. In addition, these systemic NO˙ donors can also worsen hypoxemia by increasing ventilation–perfusion mismatching.

Two approaches have been undertaken to address the nonselectivity of NO˙-donor compounds for the pulmonary vasculature: intravenous administration of NO˙-donor compounds with ultrashort half-lives (to limit exposure to the pulmonary vasculature) and aerosol administration of NO˙-donor compounds. Adrie et al. *(154)* reported that intravenous administration proline/NO˙ (PROLI/NO˙), a NO˙-donor compound with an ultrashort half-life, to lambs with U46619-induced pulmonary hypertension selectively dilated the pulmonary vasculature at low doses but caused systemic hypotension at higher doses. Several groups have reported studies of the pulmonary vasodilator effects of aerosolized NO˙-donor compounds in animal models. In pigs with U46619-induced pulmonary hypertension, Brilli et al. *(155)* observed that aerosolized NONOates, NO˙/nucleophile adducts, selectively dilated the pulmonary vasculature without causing systemic hypotension. In contrast, in lambs treated with U46619, Adrie et al. *(156)* reported that aerosolized administration of another NONOate with a short half-life, diethanolamine/NO• (DEA/NO˙), a diazeniumdiolate, was selective for the pulmonary vasculature at low doses but not at high doses. Taken together, these observations suggest that systemic administration of NO˙-donor compounds with ultrashort half-lives or aerosol delivery of NO˙-donor compounds may be useful for the treatment of patients with pulmonary hypertension; however, a narrow therapeutic index may limit the application of these drugs to a minority of patients.

As noted previously, inhalation of low concentrations of NO˙ gas selectively dilates the pulmonary vasculature without causing systemic hypotension. The two physiologic properties of NO˙, which, when delivered via inhalation, result in pulmonary selectivity, are its short half-life (seconds) and its high affinity binding to hemoglobin, which inactivates it *(157)*. When NO˙ is delivered to the alveolus, it diffuses into pulmonary VSMCs, resulting in vasodilatation. NO˙ that diffuses into the bloodstream is inactivated by binding to hemoglobin, thereby avoiding systemic vasodilatation *(18)*.

Inhaled NO˙ has been shown to decrease pulmonary hypertension selectively in a variety of clinical settings (Table 2) including hypoxic vasoconstriction *(109)*, high-altitude pulmonary edema *(158)*, CHD *(159)*, mitral valve disease *(160)*, primary pulmonary hypertension

Table 2
Potential Clinical Applications of Inhaled NO•

Condition	Reference
Hypoxic pulmonary vasoconstriction	109
High-attitude pulmonary edema	158
Congenital heart disease	159
Mitral valve disease	160
Primary pulmonary hypertension	161
Adult respiratory distress syndrome	162
Chronic obstructive lung disease	163
Persistent pulmonary hypertension of the newborn	164,165,174,175
Pulmonary hypertension secondary to collagen vascular disease	166
Pulmonary hypertension secondary to LV dysfunction	168,169
Idiopathic pulmonary fibrosis	167
Evaluation of patients for potential heart or lung transplantation	172,173

(161), adult respiratory distress syndrome *(162)*, chronic obstructive pulmonary disease *(163)*, persistent pulmonary hypertension of the newborn *(164,165)*, pulmonary hypertension secondary to collagen vascular disease *(166)*, idiopathic pulmonary fibrosis *(167)*, and pulmonary hypertension secondary to LV dysfunction *(168,169)*.

An important emerging application of inhaled NO• is in the evaluation of patients being considered for heart or lung transplantation. Pulmonary hypertension is a dominant feature of both patient populations. In patients referred for heart transplantation, it is important to demonstrate that pulmonary hypertension, if present, is at least partially reversible, because transplantation of a normal donor heart into a patient with fixed, high PVR can result in acute RV failure of the donor heart *(170)*. In one study, transplanted patients in whom PVR was not reversible to less than 2.5 Wood units had a significantly higher 3-mo mortality than did transplanted patients with low or reversible PVR *(171)*. Adatia et al. *(172)* demonstrated that inhaled NO• can be used acutely in the cardiac catheterization laboratory to assess the reversibility of pulmonary hypertension in patients being evaluated for cardiac transplantation.

In patients referred for lung transplantation because of severe pulmonary hypertension, an important determinant of the need for transplantation is the inability of the lungs to respond to vasodilators. Acute administration of intravenous NO•-donors, such as nitroprusside, is an effective method of assessing the reversibility of pulmonary vasoconstriction, but this approach is limited by the risk of severe systemic hypotension. For this reason, selective pulmonary vasodilatation with inhaled NO• is increasingly being used to assess pulmonary vasoreactivity. Sitbon et al. *(173)* demonstrated that inhaled NO• is a safe and effective screening agent for identifying responders to oral calcium channel blocker therapy in patients with primary pulmonary hypertension. Of 33 patients with primary pulmonary hypertension, 10 had a significant reduction (at least 20%) in both PA pressure and PVR to inhaled NO•, and 9 of these patients also responded to calcium channel blockers. Of the 23 patients who did not have a response to inhaled NO•, none responded to calcium channel blockers, and 9 had serious adverse reactions associated with administration of these agents. Using inhaled NO• as a screening pulmonary vasodilator may thus permit nonresponders to avoid the life-threatening systemic hypotension and impairment of RV contractility that can be associated with oral calcium channel blockers.

The beneficial effects of inhaled NO• therapy have been particularly well established for the treatment of persistent pulmonary hypertension of the newborn. Two prospective, randomized clinical trials have demonstrated that therapy with inhaled NO• produced immediate and sustained improvement in oxygenation and decreased the need for extracorporeal membrane oxygenation in infants with this condition *(174,175)*. Pending Food and Drug Administration (FDA) approval, inhaled NO• therapy is expected to become part of the standard of care for patients with persistent pulmonary hypertension of the newborn.

Most studies of inhaled NO• for patients with pulmonary hypertension have involved short-term administration to hospitalized patients. Widespread clinical applicability of inhaled NO• will require more long-term administration. To this end, Channick et al. *(176)* have described a system in which inhaled NO• can be administered chronically to patients at home via nasal prongs and a pulsed delivery system. It is likely that domiciliary-inhaled NO• therapy will become a common treatment for patients with pulmonary hypertension from many causes. For example, in patients with severe chronic obstructive pulmonary disease and pulmonary hypertension requiring domiciliary oxygen supplementation, acute administration of NO• improved oxygenation and hemodynamics (decreased PA pressure and PVR; increased CO) suggesting that chronic administration of inhaled NO• may be an important addition to the outpatient regimen of this patient population *(177)*. Inhaled NO• has also been used as an in-hospital bridge to heart–lung transplantation in patients with severe primary pulmonary hypertension *(178)*.

In patients awaiting lung transplantation, it may also be useful to combine domiciliary-inhaled NO• therapy with continuous intravenous prostacyclin infusion *(179–181)*. It remains to be demonstrated whether the beneficial effects of long-term NO• inhalation on pulmonary vascular and RV remodeling observed in animal models *(122,123,182)* will also be demonstrated in patients with primary and secondary pulmonary hypertension.

Although these experimental clinical applications of inhaled NO• for various types of pulmonary hypertension suggest a promising future therapeutic role for this agent, there have been several major limitations to the effectiveness of inhaled NO•. First, inhaled NO• does not cause pulmonary vasodilatation in all patients with pulmonary hypertension. Additionally, in those patients who respond to inhaled NO•, the pulmonary artery pressure does not usually return to normal. Moreover, the vasodilator effect is rapidly reversible after NO• inhalation is discontinued, and rebound pulmonary hypertension complicates NO• withdrawal in some patients. Other potential limitations of NO• inhalation therapy (reviewed in ref. *183*) include methemoglobinemia, which may limit oxygen transport (typically associated with inhalation of 80 ppm or more of NO•), inhibition of platelet and leukocyte functions, rebound pulmonary hypertension, exacerbation of lung injury, and, possibly, NO•-induced DNA damage *(184)*.

One approach to augment and prolong the pulmonary vasodilator effects of inhaled NO•, as well as to minimize the dose of NO• required for therapeutic efficacy, is to administer inhaled NO• in combination with a PDE inhibitor. As noted before, several classes of PDEs participate in the pulmonary catabolism of cGMP. Because they regulate the level of cGMP available to participate in vasodilatation, these enzymes play a critical role in modulating the vasodilator response to NO•. Therefore, inhibitors of specific PDE isoforms, particularly enzymes that selectively metabolize cGMP, are attractive targets for experimental and therapeutic manipulation of the vasodilator response to inhaled NO• and NO•-donating compounds. The feasibility of this approach was first demonstrated in animal models. Studying lambs with U46619-induced pulmonary hypertension, Ichinose et al. *(185)* reported that intravenous administration of zaprinast (M & B-22948; 2-o-propoxyphenyl-8-aza-purin-6-one, Rhone-Poulenc Rohrer, Essex, UK), an inhibitor of PDE5 and of PDE9 at higher doses, did not significantly augment the efficacy of inhaled NO• but markedly prolonged the duration of the vasodilator effect after NO• inhalation was discontinued (Fig. 3). Thusu et al. *(186)* reported that, in newborn lambs, zaprinast augmented both the efficacy and duration of the pulmonary vasodilatation induced by breathing NO•. More recently, Ichinose and colleagues *(187)* observed that aerosol administration of low doses of zaprinast selectively dilated the pulmonary vasculature of U46619-treated lambs. In addition, aerosolized zaprinast augmented the efficacy and duration of pulmonary vasodilatation induced by breathing NO•.

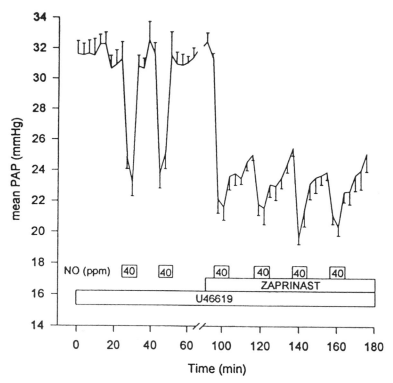

Fig. 3. Prolongation of the pulmonary vasodilator effects of inhaled NO• by PDE inhibition with zaprinast. Pulmonary hypertension was induced with U44619 in eight awake lambs. Mean pulmonary artery pressure was monitored while inhaled NO• (40 ppm) was administered intermittently before and after intravenous infusion of the cGMP-specific PDE inhibitor, zaprinast. Without zaprinast, the reduction in mean PA pressure produced by inhaled NO• persisted for only 1–2 min. With zaprinast infusion, the reduction in PA pressure was maintained for nearly 90 min with only four 4-min periods of NO• inhalation. (Reprinted from ref. *185* with permission.)

In human studies, dipyridamole, another PDE5 inhibitor, has been used to augment the efficacy of inhaled NO•. Fullerton et al. *(188)* studied 10 patients after aortic or mitral valve surgery who had pulmonary hypertension and failed to respond to inhaled NO•. They found that the combination of intravenous dipyridamole and inhaled NO• decreased PVR and PA pressure and increased CO, without changing mean arterial pressure. Kinsella and colleagues *(189)* reported that dipyridamole augmented the vasodilator effect of inhaled NO• in a child with congenital diaphragmatic hernia and severe pulmonary hypertension. Dipyridamole has also been used to facilitate the withdrawal of inhaled NO• therapy. Ivy and colleagues *(190)* reported that rebound pulmonary hypertension occurred in 7 of 23 children who were treated with inhaled NO• for pulmonary hypertension following surgery to correct congenital heart disease. In 6 of 6 children studied, intravenous administration of dipyridamole attenuated the rise in pulmonary artery pressure and deterioration in oxygenation that had been associated with NO• withdrawal.

These studies highlight the clinical utility of the combination of PDE inhibitors with inhaled NO•. However, dipyridamole inhibits adenosine transport as well as PDE5 enzyme activity, and high doses may worsen regional myocardial perfusion in patients with coronary artery disease. Unfortunately, zaprinast is not clinically available. Very recently, a highly selective PDE5 inhibitor, sildenafil, has been approved by the FDA for the treatment of male erectile dysfunction. Studies are underway to determine if sildenafil can be used to augment and prolong the efficacy of inhaled NO• for treatment of patients with pulmonary hypertension.

In addition to exposing the lung to exogenous NO˙ in the form of oral or intravenous NO˙ donors or inhaled NO˙, another approach to the treatment of pulmonary hypertension is to increase pulmonary NOS3 levels. Janssens et al. *(191)* used adenovirus-mediated gene transfer to augment pulmonary NOS3 levels. They observed that aerosol administration of a recombinant adenovirus specifying NOS3 transduced epithelial cells of large airways, alveolar lining cells, and endothelial cells of medium-sized and small pulmonary vessels. Transgene expression was maximal 5 d after adenovirus administration and was still detectable after 2 wk. These investigators examined the change in pulmonary artery pressures after exposure to 10% oxygen in rats transduced with an NOS3-specifying adenovirus and in rats transduced with a control adenovirus. They observed that hypoxic pulmonary vasoconstriction was attenuated in NOS3-transduced rats, but that systemic blood pressure did not differ between the two groups of rats. Potential disadvantages of this approach include the potential inflammatory response elicited by currently available viral vectors and the limited duration of transgene expression. There are several important advantages to gene transfer for the treatment of pulmonary hypertension. Gene transfer may permit therapy to be tailored for the pathogenesis of pulmonary hypertension (e.g., NOS3 deficiency) in an individual patient, and may allow for long-term treatment of pulmonary hypertension without the need for continuous inhalation of NO˙. As newer gene transfer techniques become available, it is likely that they will be used to increase synthesis of, or responsiveness to, vasodilators such as NO˙ in the lungs of patients with pulmonary hypertension.

CONCLUSION

The discovery of NO˙ and the elucidation of the NO˙/cGMP signal transduction pathway have increased our understanding of the pathophysiology of pulmonary hypertension. In the lung, there is complex regulation of NO˙ production by a variety of cell types. NO˙ appears to be important in the regulation of basal pulmonary vascular tone, in mediating the transition from the fetal to the neonatal circulation, in modulating the pulmonary vasoconstriction associated with acute hypoxia, and in limiting the pulmonary vascular remodeling that occurs in chronic hypoxia. Clinical studies have provided important evidence that augmenting NO˙ availability in the pulmonary vasculature is an effective approach to acutely ameliorating pulmonary hypertension in a wide variety of clinical circumstances. Future advances may include improving pulmonary vascular remodeling in chronic forms of pulmonary hypertension by the long-term administration of NO˙, NO˙ donors, and/or PDE inhibitors.

REFERENCES

1. Rich S, Brundage BH. Primary pulmonary hypertension: current update. JAMA 1984;251:2252–2254.
2. D'Alonzo GE, Barst RJ, Ayres SM, Bergofsky EH, Brundage BH, Detre KM, et al. Survival in patients with pulmonary hypertension: Results from a national prospective registry. Ann Int Med 1991;115: 343–349.
3. Pietra GG, Edwards WD, Kay JM, Rich S, Kernis J, Schloo B, et al. Histopathology of primary pulmonary hypertension. A qualitative and quantitative study of pulmonary blood vessels from 58 patients in the National Heart, Lung, and Blood Institute Primary Pulmonary Hypertension Registry. Circulation 1989;80:1198–1206.
4. Tuder RM, Lee S-D, Cool C. Histopathology of pulmonary hypertension. Chest 1998;114:1S–6S.
5. Olivari MT, Cohn JN, Weir EK, Cohn JN. Hemodynamic effects of nifedipine at rest and during exercise in primary pulmonary hypertension. Chest 1984;86:12–19.
6. Rich S, Brundage BH. High-dose calcium-channel blocking therapy for primary pulmonary hypertension: evidence of long-term reduction in pulmonary arterial pressure and regression of right ventricular hypertrophy. Circulation 1987;76:135–141.
7. Rich S, Kaufmann E, Levy PS. The effect of high doses of calcium-channel blockers on survival in primary pulmonary hypertension. N Engl J Med 1992;327:76–81.

8. Packer M, Medina N, Yushak M. Adverse hemodynamic and clinical effects of calcium channel blockade in pulmonary hypertension secondary to obliterative pulmonary vascular disease. J Am Coll Cardiol 1984;4:890–901.

9. Barst RJ, Rubin LJ, Long WA, Goon MD, Rich S, Badesch DB, et al. A comparison of intravenous epoprostenol (prostacyclin) with conventional therapy for primary pulmonary hypertension. N Engl J Med 1996;334:296–302.

10. Rubin LJ. Primary pulmonary hypertension. N Engl J Med 1997;336:111–117.

11. Haworth S. Pulmonary vascular remodeling in neonatal pulmonary hypertension: state of the art. Chest 1998;93:133S–138S.

12. Morin FC, Stenmark KR. Persistent pulmonary hypertension of the newborn. Am J Respir Crit Care Med 1995;151:2010–2032.

13. Nathan C. Nitric oxide as a secretory product of mammalian cells. FASEB J 1992;6:3051–3064.

14. Furchgott RR, Zawadski JV. The obligatory role of endothelial cells in the relaxation of arterial smooth muscle by acetylcholine. Nature 1980;288:373–376.

15. Ignarro LJ, Buga GM, Wood KS, Byrns RE, Chaudhuri G. Endothelium-derived relaxing factor produced and released from artery and vein is nitric oxide. Proc Natl Acad Sci USA 1987;84: 9265–9269.

16. Palmer RM, Ferrige AG, Moncada S. Nitric oxide release accounts for the biological activity of endothelium-derived relaxing factor. Nature 1987;327:524–526.

17. Freelisch M, Kelm M. Biotransformation of organic nitrates to nitric oxide by vascular smooth muscle and endothelial cells. Biochem Biophys Res Commun 1991;180:286–293.

18. Moncada S, Higgs A. The L-arginine-nitric oxide pathway. N Engl J Med 1993;329:2002–2012.

19. Nakane M, Arai K, Saheki S, Kuno T, Buechler W, Murad F. Molecular cloning and expression of cDNAs coding for soluble guanylate cyclase from rat lung. J Biol Chem 1990;265:16,841–16,845.

20. Vaandrager AB, deJonge HR. Signaling by cGMP-dependent protein kinases. Mol Cell Biochem 1996;157:23–30.

21. Torphy TJ. Phosphodiesterase isozymes: molecular targets for novel antiasthma agents. Am J Respir Crit Care Med 1998;157:351–370.

22. Fisher D, Smith J, Pillar J, Denis SS, Cheng J. Isolation and characterization of PDE9A, a novel human cGMP-specific phosphodiesterase. J Biol Chem 1998;273:15,559–15,564.

23. DeCatarina R, Libby P, Peng H-B, Thannickai VJ, Rajavashisth TB, Gimbrone MA, et al. Nitric oxide decreases cytokine-induced endothelial activation. J Clin Invest 1995;96:60–68.

24. Khan BV, Harrison DG, Olbrych MT, Alexander RW, Medford RM. Nitric oxide regulates vascular cell adhesion molecule 1 gene expression and redox-sensitive transcriptional events in human vascular endothelial cells. Proc Natl Acad. Sci. USA 1996;93:9114–9119.

25. Beckman JS, Beckman TW, Chen J, Marshall PA, Freeman BA. Apparent hydroxyl radical production by peroxynitrite: implications for endothelial injury from nitric oxide and superoxide. Proc Natl Acad Sci USA 1990;87:1620–1624.

26. Murad F. What are the molecular mechanisms for the antiproliferative effects of nitric oxide and cGMP in vascular smooth muscle? Circulation 1997;95:1101–1103.

27. Pollman MJ, Yamada T, Horiuchi M, Gibbons GH. Vasoactive substances regulate vascular smooth muscle cell apoptosis: countervailing influences of nitric oxide and angiotensin II. Circ Res 1996;79: 748–756.

28. Rudic RD, Shesely EG, Maeda N, Smithies O, Segal SS, Sessa WC. Direct evidence for the importance of endothelium-derived nitric oxide in vascular remodeling. J Clin Invest 1998;101:731–736.

29. Nishio E, Watanabe Y. Nitric oxide donor-induced apoptosis in smooth muscle cells is modulated by protein kinase C and protein kinase A. Eur J Pharmacol 1997;339:245–251.

30. Radomski MW, Palmer RM, Moncada S. Endogenous nitric oxide inhibits human platelet adhesion to vascular endothelium. Lancet 1987;2:1057,1058.

31. Lefer AM. Nitric oxide: nature's naturally occurring leukocyte inhibitor. Circulation 1997;95:553,554.

32. Schmidt HH, Gagne GD, Nakane M, Pollock JS, Miller MF, Murad F. Mapping of neural nitric oxide synthase in the rat suggests frequent co-localization with NADPH diaphorase but not with soluble guanylate cyclase, and novel paraneural functions for nitrinergic signal transduction. J Histochem Cytochem 1992;40:1439–1456.

33. Asano K, Chee C, Gaston B, Lilly C, Gerard C, Drazen JM, Stamler JS, et al. Constitutive and inducible nitric oxide synthase gene expression, regulation and activity in human lung epithelial cells. Proc Natl Acad Sci USA 1994;91:10,089–10,093.

34. Giaid A. Nitric oxide and endothelin-1 in pulmonary hypertension. Chest 1998;114:208S–212S.

35. Hamid Q, Springall DR, Riveros-Morena V, Chanez P, Howarth P, Redington A, et al. Induction of nitric oxide synthase in asthma. Lancet 1993;342:1510–1513.

36. Gaston B, Reilly J, Drazen JM, Fackler J, Ramdev P, Arnelle D, et al. Endogenous nitrogen oxides and bronchodilator S-nitrosothiols in human airways. Proc Natl Acad Sci USA 1993;90:10,957–10,961.

37. Tracey WR, Xue C, Klinghofer V, Barlow J, Pollock JS, Forstermann U, et al. Immunochemical detection of inducible NO synthase in human lung. Am J Physiol 1994;266:L722–L727.

38. Nakayama DK, Geller DA, Lowenstein CJ, Chern HD, Davies P, Pitt BR, Simmons L, Billiar T. Cytokines and lipopolysaccharide induce nitric oxide synthase in cultured rat pulmonary artery smooth muscle. Am J Respir Cell Mol Biol 1992.7:471–476.

39. Seidman PA, Wasserloos K, Davies P. Airway smooth muscle cells from rats exhibit transient expression of inducible nitric oxide synthase mRNA expression in response to cytokine stimulation. Am J Respir Crit Care Med 1994;149:A592.

40. Meng Q-H, Springall DR, Bishop AE, Morgan K, Evans TJ, Habib S, et al. Lack of inducible nitric oxide synthase in bronchial epithelium: a possible mechanism of susceptibility to infection in cystic fibrosis. J Pathol 1998;184:323–331.

41. Guo FH, DeRaeve HR, Rice TW, Stuehr DJ, Thunnissen FB, Erzurum SC. Continuous nitric oxide synthesis by inducible nitric oxide synthase in normal human airway epithelium in vivo. Proc Natl Acad Sci USA 1995;92:7809–7813.

42. Shaul PW, North AJ, Wu LC, Wells LB, Trannon TS, Kau KS, et al. Endothelial nitric oxide synthase is expressed in cultured human bronchiolar epithelium. J Clin Invest 1994;94:2231–2236.

43. Xue C, Johns RA. Upregulation of nitric oxide synthase correlates temporally with onset of pulmonary vascular remodeling in the hypoxic rat. Hypertension 1996;28:743–753.

44. Kobzik L, Bredt DS, Lowenstein CJ, Drazen J, Gaston B, Sugarbaker D, et al. Nitric oxide synthase in human and rat lung: immunocytochemical and histochemical localization. Am J Respir Mol Biol 1993;9:371–377.

45. Feron O, Saldana F, Michel JB, Michel T. The endothelial nitric-oxide synthase-calveolin regulatory cycle. J Biol Chem 1988;273:3125–3128.

46. Robinson LJ, Ghanouni P, Michel T. Posttranslational modifications of endothelial nitric oxide synthase. Methods Enzymol 1996.268:436–448.

47. Cosentino F, Patton S, d'Uscio L, Werner E, Werner-Felmayer G, Moreau P, et al. Tetrahydrobiopterin alters superoxide and nitric oxide release in prehypertensive rats. J Clin Invest 1998;101:1530–1537.

48. Sanders SP, Harrison SJ, Pearse DB, Maeda K, Wagner EM. Differential nitric oxide synthase activity and endothelin mRNA expression in sheep pulmonary artery, bronchial artery, and microvascular endothelial cells. Am J Respir Crit Care Med 1994;149:A438.

49. Gustafsson LE, Leone AM, Persson MG, Wiklund NP, Moncada S. Endogenous nitric oxide is present in the exhaled air of rabbits, guinea pigs and humans. Biochem Biophys Res Commun 1991;181:852–857.

50. DeSanctis GT, Mehta S, Kobzik L, Yandava C, Jiao A, Huang PL, et al. Contribution of type I NOS to expired gas NO and bronchial responsiveness in mice. Am J Physiol 1997;273;L883–L888.

51. Lundberg J, Farkas-Szallasi E, Weitzberg J, Rinder J, Lidholm J, Anggard A, et al. High nitric oxide production in human paranasal sinuses. Nat Med 1995;1:370–373.

52. Furukawa K, Harrison DG, Saleh D, Shennib H, Chagnon FP, Giaid A. Expression of nitric oxide synthase in the human nasal mucosa. Am J Respir Crit Care Med 1996;153:847–850.

53. Settergren G, Angdin M, Lundberg JO, Astudillo R, Gelinder J, Liska J, et al. Decreased pulmonary vascular resistance during nasal breathing: modulation by endogenous nitric oxide from the paranasal sinuses. Acta Physiol Scand 1998;163:235–239.

54. Dweik RA, Laskowski D, Abu-Soud HM, Kaneko F, Hutte R, Stuehr DJ, et al. Nitric oxide synthesis in the lung. Regulation by oxygen through a kinetic mechanism. J Clin Invest 1998;101:660–666.

55. Byrnes CA, Dinarevic S, Busst C, Bush A, Shinebourne EA. Is nitric oxide in exhaled air produced at airway or alveolar level? Eur Resp J 1997;10:1021–1025.

56. Moore P, Velvis H, Fineman JR, Soifer SJ, Heyman MA. EDRF inhibition attenuates the increase in pulmonary blood flow due to oxygen ventilation of fetal lambs. J Appl Physiol 1992;73:2151–2157.

57. Abman SH, Chatfield BA, Hall SL, McMurtry IF. Role of endothelium-derived relaxing factor during transition of pulmonary circulation at birth. Am J Physiol 1990;259:H1921–H1927.

58. Cornfield DN, Chatfield BA, McQueston JA, McMurtry IF, Abman SH. Effects of birth-related stimuli on L-arginine-dependent pulmonary vasodilation in ovine fetus. Am J Physiol 1992;262:H1474–H1481.

59. Fineman JR, Wong J, Morin FC, Wild LM, Soifer. SJ. Chronic nitric oxide inhibition in utero produces persistent pulmonary hypertension in newborn lambs. J Clin Invest 1994;93:2675–2683.

60. Huang PL, Fishman MC. Genetic analysis of nitric oxide synthase isoforms: targeted mutation in mice. J Mol Med 1996;74:415–421.

61. North AJ, Star RA, Brannon TS, Ujiie K, Wells LB, Lowenstein CJ, et al. Nitric oxide synthase type I and type III gene expression are developmentally regulated in rat lung. Am J Physiol 1994;266: L635–L641.

62. Kawai N, Bloch DB, Filippov G, Rapkina D, Suen H-C, Losty PD, et al. Constitutive endothelial nitric oxide synthase gene expression is regulated during lung development. Am J Physiol 1995;268: L589–L595.
63. Rairigh RL, LeCras TD, Ivy DD, Kinsella JP, Richter G, Horan MP, et al. Role of inducible nitric oxide synthase in regulation of pulmonary vascular tone in the late gestation ovine fetus. J Clin Invest 1998; 101:15–21.
64. Bloch KD, Filippov G, Sanchez LS, Nakane M, de la Monte SM. Pulmonary soluble guanylate cyclase, a nitric oxide receptor, is increased during the perinatal period. Am J Physiol 1997;272:L400–L406.
65. Sanchez LS, de la Monte SM, Filippov G, Jones RC, Zapol WM, Bloch KD. Cyclic-GMP-binding, cyclic-GMP-specific phosphodiesterase (PDE5) gene expression is regulated during rat pulmonary development. Pediatr Res 1998;43:163–168.
66. Hanson KA, Burns F, Rybalkin SD, Miller JW, Beavo J, Clarke WR. Developmental changes in lung cGMP phosphodieasterase-5 activity, protein, and message. Am J Respir Crit Care Med 1998;158: 279–288.
67. Ignarro LJ, Buga GM, Chaudhuri G. EDRF generation and release from perfused bovine pulmonary artery and vein. Eur J Pharmacol 1988;149:79–88.
68. Ignarro LJ, Byrns RE, Buga GM, Wood KS. Endothelium-derived relaxing factor from pulmonary artery and vein possesses pharmacological and chemical properties identical to those of nitric oxide. Circ Res 1987;61:866–879.
69. Cremona G, Dinh-Xuan AT, Higenbottam TW. Endothelium-derived relaxing factor and the pulmonary circulation. Lung 1991;169:185–202.
70. Dinh-Xuan AT. Endothelial modulation of pulmonary vascular tone. Eur Resp J 1992;5:757–762.
71. McMahon TJ, Hood JS, Bellan JA, Kadowitz PJ. N-Nitro-L-arginine methyl ester selectively inhibits pulmonary vasodilator responses to acetylcholine and bradykinin. J Appl Physiol 1991;71:2026–2031.
72. Archer SL, Tolins JP, Raij L, Weir EK. Hypoxic pulmonary vasoconstriction is enhanced by inhibition of the synthesis of an endothelium derived relaxing factor. Biochem Biophys Res Commun 1989;164: 1198–1205.
73. Hampl V, Weir EK, Archer SL. Endothelium-derived nitric oxide is less important for basal tone regulation in the pulmonary than the renal vessels of adult rat. J Vasc Med Biol 1994;5:22–30.
74. Hampl V, Archer SL, Nelson DP, Weir EK. Chronic EDRF inhibition and hypoxia: effects on pulmonary circulation and systemic blood pressure. J Appl Physiol 1993;75:1748–1757.
75. Perrella MA, Hildebrand FL, Margulies KB, Burnett JC. Endothelium-derived relaxing factor in regulation of basal cardiopulmonary and renal function. Am J Physiol 1991;261:R323–R328.
76. Fineman JR, Heymann MA, Soifer SJ. N-Omega-nitro-L-arginine attenuates endothelium-dependent pulmonary vasodilatation in lambs. Am J Physiol 1991;260:H1299–H1306.
77. Persson MG, Gustafsson LE, Wiklund NP, Moncada S, Hedqvist P. Endogenous nitric oxide as a probable modulator of pulmonary circulation and hypoxic pressor response in vivo. Acta Physiol Scand 1990;140:449–457.
78. Kane DW, Tesauro T, Koizumi T, Gupta R, Newman JH. Exercise-induced pulmonary vasoconstriction during combined blockade of nitric oxide synthase and beta adrenergic receptors. J Clin Invest 1994;93:677–683.
79. Archer S, Hampl V, McKenzie Z, Nelson D, Huang K, Shulz P, et al. The role of endothelial-derived nitric oxide in normal and hypertensive pulmonary vasculature. Semin Respir Med 1994;15:179–189.
80. Steudel W, Ichinose F, Huang PL, Hurford WE, Jones RC, Bevan JA, et al. Pulmonary vasoconstriction and hypertension in mice with targeted disruption of the endothelial nitric oxide synthase (NOS 3) gene. Circ Res 1997;81:34–41.
81. Stamler JS, Loh E, Roddy MA, Cirrie KE, Creager MA. Nitric oxide regulated basal systemic and pulmonary vascular resistance in healthy humans. Circulation 1994;89:2035–2040.
82. Cooper C, Landzberg M, Anderson T, Charbonneau F, Creager M, Ganz P, et al. Role of nitric oxide in the local regulation of pulmonary vascular resistance in humans. Circulation 1996;93:266–271.
83. Bradford JR, Dean HP. The pulmonary circulation. J Physiol 1894;16:34–96.
84. Nagasaka K, Bhattacharya J, Nanjo S, Gropper MA, Staub NC. Micropuncture measurement of lung microvascular pressure profile during hypoxia in cats. Circ Res 1984;54:90–95.
85. Siegel LC, Pearl RG, Shafer SL, Ream AK, Prielipp RC. The longitudinal distribution of pulmonary vascular resistance during unilateral hypoxia. Anesthesiology 1989;70:527–532.
86. Archer SL, Huang J, Henry T, Peterson D, Weir EK. A redox-based O2 sensor in rat pulmonary vasculature. Circ Res 1993;73:1100–1112.
87. Post JM, Hume JR, Archer SL, Weir EK. Direct role for potassium channel inhibition in hypoxic pulmonary vasoconstriction. Am J Physiol 1992;262:C882–C890.

88. Archer SL, Souil E, Dinh-Xuan AT, Schremmer B, Mercier J-C, Yaagoubi AE, et al. Molecular identification of the role of voltage-gated K+ channels, Kv1.5 and Kv2.1, in hypoxic pulmonary vasoconstriction and control of resting membrane potential in rat pulmonary artery myocytes. J Clin Invest 1998;101:2319–2330.

89. Cornfield DN, Stevens T, McMurtry IF, Abman SH, Rodman DM. Acute hypoxia causes membrane depolarization an calcium influx in fetal pulmonary artery smooth muscle cells. Am J Physiol 1994; 266:L469–L475.

90. Cornfield DN, Stevens T, McMurtry IF, Abman SH, Rodman DM. Acute hypoxia increases cytosolic calcium in fetal pulmonary artery smooth muscle cells. Am J Physiol 1993;265:L53–L56.

91. Weir EK, Reeve HL, Peterson DA, Michelakis ED, Nelson DP, Archer SL. Pulmonary vasoconstriction, oxygen sensing, and the role of ion channels. Chest 1998;114:17S–22S.

92. Rodman DM, Yamaguchi T, Hasunuma K, O'Brien R, McMurtry IF. Effects of hypoxia on endothelium-dependent relaxation of rat pulmonary artery. Am J Physiol 1990;258:L207–L214.

93. Demiryurek AT, Wadsworth RM, Krane KA. Effects of hypoxia on isolated intrapulmonary arteries from sheep. Pulm Pharmacol 1991;4:158–164.

94. Ogata M, Ohe M, Katayose D, Takishima T. Modulatory role of EDRF in hypoxic contraction of isolated pulmonary arteries. Am J Physiol 1992;262:H691–H697.

95. Yuan XJ, Tod ML, Rubin LJ, Blaustein MP. Contrasting effects of hypoxia on tension in rat pulmonary mesenteric arteries. Am J Physiol 1990;259:H281–H289.

96. Madden JA, Vadula MS, Kurup VP. Effects of hypoxia and other vasoactive agents on pulmonary and cerebral artery smooth muscle cells. Am J Physiol 1992;263:L384–L393.

97. Leach RM, Robertson TP, Twort CH, Ward JP. Hypoxic vasoconstriction in rat pulmonary and mesenteric arteries. Am J Physiol 1994;266:L223–L237.

98. Johns RA, Linden JM, Peach MJ. Endothelium-dependent relaxation and cGMP accumulation in rabbit pulmonary artery are selectively impaired by moderate hypoxia. Circ Res 1989;65:1508–1515.

99. Shaul PW, Wells LB, Horning KM. Acute and prolonged hypoxia attenuate endothelial nitric oxide production in rat pulmonary arteries by different mechanisms. J Cardiovasc Pharmacol 1993;22:819–827.

100. Hampl V, Cornfield DM, Cowan NJ, Archer SL. Hypoxia potentiates nitric oxide synthesis and transiently increases cytosolic calcium levels in pulmonary artery endothelial cells. Eur Resp J 1995;8: 515–522.

101. North AJ, Lau KS, Brannon TS, Wu LC, Wells LB, German Z, et al. Oxygen upregulates nitric oxide synthase gene expression in ovine fetal pulmonary artery endothelial cells. Am J Physiol 1996;270: L643–L649.

102. McQuillan LP, Leung GK, Marsden PA, Kostyk SK, Kourembanas S. Hypoxia inhibits expression of eNOS via transcriptional and post-transcriptional mechanisms. Am J Physiol 1994;267:H1921–H1927.

103. Liao JK, Zulueta JJ, Yu FS, Cote CG, Hasoun PM. Regulation of bovine endothelial constitutive nitric oxide synthase by oxygen. J Clin Invest 1995;96:2661–2666.

104. Phelan MW, Faller DV. Hypoxia decreases constitutive nitric oxide synthase transcript and protein in cultured endothelial cells. J Cell Physiol 1996;167:469–476.

105. Gess B, Schricker K, Pfeifer M, Kurtz A. Acute hypoxia upregulates NOS gene expression in rats. Am J Physiol 1997;273:R905–R910.

106. Brashers VL, Peach MJ, Rose BC. Augmentation of hypoxic pulmonary vasoconstriction in the isolated perfused rat lung by in vitro antagonists of endothelium-dependent relaxation. J Clin Invest 1988;82: 1495–1502.

107. Blitzer ML, Loh E, Reddy MA, Stamler JS, Creager MA. Endothelium-derived nitric oxide regulates systemic and pulmonary vascular resistance during acute hypoxia. J Am Coll Cardiol 1996;28: 591–596.

108. Frostell C, Fratacci MD, Wain J, Jones R, Zapol WM. Inhaled nitric oxide. A selective pulmonary vasodilator reversing hypoxic pulmonary vasoconstriction. Circulation 1991;83:2038–2047.

109. Frostell CG, Blomquist H, Hedenstierna G, Lundberg J, Zapol WM. Inhaled nitric oxide selectively reverses human hypoxic pulmonary vasoconstriction without causing systemic vasodilatation. Anesthesiology 1993;78:427–435.

110. Fishman AP. Hypoxia on the pulmonary circulation: how and where it acts. Circ Res 1976;38:221–231.

111. Voelkel NF. Mechanisms of hypoxic pulmonary vasoconstriction. Am Rev Respir Dis 1986;133: 221–231.

112. Adnot S, Raffestin B, Eddahibi S, Braquet P, Chabrier PE. Loss of endothelium-dependent relaxant activity in the pulmonary circulation of rats exposed to hypoxia. J Clin Invest 1991;87:155–162.

113. LeCras TD, Xue C, Rengasamy A, Johns RA. Chronic hypoxia upregulates endothelial and inducible NO synthase gene and protein expression in rat lung. Am J Physiol 1996;270:L164–L179.

114. Xue C, Rengasamy A, LeCras TD, Koberna PA, Dailey GC, Johns RA. Distribution of NOS in normoxic vs. hypoxic rat lung: upregulation of NOS by chronic hypoxia. Am J Physiol 1994;267:L667–L678.
115. Shaul PW, North AJ, Brannon TS, Ujiie K, Wells LB, Nisen PA, et al. Prolonged in vivo hypoxia enhances nitric oxide synthase type I and type III gene expression in adult rat lung. Am J Respir Cell Mol Biol 1995;13:167–174.
116. LeCras TD, Tyler RC, Horan MP, Morris KG, Tuder RM, McMurtry IF, et al. Effects of chronic hypoxia and altered hemodynamics on endothelial nitric oxide synthase expression in the adult rat lung. J Clin Invest 1998;101:795–801.
117. Carville C, Raffestin B, Eddahibi S, Blouquit Y, Adnot S. Loss of endothelium-dependent relaxation in proximal pulmonary arteries from rats exposed to chronic hypoxia: effects of in vivo and in vitro supplementation with L-arginine. J Cardiovasc Pharmacol 1993;22:889–896.
118. Maruyama J, Maruyama K. Impaired nitric oxide-dependent response and their recovery in hypertensive pulmonary arteries of rats. Am J Physiol 1994;266:H2476–H2488.
119. Crawley DE, Zhao L, Giembycz MA, Liu S, Barnes PJ, Winter RJ, Evans TW. Chronic hypoxia impairs soluble guanylate cyclase-mediated pulmonary arterial relaxation in the rat. Am J Physiol 1992;263:L325–L332.
120. Garg UC, Hassid A. Nitric oxide-generating vasodilators and 8-bromocyclic guanosine monophosphate inhibit mitogenesis and proliferation of cultured rat smooth muscle cells. J Clin Invest 1989;83:1774–1777.
121. Roberts JD, Roberts CT, Jones RC, Zapol WM, Bloch KD. Nitric oxide inhalation reduces hypoxic pulmonary arterial remodeling, right ventricular hypertrophy, and growth retardation in the newborn rat. Circ Res 1995;76:215–222.
122. Roos CM, Frank DU, Xue C, Johns RA, Rich GF. Chronic inhaled nitric oxide: effects on pulmonary vascular endothelial function and pathology in rats. J Appl Physiol 1996;80:252–260.
123. Kouyoumdjian C, Adnot S, Levame N, Eddahibi S, Bousbaa H. Continuous inhalation of nitric oxide protects against development of pulmonary hypertension in chronically hypoxic rats. J Clin Invest 1994;94:578–584.
124. Hassid A, Arabshahi H, Boucier T, Dhaunsi GS, Matthews C. Nitric oxide selectively amplifies FGF-2–induced mitogenesis in primary rat aortic smooth muscle cells. Am J Physiol 1994;267:H1040–H1048.
125. Bouloumie A, Bauersachs J, Linz W, Scholkens BA, Wiemer G, Fleming I, et al. Endothelial dysfunction coincides with an enhanced nitric oxide synthase expression and superoxide anion production. Hypertension 1997;30:934–941.
126. Steudel W, Scherrer-Crosbie M, Bloch KD, Weimann J, Huang PL, Jones RC, et al. Sustained pulmonary hypertension and right ventricular hypertrophy after chronic hypoxia in mice with congenital deficiency of nitric oxide synthase 3. J Clin Invest 1998;101:2468–2477.
127. Todorovich-Hunter L, Johnson DJ, Ranger P, Keeley FW, Rabinovitch M. Altered elastin and collagen synthesis associated with progressive pulmonary hypertension induced by monocrotaline. Lab Invest 1988;58:184–195.
128. Mathew R, Zeballos G, Tun H, Gewitz MH. Role of nitric oxide and endothelin-1 in monocrotaline-induced pulmonary hypertension in rats. Cardiovasc Res 1995;30:739–746.
129. Mathew R, Gloster ES, Sundararajan T, Thompson C, Zeballos GA, Gewitz MH. Role of inhibition of nitric oxide production in monocrotaline-induced pulmonary hypertension. J Appl Physiol 1997;82:1493–1498.
130. Madden JA, Keller PA, Choy JS, Alvarez TA, Hacker AD. L-Arginine-related responses to pressure and vasoactive agents in monocrotaline-treated rat pulmonary arteries. J Appl Physiol 1995;76:589–593.
131. Resta TC, Gonzales RJ, Dail WG, Sanders TC, Walker BR. Selective upregulation of arterial endothelial nitric oxide synthase in pulmonary hypertension. Am J Physiol 1997;272:H806–H813.
132. McQueston JA, Kinsella JP, Ivy DD, McMurtry IF, Abmam SH. Chronic pulmonary hypertension in utero impairs endothelium-dependent vasodilatation. Am J Physiol 1995;268:H288–H294.
133. Shaul PW, Yuhanna IS, German Z, Chen Z, Steinhorn RH, Morin FC. Pulmonary endothelial NO synthase gene expression is decreased in fetal lambs with pulmonary hypertension. Am J Physiol 1997;272:L1005–L1012.
134. Reddy VM, Wong J, Liddicoat JR, Johengen M, Chang R, Fineman JR. Altered endothelium-dependent vasoactive responses in lambs with pulmonary hypertension and increased pulmonary blood flow. Am J Physiol 1996;271:H562–H570.
135. Black SM, Fineman JR, Steinhorn RH, Bristow J, Soifer SJ. Increased endothelial NOS in lambs with increased pulmonary blood flow and pulmonary hypertension. Am J Physiol 1998;275;H1643–H1651.
136. Giaid A, Saleh D. Reduced expression of endothelial nitric oxide synthase in the lungs of patients with pulmonary hypertension. N Engl J Med 1995;333:214–221.

137. Loscalzo J. Nitric oxide and vascular disease. N Engl J Med 1995;333:251–253.
138. Xue C, Johns RA. Endothelial nitric oxide synthase in the lungs of patients with pulmonary hypertension (letter). N Engl J Med 1995;333:1642,1643.
139. Mason NA, Springall DR, Burke M, Pollock J, Mikhail G, Yacoub MH, et al. High expression of endothelial nitric oxide synthase in plexiform lesions of pulmonary hypertension. J Pathol 1998;185: 313–318.
140. Dinh-Xuan AT, Higenbottam TW, Clelland CA, Pepke-Zaba J, Cremona G, Butt AY, et al. Impairment of endothelium-dependent pulmonary-artery relaxation in chronic obstructive lung disease. N Engl J Med 1991;324:1539–1547.
141. Dinh-Xuan AT, Higenbottam TW, Clelland CA, Pepke-Zaba J, Cremona G, Wallwork J. Impairment of pulmonary endothelium-dependent relaxation in patients with Eisenmenger's syndrome. Br J Pharmacol 1990;99:9,10.
142. Palevsky HI, Long W, Crow J, Fishman AP. Prostacyclin and acetylcholine as screening agents for acute pulmonary vasodilator responsiveness in primary pulmonary hypertension. Circulation 1990;82: 2018–2026.
143. Uren NG, Ludman PF, Crake T, Oakley CM. Response of the pulmonary circulation to acetylcholine, calcitonin gene-related peptide, substance P and oral nicardipine in patients with primary pulmonary hypertension. J Am Coll Cardiol 1992;19:835–841.
144. Conraads VM, Bosmans JM, Claeys MJ, Vrints CJ, Snoeck JP, DeClerck L, et al. Paradoxic pulmonary vasoconstriction in response to acetylcholine in patients with primary pulmonary hypertension. Chest 1994;106:385–390.
145. Kaneko FT, Arroliga AC, Dweik RA, Comhair SA, Laskowski D, Oppedisano R, et al. Biochemical reaction products of nitric oxide as quantitative markers of primary pulmonary hypertension. Am J Respir Crit Care Med 1998;158:917–923.
146. Riley MS, Porszasz J, Miranda J, Engelen MP, Brundage B, Wasserman K. Exhaled nitric oxide during exercise in primary pulmonary hypertension and pulmonary fibrosis. Chest 1997;111:44–50.
147. Mehta S, Stewart DJ, Langleben D, Levy RD. Short-term pulmonary vasodilatation with L-arginine in pulmonary hypertension. Circulation 1995;92:1539–1545.
148. Mitani Y, Maruyama K, Sakurai M. Prolonged administration of L-arginine ameliorates chronic pulmonary hypertension and pulmonary vascular remodeling in rats. Circulation 1997;96:689–697.
149. Walter R, Blau N, Schaffner A, Speich R, Stocker R, Naujeck B, Schoedon G. Inhalation of the nitric oxide synthase cofactor tetrahydrobiopterin in healthy volunteers. Am J Respir Crit Care Med 1997; 156:2006–2010.
150. Adnot S, Kouyoumdjian C, Defouilloy C, Andrivet P, Sediame S, Herigault R, et al. Hemodynamic and gas exchange responses to infusion of acetylcholine and inhalation of nitric oxide in patients with chronic obstructive lung disease and pulmonary hypertension. Am Rev Respir Dis 1993;148: 310–316.
151. Gruetter CA, Gruetter DY, Lyon JE, Kadowitz PJ, Ignarro LJ. Relationship between cyclic guanosine 3':5'-monophosphate formation and relaxation of coronary arterial smooth muscle by glyceryl trinitrate, nitroprusside, nitrite and nitric oxide: effects of methylene blue and methemoglobin. J Pharmacol Exp Ther 1981;219:181–186.
152. Leier CV, Huss P, Magorien RD, Unverferth DV. Improved exercise capacity and differing arterial and venous tolerance during chronic isosorbide dinitrate therapy for congestive heart failure. Circulation 1983;67:817–822.
153. Hermiller JB, Bambach D, Thompson MJ, Huss P, Fontana ME, Magorien RD, et al. Vasodilators and prostaglandin inhibitors in primary pulmonary hypertension. Ann Intern Med 1982;97:480–489.
154. Adrie C, Hirani WM, Holzmann A, Keefer L, Zapol WM, Hurford WE. Selective pulmonary vasodilation by intravenous infusion of an ultrashort half-life nucleophile/nitric oxide adduct. Anesthesiology 1998;88:190–195.
155. Brilli RJ, Krafte-Jacobs B, Smith DJ, Passerini D, Moore L, Ballard ET. Aerosolization of novel nitric oxide donors selectively reduce pulmonary hypertension. Crit Care Med 1998;26:1390–1396.
156. Adrie C, Ichinose F, Holzmann A, Keefer L, Hurford WE, Zapol WM. Pulmonary vasodilation by nitric oxide gas and prodrug aerosols in acute pulmonary hypertension. J Appl Physiol 1998;84:435–441.
157. Rimar S, Gillis CN. Selective pulmonary vasodilation by inhaled nitric oxide is due to hemoglobin inactivation. Circulation 1993;88:2884–2887.
158. Scherrer U, Vollenweider L, Delabays A, Savcic M, Eichenberger U, Kleger GR, et al. Inhaled nitric oxide for high-altitude pulmonary edema. N Engl J Med 1996;334:624–629.
159. Roberts JD, Lang P, Bigatello LM, Vlahakes GJ, Zapol WM. Inhaled nitric oxide in congenital heart disease. Circulation 1993;87(2):447–453.

160. Girard C, Lehot J, Pannetier J, Filley S, French P, Estanove S. Inhaled nitric oxide after mitral valve replacement in patients with chronic pulmonary artery hypertension. Anesthesiology 1992;77:880–883.
161. Pepke-Zaba J, Higenbottam TW, Dinh-Xuan AT, Stone D, Wallwork J. Inhaled nitric oxide as a cause of selective pulmonary vasodilation in pulmonary hypertension. Lancet 1991;338:1173,1174.
162. Roissant R, Falke KF, Lopez F, Slama K, Pison U, Zapol WM. Inhaled nitric oxide for the adult respiratory distress syndrome. N Engl J Med 1993;328:399–405.
163. Moinard J, Manie G, Pillet O, Castaing Y. Effect of inhaled nitric oxide on hemodynamics and V/A/ Q inequalities in patients with chronic obstructive lung disease. Am J Respir Crit Care Med 1993;149: 1482–1487.
164. Roberts JD, Polaner DM, Lang P, Zapol WM. Inhaled nitric oxide in persistent pulmonary hypertension of the newborn. Lancet 1992;340:818,819.
165. Kinsella JP, Neish SR, Shaffer E, Abman SH. Low-dose inhalation nitric oxide in persistent pulmonary hypertension of the newborn. Lancet 1992;340:819,820.
166. Williamson DJ, Hayward C, Rogers P, Wallman LL, Sturgess AD, Penny R, et al. Acute hemodynamic responses to inhaled nitric oxide in patients with limited scleroderma and isolated pulmonary hypertension. Circulation 1996;94:477–482.
167. Yoshida M, Taguchi O, Gabazza EC, Yasui H, Kobayashi T, Kobayashi H, et al. The effect of low-dose inhalation of nitric oxide in patients with pulmonary fibrosis. Eur Respir J 1997;10:2051–2054.
168. Semigran MJ, Cockrill BA, Kacmarek R, Thompson BT, Zapol WM, Dec GW, et al. Hemodynamic effects of inhaled nitric oxide in heart failure. J Am Coll Cardiol 1994;24(4):982–988.
169. Loh E, Stamler JS, Hare JM, Loscalzo J, Colucci WS. Cardiovascular effects of inhaled nitric oxide in patients with left ventricular dysfunction. Circulation 1994;90:2780–2785.
170. Hunt SA. Pulmonary hypertension in severe congestive heart failure: how important is it? J Heart Lung Trans 1997;16:S13–S15.
171. Costard-Jackle A, Fowler MB. Influence of preoperative pulmonary artery pressure on mortality after heart transplantation: testing of potential reversibility of pulmonary hypertension with nitroprusside is useful in defining a high risk group. Circulation 1992;19:48–54.
172. Adatia I, Perry S, Landzberg M, Moore P, Thompson JE, Wessel DL. Inhaled nitric oxide and hemodynamic evaluation of patients with pulmonary hypertension before transplantation. J Am Coll Cardiol 1995;25:1656–1664.
173. Sitbon O, Humbert M, Jagot JL, Taravella O, Fartoukh M, Parent F, et al. Inhaled nitric oxide as a screening agent for safely identifying responders to oral calcium-channel blockers in primary pulmonary hypertension. Eur Respir J 1998;12:265–270.
174. Roberts JD, Fineman JR, Morin FC, Shaul PW, Rimar S, Schreiber MD, et al. The Inhaled Nitric Oxide Study Group. Inhaled nitric oxide and persistent pulmonary hypertension of the newborn. N Engl J Med 1997;336:605–610.
175. The Neonatal Inhaled Nitric Oxide Study Group. Inhaled nitric oxide in full-term and nearly full-term infants with hypoxic respiratory failure. N Engl J Med 1997;336:597–604.
176. Channick RN, Newhart JW, Johnson FW, Williams PJ, Auger WR, Fedullo PF, et al. Pulsed delivery of inhaled nitric oxide to patients with primary pulmonary hypertension: an ambulatory delivery system and initial clinical tests. Chest 1996;109:1545–1549.
177. Leitner C, Ziesche R, Zimpfer M, Block LH, Germann P. Low-dose inhalation therapy with nitric oxide and oxygen: implications for long-term application in patients with COPD and pulmonary hypertension. Acta Anaesth Scand 1996;109:96,97.
178. Snell GI, Salamonsen RF, Bergin P, Esmore DS, Khan S, Williams TJ. Inhaled nitric oxide used as bridge to heart-lung transplantation in a patient with end-stage pulmonary hypertension. Am J Respir Crit Care Med 1995;151:1263–1266.
179. Ichida F, Uese K, Tsubata S, Hashimoto I, Hamamichi Y, Fukahara K, et al. Additive effect of Beraprost on pulmonary vasodilatation by inhaled nitric oxide in children with pulmonary hypertension. Am J Cardiol 1997;80:662–664.
180. Jolliet P, Bulpa P, Thorens JB, Ritz M, Chevrolet JC. Nitric oxide and prostacyclin as test agents of vasoreactivity in severe precapillary pulmonary hypertension: predictive ability and consequences on haemodynamics and gas exchange. Thorax 1997;52:369–372.
181. Parker TA, Ivy DD, Kinsella JP, Torelli F, Ruyle SZ, Thilo SH, et al. Combined therapy with inhaled nitric oxide and intravenous prostacyclin in an infant with alveolar-capillary dysplasia. Am J Respir Crit Care Med 1997;155:743–746.
182. Roberts JD, Roberts CT, Jones RC, Zapol WM, Bloch KD. Continuous nitric oxide inhalation reduces pulmonary arterial remodeling, right ventricular hypertrophy, and growth retardation in the hypoxic newborn rat. Circ Res 1995;76(2):215–222.

183. Hess D, Bigatello L, Hurford WE. Toxicity and complications of inhaled nitric oxide. Respir Care Clin N Am 1997;3:487–503.
184. Szabo C, Ohshima H. DNA damage induced by peroxynitrite: subsequent biological effects. Nitric Oxide 1997;1:373–385.
185. Ichinose F, Adrie C, Hurford WE, Zapol WM. Prolonged pulmonary vasodilator action of inhaled nitric oxide by Zaprinast in awake lambs. J Appl Physiol 1995;78:1288–1295.
186. Thusu KG, Morin FC, Russell JA, Steinhorn RH. The cGMP phosphodiesterase inhibitor zaprinast enhances the effect of nitric oxide. Am J Respir Crit Care Med 1995;152:1605–1610.
187. Ichinose F, Adrie C, Hurford WE, Bloch KD, Zapol WM. Selective pulmonary vasodilation induced by aerosolized zaprinast. Anesthesiology 1998;88:410–416.
188. Fullerton DA, Jaggers J, Piedalue F, Frederick GL, McIntyre RC. Effective control of refractory pulmonary hypertension after cardiac operations. J Thorac Cardiovasc Surg 1997;113:363–370.
189. Kinsella JP, Torielli F, Ziegler JD, Ivy DD, Abman SH. Dipyridamole augmentation of response to nitric oxide. Lancet 1995;346:647,648.
190. Ivy DD, Kinsella JP, Ziegler JW, Abman SH. Dipyridamole attenuates rebound pulmonary hypertension after inhaled nitric oxide withdrawal in postoperative congenital heart disease. J Thorac Cardiovasc Surg 1998;115:875–882.
191. Janssens SP, Bloch KD, Nong Z, Gerard RD, Zoldhelyi P, Collen D. Adenovirus-mediated transfer of the human constitutive endothelial nitric oxide synthase to hypoxic rat lungs. J Clin Invest 1996;98: 317–324.

16 Nitric Oxide in Atherosclerosis

Robert T. Eberhardt and Joseph Loscalzo

INTRODUCTION

The importance of nitric oxide (NO•) in the regulation of vascular physiology and the pathophysiology of vascular diseases is now widely recognized. The discovery of NO• as a key molecule released by the endothelium to control vascular homeostasis stems from the finding of Furchgott and Zawadzki that an intact vascular endothelium is required for a vasodilator response to muscarinic agonists. These investigators found that in the presence of an intact endothelium, acetylcholine produces dose-dependent relaxation in isolated arterial segments by triggering the release of a potent vasodilator substance termed endothelium-derived relaxing factor (1). In contrast, when the endothelium is denuded, acetylcholine produces contraction owing to unopposed direct vasoconstrictor effects on vascular smooth muscle (1). Endothelium-derived relaxing factor (EDRF) was eventually identified as NO•, as both possess similar chemical and biological properties (2,3). The specific identity of EDRF has not been without controversy as it has been suggested that an S-nitrosated compound, S-nitroso-L-cysteine, is a more likely candidate molecule (4).

In vascular endothelial cells, NO• is derived from the terminal guanidino nitrogen of the precursor amino acid L-arginine during its oxidative conversion to L-citrulline (5). This reaction is catalyzed by the endothelial isoform of nitric oxide synthase (eNOS), which is constitutively expressed and regulated by calcium and calmodulin (6). Other members of this family of enzymes include an inducible isoform (iNOS), expressed in macrophages and vascular smooth muscle by exposure to cytokines, and a second constitutively expressed isoform found in neuronal cells (nNOS). NO• release is well suited for its role as a biological messenger, being a small lipid-soluble molecule that can readily diffuse across biological membranes. Furthermore, NO• is a highly reactive molecule with a short biological half-life, of the order of seconds, as a result of an unpaired electron that can readily react with oxygen, superoxide anion, or transition metals (7). Although susceptible to rapid inactivation, NO• reacts with plasma thiols in the presence of oxygen in vivo to form more stable S-nitrosothiols, which serve as a plasma NO• reservoir and prolong the biologic half-life of NO• (8).

After diffusing into the target cells, NO• activates soluble guanylyl cyclase (GC), which catalyzes the conversion of guanosine triphosphate (GTP) to cyclic guanosine monophosphate (cGMP). An increase in the cGMP level activates cGMP-dependent protein kinase leading to the phosphorylation of myosin light-chain kinase and stabilization of an inactive form of myosin (6). In addition, cGMP facilitates the transport of calcium from the cytosol and thereby alters actomyosin adenosine triphosphatase (ATPase) activity. Acting in concert, these actions serve to inhibit smooth muscle contraction. Biological responses mediated by cGMP are believed to account for the major bioactivity of NO•; however, biologic responses

From: *Contemporary Cardiology, vol. 4: Nitric Oxide and the Cardiovascular System*
Edited by: J. Loscalzo and J. A. Vita © Humana Press Inc., Totowa, NJ

by cGMP-independent mechanisms are active areas of investigation, including direct effects of NO• on potassium and calcium channel activities *(9,10)*.

By inhibiting the contractile mechanisms within vascular smooth muscle, NO• released from the vascular endothelium causes vasodilation and participates in the regulation of vascular tone. In fact, basal and stimulated release of NO• from the vascular endothelium appear to play important roles in the regulation of blood pressure and blood flow in numerous vascular beds *(11,12)*. Basal release of NO• has been shown to participate in the maintenance of resting tone and blood flow in both the peripheral and coronary circulations. Stimulation of NO• release above the basal level by various physical and biochemical stimuli results in endothelium-dependent vasodilation *(13)*. Further enhancement of NO• release occurs in response to many receptor-dependent agonists (such as acetylcholine, adenosine triphosphate, thrombin, serotonin, histamine, substance P, and bradykinin), as well as physical stimuli, including flow-induced shear stress and pulsatile stretch *(13)*. Endothelium-dependent dilation in response to these various stimuli, which are important physiological signals, appears to play a central role in the regulation of vascular tone and blood flow within numerous vascular beds.

In part through these vasodilator actions, NO• serves as a critical regulatory molecule in vascular physiology, participating in the maintenance of vascular homeostasis. NO• has also been implicated in the pathophysiology of various vascular diseases, serving as a key element in vasomotor dysfunction. In addition, endothelial-derived NO• may modulate atherothrombogenesis, in part, through antithrombotic or antiplatelet actions. A reduction in vascular NO• action, characteristic of atherosclerosis, may play an important role in the development, progression, and clinical manifestations of this common disease. This chapter reviews the role that NO• plays in vascular homeostasis and its contribution to atherogenesis.

Antiatherogenic Actions of NO•

The vascular endothelium is not simply an inert monolayer of cells lining the vessel lumen but an active vascular element important in the regulation of vascular tone and homeostasis. The endothelium may prevent thrombosis and regulate atherogenesis through actions including vasodilation, inhibition of platelet adhesion and aggregation, inhibition of leukocyte adhesion, and inhibition of smooth muscle proliferation. NO• is a key regulatory molecule released from the vascular endothelium, inhibiting many of these steps involved in the development and progression of thrombotic disorders and atherosclerosis *(14)* (Fig. 1). Furthermore, NO• produced from other sources, including circulating blood elements, vascular smooth muscle cells (VSMCs), and interstitial fibroblasts, may participate in the modulation of atherothrombogenesis.

REGULATION OF VASCULAR TONE

Vascular tone is determined largely by the contractile state of the VSMC. NO• may influence the contractile state of VSMCs by causing relaxation and thus decreasing vascular tone *(13)*. Inhibition of basal NO• generation with NOS inhibition increases tension in precontracted vessels ex vivo and constricts conductance and resistance vessels in vivo *(15–17)*. These findings support participation of basal NO• release in maintenance of resting vascular tone. In addition, the stimulation of NO• release in response to neurohormonal and physical stimuli results in vasodilation in numerous circulatory beds *(13)*. These actions of NO• may prevent excessive vasoconstriction and vasospasm, which predisposes to thrombosis.

REGULATION OF PLATELET FUNCTION

Although critical to hemostasis, platelets also play a central role in the pathogenesis of thrombosis and atherosclerosis. Early in the development of atherosclerosis, platelets adhere to the vessel wall and may form thrombi, whereas the progression of atherosclerosis is enhanced by the release of chemotactic factors and cytokines from activated platelets *(18)*.

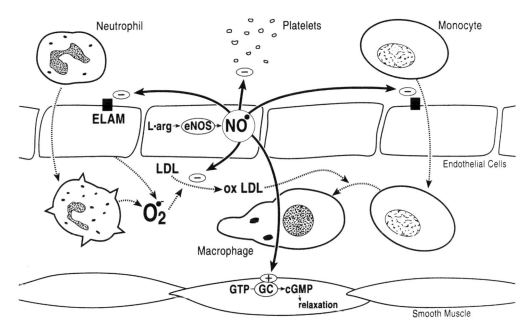

Fig. 1. The nitric oxide pathway in vascular homeostasis. Nitric oxide (NO•) is synthesized in endothelial cells by the action on eNOS during the conversion of L-arginine to L-citrulline. NO• inhibits platelet adhesion and aggregation. NO• also inhibits leukocyte and monocyte adhesion and emigration into the subendothelial space. Through this action and by inhibition of LDL oxidation, NO• may prevent the transformation of tissue macrophages into foam cells. NO• causes relaxation of vascular smooth muscle cells via the activation of guanylyl cyclase (GC) and increased cyclic guanosine monophosphate (cGMP) formation.

Endothelial antithrombotic mechanisms that prevent platelets from adhering to the vascular wall include the production and release of endothelium-derived NO• *(19)*. By influencing the platelet–endothelial interaction, endogenous NO• may participate in the regulation of the development and progression of atherosclerosis. There is evidence for the antiplatelet actions of endogenous and exogenous NO•, which inhibits platelet adhesion, activation, and aggregation, and promotes platelet disaggregation.

Exogenous NO• has been shown to inhibit multiple aspects of platelet function. Mellion and colleagues demonstrated that NO• inhibits platelet aggregation and promotes platelet disaggregation, effects that are dependent on GC activation and cGMP accumulation *(20)*. NO• and nitrovasodilators in vitro cause dose-dependent inhibition of adenosine diphosphate (ADP)-induced platelet aggregation in platelet-rich plasma as assessed by aggregometry *(20)*. Mendelsohn and colleagues found that this action of NO• is, in part, due to inhibition of platelet activation-induced exposure of the fibrinogen-binding site on the glycoprotein IIb/IIIa complex, thus inhibiting fibrinogen-dependent platelet crosslinking and aggregation *(21)*. NO• inhibits platelet activation with attenuated secretion of platelet granules and expression of activation markers. Michelson and colleagues found that NO• inhibits thrombin and thromboxane A_2 analog-induced upregulation of the α-granule protein P-selectin, the lysosomal protein CD63, and the glycoprotein IIb/IIIa complex *(22)*. In addition, exogenous NO• inhibits platelet adhesion with an attenuation of the binding of activated platelets to vascular endothelial surfaces *(23)*.

Similarly, support for the antiplatelet actions of NO• derived from vascular endothelial surfaces has been accumulating. Radomski and colleagues found that bradykinin-induced endogenous NO• production inhibits the adhesion of thrombin-stimulated human platelets to a confluent monolayer of cultured bovine endothelial cells *(23)*. Sneddon and Vane demonstrated that an intact endothelium is required for bradykinin to inhibit platelet adhesion to vascular surfaces such as bovine aorta *(24)*. Enhancing NO• production by the endothelium in vivo diminishes platelet aggregation. Yao and colleagues found that L-arginine decreases platelet aggregation and appears to eliminate cyclic reductions in blood flow caused by recurrent platelet adhesion to and accumulation in injured arteries in mongrel dogs *(25)*. In contrast, a reduction in NO• formation with inhibition of NOS enhances platelet aggregation and may induce cyclic flow variation *(25)*. These studies support the antiplatelet actions of endothelium-derived NO• with inhibition of platelet adhesion to vascular surfaces.

In addition, platelets themselves are alternative sources of endogenous NO• production that can modulate platelet reactivity, possible limiting thrombus formation and propagation. Human platelets possess both the enzyme NOS (homologous to eNOS) and a specific high-affinity L-arginine transporter, thus providing an integrated system for NO• generation *(26,27)*. Elaboration of NO• from aggregating platelets modulates platelet reactivity, inhibiting further platelet aggregation *(26)*. Radomski and colleagues found that attenuation of NO• production with NOS inhibition enhances collagen-induced platelet aggregation, whereas enhancement of NO• production with L-arginine inhibits collagen-induced platelet aggregation *(26)*. In addition, Freedman and colleagues demonstrated that NO• released from activated platelets markedly inhibits additional platelet recruitment to the growing platelet aggregate despite only modestly inhibiting platelet activation *(28)*. NOS inhibition in a primary-activated platelet population results in an increase in expression of the activation marker P-selectin on addition of a second population of platelets. Platelet-derived NO• has antiplatelet action that may limit thrombus formation and platelet recruitment to a propagating thrombus. Thus, a concerted action of endothelial- and platelet-derived NO• appears to regulate platelet function with inhibitory effects on platelet adhesion, activation, aggregation, and recruitment. These effects of NO• on platelet function may modulate atherogenesis and play a role in the management of the acute clinical manifestations of atherosclerosis.

REGULATION OF LEUKOCYTE–ENDOTHELIAL INTERACTIONS

In addition to their well-established role in the response to infectious and inflammatory diseases, leukocytes have been implicated in the development and progression of coronary artery disease (CAD) *(15)*. Neutrophil adhesion and emigration are hallmark findings of early atherosclerosis and may contribute to its development. Monocyte adhesion, migration, and transformation with focal accumulation of lipid-laden foam cells within the subintimal space are paramount in the pathogenesis of atherosclerosis *(29)*. NO• may regulate monocyte and polymorphonuclear leukocyte responses by modulating their adhesion to endothelial surfaces, thus preventing their migration from the blood stream to the subintimal space to participate in atherogenesis.

Endogenous production of NO• appears to modulate leukocyte chemotaxis and adhesion to the vascular endothelium. Bath and colleagues demonstrated that exogenous NO• inhibits basal monocyte adhesion to porcine aortic endothelial cell monolayers in culture, but has no effect on adhesion of activated monocytes stimulated with fMLP (*N*-formyl-L-methionyl-L-leucyl-L-phenylalanine) *(30)*. In contrast, NO• inhibits fMLP-stimulated monocyte migration across artificial membrane—a marker of monocyte chemotaxis *(30)*. Tsao and colleagues found that brief exposure of endothelial cells in culture to fluid flow stimulates the cells to produce NO• that alters endothelial adhesiveness to monocytes within 30 min *(31)*. In vivo, diminished basal NO• release following myocardial ischemia promotes neutrophil adhesion to coronary endothelium in a feline model of ischemia–reperfusion injury *(32)*. Further emphasizing the importance of endogenous NO• production, Kubes and colleagues found that superfusion of NOS inhibitors over feline mesenteric beds increases leukocyte adhesion 15-fold and enhances leukocyte emigration in postcapillary venules *(33)*.

NO• may regulate endothelial adhesiveness by altering the expression or activation state of adhesion molecules, and/or the secretion of chemoattractant proteins for leukocytes. The diminished adhesion of monocytes to endothelial cells during brief flow, observed by Tsao and colleagues, appears to be due to alterations in signal transduction or the activation state of endothelial adhesion molecules *(31)*. The expression of adhesion molecules intercellular adhesion molecule-1 (ICAM-1) or vascular cell adhesion molecule-1 (VCAM-1), is not influenced during this brief time period. In contrast, diminished endothelial adhesiveness during prolonged NO• exposure, either by stimulating NO• release with fluid flow or providing exogenous NO•, is associated with reduced endothelial cell expression of adhesion molecules, including ICAM-1 and VCAM-1 *(34,35)*. Further supporting regulation by NO•, the increase in leukocyte adhesion to the vascular endothelium during superfusion of NOS inhibitors is reversed with an antibody to leukocyte adhesion glycoprotein (CD11/CD18) *(33)*. In addition, Adams and colleagues found that enhancing NO• production with L-arginine supplementation reduces the adhesion of monocytes to cultures of human umbilical vein endothelial cells, which is associated with decreased expression of the adhesion molecule VCAM-1 and ICAM-1 *(36)*. NO• may also alter the expression of chemotactic factors that regulate leukocyte migration. Zeiher and colleagues found that NO• modulates the expression of monocyte chemotactic protein-1 (MCP-1), as NOS inhibition upregulates the expression of MCP-1 and enhances monocyte chemotactic activity generated by cultured human endothelial cells *(37)*.

REGULATION OF VASCULAR SMOOTH MUSCLE PROLIFERATION

VSMCs in the contractile state only rarely exhibit mitogenic activity. In contrast, excessive vascular smooth muscle proliferation with an increase in mitogenesis is another fundamental feature of atherosclerosis. Atherogenesis is characterized by migration, proliferation, and alteration of VSMC phenotype with increased production of extracellular matrix. Recent evidence supports the view that NO• may modulate aspects of VSMC function, including migration, growth, and proliferation. Endogenous NO• release from the vascular endothelium and other vascular cells may inhibit VSMC proliferation, and thus prevent the development or delay the progression of atherosclerosis.

Exogenous NO• has been shown to modulate VSMC function including migration, growth, and proliferation. Garg and Hassid demonstrated that NO•, through cGMP-dependent mechanisms, inhibits VSMC DNA synthesis *(38)*. NO• donors dose-dependently inhibit serum-induced thymidine incorporation by cultured rat aortic smooth muscle cells—an action mimicked by cGMP analogs *(38)*. In addition, NO• donors decrease proliferation of VSMC *(38)*; the antiproliferative action involves diminished activity and/or expression of several key regulators of the G_1 and S phases of the cell cycle *(39)*. NO• donors also inhibit basal and endothelin-stimulated protein synthesis and elaboration of extracellular matrix by VSMC *(40)*. In addition, Sarkar and colleagues found that NO• donors reversibly inhibit migration of smooth muscle cells following wounding of a confluent culture of rat aortic vascular smooth muscle cells. This inhibitory effect of NO• on VSMC migration is independent of antiproliferative or cytotoxic actions *(41)*.

Endogenous NO• appears to participate in the normal physiologic regulation of VSMC growth and proliferation. NO• is a critical mediator released from the endothelium that participates in the regulation of VSMC. Scott-Burden and Vanhoutte demonstrated that rat aortic smooth muscle proliferation is inhibited by coculture with bovine aortic endothelial cells *(42)*. This antiproliferative effect was, in part, due to NO•-mediated actions, as it was blunted by NOS inhibition. In addition to the endothelium, Busse and Mülsch found that production of NO• by VSMC following endothelial injury in response to cytokine induction of iNOS might modulate their growth and proliferation *(43)*. NO• production induced by interleukin-1 (IL-1) attenuates fibroblast growth factor (FGF)-induced thymidine incorporation in cultured VSMCs *(44)*. This antimitogenic effect of NO• derived from VSMC is abolished by NOS inhibition *(44)*. Thus, VSMC proliferation may be regulated by NO• derived from endogenous sources, including endothelial cells and VSMCs themselves.

MODULATION OF OXIDATIVE STRESS AND LDL OXIDATION

Superoxide anion and other reactive oxygen species are universal by-products of oxidative metabolism. Under normal physiological conditions their generation is counterbalanced by endogenous antioxidant defense mechanisms. However, excessive generation of reactive oxygen species, including superoxide anion, may cause oxidative injury to components of the blood vessel wall and facilitate the development and progression of atherosclerosis. Lawson and colleagues have demonstrated direct toxic effects of reactive oxygen species on vascular endothelial cells, resulting in endothelial cell separation, vacuolization, nuclear condensation, and blebbing (45). Another major target of oxidative stress is low-density lipoprotein (LDL), which plays a critical role in the pathogenesis of atherosclerosis (46). Once oxidized, LDL binds to scavenger receptors, facilitating LDL entry into tissue macrophages and formation of foam cells. Increased generation of reactive oxygen species has been demonstrated in models of atherosclerosis (47). Experimental and epidemiological studies suggest a benefit of antioxidants in the suppression of atherosclerosis, thus supporting oxidative stress in the pathogenesis of atherosclerosis (46).

NO• may participate in the modulation of oxidative injury, acting as a chain-breaking antioxidant capable of scavenging reactive oxygen species and free radicals. In addition, NO• may attenuate direct cellular damage from reactive oxygen species and prevent subsequent oxidation of LDL (46). NO• may attenuate cellular toxicity by limiting the generation and enhancing the inactivation of superoxide anion. In equimolar amounts, NO• reacts with superoxide to form peroxynitrite, which at low concentrations retains some of the antiplatelet and vasodilator properties of NO• (48,49). In addition, Hogg and colleagues found that continuous NO• generation directly inhibits LDL oxidation (50). Furthermore, NO• may attenuate subintimal LDL oxidation by altering vascular permeability and decreasing the flux of LDL into the subintimal space (51). However, there is considerable controversy regarding the exact role that NO• and NOS play in modulating oxidative stress and LDL oxidation.

Although NO• may attenuate oxidative stress, a potential detrimental role of NO• and NOS in atherogenesis has been suggested, in part, resulting from heightened generation of reactive oxygen species. NO• may directly contribute to oxidative injury, whereas NOS may contribute to further generation of reactive oxygen species. NO• may cause direct toxic effects with nitration and nitrosation of proteins, ADP ribosylation, and DNA damage. In addition, in the presence of superoxide anion or at a low pH in the presence of oxygen, NO• directly enhances LDL oxidation (52). Excessive amounts of NO•, produced via iNOS, may combine with superoxide to increase the production of peroxynitrite. At high concentrations, peroxynitrite may exacerbate oxidative damage leading to increased LDL oxidation and lipid peroxidation (53). High concentrations of peroxynitrite have also been shown to promote platelet aggregation and blunt coronary vasodilator responses (47,48). These findings have led to the suggestion that excessive NO• production may play a deleterious role and contribute to atherogenesis. Furthermore, increased generation of reactive oxygen species by NOS itself may occur under select conditions, such as inadequate tetrahydrobiopterin (BH_4) or L-arginine stores (54).

A potential dual role of NO• in the modulation of oxidative stress has been suggested with basal NO• production reducing oxidative stress, and excessive NO• production exacerbating oxidative stress. This potential dual role of NO• may be relevant within the vascular wall: prevention of lipid oxidation may provide early protection against atherosclerosis, whereas enhanced lipid oxidation within an established plaque may contribute to late progression.

NO• REGULATION OF APOPTOSIS IN ATHEROSCLEROSIS

Evidence is accumulating in support of the participation of apoptosis, or programmed cell death, in the pathogenesis of atherosclerosis. Apoptosis of VSMCs has been demonstrated in atherosclerotic plaques, especially in those containing immune cells, e.g., macrophages and T lymphocytes *(55)*. Apoptosis occurs in SMCs localized to the fibrous cap and the underlying media, raising the possibility that this contributes to plaque instability and rupture. Activation of the Fas death-signaling pathway appears to contribute to apoptosis of VSMCs exposed to inflammatory cytokines *(56)*. In addition, Hegyi and colleagues found that apoptosis contributes to foam cell death at the edge of the lipid core, suggesting that this process might play a role in the formation and enlargement of the lipid core *(57)*. Expansion of the acellular lipid core and weakened integrity of the fibrous cap, in part due to apoptosis of foam cells and VSMCs during vascular remodeling, may predispose to plaque rupture and subsequent myocardial infarction.

NO• has been demonstrated to induce apoptosis in several vascular cells including vascular smooth cells, tissue macrophages, and even vascular endothelial cells. Fukuo and colleagues found that macrophage-derived cytokines induce apoptosis of VSMCs through an NO•-dependent mechanism *(58)*. An inhibitor of NOS inhibited the upregulation of Fas induced by cytokines in VSMCs *(59)*. Similarly, Shimaoka and colleagues found that an exogenous NO•-releasing compound, NOC-18, induced apoptosis of macrophages in a dose-dependent fashion *(60)*. Apoptosis of activated macrophages by oxidized LDL is diminished by inhibition of NO• generated by iNOS *(61)*. It appears that NO• production via iNOS may lead to apoptosis of VSMCs and macrophages and may participate in the pathogenesis of atherosclerosis. The precise role that apoptosis plays in atherogenesis remains uncertain; however, it appears that NO• is an important element in its regulation.

NO• IN THE PATHOGENESIS OF ATHEROSCLEROSIS

Impact of Atherosclerosis on NO•

Atherosclerosis is accompanied by endothelial dysfunction with impairment in endothelium-dependent relaxation in animal models and clinical investigations. This defect in endothelial function, as demonstrated in experimental models, is primarily a result of impaired NO•-mediated bioaction. Animals such as rabbits fed a diet rich in cholesterol begin to manifest early atherosclerotic changes with formation of fatty streaks within 8 wk. Atherosclerotic vessels from rabbits fed this atherogenic diet manifest impaired endothelial function *(62)*. Precontracted aortic rings from cholesterol-fed animal have impaired endothelium-dependent relaxation to acetylcholine (ACh) despite preservation of endothelium-independent relaxation to nitroglycerin *(62)* (Fig. 2). Bossaller and colleagues found that this defect in endothelium-dependent relaxation is associated with diminished muscarinic agonist-induced cGMP accumulation in aortic strips from rabbits with diet-induced atherosclerosis *(63)*. This diminished cGMP accumulation supports an attenuation of biologically active NO• in atherosclerosis. Similar findings of impaired endothelium-dependent relaxation induced by ACh, bradykinin, thrombin, A23187, adenosine diphosphate (ADP), and/or 5-hydroxytryptamine have been reported in pigs, monkeys, and humans with hypercholesterolemia and atherosclerosis *(63–65)*. Impairment in endothelial function with attenuated endothelium-dependent vasodilation has also been demonstrated in vivo in atherosclerosis. Humans with atherosclerosis demonstrate abnormal endothelial function with paradoxical vasoconstriction of epicardial vessels to ACh *(66)*. This defect in endothelial function appears to be systemic in nature with impairment of endothelium-dependent relaxation extending into the microcirculation and peripheral vasculature in humans with atherosclerosis *(67)*.

Endothelial dysfunction plays an active role in atherogenesis serving as an early marker of atherosclerosis and not simply a consequence of atherosclerosis. Endothelial dysfunction occurs in response to vascular insult, appearing early in the progression of atherosclerosis *(15)*. Verbeuren and colleagues found progressive impairment in endothelium-dependent relaxation in cholesterol-fed rabbits with increasing fatty streak formation *(62)*. Similarly, McLenachan and colleagues found that the loss of ACh-induced or flow-induced, endothelium-dependent

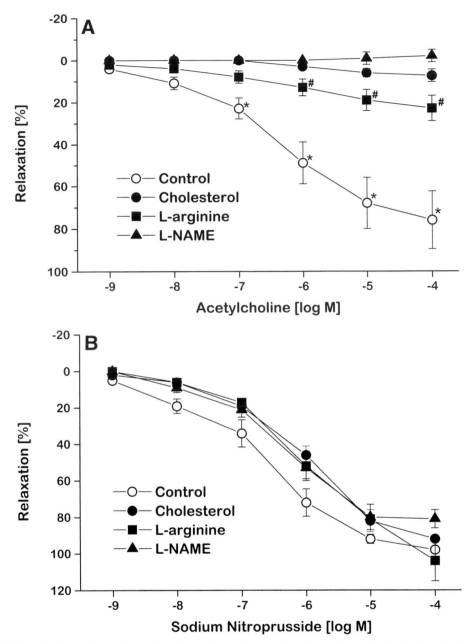

Fig. 2. Endothelium-dependent relaxation induced by acetylcholine (**A**), and endothelium-independent relaxation induced by sodium nitroprusside (**B**), of isolated aortic rings ex vivo from rabbits fed a normal diet (Control), or a cholesterol-enriched diet (Cholesterol), or cholesterol-enriched diet plus L-arginine (L-arginine) or plus L-NAME (L-NAME). Values represent means ± SEM of 4 rings from 8 rabbits per group (4 rabbits in the control group). *$p < 0.05$ for control vs. cholesterol-fed. #$p < 0.05$ vs. cholesterol-fed. Reprinted with the permission of Elsevier Science from Böger et al., Atherosclerosis 1995;117:273.

vasodilation occurs early in the course of atherosclerosis in cholesterol-fed monkeys *(68)*. Iliac arteries devoid of luminal narrowing, with only intimal thickening, fail to dilate to a doubling of flow induced by adenosine and constrict in response to ACh *(68)*. Furthermore, Cohen and colleagues found that impairment in endothelium-dependent coronary vasodilation in cholesterol-fed pigs occurs prior to the onset of histological atherosclerotic changes *(65)*. Similar findings have been observed in humans: endothelium-dependent vasomotor function is impaired in subjects with risk factors for atherosclerosis prior to the development of any observable changes in the vessel intima, as assessed by angiography and intravascular ultrasound *(69,70)*. Otsuji and colleagues found that progressive impairment in endothelium-dependent coronary vasodilation correlates with the progression of atherosclerosis and suggested that endothelial dysfunction with diminished NO• action is an early marker of coronary atherogenesis *(71)*. This impairment in endothelial function with diminished NO• vasodilator function prior to the appearance of overt atherosclerotic changes is consistent with the participation of this abnormality in the pathogenesis of atherosclerosis.

Mechanisms of Impaired NO• Bioaction

Mechanisms that may account for the impairment in NO•-mediated bioactivity in atherosclerosis include a decrease in NO• production, an increase in NO• inactivation, and a decrease in sensitivity to NO•. Blood vessels with early atherosclerosis do not have a generalized impairment in vasodilator function due to diminished compliance or an increased barrier to diffusion. The vasodilator response to endothelium-independent vasodilators is largely preserved in atherosclerotic vessels *(62–65)*. Sensitivity to NO• appears normal, and possibly heightened, in atherosclerosis, as vessels from cholesterol-fed rabbits relax equally on exposure to the NO• donor nitroglycerin and the direct NO• donor-acidified nitrite *(62,72)*. Because the responsiveness to exogenous NO• is preserved, a disturbance in either endogenous NO• synthesis or accelerated NO• breakdown has been suggested to account for the diminished bioaction of NO• in atherosclerosis. More recent experimental evidence suggests diminished sensitivity to NO• in atherosclerosis despite preserved response to NO• donors. Atherosclerotic vessels from ApoE knockout mice demonstrate impaired response to NO• despite preserved response to sodium nitroprusside *(73)*.

There is support for impairment of NO• production and/or release in atherosclerosis. Verbeuren and colleagues demonstrated diminished relaxation of detector control vessels when atherosclerotic donor vessels are stimulated with ACh to release NO•, compared with donor control vessels *(74)*. Diminished NO• formation may result from inhibition of NOS activity or limitation of substrate availability in atherosclerotic vessels. This conclusion is supported by the findings of Böger and colleagues that urinary nitrite excretion is decreased in hypercholesterolemia *(75)*. This effect of hypercholesterolemia on nitrite excretion is potentiated by NOS inhibition and attenuated by L-arginine *(75)*. Limited substrate availability may be a consequence of a limited capacity of inducers of iNOS to stimulate y^+ carrier-mediated L-arginine transport into VSMCs *(76)*. However, the concentration of intracellular L-arginine in endothelial cells far exceeds the K_m value for eNOS, thus it is unlikely that the extracellular L-arginine concentration is the rate-limiting step in endothelial NO• generation *(77)*. Bode-Böger and colleagues found a relative increase in the endogenous NOS inhibitor asymmetric dimethyl L-arginine in atherosclerosis *(78)*. They suggested that this increase may lead to the diminished production of NO• *(78)*. In addition, there is reduced transcription and enhanced breakdown of NOS transcripts by increasing concentrations of oxidized LDL *(79)*. Thus, diminished NO• production may result from inhibition, inactivation, and/or decreased production of NOS.

Alternatively, there is evidence for inactivation of NO• in atherosclerosis. The principal mechanism contributing to the inactivation of NO• is oxidative degradation. Supporting this view is the finding that superoxide production is increased in atherosclerotic and preatherosclerotic vessels *(47,75)*. Ohara and colleagues found that superoxide production is increased threefold in vessels from cholesterol-fed rabbits *(47)*. Gryglewski and colleagues demonstrated that superoxide anion is involved in the breakdown of biologically active NO• *(80)*.

The increased superoxide production may overcome the intrinsic vascular antioxidant protective mechanisms and lead to inactivation of NO• prior to or immediately after release. Supporting this conclusion are the findings that enhancing antioxidant defense mechanisms markedly improve endothelium-dependent relaxation in animal models of atherosclerosis *(81,82)*. Mügge and colleagues found that injection of polyethelene-glycolated-superoxide dimutase (SOD) improves ACh-induced relaxation in vessels from hypercholesterolemic rabbits *(81)*. Similarly, the use of antioxidant vitamin supplementation improved endothelium-dependent relaxation in rabbits with diet-induced atherosclerosis *(82)*. Furthermore, diminished antioxidant defense mechanisms, including glutathione peroxidase and glutathione reductase, have been shown in atherosclerotic lesions *(83)*. In addition, NOS activity may be increased rather than decreased in atherosclerosis, as Minor and colleagues found that basal and stimulated NO• release is increased in aortic segments from hypercholesterolemic rabbits despite diminished NO• bioactivity *(84)*. Thus, an imbalance between pro-oxidant and antioxidant activities in atherosclerosis may lead to a deficiency of biologically active NO•.

Superoxide anion and other reactive oxygen species may be generated from several potential sources in atherosclerosis including xanthine oxidase, NADH/NADPH (nicotinamide adenine dinucleotide phosophate) oxidase, and NOS itself (especially when substrate or cofactors are limiting) *(47,54,85,86)*. Ohara and colleagues found that inhibition of xanthine oxidase with oxypurinol normalizes superoxide anion production and restores endothelium-dependent relaxation in vessels from hypercholesterolemic rabbits *(47)*. Increased superoxide anion production may be driven by activation of membrane-bound NADH/NADPH oxidase, as found in a model of hypertension induced by angiotensin *(86)*. In contrast, Pritchard and colleagues found that NOS inhibition largely prevents the release of superoxide from endothelial cells incubated with LDL *(87)*. Both L-arginine and BH_4 supplementation are effective in restoring endothelium-dependent vasodilation in hypercholesterolemia *(54)*. Thus, in various models of atherosclerosis, and in the presence of risk factors for atherosclerosis, an increase in superoxide anion production has been demonstrated to be dependent on xanthine oxidase, NADH/NADPH oxidase, and/or NOS activity.

Consequences of Impaired NO• Bioaction

Impaired NO• bioactivity creates an environment that strongly favors the development and progression of atherosclerosis. Enhancement of platelet adhesion and aggregation in hypercholesterolemia favors atherothrombogenesis. Tsao and colleagues found that ADP-induced platelet aggregation is greater in hypercholesterolemic rabbits compared with control rabbits *(88)*. Enhancing endogenous NO• production with L-arginine supplementation attenuates this increase in platelet reactivity *(88)*. Adhesion of circulating platelets triggers the formation of platelet aggregates and increases the propensity toward thrombus formation. Activated platelets may then release chemotactic and growth factors that perpetuate the cascade of events involved in atherogenesis.

This response contributes to the enhancement of neutrophil and monocyte adhesion to the vascular endothelium. Lefer and Ma found that decreased basal NO• release is associated with a threefold increase in neutrophil adhesion to the coronary endothelium in hypercholesterolemic rabbits *(89)*. Tsao and colleagues found that exogenous NO• inhibits the binding of monocytes to the thoracic aorta of hypercholesterolemic rabbits, an effect attenuated by L-arginine and enhanced by NOS inhibition *(90)*. Similarly, Adams and colleagues found that enhancing endogenous NO• production with L-arginine supplementation in human subjects with coronary artery disease reduces ex vivo adhesion of monocytes to human umbilical vein endothelial cells in culture *(91)*. Diminished biologically active NO• in atherosclerosis promotes the adhesion of circulating monocytes to the endothelium with subsequent migrate into the subintima and transformation into tissue macrophages and foam cells.

Enhanced uptake of LDL into the subintimal space with subsequent oxidative modification further contributes to foam cell formation. Increased generation of reactive oxygen species is seen in atherosclerosis with enhanced basal and stimulated superoxide anion production in hypercholesterolemic animals (75). This increase in reactive oxygen species, including superoxide anion and peroxynitrite, promotes the oxidation of LDL. Oxidatively modified LDL induces endothelial cells to express chemotactic and adhesion molecules, including MCP-1 and macrophage colony-stimulating factor, leading to further monocyte recruitment (46). Monocytes undergo differentiation to tissue macrophages with uptake of oxidized LDL by scavenger receptors and subsequent transformation into foam cells.

Both superoxide anion and oxidized LDL contribute to the further inactivation of NO• by direct and indirect mechanisms, thus perpetuating the defect in endothelial function (80,92). Increased oxidized LDL decreases the expression of eNOS and promotes further generation of superoxide anion from the residual eNOS (79,87). Diminished NO• production leads to nuclear factor κ-B (NF-κB) activation, which is a transcription factor that initiates a proinflammatory cascade: genes normally suppressed by NF-κB become activated with increased generation of adhesion molecules, cytokines, and growth factors. In addition, diminished NO• bioactivity leads to increased VSMC migration and proliferation, as supported by Koglin and colleagues who showed that smooth muscle proliferation contributes to an exacerbation of transplant atherosclerosis in iNOS deficient mice (93). VSMCs are stimulated to produce and release extracellular matrix, which accumulates as the plaque evolves. Thus, conditions within an atherosclerotic plaque favor further depletion of NO• and generation of excessive reactive oxygen species, which may accelerate atherosclerosis.

Impairment in NO•-mediated actions also contributes to the clinical expression of atherosclerosis and manifestations of CAD, including myocardial ischemia, coronary vasospasm, and myocardial infarction. This is particularly relevant in the coronary circulation, as diminished NO• bioactivity contributes to the dysregulation of coronary blood flow and limitation to coronary flow reserve in patients with CAD (94). Decreased basal and stimulated NO• release for the vascular endothelium increases vascular tone and predisposes toward vasospasm. Attenuated endothelium-dependent vasodilation of epicardial vessels in response to the stimulus of increased flow during exercise or mental stress may contribute to limiting coronary blood flow to regions of myocardium supplied by stenotic vessels (95–98). This impairment in NO• release extends into the coronary microcirculation, influencing the regulation of coronary blood flow and further limiting flow reserve (99,100). This may limit the increase in coronary blood flow during times of increased metabolic demand, thus contributing to myocardial ischemia (94,100). Furthermore, a propensity toward vasospasm with paradoxical vasoconstriction due to a loss of NO• vasodilatory actions occurs in vessels with atherosclerosis (66). Diminished NO• actions near atherosclerotic plaques predisposes toward thrombosis and infarction accompanying plaque instability, heightened platelet aggregability, vasoconstriction, and vasospasm. Yao and colleagues demonstrated that enhancing endogenous NO• production with L-arginine supplementation delays intracoronary thrombus formation in injured canine coronary arteries (101). In addition, diminished NO• release during a myocardial infarction may contribute to difficulty achieving successful thrombolysis and vulnerability to reocclusion. Adrie and colleagues demonstrated that inhaled NO• administered during thrombolysis increases coronary patency (102).

Modulation of Atherogenesis by NO•

Experimental models of atherosclerosis have been utilized to determine the role NO• plays in atherogenesis. The bioavailability of NO• may be heightened with an increase in endogenous NO• production by providing the precursor L-arginine or augmenting NOS production, or reduced with a decrease in endogenous NO• production by inhibiting NOS. Evaluation of the impact that manipulating NO• production has on vascular reactivity and atherosclerotic lesion formation may provide insight into the role of NO• in atherogenesis.

Enhancing endogenous NO• production has beneficial effects on vascular endothelial function in experimental models of hypercholesterolemia. Exogenous L-arginine augments endothelium-dependent vasodilation of hind limb resistance vessels in cholesterol-fed rabbits in vivo *(103)*. Girerd and colleagues found that infusion of L-arginine potentiates the blunted vasodilator response in cholesterol-fed animals to graded concentrations of ACh, suggesting a restoration of endothelial function *(103)* (Fig. 3). Infusion of L-arginine does not alter the vasodilator response to the endothelium-independent agent nitroprusside *(103)*. In contrast, brief exposure of excised aorta from cholesterol-fed rabbits to L-arginine in vitro failed to restore endothelium-dependent relaxation *(104)*. However, Cooke and colleagues found that in vivo exposure to L-arginine administered by intravenous infusion for 70 min potentiates endothelium-dependent relaxation to ACh in isolated thoracic aorta from hypercholesterolemic rabbits ex vivo *(105)*. Augmented vasodilation to ACh is stereospecific for L-arginine, as these effects are not duplicated by D-arginine *(105)*. This improvement in endothelium-dependent vasodilation is not accompanied by an improvement in endothelium-independent relaxation, as the response to sodium nitroprusside is unaltered *(105)*. The restoration in endothelial function with L-arginine appears to be caused by an enhancement in NO• production, as supported by an increase in urinary nitrite/nitrate excretion *(75)*.

In addition to improving endothelium-dependent vasodilation, enhanced NO• production and bioaction appears to limit atherogenesis in animal models of atherosclerosis. Supplementation with L-arginine is associated with a delay in the formation and progression of atherosclerotic lesions in animal models with diet-induced atherosclerosis. Cooke and colleagues found that chronic oral L-arginine supplementation reduces atheromatous lesion formation with a 50–75% reduction in lesion surface area and intimal thickness in the aortas of cholesterol-fed rabbits *(106)*. These effects on atherogenesis are observed in the absence of a change in the serum cholesterol or blood pressure *(106)*. Treatment with L-arginine modulates atherogenesis, in part by influencing macrophage accumulation, as supported by a near absence of adherent monocytes and tissue macrophages in the coronary arteries of cholesterol-fed rabbits. These results are associated with almost no progression of intimal thickening in the coronary arteries *(107)*. Similarly, L-arginine is effective in decreasing plaque area by approx 78% in the carotid arteries of cholesterol-fed rabbits *(75)*. Furthermore, despite subtle changes in vascular reactivity, Singer and colleagues found that L-arginine administration has a marked effect on atheroma formation with an eightfold reduction in intimal thickness in hypercholesterolemic rabbits *(108)*. Thus, L-arginine appears to reverse hypercholesterolemia-induced impairment in endothelium-dependent relaxation and to inhibit atherosclerotic lesion formation in cholesterol-fed animals.

Endogenous NO• may promote the regression of atheroma, as well as delay the progression of atherosclerosis. Candipan and colleagues found that L-arginine improves endothelium-dependent relaxation and reduces preexisting intimal lesions in the aorta of cholesterol-fed rabbits *(109)*. Despite continued intake of a cholesterol-rich diet, oral L-arginine supplementation for 8 wk tends to reduce the lesion surface area and intima-media ratio in the aortas from rabbits previously on a high-cholesterol diet alone for 10 wk *(109)* (Table 1). The improvement in endothelial function during L-arginine supplementation is associated with a significant increase in the vascular elaboration of NO•, whereas the elaboration of superoxide anion is significantly reduced *(109)*. Similarly, Böger and colleagues found that L-arginine blocks the progression of carotid intimal plaques and reduces aortic intimal thickening in association with partial restoration of urinary excretion of nitrite/nitrate and cGMP *(110)*. This suggests that the mechanism of protection by L-arginine includes increased substrate availability for NOS with generation of NO•, which reacts with superoxide anion to form peroxynitrite. In fact, measurable levels of superoxide anion are diminished during L-arginine

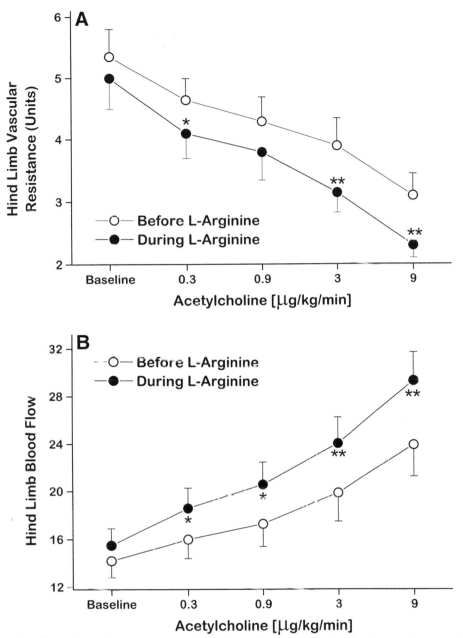

Fig. 3. The effect of L-arginine on endothelium-dependent vasodilation in vivo in cholesterol-fed rabbits ($n = 8$), manifested by a greater decrease in hind limb vascular resistance (**A**) and increase in hind limb blood flow (**B**) in response to graded-dose of ACh. Data are mean ± SEM. Significant differences between conditions at specific doses are indicated. $*p < 0.05$, $**p < 0.01$. Reproduced with permission of the American Heart Association from Girerd et al., Circ Res 1990;67:1301.

supplementation *(110)*. These findings support the view that restoration of bioactive NO• promotes regression of atherosclerotic lesions.

Inhibition of endogenous NO• production has a detrimental effect on endothelium-dependent vasomotor function and accelerates atherogenesis in animal models with diet-induced and immune-mediated vascular injury. Cayatte and colleagues found that inhibition of NOS in hypercholesterolemic rabbits results in further impairment of endothelium-dependent

Table 1
The Effect of L-Arginine on Atherosclerosis Progression

Week	Intima, mm^2		Media, mm^2		Intima—media ratio	
	Chol	Arg	Chol	Arg	Chol	Arg
10	0.92 ± 0.36	0.98 ± 0.16	3.14 ± 0.18	3.54 ± 0.35	0.28 ± 0.11	0.28 ± 0.05
14	1.80 ± 0.37	2.33 ± 1.36	3.53 ± 0.27	3.42 ± 0.53	0.50 ± 0.07	0.51 ± 0.24
18	3.58 ± 0.71	$1.51 \pm 0.64^*$	3.91 ± 0.35	3.56 ± 0.42	1.0 ± 0.27	$0.35 \pm 0.12^*$

Histomorphologic analysis of vessels from cholesterol-fed rabbits evaluating the impact of L-arginine supplementation on atherosclerotic lesion progression. Cholesterol feeding was initiated 10 wk prior to L-arginine supplementation to allow for "preexisting" atheroma formation. Analysis was performed 4 and 8 wk following initiation of L-arginine supplementation (Arg) with comparison to continued cholesterol feeding (Chol) *$p < 0.05$, significant difference from Chol values at the same point in time. Reproduced with permission of the American Heart Association from Candipan et al. Arterioscler Thromb Vasc Biol 1996;16:44.

relaxation to ACh in isolated aortic rings (111). This effect is associated with diminished ACh-induced cGMP accumulation in arterial segments (111). Naruse and colleagues found that long-term NOS inhibition with oral administration of N^G-nitro-L-arginine methyl ester (L-NAME) for 8–12 wk markedly enlarges the intimal atherosclerotic area and increases lipid accumulation in cholesterol-fed animals (112). However, under these conditions there is an augmentation in the serum cholesterol values, which may play a role in the atherogenic response. Similarly, Cayatte and colleagues observed that chronic NOS inhibition with subcutaneous infusion of L-NAME for 4 wk accelerates neointimal formation with a significant increase in the lesion area and intima to media ratio (111). In contrast, these effects on early atherogenesis could not be attributed to differences in cholesterol metabolism or arterial blood pressure (111). These results support the view that NO• generation modulates the detrimental effects of hypercholesterolemia, as NOS inhibition further impairs endothelium-dependent relaxation and promotes and accelerates atherogenesis.

More recently, the role that isotypes of NOS play in atherogenesis has undergone exploration. Buttery and colleagues found increased iNOS expression in human atherosclerotic coronary arteries (113). Similarly, Ravalli and colleagues found increased iNOS expression and activity in neointimal lesions in human coronary vessels with transplant atherosclerosis (114). This increase is associated with extensive nitration of protein tyrosines, thus suggesting that iNOS induction is accompanied by excessive peroxynitrite formation and enhanced transplant arteriosclerosis (114). In contrast, Koglin and colleagues found a possible protective role of iNOS in transplant arteriosclerosis (93). As recipients in a chronic cardiac rejection model, mice lacking the iNOS gene display accelerated arteriosclerosis with increased neointimal proliferation compared with wild-type recipients (93) (Fig. 4). Within the neointimal lesions, there is an increase in SMC accumulation, supporting a role for iNOS in suppression of smooth muscle proliferation following vascular injury (93).

PARTICIPATION OF NO• IN THE PATHOGENESIS OF RESTENOSIS

Percutaneous peripheral and coronary angioplasty disrupts the normal protective endothelial barrier eliciting a series of responses that may lead to restenosis. Exposure of subendothelial matrix elements with denuding of the endothelium results in platelet adhesion and activation with the release of chemotactic and mitogenic factors. Adhesion and migration of leukocytes releases additional growth factors, leading to migration and proliferation of VSMCs and myofibroblasts with neointima formation. NO• can modulate the response to acute vascular injury accompanying angioplasty by inhibition of several key components

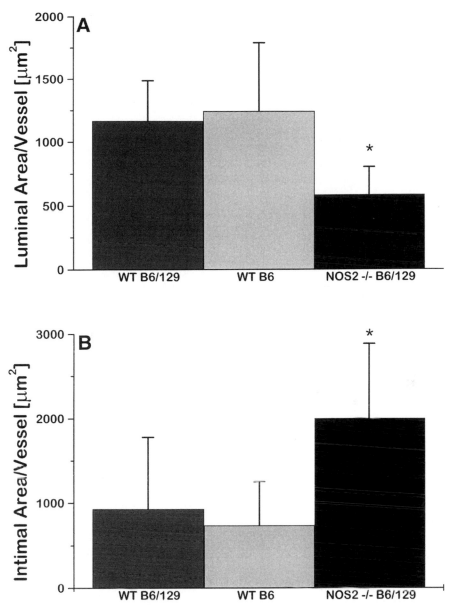

Fig. 4. The effect of NOS2 on transplant arteriosclerosis. Morphometric analysis revealed a decrease in mean luminal area (**A**), an increase in mean intimal area (**B**), and unchanged mean medial area.

in the process of intimal hyperplasia, including platelet adhesion and aggregation, leukocyte adhesion, and SMC proliferation. Further decrease in NO• release as a consequence of endothelial injury is superimposed on the already-diminished basal NO• action in atherosclerosis and contributes to neointimal proliferation and the development of restenosis.

Dysfunction of the NO• pathway as a result of endothelial damage has been demonstrated following arterial injury in experimental models. Balloon angioplasty performed on arterial blood vessels results in complete loss of the endothelial surface assessed by microscopy. This denudation of the endothelium is associated with loss of endothelium-dependent relaxation in response to ACh and the calcium ionophore A23187 in isolated vessels ex vivo *(115)*. This impairment in endothelium-dependent relaxation persists beyond 4 wk despite regeneration

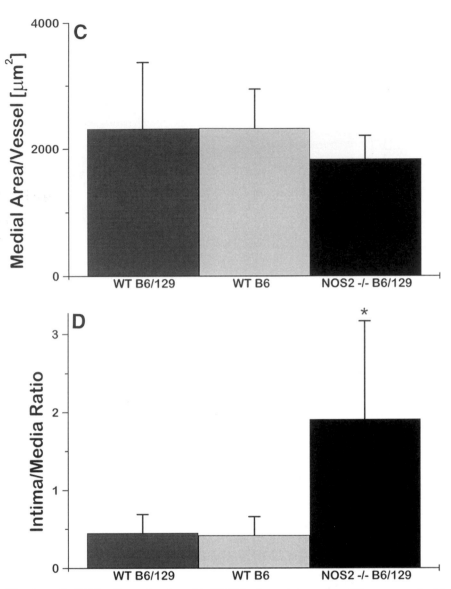

Fig. 4. (Continued). (**C**) in allografts placed in NOS2 –/– recipients (*n* = 13) compared with those placed into B6 (*n* = 8) and B6/129 (*n* = 7) wild-type controls. This results in increased mean intima/media ratio (**D**) and mean % luminal occlusion.

of morphologically altered endothelial cells within 2 wk *(115)*. Persistent dysfunction of the NO• pathway following arterial injury, despite neoendothelial surface formation, may contribute to neointimal hyperplasia and the development of restenosis.

Studies that manipulate endogenous NO• production or provide exogenous NO• may provide insight into the role of NO• in restenosis following vascular injury. Enhancement of endogenous NO• production with L-arginine supplementation improves endothelial function following arterial injury. This is characterized by an improvement in ACh-induced vasorelaxation in isolated iliac arteries from normocholesterolemic rabbits following balloon-induced injury *(116,117)*. The improvement in endothelial function with L-arginine supplementation is associated with decreased neointima formation with reduced intimal thickness and area *(117)*. In

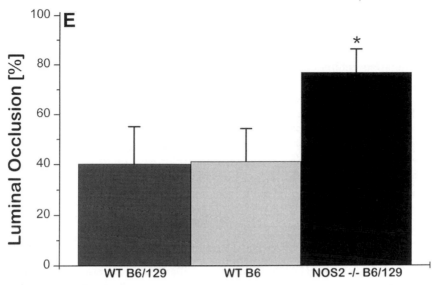

Fig. 4. (Continued). (**E**) in allografts from NOS2-deficient recipients. Mean area (μm^2) and % luminal occlusion from all captured vessels reported as mean ± SD for all grafts in each recipient group. *$p < 0.01$. Reproduced with permission of the American Heart Association from Koglin et al., Circulation 1998;97:2059.

addition, systemic delivery of organic NO• donor compounds such as molsidomine inhibits platelet adhesion and SMC proliferation following balloon-induced carotid artery injury in pigs (118). Similarly, we observed that local delivery of a stable protein S nitrosothiol reduces platelet deposition and inhibits neointimal proliferation after vascular arterial balloon injury (119). The ACCORD study suggested that administration of the NO• donors linsidomine and molsidomine to patients undergoing coronary angioplasty led to a modest improvement in the immediate angiographic outcome, with a greater minimal luminal diameter (120). At the 6-mo angiographic follow up, this modest improvement is sustained, although there is no protection against late luminal loss (120). Thus, following arterial injury, augmenting NO• production or providing exogenous NO• reduces intimal hyperplasia in animal models, however the benefit in human subject remains questionable.

Enhancing endogenous NO• production using molecular strategies inhibits neointimal proliferation. Von der Leyen and colleagues found a 70% reduction in neointima formation 14 d after balloon-induced injury in rat carotid arteries by overexpression of bovine eNOS (121). Transfection with eNOS improves vascular NO• production with restoration of endothelium-dependent relaxation in response to the calcium ionophore A23187 (121). Similar findings occur with transfection of human eNOS with restoration of vascular NO• production and preservation of vascular cGMP levels (123). This enhanced NO• production is associated with an inhibition of neointimal formation with a reduction in the intima-to-media ratio (122). Furthermore, Janssens and colleagues found that eNOS expression inhibits DNA synthesis and reduces VSMC proliferation following arterial injury (122). There is a 28% reduction in 5'-bromodeoxyuridine incorporation in vitro and a 35% reduction in 5'-bromodeoxyuridine labeling in vivo (122). Miyagishima and colleagues found that intraluminal iNOS gene transfer effectively inhibits intimal hyperplasia following arterial injury in rats and pigs (123). This inhibition of neointimal proliferation by NOS gene transfer is, in part, the result of its antiproliferative actions on VSMCs (123). Taken together, these studies support the role of the NO• pathway in modulating the response to vascular injury and regulating intimal hyperplasia.

SUMMARY

NO• plays a critical role in the regulation of vascular homeostasis, exerting numerous antiatherogenic actions including vasodilation, inhibition of platelet function, inhibition of VSMC proliferation, inhibition of leukocyte adhesion and migration, and modulation of oxidative stress. There are potential proatherogenic effects of excessive amount of NO•, generated by iNOS, as a consequence of oxidative damage. However, in atherosclerosis, there is diminished biological activity of endogenously derived NO•, in part due to its inactivation by reactive oxygen species. NO• modulates the development and progression of atherosclerosis in experimental models of atherosclerosis induced by hypercholesterolemia. In these studies, impairing NO• production promotes atherosclerosis, whereas augmenting NO• production inhibits atherogenesis. Such findings provide a strong link between NO• and atherosclerosis, and suggest that NO• may be a crucial regulator of atherogenesis.

REFERENCES

1. Furchgott RF, Zawadzki JV. The obligatory role of endothelial cells in the relaxation of arterial smooth muscle by acetylcholine. Nature 1980;288:373–376.
2. Ignarro LJ, Byrns RE, Buga GM, Wood KS. Endothelium-derived relaxing factor from pulmonary artery and vein possess pharmacologic and chemical properties identical to those of nitric oxide radical. Circ Res 1987;61:866–879.
3. Palmer RM, Ferrige AG, Moncada S. Nitric oxide release accounts for the biological activity of endothelium-derived relaxing factor. Nature 1987;327:524–526.
4. Myers PR, Minor RL, Guerra R, Bates JN, Harrison DG. Vasorelaxant properties of the endothelium-derived relaxing factor more closely resembles S-nitrosocysteine than nitric oxide. Nature 1990;345: 161–163.
5. Palmer RM, Ashton DS, Moncada S. Vascular endothelial cells synthesize nitric oxide from L-arginine. Nature 1988; 333:664–666.
6. Loscalzo J, Welch G. Nitric oxide and its role in the cardiovascular system. Progr Cardiovasc Dis 1995; 38:87–104.
7. Stamler JS, Singel DJ, Loscalzo J. Biochemistry of nitric oxide and its redox-activated forms. Science 1992;258:1898–1902.
8. Stamler J, Simon DI, Osborne JA, Mullins ME, Jaraki O, Michel T, et al. S-nitrosylation of proteins with nitric oxide: synthesis and characterization of biologically active compounds. Proc Natl Acad Sci USA 1992;89:444–448.
9. Najibi S, Cohen RA. Enhanced role of K+ channels in relaxation of hypercholesterolemic rabbit carotid artery to NO. Am J Physiol 1995;269:H805–H811.
10. Xu L, Eu JP, Meissner G, Stamler JS. Activation of the cardiac calcium release channel (ryanodine receptor) by poly-S-nitrosylation. Science 1998;279:234–237.
11. Vallance P, Collier J, Moncada S. Effects of endothelium-derived nitric oxide on peripheral arteriolar tone in man. Lancet 1989;2:997–1000.
12. Rees DD, Palmer RM, Moncada S. Role of endothelium-derived nitric oxide in the regulation of blood pressure. Proc Natl Acad Sci USA 1989;86:3375–3378.
13. Busse R, Mülsch A, Fleming I, Hecker M. Mechanisms of nitric oxide release from the vascular endothelium. Circulation 1993;87:V18–V25.
14. Cooke JP, Tsao PS. Is NO an endogenous antiatherogenic molecule? Arterioscler Thromb 1994;14: 653–655.
15. Chester AH, O'Neil GS, Moncada S, Tadjkarimi S, Yacoub MH. Low basal and stimulated release of nitric oxide in atherosclerotic epicardial coronary arteries. Lancet 1990;336:897–900.
16. Lefroy DC, Crake T, Uren NG, Davies GJ, Maseri A. Effect of inhibition of nitric oxide synthesis on epicardial coronary artery caliber and coronary blood flow in humans. Circulation 1993;88:43–54.
17. Kelm M, Schrader J. Control of coronary vascular tone by nitric oxide. Circ Res 1990;66:1561–1575.
18. Ross R. The pathogenesis of atherosclerosis: a perspective for the 1990's. Nature 1993;362:801–808.
19. Ware JA, Heistad DD. Seminars in medicine of the Beth Israel Hospital, Boston. Platelet-endothelium interactions. N Engl J Med 1993;328:628–635.
20. Mellion BT, Ignarro LJ, Ohlstein EH, Pontecorvo EG, Hyman AL, Kadowitz PJ. Evidence for the inhibitory role of guanosine 3', 5'-monophosate in ADP-induced human platelet aggregation in the presence of nitric oxide and related vasodilators. Blood 1981;57:946–955.

21. Mendelsohn ME, O'Neill S, George D, Loscalzo J. Inhibition of fibrinogen binding to human platelets by S-nitroso-N-acetylcysteine. J Biol Chem 1990;265:19,028–19,034.

22. Michelson AD, Benoit SE, Furman MI, Breckwoldt WL, Rohrer MJ, Barnard MR, et al. Effects of nitric oxide/EDRF on platelet surface glycoproteins. Am J Physiol 1996;270:H1640–H1648.

23. Radomski MW, Palmer RM, Moncada S. Endogenous nitric oxide inhibits human platelet adhesion to vascular endothelium. Lancet 1987;2:1057,1058.

24. Sneddon JM, Vane JR. Endothelium-derived relaxing factor reduces platelet adhesion to bovine endothelial cells. Proc Natl Acad Sci USA 1988;85:2800–2804.

25. Yao SK, Ober JC, Krishnaswami A, Ferguson JJ, Anderson HV, Golino P, et al. Endogenous nitric oxide protects against platelet aggregation and cyclic flow variations in stenosed and endothelium-injured arteries. Circulation 1992;86:1302–1309.

26. Radomski MW, Palmer RM, Moncada S. An L-arginine/nitric oxide pathway present in human platelets regulates aggregation. Proc Natl Acad Sci USA 1990;87:5193–5197.

27. Vasta, V, Meacci, E, Farnararo, M, Bruni, P. Identification of a specific transport system for L-arginine in human platelets. Biochem Biophys Res Commun 1995;206:878–884.

28. Freedman JE, Loscalzo J, Barnard MR, Alpert C, Keaney JF Jr, Michelson AD. Nitric oxide released from activated platelets inhibits platelet recruitment. J Clin Invest 1997;100:350–356.

29. Gimbrone MA Jr. Vascular endothelium: an integrator of pathophysiologic stimuli in atherosclerosis. Am J Cardiol 1995;75:67B–70B.

30. Bath PM, Hassall DG, Gladwin AM, Palmer RM, Martin JF. Nitric oxide and prostacyclin. Divergence of inhibitory effects on monocyte chemotaxis and adhesion to endothelium in vitro. Arteroscler Thromb 1991;11:254–260.

31. Tsao PS, Lewis NP, Alpert S, Cooke JP. Exposure to shear stress alters endothelial adhesiveness. Role of nitric oxide. Circulation 1995;92:3513–3519.

32. Ma X, Weyrich AS, Lefer DJ, Lefer AM. Diminished basal nitric oxide release after myocardial ischemia and reperfusion promotes neutrophil adherence to coronary endothelium. Circ Res 1993;72:403–412.

33. Kubes P, Suzuki M, Granger DN. Nitric oxide: an endogenous modulator of leukocyte adhesion. Proc Natl Acad Sci USA 1991;88:4651–4655.

34. Tsao PS, Buitrago R, Chan JR, Cooke JP. Fluid flow inhibits endothelial adhesiveness. Nitric oxide and transcriptional regulation of VCAM-1. Circulation 1996;94:1682–1689.

35. Lefer DJ, Klunk DA, Lutty GA, Merges C, Schleimer RP, Bochner BS, et al. Nitric oxide donors reduce basal ICAM-1 expression on human aortic endothelial cells. Circulation 1993;88:I-565.

36. Adams MR, Jessup W, Hailstones D, Celermajer DS. L-arginine reduces human monocyte adhesion to vascular endothelium and endothelial expression of cell adhesion molecules. Circulation 1997;95:662–668.

37. Zeiher AM, Fisslthaler B, Schray-Utz B, Busse R. Nitric oxide modulates the expression of monocyte chemoattractant protein 1 in cultured human endothelial cells. Circ Res 1995;76:980–986.

38. Garg UC, Hassid A. Nitric oxide-generating vasodilators and 8-bromo-cyclic guanosine monophosphate inhibit mitogenesis and proliferation of cultured rat vascular smooth muscle cells. J Clin Invest 1989;83:1774–1777.

39. Guo K, Andres V, Walsh K. Nitric oxide-induced downregulation of cdk2 activity and cyclin A gene transcription in vascular smooth muscle cells. Circulation 1998;97:2066–2072.

40. Rizvi MA, Myers PR. Nitric oxide modulates basal and endothelin-induced coronary artery vascular smooth muscle cell proliferation and collagen levels. J Mol Cell Cardiol 1997;29:1779–1789.

41. Sarkar R, Meinberg EG, Stanley JC, Gordon D, Webb RC. Nitric oxide reversibly inhibits the migration of cultured vascular smooth muscle cells. Circ Res 1996;78:225–230.

42. Scott-Burden T, Vanhoutte PM. The endothelium as a regulator of vascular smooth muscle cell proliferation. Circulation 1993;87:V51–V55.

43. Busse R, Mülsch A. Induction of nitric oxide synthase by cytokines in vascular smooth muscle cells. FEBS Lett 1990;275:87–90.

44. Scott-Burden T, Schini VB, Elizondo E, Junquero DC, Vanhoutte PM. Platelet-derived growth factor suppresses and fibroblast growth factor enhances cytokine-induced production of nitric oxide by cultured smooth muscle cells. Circ Res 1992;71:1088–1100.

45. Lawson DL, Mehta JL, Nichols WW, Mehta P, Donnelly WH. Superoxide radical-mediated endothelial injury and vasoconstriction of rat thoracic aortic rings. J Lab Clin Med 1990;115:541–548.

46. Keaney JF Jr, Vita JA. Atherosclerosis, oxidative stress and antioxidant protection in endothelium-derived relaxng factor action. Prog Cardiovasc Dis 1995;38:129–154.

47. Ohara Y, Peterson TE, Harrison DG. Hypercholesterolemia increases endothelial superoxide anion production. J Clin Invest 1993;91:2546–2551.
48. Moro MA, Darley-Usmar VM, Goodwin DA, Read NG, Zamora-Pino R, Feelisch M, et al. Paradoxical fate and biological action of peroxynitrite on human platelets. Proc Natl Acad Sci USA 1994;91: 6702–6706.
49. Villa LM, Salas E, Darley-Usmar VM, Radomski MW, Moncada S. Peroxynitrite induces both vasodi- lation and impaired vascular relaxation in the isolated perfused rat heart. Proc Natl Acad Sci USA 1994; 91:12,383–12,387.
50. Hogg N, Kalyanaraman B, Joseph J, Struck A, Parthasarathy S. Inhibition of low-density lipoprotein oxidation by nitric oxide: potential role in atherogenesis. FEBS Lett 1993;334:170–174.
51. Cardona-Sanclemente LE, Born GV. Effect of inhibition of nitric oxide synthesis on the uptake of LDL and fibrinogen by arterial walls and other organs of the rat. Br J Pharmacol 1995;114:1490–1494.
52. Chang GJ, Woo P, Honda HM, Ignarro LJ, Young L, Berliner JA, et al. Oxidation of LDL to a biologically active form by derivatives of nitric oxide and nitrite in the absence of superoxide. Arterio- scler Thromb 1994;14:1808–1814.
53. Beckman JS, Beckman TW, Chen J, Marshall PA, Freeman BA. Apparent hydroxyl radical production by peroxynitrite: implications for endothelial injury from nitric oxide and superoxide. Proc Natl Acad Sci USA 1990;87:1620–1624.
54. Wever RMF, Lüscher TF, Cosentino F, Rabelink TJ. Atherosclerosis and the two faces of endothelial nitric oxide synthase. Circulation 1998;97:108–112.
55. Bjorkerud S, Bjorkerud B. Apoptosis is abundant in human atherosclerotic lesions, especially in inflammatory cells (macrophages and T cells), and may contribute to the accumulation of gruel and plaque instability. Am J Pathol 1996;149:367–380.
56. Geng YJ, Henderson LE, Levesque EB, Muszynski M, Libby P. Fas is expressed in human atheroscle- rotic intima and promotes apoptosis of cytokine-primed human vascular smooth muscle cells. Arterio- scler Thromb Vasc Biol 1997;17:2200–2208.
57. Hegyi L, Skepper JN, Cary NR, Mitchinson MJ. Foam cell apoptosis and the development of the lipid core of human atherosclerosis. J Pathol 1996;180:423–429.
58. Fukuo K, Inoue T, Morimoto S, Nakahashi T, Yasuda O, Kitano S, et al. Nitric oxide mediates cytotoxity and basic fibroblast growth factor release in culutred vascular smooth muscle cells. A possible mechanism of neovascularization in atherosclerotic plaques. J Clin Invest 1995;95:669–676.
59. Fukuo K, Nakahashi T, Nomura S, Hata S, Suhara T, Shimizu M, et al. Possible participation of Fas- mediated apoptosis in the mechanism of atherosclerosis. Gerontology 1997;43:35–42.
60. Shimaoka M, Iida T, Ohara A, Taenaka N, Mashimo T, Honda T, et al. NOC, a nitric-oxide-releasing compound, induces dose dependent apoptosis in macrophages. Biochem Biophys Res Commun 1995; 209:519–526.
61. Yang X, Galeano NF, Szabolcs M, Sciacca RR, Cannon PJ. Oxidized low density lipoproteins alter macrophage lipid uptake, apootosis, viability and nitric oxide synthesis. J Nutr 1996;126:1072S–1075S.
62. Verbeuren TJ, Jordaens FH, Zonnekeyn LL, Van Hove CE, Coene MC, Herman AG. Effect of hyper- cholesterolemia on vascular reactivity in the rabbit. I. Endothelium-dependent and endothelium-inde- pendent contractions and relaxations in isolated arteries of control and hypercholesterolemic rabbits. Circ Res 1986;58:552–564.
63. Bossaller C, Habib GB, Yamamoto H, Williams C, Wells S, Henry PD. Impaired muscarinic endo- thelium-dependent relaxation and cyclic guanosine 5'-monophosphate formation in atherosclerotic human coronary artery and rabbit aorta. J Clin Invest 1987;79:170–174.
64. Freiman PC, Mitchell GC, Heistad DD, Armstrong ML, Harrison DG. Atherosclerosis impairs endo- thelium-dependent vascular relaxation to acetylcholine and thrombin in primates. Circ Res 1986;58: 783–789.
65. Cohen RA, Zitnay KM, Haudenschild CC, Cunningham LD. Loss of selective endothelial cell vaso- active functions caused by hypercholesterolemia in pig coronary arteries. Circ Res 1988;63:903–910.
66. Ludmer PL, Selwyn AP, Shook TL, Wayne RR, Mudge GH, Alexander RW, et al. Paradoxical vaso- constriction induced by acetylcholine in atherosclerotic coronary arteries. N Engl J Med 1986;315: 1046–1051.
67. Anderson TJ, Gerhard MD, Meredith IT, Charbonneau F, Delagrange D, Creager MA, et al. Systemic nature of endothelial dysfunction in atherosclerosis. Am J Cardiol 1995;75:71B–74B.
68. McLenachan JM, Williams JK, Fish RD, Ganz P, Selwyn AP. Loss of flow-mediated endothelium- dependent dilation occurs early in the development of atherosclerosis. Circulation 1991;84:1273–1278.
69. Vita JA, Treasure CB, Nabel EG, McLenachan JM, Fish RD, Yeung AC, et al. Coronary vasomotor response to acetylcholine relates to risk factors for coronary artery disease. Circulation 1990;81:491–497.

70. Reddy KG, Nair R, Sheehan HM, Hodgson JM. Evidence that selective endothelial dysfunction may occur in the absence of angiographic or ultrasound atherosclerosis in patients with risk factors for atherosclerosis. J Am Coll Cardiol 1994;23:833–843.
71. Otsuji S, Nakajima O, Waku S, Kojima S, Hosokawa H, Kinoshita I, et al. Attenuation of acetylcholine-induced vasoconstriction by L-arginine is related to the progression of atherosclerosis. Am Heart J 1995;129:1094–1100.
72. Osborne JA, Siegman MJ, Sedar AW, Mooers SU, Lefer AM. Lack of endothelium-dependent relaxation in coronary resistance arteries of cholesterol-fed rabbits. Cell Physiol 1989;25:C591–C597.
73. Yaghoubi M, Cayatte AJ, Cohen RA. Decreased nitric oxide response precedes impaired endothelium-dependent relaxation of hypercholesterolemic ApoE knockout mouse aorta. Circulation 1998;98:I44.
74. Verbeuren TJ, Jordaens FH, Van Hove CE, Van Hoydonck AE, Herman AG. Release and vascular activity of endothelium-derived relaxing factor in atherosclerotic rabbit aorta. Eur J Pharmacol 1990; 191:173–184.
75. Böger RH, Bode-Böger SM, Mügge A, Kienke S, Brandes R, Dwenger A, et al. Supplementation of hypercholesterolaemic rabbits with L-arginine reduces the vascular release of superoxide anions and restores NO production. Atherosclerosis 1995;117:273–284.
76. Durante W, Liao L, Schafer AI. Differential regulation of L-arginine transport and inducible NOS in cultured vascular smooth muscle cells. Am J Physiol 1995;268:H1158–H1164.
77. Arnal JF, Munzel T, Venema RC, James NL, Bai CL, Mitch WE, et al. Interactions between L-arginine and L-glutamine change endothelial NO production: an effect independent of NO synthase substrate availability. J Clin Invest 1995;99:433–438.
78. Bode-Böger SM, Böger RH, Kienke S, Junker W, Frölich JC. Elevated L-arginine/dimethylarginine ratio contributes to enhanced systemic NO production by dietary L-arginine in hypercholesterolemic rabbits. Biochem Biophys Res Commun 1996;219:598–603.
79. Liao JK, Shin WS, Lee WY, Clark SL. Oxidized low-density lipoprotein decreases the expression of endothelial nitric oxide synthase. J Biol Chem 1995;270:319–324.
80. Gryglewski RJ, Palmer RM, Moncada S. Superoxide anion is involved in the breakdown of endothelium-derived vascular relaxing factor. Nature 1986;320:454–456.
81. Mügge A, Elwell JH, Peterson TE, Hofemeyer TG, Heistad DD, Harrison DG. Chronic treatment with polyethylene glycolated superoxide dismutase partially restores endothelium-dependent vascular relaxations in cholesterol-fed rabbits. Circ Res 1991;69:1293–1300.
82. Keaney JF Jr, Gaziano JM, Xu A, Frei B, Curran-Cellentano J, Shwaery GT, et al. Dietary antioxidants preserve endothelium-dependent vessel relaxation in cholesterol-fed rabbits. Proc Natl Acad Sci USA 1993;90:11,880–11,884.
83. Lapenna D, de Gioia S, Ciofani G, Mezzetti A, Ucchino S, Calafiore AM, et al. Glutathione-related antioxidant defenses in human atherosclerotic plaques. Circulation 1998;97:1930–1934.
84. Minor RL, Meyers PR, Guerra R Jr, Bates JN, Harrison DG. Diet-induced atherosclerosis increases the release of nitrogen oxides from rabbit aorta. J Clin Invest 1990;86:2109–2116.
85. Clancy RM, Leszcynska-Piziak J, Abramson SB. Nitric oxide, an endothelial cell relaxation factor, inhibits neutrophil superoxide anion production via a direct action on the NADPH oxidase. J Clin Invest 1992;90:1116–1121.
86. Rajagopalan S, Kurz S, Munzel T, Tarpey M, Freeman BA, Griendling KL, et al. Angiotensin II-mediated hypertension in the rat increases vascular superoxide production via membrane NADH/NADPH oxidase activation. Contribution to alteration of vasomotor tone. J Clin Invest 1996;97:1916–1923.
87. Pritchard KA, Groszek L, Smalley DM, Sessa WC, Wu M, Villalon P, et al. Native low density lipoprotein increases endothelial cell nitric oxide synthase generation of superoxide anion. Circ Res 1995;77:510–518.
88. Tsao PS, Theilmeier G, Singer AH, Leung LL, Cooke JP. L-arginine attenuates platelet reactivity in hypercholesterolemic rabbits. Arterioscler Thromb 1994;14:1529–1533.
89. Lefer AM, Ma X. Decreased basal nitric oxide release in hypercholesterolemia increases neutrophil adherence to rabbit coronary artery endothelium. Arterioscler Thromb 1993;13:771–776.
90. Tsao PS, McEvoy LM, Drexler H, Butcher EC, Cooke JP. Enhanced endothelial adhesiveness in hypercholesterolemia is attenuated by L-arginine. Circulation 1994;89:2176–2182.
91. Adams MR, McCredie R, Jessup W, Rodinson J, Sullivan D, Celermajer DS. Oral L-arginine improves endothelium-dependent dilatation and reduces monocyte adhesion to endothelial cells in young men with coronary artery disease. Atherosclerosis 1997;129:261–269.
92. Chin JH, Azhar S, Hoffman BB. Inactivation of endothelium derived relaxing factor by oxidized lipoproteins. J Clin Invest 1992;89:10–18.

93. Koglin J, Glysing-Jensen T, Mudgett JS, Russell ME. Exacerbated transplant arteriosclerosis in inducible nitric oxide-deficient mice. Circulation 1998;97:2059–2065.

94. Meredith IT, Yeung AC, Weidinger FF, Anderson TJ, Uehata A, Ryan TJ, et al. Role of impaired endothelium–dependent vasodilation in ischemic manifestations of coronary artery disease. Circulation 1993;87:V56–V66.

95. Cox DA, Vita JA, Treasure CB, Fish RD, Alexander RW, Ganz P, et al. Impairment of flow-mediated coronary dilation by atherosclerosis in man. Circulation 1989;80:458–465.

96. Nabel EG, Selwyn AP, Ganz P. Large coronary arteries in humans are responsive to changing blood flow: an endothelium-dependent mechanism that fails in patients with atherosclerosis. J Am Coll Cardiol 1990;16:349–356.

97. Gordon JB, Ganz P, Nabel EG, Fish RD, Zebede J, Mudge GH, et al. Atherosclerosis influences the vasomotor response of epicardial coronary arteries to exercise. J Clin Invest 1989;83:1946–1952.

98. Yeung AC, Vekshtein VI, Krantz DS, Vita JA, Ryan TJ Jr, Ganz P, et al. The effect of atherosclerosis on the vasomotor response of coronary arteries to mental stress. N Engl J Med 1991;325:1551–1556.

99. Zeiher AM, Drexler H, Wollschlager H, Just H. Endothelial dysfunction of the coronary microvasculature is associated with impaired coronary blood flow regulation in patients with early atherosclerosis. Circulation 1991;84:1984–1992.

100. Quyyumi AA, Dakak N, Andrews NP, Gilligan DM, Panza JA, Cannon RO 3rd. Contribution of nitric oxide to metabolic coronary vasodilation in the human heart. Circulation 1995;92:320–326.

101. Yao SK, Akhtar S, Scott-Burden T, Ober JC, Golino P, Buja LM, et al. Endogenous and exogenous nitric oxide protect against intracoronary thrombosis and reocclusion after thrombolysis. Circulation 1995;92:1005–1010.

102. Adrie C, Bloch KD, Moreno PR, Hurford WE, Guerrero JL, Holt R, et al. Inhaled nitric oxide increases coronary artery patency after thrombolysis. Circulation 1996;94:1919–1926.

103. Girerd XJ, Hirsch AT, Cooke JP, Dzau VJ, Creager MA. L-arginine augments endothelium-dependent vasodilation in cholesterol-fed rabbits. Circ Res 1990;67:1301–1308.

104. Mügge A, Harrison DG. L-arginine does not restore endothelial dysfunction in atherosclerotic rabbit aorta in vitro. Blood Vessels 1991;28:354–357.

105. Cooke JP, Andon NA, Girerd XJ, Hirsch AT, Creager MA. Arginine restores cholinergic relaxation of hypercholesterolemic rabbit thoracic aorta. Circulation 1991;83:1057–1062.

106. Cooke JP, Singer AH, Tsao P, Zera P, Rowan RA, Billingham ME. Antiatherogenic effects of L-arginine in the hypercholesterolemic rabbit. J Clin Invest 1992;90:1168–1172.

107. Wang BY, Singer AH, Tsao PS, Drexler H, Kosek J, Cooke JP. Dietary arginine prevents atherogenesis in the coronary artery of the hypercholesterolemic rabbit. J Am Coll Cardiol 1994;23:452–458.

108. Singer AH, Tsao PS, Wang BY, Bloch DA, Cooke JP. Discordant effects of dietary L-arginine on vascular structure and reactivity in hypercholesterolemic rabbits. J Cardiovasc Pharmacol 1995;25:710–716.

109. Candipan RC, Wang B, Buitrago R, Tsao PS, Cooke JP. Regression or progression. Dependency on vascular nitric oxide. Arterioscler Thromb Vasc Biol 1996;16:44–50.

110. Böger RH, Bode-Böger SM, Brandes RP, Phivthong-ngam L, Bohme M, Nafe R, et al. Dietary L-arginine reduces the progression of atherosclerosis in cholesterol-fed rabbits: comparison with lovastatin. Circulation 1997;96:1282–1290.

111. Cayatte AJ, Palacino JJ, Horten K, Cohen RA. Chronic inhibition of nitric oxide production accelerates neointimal formation and impairs endothelial function in hypercholesterolemic rabbits. Arterioscler Thromb 1994;14:753–759.

112. Naruse K, Shimizu K, Muramatsu M, Toki Y, Miyazaki Y, Okumura K, et al. Long-term inhibition of NO synthesis promotes atherosclerosis in the hypercholesterolemic rabbit thoracic aorta. PGH2 does not contribute to impaired endothelium-dependent relaxation. Arterioscler Thromb 1994;14:746–752.

113. Buttery LD, Springall DR, Chester AH, Evans TJ, Standfield N, Parums DV, et al. Inducible nitric oxide synthase is present within human atherosclerotic lesions and promotes the formation and activity of peroxynitrite. Lab Invest 1996;75:77–85.

114. Ravalli S, Albala A, Ming M, Szabolcs M, Barbone A, Michler RE, et al. Inducible nitric oxide synthase expression in smooth muscle cells and macrophages of human transplant coronary artery disease. Circulation 1998;97:2338–2345.

115. Weidinger FF, McLenachan JM, Cybulsky MI, Jordan JB, Rennke HG, Hollenberg NK, et al. Persistent dysfunction of regenerated endothelium after balloon angioplasty of rabbit iliac artery. Circulation 1990;81:1667–1679.

116. Tarry WC, Makhoul RG. L-arginine improves endothelium-dependent vasorelaxation and reduces intimal hyperplasia after balloon angioplasty. Arterioscler Thromb 1994;14:938–943.

117. Hamon M, Vallet B, Bauters C, Wernert N, McFadden EP, Lablanche JM, et al. Long-term oral administration of L-arginine reduces intimal thickening and enhances neoendothelium-dependent acetycholine-induced relaxation after arterial injury. Circulation 1994;90:1357–1362.

118. Groves PH, Banning AP, Penny WJ, Newby AC, Cheadle HA, Lewis MJ. The effects of exogenous nitric oxide on smooth muscle cell proliferation following porcine carotid angioplasty. Cardiovasc Res 1995;30:87–96.

119. Marks DS, Vita JA, Folts JD, Keaney JF Jr, Welch GN, Loscalzo J. Inhibition of neointimal proliferation in rabbits after vascular injury by a single treatment with a protein adduct of nitric oxide. J Clin Invest 1995;96:2630–2638.

120. Lablanche JM, Grollier G, Lusson JR, Bassand JP, Drobinski G, Bertrand B, et al. Effect of the direct nitric oxide donors linsidomine and molsidomine on angiographic restenosis after coronary balloon angioplasty. The ACCORD Study (Angioplastic Coronaire Corvasal Diltiazem). Circulation 1997;95: 83–89.

121. von der Leyen HE, Gibbons GH, Morishita R, Lewis NP, Zhang L, Nakajima M, et al. Gene therapy inhibiting neointimal vascular lesion: in vivo transfer of endothelial cell nitric oxide synthase gene. Proc Natl Acad Sci USA 1995;92:1137–1141.

122. Janssens S, Flaherty D, Nong Z, Varenne O, van Pelt N, Haustermans C, et al. Human endothelial nitric oxide synthase gene transfer inhibits vascular smooth muscle cell proliferation and neointima formation after balloon injury in rats. Circulation 1998;97:1274–1281.

123. Miyagishima M, Tzeng E, Shears LJ, Kawaharada N, Watkins S, Billiar TR. Perivascular iNOS gene transfer using a novel non-occlusive gene delivery device inhibits intimal hyperplasia. Circulation 1997;96:I13.

17

Thrombotic Disorders and Nitric Oxide Insufficiency

Jane E. Freedman and Joseph Loscalzo

BACKGROUND

Thrombus formation within a coronary vessel is the precipitating event in myocardial infarction and unstable angina as shown in angiographic *(1)* and pathologic *(2)* studies. The angiographic severity of coronary stenoses does not adequately predict sites of subsequent acute coronary syndromes. For this reason, rupture of atheromatous plaque in relatively mildly stenosed vessels and subsequent thrombus formation is believed to underlie the majority of acute coronary syndromes *(3,4)*. Both superficial and intimal injury caused by endothelial denudation and deep intimal injury caused by plaque rupture expose collagen and von Willebrand factor to platelets *(4)*. Platelets then adhere directly to collagen or indirectly via the binding of von Willebrand factor to glycoprotein (GP) Ib/IX and to the matrix. Local platelet activation by tissue factor-mediated thrombin generation or by collagen stimulates further thrombus formation and additional platelet recruitment by supporting cell-surface thrombin formation and releasing adenosine diphosphate (ADP), serotonin, and thromboxane A_2 *(5)*. Thrombus forms as platelets aggregate via the binding of bivalent fibrinogen to GPIIb/IIIa. In support of these mechanisms, increased platelet derived thromboxane and prostaglandin metabolites have been detected in patients with acute coronary syndromes *(6)*. The importance of platelet activation in acute coronary syndromes is further supported by the clear clinical benefit of treatment with aspirin for both primary and secondary prevention strategies *(7,8)*. In addition, patients with coronary atherosclerosis have impaired bioactivity of endothelial nitric oxide (NO•), a known vasodilator and inhibitor of platelet function. In this chapter, the role of NO• insufficiency in experimental and clinical thrombotic disorders is explored.

VASCULAR NO• PRODUCTION AND PLATELET FUNCTION

The role of NO• in platelet function is briefly reviewed. For an extensive discussion of this topic, the reader is referred to Chapter 8.

NO• inhibits platelet function by stimulating soluble guanylyl cyclase (GC) to produce cyclic guanosine monophosphate (cGMP). This results in the stimulation of cGMP-dependent protein kinase that leads to a reduction in fibrinogen binding to GPIIb/IIIa and modulation of phospholipase A_2- and C-mediated responses *(9)*. In addition, NO• attenuates the oxidation of arachidonate *(10)* and inhibits the agonist-dependent increase in platelet cytosolic-free calcium in a cGMP-dependent manner *(11)*.

From: *Contemporary Cardiology, vol. 4: Nitric Oxide and the Cardiovascular System*
Edited by: J. Loscalzo and J. A. Vita © Humana Press Inc., Totowa, NJ

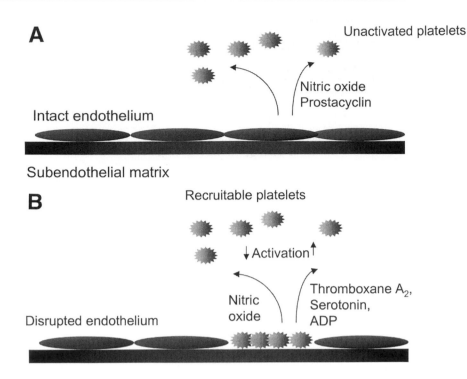

Fig. 1. In the intact vessel (**A**), production of prostacyclin and NO• by the endothelium prevents adherence and activation of platelets to the vessel surface. In the disrupted endothelium (**B**), platelets adhere to the subendothelial matrix, become activated, and release the prothrombotic substances thromboxane A_2, serotonin, and ADP that recruit additional platelets to the growing thrombus. This process may be limited by the release of NO• by the activated platelet.

Activation and recruitment of platelets is tightly regulated. Adhesion of platelets to the endothelium is prevented by several mechanisms, including endothelial cell production of prostacyclin and NO• (Fig. 1A) *(12,13)*. NO• inhibits platelet activation *(14,15)* and prevents thrombosis *(16)*. Exogenous NO• has been shown to inhibit the normal activation-dependent increase in the expression of platelet surface GPs, including P-selectin and the integrin GPIIb–IIIa complex *(17)*.

In addition to the effects of endothelium-derived NO•, constitutive nitric oxide synthase (cNOS) has been identified in both human platelets and megakaryoblastic cells *(18,19)*. Platelet aggregation is enhanced by incubation with inhibitors of cNOS and inhibited by incubation with the cNOS substrate L-arginine *(20)*. In vivo, systemic infusion of the cNOS inhibitor L-N^G-monoethyl arginine citrate (L-NMMA) causes a reduction in bleeding time without a change in vessel tone *(21)* and enhanced platelet reactivity to various agonists *(22)*. Interestingly, studies report NO• release from resting *(23)* and aggregating platelets *(24,25)*. NO• release from activated human platelets has been indirectly measured and estimated to be 11.2 pmol NO•/min/10^8 cells, indicating that the amount of NO• released by platelets may be comparable to that of endothelial cells *(23)*. In addition, platelet NO• release inhibits platelet recruitment to the growing thrombus (Fig. 1B) *(26)*.

NO• AND VESSEL PATENCY

Although there are limited studies evaluating the effect of endogenous NO• production on thrombosis, the role of the vascular endothelium, which mediates vasomotor tone, in part,

Table 1
Thrombotic Diseases Associated with NO• Deficiency in Experimental Models

Disease	Animal model
Unstable coronary syndromes	Dog model of coronary artery occlusion (31,56)
Thrombotic cerebrovascular disease	Rat model of thromboembolic stroke (33)
Renal thrombosis	Endotoxin-induced model of glomerular thrombosis (16)
Mesenteric thrombosis	Rabbit model of mesenteric arteriole and venule occlusion (35)

through NO• release, has been extensively characterized. As reviewed in Chapter 13, endothelium-dependent dilation is impaired in animal models of atherosclerosis and in isolated human atherosclerotic human coronary arteries (27). In addition, it is well established that cardiovascular disease and coronary risk factors, including cholesterol level, male gender, family history, and age, are associated with impaired endothelium-dependent vasodilation in coronary arteries (28). Endothelium-dependent dilation of systemic arteries is also impaired in patients with cardiovascular disease as well as adults and children with risk factors for atherosclerosis (29,30). Although NO• is not directly measured in these studies, the reported abnormalities in vascular reactivity imply that the normal NO•-dependent antithrombotic properties of the vessel are attenuated as well.

Thrombosis in Experimental Models of NO• Insufficiency

Most experimental models of NO• insufficiency utilize inhibitors of NO• synthase (NOS). Because these inhibitors have nonspecific effects on the three NOS isoforms and affect platelets and the vessel wall, many of the pathophysiological findings are also nonspecific. Therefore, in studies using NOS inhibitors and the NOS substrate L-arginine to examine the effect of NO• production on thrombosis, it may be difficult to determine whether findings are attributable to altered vascular reactivity, platelet activation, or a combination of both. Despite these limitations, the role of NO• insufficiency has been examined in many experimental models in an attempt to characterize a variety of thrombotic disorders (Table 1).

NO• AND THROMBOSIS FORMATION
IN EXPERIMENTAL MODELS OF VASCULAR OCCLUSION

We evaluated the effect of NO• on blood flow in the injured, stenosed dog coronary artery. Using the Folts model, which manifests cyclic reductions in coronary flow as a consequence of transient platelet occlusion (31), we showed that the NO• donor S-nitroso-bovine serum albumin dramatically reduced the frequency of flow cycles. The IC_{50} for inhibiting cyclic platelet-dependent occlusion was 1 nmol/kg in these animals (31). Importantly, these effects on coronary flow occurred at concentrations of the NO• donor that had no or minimal effects on mean arterial blood pressure: at 1 nmol/kg S-nitroso-serum albumin we observed no effect on mean arterial pressure, and at 100 nmol/kg we observed not more than a 10% decrease in mean arterial pressure. These observations suggest that the antiplatelet, antithrombotic effects of this NO• donor are comparatively selective in this model of platelet-mediated coronary thrombosis.

The effect of NOS inhibitors on intracoronary thrombosis and reocclusion has been characterized in a dog model of coronary occlusion. Yao and colleagues showed that thrombus formation in the coronary artery could be delayed by an L-arginine infusion (32). In addition, lysis of thrombus in the coronary arteries could be hastened by infusion of L–arginine (32). In this study, ex vivo platelet aggregations were also inhibited after animals were treated with L-arginine, suggesting that increasing NO• production inhibits platelet function and attenuates thrombus formation.

Thrombosis also appears to be regulated by the bioactivity of NO• in the cerebrovascular system. In a rat model of thromboembolic stroke, infusion of the NOS inhibitor N^G-nitro-L-arginine methyl ester (L-NAME) caused both an increase in platelet deposition and a reduction in global flow *(33)*, suggesting that both hemodynamic and thrombotic determinants contributed to the enhanced cerebral deficits in these animals.

The effect of NO• on glomerular thrombosis has also been investigated. To determine the role of endogenous NO• production in the development of glomerular thrombosis associated with septic shock, Shultz and colleagues studied an endotoxin-induced model of renal thrombosis *(16)*. NO• production was increased by endotoxin injection and this effect was prevented by infusion of L-NAME. Most importantly, examination of kidneys from rats given endotoxin and L-NAME revealed thrombosis in 55% of glomeruli as compared with <5% of the glomeruli from rats given either endotoxin or L-NAME alone. These investigators concluded that NO• is critical in preventing renal thrombosis resulting from septic shock.

As with septic shock, NO• synthesis is enhanced in glomerulonephritis. In a model of nephrotoxic nephritis, rats depleted of plasma L-arginine by an infusion of arginase developed systemic hypertension and glomerular thrombosis, suggesting that the enhanced production of NO• in this condition prevents further acute glomerular injury *(34)*.

In a study of rabbit mesenteric arterioles and venules, inhibition of NOS with a NOS inhibitor increased the duration of embolization and the number of emboli in venules but not the arterioles *(35)*. Infusion of L-arginine but not D-arginine reversed the increase in venous embolization.

ANTIOXIDANTS AND ANTIOXIDANT
DEPLETION IN NO•-DEPENDENT THROMBOSIS

A prominent feature of both abnormal platelet function and dysfunctional endothelium-dependent vasodilation in the setting of cardiovascular and thrombotic disease is oxidative stress. Superoxide anion is an important source of oxidative stress and limits the biological activity of NO•.

Evidence also suggests that oxidative stress normally accompanies platelet activation. Platelet aggregation is associated with a burst of oxygen consumption *(36)* and a marked rise in glutathione disulfide *(37)*. Although dramatic changes in platelet redox status occur during normal aggregation, conditions that provoke oxidative stress without inducing a florid aggregation response have also been shown to be prothrombotic. Reactive oxygen species contribute causally to many pathophysiologic conditions, and superoxide, in particular, is known to augment platelet aggregation responses *(38)*. Superoxide and NO• readily combine to form peroxynitrite (OONO$^-$) with a rate constant of $6.9 \times 10^9\ M^{-1}/s^{-1}$, suggesting that this reaction is essentially a diffusion-limited process that competes kinetically favorably with the dismutation reaction catalyzed by the antioxidant enzyme superoxide dismutase (SOD) *(39)*.

Antioxidants may indirectly inhibit platelets through metabolism of reactive oxygen species, many of which alter platelet function. Hydroperoxides produced by the platelet (prostaglandin G$_2$, 12-hydroperoxy-eicosatetraenoic acid, and phospholipid hydroperoxides) are metabolized by the cytosolic selenium-dependent enzyme cellular glutathione peroxidase. Cellular glutathione peroxidase (cGPx) is tightly coupled to the hexose monophosphate shunt through reduced nicotinamide adenine dinucleotide phosphate (NADPH), which restores reduced glutathione (GSH) concentrations and reestablishes the platelet thiol redox state via glutathione reductase. Glutathione depletion in platelets leads to attenuated cGPx activity and increased lipid peroxidation *(40)*. Increased lipid peroxides, in turn, lead to an increased likelihood of lipid peroxyl radical formation (LOO•), which can react with and inactivate NO• by forming lipid peroxynitrites (LOONOx). The antioxidant enzyme glutathione peroxidase potentiates the inhibition of platelet function by NO• by reducing LOOH and derivative LOONOs.

Experimental evidence suggests that antioxidant status is important in normal platelet function and the prevention of thrombosis. Studying cyclic flow variations in rabbit carotid arteries, Meng and colleagues showed that platelet-mediated thrombosis can be attenuated by an intravenous infusion of superoxide dismutase *(41)*. Infusion of the NOS inhibitor N^G-monomethyl L-arginine (L-NMMA) restored the cyclic thrombotic response. These findings were accompanied by decreases in cyclic guanosine 5'-monophosphate (cGMP) levels in platelets isolated from these animals. This study suggests that dismutation of superoxide decreases platelet-dependent thrombus formation by potentiation of endogenous NO• activity.

Consistent with these observations, in a model of endothelium-injured canine coronary arteries, Ikeda and colleagues demonstrated that cyclic flow variation was attenuated by intravenous infusion of SOD and catalase *(42)*. However, an infusion of xanthine and hypoxanthine or hydrogen peroxide significantly increased cyclical flow variation. These data suggest that reactive oxygen species contribute to platelet activation and thrombosis.

NO•-DEPENDENT HEMOSTASIS IN ENOS-DEFICIENT MICE

As discussed, endothelial nitric oxide synthase (eNOS) has been identified in human platelets and is the source of NO• released following platelet activation. Most experimental models of NO• insufficiency utilize inhibitors of NOS. Because these inhibitors have nonspecific effects on the three NOS isoforms and affect both platelets and the vessel wall, many of the pathophysiological findings are also nonspecific. To specifically define the role of eNOS in platelet function and hemostasis, we studied mice lacking a functional eNOS gene (*NOS3* knockout mice) *(43)*. In eNOS-deficient mice, *NOS3* mRNA derived from megakaryocytes was absent in bone marrow but present in wild-type mice by RT-PCR. In addition, adenosine triphosphate (ADP) stimulated platelets from eNOS-deficient mice released no measurable NO• in contrast to platelets from wild-type mice (0.0 vs 15.9 pmol/10^8 platelets, respectively) *(43)*. To determine the relative contribution of endothelial- and platelet-derived NO• to the bleeding time, platelets from eNOS-deficient or wild-type mice were isolated, transfused into thrombocytopenic eNOS-deficient mice, and the bleeding time measured. Compared with the thrombocytopenic controls, bleeding times in mice transfused with eNOS-deficient platelets were decreased to a significantly greater extent than those transfused with wild-type platelets ($\Delta BT = 24.6 \pm 9$ s vs 3.4 ± 5 s, $p < 0.04$). Because the bleeding time was significantly shortened even after controlling for endothelial NO• production, these findings support a role for platelet-derived NO• in platelet-dependent thrombus formation and in vivo hemostasis.

NO• INSUFFICIENCY AND CLINICAL THROMBOTIC DISORDERS

Background

Several clinical disorders have been reported in which an insufficiency of endogenous NO• production is believed to contribute to a thrombotic event (Table 2). Human in vivo studies suggest that the regulation of endogenous NO• production influences vessel patency. Endothelial cell NO• production modulates platelet function *(13)* and may also affect the process of platelet recruitment in the growing thrombus. In a recent study, oral L-arginine supplementation in healthy adult males inhibited platelet aggregation, and this effect could be reversed by ex vivo incubation with the NO• synthase inhibitor L-NMMA *(44)*. In that study *(44)*, no change was observed in endothelium-dependent dilation of the brachial artery, suggesting that oral L-arginine principally caused a platelet-specific increase in NO• production to account for the inhibition of aggregation. In vivo, systemic infusion of a NOS inhibitor into normal subjects causes a reduction in bleeding time without changing vessel tone *(21)* and enhances platelet reactivity to various agonists *(22)*, supporting the clinical relevance of platelet-derived NO•. Thus, in addition to NO• produced by the vascular endothelium, NO•

Table 2
**Clinical Thrombotic Disorders
Associated with Impaired NO• Production**

Clinical thrombotic disorder
Thrombotic microangiopathy *(50)*
Hemolytic uremic syndrome
Thrombotic thrombocytopenic purpura
Atrial fibrillation *(47)*
Unstable coronary syndromes *(45)*
Acute myocardial infarction
Unstable angina
Pregnancy and preeclampsia *(49)*
Pediatric thromboembolic cerebrovascular disease *(54)*

production by the platelet may contribute to the prevention of thrombotic episodes. In the clinical studies as well as the experimental models, the source of NO• and mechanism(s) of action are often difficult to determine.

NO• DEFICIENCY AND CLINICAL THROMBOTIC DISORDERS

As shown in Table 2, the thrombotic mechanism underlying many clinical disorders has been attributed to deficient production of NO•. It is well established that thrombosis is the usual cause of unstable angina and myocardial infarction *(1,2)*, and, importantly, activated platelets from patients with these acute coronary syndromes produce significantly less NO• as compared to patients with stable coronary artery disease *(45)*. This decrease in NO• production in significant even after controlling for cardiovascular risk factors and the extent of atherosclerotic disease (Fig. 2). This observation suggests that impaired platelet-derived NO• may contribute to the development of acute coronary syndromes by influencing platelet function or recruitment and consequent thrombus formation.

Supportive of these observations is a recent study showing that platelets from patients with acute myocardial infarction and unstable angina, despite aspirin treatment, are still partially activated as measured by platelet surface expression of P-selectin and active GPIIb/IIIa *(46)*. For patients with both atrial fibrillation and unstable angina or acute myocardial infarction, surface expression of P-selectin and active GPIIb/IIIa was reduced by treatment with NO• donors, including nitroglycerin or *S*-nitrosoglutathione.

Patients with atrial fibrillation, a condition associated with increased cardiac thrombosis and embolism, have decreased plasma levels of nitrite and nitrate as well as lower levels of platelet cGMP *(47)* suggesting that there may be decreased levels of bioavailable NO• in this setting. In this study, there was no significant differences in levels of tissue-type plasminogen activator or plasminogen activator inhibitor type 1. The precise mechanism for the decreased NO• levels associated with atrial fibrillation is currently unknown, however, turbulent flow conditions have been associated with decreased NOS activity *(48)*.

Thrombosis has also been attributed to NO• deficiency in noncardiac clinical disorders. In women with preeclampsia, a disease state associated with hypertension, and intrarenal thrombosis and vasospasm, cGMP levels were depressed *(49)*. In patients with recurrent forms of thrombotic microangiopathy, including hemolytic uremic syndrome and thrombotic thrombocytopenic purpura, there is evidence that endothelial damage is a crucial feature in the development of microvascular thrombosis. Patients with these disease states manifest elevated plasma concentrations of NO• metabolites, and serum from these patients enhances NO• release when incubated with cultured endothelial cells. Importantly, superoxide production and lipid peroxidation are also enhanced *(50)*, suggesting that the interaction of these

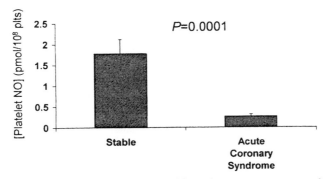

Fig. 2. Platelet NO• production in patients with stable and acute coronary syndromes. Platelet NO• production following activation with 5 μM ADP was significantly decreased ($p < 0.0001$) in patients with acute coronary syndromes as compared to patients with stable disease. Reprinted with permission of Lippincott Williams & Wilkins from Freedman et al., Circulation 1998;45:1481–1486.

reactive oxygen species with NO• reduces its bioactivity by increasing its oxidative state, potentially leading to enhanced thrombus formation.

NO•, ANTIOXIDANTS, AND REACTIVE OXYGEN SPECIES IN CLINICAL THROMBOTIC DISORDERS

As previously discussed, a prominent feature of both abnormal platelet function and dysfunctional endothelium-dependent vasodilation in the setting of cardiovascular and thrombotic disease is oxidative stress. Superoxide anion, an important source of oxidative stress, limits the biological activity of NO•. Excessive vascular superoxide production has been demonstrated in hypercholesterolemia as well as other disease states associated with endothelial dysfunction *(51)*.

There is ample clinical evidence to suggest that antioxidant status is important in normal platelet function and the prevention of thrombosis. For example, in patients with coronary artery disease, decreased plasma and platelet antioxidant activity is associated with increased platelet aggregability *(52)*.

As discussed, antioxidants may indirectly inhibit platelets through metabolism of reactive oxygen species, many of which alter platelet function. The antioxidant enzyme glutathione peroxidase potentiates the inhibition of platelet function by NO• by reducing LOOH concentrations *(53)*. Impairment of this process can lead to a clinical thrombotic disorder as shown in brothers with thrombotic strokes in childhood *(54)*. In these children, aggregometry and flow cytometry studies showed that their platelets were hyperreactive due to an abnormality in their plasma. In the presence of their plasma, NO• failed to inhibit aggregation or surface expression of P-selectin on normal platelets (Fig. 3). The decrease in plasma cGMP levels in these patients was secondary to reduced bioactive NO• as plasma glutathione peroxidase activity was decreased by approximately one-half in the probands. Importantly, sensitivity of the platelets to inhibition by NO• was restored by adding exogenous glutathione peroxidase to their plasma (Fig. 4). We recently reported a similar deficiency in four other families with childhood stroke *(55)*. This important antioxidant role of plasma glutathione peroxidase (PGPx) may be of broader relevance than this rare thrombotic disorder in children. GPx is a selenium-containing enzyme, and selenium deficiency has been reported in patients with acute myocardial infarction and coronary atherothrombotic disease *(56)*.

Supporting the role of antioxidant status in thrombosis are clinical studies indicating that vitamin E (α-tocopherol) exerts a beneficial effect on cardiovascular disease *(57)*. By examining plasma α-tocopherol concentration in 87 consecutive patients undergoing coronary angiography, we also determined that α-tocopherol is associated with platelet release of NO•

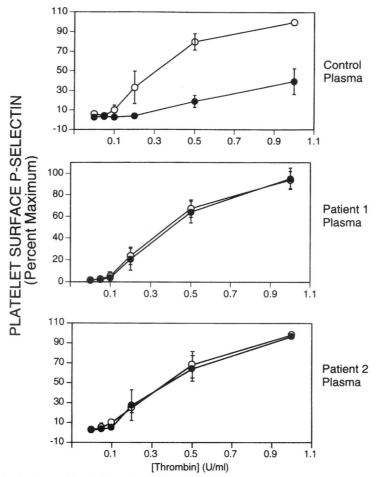

Fig. 3. NO• inhibits thrombin-induced platelet degranulation in the presence of control plasma, but not in the presence of plasma from patients 1 or 2. Washed platelets from normal donors were incubated with thrombin in the presence (closed circles) or absence (open circles) of 10 μM S-nitroso-N-acetylcysteine, and in the presence of control plasma (**top**), patient 1 plasma (**middle**), or patient 2 plasma (**bottom**). Samples were fixed and analyzed by flow cytometry with a P-selectin-specific monoclonal antibody. (Data are expressed as mean + SEM $n = 3$ experiments; $p < 0.05$ for control plasma). Reproduced with permission from the Journal of Clinical Investigation from Freedman et al., 1996;54:979–987.

(58). α-Tocopherol levels were 21.6 ± 3.2 μM and 12.2 ± 12 μM in patients in the highest quartile and lower three quartiles of platelet NO• production, respectively ($p < 0.01$). Platelet NO• production correlated with plasma α-tocopherol concentration ($R = 0.5$; $p < 0.01$) and this effect was independent of aspirin and nitrate treatment. Therefore, in patients with unstable coronary syndromes, α-tocopherol levels are associated with platelet-derived NO• release. These observations suggest a potential mechanism for the beneficial effect of α-tocopherol in patients with cardiovascular disease.

CONCLUSIONS

NO• is an important endogenous inhibitor of platelet activation and hemostasis. A deficiency of NO• supports and sustains platelet-mediated thrombotic responses, and this mechanism may underlie a broad range of thrombotic disorders from childhood stroke to coronary atherothrombotic disease.

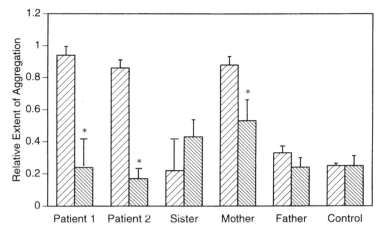

Fig. 4. The effect of glutathione peroxidase on platelet inhibition by S-nitrosoglutathione. Gel-filtered platelets from a normal adult donor were incubated with plasma from a family member or from a pooled pediatric control. S-nitrosoglutathione (5 μM) was added for 1 min and aggregation induced with ADP. Relative extent of platelet aggregation was determined in the presence (second set of bars) or absence (first set of bars) of glutathione peroxidase (5 U/mL). Data are expressed as a percent of control aggregation for each subject with ADP alone. (For patient 1, patient 2, and mother, $p < 0.05$ for incubation with glutathione peroxidase compared to aggregation with S-nitrosoglutathione alone; error bars represent standard error of the mean for $n = 3$ experiments). Reproduced with permission from the Journal of Clinical Investigation from Freedman et al., 1996; 54:979–987.

REFERENCES

1. DeWood MA, Spores J, Notske R, Mouser LT, Burroughs R, Golden MS et al. Prevalence of total coronary occlusion during the early hours of transmural myocardial infarction. N Engl J Med 1980;303: 897–902.
2. Falk E. Unstable angina with fatal outcome: dynamic coronary thrombosis leading to infarction and/or sudden death. Autopsy evidence of recurrent mural thrombosis with peripheral embolization culminating in total vascular occlusion. Circulation 1985;71:699–708.
3. Falk E. Plaque rupture with severe pre-existing stenosis precipitating coronary thrombosis. Characteristics of coronary atherosclerotic plaques underlying fatal occlusive thrombi. Br Heart J 1983;50:127–134.
4. Davies MJ, Thomas AC. Thrombosis and acute coronary-artery lesions in sudden cardiac ischemic death. N Engl J Med 1984;310:1137–1140.
5. Santos MT, Valles J, Marcus AJ, Safier LB, Brockman J, Islam N, et al. Enhancement of platelet reactivity and modulation of eicosanoid production by intact erythrocytes. A new approach to platelet activation and recruitment. J Clin Invest 1991;87:571–580.
6. Fitzgerald DJ, Roy L, Catella F, FitzGerald A. Platelet activation in unstable coronary disease. N Engl J Med 1986;315:983–989.
7. The RISC Group. Risk of myocardial infarction and death during treatment with low dose aspirin and intravenous heparin in men with unstable coronary artery disease. Lancet 1990;336:827–830.
8. Antiplatelet Trialist Collaboration. Collaborative overview of randomised trials of antiplatelet therapy: 1: Prevention of death, myocardial infarction, and stroke by prolonged antiplatelet therapy in various categories of patients. Br Med J 1994;308:81–106.
9. Radomski MW, Moncada S. Regulation of vascular homeostasis by nitric oxide. Thromb Haemost 1993;70:36–41.
10. Wirthumer-Hocke C, Silberbauer K, Sinzinger H. Effect on nitroglycerin and other organic nitrates on the in vitro biosynthesis of arachidonic acid-metabolites in washed human platelets. Prostaglandins Leukot Med 1984;15:317–323.
11. Negrescu EV, Sazonova LN, Baldenkov GN, Mazaev AV, Tkachuk VA. Relationship between the inhibition of receptor-induced increase in cytosolic free calcium concentration and the vasoldilator effects of nitrates in patients with congestive heart failure. Int J Cardiol 1990;26:175–184.

12. de Graaf JC, Banga JD, Moncada S, Palmer RM, de Groot PG, et al. Nitric oxide functions as an inhibitor of platelet adhesion under flow conditions. Circulation 1992;85:2284–2290.

13. Radomski MW, Palmer RM, Moncada S. The role of nitric oxide and cGMP in platelet adhesion to vascular endothelium. Biochem Biophys Res Commun 1987;148:1482–1489.

14. Stamler J, Mendelsohn ME, Amarante P, Smick D, Andon N, Davies JP, et al. N-acetylcysteine potentiates platelet inhibition by endothelium-derived relaxing factor. Circ Res 1989;65:789–795.

15. Cooke JP, Stamler J, Andon N, Davies PF, McKinley G, Loscalzo J. Flow stimulates endothelial cells to release a nitrovasodilator that is potentiated by reduced thiol. Am J Physiol 1990;259:H804–H812.

16. Shultz PJ, Raij L. Endogenously synthesized nitric oxide prevents endotoxin-induced glomerular thrombosis. J Clin Invest 1992;90:1718–1725.

17. Michelson AD, Benoit SE, Furman MI, Breckwoldt WL, Rohrer MJ, Bamard MR, et al. Effects of nitric oxide/endothelium-derived relaxing factor on platelet surface glycoproteins. Am J Physiol 1996;270: H1640–H1648.

18. Mehta JL, Chen LY, Kone BC, Mehta P, Turner P. Identification of constitutive and inducible forms of nitric oxide synthase in human platelets. J Lab Clin Med 1995;125:370–377.

19. Sase K, Michel T. Expression of constitutive endothelial nitric oxide synthase in human blood platelets. Life Sci 1995;57:2049–2055.

20. Chen LY, Mehta JL. Variable effects of L-arginine analogs on L-arginine-nitric oxide pathway in human neutrophils and platelets may relate to different nitric oxide synthase isoforms. J Pharmacol Exp Therap 1996;276:253–257.

21. Simon DI, Stamler J, Loh E, Loscalzo J, Francis SA, Creager MA. Effect of nitric oxide synthase inhibition on bleeding time in humans. J Cardiovasc Pharmacol 1995;26:339–342.

22. Bodzenta-Lukaszyk A, Gabryelewicz A, Lukaszyk A, Bielawiec M, Konturek JW, Domschke W. Nitric oxide synthase inhibition and platelet function. Thromb Res 1994;75:667–672.

23. Zhou Q, Hellermann GR, Solomonson LP. Nitric oxide release from resting human platelet. Thromb Res 1995;77:87–96.

24. Malinski T, Radomski MW, Taha Z, Moncada S. Direct electrochemical measurement of nitric oxide released from human platelets. Biochem Biophys Res Commun 1993;194:960–965.

25. Radomski MW, Palmer RM, Moncada S. An L-arginine/nitric oxide pathway present in human platelets regulates aggregation. Proc Natl Acad Sci USA 1990;87:5193–5197.

26. Freedman JE, Loscalzo J, Barnard MR, Alpert C, Keaney JF Jr, Michelson A. Nitric oxide released from activated platelets inhibits platelet recruitment. J Clin Invest 1997;100:350–356.

27. Bossaller C, Habib GB, Yamamoto H, Williams C, Wells S, Henry PD. Impaired muscarinic endothelium-dependent relaxation and cyclic guanosine 5'monophosphate formation in atherosclerotic human coronary artery and rabbit aorta. J Clin Invest 1987;79:170–174.

28. Vita JA, Treasure CB, Nabel EG, McLenachan JM, Fish RD, Yeung AC, et al. Coronary vasomotor response to acetylcholine relates to risk factors for coronary artery disease. Circulation 1990;81:491–497.

29. Celermajer DS, Sorensen KE, Gooch VM, Spiegelhalter DJ, Miller OI, Sullivan LD, et al. Non-invasive detection of endothelial dysfunction in children and adults at risk of atherosclerosis. Lancet 1992;340: 1111–1115.

30. Celermajer DS, Sorensen KE, Bull C, Robinson J, Deanfield JE. Endothelium-dependent dilation in the systemic arteries of symptomatic subjects relates to coronary risk factors and their interaction. J Am Coll Cardiol 1994;24:1468–1474.

31. Folts JD, Stamler J, Loscalzo J. Intravenous nitroglycerin infusion inhibits periodic platelet thrombus formation in stenosed dog coronary arteries. Circulation 1991;83:2122–2127.

32. Yao SH, Ober JC, Krishnaswami A, Ferguson JJ, Anderson HV, Golino P, et al. Endogenous nitric oxide protects against platelet aggregation and cyclic flow variations in stensosed and endothelium-injured arteries. Circulation 1992;86:1302–1309.

33. Stagliano N, Zhao W, Prado R, Dewanjee M, Ginsberg M, Dietrich W. The effect of nitric oxide synthase inhibition on acute platelet accumulation and hemodynamic depression in a rat model of thromboembolic stroke. J Cereb Blood Flow Metab 1997;17:1182–1190.

34. Waddington S, Cook HT, Reaveley D, Jansen A, Cattell V. L-arginine depletion inhibits glomerular nitric oxide synthesis and exacerbates rat nephrotoxic nephritis. Kidney Int 1996;49:1090–1096.

35. Broeders MA, Tangelder GJ, Slaaf DW, Reneman RS, oude Egbrink MG. Endogenous nitric oxide protects against thromboembolism in venules but not in arterioles. Arterio Thromb Vasc Biol 1998;18: 139–145.

36. Bressler NM, Broekman MJ, Marcus AJ. Concurrent studies of oxygen consumption and aggregation in stimulated human platelets. Blood 1979;53:167–178.

37. Burch J, Burch P. Glutathione disulfide production during arachidonic acid oxygenation in human platelets. Prostaglandins 1990;39:123–134.
38. Handin RI, Karabin R, Boxer GJ. Enhancement of platelet aggregation by superoxide anion. J Clin Invest 1987;59:959–965.
39. Huie RE, Padmaja S. The reaction of NO with superoxide. Free Rad Res Commun 1993;18:195–199.
40. Calzada C, Verice E, Lagarde M. Decrease in platelet reduced glutathione increases lipoxygenase activity and decreases vitamin E. Lipids 1991;26:696–699.
41. Meng YY, Trachtenburg J, Ryan US, Abendschein DR. Potentiation of endogenous nitric oxide with superoxide dismutase inhibits platelet-mediated thrombosis in injured stenotic arteries. J Am Coll Cardiol 1995;25:269–275.
42. Ikeda H, Koga Y, Oda T, Kuwano K, Nakayama H, Ueno T, et al. Free oxygen radicals contribute to platelet aggregation and cyclic flow variations in stenosed and endothelium-injured canine coronary arteries. J Am Coll Cardiol 1994;24:1749–1756.
43. Freedman JE, Sauter R, Battinelli E, Ault K, Knowles C, Huang P, et al. Deficient platelet-derived nitric oxide and enhanced hemostasis in mice lacking the NOS3 gene. Circulation 1998;98:I-4.
44. Adams MR, Forsyth CJ, Jessup W, Robinson J, Celermajer DS. Oral L-arginine inhibits platelet aggregation but does not enhance endothelium-dependent dilation in healthy young men. J Am Coll Cardiol 1995;26:1054–1061.
45. Freedman JE, Ting B, Hankin B, Loscalzo J, Keaney JF Jr, Vita JA. Impaired platelet production of nitric oxide in patients with unstable angina. Circulation 1998;98:1481–1486.
46. Langford EJ, Wainwright RJ, Martin J. Platelet activation in acute myocardial infarction and unstable angina is inhibited by nitric oxide donors. Arterio Thromb Vasc Biol 1996;16:51–55.
47. Minamino T, Kitakaze M, Sato H, Asanuma H, Funaya H, Koretsune Y, et al. Plasma levels of nitrite/nitrate and platelet cGMP levels are decreased in patients with atrial fibrillation. Arterio Thromb Vasc Biol 1997;17:3191–3195.
48. Noris M, Morigi M, Donadelli R, Aiello S, Foppolo M, Todeschini M, et al. Nitric oxide synthesis by cultured endothelial cells is modulated by flow conditions. Circ Res 1995;76:536–543.
49. Clark BA, Ludmir J, Epstein FH, Alvarez J, Tavara L, Bazul J, et al. Urinary cyclic GMP, endothelin, and prostaglandin E2 in normal pregnancy and preeclampsia. Am J Perinat 1997;14:559–562.
50. Noris M, Ruggenenti P, Todeschini M, Figliuzzi M, Macconi D, Zoja, C, et al. Increased nitric oxide formation in recurrent thrombotic microangiopathies: a possible mediator of microvasclar injury. Am J Kidney Dis 1996;27:790–796.
51. Ohara Y, Peterson TE, Harrison DG. Hypercholesterolemia increases endothelial superoxide anion production. J Clin Invest 1993;91:2546–2551.
52. Buczynski A, Wachowicz B, Kedziora-Konatowska K, Tkaczewski W, Kedziora J. Changes in antioxidant enzyme activities, aggregability and malonyldialdehyde concentration in blood platelets from patients with coronary heart disease. Atherosclerosis 1993;100:223–228.
53. Freedman JE, Frei B, Welch GN, Loscalzo J. Glutathione peroxidase potentiates the inhibition of platelet function by S-nitrosothiols. J Clin Invest 1995;96:394–400.
54. Freedman JE, Loscalzo J, Benoit SE, Valeri CR, Barnard MR, Michelson AD. Decreased platelet inhibition by nitric oxide in two brothers with a history of arterial thrombosis. J Clin Invest 1996;97:979–987.
55. Kenet G, Freedman J, Shenkman B, Regina E, Brok-Simoni F, Holzman F, et al. Plasma glutathione peroxidase deficiency and platelet insensitivity to nitric oxide in children with familial stroke. Arterio Thromb Vasc Biol 1999;19:2017–2023.
56. Salonen JT, Alfthan G, Huttenen JK, Pikkarainen J, Puska P. Association between cardiovascular death and myocardial infarction and serum selenium in a matched-pair longitudinal study. Lancet 1982;2:175–179.
57. Rimm E, Stampfer MJ, Ascherio A, Giovannucci E, Colditz GA, Willet WC. Vitamin E consumption and the risk of coronary heart disease in men. N Engl J Med 1993;328:1450–1456.
58. Freedman J, Li L, Vita J, Keaney JF Jr. Alpha-tocopherol levels are associated with platelet release of nitric oxide. J Am Coll Cardiol 1999;Abstract, in press.

18 Myocardial Nitric Oxide in Heart Failure

Douglas B. Sawyer and Wilson S. Colucci

INTRODUCTION

Over the past decade, evidence has emerged that nitric oxide (NO•) may play a role in the pathogenesis of myocardial failure. The effects of NO• in myocardial failure, as in other clinical situations, may be either beneficial or deleterious. NO• at relatively low levels appears to modulate the response of the myocardium to potentially deleterious stimuli, and thus in some situations may offset the progression of myocardial failure. On the other hand, at higher levels NO• has the ability to impair normal myocardial function and to exert direct toxic effects in the myocardium, as it can in other tissues. The effects of higher levels of NO• may be relevant to a variety of situations in which myocardial NO• is increased. These include conditions in which there is a clear inflammatory reaction such as sepsis, myocarditis, transplant rejection or acute infarction. There is now evidence that NO• production is also increased above physiologic levels in the myocardium of patients with chronic heart failure. These observations have led to the concern that with increasing levels, NO• may contribute to the pathogenesis of myocardial failure, and thus change from a friend to a foe.

NITRIC OXIDE SYNTHASES (NOS) IN THE MYOCARDIUM

Constitutive NOS in the Normal and Failing Myocardium

NO• is a ubiquitous signaling molecule synthesized in the conversion of L-arginine to L-citrulline by a family of NOSs (1). Both constitutive (NOS3) and inducible (NOS2) NOSs are present in the myocardium, and there appear to be changes in the activity of both of these enzymes in the setting of myocardial failure.

Under normal circumstances, myocardial NO• is produced only by NOS3. The activity of this enzyme, which is present constitutively in virtually all cell types in the myocardium, including cardiac myocytes, fibroblasts and endothelial cells, is regulated by a calcium-sensitive interaction with calmodulin in response to signals that increase intracellular calcium. Pinsky and colleagues have used a porphyrinic NO• sensitive microelectrode in the intact normal heart and found that there are beat-to-beat changes in the amount of NO• present (2). These changes in NO• on a short time scale may work to control energy utilization and instantaneous myocardial function. The same technique has not been applied to the failing heart. However, with the abnormalities in calcium handling that exist in heart failure (3), one might expect that NOS3 activity would be increased, at least in cardiac myocytes, because of the consistently higher calcium concentrations. Using the same technique in isolated ventricular myocytes, Malinski and colleagues (4) were able to demonstrate a transient increase in NO•

From: *Contemporary Cardiology, vol. 4: Nitric Oxide and the Cardiovascular System*
Edited by: J. Loscalzo and J. A. Vita © Humana Press Inc., Totowa, NJ

after stimulation with a β-adrenergic agonist. However longer periods of exposure to elevated levels of cyclic adenosine monophosphate (cAMP) or phosphodiesterase inhibitors decreases the expression of NOS3 mRNA as well as the activity of the enzyme in isolated cardiac myocytes *(5)*.

Inducible NOS in the Failing Myocardium

In the presence of hypoxia or increased levels of inflammatory cytokines, endothelial cells, myocytes, and infiltrating macrophages can markedly increase their production of NO$^\bullet$ via the induction of NOS2. This enzyme is not expressed in the myocardium under normal conditions. However, after exposure to cytokines, hypoxia, and perhaps other stimuli there is rapid expression of NOS2 due to activation of specific transcription factors *(6)*. Although NOS2 can produce low levels of NO$^\bullet$ that may exert a modulatory function, when fully induced NOS2 more typically produces much higher, "pathologic" levels of NO$^\bullet$ that may be deleterious. This capacity to damage cells should come as no surprise, since it is by the generation of high levels of NO$^\bullet$ that NOS2 serves as the effector arm of the immunologic response to certain pathogens *(7,8)*.

Some investigators have found that the expression and activity of NOS2 are increased in the myocardium of patients with both idiopathic and ischemic dilated cardiomyopathies *(9, 10)*. However, this finding has not been universal, and other studies have found elevations of NOS2 only in patients with sepsis *(11)*. Several animal models of heart failure show elevations of NOS2 activity, including models of myocardial infarction *(12)* and autoimmune myocarditis *(13)*. The mediators of the increase in NOS2 expression appear to include a combination of factors, including cytokines and adrenergic agonists. The levels of circulating proinflammatory cytokines are elevated systemically *(14,15)* and in the myocardium *(16)* of patients with idiopathic and ischemic dilated cardiomyopathies, as is the level of adrenergic agonists *(17)*. Proinflammatory cytokines including interleukin-1β (IL-1β) and tumor necrosis factor-α (TNF-α) have been shown to induce the expression of NOS2 in isolated cardiac myocytes, as well as microvascular endothelial cells from the heart *(18,19)*. Although norepinephrine does not directly induce NOS2, it potentiates the expression of cytokine-stimulated NOS2 by stabilizing its mRNA *(20)*. Thus, increased NO$^\bullet$ production in failing myocardium is most likely due to the expression of NOS2. There is very little information about NOS3 expression in failing myocardium.

EFFECTS OF NO$^\bullet$ ON MYOCARDIAL FUNCTION

Effect of NO$^\bullet$ on Myocardial Contractility

NO$^\bullet$ appears to play an important role in determining the myocardial response to both sympathetic and parasympathetic stimulation. In particular, the increase in myocardial NO$^\bullet$ may account, in part, for the blunted adrenergic responsiveness that occurs in heart failure. Gulick et al. showed that in isolated cardiac myocytes the contractile response to isoproterenol was attenuated by exposure to media conditioned by monocytes activated by lipopolysaccharide *(21)*. Balligand et al. *(22)* showed that inhibitors of NOS potentiate the positive inotropic response to β-adrenergic stimulation in single myocytes treated with inflammatory cytokines. These investigators and others have gone on to show that conditioned media and cytokines can induce the expression of NOS2 in myocytes *(19,23)*, with an increase in NO$^\bullet$ produced by single myocytes as detected by an NO$^\bullet$-sensitive microelectrode *(18)*.

Similar observations have been made in the intact heart. We found that in closed-chest dogs the intracoronary infusion of NOS inhibitors had no effect on basal contractility (as assessed by measurement of +*dP/dt*), but significantly augmented the positive inotropic response to β-adrenergic stimulation *(24)*. Similarly, in patients with various degrees of left ventricular (LV) dysfunction we found that the intracoronary infusion of the NOS inhibitor

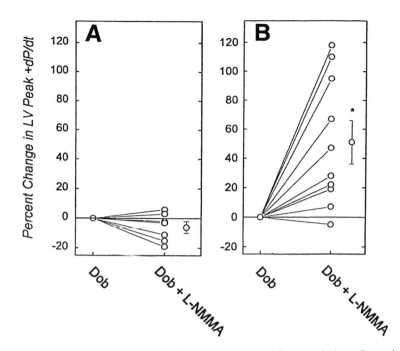

Fig. 1. Increased sensitivity to NOS inhibition in patients with heart failure. In patients with or without left ventricular failure, the β-adrenergic agonist dobutamine (Dob) was infused systemically with and without concurrent infusion of the NOS inhibitor L-NMMA directly into the left coronary artery. Infusion of L-NMMA increased the positive inotropic response (measured as LV +*dP/dt*) to dobutamine in patients with heart failure (**B**), but not in control subjects with normal left ventricular function (**A**). Reproduced with permission from ref. *26*.

N^G-monomethyl-L-arginine (L-NMMA) potentiated the positive inotropic response to dobutamine *(25)*. More recently, we found that intracoronary infusion of L-NMMA potentiated the positive inotropic response to dobutamine in patients with clinical heart failure caused by systolic LV dysfunction, but had no effect in subjects with normal LV function (Fig. 1) *(26)*. These results are consistent with the in vitro experiments showing that NO' impairs β-adrenergic responsiveness and suggest that the expression of myocardial NO' is increased in patients with myocardial failure.

It is unclear whether this inhibitory effect of NO' on the inotropic responses to β-adrenergic stimulation in patients with heart failure is adaptive or maladaptive. Since β-adrenergic stimulation is a short-term adaptation that serves to support cardiac function, a negative inotropic action of myocardial NO' might promote further LV dysfunction and thereby worsen the severity of heart failure. However, there is also evidence that *chronic* β-adrenergic activation may be deleterious by causing progression of myocardial failure. This view is supported by the demonstration that β-blockers can decrease the rate of disease progression and improve functional class and survival in patients with chronic stable heart failure *(27,28)*. In this context, inhibition of β-adrenergic responsiveness by NO' could be considered adaptive. NO' might thus have beneficial effects similar to β-adrenergic receptor blockade. Some of these beneficial effects are possibly due to inhibition of adrenergic mediated remodeling (*see* following).

Role of NO' in Mediating Parasympathetic Actions

The negative chronotropic and inotropic effects of parasympathetic stimulation may be mediated, in part, via NO'. In isolated spontaneously beating ventricular myocytes, inhibition

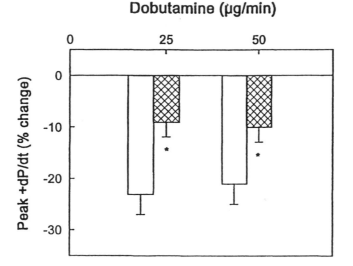

Fig. 2. Role of NO· in mediating the negative inotropic action of vagal nerve stimulation in dogs. In closed-chest dogs, bilateral stimulation of the vagal nerves in neck decreased the positive inotropic response (measured as LV +dP/dt) to intracoronary dobutamine infusion (clear bars). When the NOS inhibitor L-NMMA was infused into the left coronary artery, the negative inotropic effect of vagal nerve stimulation was attenuated (hatched bars), suggesting that NO· plays a role in mediating the effects of parasympathetic nerve stimulation on the heart. Reproduced with permission from ref. *31.*

of NOS prevents the negative chronotropic action of muscarinic cholinergic stimulation *(29).* This effect of NO· appears to be mediated by activation of guanylate cyclase resulting in cGMP-dependent phosphorylation of the L-type calcium channel *(30).* Similarly, the effects of vagal stimulation on cardiac function in vivo are attenuated by inhibition of NOS. For example, in closed-chest dogs muscarinic cholinergic actions caused by direct stimulation of the vagus nerve attenuate the positive inotropic effect of dobutamine *(31).* We found that this inhibitory effect of vagal stimulation depends, in part, on NO·, as the intracoronary infusion of L-NMMA reduced the inhibitory effect of vagal stimulation by 60%, and the subsequent infusion of L-arginine restored the inhibitory effect (Fig. 2). Thus, NO· plays an important modulatory role in the myocardium by inhibiting the response to sympathetic stimulation and mediating the action of parasympathetic stimulation (Fig. 3).

Direct Negative Inotropic Effects of NO·

There is evidence, both in vitro and in vivo, that cytokine-induced increases in NO· production by NOS2 may be sufficient to decrease basal ventricular contractile function (i.e., in the unstimulated state). For example, Finkel et al. showed that inflammatory cytokines cause direct negative inotropic effects in isolated papillary muscles that are prevented by NOS inhibition *(32).* Similarly, Brady et al. found that basal contractile function was reduced in myocytes exposed to systemic endotoxin for 4 h *(23).* Inhibition of NOS with L-NMMA in the media caused an improvement in myocyte function that was overcome by L-arginine, suggesting that the negative inotropic effect of endotoxemia was mediated by NO·. In intact animals, Pagani et al. found that infusion of TNF-α in dogs for 24-48 h caused a decrease in left ventricular systolic and diastolic function over 24-48 h that was prevented by inhibitors of NOS *(33).*

The mechanism by which NO· can depress basal contractile function is not known, but may simply reflect a more profound inhibition of voltage-dependent calcium channels by

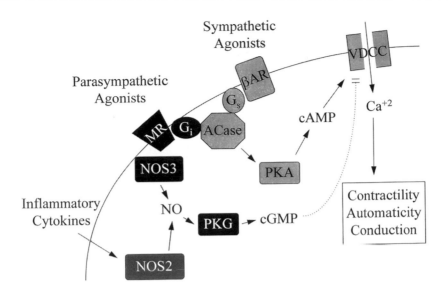

Fig. 3. Postulated role of NO· in regulating sympathetic and parasympathetic autonomic responses in the myocardium. Data from in vitro and in vivo studies suggest that NO· derived from either NOS3 or NOS2 can inhibit the positive inotropic response to β-adrenergic stimulation in the myocardium. NOS2 may be elevated in the myocardium under pathologic circumstances such as inflammation and with chronic heart failure. NOS3, which is normally present in the myocardium, may be coupled to muscarinic cholinergic receptors, and thus mediate the inhibitory effect of parasympathetic nerve stimulation. The negative inotropic effects of NO· appear to be mediated via cGMP-dependent inhibition of calcium channel influx. (Dashed line indicates inhibition.)

high levels of cGMP. Alternatively, it might be due to inhibition of mitochondrial respiration resulting in reduced adenosine triphosphate (ATP) availability. In cultured rat ventricular myocytes, stimulation with the cytokine interleukin-1β caused a reversible decrease in mitochondrial respiration that was prevented by an NOS inhibitor *(34)*. It is also possible that reduced contractility is due to the modification of thiol groups on proteins involved in excitation-contraction coupling, with subsequent alteration in protein function *(35,36)*.

EFFECTS ON NO· ON VENTRICULAR REMODELING

Myocyte Protective Effects of NO· In Vitro

The modulatory or beneficial effects of NO· on adrenergic responses in the heart go beyond their effects on contractility. Chronic adrenergic stimulation has been implicated in ventricular remodeling and the progression of myocardial failure. In animal models, chronic adrenergic stimulation leads to myocardial hypertrophy *(37,38)*, altered gene expression with downregulation of genes involved in excitation-contraction coupling *(39)*, and programmed cell death of cardiac myocytes *(40)*. In cardiac myocytes and fibroblasts in vitro, we found that many of the effects of adrenergic stimulation can be attenuated with NO· donors in a concentration-dependent manner *(41)*. For example, in cardiac myocytes the NO· donor *S*-nitroso-*N*-acetyl-D,L-penicillamine (SNAP) attenuated the ability of norepinephrine to stimulate protein synthesis, whereas addition of a NOS inhibitor augmented the response to norepinephrine (Fig. 4). The effects of NO· were mimicked by cGMP, indicating that this action of NO· is likely mediated via a cGMP-dependent pathway.

Cytokines, such as IL-1β, can also induce hypertrophy and altered gene expression in isolated cardiac myocytes *(42)*. Although cytokines are potent stimulators of NOS2 expression and

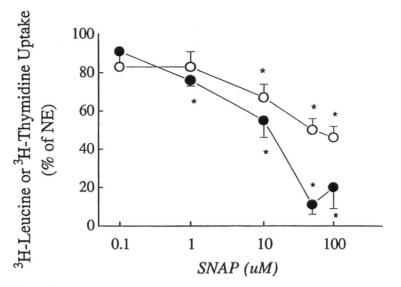

Fig. 4. Inhibition of the growth-stimulating effects of norepinephrine in cardiac myocytes and fibroblasts in vitro. Norepinephrine stimulated protein and DNA synthesis in myocytes (open circles) and fibroblasts (closed circles) cultured from neonatal rats. The addition of the NO• donor SNAP inhibited protein synthesis in the myocytes and DNA synthesis in the fibroblasts in a concentration-dependent manner. Thus, NO• may counteract the growth promoting effects of sympathetic stimulation in the heart. Reproduced with permission from ref. *41*.

activity *(19)*, the hypertrophic response of myocytes to IL-1β appears not to be attenuated by NO•, perhaps reflecting differences in the signaling pathways used by norepinephrine and IL-1β.

NO• Attenuates Stretch-Induced Apoptosis in Cardiac Myocytes

A variety of exogenous stimuli, including mechanical stretch and norepinephrine, have been found to increase the rate of apoptosis in cardiac myocytes in vitro. Cheng et al. stretched isolated papillary muscles by 20% for 4 h *(43)*. Under these conditions, mechanical stretch induced apoptosis in myocytes, and this effect was inhibited completely by the addition of an NO• donor. The mechanism by which NO• protects myocytes remains to be elucidated. However, in other cell types, it appears that NO• can inhibit apoptosis by inhibiting specific enzymes in the programmed cell death pathway *(44)*. Of note, Cheng et al. *(43)* found that the protective effect of NO• correlated with its ability to decrease the level of superoxide in the myocardium, suggesting that it might exert its beneficial action by scavenging superoxide generated by mechanical stretch.

Myocardial Toxicity of NO•

Experiments in vitro show direct toxic effects of high concentrations of NO• on cardiac myocytes. Pinsky et al. demonstrated that adult rat ventricular myocytes in culture died in response to stimulation with cytokines (IL-1β, interferon-γ [IFN-γ], and TNF-α) *(45)* (Fig. 5). This effect of the cytokines could be prevented by inhibition of NOS with L-NMMA, suggesting that NO• played an important role. Recently, we have found that NO• donors that result in high levels of NO• cause apoptosis of cardiac myocytes in vitro (our unpublished data). This observation raises the intriguing possibility that in failing myocardium, high levels of NO• produced by NOS2 may contribute to progressive myocardial failure by causing apoptosis *(46)*.

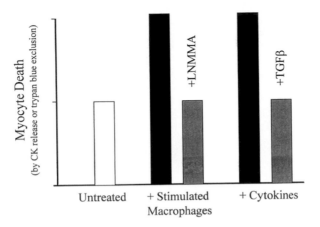

Fig. 5. Direct toxic actions of NO' in vitro. Adult ventricular myocytes treated with stimulated macrophages or a combination of inflammatory cytokines show an increase in cell death as evidenced by reduced number of cells able to exclude trypan blue as well the release of creatine kinase into the media. These effects can be inhibited by either L-NMMA, an inhibitor of NOS, or TGF-β, a cytokine known to inhibit the induction of NOS2 in myocytes. After Pinsky et al. *(45)* with permission.

The mechanism by which NO' causes myocyte apoptosis remains to be learned. One possibility is the formation of reactive oxygen and nitrogen species when NO' is produced at extremely high levels. NO' is a free radical gas that is buffered in the cell by reactions with glutathione. Through chemical reactions with other oxygen species, NO' can either decrease or increase the oxidative state of a cell or tissue. On the one hand, NO' may reduce the level of oxidative stress by buffering low levels of reactive oxygen species (ROS). Alternatively, higher levels of NO' may increase oxidative stress by, among other means, reacting with superoxide anion (O_2^-) to generate peroxynitrite ($ONOO^-$), a free radical that may be more toxic and long-lived than either NO' or O_2^- *(47)*. $ONOO^-$ can react with tyrosine residues of susceptible proteins, in some cases causing irreversible inactivation *(48)*.

Based on the relative rate constants of O_2^- with superoxide dismutase (SOD) and NO', the formation of $ONOO^-$ is favored when the levels of O_2^- or NO' are high, or the level of SOD is low *(49)*. Moreover, Xia and Zweier have shown that under appropriate conditions of substrate deficiency NOS2 is capable of directly catalyzing the formation of O_2^- *(50)*. Interestingly, Singal and colleagues have shown that the activity of antioxidant enzymes, including SOD, is reduced in two models of heart failure *(51,52)*, and might thus account for increased levels of O_2^- and $ONOO^-$. It is therefore interesting that myocardial $ONOO^-$ formation is increased in autopsy samples of patients who died of sepsis or myocarditis, as evidenced by increased staining for nitrotyrosine *(53)*. One target of $ONOO^-$ is manganese-superoxide dismutase (MnSOD), which is irreversibly inactivated by nitrosylation *(54)*. Inactivation of MnSOD could, in turn, further increase oxidative stress (Fig. 6).

Animal models of autoimmune and viral myocarditis implicate a direct toxic effect of NO' and $ONOO^-$ in vivo. In these models there is massive inflammation in the heart that results in overt myocyte necrosis. Ishiyama et al. were able to reduce the amount of necrotic myocardium as well as the elevation of creatine kinase in rats with experimental autoimmune myocarditis using aminoguanidine, an inhibitor of NOS2 *(13)*. Interestingly, in that system treatment with aminoguanidine also decreased the amount of superoxide anion formed. The source of superoxide anion in that model was not determined. Although it is possible that superoxide anion was formed by NOS2 in this system, equally likely is that an increase in superoxide anion resulted from the inactivation of MnSOD by $ONOO^-$.

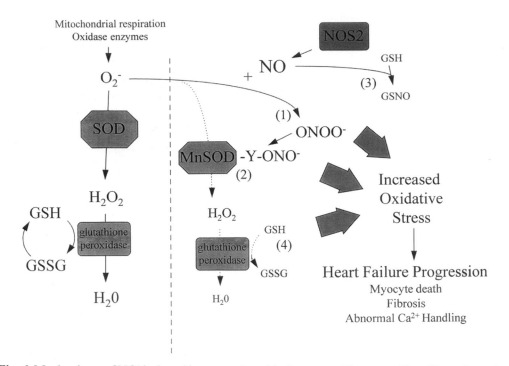

Fig. 6. Mechanisms of NO• induced increases in oxidative stress. The normal handling of reactive oxygen species (left) can be altered by large increases in NO• that may occur in heart failure resulting from induction of NOS2 activity, leading to increases in oxidative stress. NO• can react directly with O_2^- directly to form the ONOO⁻ (1). ONOO⁻ formation may lead to inactivation of MnSOD through nitrotyrosine formation (2), thus further increasing the levels of O_2^-. NO• reacts with glutathione (GSH) to form GSNO (3), thus depleting reduced glutatione, an important cellular antioxidant. GSH is a necessary cofactor for the activity of glutathione peroxidase, and thus depletion of GSH will lead to increased levels of peroxides, with increased formation of hydroxyl radicals as well (4).

Mikama et al. were able to reveal both protective and toxic effects of NO• when they examined the effect of inhibition of NO• synthesis with N^G-nitro-L-arginine methyl ester (L-NAME) on the mortality and the extent of myocardial injury in a murine model of viral myocarditis *(55)*. Mice were infected with coxsackie virus B3 in the presence of increasing doses of L-NAME. At the highest dose of L-NAME, survival was markedly worse in the infected but untreated mice. At a low dose, however, L-NAME improved survival and reduced the severity of heart failure and area of myocardial necrosis. This is consistent with a dual action of NO•, where some NO• (low concentrations of L-NAME) is better than too much NO• (no L-NAME), and no NO• (high concentrations of L-NAME) is worst of all. Further insight into the mechanisms by which NO• exerts these opposing actions will be needed before rational therapies can be designed.

It is unlikely that NO• and reactive nitrogen species can explain all of the effects of the inflammatory cytokines in the heart. For example, in the murine model of cardiac myosin-induced autoimmune myocarditis, Bachmaier et al. were able to show that NOS2 expression was present in the heart in both inflammatory macrophages as well as cardiomyocytes *(56)*. Autoimmune heart disease was accompanied by formation of the ONOO⁻ reaction product nitrotyrosine in inflammatory macrophages as well as in cardiomyocytes. Mice defective for the interferon regulatory transcription factor-1 (IRF-1(−/−) after gene targeting failed to induce NOS2 expression and nitrotyrosine formation in the heart, but developed cardiac myosin-induced myocarditis at prevalence and severity similar to those of heterozygous littermates.

SUMMARY

NO• plays a central role in normal myocardial physiology. In addition, NO• has the ability to exert either beneficial or deleterious effects on the myocardium. At lower concentrations, NO• may protect from deleterious stimuli such as mechanical stress and norepinephrine. At higher concentrations, NO• may change to a pathogen capable of stimulating the loss of myocytes. The mechanism by which NO• exerts these contrasting effects may involve decreases and increases in oxidative stress, respectively. A better understanding of the role that NO• plays in the development and progression of myocardial failure may lead to new treatment strategies.

REFERENCES

1. Nathan C. Natural resistance and nitric oxide. Cell 1995;82:873–876.
2. Pinsky DJ, Patton S, Mesaros S, Brovkovych V, Kubaszewski E, Grunfeld S, et al. Mechanical transduction of nitric oxide synthesis in the beating heart. Circ Res 1997;81:372–379.
3. Gwathmey JK, Copelas L, MacKinnon R, Schoen FJ, Feldman MD, Grossman W, et al. Abnormal intracellular calcium handling in myocardium from patients with end-stage heart failure. Circ Res 1987; 61:70–76.
4. Kanai AJ, Mesaros S, Finkel MS, Oddis CV, Birder LA, Malinski T. Beta-adrenergic regulation of constitutive nitric oxide synthase in cardiac myocytes. Am J Physiol 1997;273:C1371–C1377.
5. Belhassen L, Kelly RA, Smith TW, Balligand JL. Nitric oxide synthase (NOS3) and contractile responsiveness to adrenergic and cholinergic agonists in the heart. Regulation of NOS3 transcription in vitro and in vivo by cyclic adenosine monophosphate in rat cardiac myocytes. J Clin Invest 1996;97:1908–1915.
6. Singh K, Balligand JL, Fischer TA, Smith TW, Kelly RA. Regulation of cytokine-inducible nitric oxide synthase in cardiac myocytes and microvascular endothelial cells. Role of extracellular signal-regulated kinases 1 and 2 (ERK1/ERK2) and STAT1 alpha. J Biol Chem 1996;271:1111–1117.
7. Macmicking JD, North RJ, LaCourse R, Mudgett JS, Shah SK, Nathan CF. Identification of nitric oxide synthase as a protective locus against tuberculosis. Proc Natl Acad Sci USA 1997;94:5243–5248.
8. Wheeler MA, Smith SD, Garcia-Cardena G, Nathan CF, Weiss RM, Sessa WC. Bacterial infection induces nitric oxide synthase in human neutrophils. J Clin Invest 1997;99:110–116.
9. Haywood GA, Tsao PS, von der Leyen HE, Mann MJ, Keeling PJ, Trindade PT, et al. Expression of inducible nitric oxide synthase in human heart failure. Circulation 1996;93:1087–1094.
10. Habib FM, Springall DR, Davies GJ, Oakley CM, Yacoub MH, Polak JM. Tumour necrosis factor and inducible nitric oxide synthase in dilated cardiomyopathy. Lancet 1996;347:1151–1155.
11. Thoenes M, Forstermann U, Tracey WR, Bleese NM, Nussler AK, Scholz H, et al. Expression of inducible nitric oxide synthase in failing and non-failing human heart. J Mol Cell Cardiol 1996;28:165–169.
12. Wildhirt SM, Dudek RR, Suzuki H, Bing RJ. Involvement of inducible nitric oxide synthase in the inflammatory process of myocardial infarction. Int J Cardiol 1995;50:253–261.
13. Ishiyama S, Hiroe M, Nishikawa T, Abe S, Shimojo T, Ito H, et al. Nitric oxide contributes to the progression of myocardial damage in experimental autoimmune myocarditis in rats. Circulation 1997;95: 489–496.
14. MacGowan GA, Mann DL, Kormos RL, Feldman AM, Murali S. Circulating interleukin-6 in severe heart failure. Am J Cardiol 1997;79:1128–1131.
15. Torre-Amione G, Kapadia S, Benedict C, Oral H, Young JB, Mann DL. Proinflammatory cytokine levels in patients with depressed left ventricular ejection fraction: a report from the studies of left ventricular dysfunction (SOLVD). J Am Coll Cardiol 1996;27:1201–1206.
16. Torre-Amione G, Kapadia S, Lee J, Durand J, Bies RD, Young JB, et al. Tumor necrosis factor-α and tumor necrosis factor receptors in the failing human heart. Circulation 1996;93:704–711.
17. Cohn JN, Levine TB, Olivari MT, Garberg V, Lura D, Francis GS, et al. Plasma norepinephrine as a guide to prognosis in patients with chronic congestive heart failure. N Engl J Med 1984;311:819–823.
18. Balligand JL, Ungureanu-Longrois D, Simmons WW, Pimental D, Malinski TA, Kapturczak M, et al. Cytokine-inducible nitric oxide synthase (iNOS) expression in cardiac myocytes. Characterization and regulation of iNOS expression and detection of iNOS activity in single cardiac myocytes in vitro. J Biol Chem 1994;269:27,580–27,588.
19. Balligand JL, Ungureanu-Longrois D, Simmons WW, Kobzik L, Lowenstein CJ, Lamas S, et al. Induction of NO synthase in rat cardiac microvascular endothelial cells by IL-1 beta and IFN-gamma. Am J Physiol 1995;268:H1293–H303.

20. Oddis CV, Simmons RL, Hattler BG, Finkel MS. Chronotropic effcts of cytokines and the nitric oxide synthase inhibitor, L-NMMA, on cardiac myocytes. Biochem Biophys Res Commun 1994;205:992–997.

21. Gulick T, Pieper SJ, Murphy MA, Lange LG, Schreiner GF. A new method for assessment of cultured cardiac myocyte contractility detects immune factor-mediated inhibition of beta-adrenergic responses. Circulation 1991;84:313–321.

22. Balligand JL, Ungureanu D, Kelly RA, Kobzik L, Pimental D, Michel T, et al. Abnormal contractile function due to induction of nitric oxide synthesis in rat cardiac myocytes follows exposure to activated macrophage-conditioned medium. J Clin Invest 1993;91:2314–2319.

23. Brady AJ, Warren JB, Poole-Wilson PA, Williams TJ, Harding SE. Nitric oxide attenuates cardiac myocyte contraction. Am J Physiol 1993;265:H176–H186.

24. Keaney JF Jr, Hare JM, Balligand JL, Loscalzo J, Smith TW, Colucci WS. Inhibition of nitric oxide synthase augments myocardial contractile responses to beta-adrenergic stimulation. Am J Physiol 1996; 271:H2646–H2652.

25. Hare JM, Loh E, Creager MA, Colucci WS. Nitric oxide inhibits the positive inotropic response to beta-adrenergic stimulation in humans with left ventricular dysfunction. Circulation 1995;92:2198–2203.

26. Hare JM, Givertz MM, Creager MA, Colucci WS. Increased sensitivity to nitric oxide synthase inhibition in patients with heart failure. Potentiation of β-adrenergic inotropic responsiveness. Circulation 1998;97:161–166.

27. Packer M, Colucci WS, Sackner-Bernstein JD, Liang CS, Goldscher DA, Freeman I, et al. Double-blind, placebo-controlled study of the effects of carvedilol in patients with moderate to severe heart failure. The PRECISE Trial. Prospective Randomized Evaluation of Carvedilol on Symptoms and Exercise. Circulation 1996;94:2793–2799.

28. Colucci WS, Packer M, Bristow MR, Gilbert EM, Cohn JN, Fowler MB, et al. Carvedilol inhibits clinical progression in patients with mild symptoms of heart failure. US Carvedilol Heart Failure Study Group. Circulation 1996;94:2800–2806.

29. Balligand JL, Kelly RA, Marsden PA, Smith TW, Michel T. Control of cardiac muscle cell function by an endogenous nitric oxide signaling system. Proc Natl Acad Sci USA 1993;90:347–351.

30. Han X, Kobzik L, Balligand J-L, Kelly RA, Smith TW. Nitric oxide synthase (NOS3)-mediated cholinergic modulation of $Ca2+$ current in adult rabbit atrioventricular nodal cells. Circ Res 1996;78:998–1008.

31. Hare JM, Keaney JF Jr, Balligand JL, Loscalzo J, Smith TW, Colucci WS. Role of nitric oxide in parasympathetic modulation of beta-adrenergic myocardial contractility in normal dogs. J Clin Invest 1995;95:360–366.

32. Finkel MS, Oddis CV, Jacob TD, Watkins SC, Hattler BG, Simmons RL. Negative intropic effects of cytokines on the heart mediated by nitric oxide. Science 1992;257:387–389.

33. Pagani FD, Baker LS, Hsi C, Knox M, Fink MP, Visner MS. Left ventricular systolic and diastolic dysfunction after infusion of tumor necrosis factor-alpha in conscious dogs. J Clin Invest 1992;90:389–398.

34. Oddis CV, Finkel MS. Cytokine-stimulated nitric oxide production inhibits mitochondrial activity in cardiac myocytes. Biochem Biophys Res Commun 1995;213:1002–1009.

35. Campbell DL, Stamler JS, Strauss HC. Redox modulation of L-type calcium channels in ferret ventricular myocytes. Dual mechanism regulation by nitric oxide and S-nitrosothiols. J Gen Physiol 1996;108: 277–293.

36. Xu L, Eu JP, Meissner G, Stamler JS. Activation of the cardiac calcium release channel (Ryanodine receptor) by poly-S-nitrosylation. Science 1998;279:234–237.

37. Malik AB, Geha AS. Role of adrenergic mechanisms in the development of cardiac hypertrophy. Proc Soc Exp Biol Med 1975;150:796–800.

38. Kudej RK, Iwase M, Uechi M, Vatner DE, Oka N, Ishikawa Y, et al. Effects of chronic beta-adrenergic receptor stimulation in mice. J Mol Cell Cardiol 1997;29:2735–2746.

39. Stein B, Bartel S, Kirchhefer U, Kokott S, Krause EG, Neumann J, et al. Relation between contractile function and regulatory cardiac proteins in hypertrophied hearts. Am J Physiol 1996;270:H2021–H2028.

40. Communal C, Singh K, Pimentel DR, Colucci WS. Norepinephrine stimulates apoptosis in adult rat ventricular myocytes by activation of the β-adrenergic pathway. Circulation 1998;98:1329–1334.

41. Calderone A, Thaik CM, Takahashi N, Chang DLF, Colucci WS. Nitric oxide, atrial natriuretic peptide, and cGMP inhibit the growth-promoting effects of norepinephrine in cardiac myocytes and fibroblasts. J Clin Invest 1998;101:812–818.

42. Thaik CM, Calderone A, Takahashi N, Colucci WS. Interleukin-1β modulates the growth and phenotype of neonatal rat cardiac myocytes. J Clin Invest 1995;96:1093–1099.

43. Cheng W, Li B, Kajstura J, Li P, Wolin MS, Sonnenblick EH, et al. Stretch-induced programmed myocyte cell death. J Clin Invest 1995;96:2247–2259.

44. Mannick JB, Miao XQ, Stamler JS. Nitric oxide inhibits Fas-induced apoptosis. J Biol Chem 1997; 272:24,125–24,128.

45. Pinsky DJ, Cai B, Yang X, Rodriguez C, Sciacca RR, Cannon PJ. The lethal effects of cytokine-induced nitric oxide on cardiac myocytes are blocked by nitric oxide synthase antagonism or transforming growth factor b. J Clin Invest 1995;95:677–685.

46. Olivetti G, Abbi R, Quaini F, Kajstura J, Cheng W, Nitahara JA, et al. Apoptosis in the failing human heart. N Engl J Med 1997;336:1131–1141.

47. Radi R, Beckman JS, Bush KM, Freeman BA. Peroxynitrite oxidation of sulfhydryls. The cytotoxic potential of superoxide and nitric oxide. J Biol Chem 1991;266:4244–4250.

48. Ischiropoulos H, Zhu L, Chen J, Tsai M, Martin JC, Smith CD, et al. Peroxynitrite-mediated tyrosine nitration catalyzed by superoxide dismutase. Arch Biochem Biophys 1992;298:431–437.

49. Beckman JS, Koppenol WH. Nitric oxide, superoxide, and peroxynitrite: the good, the bad, and ugly. Am J Physiol 1996;271:C1424–C1437.

50. Xia Y, Zweier JL. Superoxide and peroxynitrite generation from inducible nitric oxide synthase in macrophages. Proc Natl Acad Sci USA 1997;94:6954–6958.

51. Dhalla AK, Singal PK. Antioxidant changes in hypertrophied and failing guinea pig hearts. Am J Physiol 1994;266:H1280–H1285.

52. Hill MF, Singal PK. Right and left myocardial antioxidant responses during heart failure subsequent to myocardial infarction. Circulation 1997;96:2414–2420.

53. Kooy NW, Lewis SJ, Royall JA, Ye YZ, Kelly DR, Beckman JS. Extensive tyrosine nitration in human myocardial inflammation: evidence for the presence of peroxynitrite. Crit Care Med 1997;25:812–819.

54. MacMillan-Crow LA, Crow JP, Kerby JD, Beckman JS, Thompson JA. Nitration and inactivation of manganese superoxide dismutase in chronic rejection of human renal allografts. Proc Natl Acad Sci USA 1996;93:11,853–11,858.

55. Mikami S, Kawashima S, Kanazawa K, Hirata K, Hotta H, Hayashi Y, et al. Low-dose N omega-nitro-L-arginine methyl ester treatment improves survival rate and decreases myocardial injury in a murine model of viral myocarditis induced by coxsackievirus B3. Circ Res 1997;81:504–511.

56. Bachmaier K, Neu N, Pummerer C, Duncan GS, Mak TW, Matsuyama T, et al. iNOS expression and nitrotyrosine formation in the myocardium in response to inflammation is controlled by the interferon regulatory transcription factor 1. Circulation 1997;96:585–591.

19 Shock States and Nitric Oxide

*Hartmut Ruetten
and Christoph Thiemermann*

INTRODUCTION

Septic Shock

GENERAL OVERVIEW OF SEPTIC SHOCK

Septic shock is the life-threatening complication of an overwhelming systemic infection in which the immune system releases inflammatory mediators resulting in pathophysiological vasodilatation, hematological abnormalities, and organ dysfunction and failure. Sepsis affects 300,000–500,000 patients annually in the United States *(1)*. The prevalence of sepsis in hospitalized patients appears to have significantly increased over the past decade. Data from the Center for Disease Control and Prevention's National Hospital Discharge Survey show a 139% increase in the discharge diagnosis of sepsis from 1977–1987 *(2)*. The increase was especially marked for patients over 65 yr of age (162%). Despite improvements in intensive care management of critically ill patients, new antibiotics, and extensive research into the etiology of sepsis, the mortality of septic shock ranges from 20–55% *(3,4)*. Mortality increases to 77–90% when shock occurs *(5,6)*.

Septic shock represents the combined effect of a variety of inflammatory and hormonal systems. A paradox of this disease entity is that the same inflammatory system responsible for defending us against the microbial invasion of tissues may produce shock when it is excessively activated. The initial clinical presentation of sepsis usually consists of fever, tachycardia, peripheral vasodilatation, hypotension, and oliguria. However, the key symptom of shock is a severe fall in blood pressure that is often associated with the dysfunction or failure of several important organs including lung, kidney, liver, and brain. Despite the observed increase in cardiac output, blood pressure is not maintained because of excessive vasodilatation. Treatment includes respiratory support to optimize tissue oxygenation, intravenous fluid administration, broad spectrum antimicrobial therapy, and vasopressor support.

The definition of septic shock is independent of the presence or absence of a multiple organ failure syndrome (MODS), which is defined as impaired organ function such that homeostasis cannot be maintained without intervention *(7)*. Primary MODS is a direct result of a well-defined insult to a specific organ. Secondary MODS occurs as a consequence of an exaggerated host response, termed systemic inflammatory response syndrome (SIRS). The natural history of septic shock is often as follows: about 75% of deaths occur within hours to days after the onset of shock and are caused by therapy-resistant hypotension leading to the conclusion that peripheral vascular failure is the predominant factor that determines outcome *(8)*.

From: *Contemporary Cardiology, vol. 4: Nitric Oxide and the Cardiovascular System*
Edited by: J. Loscalzo and J. A. Vita © Humana Press Inc., Totowa, NJ

The rest of the deaths occur days or weeks after the patient has recovered from hypotension, and the cause of death is multiple organ failure *(9)*. Adult respiratory-distress syndrome (ARDS), followed by renal and hepatic failure is the most common sequence of events.

Septic shock is primarily initiated by components of the cell wall of Gram-positive or Gram-negative bacteria *(10)*, but structural components of many other microorganisms generate a very similar spectrum of biological activities. Among the most studied are the peptidoglycans, a ubiquitous component of all bacterial cell walls, but particularly concentrated in Gram-positive organisms *(11)*. In addition, peptidoglycan and lipoteichoic acid from *Staphylococcus aureus* act in synergy to cause shock and multiple organ failure *(12)*. Trehalose diesters produced by mycobacteria and corynebacteria and other Gram-positive bacterial products including lipomannans also cause lipopolysaccharide (LPS)-like effects *(13,14)*.

The Cytokine Network

Cytokines are a heterogeneous group of hormonelike proteins, produced by all organs and many cell types of the body that establish a communication network between various cells of each organ. Activation of the cytokine network follows a lag phase and is preceded by the activation of, e.g., the complement and kallikrein system. The study and the understanding of the cytokine network is complicated by the facts that (1) cytokines often induce the secretion of additional cytokines, (2) cytokines modulate the effects of other cytokines, resulting in additional, synergistic or inhibitory effects, or even a novel effect not seen with individual cytokines alone, (3) the sequence of cytokine exposure can influence target cell responses, and (4) cytokine effects may be dose-related with qualitatively different biologic effects seen at different doses *(15)*.

The proinflammatory cytokines tumor necrosis factor-α (TNF-α) and interleukin-1β (IL-1β) have been implicated in the pathophysiology of many cardiovascular disorders *(16–18)* including circulatory shock *(19–23)*. Administration of TNF-α alone, or in combination with low doses of endotoxin mimics several features of the pathophysiology of circulatory shock including hypotension and organ injury *(20,21)*. Intravenous administration of IL-1 either alone, or in combination with low doses of LPS or TNF-α, also produces a shocklike state *(19)*. Pronounced rises in the serum levels of TNF-α and IL-1β occur in experimental endotoxemia *(21–25)*. More importantly, enhanced serum concentrations of TNF-α and IL-1β have been documented in human subjects with sepsis and septic shock *(26)*, particularly in the early phase of shock. Moreover, TNF-α and IL-1β are secreted from the most severely affected organs (e.g. lung and liver) in patients with sepsis-related MODS *(27)*. Higher concentrations of TNF-α and IL-1β are associated, not only with an increase in mortality rate, but also with an increased risk for subsequent ARDS and MODS *(28)*. In addition, antibodies directed against TNF-α or IL-1β as well as agents which inhibit the release of TNF-α, such as pentoxyfilline *(29)*, or IL-1β exert protective effects in various animal models of endotoxin shock *(30,31)*. In contrast, clinical trials aimed at demonstrating a reduction in 28-d mortality with such interventions have so far not met with the expected success. For instance, there is no convincing evidence that interventions aimed at reducing the effects of TNF-α (e.g., antibodies against TNF-α, soluble TNF-α receptors, and so on) cause a significant reduction in 28-d mortality in patients with septic shock *(32–35)*. Most notably, there is one recent report documenting that the treatment of septic patients with the TNF receptor: Fc fusion protein causes a dose-related increase in mortality *(36)*. Similarly, clinical trials evaluating the effects of the IL-1 receptor antagonists have not resulted in a significant reduction in 28-d mortality *(37,38)*.

Although the aforementioned trials failed to provide evidence that any of the anticytokine interventions used caused a significant reduction in 28-d mortality, these studies nevertheless support the view that both TNF-α as well as IL-1 play a role in the pathophysiology of septic shock and indicate that anticytokine therapy may well be of benefit for certain groups of patients. The IL-1ra Phase III Sepsis Syndrome Group has recently reported that (1) there is a direct relationship between a patient's predicted risk of mortality at study entry and the efficacy of the IL-1 receptor antagonist (Il-1ra) in that (2) patients with a predicted risk of mortality of <24% derived little benefit, whereas (3) IL-1ra reduced the risk of death in the first 2 d for patients with a predicted risk of mortality of >24% *(38)*. The reasons for the discrepancy in outcome between animal experiments and clinical trials are not entirely clear, but may include (1) relatively late intervention in clinical trials (vs. pretreatment in animal studies), (2) inhomogeneity of patients (e.g. differences in age, gender, causes of shock, severity of disease), or (3) the pharmacology (dose regimen, time of intervention, length of treatment) of the intervention chosen.

One could also argue that the pathophysiology leading to the circulatory failure, organ dysfunction and ultimately death in patients with septic shock is multifactorial and, hence, that interventions aimed at eliminating the detrimental effects of a single mediator ("single-bullet approach to the therapy of shock")—although useful in some acute animal models—are less likely (if not unlikely) to cause a significant reduction in 28-d mortality. Indeed, there is some evidence that the prevention of the formation of both TNF-α and IL-1β (e.g., with interferon-γ or IL-10) is superior to prevention of the formation of either one of these cytokines in reducing mortality in rodent models of endotoxemia *(39)*. Moreover, the reduction in survival afforded by a combination immunotherapy (antibody against TNF-α, J5 antiserum against endotoxin, and a *Pseudomonas* O-serotype-specific opsonophagocytic monoclonal antibody) was greater than the one afforded by any combination of two antibodies or single antibody therapy *(40)*. Recently, we demonstrated in a rat model of endotoxaemia that (1) coadministration of two polyclonal antibodies directed against either TNF-α or IL-1 or (2) neutralization of the effects of either TNF-α or IL-1 with one polyclonal antibody directed against both cytokines is superior in reducing the circulatory failure and MODS caused by endotoxin in the rat than a therapy with a single antibody directed against either cytokine *(41)*. Having stated that some anticytokine therapies have caused an increase in mortality in patients with septic shock *(38)*, it should also be noted that there may be potential hazards of combination immunotherapy. For instance, coadministration of IL-1ra and TNF-binding protein caused an increase in mortality in neutropenic rats with sepsis caused by *Pseudomonas aeruginosa (42)*. Thus, further studies are warranted to gain a better understanding of the beneficial and adverse effects of combination immunotherapy in experimental endotoxemia and sepsis.

Another proinflammatory cytokine, interferon-γ (IFN-γ), is known as a mediator of septic shock. IFN-γ is produced by activated lymphocytes and is a strong potentiator of the effect of TNF-α, IL-1β, or LPS in vitro and in vivo. Moreover, neutralization of IFN-γ in mice prevents LPS-induced lethality *(43)*.

NITRIC OXIDE

General

Nitric oxide (NO•) is one of the smallest, biologically active messenger molecules. It is also a gaseous biological messenger, with a wide range of physiological and pathophysiological actions. The formation of NO• from the guanidino nitrogen group of L-arginine is catalyzed by a group of isoenzymes termed nitric oxide synthases (NOSs) *(44,45)*. Although the three isoforms, endothelial cell NOS (ecNOS or NOS III), brain NOS (bNOS or NOS I), and inducible NOS (iNOS or NOS II), have different molecular weights and variable cofactor requirements, all of them are dependent on nicotinamide adenosine dinucleotide phosphate (NADPH), show similarities with cytochrome P_{450} reductase and also with the bacterial enzymes sulphite reductase and cytochrome P_{450} BM3. The formation of NO• by NOS is linked to incorporation of molecular oxygen into the molecule *(46)*. NOSs, in general, have the following catalytic activities: arginine, N^{ω}-hydroxylase, N^{ω}-hydroxyarginine, monooxygenase, NADPH oxidase, cytochrome c reductase, and dihydropterine reductase. NOS has been proposed to form NO• and L-citrulline in two steps, the first step being the formation of N^{G}-hydroxy-L-arginine, and the second, its three-electron oxidation. Both steps may utilize different heme-based oxidants, i.e., a perferryl species, $[FeO]^{3+}$, for the first step and a peroxoiron species, $[FeOO]^{+}$, for the second step. Both of these are produced when heme reacts with molecular oxygen *(47,48)*. All forms of NOS contain four prosthetic groups; flavin–adenine dinucleotide (FAD), flavin mononucleotide (FMN), tetrahydrobiopterin (BH_4), and a heme complex, iron protoporphyrin IX. They are all dependent on calmodulin; in the inducible isoform calmodulin is already present in a tightly bound form.

All of the NOS isoforms can be inhibited to a variable degree, with N^{G}-substituted L-arginine analogs, e.g., N^{G}-monomethy-L-arginine (L-NMMA). Some NOS inhibitors show some isoform selectivity; e.g., calmodulin-binding agents such as trifluoperazine do not inhibit the calmodulin-independent (iNOS) isoform. For reasons that are not entirely understood, some of the L-arginine analog NOS inhibitors also show limited isoform selectivity: N^{G}-cyclopropyl-L-arginine, N^{G}-nitro-L-arginine, and its methyl ester, L-NAME (after hydrolysis), show some selectivity toward the constitutive NOS, whereas L-NMMA, N^{G}-amino-L-homoarginine and N^{G}-amino-L-arginine are approximately equipotent inhibitors of ecNOS and iNOS activity *(49,50)*. Moreover, prolonged exposure of NOS to L-NMMA results in an irreversible inactivation of the enzyme, and this is preceded by an NADPH-independent hydroxylation of the inhibitor *(51)*.

The inducible isoform of NOS (iNOS) is, under physiological conditions, absent from mammalian cells, but is induced by proinflammatory stimuli, such as bacterial lipopolysaccharide or the cytokines TNF-α, IL-1β, or IFN-γ, as well as their combination. In contrast to ecNOS and bNOS, however, iNOS tightly binds calmodulin to exert its full biological activity. Thus, iNOS is not regulated by intracellular calcium levels and produces a long-lasting generation of large amounts of NO• (in the n*M* range) *(52,53)*. In contrast to ecNOS or bNOS, the availability of extracellular L-arginine can be rate limiting to obtain a maximal generation of NO• by iNOS *(54)*.

Since the discovery in 1990 that an enhanced formation of endogenous NO• contributes to (1) the hypotension caused by endotoxin and TNF-α *(55,56)*, (2) the vascular hyporesponsiveness to vasoconstrictor agents (also termed "vasoplegia") *(57,58)*, and (3) the protection of liver integrity in rodents with sepsis *(59)*, there has been an increasing interest in the role of NO• in the pathophysilogy of animal and humans with septic shock. In addition to endotoxic shock, an enhanced formation of NO• also occurs in other types of shock including Gram-positive, hemorrhagic, traumatic, and anaphylactic shock *(60)*. The overproduction of NO• in animal models of circulatory shock is due to an early activation of ecNOS (which is transient) and the delayed induction of iNOS activity in macrophages (host defense) and vascular smooth muscle cells (hypotension, vascular hyporeactivity, maldistribution of blood flow) *(61)*. The finding that inhibitors of NOS activity (e.g., L-NAME, L-NMMA) attenuate the hypotension and vasoplegia caused by endotoxin in animals *(56,58)*, together with the discovery that mice that are deficient in iNOS (iNOS knockout mice) exhibit only a minor fall in blood pressure when challenged with endotoxin *(62,63)*, support the hypothesis that an overproduction of NO• by iNOS contributes to the circulatory failure in septic shock. It is, however, less clear, whether increased formation of NO• also contributes to the organ injury and dysfunction caused by endotoxin. These data support the view that reducing the enhanced formation of NO• by iNOS may become a useful therapeutic approach in sepsis/septic shock. In principle, there are two approaches to achieve this goal, i.e., inhibition of iNOS induction and/or inhibition of the activity of iNOS, by inhibiting the enzyme itself or one of its cofactors.

Inhibition of the Induction of iNOS

The mechanism of iNOS induction is not fully understood. It clearly involves the transcription of mRNA and novel protein biosynthesis. The sequencing of the DNA regions upstream to the NOS gene (i.e., the promoter region) revealed separate promoter regions for the induction of iNOS by LPS and IFN-γ *(64)*. There is increasing evidence for the involvement of the nuclear transcription factor NF-κB *(65,66)*, tyrosine kinase activation *(67–69)*, microtubule depolimerization, and protein kinase C-epsilon *(70)* in the induction process.

Induction of iNOS can be inhibited by numerous agents including glucocorticoids, thrombin, or ethanol; macrophage deactivation factor and transforming growth factor β (TGF-β), platelet-derived growth factor, endothelin-1, IL-4, IL-8, IL-10, and IL-13 *(53,71–75)*. Inhibitors of protein kinase C (PKC), or of protein tyrosine kinase *(68,69,76)*, or of the activation of NF-κB *(66,77)* can also inhibit the induction of iNOS. An increase in cyclic adenosine monophosphate (cAMP) induces iNOS in vascular smooth muscle cells (VSMCs) and rat renal mesangial cells *(78,79)*, whereas prolonged elevation in intracellular cAMP levels in macrophages inhibits iNOS induction *(80)*. NO• itself can also regulate its activity, both by inhibiting iNOS activity *(81)* and by downregulating iNOS mRNA *(82)*.

INHIBITION OF PROTEIN TYROSINE KINASE

Phosphorylation of proteins on tyrosine residues by protein tyrosine kinases plays an important role in the regulation of cell proliferation, cell differentiation, and signaling processes in cells of the immune system. The receptor tyrosine kinases participate in transmembrane signaling, whereas the intracellular tyrosine kinases take part in the signal transduction to the nucleus. Enhanced activity of tyrosine kinases has been implicated in the pathophysiology of many diseases associated with local (atherosclerosis, psoriasis) or systemic inflammation including sepsis and septic shock *(83)*.

Endotoxin LPS causes the phosphorylation of tyrosine kinases in macrophages (and other target cells) *(84)*, resulting in the release of proinflammatory cytokines including TNF-α, IL-1, and IFN-γ. In human monocytes activated with LPS, inhibition of tyrosine kinase activity with genistein or herbimycin A attenuates the expression of the mRNA's for IL-1, TNF-α, and IL-6 *(85)*. TNF-α and IL-1 also induce the phosphorylation of tyrosine in target cells *(86,87)* and when given to animals mediate many of the effects of LPS (*see* ref. *23*). Inhibition of the activity of tyrosine kinases by tyrphostin AG126 prevents (when given 2 h prior to LPS) the mortality caused by LPS in mice, but is less effective when given together with LPS *(88)*. Tyrphostin AG556, which is more lipophilic than AG126, prevents the mortality caused by endotoxin in mice when given as late as 2 h after injection of endotoxin *(89)*. The mechanism(s) of these beneficial effects of tyrosine kinase inhibitors in shock is largely unknown. We demonstrated that several chemical distinct tyrphostins, i.e., AG126, AG490, AG556, AG1641, or A1 or the isoflavone genistein prevent (1) the circulatory failure (hypotension and vascular hyporeactivity to noradrenaline), (2) the multiple organ dysfunction (liver and pancreatic dysfunction/injury, lactacidosis, hypoglycemia) (Fig. 1), as well as (3) the induction of iNOS protein and activity in rats with endotoxic shock. The mechanism(s) by which the tyrosine kinase inhibitors exert the beneficial effects in shock warrants further investigation, but may involve the prevention of the formation of TNF-α and the expression of iNOS protein *(76)*.

INHIBITION OF THE NUCLEAR TRANSCRIPTION FACTOR NF-κB

The expression of inducible genes in eukaryocytes is largely controlled by proteins, such as NF-κB, which activate transcription *(90,91)*. NF-κB is itself activated by the exposure of cells to endotoxin or TNF-α, IL-1, IL-2, or phorbol 12-myristate 13-acetate (PMA) *(92–95)*. NF-κB is a family of dimers, all of which are composed of members of the Rel/NF-κB family

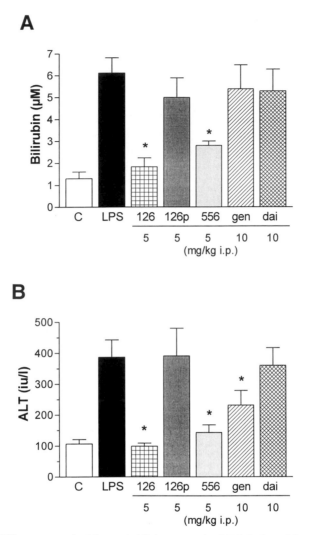

Fig. 1. Effect of different tyrosin kinase inhibitors on the LPS-induced increases in the serum concentrations of (**A**) bilirubin, and (**B**) ALT (indicator of liver injury) at 6 h after the injection of *E. coli* lipopolysaccharide (LPS; 10 mg/kg iv). Different groups of rats received (1) vehicle (50% DMSO/PBS, 1 ml/kg ip) rather than LPS (C, $n = 4$), (2) vehicle (50% DMSO/PBS, 1 ml/kg ip) plus LPS (LPS; $n = 6$), (3) LPS plus tyrphostin AG126 (126; $n = 6$), (4) LPS plus delayed administration of tyrphostin AG126 (126p; $n = 4$), (5) LPS plus tyrphostin AG556 (556; $n = 6$), (6) LPS plus genistein (gen; $n = 6$), or (7) LPS plus daidzein (dai; $n = 5$). Data are expressed as mean ± SEM of n observations. *$p < 0.05$ represents significant difference when compared to LPS controls.

of polypeptides. The most frequent form of NF-κB is a dimer composed of two DNA-binding proteins, i.e., NF-κB1 (or p50) and RelA (or p65), although other dimeric combinations also exist *(96)*. Under physiological conditions, NF-κB is held (in an inactive form) in the cytoplasm by the inhibitory protein IκB-α, which avidly binds to most heterodimers including the NF-κB1/Rel A heterodimer. This inhibitory subunit can be considered to be a cytoplasmatic anchor, as it prevents the nuclear uptake of NF-κB. Activation of NF-κB involves the release of the inhibitory subunit IκB-α from a cytoplasmic complex, which IκB forms together with the DNA-binding subunit RelA and NF-κB1 *(97,98)*. Activation of NF-κB allows NF-κB to translocate to the nucleus and to induce the expression of specific genes. The cascade of events

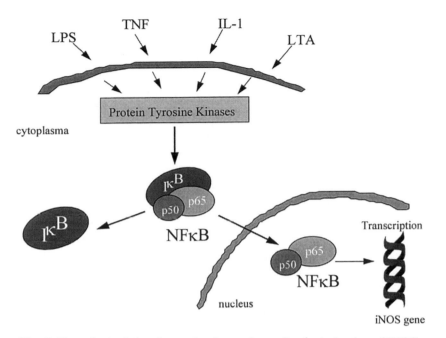

Fig. 2. Hypothetical signal transduction pathway for the induction of iNOS.

leading to the activation of NF-κB involves the signal-induced phosphorylation of IκB-α, resulting in its proteolytic degradation and the release of NF-κB from its cytoplasmatic anchor. NF-κB then translocates into the nucleus, where it binds to different gene promotors and, hence, induces a large number of genes *(99,100)*. The proteolytic degradation of IκB-α is inhibited by the cysteine protease inhibitor calpain inhibitor I, but not by other inhibitors of serine and cysteine proteases, such as chymostatin or leupeptin *(101)*.

There is evidence that the expression of the gene for iNOS involves the activation of NF-κB (Fig. 2), and the expression of iNOS in vitro caused by LPS or lipoteichoic acid is prevented by several agents that interfere with the activation of NF-κB, such as the radical scavanger rotenone, butylated hydroxyanisole, and pyrroidine dithiocarbamate (PDTC) *(66,77)*. More-over, aspirin, sodium salicylate, and N-acetylcysteine attenuate the activation of NF-κB by a mechanism that involves antioxidant effects of these agents. Interestingly, IL-10 (which has been reported to improve survival in animal models of endotoxin shock) also prevents the activation of NF-κB *(102)*. Recently, we demonstrated that inhibition of the activation of NF-κB in vivo by calpain inhibitor I and dexamethasone, but not the serine and cysteine protease inhibitor chymostatin, attenuate (1) the circulatory failure (hypotension and vascular hyporeactivity to noradrenaline), (2) the multiple organ dysfunction (liver and pancreatic injury/dysfunction, increase in lactate, hypoglycemia), and (3) the induction of iNOS protein and activity (in lung and liver) of rats with endotoxic shock (Figs. 3 and 4). We proposed that the reduction of the expression of iNOS contributes to the beneficial effects of calpain inhibitor I. These results support the view that attenuation or prevention of the activation of NF-κB with calpain inhibitor I may be useful in the therapy of circulatory shock or of disorders associated with local or systemic inflammation *(103)*.

It should be noted that the molecular mechanism by which dexamethasone, an agent that is well known to inhibit the endotoxin-mediated induction of iNOS in vitro and in vivo *(104)*, exerts beneficial effects in endotoxin shock, is not well understood, but there is recent evidence that glucocorticoids inhibit the action of the transcription factors AP-1 and NF-κB *(102)*. Interestingly, there is recent evidence that there is a protein–protein interaction between the

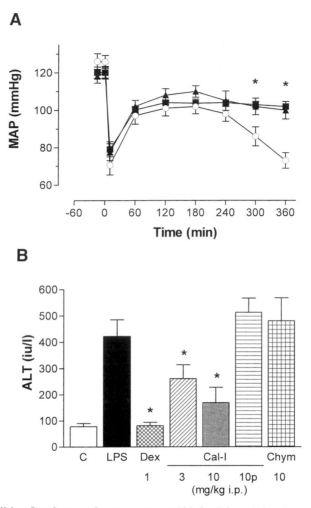

Fig. 3. Calpain inhibitor I or dexamethasone prevent (**A**) the delayed circulatory failure (fall in mean arterial blood pressure; MAP) and (**B**) liver failure (increase in alanine aminotransferase; ALT) in rats with septic shock. Different groups of animals received vehicle for *E. coli* lipopolysaccharide (LPS) (C, $n = 4$), LPS alone (LPS, 10 mg/kg iv, $n =10$, open circles), LPS plus 1 mg/kg ip dexamethasone (Dex, $n = 6$; filled squares), LPS plus 3 mg/kg ip of calpain inhibitor I (Cal-I, 3; $n = 6$), LPS plus 10 mg/kg ip of calpain inhibitor I (Cal-I, 10; $n = 7$, filled triangles), LPS plus late administration at 2 h after LPS of 10 mg/kg ip of calpain inhibitor I (Cal-I, 10p; $n = 4$) or LPS plus chymostatin (Chym; $n = 5$). Data are expressed as mean ± SEM of n observations. *$p < 0.05$ represents significant difference when compared to LPS controls.

activated glucocorticoid receptor and NF-κB, resulting in prevention of its binding to the κB consensus motif on the promotor of its target genes. In addition, glucocorticoids enhance the formation of IκBα, which results in an excess of this inhibitory factor in the nucleus and cytosol. Thus, activated NF-κB when "travelling" to the nucleus meets with and binds to IκB to form its "dormant" (inactive) cytosolic form (for a detailed review, *see* ref. *102*).

Although there is good evidence that TNF-α (and other proinflammatory cytokines) cause the activation and translocation of NF-κB into the nucleus, there is also evidence that (1) tyrosine phosphorylation itself plays an important role in the activation of NF-κB and that (2) tyrosine kinase inhibitors diminish the activation of NF-κB. For instance, higher concentrations of genistein (100 μ*M*) attenuate the translocation of NF-κB in rat pancreatic beta cells activated with IL-1 *(105)*. Herbimycin A also suppresses the activation of NF-κB and the

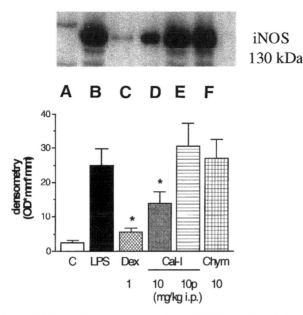

Fig. 4. Effect of calpain inhibitor I on the expression of iNOS protein in lung homogenates at 6 h after administration of endotoxin. Different groups of animals received vehicle (C) for *E. coli* lipopolysaccharide (LPS; lane A), LPS alone (LPS; lane B), LPS plus 1 mg/kg ip dexamethasone (Dex; lane C), LPS plus 10 mg/kg ip of calpain inhibitor I (Cal-I; lane D), LPS plus late administration at 2 h after LPS of 10 mg/kg ip of calpain inhibitor I (Cal-I; lane E) or LPS plus chymostatin (Chym; lane F). Similar results of the Western blots were seen using tissue extracts from two other animals with the same treatment. *$p < 0.05$ represents significant difference when compared to LPS controls.

phosphorylation of Janus kinase 2 (JAK2) caused by LPS and interferon-γ in C6 glial cells, respectively *(106)*. Herbimycin A also reduces the activation of NF-κB caused by IL-1 and phorbol 12-myristate 13-acetate (PMA) in thymoma cells or by PMA in Jurkat T cells. However, the inhibition of the activation of NF-κB by herbimycin A is secondary to a modification of the p50 subunit on cysteine 62 in the NF-κB complex, but is independent of the inhibition of tyrosine kinase activity *(107)*. The expression of matrix metalloproteinase-9 (MMP-9) caused by IL-1 in glomerular mesangial cells is also (at least in part) attributable to tyrosine kinase-mediated activation of NF-κB *(108)*. The prevention by genistein and herbimycin A of the expression of COX-2 in rat mesangial cells is not caused by inhibition of the activation of NF-κB, suggesting that an upstream tyrosine kinase pathway may not be required for the IL-1-induced activation of NF-κB in these cells *(109)*. Most notably, stimulation of Jurkat T cells with the protein tyrosine phosphatase inhibitor and T-cell activator pervanadate leads to activation of NF-κB resulting from tyrosine phosphorylation, but not degradation of I-κBα. It has therefore been suggested *(110)* that the tyrosine phosphorylation of I-κBα represents a proteolysis-independent mechanism of NF-κB activation that directly couples NF-κB to cellular tyrosine kinase. Thus, it is possible that the tyrosine kinase inhibitors prevent the activation of NF-κB either by an indirect (e.g., prevention of the formation of TNF-α) or by a direct effect. Suppression of the activation of NF-κB by tyrosine kinase inhibitors may well result in a reduced expression of enzymes (e.g., iNOS, COX-2, cPLA$_2$, and so forth), cytokines (TNF-α, IL-1β, IL-6, and so on), chemokines (IL-8, RANTES, and the like) or adhesion molecules (ICAM-1, VCAM-1, E-selectin) known to play an important role in the pathophysiology of endotoxin shock *(111)*.

It should be stressed, however, that all of the foregoing therapeutics must be administered prior to the application of endotoxin or at least prior to the induction of iNOS (e.g., approx

Table 1
Possible Effects of Administration of NOS Inhibitors in Septic Shock

Beneficial	Adverse
Increased blood pressure	Excessive vasoconstriction
Restores responsiveness to pressor agents	Pulmonary hypertension
Cardiac output return to baseline values	Fall in cardiac output
Decreased production of peroxynitrite	Increased platelet adhesiveness
Attenuation of inhibition of mitochondrial respiration	Increased neutrophil adhesion
Improved organ function	Worsened organ function
Improved survival	Reduction in survival

2 h after endotoxin) to prevent the severe delayed circulatory failure, the MODS as well as the induction of iNOS caused by endotoxin in animal models of SIRS. For example, the administration of dexamethasone, calpain inhibitor I, or tyrosine kinase inhibitors to rats 2 h after the injection of endotoxin neither exerts beneficial effects on hemodynamic or organ injury nor inhibits the induction of iNOS *(76,103,112,113)*. As for the cytokine antibodies, the timely administration of inhibitors of the induction of iNOS will be crucial to achieve beneficial effects in patients with severe sepsis. Practically, one needs to determine the time between the induction of iNOS (or early phases of the syndrome) and the administration of the inhibitors of iNOS induction. This supports the view that drugs that directly inhibit iNOS activity are useful tools, whereas the use of agents that inhibit the induction of iNOS may be less useful.

Inhibition of NOS Activity

Since the discovery in 1990 that an enhanced formation of endogenous NO• resulting from the induction of iNOS contributes to the hypotension caused by endotoxin and TNF-α *(56)* and vascular hyporesponsiveness to vasoconstrictor agents (vasoplegia) *(57)* and the finding that inhibitors of NOS activity attenuate the hypotension and vasoplegia in endotoxemia, together with the discovery that mice, in which the iNOS gene has been inactivated by gene-targeting (iNOS knockout mice), exhibit only a minor fall in blood pressure when challenged with endotoxin *(62,63)* support the hypothesis that an overproduction of NO• by iNOS contributes to the circulatory failure in septic shock. It is, however, less clear whether increased formation of NO• caused by the induction of iNOS may cause cellular damage in a paracrine or autocrine fashion *(114,115)*, and, hence, also contributes to the organ injury and dysfunction caused by endotoxin in septic shock. It is noteworthy that the formation of NO• by eNOS and potentially also by iNOS also exerts beneficial effects in shock including vasodilatation, prevention of platelet and leukocyte adhesion, maintenance of microcirculatory blood flow, and augmentation of host defense. Thus, it is not surprising that basic and clinical scientists have advocated the use of contrasting therapeutic approaches including inhibition of NOS activity, enhancement of the availability of NO• (NO• donors, NO• inhalation) or a combination of both approaches (for review *see* refs. *60,61,* and *116*). The following paragraphs highlight some of the effects and side effects of inhibitors of NOS activity (Table 1) in animal models of septic shock.

INHIBITION OF NOS ACTIVITY IN ANIMAL MODELS OF SHOCK: EFFECTS AND SIDE EFFECTS

Although there is good evidence that endotoxemia or sepsis in rodents results in the induction of iNOS (in various tissues) leading to an increase in the plasma levels of nitrite/nitrate (from 20 up to 600 μM) *(149)*, there is limited information regarding the time-course of iNOS induction, the degree of iNOS activity (in tissues) or even the plasma levels of nitrite/nitrate in large animal models (pig, dog, sheep, baboon) of shock or in humans with sepsis and septic shock. Clearly, sepsis (or endotoxemia) results in an increase in the plasma levels of nitrite/nitrate in these species. Thus, when evaluating the role of NO• or elucidating the effects of NOS inhibitors in animal models of shock, one needs to consider that (1) many of the models used are acute, nonresuscitated, hypodynamic models of shock, (2) the effects (and side effects) of nonselective inhibitors of NOS activity will greatly vary depending on the degree of iNOS induction in the species, and (3) any observed effects of the respective NOS inhibitor used will obviously depend on the chosen dose regimen and timing of the intervention.

The N-substituted L-arginine analog L-NMMA was the first agent reported to inhibit NOS activity. Following the discovery in 1990 that L-NMMA exerts beneficial hemodynamic effects in animal models of endotoxemia (55,56), many subsequent studies aimed at elucidating the role of NO• in septic shock have used the NOS inhibitor L-NAME rather than L-NMMA, as L-NAME is cheap and readily available. In contrast to L-NMMA, L-NAME is a relatively selective inhibitor of eNOS rather than iNOS activity (117). Hence, higher doses of this agent may cause excessive vasoconstriction (particularly in the pulmonary, renal, and myocardial vascular bed) and enhance the incidence of both microvascular thrombosis and neutrophil adhesion in the endothelium. Thus, L-NAME reduces oxygen delivery and exacerbates organ injury in (many, but not all) animal models of endotoxic shock (136). These results are not necessarily solely due to the use of very large amounts of L-NAME, but rather a reflection of the fact that L-NAME is a more selective inhibitor of eNOS than iNOS activity. In rats with endotoxemia, infusion of very low doses of L-NAME (e.g., 0.03–0.3 mg/kg/h) results in a dose-related increase in blood pressure (because of inhibition of eNOS activity) without reducing the rise in the plasma levels of nitrite/nitrate (an indicator of NOS activity) or the organ injury caused by endotoxin (118) (Fig. 5). However, it should be noted that in the kidney, eNOS may have protective (antithrombotic) actions in some models of LPS-induced renal damage (146). Indeed, infusion of very low doses (30–50 μg/kg/min) of L-NAME cause (1) a reduction in renal cortical blood flow without causing an increase in blood pressure in the rat (119), and (2) a significant increase in pulmonary vascular resistance caused by endotoxin in the pig (120). Although L-NAME may be suitable to inhibit the generation of NO• by all three isoforms of NOS, this agent should not be used as a therapeutic intervention in such diseases as septic shock, where an overproduction of NO• by iNOS has been implicated as an underlying cause of the pathology.

In contrast to L-NAME, L-NMMA is an endogenous substance present in the urine of both animals and humans. Although L-NMMA inhibits all isoforms of NOS to a variable degree, it is a more potent inhibitor of iNOS than eNOS activity. L-NMMA is a competitive inhibitor of the binding of L-arginine to NOS and, hence, excess of L-arginine reverses the inhibition of NOS activity by L-NMMA. The effects of L-NMMA in models of shock vary from "very beneficial" to "moderately beneficial with some adverse effects" to "detrimental" (often caused by marked inhibition of eNOS activity) (117,136). Clearly, the observed results depend on the dose of L-NMMA as well as the model of shock used. When given after the onset of hypotension, infusions of relatively low doses of L-NMMA (3–10 mg/kg/h) have been convincingly demonstrated to exert beneficial hemodynamic effects in rodents, sheep, dogs, and baboon models of endotoxemia and sepsis. For instance, in conscious baboons, administration of live *Escherichia coli* bacteria resulted in a significant increase in the serum levels of biopterin, neopterin, and nitrate, suggesting an induction of guanosine triphosphate (GTP) cyclohydrolase I and iNOS. In this model, infusion of L-NMMA (5 mg/kg/h) attenuated the rise in the serum levels of nitrate and creatinine, the hypotension and fall in peripheral vascular resistance and the substantial 7-d mortality caused by severe sepsis in this species (Daryl Rees and Heinz Redl, personal communication). These findings clearly document that the circulatory failure caused by septic shock in baboons is largely mediated by an enhanced formation of NO• by iNOS and that inhibition of iNOS with L-NMMA improves outcome in this model.

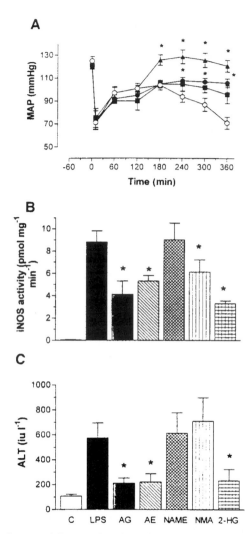

Fig. 5. (A) Effect of aminoguanidine (AG, $n = 8$; filled squares), or aminoethyl-isothiurea (AE, $n = 8$; filled circles) or N^{ω}-nitro-L-arginine methyl ester (L-NAME, $n = 6$; filled triangles) on the fall in mean arterial blood pressure (MAP) caused by *E. coli* lipopolysaccharide (LPS; 10 mg/kg iv) in the anesthetized rat. The alterations in MAP (over time) of rats that were pretreated with vehicle (for the drugs) and then received LPS are also shown (LPS control, $n = 10$; open circles). **(B)** Effect of different NOS inhibitors on the increase in iNOS activity and **(C)** the serum concentration of alanine aminotransferase (ALT) in rats with septic shock. Different groups of LPS rats were infused for 4 h with vehicle ($n = 10$), AG ($n = 8$), AE ($n = 8$), N^{ω}-nitro-L-arginine methyl ester (NAME, $n = 6$), N^{G}-methyl-L-arginine (NMA, $n = 6$) or 1-amino-2-hydroxy-guanidine (2-HG, $n = 10$). The infusion of drug or vehicle was started at 2 h after LPS. Data are expressed as mean ± SEM of n observations. $*p < 0.05$ represents a significant reduction in concentration/activity when compared to LPS rats.

The observed beneficial effects of L-NMMA in animal models of septic shock stimulated the search for selective inhibitors of iNOS activity. In the last years, several compounds including aminoguanidine, certain isothiurea derivates (e.g., aminoethyl-isothiurea), acetamidines (e.g., 1400W) and amino acid analogs (L-NIL). Aminoguanidine was the first relatively selective inhibitor of iNOS activity discovered *(121)*. Although aminoguanidine is a more potent inhibitor of iNOS than of eNOS activity in vitro and in vivo, aminoguanidine is not a very potent inhibitor of iNOS activity. Aminoguanidine attenuates the delayed hypotension in rats *(122)* and rabbits *(123)* with endotoxin shock and improves survival in mice challenged with endotoxin *(122)*. Aminoguanidine and its analog 1-hydroxy-2-guanidine also attenuate the liver injury and hepatocellular dysfunction caused by endotoxin in the rat *(122,124)* (Fig. 5). In rats with endotoxic shock, aminoguanidine also reduces the increase in pulmonary transvascular flux *(125)*. The interpretation of the mechanism(s) by which aminoguanidine exert these beneficial effects is difficult, as aminoguanidine is not a specific inhibitor of iNOS activity but has many other pharmacological properties including inhibition of (1) histamine metabolism, (2) polyamine catabolism, (3) the formation of advanced glycosylation end products, and (4) catalase activity (as well as other copper- or iron-containing enzymes) *(126–129)*. Interestingly, aminoguanidine also prevents the expression of iNOS protein by a hitherto-unknown mechanism *(130)*. Thus, aminoguanidine has to be regarded as an agent that (1) is a relatively selective, but not very potent inhibitor of iNOS activity, (2) reduces the formation of NO• by two distinct mechanisms, i.e., prevention of the expression of iNOS protein and inhibition of iNOS activity, and (3) exerts many other effects, which appear to be unrelated to the inhibition of iNOS activity (nonspecific effects).

S-substituted isothioureas (ITUs) are non-amino acid analogs of L-arginine and also potent inhibitors of iNOS activity with variable isoform selectivity *(131–133)*. For instance, *S*-ethyl-ITU is a potent competitive inhibitor of all isoforms of human NOS, whereas *S*-aminoethyl-ITU and *S*-methyl-ITU are more selective inhibitors of iNOS than of eNOS activity *(132)*. In 1994, we demonstrated that *S*-methyl-ITU reverses the circulatory failure caused by endotoxin in the rat. The beneficial hemodynamic effect of *S*-methyl-ITU was associated with an attenuation of the liver injury and hepatocellular dysfunction caused by endotoxin in rats as well as an increase in the survival rate of mice challenged with high dose of endotoxin *(131)*. Similarly, administration of aminoethyl-ITU (1 mg/kg/h commencing 2 h after injection of endotoxin) results in beneficial hemodynamic effects and attenuates the degree of liver injury/dysfunction caused by endotoxin in the rat *(134)* (Fig. 5). In pigs with endotoxemia, injection of aminoethyl-ITU (10 mg/kg iv at 3 h after endotoxin) restores hepatic arterial blood flow (from reduced to normal levels) and increases hepatic oxygen consumption, without affecting cardiac output *(135)*. Some of the beneficial effects of aminoguanidine in shock may not be due to its ability to inhibit iNOS activity. For instance, aminoethyl-ITU is a scavenger of peroxynitrite and exerts beneficial effects on models of disease/pathology known to be mediated by oxygen-derived free radicals *(136)*. Interestingly, dimethyl-ITU (which does not inhibit iNOS activity) is a weak radical scavenger that inhibits the activation of the transcription factor NF-κB. In rats challenged with either endotoxin or live *Salmonella typhimurium*, dimethyl-ITU attenuates the formation of TNF-α and improves survival *(137)*. It is conceivable that other S-substituted isothioureas will also prevent the activation of NF-κB. This property may well explain why aminoethyl-ITU prevents the expression of iNOS protein caused by endotoxin in cultured macrophages and in the rat in vivo *(130)*.

Recently, an analog of acetamidine termed 1400W [*N*-(3-(aminomethyl)benzyl) acetamidine], has been reported to be an approx 5000-fold more potent inhibitor of iNOS activity than eNOS activity (human). The inhibition by 1400W of the activity of human iNOS is potent (K_d value approx 7 nM), dependent on the cofactor NADPH and either irreversible or extremely slowly reversible. In a rat model of vascular injury caused by endotoxin, 1400W is 50-fold more potent as an inhibitor of iNOS than eNOS activity and attenuates the vascular leak syndrome *(138)*. Surprisingly, in a rat model of severe sepsis, 1400W has been demonstrated to prevent the delayed circulatory failure, but not the liver injury/dysfunction caused by endotoxin. This finding supports the view that selective inhibition of iNOS activity might a useful approach in the restoration of blood pressure in patients with septic shock. Most notably, however, these data are consistent with the notion that—as in the case of iNOS knockout mice challenged with endotoxin *(62)*—enhanced formation of NO• by iNOS primarily contributes to the circulatory failure, but not to the liver injury/dysfunction caused by endotoxin.

Inhibition of NOS Activity
in Humans with Septic Shock

Although our understanding of the role of NO• in animal models of circulatory shock has improved substantially over the past years, our knowledge regarding the biosynthesis and importance of NO• in the pathophysiology of patients with SIRS or septic shock is still very limited. There is evidence that endotoxin and cytokines (when given in combination) cause the expression of iNOS as well as the formation of NO• (nitrite/nitrate) in various human cells (primary or cell lines) including hepatocytes, mesangial cells, retinal pigmented epithelial cells, and lung epithelial cells *(139,140)*. Elevated plasma levels and urine levels of nitrite/ nitrate have been reported in adults and children with severe sepsis as well as in patients with burns who subsequently developed sepsis *(147,148)*. Moreover, elevated plasma levels of nitrite/ nitrate occur in patients receiving IL-2 chemotherapy *(140)*. Interestingly, the increase in iNOS activity in leukocytes obtained from patients with sepsis appear to correlate with the number of failing organs, but not with blood pressure. Taken together, these studies support the view that severe sepsis/septic shock in humans is associated with an enhanced formation of NO•. However, it appears that the rise in the plasma levels of nitrite/nitrate in vivo in humans with septic shock is much smaller than in rodents (10-fold). Moreover, our understanding of (1) the biosynthesis of NO•, (2) the regulation of and the mechanism involved in the expression of iNOS, and (3) the role of NO• in MODS in shock are largely based on animal experiments of septic shock in rodents. In contrast, relatively little is known about the role of NO• in patients with septic and other forms of circulatory shock.

Early reports of beneficial hemodynamic effects of L-NMMA in humans with septic shock *(141–144)* stimulated a phase I, multicenter, open-label, dose-escalation (1, 2.5, 5, 10, or 20 mg/kg/h for up to 8 h) study using L-NMMA (546C88) in 32 patients with septic shock. In that study, L-NMMA sustained blood pressure and enabled a reduction in vasopressor (norepinephrine) support. The cardiac index fell to baseline values (possible due to an increase in peripheral vascular resistance) and left ventricular function was well maintained. Moreover, L-NMMA increased oxygen extraction, whereas pulmonary shunt was not worsened *(145)*. A recent, placebo-controlled multicenter study involving 312 patients with septic shock has evaluated the effects of L-NMMA on the resolution of shock at 72 h (primary endpoint) *(150)*. The severity of illness according to the SAPS II score was similar between placebo and the L-NMMA group. Infusion of L-NMMA enhanced mean arterial blood pressure and systemic vascular resistance index and decreased cardiac output (from elevated toward normal levels). L-NMMA had no effect on left ventricular systolic work index, indicating that the fall in cardiac output was not caused by an impairment in cardiac contractility. In patients treated with L-NMMA, there was a transient increase in mean pulmonary artery pressure. Interestingly, L-NMMA did not affects the thrombocytopenia or renal dysfunction caused by sepsis. Most notably, 41% of patients treated with L-NMMA, but only 21% of patients treated with placebo, recovered from shock within 72 h. There was a strong trend for a reduction in mortality (at d 14) in patients treated with L-NMMA.

In 1997, Glaxo Wellcome started a phase III clinical trial evaluating the effect of 546C88 (targinine, L-NMMA) in patients with septic shock. That trial was stopped by the company (after an interim analysis) in spring 1998, because of *"concerns about a higher mortality in the treated group than in the placebo group."* The trial, which involved 177 centers from 26 countries, started in June 1997 and had enrolled 797 patients at the time of suspension. The interim analysis included data from 522 patients, 309 of whom had received 546C88. The data and safety-monitoring committee reported a trend toward increased mortality in the active treatment group and thus recommended stopping the trial because of patient safety concerns. The trial will not be resumed, and it is unlikely that development of the drug will continue (SCRIP, 1998; No. 2330, p. 21).

CONCLUDING REMARKS

Since 1990, numerous studies have documented an enhanced formation of NO• in various animal models of endotoxin and septic shock. Similarly, patients with septic shock exhibit elevated plasma levels of nitrite/nitrate. Although the enhanced formation of NO• in animals and humans with septic shock contributes to hypotension and hyporeactivity of the vasculature to vasoconstrictor agents (vasoplegia), it is still unclear whether NO• (from iNOS) contributes to the organ dysfunction/failure syndrome associated with severe septic shock. The finding that the highly selective inhibitor of iNOS activity, 1400W, attenuates the delayed hypotension, but does not affect the multiple organ dysfunction caused by endotoxin in the rat, supports the view that an enhanced formation of NO• within the vasculature contributes to the circulatory failure, but does not directly contribute to the development of organ injury. This notion is supported by the finding that iNOS knockout mice elicit less hypotension but do develop liver injury when challenged with endotoxin.

Although there is evidence that human cells/tissue can, in principle, induce iNOS protein and activity (when challenged with endotoxin and cytokines), the degree of iNOS activity in patients with septic shock appears to be substantially lower than in some animal species (e.g., rodents). The finding that inhibition of NOS activity with L-NMMA in patients with septic shock exerted beneficial hemodynamic effects but did not affect, or even tended to increase, mortality rate is somewhat not surprising, as L-NMMA is only a moderately selective inhibitor of iNOS activity. Whether highly selective inhibitors of iNOS activity do not only exert beneficial hemodynamic effects but also decrease mortality rate in patients with septic shock deserves further investigations.

There is increasing evidence—derived primarily from in vitro studies—that the activation of the transcription factor NF-κB plays a pivotal role in local or systemic inflammation. The finding that inhibition of the activation of NF-κB by calpain inhibitor I attenuates the circulatory failure and the multiple organ dysfunction syndrome caused by endotoxin in the rat may represent a novel approach for the therapy of circulatory shock.

REFERENCES

1. Parrillo JE. Septic shock in humans: clinical evaluation, pathogenesis, and therapeutic approach. In: Shoemaker W, Ayres S, Grenuik A, Holbrook P, Thompson W, ed. Textbook of Critical Care, 2nd ed. Saunders, Philadelphia, 1989, p. 1006.
2. Morbidity and Mortality Weekly Report. Increase in national hospital discharge survey rates for septicemia—United States. 1979–1987. MMWR 1988;89:31–34.
3. Dunn D. Immunotherapeutic advances in the treatment of gram-negative sepsis. World J Surg 1987; 11:233–240.
4. Young L. Gram negative sepsis. In: Mandell GL, et al., eds. Principles and Practice of Infectious Disease. Churchill Livingston, New York, 1990, pp. 611–636.
5. Parker M, Parrillo JE. Septic shock: hemodynamics and pathogenesis. JAMA 1983;250:3324–3327.
6. Sprung CL, Caralis PV, Marcial EH, Pierce M, Gelbard MA, Long WM, et al. The effects of high-dose corticosteroids in patients with septic shock. A prospective, controlled study. N Engl J Med 1984;311: 1137–1143.
7. Baue AE. The multiple organ or system failure syndrome. In: Schlag G, Redl H, eds. Pathophysiology of Shock, Sepsis, and Organ Failure. Springer Verlag, Berlin, 1993, pp. 1004–1018.
8. Groeneveld AB, Nauta JJ, Thijs LG. Peripheral vascular resistance in septic shock: its relation to outcome. Intensive Care Med 1988;14:141–147.
9. Dal Nogare AR. Southwestern internal medicine conference: septic shock. Am J Med Sci 1991;302: 50–65.
10. Rietschel ET, Brade H. Bacterial endotoxins. Sci Am 1992;267:54–61.
11. Springer TA. Adhesion receptors of the immune system. Nature 1990;346:425–434.
12. De Kimpe SJ, Kengatharan M, Thiemermann C, Vane JR. The cell wall components peptidoglycan and lipoteichoic acid from Staphylococcus aureus act in synergy to cause shock and multiple organ failure. Proc Natl Acad Sci USA 1995;92:10,359–10,363.

13. Wicken AJ, Knox KW. Bacterial cell surface amphiphiles. Biochim Biophys Acta 1980;604:1–26.

14. Barnes PF, Chatterjee D, Abrams JS, Lu S, Wang E, Yamamura M, et al. Cytokine production induced by Mycobacterium tuberculosis lipoarabinomannan. Relationship to chemical structure. J Immunol 1992;149:541–547.

15. Deitsch EA. Multiple organ failure: pathophysiology and potential future therapy. Ann Surg 1992;216: 117–134.

16. Latini R, Bianchi M, Correale E, Dinarello CA, Fantuzzi G, Fresco C, et al. Cytokines in acute myocardial infarction: selective increase in circulating tumor necrosis factor, its soluble receptor, and interleukin-1 receptor antagonist. J Cardiovasc Pharmacol 1994;23:1–6.

17. McKenna RM, Macdonald C, Bernstein KN, Rush DN. Increased production of tumor necrosis factor activity by hemodialysis but not peritoneal dialysis patients. Nephron 1994;67:190–196.

18. Testa M, Yeh M, Lee P, Fanelli R, Loperfido F, Berman JW, et al. Circulating levels of cytokines and their endogenous modulators in patients with mild to severe congestive heart failure due to coronary artery disease or hypertension. J Am Coll Cardiol 1996;28:964–971.

19. Okusawa S, Gelfand JA, Ikejima T, Connolly RJ, Dinarello CA. Interleukin 1 induces a shock-like state in rabbits. Synergism with tumor necrosis factor and the effect of cyclooxygenase inhibition. J Clin Invest 1988;81:1162–1172.

20. Tracey KJ. Tumor necrosis factor (cachectin) in the biology of septic shock syndrome. Circ Shock 1991;35:123–128.

21. Billiau A, Vandekerckhove F. Cytokines and their interactions with other inflammatory mediators in the pathogenesis of sepsis and septic shock. Eur J Clin Invest 1991;21:559–573.

22. Mozes T, Ben-Efraim S, Tak CJ, Heiligers JP, Saxene PR, Bonta IL. Serum levels of tumor necrosis factor determine the fatal or non-fatal course of endotoxic shock. Immunol Lett 1991;27:157–162.

23. Dinarello CA. Cytokines as mediators in the pathogenesis of septic shock. Curr Top Micobiol Immunol 1996;216:133–165.

24. Beutler B, Milsark IW, Cerami AC. Passive immunization against cachectin/tumor necrosis factor protects mice from lethal effect of endotoxin. Science 1985;229:869–871.

25. Fletcher DS, Agarwal L, Chapman KT. A synthetic inhibitor of interleukin-1 beta converting enzyme prevents endotoxin-induced interleukin-1 beta production in vitro and in vivo. J Interferon Cytokine Res 1995;15:243–248.

26. Stuber F, Petersen M, Bokelmann F, Schade UA. Genomic polymorphism within the tumor necrosis factor locus influences plasma tumor necrosis factor-alpha concentrations and outcome of patients with severe sepsis. Crit Care Med 1996;24:381–384.

27. Douzinas EE, Tsidemiadou PD, Pitaridis MT, Andrianakis I, Bobota-Chloraki A, Katsouyanni K, et al. The regional production of cytokines and lactate in sepsis-related multiple organ failure. Am J Respir Crit Care Med 1997;155:53–59.

28. Roumen RM, Hendriks T, van der Ven-Jongekrijg J, Nieuwenhuijzen GA, Sauerwein RW, van der Meer JW, et al. Cytokine patterns in patients after major vascular surgery, hemorrhagic shock, and severe blunt trauma. Relation with subsequent adult respiratory distress syndrome and multiple organ failure. Ann Surg 1993;218:769–776.

29. Schade UF. Pentoxifylline increases survival in murine endotoxin shock and decreases formation of tumor necrosis factor. Circ Shock 1990;31:171–181.

30. Tracey KJ, Fong Y, Hesse DG, Manogue KR, Lee AT, Kuo GC, et al. Anti-cachectin/TNF monoclonal antibodies prevent septic shock during lethal bacteraemia. Nature 1987;330:662–664.

31. Wakabayashi G, Gelfand JA, Burke JF, Thompson RC, Dinarello CA. A specific receptor antagonist for interleukin 1 prevents Escherichia coli-induced shock in rabbits. FASEB J 1991;5:338–343.

32. Abraham E, Wunderink R, Silverman H, Perl TM, Nasraway S, Levy H, et al. Efficacy and safety of monoclonal antibody to human tumor necrosis factor-alpha in patients with sepsis syndrome. A randomized, controlled, double-blind, multicenter trial. TNF-alpha Mab Sepsis Study Group. JAMA 1995;273:934–941.

33. Dhainaut JF, Vincent JL, Richard C, Lejeune P, Martin C, Fierobe L, et al. CDP571, a humanized antibody to tumor necrosis factor-alpha safety, pharmacokinetics, immune response, and influence of the antibody on cytokine concentrations in patients with septic shock. CPD571 Sepsis Study Group. Crit Care Med 1995;23:1461–1469.

34. Cohen J, Carlet J. INTERSEPT: an international, multicenter, placebo-controlled trial of monoclonal antibody to human tumor necrosis factor-alpha in patients with sepsis. International Sepsis Trial Study Group. Crit Care Med 1996;24:1431–1440.

35. Reinhart K, Wiegand-Lohnert C, Grimminger F, Kaul M, Withington S, Treacher D, et al. Assessment of the safety and efficacy of the monoclonal anti-tumor necrosis factor antibody-fragment, MAK 195F,

in patients with sepsis and septic shock: a multi-center, randomized, placebo-controlled, dose-ranging study. Crit Care Med 1996;24:733–742.

36. Fisher CJ Jr, Agosti JM, Opal SM, Lowry SF, Balk RA, Sadoff JC, et al. Treatment of septic shock with the tumor necrosis factor receptor:Fc fusion protein. The soluble TNF Receptor Sepsis Study Group. N Engl J Med 1996;334:1697–1702.

37. Fisher CJ Jr, Dhainaut JF, Opal SM, Pribble JB, Balk RA, Slotman GJ, et al. Recombinant human interleukin 1 receptor antagonist in the treatment of patients with sepsis syndrome. Results from a randomized, double-blind, placebo controlled trial. Phase III rhIL-1ra Sepsis Syndrome Study Group. JAMA 1994;271:1836–1843.

38. Knaus WA, Harrell FE Jr, LaBrecque JF, Wagner DP, Pribble JP, Draper EA, et al. Use of predicted risk of mortality to evaluate the efficacy of anti-cytokine therapy in sepsis. The rhIL-1ra Phase III Sepsis Syndrome Study Group. Crit Care Med 1996;24:46–56.

39. Smith SR, Calzetta A, Bankowski J, Kenworthy-Bott L, Terminelli C. Lipopolysaccharide-induced cytokine production and mortality in mice treated with Corynebacterium parvum. J Leukoc Biol 1993; 54:23–29.

40. Cross AS, Opal SM, Palardy JE, Bodmer MW, Sadoff JC. The efficacy of combination immunotherapy in experimental Pseudomonas sepsis. J Infect Dis 1993;167:112–118.

41. Ruetten H, Thiemermann C. Combination immunotherapy which neutralises the effects of TNF alpha and IL-1 beta attenuates the circulatory failure and multiple organ dysfunction caused by endotoxin in the rat. J Physiol Pharmacol 1997;48:605–621.

42. Opal SM, Cross AS, Jhung JW, Young LD, Palardy JE, Parejo NA, et al. Potential hazards of combination immunotherapy in the treatment of experimental septic shock. J Infect Dis 1996;173: 1415–1421.

43. Heinzel FP. The role of IFN-gamma in the pathology of experimental endotoxemia. J Immunol 1990; 145:2920–2924.

44. Moncada S, Palmer RM, Higgs EA. Nitric oxide: physiology, pathophysiology, and pharmacology. Pharmacol Rev 1991;43:109–142.

45. Forstermann U, Pollock JS, Schmidt HH, Heller M, Murad F. Calmodulin-dependent endothelium-derived relaxing factor/nitric oxide synthase activity is present in the particulate and cytosolic fraction of bovine aortic endothelial cells. Proc Natl Acad Sci USA 1991;88:1788–1792.

46. Leone AM, Palmer RM, Knowles RG, Francis P, Ashton DS, Moncada S. Constitutive and inducible nitric oxide synthases incorporate molecular oxygen into both nitric oxide and citrulline. J Biol Chem 1991;266:23,790–23,795.

47. Marletta MA. Nitric oxide synthase structure and mechanism. J Biol Chem 1993;268:12,231–12,334.

48. Feldman PL, Griffith OW, Stuehr DJ. The surprising life of nitric oxide. Chem Eng News 1993; Dec. 20:26–38.

49. Gross SS, Stuehr DJ, Aisaka K, Jaffe EA, Levi R, Griffith OW. Macrophage and endothelial cell nitric oxide synthesis: cell-type selective inhibition by N^G-aminoarginine, N^G-nitroarginine and N^G-methylarginine. Biochem Biophys Res Commun 1990;170:96–103.

50. Lambert LE, French JF, Whitten JP, Baron BM, McDonald IA. Characterization of cell selectivity of two novel inhibitors of nitric oxide synthesis. Eur J Pharmacol 1992;216:131–134.

51. Feldman PL, Griffith OW, Hong H, Stuehr DJ. Irreversible inactivation of macrophage and brain nitric oxide synthase by L-NG-methylarginine requires NADPH-dependent hydroxylation. J Med Chem 1993;36:491–496.

52. Nathan C. Nitric oxide as a secretory product of mammalian cells. FASEB J 1992;6:3051–3064.

53. Green SF, Nacy CA. Antimicrobial and immunophatologic effects of cytokine-induced nitric oxide synthesis. Curr Opin Infect Dis 1993;6:384–396.

54. Schott CA, Gray GA, Stoclet JC. Dependence of endotoxin-induced vascular hyporeactivity ON extracellular L-arginine. Br J Pharmacol 1993;108:38–43.

55. Kilbourn RG, Jubran A, Gross SS, Griffith OW, Levi R, Adams J, et al. Reversal of endotoxin-mediated shock by NG-methyl-L-arginine, an inhibitor of nitric oxide synthesis. Biochem Biophys Res Commun 1990;172:1132–1138.

56. Thiemermann C, Vane JR. Inhibition of nitric oxide synthesis reduces the hypotension induced by bacterial lipopolysaccharide in the rat in vivo. Eur J Pharmacol 1990;182:591–595.

57. Julou-Schaeffer G, Gray GA, Fleming I, Schott C, Parratt JR, Stoclet JC. Loss of vascular responsiveness induced by endotoxin involves the L-arginine pathway. Am J Physiol 1990;259:H1038–H1043.

58. Rees DD, Cellek S, Palmer RM, Moncada S. Dexamethasone prevents the induction by endotoxin of nitric oxide synthase and the associated effects on vascular tone: an insight into endotoxin shock. Biochem Biophys Res Commun 1990;173:541–547.

59. Billiar TR, Curran RD, Harbrecht BG, Stuehr DJ, Demetris AJ, Simmons RL. Modulation of nitrogen oxide synthesis in vivo: NG-monomethyl-L-arginine inhibits endotoxin-induced nitrate/nitrate biosynthesis while promoting hepatic damage. J Leukoc Biol 1990;48:565–569.

60. Szabo C, Thiemermann C. Regulation of the expression of the inducible isoform of nitric oxide synthase. Adv Pharmacol 1995;34:113–153.

61. Thiemermann C. The role of the L-arginine: nitric oxide pathway in circulatory shock. Adv Pharmacol 1994;28:45–79.

62. MacMicking JD, Nathan C, Hom G, Chartrain N, Fletcher DS, Trumbauer M, et al. Altered responses to bacterial infection and endotoxic shock in mice lacking inducible nitric oxide synthase. Cell 1995; 81:641–650.

63. Wei XQ, Charles IG, Smith A, Ure J, Feng GJ, Huang FP, et al. Altered immune responses in mice lacking inducible nitric oxide synthase. Nature 1995;375:408–411.

64. Xie Q, Whisnant R, Nathan C. Promotor of the mouse gene encoding calcium-independent nitric oxide synthase confers inducibility by interferon gamma and bacterial lipopolysaccharide. J Exp Med 1993; 177:1779–1784.

65. Sherman MP, Aeberhard EE, Wong VZ, Griscavage JM, Ignarro LJ. Pyrrolidine dithiocarbamate inhibits induction of nitric oxide synthase activity in rat alveolar macrophages. Biochem Biophys Res Commun 1993;191:1301–1308.

66. Griscavage JM, Wilk S, Ignarro LJ. Serine and cysteine proteinase inhibitors prevent nitric oxide production by activated macrophages by interfering with transcription of the inducible NO synthase gene. Biochem Biophys Res Commun 1995;215:721–729.

67. Dong Z, Qi X, Fidler IJ. Protein tyrosine kinase inhibitors decrease the induction of nitric oxide synthase activity in lipopolysaccharide-responsive and non-responsive murine macrophages. J Immunol 1993; 151:2717–2724.

68. Salzman A, Denenberg AG, Ueta I, O'Conner M, Linn SC, Szabo C. Induction and activity of nitric oxide synthase in cultured human intestinal epithelial monolayers. Am J Physiol 1996;270: G565–G573.

69. Joly GA, Ayres M, Kilbourn RG. Potent inhibition of inducible nitric oxide synthase by geldanamycin, a tyrosine kinase inhibitor, in endothelial, smooth muscle cells, and in rat aorta. FEBS Lett 1997; 403:40–44.

70. Diaz-Guerra MJ, Bodelon OG, Velasco M, Whelan R, Parker PJ, Bosca L. Up-regulation of protein kinase C-epsilon promotes the expression of cytokine-inducible nitric oxide synthase in RAW 264.7 cells. J Biol Chem 1996;271:32,028–32,033.

71. Radomski MW, Palmer RM, Moncada S. Characterization of the L-arginine: nitric oxide pathway in human platelets. Br J Pharmacol 1990;101:325–330.

72. Schini VB, Catovski S, Scott-Burden T, Vanhoutte P. The inducible nitric oxide synthase is impaired by thrombin in vascular smooth muscle cells. J Cardiovasc Pharmacol 1992;20:S142–S144.

73. Doyle AG, Herbein G, Montaner LJ, Minty AJ, Caput D, Ferrara P, et al. Interleukin-13 alters the activation state of murine macrophages in vitro: comparison with interleukin-4 and interferon-gamma. Eur J Immunol 1994;24:1441–1445.

74. Hirahashi J, Nakaki T, Hishikawa K, Marumo T, Yasumori T, Hayashi M, et al. Endothelin-1 inhibits induction of nitric oxide synthase and GTP cyclohydrolase I in rat mesangial cells. Pharmacology 1996;53:241–249.

75. Saura M, Martinez-Dalmau R, Minty A, Perez-Sala D, Lamas S. Interleukin-13 inhibits inducible nitric oxide synthase expression in human mesangial cells. Biochem J 1996;313:641–646.

76. Ruetten H, Thiemermann C. Effects of tyrphostins and genistein on the circulatory failure and organ dysfunction caused by endotoxin in the rat: a possible role for protein tyrosine kinase. Br J Pharmacol 1997;122:59–70.

77. Xie Q, Kashiwabara Y, Nathan C. Role of transcription factor NF-(B/Rel) in induction of nitric oxide. J Biol Chem 1994;269:4705–4708.

78. Koide M, Kawahara Y, Nakayama I, Tsuda T, Yokoyama M. Cyclic AMP-elevating agents induce an inducible type of nitric oxide synthase in cultured vascular smooth muscle cells. Synergism with the induction elicited by inflammatory cytokines. J Biol Chem 1993;268:24,959–24,966.

79. Kunz D, Walker G, Wiesenberg I, Pfeilschifter J. Inhibition by tetranactin of interleukin 1 beta- and cyclic AMP-induced nitric oxide synthase expression in rat renal mesangial cells. Br J Pharmacol 1996;118:1621–1626.

80. Bulut V, Severn A, Liew FY. Nitric oxide production by murine macrophages is inhibited by prolonged elevation of cyclic AMP. Biochem Biophys Res Commun 1993;195:1134–1138.

81. Assreuy J, Cunha FQ, Liew FY, Moncada S. Feedback inhibition of nitric oxide synthase activity by nitric oxide. Br J Pharmacol 1993;108:833–837.

82. Nussler AK, Billiar TR. Inflammation, immunoregulation, and inducible nitric oxide synthase. J Leukoc Biol 1993;54:171–178.

83. Levitzki A, Gazit A. Tyrosine Kinase inhibition: an approach to drug development. Science 1995; 267:1782–1788.

84. Weinstein SL, Gold MR, De Franco AL. Bacterial lipopolysaccharide stimulates protein tyrosine phosphorylation in macrophages. Proc Natl Acad Sci USA 1991;88:4148–4152.

85. Geng Y, Zhang B, Lotz M. Protein tyrosine kinase activation is required for lipopolysaccharide induction of cytokines in human blood monocytes. J Immunol 1993;151:6692–6700.

86. Evans JPM, Mire-Sluis AR, Hoffbrand AV, Wickremasinghe RG. Binding of G-CSF, GM-CSF, tumor necrosis factor-alpha and gamma-interferon to cell surface receptors on human myeloid leukemia cells triggers rapid tyrosine and serine phosphorylation of a 75-Kd protein. Blood 1990;75:88–95.

87. Kohno M, Nishizawa N, Tsujimoto M, Nomoto H. Mitogenic signalling pathway of tumor necrosis factor involves the rapid tyrosine phosphorylation of 41000-M(r) and 43000-M(r) cytosol proteins. Biochem J 1990;267:91–98.

88. Novogrodsky A, Vanichkin A, Patya M, Gazit A, Osherov N, Levitzki A. Prevention of lipopolysaccharide-induced lethal toxicity by tyrosine kinase inhibitors. Science 1994;264:1319–1322.

89. Vanichikin A, Patya M, Gazit A, Levitzki A, Novogrodsky A. Late administration of a lipophylic tyrosine kinase inhibitor prevents lipopolysaccharide and Escherichia coli-induced lethal toxicity. J Infect Dis 1996;173:927–933.

90. Nabel G, Baltimore D. An inducible transcription factor activates expression of human immunodeficiency virus in T cells. Nature 1987;326:711–713.

91. Grimm S, Bauerle PA. The inducible transcription factor NF-kappa B: structure function relationship of its protein subunit. Biochem J 1993;290:297–308.

92. Sen R, Baltimore D. Inducibility of kappa immunoglobulin enhancer binding protein NF-kappa B by a posttranslation mechanism. Cell 1986;47:921–928.

93. Lowenthal JW, Ballard DW, Boehnlein E, Greene WC. Tumor necrosis factor alpha induces proteins that bind specifically to kappa B-like enhancer elements and regulate interleukin 2 receptor alpha-chain gene expression in primary human T lymphocytes. Proc Natl Acad Sci USA 1989;86:2331–2335.

94. Arima N, Kuziel WA, Gardine TA, Greene WC. Il-2-induced signal transduction involves the activation of nuclear NF-kappa B expression. J Immunol 1992;149:83–91.

95. Henkel T, Machleidt T, Alkalay I, Kroenke M, Ben-Neriah Y, Bauerle PA. Rapid proteolysis of IκB-α is necessary for activation of transcription factor NF κB. Nature 1993;365:182–185.

96. Siebenlist U, Franzoso G, Brown K. Structure, regulation and function of NF-kappa B. Annu Rev Cell Biol 1994;10:405–455.

97. Baeuerle PA, Baltimore D. Activation of DNA binding activity in an apparently cytoplasmic precursor of the NF-kappa B transcription factor. Cell 1988;53:211–217.

98. Baeuerle PA, Baltimore D. I kappa B: a specific inhibitor of the NF-kappa B transcription factor. Science 1988;242:540–546.

99. Sun SC, Ganchi PA, Ballard DW, Greene WC. NF-kappa B controls expression of inhibitor I kappa B alpha: evidence for an inducible autoregulatory pathway. Science 1993;259:1912–1915.

100. Miyamoto S, Maki M, Schmitt MJ, Hatanaka M, Verma IM. Tumor necrosis factor α-induced phosphorlyation of IκB-α is a signal for its degradation but not dissociation from NF-κB. Proc Natl Acad Sci USA 1994;91:12,740–12,744.

101. Lin YC, Brown K, Siebenlist U. Activation of NFκB requires proteolysis of the inhibitor IκB-α: signal-induced phosphorylation of IκB-α alone does not release active NFκB. Proc Natl Acad Sci USA 1995;92:552–556.

102. Barnes PJ, Karin M. Nuclear factor-kappaB: a pivotal transcription factor in chronic inflammatory diseases. N Engl J Med 1997;336:1066–1071.

103. Ruetten H, Thiemermann C. Attenuation by calpain inhibitor 1, an inhibitor of the proteolysis of IκB, of the circulatory failure and multiple organ dysfinction caused by endotoxin in the rat. Br J Pharmacol 1997;121:695–704.

104. Radomski MW, Palmer RM, Moncada S. Glucocorticoids inhibit the expression of an inducible, but not the constitutive, nitric oxide synthase in vascular endothelial cells. Proc Natl Acad Sci USA 1990; 87:10,043–10,047.

105. Kwon G, Corbett JA, Rodi CP, Sullivan P, McDaniel ML. Interleukin-1 beta-induced nitric oxide synthase expression by rat pancreatic beta-cells: evidence for the involvement of nuclear factor kappa B in the signaling mechanism. Endocrinology 1995;136:4790–4795.

106. Nishiya T, Uehara T, Nomura Y. Herbimycin A suppresses NF-kappa B activation and tyrosine phosphorylation of JAK2 and the subsequent induction of nitric oxide synthase in C6 glioma cells. FEBS Lett 1995;371:333–336.

107. Mahon TM, O'Neill LA. Studies into the effect of the tyrosine kinase inhibitor herbimycin A on NF-kappa B activation in T lymphocytes. Evidence for covalent modification of the p50 subunit. Biochem J 1995;270:28,557–28,564.

108. Yokoo T, Katamura M. Dual regulation of IL-1 beta-mediated matrix metalloproteinase-9 expression in mesangial cells by NF-kappa B and AP-1. Am J Physiol 1996;270:F123–F130.

109. Tetsuka T, Srivastava SK, Morrison AR. Tyrosine kinase inhibitors, genistein and herbimycin A, do not block interleukin-1 beta-induced activation of NF-kappa B in rat mesangial cells. Biochem Biophys Res Commun 1996;26:808–812.

110. Imbert V, Rupec RA, Livolsi A, Pahl HL, Traenckner EB, Mueller-Dieckmann C, et al. Tyrosine phosphorylation of I kappa B-alpha activates NF-kappa B without proteolytic degrdation of I kappa B-alpha. Cell 1996;86:787–798.

111. Barnes PJ, Adcock IM. NF-κB: a pivotal role in asthma and a new target for therapy. TIPS 1997;18: 46–50.

112. Wright CE, Rees DD, Moncada S. Protective and pathological roles of nitric oxide in endotoxin shock. Cardiovasc Res 1992;26:48–57.

113. Paya D, Gray GA, Fleming I, Stoclet JC. Effect of dexamethasone on the onset and persistence of vascular hyporeactivity induced by E. coli lipopolysaccharide in rats. Circ Shock 1993;41:103–112.

114. Estrada C, Gomez C, Martin C, Moncada S, Gonzalez C. Nitric oxide mediates tumor necrosis factor-alpha cytotoxicity in endothelial cells. Biochem Biophys Res Commun 1992;186:475–482.

115. Palmer RM, Bridge L, Foxwell NA, Moncada S. The role of nitric oxide in endothelial cell damage and its inhibition by glucocorticoids. Br J Pharmacol 1992;105:11,12.

116. Morris SM Jr, Billiar TR. New insights into the regulation of inducible nitric oxide synthesis. Am J Physiol 1994;266:E829–E839.

117. Southan GJ, Szabo C. Selective pharmacological inhibition of distinct nitric oxide synthase isoforms. Biochem Pharmacol 1996;51:383–394.

118. Wu CC, Ruetten H, Thiemermann C. Comparison of the effects of aminoguanidine and N$^\omega$-nitro-L-arginine methyl ester on the multiple organ dysfunction caused by endotoxaemia. Eur J Pharmacol 1996;300:99–104.

119. Walder CE, Thiemermann C, Vane JR. The involvement of endothelium-derived relaxing factor in the regulation of renal cortical blood flow in the rat. Br J Pharmacol 1991;102:967–973.

120. Robertson FM, Offner PJ, Ciceri DP, Becker WK, Pruitt BA Jr. Detrimental hemodynamic effects of nitric oxide synthase inhibition in septic shock. Arch Surg 1994;129:149–156.

121. Corbett JA, Tilton RG, Chang K, Hasan KS, Ido Y, Wang JL, et al. Aminoguanidine, a novel inhibitor of nitric oxide formation, prevents diabetic vascular dysfunction. Diabetes 1992;41:552–556.

122. Wu CC, Chen SJ, Szabo C, Thiemermann C, Vane JR. Aminoguanidine attenuates the delayed circulatory failure and improves survival in rodent models of endotoxic shock. Br J Pharmacol 1995;114: 1666–1672.

123. Seo HG, Fujiwara N, Kaneto H, Asahi M, Fujii J, Taniguchi N. Effect of a nitric oxide synthase inhibitor, S-ethylisothiourea, on cultured cells and cardiovascular functions of normal and lipopolysaccharide-treated rabbits. J Biochem (Tokyo) 1996;119:553–558.

124. Ruetten H, Southan GJ, Abate A, Thiemermann C. Attenuation of endotoxin-induced multiple organ dysfunction by 1-amino-2-hydroxy-guanidine, a potent inhibitor of inducible nitric oxide synthase. Br J Pharmacol 1996;118:261–270.

125. Arkovitz MS, Wispe JR, Garcia VF, Szabo C. Selective inhibition of the inducible isoform of nitric oxide synthase prevents pulmonary transvascular flux during acute endotoxemia. J Pediatr Surg 1996; 31:1009–1015.

126. Bieganski T, Kusche J, Lorenz W, Hesterberg R, Stahlknecht CD, Feussner KD. Distribution and properties of human intestinal diamine oxidase and its relevance for the histamine catabolism. Biochim Biophys Acta 1983;756:196–203.

127. Seiler N, Bolkenius FN, Knodgen B. The influence of catabolic reactions on polyamine excretion. Biochem J 1985;225:219–226.

128. Edelstein D, Brownlee M. Aminoguanidine ameliorates albuminuria in diabetic hypertensive rats. Diabetologia 1992;35:96,97.

129. Ou P, Wolff SP. Aminoguanidine: a drug proposed for prophylaxis in diabetes inhibits catalase and generates hydrogen peroxide in vitro. Biochem Pharmacol 1993;46:1139–1144.

130. Ruetten H, Thiemermann C. Prevention of the expression of inducible nitric oxide synthase by aminoguanidine or aminoethyl-isothiourea in macrophages and in the rat. Biochem Biophys Res Commun 1996;225:525–530.

131. Szabo C, Southan GJ, Thiemermann C. Beneficial effects and improved survival in rodent models of shock with S-methyl-isothiourea, a novel, potent and selective inhibitor of inducible nitric oxide synthase. Proc Natl Acad Sci USA 1994;91:12,472–12,476.
132. Southan GJ, Szabo C, Thiemermann C. Isothioureas: potent inhibitors of nitric oxide synthases with variable isoform selectivity. Br J Pharmacol 1995;114:510–516.
133. Garvey EP, Oplinger JA, Tanoury GJ, Sherman PA, Fowler M, Marshall S, et al. Potent and selective inhibition of human nitric oxide synthases. Inhibition by non-amino acid isothioureas. J Biol Chem 1994;269:26,669–26,676.
134. Thiemermann C, Ruetten H, Wu CC, Vane JR. The multiple organ dysfunction syndrome caused by endotoxin in the rat: attenuation of liver dysfunction by inhibitors of nitric oxide synthase. Br J Pharmacol 1995;116:2845–2851.
135. Saetre T, Gundersen Y, Thiemermann C, Lilleaasen P, Aasen AO. Aminoethyl-isothiourea, a selective inhibitor of inducible nitric oxide synthase activity, improves liver circulation and oxygen metabolism in a porcine model of endotoxemia. Shock 1998;9:109–115.
136. Thiemermann C. Nitric oxide and septic shock. Gen Pharmacol 1997;29:159–166.
137. Sprong RC, Aarsman CJ, van Oirschot JF, van Asbeck BS. Dimethylthiourea protects rats against gram-negative sepsis and decreases tumor necrosis factor and nuclear factor kappaB activity. J Lab Clin Med 1997;129:470–481.
138. Garvey EP, Oplinger JA, Furfine ES, Kiff RJ, Laszlo F, Whittle BJ, et al. 1400W is a slow, tight binding, and highly selective inhibitor of inducible nitric-oxide synthase in vitro and in vivo. J Biol Chem 1997;272:4959–4963.
139. Morris SM Jr, Billiar TR. New insights into the regulation of inducible nitric oxide synthesis. Am J Physiol 1994;266:E829–E839.
140. Preiser JC, Vincent JL. Nitric oxide involvement in septic shock: Do human beings behave like rodents? In Vincent JL, ed. Yearbook of Intensive Care and Emergency Medicine. Springer Verlag, Berlin, 1996, pp. 358–365.
141. Petros A, Bennett D, Vallance P. Effect of nitric oxide synthase inhibitors on hypotension in patients with septic shock. Lancet 1991;338:1557,1558.
142. Schilling J, Cakmakci M, Battig U, Geroulanos S. A new approach in the treatment of hypotension in human septic shock by NG-monomethyl-L-arginine, an inhibitor of the nitric oxide synthetase. Intensive Care Med 1993;19:227–231.
143. Lorente JA, Landin L, De Pablo R, Renes E, Liste D. L-arginine pathway in the sepsis syndrome. Crit Care Med 1993;21:1287–1295.
144. Petros A, Lamb G, Leone A, Moncada S, Bennett D, Vallance P. Effects of a nitric oxide synthase inhibitor in humans with septic shock. Cardiovasc Res 1994;28:34–39.
145. Watson D, Donaldson J, Grover R, Mottola D, Guntipalli K, Vincent JL. The cardiopulmonary effects of 546C88 in human with septic shock. Int Care Med 1995;21:S117.
146. Shultz PJ, Raij I. Endogenously synthesized nitric oxide prevents endotoxin-induced glomerular thrombosis. J Clin Invest 1992;90:1718–1725.
147. Doughty LA, Kaplan SS, Carcillo JA. Inflammatory cytokine and nitric oxide responses in pediatric sepsis and organ failure. Crit Care Med 1996;24:1137–1143.
148. Preiser JC, Reper P, Vlasselaer D, Vray B, Zhang H, Metz G, et al. Nitric oxide production is increased in patients after burn injury. J Trauma 1996;40:368–371.
149. Tracey WR, Tse J, Carter G. Lipopolysaccharide-induced changes in plasma nitrite and nitrate concentrations in rats and mice: pharmacological evaluation of nitric oxide synthase inhibitors. J Pharmacol Exp Ther 1995;272:1011–1015.
150. Grover R, Zaccardelli D, Colice G, Guntupali K, Watson D, Vincent JL. An open-label dose escalation study of the nitric oxide synthase inhibitor, N(G)-methyl-L-arginine hydrochloride (546188), in patients with septic shock. Crit Care Med 1999;27:913–922.

Stroke and Nitric Oxide

Nancy E. Stagliano and Paul L. Huang

INTRODUCTION

Nitric oxide (NO•) is produced by many different cell types in the brain, including neurons, vascular endothelial cells, glial cells, and astrocytes. Although the neuronal nitric oxide synthase (nNOS) isoform accounts for the majority of NOS in the brain, all three isoforms are present and serve as potential sources of NO• production under physiological and pathological conditions *(1,2)*. Therefore, precise tools and carefully designed experiments are necessary to elucidate the functions and effects of this ubiquitous molecule. In this chapter, we summarize the evidence to date that NO• and NOS isoforms play important roles in the pathophysiology of cerebral ischemia.

NO• PRODUCTION IN THE BRAIN

Discovery of NO• in the Brain

Long before the discovery that NO• is produced by the brain, there were hints regarding its roles in neuronal function. The excitatory neurotransmitter glutamate, acting by binding to the *N*-methyl-D-aspartate (NMDA) receptor, elevates the levels of cyclic guanosine monophosphate (c-GMP) that mediates the downstream effects of excitatory neurotransmission. However, the molecular events between NMDA receptor binding and cGMP production were unknown. Two key discoveries provided the missing pieces of this puzzle. The first was the discovery that cerebellar cells stimulated by NMDA generate NO• *(3)*. The second was the identification and purification of nNOS from the brain *(4)*. Neuronal NOS (nNOS, type I NOS) is distinct from endothelial NOS (eNOS, type III NOS) and inducible or macrophage NOS (iNOS, type II NOS). Like eNOS, nNOS is calcium sensitive and it is activated by increases in intracellular calcium concentration caused by NMDA receptor binding. With these two discoveries, it became clear that NO• is an important intermediate that links NMDA receptor binding to activation of soluble guanylyl cyclase (GC) and increases cGMP production.

NADPH Diaphorase Positive Neurons

Another hint as to the role of NO• in the brain comes from nicotinamide adenine dinucleotide phosphate (NADPH) diaphorase staining, a histochemical technique first described in 1964 *(5)*. Diaphorase staining involves incubating fixed tissues with the dye nitroblue tetrazolium (NBT). In the presence of NADPH, diaphorase positive cells convert the dye from a pale yellow color to a dark blue. The enzymatic activity responsible for this reaction is resistant to formaldehyde fixation, whereas other enzymatic activities that may cause nonspecific staining are inactivated by formaldehyde. Only a specific population of neurons in

From: *Contemporary Cardiology, vol. 4: Nitric Oxide and the Cardiovascular System*
Edited by: J. Loscalzo and J. A. Vita © Humana Press Inc., Totowa, NJ

Table 1
Physiological Functions of NO• in the Brain

Mediation of excitatory glutamate neurotransmission
Regulation of basal CBF
Coupling of CBF to neuronal metabolism
Signaling as retrograde messenger

the brain are NADPH diaphorase positive. Interestingly, these neurons are resistant to ische-mia, toxicity, and neurodegeneration *(6)*. Once nNOS was localized to the brain, it became apparent that the staining pattern for nNOS and NADPH diaphorase are similar and the two colocalize *(7)*. Furthermore, purified cloned nNOS protein possesses NADPH diaphorase activity, proving that the two activities reside in the same molecule *(8)*. The fact that these neurons generate NO• and their neighbors die under conditions of ischemia, toxicity, or neurodegeneration suggested that NADPH diaphorase/nNOS positive neurons may actually kill their neighbors by producing excessive NO•. Why would the nNOS neurons themselves be resistant to NO• toxicity? One possible molecular basis for resistance to oxidative insults is their high level of manganese superoxide dismutase (MnSOD) expression *(9)*. By remov-ing superoxide anion from the NADPH diaphorase positive neurons, MnSOD would prevent the formation of toxic peroxynitrite anion, providing protection from neurotoxicity. Neigh-boring cells with less MnSOD would lack this resistance, form peroxynitrite by the reaction of superoxide with NO•, and die.

NOS Isoforms in the Brain

All three NOS isoforms are present in the brain and can potentially contribute to the toxicity and vascular effects of NO•. As evidenced by quantitative in vitro [3H]L-N^G-argi-nine autoradiography, the majority of NOS-positive cells in the brain contain the neuronal isoform (44). These cells are typically neurons, although they represent only 1–2% of the total neurons in the brain. Despite this, the extensive processes of nNOS-positive neurons allow the NO• produced by these neurons to reach most regions of the brain by diffusion. Endothelial NOS is found in the endothelium of most cerebral vessels and can also be detected in some hippocampal neurons. The NO• derived from eNOS is thought to act locally as a perivascular signaling molecule that mediates vasorelaxation and cGMP production. Upon stimulation, iNOS can be detected in brain glial cells. After injury, these cells migrate into brain tissue and release high levels of NO•.

FUNCTIONS OF NO• IN THE BRAIN

The normal functions served by NO• in the brain include mediation of glutamate responses, regulation of cerebral blood flow (CBF), and retrograde messenger signaling in long-term potentiation (LTP) and long-term depression (LTD) (Table 1).

Regulation of Cerebral Blood Flow

In the brain, as in other tissues, NO• plays an important role in controlling blood flow. NOS is present not only within populations of neurons, but also within endothelial cells and NOS-positive nerve fibers that encircle blood vessels in the brain *(10)*. Thus, several potential sources of NO• are anatomically arranged so they may regulate CBF. Treatment of rats with the NOS inhibitor N^G-monomethyl-L-arginine (L-NMMA) significantly reduces absolute blood flow to all cortical and subcortical regions *(11)*. Upregulation of eNOS mRNA levels by -coenzyme A (hydroxymethylglutaryl [HMG]-CoA) reductase inhibitors increases abso-lute CBF in several regions of the brain *(12)*, implicating eNOS in the regulation of basal CBF.

In contrast, the nNOS isoform appears involved in the coupling of local neuronal activity in the brain to CBF, a relationship that is the basis for functional imaging techniques such as positron emission tomography (PET) scanning. This coupling may involve multiple mediators, including products of neuronal metabolism (H+ and adenosine), ions released following neuronal activation, or neurotransmitters released adjacent to blood vessels. NO$^\bullet$ is well suited to couple CBF to brain metabolism because it diffuses freely across cell membranes and has a short biological half-life *(13–15)*. Two experimental models of blood flow–metabolism coupling are the general CBF increase in response to hypercapnia, and the local blood flow increase over cortical barrels caused by whisker stimulation.

In many species, including humans, CBF increases in response to hypercapnia. These changes are accompanied by increases in NO$^\bullet$ production, blocked by the general NOS inhibitor nitroso-L-arginine (L-NA) and the nNOS specific inhibitor 7-nitroindazole *(16,17)*, and have been demonstrated in humans *(18)*. In mice, the response of CBF to moderate hypercapnia (5% CO_2) is blocked by NOS inhibitors such as L-NA and N^G-nitroso-L-arginine methyl ester (L-NAME). However, NO$^\bullet$ is not the only vasoactive agent involved, as NOS inhibitors can only block the response within a range of CO_2 levels, and even in the most susceptible range, there is residual vasodilation. Mice lacking nNOS have equivalent responses to 5% CO_2 as wild-type mice. However, although topical L-NA blocks the response of wild-type mice, it has no effect on nNOS mutant mice *(19)*. Thus, the response of nNOS mutant mice is not due to eNOS or another NOS isoform. Mediators other than NO$^\bullet$ must therefore mediate the response in nNOS mutant mice. These same mediators participate in wild-type animals, as NOS inhibition blocks the relative CBF (rCBF) response only over a very narrow range of $PaCO_2$. Thus, nNOS plays a role in hypercapnic hyperemia in the wild-type animal, but in the chronic absence of nNOS in the nNOS mutant mice, other mechanisms compensate to maintain a quantitatively normal response.

A second model of CBF coupling to neuronal metabolism is the cortical barrel blood flow response to whisker stimulation. In rodents, mechanical stimulation of whiskers at 2–3 Hz for 60 s results in a predictable increase in rCBF over the cortical barrels in the brain that correspond to those whiskers. This response can be attenuated by either systemic treatment or topical superfusion with L-NA, suggesting that NO$^\bullet$ serves as a mediator inducing vasodilation. nNOS inhibition abolishes the coupling between whisker stimulation and rCBF increase in the second-order relay stations of the trigeminal relay *(20)*. In nNOS knockout animals, the response to whisker stimulation is very similar to wild-type animals, but topical L-NA has no effect *(21)*. Endothelium-dependent relaxation, as assessed by pial dilation to acetylcholine, is the same in wild-type and nNOS knockout mice. These results indicate that endothelial NOS does not mediate the whisker response in nNOS knockout mice, and that the effect of L-NA in wild-type mice is due to nNOS inhibition. In addition, they suggest that NO$^\bullet$-independent mechanisms couple rCBF with metabolism in nNOS knockout mice. In separate studies, eNOS knockout mice have a response indistinguishable from wild-type, including sensitivity to L-NA, confirming that nNOS mediates blood flow responses in the cortical barrel fields *(22)*. Inhibition of nNOS also reduces the blood flow increases in the cerebellar cortex induced by parallel fiber simulation of cerebellar granule cells *(23)*. Thus, neuronally derived NO$^\bullet$ appears to couple blood flow to somatosensory activation in a region-dependent manner.

Overall, these results indicate that the nNOS isoform, not the eNOS isoform, mediates the coupling of CBF to neuronal metabolism. nNOS-derived NO$^\bullet$ acts in parallel with other vasodilators, as NOS inhibition attenuates, but does not obliterate, these responses. In the nNOS knockout mice, redundant vasodilatory mechanisms compensate for the chronic absence of nNOS expression, and the response is preserved, but no longer L-NA sensitive. The nNOS knockout mice also demonstrate other examples of physiological compensation in minimum alveolar concentration of anesthetics *(24)* and nociception *(25)*.

Retrograde Messenger Functions of NO•

Long-term potentiation (LTP) and long-term depression (LTD), electrophysiological correlates of learning and memory in the central nervous system (CNS), are examples of synaptic plasticity. Repetitive, timed firing of presynaptic neurons results in a strengthening of some synapses and weakening of others. These changes are the result of both postsynaptic changes, e.g., changes in receptor number, and presynaptic changes, e.g., changes in neurotransmitter release. This latter, presynaptic component necessitates a retrograde messenger to provide a feedback signal to presynaptic nerve terminals. The identity of the retrograde messenger(s) has been elusive to date.

NO• has unique properties that would allow it to serve as a retrograde messenger. NO• diffuses freely across cell membranes and has a short biological half-life, limiting its sphere of influence to a precise volume in space *(13,26)*. NO• acts at both pre- and postsynaptic nerve terminals in the CNS *(27)*. Preexisting NOS in the postsynaptic neuron can easily be activated by receptor-mediated calcium influx that occurs on stimulation. In the hippocampus, the site of LTP, NO•-sensitive GC, exists in presynaptic nerve terminals and NO• elicits neurotransmitter release. In postsynaptic hippocampal neurons, NOS staining is present in dendrites.

Inhibitors of NOS and scavengers of NO• block LTP, and application of exogenous NO• produces activity-dependent enhancement of synaptic transmission *(26,28–30)*, indicating that NO• is required for LTP. However, there has been considerable controversy over the role of NO• in neuronal plasticity owing to several conflicting results. First, L-NAME fails to inhibit LTP and spatial learning in vivo *(31,32)*. Second, the nNOS isoform could not be detected in the appropriate cells, the hippocampal pyramidal neurons. The nNOS mutant mice show preserved LTP, suggesting that the nNOS isoform may not be exclusively responsible for LTP *(33)*. Immunohistochemical studies localized eNOS to pyramidal cells *(33,34)*, raising the possibility that eNOS might generate NO• as the retrograde messenger. Later studies demonstrated that using gentler methods of fixation, the nNOS isoform can, indeed, be detected in pyramidal cells *(35)*, so both nNOS and eNOS could be involved in LTP. Double mutant mice that lack both nNOS and eNOS mice show reduced LTP in the stratum radiatum, whereas mice lacking nNOS or eNOS alone did not *(36)*. Thus, both nNOS and eNOS isoforms are involved in LTP, and each can compensate for the absence of the other.

Tsien and coworkers could not induce LTD in cerebellar slices from nNOS knockout mice *(37)*, confirming that nNOS is required for LTD. However, caged compounds designed to deliver NO• and cGMP inside Purkinje cells could not rescue the nNOS knockout mice, even though these compounds can circumvent pharmacologic inhibition of NO• synthesis or GC in wild-type mice. Thus, chronic absence of nNOS in the mutant mice may have allowed "atrophy" of the signalling pathways downstream of cGMP.

NO• SYNTHESIS IN CEREBRAL ISCHEMIA

Generation of NO• Following Ischemia

Using a porphyrinic microsensor to measure NO• levels in tissues, Malinski and colleagues found that NO• normally exists in the brain in nanomolar quantities. However, during and after cerebral ischemia, NO• levels increase dramatically from baseline to micromolar levels *(38)*. These elevated levels are correlated with increases in cGMP levels measured by microdialysis *(39)*. Radiometric determinations of regional NOS enzymatic activity reveal changes in NOS catalytic activity, including dramatic increases up to 3 h after middle cerebral artery (MCA) occlusion and moderate decreases in other models of stroke *(40,41)*.

The source of the early increase in NO• production appears to be the nNOS isoform. Electron spin trapping techniques show NO• production at baseline in the mouse brain, which increases significantly with ischemia. These changes are correlated with increases in brain cGMP production. However, nNOS knockout mice have no detectable NO• by electron spin trapping either at baseline or following ischemia. They have lower basal cGMP levels than do wild-type animals, and no increase in cGMP levels following ischemia (42). The early increase in neuronal production of NO• is attributable, in part, to activation of preexisting nNOS enzyme by increased intracellular calcium concentrations caused by NMDA receptor activation and loss of ion homeostasis. However, there is also upregulation of nNOS mRNA and protein following ischemia, as well. The level of nNOS mRNA increases as early as 15 min after middle cerebral artery occlusion (MCAO) and peaks at 1 h, whereas nNOS-containing neurons peak in number 4 h later (43,44). Similarly, [^{3}H]-L-NA binding to brain sections increases by up to 250% after MCAO. The expression of the eNOS isoform, as detected by immunohistochemistry, increases in cerebral microvessels after MCAO as well (45).

Continued expression and function of eNOS isoform appears to be important for regulation of CBF in the setting of ischemia. Thus, nNOS and eNOS, which have been viewed as constitutive NOS isoforms, are induced in the brain following cerebral ischemia. A second wave of NO• production occurs later after the acute ischemic event due to induction and activation of the iNOS isoform. In spontaneously hypertensive rats, iNOS activity peaks 2 d after MCAO (40), and temporally correlates with an infiltration of macrophages into the infarct zone. Similarly, iNOS messenger RNA levels peak 2 d after focal ischemia in C57BL/6 mice (46,47).

Studies Using NOS Inhibitors

Pharmacologic inhibition of NOS by nonselective inhibitors during ischemia have led to conflicting results. This topic has been comprehensively reviewed (48,49). Depending on the type and dose of inhibitor used, the ischemia model tested, the route and timing of drug administration, and the species studied, the effects of NOS inhibition on outcome of cerebral ischemia were highly variable. Two factors may account for this variability. First, the redox state of NO• influences its biological effects (50). Free NO• radical combines with superoxide to form peroxynitrite, which is neurotoxic. However, nitrosonium ion (NO+) S-nitrosylates the NMDA receptor, downregulating its activity and protecting against excitotoxicity. Second, all three NOS isoforms are present and may generate NO• following ischemia. NO• from these sources can have separate, and in some cases, opposing biological effects (49). Neuronal overproduction of NO• can contribute to cellular damage following ischemia by formation of peroxynitrite anion, activation of poly-ADP ribose polymerase (PARP), and inhibition of mitochondrial energy metabolism. In contrast, eNOS is important for the maintenance of normal vascular tone, and during and after an ischemic event, may play important roles in attempting to restore or maintain blood flow to ischemic regions. Inducible NOS in astrocytes, macrophages, and microglia also generates NO• following ischemia. Owing to these multiple effects, blockade of NOS by nonselective inhibitors might yield different results depending on which NOS isoforms are inhibited and to what extent.

There are now relatively selective inhibitors of nNOS. For example, 7-nitroindazole blocks both nNOS and eNOS in vitro, but its tissue distribution makes it selective for the nNOS isoform in vivo. 7-Nitroindazole and other nNOS-specific inhibitors reduce infarct size in rats and mice using models of focal ischemia, consistent with the hypothesis that nNOS contributes to toxicity and cellular damage following ischemia (51–53). Among NOS isoforms, aminoguanidine is relatively selective for iNOS, although it has other unrelated biological activities. Aminoguanidine blocks delayed neuronal damage following ischemia, consistent with a toxic role of iNOS (54,55).

Studies Using NOS Knockout Mice

The genetic approach of disrupting the genes for the NOS isoforms complements the pharmacologic approach of inhibiting NOS enzyme activity. Mice that lack each NOS isoform are viable and fertile. Neuronal NOS knockout mice display enlarged stomachs as a result of the absence of the nNOS isoform in the myenteric plexus of the stomach and pylorus

(56,57). They serve as the first animal model for the human disorder infantile hypertrophic pyloric stenosis. Endothelial NOS knockout mice are hypertensive and lack endothelium-dependent relaxing factor *(58)*. Inducible NOS knockout mice are resistant to the hypotensive effects of lipopolysaccharide and endotoxin *(59–61)*. All of the NOS knockout mice have normal neuroanatomy and cerebrovascular anatomy, important prerequisites for their use in studies of cerebrovascular ischemia.

Primary neuronal cultures grown from nNOS knockout mice are resistant to both NMDA-induced neurotoxicity and oxygen–glucose deprivation *(62)*. On the other hand, these cells are as vulnerable to kainate toxicity as wild-type neurons. These data support the roles of NMDA stimulation and nNOS activation in excitotoxic neuronal injury. Neuronal NOS mutant mice are resistant to both global and focal ischemia in vivo. MCA occlusion using an intraluminal filament model causes less morphological damage and smaller infarcts in nNOS knockout mice than in their wild-type counterparts *(42)*. The nNOS knockout mice also have better functional neurologic outcome. The neuroprotection is independent of changes in relative CBF (rCBF) reductions as measured by laser Doppler flowmetry, indicating that the primary ischemic insult is unchanged. Both transient and permanent models of MCAO show protection in the nNOS knockout mice *(63)*. Protection is also observed in global ischemia models. Ten minutes of bilateral common carotid artery occlusion, which usually results in severe CA1 hippocampal damage and behavioral deficits, has only minor effects on nNOS knockout mice *(64)*. These data confirm that neuronally produced NO• contributes to cellular damage following cerebral ischemia, in agreement with the pharmacological data showing a benefit from nNOS inhibition.

In contrast, eNOS knockout mice develop larger infarcts and more severe neurological deficits from MCAO than wild-type animals *(65)*. These infarcts correlate with more severe reductions in blood flow measured by laser Doppler flowmetry and by functional CT imaging *(66)*. Inhibition of the remaining eNOS isoform in nNOS knockout mice also results in worsening of the outcome. These results confirm that the eNOS isoform serves important protective roles in maintaining blood flow following ischemia. Because many pharmacological NOS inhibitors target eNOS as well as nNOS, these results are consistent with the aggravation of outcome found with nonspecific NOS inhibition.

Like nNOS knockout mice, iNOS knockout mice develop smaller infarcts following MCAO when observed at a later time point *(67)*. Other markers for severity of ischemic injury, such as rCBF reduction, neutrophil accumulation, and astrocytic proliferation, were comparable between the knockouts and their wild-type littermates, indicating that the ischemic resistance of the mice is caused by lack of iNOS and that iNOS contributes to late neurotoxicity following ischemia.

Thus, nNOS and iNOS are important mediators of early and late toxicity following ischemia, whereas eNOS serves important vascular protective roles. These results suggest that selective blockade of nNOS and iNOS and, potentially, the augmentation of eNOS might be beneficial in the treatment of stroke. Although the genetic manipulation of the NOS isoforms has served to clarify the roles of NO• in stroke, the precise molecular mechanisms by which NO• can protect and injure the brain are still being defined.

Implications for the Manipulation of NO• in the Clinical Setting

Although no clinically available nNOS inhibitors exist, other targets are being pursued that can prevent or interrupt neuronal NO• synthesis and the injury that it produces. NMDA-receptor activation is a key mediator in the ischemic injury cascade, which is upstream of NOS activation. The link between NMDA–receptor stimulation and NO• production is clear *(3)*. Several lines of evidence indicate that NMDA antagonism, most typically by MK-801 (dizocilpine) before, during, and after both focal and global experimental ischemia, is neuroprotective *(95,98,99)*. Although the antagonism of this glutamate receptor subtype can reduce

Table 2
Toxic Effects of NO$^\bullet$

Formation of peroxynitrite anion (OONO$^-$)
   DNA strand breakage
   Lipid peroxidation
   Hydroxyl radical formation
   Nitrosylation of tyrosine residues
Activation of poly ADP-ribose polymerase (PARP)
   Depletion of cellular energy stores
   Apoptosis and necrosis
Direct induction of apoptosis
   Nitrosylation of caspases
   cGMP-dependent modulation of caspase function

ischemic damage in the experimental setting, the clinical usage of these agents has proved difficult. Tolerance of NMDA antagonists, because of their psychostimulatory properties, was low in patients *(97)* and trials using these drugs failed to demonstrate therapeutic efficacy in ischemia *(96)*. Treatment strategies directed at downstream mediators of NO$^\bullet$-mediated toxicity such as PARP (*see* "Activation of PARP" following) have also been considered *(68,69)*.

The benefit of eNOS augmentation may extend beyond the domain of stroke treatment to the understudied area of stroke prophylaxis, ideally in patients who are at high-risk for an ischemic insult. In several large clinical studies, the use of HMG–CoA reductase inhibitors, commonly known as "statins," was associated with reductions in the incidence of stroke, even independent of cholesterol-lowering effects *(70,71)*. In experimental animals, simvastatin and lovastatin protect against cerebral infarction and neurologic dysfunction after MCAO *(12)*. One of the mechanisms for these effects may involve modulation of eNOS expression. In cultured endothelial cells and in the heart, aorta, and brain of mice, the statins increase eNOS messenger RNA (mRNA) and protein levels by stabilization of eNOS mRNA *(72)*. The beneficial effect of the statins is absent in eNOS mutant mice, indicating that the protection is predominantly the result of the apparent stabilization of eNOS mRNA *(12)*. These effects are functionally significant because statin treatment augments CBF both at baseline and following ischemia in the MCA core and penumbra.

TOXIC MECHANISMS OF NO$^\bullet$

Neuronal NO production markedly increases following cerebral ischemia due to both stimulation of pre-existing nNOS by elevated intracellular calcium levels and induction of new nNOS synthesis. Increased NO$^\bullet$ levels may be toxic by formation of peroxynitrite anion, activation of PARP, induction of programmed cell death, and inhibition of mitochondrial complexes (*see also* Table 2).

Formation of Peroxynitrite

NO$^\bullet$ reacts with superoxide to form peroxynitrite anion in an extremely rapid reaction. The rate constant for the reaction of superoxide with NO$^\bullet$ is 6.7×10^9 *M*/s, as compared with the rate constant for superoxide dismutase (SOD), which is 2.0×10^9 *M*/s *(73,74)*. Thus, superoxide reacts quicker with NO$^\bullet$ than it can be scavenged by SOD. In addition, NOS can generate superoxide as well as NO$^\bullet$, providing both reactants for the formation of peroxynitrite. Peroxynitrite has many potentially dangerous actions, including DNA strand breakage, PARP activation, lipid peroxidation, and hydroxyl radical formation *(74)*. Peroxynitrite reacts specifically with the ortho position of tyrosine residues of proteins to form 3-nitro-

Table 3
Protective Effects of NO$^\bullet$

Preservation of CBF
Scavenging of superoxide and other reactive oxygen species (with formation of peroxynitrite, however)
Reduced platelet aggregation and activation
Reduced leukocyte adhesion and activation

tyrosine. Neurofilament is one of the major proteins nitrosylated after ischemia *(75)* and nitrosylation interferes with the normal function of tyrosine phosphorylation *(76)*.

NO$^\bullet$ itself does not nitrosylate tyrosine residues. Rather, peroxynitrite yields the nitrated tyrosine product, and nitrotyrosine is therefore a specific marker for peroxynitrite formation. Immunohistochemistry for protein-bound nitrotyrosine and high-performance liquid chromatography (HPLC) quantification of free nitrotyrosine are two techniques used to detect peroxynitrite. Peroxynitrite is formed in brains subjected to excitotoxicity and ischemia/reperfusion injury *(77–79)*. Nitrotyrosine levels were significantly reduced in these model systems with either NOS inhibition or nNOS deletion, indicating that neuronally derived NO$^\bullet$ is required for the formation of peroxynitrite.

Activation of PARP

NO$^\bullet$-induced formation of peroxynitrite promotes DNA single-strand breakage and subsequent activation of the nuclear DNA-repair enzyme, PARP. This early activation of PARP has been coined the "PARP suicide hypothesis" in that it plays a pivotal role in the rapid cellular energy depletion, which contributes to cell death in ischemia and other injuries *(80)*. Following MCAO, PARP becomes maximally activated at 5 min of reperfusion, reducing NAD+ levels and slowing electron transport, glycolysis, and ATP-formation *(68)*. Pharmacological inhibition of PARP and genetic deletion of PARP are neuroprotective in stroke *(69,81)*. In nNOS knockout mice, PARP formation in the parietal cortex is reduced after focal ischemia.

Induction of Apoptosis

Cell death as a result of a massive surge in NO$^\bullet$ synthesis can initiate apoptosis in a variety of cell types. In cerebellar granule cells, NO$^\bullet$ donors elicit apoptosis by a mechanism that involves excitotoxic mediators, calcium overload, and activation of caspases. In endothelial cells, NO$^\bullet$ in large quantities induces apoptosis, whereas in small amounts it protects against apoptotic-inducing stimuli *(82)*. NO$^\bullet$ inhibits the activation of caspase-3 via a cGMP-dependent mechanism *(83)*, and directly inhibits the activity of several members of the caspase family by *S*-nitrosylation of reactive cysteine residues *(84,85)*.

PROTECTIVE MECHANISMS OF NO$^\bullet$ IN ISCHEMIC INJURY

The vast majority of strokes in humans are of thromboembolic origin *(86)*. Occlusion of cerebral vessels by circulating platelet emboli or dislodged vascular plaques injures both the vasculature and the parenchyma. Therefore, the hemodynamic actions of NO$^\bullet$ are very important in the restoration of CBF and in the direct and indirect prevention of platelet and leukocyte adhesion during reperfusion (*see* Table 3).

Effects on Vascular Tone and Perfusion

The immediate goal during an ischemic crisis is to restore adequate blood flow to the deprived tissue. Because endothelial NO$^\bullet$ regulates basal vascular tone, augmentation of

Table 4
Toxic and Protective Effects of NO$^•$ in Ischemia

	Toxic roles	Beneficial effects

Type I NOS—nNOS	Formation of OONO$^-$
	DNA deamination
	Inhibition of mitochondrial
	   respiratory enzymes
	   (acute injury)
		Scavenging of O$_2$ radicals
		NMDA–receptor nitrosylation
		   and inactivation

Type II NOS—iNOS	Formation of OONO$^-$ (late injury)	

Type III NOS—eNOS		Vasodilation and improved blood flow
		Inhibition of platelet adhesion and
		   aggregation
		Inhibition of leukocyte adhesion and
		   migration

endothelial NO$^•$ production would directly target this goal. Indeed, experimentally induced cerebral ischemia followed by intravascular NO$^•$-donor infusion or by L-arginine supplementation results in less severe tissue damage than if left untreated (87). Conversely, inhibition of eNOS in many models of stroke aggravates tissue damage and hypoperfusion, induces platelet aggregation, and worsens behavioral outcome.

Effects on Platelets and Leukocytes

NO$^•$ has effects on circulating platelets and leukocytes. Platelets contain soluble GC that mediates decreased platelet activation and aggregability following exposure to NO$^•$ (88). NO$^•$ blocks leukocyte adhesion, which would reduce the recruitment of inflammatory cells to the region. The expression of the intercellular adhesion molecule-1 (89,90) and the chemokines macrophage inflammatory protein-1a and monocyte chemoattractant protein-1 (91) are upregulated following focal ischemia and may play a role in recruitment of leukocytes and postischemic inflammatory processes. NO$^•$ may also be protective by inhibiting calcium fluxes through NMDA receptors (92).

SUMMARY

As in other organ systems, NO$^•$ plays multiple roles in normal brain physiology and in the pathophysiology of cerebral ischemia (see Table 4). Physiological roles of NO$^•$ in the brain include mediation of excitatory glutamate responses (nNOS), regulation of basal CBF (eNOS), coupling of local blood flow to neuronal metabolism (nNOS), and mediation of retrograde neurotransmission in synaptic plasticity (nNOS and eNOS). Under conditions of cerebral ischemia, NO$^•$ production from each of the three isoforms increases, although NO$^•$ generated early by nNOS and later by iNOS appears to contribute to neurotoxicity, whereas continued eNOS function appears important for minimizing ischemic damage. Toxic mechanisms of NO$^•$ include the formation of peroxynitrite, activation of PARP, and induction of apoptosis. Protective mechanisms of NO$^•$ include vasodilation and preservation of CBF, inhibition of platelet aggregation, and inhibition of leukocyte activation. These concepts have been demonstrated both in intact animals and in culture models, using a combination of pharmacological and genetic approaches. Understanding the precise contributions of each NOS isoforms to toxicity and protection in cerebral ischemia may allow the modulation of these responses by NO$^•$ donors, NOS inhibitors, and modulators of NOS expression such as the statins.

REFERENCES

1. Bredt DS, Snyder SH. Nitric oxide: a physiologic messenger molecule. Ann Rev Biochem 1994;63: 175–195.
2. Dawson TM, Dawson VL, Snyder SH. A novel neuronal messenger molecule in brain: the free radical, nitric oxide. Ann Neurol 1992;32(3): 297–311.
3. Garthwaite J, Charles SL, Chess-Williams R. Endothelium-derived relaxing factor release on activation of NMDA receptors suggests role as intercellular messenger in the brain. Nature 1988;336:385–388.
4. Bredt DS, Snyder SH. Isolation of nitric oxide synthetase, a calmodulin-requiring enzyme. Proc Natl Acad Sci USA 1990;87:682–685.
5. Thomas E, Pearse AG. The solitary active cells. Histologic demonstration of damage-resistant nerve cells with a TPN-diaphorease reaction. Acta Neuropathol 1964;3:238–249.
6. Vincent SR, Hope BT. Neurons that say NO. Trends Neurosci 1992;15:108–113.
7. Bredt DS, Glatt CE, Hwang PM, Fotuhi M, Dawson TM, Snyder SH. Nitric oxide synthase protein and mRNA are discretely localized in neuronal populations of the mammalian CNS together with NADPH diaphorase. Neuron 1991;7:615–624.
8. Dawson TM, Bredt DS, Fotuhi M, Hwang PM, Snyder SH. Nitric oxide synthase and neuronal NADPH diaphorase are identical in brain and peripheral tissues. Proc Natl Acad Sci USA 1991;88:6368–6371.
9. Gonzalez ZM, Ensz LM, Mukhina G, Lebovitz RM, Zwacka RM, Engelhardt JF, et al. Manganese superoxide dismutase protects nNOS neurons from NMDA and nitric oxide-mediated neurotoxicity. J Neurosci 1998;18(6):2040–2055.
10. Bredt DS, Hwang PM, Snyder SH. Localization of nitric oxide synthase indicating a neural role for nitric oxide. Nature 1990;347:768–770.
11. Tanaka K, Gotoh F, Gomi S, Takashima S, Mihara B, Shirai TNS, et al. Inhibition of nitric oxide synthesis induces a significant reduction in local cerebral blood flow in the rat. Neurosci Lett 1991;127:129–132.
12. Endres M, Laufs U, Huang Z, Nakamura T, Huang P, Moskowitz MA, et al. Stroke protection by 3-hydroxy-3-methylglutaryl (HMG)-CoA reductase inhibitors mediated by endothelial nitric oxide synthase. Proc Natl Acad Sci USA 1998;95:8880–8885.
13. Edelman GM, Gally JA. Nitric oxide: linking space and time in the brain. Proc Natl Acad Sci USA 1992; 89(24):11,651,11,652.
14. Dirnagl U, Niwa K, Lindauer U, Villringer A. Coupling of cerebral blood flow to neuronal activation: role of adenosine and nitric oxide. Am J Physiol 1994;267(1 Pt 2):H296–H301.
15. Northington FJ, Tobin JR, Koehler RC, Traystman RJ. In vivo production of nitric oxide correlates with NMDA-induced cerebral hyperemia in newborn sheep. Am J Physiol 1995;269(1 Pt 2):H215–H221.
16. Iadecola C, Xu X. Nitro-L-arginine attenuates hypercapnic cerebrovasodilation without affecting cerebral metabolism. Am J Physiol 1994;266(2 Pt 2):R518–R525.
17. Harada M, Fuse A, Tanaka Y. Measurement of nitric oxide in the rat cerebral cortex during hypercapnea. Neuroreport 1997;8(4):999–1002.
18. Schmetterer L, Findl O, Strenn K, Graselli U, Kastner J, Eichler HG, et al. Role of NO in the O2 and CO2 responsiveness of cerebral and ocular circulation in humans. Am J Physiol 1997;273:R2005–R2012.
19. Irikura K, Huang PL, Ma J, Lee WS, Dalkara T, Fishman MC, et al. Cerebrovascular alterations in mice lacking neuronal nitric oxide synthase gene expression. Proc Natl Acad Sci USA 1995;92(15):6823–6827.
20. Cholet N, Seylaz J, Lacombe P, Bonvento G. Local uncoupling of the cerebrovascular and metabolic responses to somatosensory stimulation after neuronal nitric oxide synthase inhibition. J Cereb Blood Flow Metab 1997;17(11):1191–1201.
21. Ma J, Ayata C, Huang PL, Fishman MC, Moskowitz MA. Regional cerebral blood flow response to vibrissal stimulation in mice lacking type I NOS gene expression. Am J Physion 1996;270:H1085–H1090.
22. Ayata C, Ma J, Meng W, Huang P, Moskowitz MA. L-NA-sensitive ICBF augmentation during vibrissal stimulation in type In nitric oxide synthase mutant mice. J Cereb Blood Flow Metab 1996;16:539–541.
23. Li J, Iadecola C. Nitric oxide and adenosine mediate vasodilation during functional activation in cerebellar cortex. Neuropharmacology 1994;33(11):1453–1461.
24. Ichinose F, Huang PL, Zapol WM. Effects of targeted neuronal nitric oxide synthase gene disruption and nitroG-L-arginine methylester on the threshold for 10 isoflurane anesthesia. Anesthesiology 1995; 83(1):101–108.
25. Crosby G, Marota JJ, Huang PL. Intact nociception-induced neuroplasticity in transgenic mice deficient in neuronal nitric oxide synthase. Neuroscience 1995;69:1013–1017.
26. O'Dell TJ, Hawkins RD, Kandel ER, Arancio O. Tests of the roles of two diffusable substances in long-term potentiation: evidence for nitric oxide as a possible early retrograde messenger. Proc Natl Acad Sci USA 1991;88:11,285–11,289.

27. Holscher C. Nitric oxide, the enigmatic neuronal messenger: its role in synaptic plasticity. Trends Neurosci 1997;20(7):298–303.
28. Bohme GA, Bon C, Lemaire M, Reibaud M, Piot O, Stutzmann JM, et al. Altered synaptic plasticity and memory formation in nitric oxide synthase inhibitor-treated rats. Proc Natl Acad Sci USA 1993;90(19): 9191–9194.
29. Schuman EM, Madison DV. A requirement for the intercellular messenger nitric oxide in long-term potentiation. Science 1991;254:1503–1506.
30. Haley JE, Wilcox GL, Chapman PF. The role of nitric oxide in hippocampal long-term potentiation. Neuron 1992;8:211–216.
31. Bannerman DM, Chapman PF, Kelly PA, Butcher SP, Morris RG. Inhibition of nitric oxide synthase does not prevent the induction of long-term potentiation in vivo. J Neurosci 1994;14(12):7415–7425.
32. Bannerman DM, Chapman PF, Kelly PA, Butcher SP, Morris RG. Inhibition of nitric oxide synthase does not impair spatial learning. J Neurosci 1994;14(12):7404–7414.
33. O'Dell TJ, Huang PL, Dawson TM, Dinerman JL, Snyder SH, Kandel ER, et al. Endothelial NOS and the blockade of LTP by NOS inhibitors in mice lacking neuronal NOS. Science 1994;265(5171):542–546.
34. Dinerman JL, Dawson TM, Schell MJ, Snowman A, Snyder SH. Endothelial nitric oxide synthase localized to hippocampal pyramidal cells: implications for synaptic plasticity. Proc Natl Acad Sci USA 1994;91(10):4214–4218.
35. Wendland B, Schweizer FE, Ryan TA, Nakane M, Murad F, Scheller RH, et al. Existence of nitric oxide synthase in rat hippocampal pyramidal cells. Proc Natl Acad Sci USA 1994;91:2151–2155.
36. Son H, Hawkins RD, Martin K, Kiebler M, Huang PL, Fishman MC, et al. Long-term potentiation is reduced in mice that are doubly mutant in endothelial and neuronal nitric oxide synthase. Cell 1996;87: 1015–1023.
37. Lev-Ram V, Nebyelul Z, Ellisman MH, Huang PL, Tsien RY. Absence of cerebellar long-term depression in mice lacking neuronal nitric oxide synthase. Learning Memory 1997;3:169–177.
38. Malinski T, Bailey F, Zhang ZG, Chopp M. Nitric oxide measured by a porphyrinic microsensor in rat brain after transient middle cerebral artery occlusion. J Cereb Blood Flow Metab 1993;13(3):355–358.
39. Globus M-T, Prado R, Sanchez-Ramos J, Dietrich WD, Ginsberg MD, Busto R. Excitotoxic and ischemic damage: role of nitric oxide. In: Krieglstein J, Oberpichler-Schwenk H, eds. Pharmacology of Cerebral Ischemia. Wissenschaftliche Verlagsgesellschaft, Stuttgart, Germany, 1994, pp. 363–373.
40. Iadecola C, Xu X, Zhang F, el-Fakahany EE, Ross ME. Marked induction of calcium-independent nitric oxide synthase activity after focal cerebral ischemia. J Cereb Blood Flow Metab 1995;15(1):52–59.
41. Stagliano N, Dietrich WD, Prado R, Green EJ, Busto R. The role of nitric oxide in the pathophysiology of thromboembolic stroke in the rat. Brain Res 1997;759(1):32–40.
42. Huang Z, Huang PL, Panahian N, Dalkara T, Fishman MC, Moskowitz MA. Effects of cerebral ischemia in mice deficient in neuronal nitric oxide synthase. Science 1994;265(5180):1883–1885.
43. Hara H, Ayata C, Huang PL, Waeber C, Ayata G, Fujii M, et al. [3H]L-NG-nitroarginine binding after transient focal ischemia and NMDA-induced excitotoxicity in type I and type III nitric oxide synthase null mice. J Cereb Blood Flow Metab 1997;17:515–526.
44. Zhang ZG, Chopp M, Bailey F, Malinski T. Nitric oxide changes in the rat brain after transient middle cerebral artery occlusion. J Neurol Sci 1995;128(1):22–27.
45. Zhang ZG, Chopp M, Zaloga C, Pollock JS, Forstermann U. Cerebral endothelial nitric oxide synthase expression after focal cerebral ischemia in rats. Stroke 1993;24(12):2016–2121.
46. Iadecola C, Zhang F, Casey R, Clark HB, Ross ME. Inducible nitric oxide synthase gene expression in vascular cells after transient focal cerebral ischemia. Stroke 1996;27(8):1373–1380.
47. Iadecola C, Zhang F, Casey R, Nagayama M, Ross M. Delayed reduction of ischemic brain injury and neurological deficits in mice lacking the inducible nitric oxide synthase gene. J Neurosci 1997;17(23): 9157–9164.
48. Iadecola C, Pelligrino DA, Moskowitz MA, Lassen NA. Nitric oxide synthase inhibition and cerebrovascular regulation. J Cereb Blood Flow Metab 1994;(2):175–192.
49. Iadecola C. Bright and dark sides of nitric oxide in ischemic brain injury. Trends Neurosci 1997;20: 132–139.
50. Lipton SA, Choi YB, Pan ZH, Lei SZ, Chen HS, Sucher NJ, et al. A redox-based mechanism for the neuroprotective and neurodestructive effects of nitric oxide and related nitroso-compounds. Nature 1993;364(6438):626–632.
51. Yoshida T, Limmroth V, Irikura K, Moskowitz MA. The NOS inhibitor, 7-nitroindazole, decreases focal infarct volume but not the response to topical acetylcholine in pial vessels. J Cereb Blood Flow Metab 1994;14:924–929.

52. Nagafuji T, Sugiyama M, Muto A, Makino T, Miyauchi T, Nabata H. The neuroprotective effect of a potent and selective inhibitor of type I NOS (L-MIN) in a rat model of focal cerebral ischaemia. Neuroreport 1995;6:1541–1545.

53. Zhang ZG, Reif D, Macdonald J, Tang WX, Kamp DK, Gentile RJ, et al. ARL 17477, a potent and selective neuronal NOS inhibitor decreases infarct volume after transient middle cerebral artery occlusion in rats. J Cereb Blood Flow Metab 1996;16:599–604.

54. Iadecola C, Zhang F, Xu X. Inhibition of inducible nitric oxide synthase ameliorates cerebral ischemic damage. Am J Physiol 1995;268(1 Pt 2):R286–R292.

55. Zhang F, Casey RM, Ross ME, Iadecola C. Aminoguanidine ameliorates and L-arginine worsens brain damage from intraluminal middle cerebral artery occlusion. Stroke 1996;27(2):317–323.

56. Huang PL, Dawson TM, Bredt DS, Snyder SH, Fishman MC. Targeted disruption of the neuronal nitric oxide synthase gene. Cell 1993;75(7):1273–1286.

57. Mashimo H, He XD, Huang PL, Fishman MC, Goyal RK. Neuronal constitutive nitric oxide synthase is involved in murine enteric inhibitory neurotransmission. J Clin Invest 1996;98:8–13.

58. Huang PL, Huang Z, Mashimo H, Bloch KD, Moskowitz MA, Bevan JA, et al. Hypertension in mice lacking the gene for endothelial nitric oxide synthase. Nature 1995;377(6546):239–242.

59. MacMicking JD, Nathan C, Hem G, Chartrain N, Fletcher DS, Trumbauer M, et al. Altered responses to bacterial infection and endotoxic shock in mice lacking inducible nitric oxide synthase. Cell 1995; 81(4):641–650.

60. Laubach VE, Shesely EG, Smithies O, Sherman PA. Mice lacking inducible nitric oxide synthase are not resistant to lipopolysaccaride-induced death. Proc Natl Acad Sci USA 1995;92:10,688–10,692.

61. Wei XQ, Charles IG, Smith A, Ure J, Feng GJ, Huang FP, et al. Altered immune responses in mice lacking inducible nitric oxide synthase. Nature 1995;375(6530):408–411.

62. Dawson VL, Kizushi VM, Huang PL, Snyder SH, Dawson TM. Resistance to neurotoxicity in cortical cultures from neuronal nitric oxide synthase-deficient mice. J Neurosci 1996;16(8):2479–2487.

63. Hara H, Huang PL, Panahian N, Fishman MC, Moskowitz MA. Reduced brain edema and infarction volume in mice lacking the neuronal isoform of nitric oxide synthase after transient MCA occlusion. J Cereb Blood Flow Metab 1996;16:605–611.

64. Panahian N, Yoshida T, Huang PL, Hedley-Whyte ET, Fishman MC, Moskowitz MA. Attenuated hippocampal damage after global cerebral ischemia in mice mutant in neuranal nitric oxide synthase. Neuroscience 1996;72:343–354.

65. Huang Z, Huang PL, Ma J, Meng W, Ayata C, Fishman MC, et al. Enlarged infarcts in endothelial nitric oxide synthase knockout mice are attenuated by nitro-L-arginine. J Cereb Blood Flow Metab1996;16: 981–987.

66. Lo E, Hara H, Rogowska J, Trocha M, Pierce AR, Huang PL, et al. Temporal correlation mapping analysis of the hemodynamic penumbra in mutant mice deficient in endothelial nitric oxide synthase gene expression. Stroke 1996;27:1381–1385.

67. Iadecola C, Zhang F, Casey R, Nagayama M, Ross ME. Delayed reduction of ischemic brain injury and neurological deficits in mice lacking the inducible nitric oxide synthase gene. J Neurosci 1997;17: 9157–9164.

68. Endres M, Scott G, Namura S, Salzman AL, Huang PL, Moskowitz MA, et al. Role of peroxynitrite and neuronal nitric oxide synthase in the activation of poly(ADP-ribose) synthetase in a murine model of cerebral ischemia-reperfusion. Neurosci Lett 1998;248:41–44.

69. Endres M, Scott GS, Salzman AL, Kun E, Moskowitz MA, Szabo C. Protective effects of 5-iodo-6-1,2-benzopyrone, an inhibitor of poly(ADP-ribose) synthetase against peroxynitrite-induced glial damage and stroke development. Eur J Pharmacol 1998;351:377–382.

70. Sacks FM, Pfeffer MA, Moye LA, Rouleau JL, Rutherford JD, Cole TG, et al. The effect of pravastatin on coronary events after myocardial infarction in patients with average cholesterol levels. Cholesterol and recurrent events trial investigators. N Engl J Med 1996;335:1001–1009.

71. Blauw GJ, Lagaay AM, Smelt AH, Westendorp RG. Stroke, statins, and cholesterol. A meta-analysis of randomized, placebo-controlled double-blind vials with HMG-CoA reduclase inhibitors. Stroke 1997; 28:946–950.

72. Laufs U, Fata VL, Liao JK. Inhibition of 3-hydroxy-3-methylglutaryl (HMG)-CoA reductase blocks hypoxia-mediated down-regulation of endothelial niuic oxide synthase. J Biol Chem 1997;272: 31,725–31,729.

73. Beekman JS, Ye YZ, Anderson PG, Chen J, Accavitti MA, Tarpey MM, et al. Extensive nitration of protein tyrosines in human atherosclerosis detected by immunohistochemistry. Biol Chem Hoppe-Seyler 1994;375:81–88.

74. Beckman JS, Chen J, Ischiropoulos H, Crow JP. Oxidative chemistry of peroxynitrite. Methods Enzymol 1994;233:229–240.
75. Crow JP, Ye YZ, Strong M, Kirk M, Barnes S, Beckman JS. Superoxide dismutase catalyzes nitration of tyrosines by peroxynitrite in the rod and head domains of neurofilament-L. J Neurochem 1997;69: 1945–1953.
76. Li X, De Sarno P, Song L, Beckman JS, Jope RS. Peroxyniuite modulates tyrosine phosphorylation and phosphoinositide signalling in human neuroblastoma SH-SY5Y cells: attenuated effects in human 1321N1 astrocytoma cells. Biochem J 1998;331:599–606.
77. Ayata C, Ayata G, Hara H, Matthews RT, Beal MF, Ferrante RJ, et al. Mechanisms of reduced striatal NMDA excitotoxicity in type I nitric oxide synthase knock-out mice. J Neurosci 1997;17:6908–6917.
78. Forman LJ, Liu P, Nagele RG, Yin K, Wong PY. Augmentation of nitric oxide, superoxide, and peroxynitrite production during cerebral ischemia and reperfusion in the rat. Neurochem Res 1998;23(2): 141–148.
79. Fukuyama N, Takizawa S, Ishida H, Hoshiai K, Shinohara Y, Nakazawa H. Peroxynitrite formation in focal cerebral ischemia-reperfusion in rats occurs predominantly in the peri-infarct region. J Cereb Blood Flow Metab 1998;18:123–129.
80. Endres M, Wang ZQ, Namura S, Waeber C, Moskowitz MA. Ischemic brain injury is mediated by the activation of poly(ADP-ribose) polymerase. J Cereb Blood Flow Metab 1997;17:1143–1151.
81. Eliasson MJ, Sampei K, Mandir AS, Hurn PD, Traystman RJ, Bao J, et al. Poly(ADP-ribose) polymerase gene disruption renders mice resistant to cerebral ischemia. Nat Med 1997;3:1089–1095.
82. Shen YH, Wang XL, Wilcken DEL. Nitric oxide induces and inhibits apoptosis through different pathways. FEBS Lett 1998;433:125–131.
83. Kim YM, Talanian RV, Billiar TR. Nitric oxide inhibits apoptosis by preventng increases in caspase-3-lile activity bia two distinct mechanisms. J Biol Chem 1997;272:31,138–31,148.
84. Haendeler J, Weiland U, Zeiher AM, Dimmeler S. Effects of redoxrelated congeners of NO on apoptosis and caspase-3 activity. Nitric Oxide 1997;1:284–293.
85. Li J, Billiar TR, Talanian RV, Kim YM. Nitric oxide reversibly inhibits seven members of the caspase family via S-nitrosylation. Biochem Biophys Res Commun 1997;240:419–424.
86. Camarata PJ, Heros RC, Latchaw RE. "Brain attack": the rationale for treating stroke as a medical emergency. Neurosurgery 1994;34:144–158.
87. Zhang F, White JG, Iadecola C. Nitric oxide donors increase blood flow and reduce brain damage in focal ischemia: evidence that nitric oxide is beneficial in the early stages of cerebral ischemia. J Cereb Blood Flow Metab 1994;14(2):217–226.
88. Radomski MW, Palmer RM, Moncada S. Modulation of platelet aggregation by an L-arginine-nitric oxide pathway. Trends Pharmacol Sci 1991,12:87,88.
89. Zhang RL, Chopp M, Zaloga C, Zhang ZG, Jiang N, Gautam SC, et al. The temporal profiles of ICAM-I protein and mRNA expression after transient MCA occlusion in the rat. Brain Res 1995;682(1–2): 182–188.
90. Zhang RL, Chopp M, Jiang N, Tang WX, Prostak J, Manning AM, et al. Anti-intercellular adhesion molecule-i antibody reduces ischemic cell damage after transient but not permanent middle cerebral artery occlusion in the Wistar rat. Stroke 1995;26(8):1438–1442.
91. Kim JS, Gautam SC, Chopp M, Zaloga C, Jones ML, Ward PA, et al. Expression of monocyte chemoattractant protein-1 and macrophage inflammatory protein-1 after focal cerebral ischemia in the rat. J Neuroimmunol 1995;56(2):127–134.
92. Lipton SA, Singel DJ, Stamler JS. Neuroprotective and neurodestructive effects of nitric oxide and redox congeners. Ann NY Acad Sci 1994;738:382–387.

21   The Role of Nitric Oxide in Ischemia-Reperfusion

Allan M. Lefer and Reid Hayward

PATHOPHYSIOLOGY OF ISCHEMIA-REPERFUSION

Considering the prevalence of ischemic cardiovascular disorders and the advent of thrombo-lytic therapies, percutaneous transluminal angioplasty, vascular bypass, and organ transplantation, ischemia and reperfusion of a vascular bed have become routine in the development, progression, and treatment of numerous cardiovascular disease states. The possibility that the reestablishment of blood flow in a previously ischemic region might injure cells that were viable at the time of reperfusion was suggested in the late 1970s (1) and later defined by Rosenkranz and Buckberg (2), and Braunwald and Kloner (3). Since that time, the patho-physiology of ischemia-reperfusion has been studied intensively and the series of events involved in this phenomenon are now more clearly defined. Ischemia-reperfusion produces tissue injury that is apparent within several hours of reperfusion and involves two distinct yet interrelated phases. These have been described as an endothelial triggering phase and a neutrophil amplification phase (4), both of which are closely linked to endothelium-derived nitric oxide (NO•).

Very early in the reperfusion period (i.e., within 2.5–5 min) (5) the endothelium becomes dysfunctional (i.e., endothelial triggering), characterized by an impaired elaboration of endo-thelium-dependent vasodilators (i.e., reduced endothelium-derived NO•). This is followed by an increased adhesiveness for leukocytes about 20 min after reperfusion. The resulting interactions between endothelial cells and leukocytes lead to neutrophil adherence to the endothelium and subsequent transmigration of many of them across the endothelium into the target tissue (Fig. 1). Activated neutrophils are capable of releasing numerous cytotoxic and chemotactic substances that serve to injure surrounding cells and attract still more neutro-phils (i.e., neutrophil amplification). In this process, endogenous NO• plays a key defensive role, as basal release of endothelium-derived NO• provides numerous beneficial effects to the vasculature. In situations such as ischemia-reperfusion, endothelial release of biologically active NO• is inhibited compromising the integrity and normal function of the endothelium.

Endothelial Dysfunction

The normal endothelium serves a variety of major homeostatic functions, all of which can be dramatically affected by ischemia-reperfusion. These functions include providing a non-thrombotic surface for blood flow, regulating vascular permeability, controlling vascular tone, and regulating leukocyte traffic. The endothelium is highly susceptible to functional alterations following ischemia-reperfusion and attenuation of endothelium-dependent vaso-dilation is a sensitive and early marker of endothelial dysfunction (5–7). This dysfunction has been shown to occur in the coronary (5–10), mesenteric (11), renal (12), cerebral (13), as well

From: *Contemporary Cardiology, vol. 4: Nitric Oxide and the Cardiovascular System*
Edited by: J. Loscalzo and J. A. Vita © Humana Press Inc., Totowa, NJ

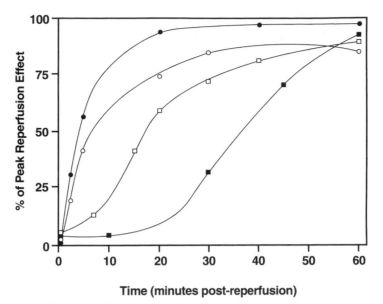

Fig. 1. Time course of key variables in splanchnic ischemia-reperfusion, including endothelial dysfunction, which occurs within 5 min of reperfusion; endothelial cell surface P-selectin expression, which closely follows endothelial dysfunction; PMN adherence, which occurs within 20 min post-reperfusion; and PMN accumulation in the reperfused tissue, which increases by 30 min postreperfusion. (Adapted from Hayward and Lefer [*11*].)

as limb *(14)* circulations. Ischemia for periods of up to 2–3 h with no reperfusion results in little change in the vascular response to endothelium-dependent vasodilators *(11,15)*, and there appears to be no histological evidence of significant endothelial injury until 4–6 h after ischemia *(15,16)*. However, if the ischemic vasculature is reperfused, endothelial dysfunction is an early and severe event. In a series of studies by our group, an impaired relaxation response to the endothelium-dependent vasodilator acetylcholine (ACh) was demonstrated as early as 2.5 min following reperfusion of the cat *(5)* and rat *(9)* coronary circulations as well as that of the rat mesenteric circulation *(11,17)*. In each of these studies, maximal endothelial dysfunction was observed by 20 min after reperfusion with no restoration of endothelial function noted at 270 min.

The key event in the development of endothelial dysfunction appears to be the generation of oxygen-derived free radicals, which can be produced by either the ischemic tissue or the activated leukocytes accumulating in the reperfused tissue. Although endothelial dysfunction occurs early in the reperfusion phase, this event is most likely preceded by the production of free radicals *(18)*. Possible sources of free radical production include pathways of catecholamine degradation *(19)*, prostaglandin synthesis *(20)*, and oxygen utilization by mitochondria *(21)*. However, it appears as though the primary source of these free radicals may be xanthine oxidase on the endothelial cell surface *(22–24)*. During ischemia, adenosine triphosphate (ATP) is degraded to hypoxanthine, and xanthine dehydrogenase is converted to xanthine oxidase. Upon reperfusion, xanthine oxidase catalyzes the conversion of hypoxanthine to uric acid, and superoxide is produced as a by-product *(25,26)*. Regardless of the chemical source of free-radical production, it is clear that large amounts of these substances are produced by the reperfused tissues *(27,28)* and subsequently contribute to endothelial dysfunction *(29,30)*.

Several studies have demonstrated that although free-radical production by the reperfused tissue does not account for all of the oxyradical-induced endothelial dysfunction following ischemia-reperfusion, it is a major contributor. Cultured endothelial cells from the bovine pulmonary artery *(31)*, rat brain capillary *(32)*, and human umbilical vein *(33)* exhibit signs of cellular injury following hypoxia and reoxygenation that were significantly attenuated by the addition of free radical scavengers. In an in vivo model of intestinal ischemia-reperfusion, the reperfused intestine was capable of producing free radicals even when perfused with lactated Ringer's solution devoid of blood cells *(34)*. The free radicals produced by reperfused tissue appears to be quite capable of causing severe endothelial dysfunction in the absence of other free-radical-producing cells such as neutrophils. This was demonstrated in rat hearts subjected to ischemia-reperfusion perfused with oxygenated buffer lacking blood cells *(9)*. The reperfused myocardium was shown to produce large amounts of superoxide radicals *(18)*, which leads to the development of severe endothelial dysfunction as evidenced by a depressed endothelium-dependent dilation (e.g., to ACh) to approx 25–30% of control values *(9,18)*. In each of these studies, endothelial dysfunction was attenuated by the administration of recombinant human superoxide dismutase (rhSOD). Thus, it appears as though superoxide radicals produced by the endothelium feed back directly on the endothelium where they inhibit vaso-relaxation by either quenching NO˙, reacting with it to produce peroxynitrite, or by inhibiting the ability of the endothelium to generate NO˙ *(35)*.

Neutrophil Involvement

Neutrophils have received considerable attention as a major component of the tissue injury associated with ischemia-reperfusion, as strategies designed to limit neutrophil activation and recruitment are quite effective at limiting tissue injury. Several investigators have demonstrated that by depletion of circulating leukocytes, the extent of cellular injury is substantially reduced following ischemia-reperfusion *(36–38)*. Once the endothelial cells have become dysfunctional, they demonstrate an increased adhesiveness for neutrophils, thus promoting neutrophil–endothelial cell interactions and exacerbating endothelial dysfunction *(39,40)*. Activation of the endothelium promotes the release of inflammatory mediators, such as oxygen-derived free radicals and platelet-activating factor (PAF), which in turn activate circulating neutrophils. Because unactivated neutrophils do not contribute to endothelial dysfunction, neutrophil activation is an important step in this sequence of events *(40, 41)*. Activated neutrophils are capable of releasing cytokines, proteases, leukotrienes, and oxygen-derived free radicals, all of which are capable of provoking tissue injury associated with ischemia-reperfusion.

One important proinflammatory mediator released by neutrophils is leukotriene B_4 (LTB$_4$), which is a potent chemotactic eicosanoid that activates neutrophils and promotes their adherence to the vascular endothelium *(42)*. Several studies have shown that LTB$_4$ antagonists attenuate neutrophil-mediated injury following ischemia-reperfusion in rat *(43)* and cat *(44)* intestine. Activated neutrophils are also capable of releasing proteases, such as elastase and cathepsin G, which are thought to mediate a significant degree of tissue injury. Elastase is capable of cleaving peptides from proteins that may promote leukocyte rolling and adherence. This serine protease also contributes to the degradation of structural components of the vasculature *(45,46)* allowing neutrophils and other leukocytes to extravasate through the endothelial barrier and accumulate within the reperfused tissue. Cathepsin G also contributes to tissue injury by enhancing the activity of elastase *(47)*, and by stimulating the release of factors involved in neutrophil chemotaxis, such as PAF and LTB$_4$, from activated neutrophils *(48)*. Inhibition of LTB$_4$ *(43)* or PAF *(49)* also preserves endothelial function and maintains NO˙ release by the endothelium. Moreover, inhibition of proteases including elastase and cathepsin G have been shown to be effective at limiting neutrophil accumulation in the reperfused myocardium *(50,51)* and intestine *(52)*.

Oxygen-derived free radicals can exert a wide range of effects on both intracellular and extracellular components of reperfused tissues, thus altering structural and functional characteristics following reperfusion *(53)*. Neutrophil-derived free radicals can initiate lipid peroxidation, alter membrane permeability, and inactivate endothelium-derived NO$^\bullet$. In addition, free radicals may impair sarcolemmal or sarcoplasmic reticular function and lead to alterations in calcium handling, which could subsequently enhance injury by eliciting cellular dysfunction. We have studied the effects of rhSOD and N-(2-mercaptoproprionyl)-glycine (MPG), superoxide and hydroxyl radical scavengers, respectively, following ischemia-reperfusion of the myocardium *(5,9,54)*. rhSOD consistently provides a significant degree of tissue protection as evidenced by a preservation of endothelial function and an attenuation in myocardial necrosis or intestinal injury *(5,55,56)*. In contrast, MPG did not result in cardioprotection in either the isolated perfused rat heart *(9)* or the in vivo cat heart *(5)* suggesting that superoxide, and not hydroxyl radical, plays a primary role in eliciting tissue injury following ischemia-reperfusion.

Endogenous NO$^\bullet$

Endogenous NO$^\bullet$ is produced by endothelial cells at basal concentrations of about 1–10 nM *(57,58)* and has a half-life of only 10–20 s in physiological solutions *(59,60)*. NO$^\bullet$ is a highly soluble gas capable of diffusing readily across cell membranes to adjacent cells as well as into the vascular space. Upon reaching its target, NO$^\bullet$ exerts a variety of physiological effects that contribute to vascular homeostasis as reviewed in detail throughout the book. These effects include the physiologic regulation of vascular tone, inhibition of platelet aggregation, attenuation of leukocyte adherence to the endothelium, scavenging oxygen-derived free radicals, maintenance of normal vascular permeability, inhibition of smooth muscle proliferation, and stimulation of endothelial cell regeneration *(58,61)*. Endogenous NO$^\bullet$ release from constitutive NO$^\bullet$ synthase located in endothelial cells (eNOS) can be accomplished by two mechanisms. First, pulselike NO$^\bullet$ release from can be stimulated by any of several agonists including ACh, ATP, adenosine diphosphate (ADP), thrombin, bradykinin, substance P, and the calcium ionophore A23187 *(58,62,63)*. Second, low amounts of NO$^\bullet$ are continuously released under basal conditions *(57,58)*, which appears to be the primary mode of endogenous NO$^\bullet$ release and is the major factor regulating vascular tone and leukocyte–endothelial cell interaction. This is demonstrated by the use of NOS inhibitors, such as N^G-nitro-L-arginine-methyl ester (L-NAME) or N^G-monomethyl-L-arginine (L-NMMA), which results in increases in mean arterial blood pressure in vivo, or vasoconstriction of isolated vascular rings *(64)*, and increased leukocyte rolling and adherence in vivo *(65)*.

It is now well established that ischemia-reperfusion results in severe dysfunction of the affected endothelium characterized by a reduction in the release of NO$^\bullet$ resulting in a significantly attenuated vasodilator response following stimulation with several endothelium-dependent vasodilators. Classic studies by Tsao et al. *(5)*, Mehta et al. *(7)*, and Van Benthuysen et al. *(10)* showed that following myocardial ischemia-reperfusion, vascular relaxation was significantly blunted in response to several endothelium-dependent vasodilators. These studies demonstrated an inability of eNOS to release NO$^\bullet$ in response to selected stimuli. However, what may be of greater importance following ischemia-reperfusion is a diminution in the basal release of NO$^\bullet$. Ma et al. *(66)* demonstrated that not only did coronary artery rings isolated from cats subjected to ischemia-reperfusion exhibit a blunted relaxation to acetylcholine, but these artery rings also failed to constrict significantly when incubated with the NOS inhibitor L-NAME. The fact that L-NAME resulted in markedly reduced vasoconstriction suggests that there is a significant reduction in basal NO$^\bullet$ release from these ischemic-reperfused coronary vessels.

The mechanisms responsible for the inhibition of NO$^\bullet$ production from the endothelium following ischemia-reperfusion are still uncertain, although several possibilities exist to explain this phenomenon. First, exogenous administration of L-arginine, the substrate utilized by NOS to synthesize NO$^\bullet$, was shown to provide protective effects following ischemia-reperfusion. Weyrich et al. *(67)* reported that intravascular administration of L-arginine preserved endothelial function and attenuated neutrophil-mediated myocardial injury in feline ischemia-reperfusion. At the same time, others *(62)* reported similar findings in dogs subjected to myocardial ischemia-reperfusion. Moreover, administration of D-arginine, the stereoisomer of L-arginine, was ineffective under the same conditions. These data are supported by the work of Kubes et al. *(68)*, who demonstrated that leukocyte adherence to postcapillary venular endothelium is increased up to 15-fold with the administration of L-NAME and that this response is completely reversed with the simultaneous administration of L-arginine. This has been confirmed for leukocyte adherence and extended to leukocyte rolling by Davenpeck et al. *(65)*. Second, production of oxygen-derived free radicals may account for much of the decrease in endothelial production of NO⁺ following ischemia-reperfusion. The large burst of free radicals generated from reperfused tissues *(7,35)* or localized neutrophils *(9,69)* could combine with endogenous NO⁺, rendering it inactive by quenching *(35,69)*. Third, the formation of NO⁺ via NOS requires several cofactors including nicotinamide adenine dinucleotide phosphate (NADPH), Ca^{2+}/calmodulin, flavin nucleotides, and tetrahydrobiopterin (BH_4), the availability of which may be compromised following ischemia-reperfusion. In this connection, Tiefenbacher et al. *(70)* observed the effects of the precursor to BH_4, sepiapterin, or a synthetic BH_4, 6-methyltetrahydropterin (MH_4), on left anterior descending coronary artery endothelial function following ischemia-reperfusion. Their results showed that endothelium-dependent relaxation was preserved when isolated rings were incubated with either sepiapterin or MH_4, and this response was completely reversed after the washout of either substance *(70)*. Thus, there are several means available to preserve NO⁺ formation following ischemia and reperfusion.

The consequences of a loss of endogenous NO⁺ production following ischemia-reperfusion could be diverse and far reaching. Decreased NO⁺ can promote severe vasoconstriction *(66)* and vasospasm *(41,71)*, which may contribute to the no-reflow phenomenon observed following ischemia-reperfusion. The loss of NO⁺ production also promotes the release of platelet-derived proinflammatory mediators, such as thromboxane A_2 and PAF, and facilitates platelet aggregation. In addition, reduced NO⁺ production following ischemia-reperfusion leads to an increase in neutrophil adherence to the coronary or mesenteric vascular endothelium *(66,72)*. Thus, the loss of endogenous NO⁺ production leads to a series of events that results in endothelial dysfunction and neutrophil-mediated tissue injury.

ROLE OF NO⁺ IN LEUKOCYTE–ENDOTHELIUM INTERACTION

Since endothelium-derived relaxing factor was identified as NO⁺ or a NO⁺ carrying nitroso-substance *(59,73)*, considerable attention has focused on the biological properties of NO⁺, particularly in relation to leukocyte–endothelial cell interactions. The migration of polymorphonuclear neutrophils (PMN) from the circulation to inflammatory sites has been described as a three-step process *(74)*. First, the vascular endothelium must recognize and capture circulating leukocytes, which results in the characteristic rolling action along the endothelial surface. While rolling, leukocytes strengthen their adhesive forces with the endothelium and subsequently become firmly adherent to endothelial cells. Finally, many of the adherent PMNs subsequently diapedese between endothelial cells in the endothelial monolayer and come in close proximity to the target tissue where they are able to produce their injurious effects. In this connection, both endogenous and exogenous NO⁺ sources have the potential to act as powerful anti-inflammatory agents at various levels in the processes underlying ischemia-reperfusion, from the inhibition of adhesion molecule function to the downregulation of specific genes that encode for adhesion molecules and cytokines.

Leukocyte Rolling and Adherence

Leukocyte rolling along the endothelium is primarily regulated by the selectin family of adhesion molecules, designated as P-, E-, and L-selectin. Following ischemia-reperfusion of the feline myocardium, maximal surface expression of endothelial P-selectin occurs approx 10–20 min following reperfusion and remains elevated, although at subpeak levels for as long as 270 min (75). Similar results have been shown following intestinal ischemia-reperfusion with increases in P-selectin expression occurring as early as 5–10 min following reperfusion and elevated levels seen as long as 120 min postreperfusion (11). Neutrophils stimulated with chemotactic agents such as those generated during ischemia-reperfusion result in a rapid increase in the binding affinity of surface expressed L-selectin, which is followed by a shedding of L-selectin from the cell surface (76,77). The relative importance of P- and L-selectin in the development and progression of the inflammatory response to ischemia-reperfusion is becoming increasingly recognized. Kubes et al. (78) studied the relative contribution of P- and L-selectin to leukocyte rolling in the postischemic vasculature. Their results showed monoclonal antibodies (MAbs) directed against either P- or L-selectin attenuated leukocyte rolling to a similar degree in ischemia-reperfusion. However, this effect was not additive with simultaneous administration of mAbs, suggesting that these adhesion molecules may serve as reciprocal ligands for one another. E-selectin is not constitutively expressed and is not significantly upregulated on endothelial cells until 4–6 h following reperfusion (75). The majority of evidence suggests that E-selectin plays little or no role in the first several hours of reperfusion.

Leukocyte adherence to the endothelium is largely governed by the interaction between integrins and members of the immunoglobulin (Ig)-like family of adhesion proteins. The primary integrin responsible for firm leukocyte adhesion to the endothelium is the CD11/CD18 complex coupled to intercellular adhesion molecule-1 (ICAM-1). CD18 exists as a low-affinity adhesion molecule under basal conditions, and on stimulation, undergoes a conformational change that produces a high-affinity state. Leukocyte rolling in postcapillary venules is not affected by the administration of a CD18-specific MAb, yet the antibody is effective at reducing leukocyte adherence to venular endothelium at a variety of shear rates (79–81). Kubes et al. (68) demonstrated that a CD18 MAb was not only capable of reducing adherence in the mesenteric microvasculature, but in the setting of ischemia-reperfusion, administration of CD18-specific MAb also results in a significant attenuation in leukocyte adherence and prevents the accumulation of neutrophils in the reperfused myocardium (82).

Of the Ig-like adhesion molecules, ICAM-1 and platelet-endothelial cell adhesion molecule (PECAM-1) play a primary role in the pathophysiology of ischemia-reperfusion. Anti-ICAM-1 Abs have been shown to limit leukocyte-mediated tissue injury following ischemia-reperfusion of the liver (83), kidney (84), mesentery (85), cremaster muscle (86), and heart (87,88). Anti-PECAM-1 Abs are also effective at inhibiting leukocyte accumulation in inflamed tissues, primarily by limiting the process of diapedesis or transmigration through the vasculature (89,90). Intravital microscopy studies of the mesenteric vasculature have shown that the large increases in leukocyte rolling and adherence that follow stimulation with tumor necrosis factor-α (TNF-α) (90), L-NAME, or hydrogen peroxide (H_2O_2) (91) were unaffected by pretreatment with an anti-PECAM-1 Ab. However, pretreatment with the anti-PECAM-1 Ab was effective at inhibiting the transmigration of leukocytes. Electron microscopic analysis of vascular segments showed that although leukocytes were able to penetrate interendothelial cell junctions, they were unable to traverse the basement membrane (90). Moreover, antibodies directed against PECAM-1 have been shown to protect the ischemic, reperfused myocardium against reperfusion injury (92,93).

NO• and Cell Adhesion Molecules

Both endogenous and exogenous NO• are capable of exerting powerful effects on the suppression of the inflammatory process, which are mediated in large part by the regulation of adhesion molecule function and expression. There is ample evidence demonstrating that NO• regulates cell adhesion molecule expression in the first few minutes following reperfusion as well as over several hours. In the short term (i.e., minutes), NO• can downregulate the surface expression of several adhesion molecules, suggesting that there is a direct effect of NO• on either the signaling pathway or the translocation of these molecules to the cell surface, whereas in the longer term (i.e., hours) NO• can inhibit the function of transcription factors that encode for proteins involved in the inflammatory process.

Ischemia-reperfusion of the mesenteric circulation, which reduces endothelial NO• production, increases the number of rolling and adherent leukocytes during the first 30 min following reperfusion (94). In addition, immunohistochemical analysis of the mesenteric microcirculation shows a progressive increase in the surface expression of P-selectin during this time period (11). Therefore, during reperfusion, when NO• production is severely compromised, P-selectin surface expression is markedly upregulated, and this response may be at least partially caused by a net production of free radicals. Under these conditions, Gauthier et al. (72) demonstrated that administration of the NO• donor S-nitroso-N-acetyl penicillamine (SNAP) completely eliminated the ischemia-reperfusion-induced increase in leukocyte rolling and adherence in the mesenteric microvasculature. In addition, SNAP treatment decreased the surface expression of P-selectin on the postcapillary venular endothelium. Davenpeck et al. (65) demonstrated that superfusion of the mesenteric circulation with L-NAME simulated the effects of ischemia-reperfusion. L-NAME increased leukocyte rolling, leukocyte adherence, as well as in P-selectin expression, and these effects were markedly attenuated by the coadministration of L-arginine but not of D-arginine. Similar beneficial effects of NO• donors have been reported in cats undergoing regional myocardial ischemia-reperfusion of the left anterior descending coronary artery (LAD). Occlusion of the LAD for 90 min resulted in a rapid increase in P-selectin expression (75) along with a 3-fold increase in neutrophil adherence to the ischemic-reperfused LAD (66) 20 min following reperfusion. Moreover, administration of an NO• donor just prior to reperfusion inhibited neutrophil adherence to the ischemic-reperfused LAD and reduced the number of myocardial microvessels expressing surface P-selectin (50).

NO• also appears to exert control over both constitutively expressed ICAM-1 as well as ICAM-1 expression upregulated during reperfusion. Biffl et al. (95) reported that approx 20% of cultured human endothelial cells positively expressed ICAM-1 under basal normoxic conditions. However, incubation of these cells with the NO• donor 3-morpholinosydnonimine reduced the number of ICAM-1 positive cells by 50%. When NO• production is inhibited, such as in ischemia-reperfusion, hypoxia-reoxygenation, or the administration of NOS inhibitors, surface expressed ICAM-1 is upregulated (75,91,96). Kupatt et al. (97) recently described the role of NO• in regulating ICAM-1 surface expression. They showed that the incubation of endothelial cells during hypoxia-reoxygenation with the NOS inhibitor nitro-L-arginine exacerbated both the increase in ICAM-1 expression and the free radical production observed following hypoxia-reoxygenation. However, incubation of cells with SNAP during hypoxia-reoxygenation resulted in a 50% reduction in surface expression of ICAM-1 and a 35% reduction in the production of free radicals compared to cells undergoing hypoxia-reoxygenation in the absence of SNAP. Thus, numerous studies demonstrate an inverse relationship between NO• levels and adhesion molecule expression, such that reduced NO• upregulates cell adhesion molecules, whereas increased NO• downregulate these CAMs.

The mechanisms involved in the regulation of cell adhesion molecules by NO• in the first hour of reperfusion are attributable in large part to interactions with oxygen-derived free radicals and their cell-signaling processes. Oxygen derived free radicals are potent stimulators of adhesion molecule expression on neutrophils (98,99) and endothelial cells (100–102), and free radical production is dramatically increased following ischemia- reperfusion (9, 18,24,28). Under normal conditions, NO• acts as an endogenous inhibitor of free radicals, thereby attenuating the upregulation of adhesion molecules and limiting leukocyte–endothelial cell interactions. However, under conditions such as ischemia-reperfusion, when there is marked oxidant stress, net NO• production is substantially reduced. When the production of NO• is compromised, cell adhesion molecules are upregulated and leukocyte–endothelial cell interactions are enhanced. This is exemplified by the fact that inhibition of NO• synthesis increases leukocyte–endothelial cell interactions and adhesion molecule expression, whereas administration of rhSOD completely eliminates L-NAME-induced increased rolling, adherence, and P-selectin expression (65). Similarly, reducing the production of free radicals generated following hypoxia-reoxygenation attenuated ICAM-1 expression on microvascular endothelial cells (97). These data, along with those from many other studies, are consistent with the concept that free radical generation is responsible for the upregulation of cell adhesion molecules on the endothelium, and that NO• plays an integral role in modulating upregulation of adhesion molecules.

Protein kinase C (PKC) is a cytosolic enzyme involved in the pathway of translocation of P-selectin to the cell surface and has been shown to be regulated by NO•. Activation of PKC promotes the rapid upregulation of surface expressed P-selectin on platelets (103) and endothelial cells (104), which, in turn, leads to an increase in cell–cell interactions (103,104). NO• may directly inhibit PKC activity by S-nitrosation of protein thiols (105) or by the stimulation of soluble guanylyl cyclase to produce cyclic guanosine monophosphate (cGMP) (106). Murohara et al. (103) demonstrated that either SNAP or the stable cGMP analog 8-bromo-guanosine 3',5'-cyclic monophosphate (8-Br-cGMP) inhibits P-selectin expression and neutrophil adherence under conditions in which endogenous NO• production was compromised. In addition, a specific PKC inhibitor inhibited P-selectin expression and neutrophil adherence to a similar degree as SNAP and 8-Br-cGMP. Data corroborating these in vitro studies has been obtained in vivo. The simultaneous superfusion of the mesenteric microcirculation with L-NAME and 8-Br-cGMP attenuates leukocyte rolling, leukocyte adherence, as well as the number of venules staining positively for P-selectin (65). Moreover, administration of low doses of the PKC inhibitor N,N,N-trimethylsphingosine (TMS) inhibited L-NAME-induced leukocyte rolling and adherence in the mesenteric microvasculature and attenuated P-selectin expression on platelets and endothelial cells (107). TMS also attenuated the in vivo neutrophil accumulation in the left ventricular free wall following regional myocardial ischemia-reperfusion suggestive of an inhibition in leukocyte–endothelial cell interaction via an inhibition of P-selectin expression (107).

Although there is considerable evidence linking NO• and P-selectin in the process of leukocyte–endothelial cell interactions, recent data suggest PECAM-1 may also be closely regulated by NO•. Our group recently (91) demonstrated that PECAM-1 may be upregulated in inflammatory states relevant to ischemia-reperfusion. Thus, it appears that NO• is prominently involved in the control of PECAM-1 in the microvasculature.

NO• Regulation of Endothelial Gene Expression

The presence of NO• clearly acts as a powerful antioxidant and interrupts cellular-signaling processes, both of which are involved in the rapid upregulation of cell adhesion molecules. Because adhesion molecules are upregulated and cytokines are released during the hours following reperfusion of an ischemic vascular bed, their long-term function depends on de novo protein synthesis. Liao and coworkers (108–110) have demonstrated that NO• is a primary regulatory factor for the synthesis of several proinflammatory proteins. Their studies showed that following stimulation, cultured endothelial cells incubated with one of several NO• donors demonstrate an attenuation in vascular cellular adhesion molecule-1 (VCAM-1) expression by up to 55%, whereas the inhibition of endogenous NO• with (L-NMMA) markedly increased VCAM-1 expression (108). Moreover, addition of an NO• donor resulted in a reduction in VCAM-1 mRNA, which translated into a decrease in monocyte adherence to stimulated endothelial cells. Similarly, Spiecker et al. (110) showed that several NO• donors

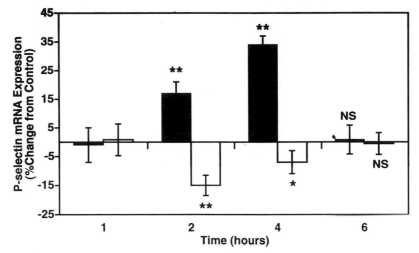

Fig. 2. The effect of L-NAME (3 m*M*) and the NO• donor SPM-5185 (10 μ*M*) on P-selectin mRNA expression in cultured human internal iliac vein endothelial cells at 1, 2, 4, and 6 h. Inhibition of endogenous NO• by L-NAME markedly increased P-selectin mRNA, whereas SPM-5185 attenuated P-selectin mRNA. (Modified from Armstead et al. [*111*].)

attenuate surface expression of ICAM-1, VCAM-1, and E-selectin following stimulation with TNF-α. We have demonstrated that NO• is also involved in the regulation of P-selectin protein synthesis and surface expression on human cultured iliac vein endothelial cells (*111*). Cells incubated with L-NAME showed an increase in P-selectin mRNA expression as well as an increase in P-selectin protein synthesis, both of which were reversed by the addition of L-arginine or an NO• donor. Similar results have been obtained in cultured endothelial cells stimulated by hypoxia-reoxygenation or TNF-α in which the administration of NOS inhibitors enhanced the accumulation of VCAM-1 and ICAM-1 mRNA (*97,112*). Eppihimer et al. (*113*) observed increases in P-selectin expression and P-selectin mRNA in the small intestine following 20 min of ischemia and variable periods of reperfusion. Their results showed that P-selectin expression was increased at 10 and 30 min following reperfusion with maximal expression observed at 5 h and a return to baseline levels at 24 h. The maximal increase in expression observed at 5 h could be attenuated by an NO• donor. In addition, P-selectin mRNA demonstrated a linear increase up to 5 h following reperfusion (Fig. 2). These data suggest that the sustained surface expression of P-selectin during the hours following reperfusion is dependent on the synthesis of new protein, and that this process is regulated in large part by NO•.

With this background, it is clear that NO• is a key factor influencing the synthesis of proinflammatory proteins and it follows that NO• may be exerting its effects at the transcriptional level most likely by regulation of transcription factors. Protein synthesis is regulated by a host of transcription factors that serve as molecular switches and regulators of various cellular actions, such as gene expression, cytokine production, and the production of other regulatory substances. One of these transcription factors is nuclear factor-κB (NF-κB), which regulates the expression of several genes that are involved in the inflammatory processes of ischemia-reperfusion. NF-κB induces the rapid expression of TNF-α and -β, several interleukins (IL) (IL-1β, IL-2, IL-6, IL-11, IL-12, IL-17), chemokines (IL-8, MIP-1, MCP-1, RANTES), enzymes (inducible nitric oxide synthase, inducible cyclooxygenase), and adhesion molecules (ICAM-1, VCAM-1, E-selectin, P-selectin) (*114,115*). Although NF-κB is regulated by several factors in the setting of ischemia-reperfusion, it appears that reoxygenation is the key stimulus. Ischemia or hypoxia alone is not a sufficient stimulus for the upregulation of NF-κB, as neither 90 min of ischemia in vivo *(75)* nor 20 h of hypoxia in vitro *(97)* were capable of upregulating surface expression of ICAM-1. This suggestion is supported by observations that hypoxia alone resulted in minimal activation of NF-κB and ICAM-1 mRNA, whereas marked increases in NF-κB and ICAM-1 mRNA were observed as early as 30–60 min following reoxygenation *(97)*.

Several studies suggests that NO· regulates expression of these proteins via interactions with the NF-κB transcription factor and its related proteins. Lander et al. *(116)* demonstrated that NO· activates protein phosphatases, suggesting that NO· inhibits NF-κB activation by preventing the phosphorylation of the inhibitory protein IκBα and its subsequent dissociation from NF-κB. By maintaining the interaction between the inhibitory protein IκBα and NF-κB, upregulation of adhesion molecules is inhibited. Cultured coronary endothelial cells incubated with *N*-acetyl-leucinyl-leucinyl-norleucinal, a proteasome inhibitor that blocks the degradation of IκBα, exhibited reduced ICAM-1 expression following hypoxia-reoxygenation *(97)*. Similarly, stimulation of endothelial cells with proinflammatory cytokines increases NF-κB activity, IκBα degradation, and surface expression of ICAM-1, VCAM-1, and E-selectin *(110)*. However, an NO· donor decreased NF-κB activity, prevented IκBα degradation, attenuated ICAM-1 expression, and completely eliminated the surface expression of VCAM-1 and E-selectin *(110)*.

Oxygen-derived free radicals have been shown to stimulate protein kinase C activity and activate NF-κB *(117,118)*. Cultured cells exposed to hypoxia-reoxygenation produce large amounts of free radicals, which correlates well with NF-κB activation and this response can be markedly attenuated with an NO· donor *(97)*. Moine et al. *(119)* showed that blocking xanthine oxidase activity not only prevented NF-κB activation by directly inhibiting the generation of oxygen-derived free radicals, but this treatment also increased IκBα. In addition, Peng et al. *(109)* demonstrated that NO· stabilized IκBα preventing its dissociation from NF-κB and increased the expression of IκBα, in essence making more inhibitor available to bind to NF-κB. These investigators *(109)* further demonstrated that inhibition of endogenous production of NO· resulted in a significant increase in NF-κB activation. Thus, since NO· has been shown to inactivate oxygen-derived free radicals and either directly or indirectly increase levels of inhibitory proteins, NO· prevents the formation of substances that activate NF-κB, as well as enhancing the activity of proteins that inhibit NF-κB. It appears that a diminution in NO· production, which occurs within min following ischemia-reperfusion, leads to a dissociation of IκBα from NF-κB and a decrease in the synthesis of the IκBα, promoting the synthesis of endothelium-derived proinflammatory proteins including enzymes, cytokines, and adhesion molecules.

ADMINISTRATION
OF NO· IN REPERFUSION INJURY

As enunciated at the beginning of this chapter, it is very clear there is a marked functional deficit in endothelium-derived nitric oxide (EDNO) following reperfusion of an ischemic vasculature. Therefore, one must conclude that a functional deficit exists in releasable NO· by the endothelium. That being the situation, we hypothesized that replacement of physiological levels of NO· could ameliorate the well-known reperfusion injury observed on reestablishment of flow following total occlusion of the left anterior descending (LAD) branch of the left coronary artery (MI/R) or of the splanchnic vasculature (SAO/R). These experiments were started in 1990 and led to a new paradigm in assessing reperfusion injury. Thus, the role of NO· in reperfusion injury will be analyzed in the following ways: (1) addition of authentic NO·; (2) use of NO· donating compounds (i.e., NO· donors); (3) administration of precursors of NO· (L-arginine); (4) use of NO· metabolites (peroxynitrite); and (5) inhibition of nitric oxide synthases (NOS).

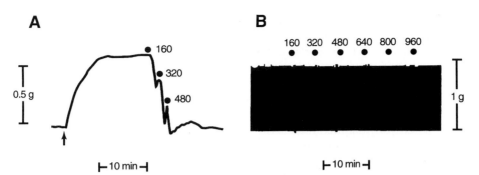

Fig. 3. Representative recordings of the response to solutions of NO• of an isolated cat coronary artery ring and an isolated cat papillary muscle, both isolated from the same heart. The numbers above the dots indicate the concentration of NO• in nM. The coronary artery ring was precontracted with 100 nM U-46619 (arrow) and the papillary muscle was electrically paced at 1 Hz with pulses of 5-ms duration. Calibrations are 0.5 g of force and 10 min time. At 480 nM, NO• completely relaxed the coronary artery ring, whereas 960 nM NO• did not produce any decrease in cardiac contractile force. (From Weyrich et al. [*125*].)

Authentic NO•

The first study to show that NO• could protect against reperfusion injury was reported by Aoki et al. (*120*), who infused authentic NO• gas into cats subjected to occlusion of the celiac, superior mesenteric, and inferior mesenteric arteries for 120 min. The NO• gas was dissolved in saline and infused close to the site of ischemia starting 5 min prior to reperfusion. NO• markedly attenuated postreperfusion hypotension, lysosomal disruption, enhanced plasma proteolysis, and formation of a cardiotoxic peptide known as MDF (*120,121*). These salutary effects of physiologic levels of NO• led to a significant improvement in survival time and a clear moderation of splanchnic ischemia shock. Shortly thereafter, Johnson et al. (*122*) extended these findings to feline myocardial ischemia reperfusion. In these experiments, NO• gas in solution was infused intravascularly following 80 min of a 90-min LAD occlusion, and continuing over the 4.5-h reperfusion period. The NO• solution was also bioassayed on isolated cat aortic rings for vasorelaxant activity to ensure that active NO• was infused throughout the reperfusion period. The NO• infusion did not significantly alter mean arterial blood pressure or heart rate. The beneficial effects of NO• infusion included a marked attenuation of cardiac necrosis and reduced neutrophil infiltration (*122*). NaNO$_2$ at pH 7.4, used as a control, was ineffective in these indices of cardioprotection.

One of the concerns of administering NO• gas to animals in myocardial ischemia is the purported negative inotropic effect of NO• (*123*). However, this effect is quite small, only constituting a 5–7% decrease in cardiac contractility (*123,124*). Moreover, these studies were done with NOS inhibitors or NO• donors. When authentic NO• gas was given to cat or rat papillary muscles, virtually no negative inotropic effect was observed (*125*). Only when these cardiac muscle preparations were maximally stimulated with norepinephrine was a modest (i.e., 5–7%) negative inotropic effect observed. This lack of inotropicity of NO• has been confirmed in the intact animal (*126,127*) using NO• donors. The major reason for this lack of effect of NO• on cardiac muscle presumably is the high myoglobin levels in cardiac myocytes that soak up the NO• before it can exert an inotropic effect.

Figure 3 illustrates the effect of NO• on a coronary artery ring and a right ventricular papillary muscle obtained from the same cat heart. At a NO• concentration of 480 nM, complete vasorelaxation of the coronary artery occurred, whereas NO• concentrations from 160–980 nM failed to decrease contractility of the cat papillary muscle at all (*125*).

Similarly, a variety of NO• donors also failed to reduce cardiac contractility in these right ventricular cat papillary muscles as well as in left ventricular rat papillary muscles. A similar lack of inotropic effect for these agents was observed in electrically stimulated isolated cardiomyocytes *(125)* clearly showing that diffusion distance is not the explanation for the lack of inotropic effect of NO• in papillary muscles.

Although isolated cardiac muscle preparations are useful for illustrating direct inotropicity, many cardiovascular investigators prefer to employ the intact heart *in situ*. Several well-executed and carefully controlled studies show that NO• or NO• donors do not exert any measurable negative inotropic effect in dogs *(126,127)*. In fact, inhibition of NO• synthesis exacerbates cardiac stunning in the conscious dog *(128)*. Thus, use of reasonable doses of NO• or of NO• donors in myocardial ischemia-reperfusion should not result in cardiodepression. If that were the case, nitroglycerin and nitroprusside would be hazardous in myocardial ischemia rather than therapeutic in these situations.

In addition to using NO• dissolved in aqueous media, NO• gas can be inhaled. Zapol and colleagues *(129)* have pioneered the use of inhaled NO• at low concentrations (i.e., 20–80 ppm) as a selective pulmonary vasodilator in hypoxic pulmonary hypertension. More recently, inhaled NO• was found to enhance coronary artery patency in dogs subjected to traumatic stenosis resulting in cyclic flow variations (CFW) followed by thrombolysis. No systemic hemodynamic effects occurred in NO•-treated dogs. More recently, inhaled NO• has been found to exert significant antileukocyte adherence effects in distant nonischemic microvascular beds in ischemia-reperfusion in the cat *(130)*. Thus, inhaled NO• gas may be an opportune method for delivering physiologically useful concentrations of NO• to the heart and lungs. Presumably, the NO• nitrosates plasma proteins and is transported in that manner to the site of action *(131)*.

NO• Donors

There are wide variety of nitrogenous compounds that can release NO• in solution. These NO•-generating compounds are collectively known as NO• donors. Almost all of them are organic nitrates, but a substance as simple as $NaNO_2$ at acidic pH (i.e., pH 2.0) can spontaneously release significant quantities of free NO• in solution. The major classes of organic NO• donors are the sydnonimines (e.g., SIN-1), cysteine-containing NO• donors (e.g., SPM-5185), the NONOates (e.g., DEA/NO•, SPER/NO•), and, of course, the well-known organic nitrates widely used for many years (e.g., nitroglycerin, sodium nitroprusside). The use of these NO• donors in cardiovascular disease has been reviewed recently *(132)*.

The earliest study showing that a NO• donor can work in myocardial ischemia is that of Johnson et al. *(133)* who employed acidified $NaNO_2$ in a feline model of myocardial ischemia/reperfusion. The $NaNO_2$ significantly attenuated reperfusion induced myocardial necrosis and cardiac infiltration of PMNs (e.g., to reduced cardiac myeloperoxidase (MPO) activity). The effective doses of $NaNO_2$ also inhibited cat platelet aggregation in vitro. One problem with this study was that no control compound lacking NO•-releasing ability was employed as a control. However, this was followed up by a seminal study *(134)* employing two SIN-1 NO• donors including a control substance (i.e., the same organic backbone of the NO• donor molecule minus the NO• moiety). These NO• donors (i.e., SIN-1, C87-3754) both attenuated cardiac necrosis by 65–70% in cats subjected to MI/R compared to the parent compound lacking the NO• moiety. Moreover, the cardioprotective effect occurred at infusion rates that did not affect systemic hemodynamics. Furthermore, both SIN-1 and C87-3754 preserved the coronary endothelium, significantly attenuating the endothelial dysfunction observed in untreated MI/R cats *(134)*. As a further investigation into the mechanism of this cardioprotection *(135)*, these NO• donors were found to blunt the coronary vasoconstriction produced by activated PMNs by preventing their release of superoxide and the subsequent inactivation of endothelium-derived NO• *(41)*. These results were confirmed in a follow-up study with a cysteine-containing NO• donor (i.e., SPM-5185) and its non-NO• containing control (i.e., SPM-5267) *(136)*.

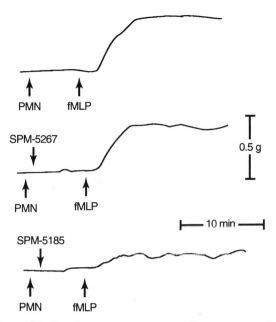

Fig. 4. Typical recordings of isolated cat coronary artery rings contracted with 5×10^5 activated PMN leukocytes. Prior to activation with formyl-methionyl-leucyl-phenylalanine (fMLP) PMNs were incubated with either Krebs–Henseleit solution, the NO• donor SPM-5185 (500 nM), or the non-NO• donating control compound, SPM-5267 (500 nM). Calibrations are 0.5 g of force and 10 min time. SPM-5185, significantly inhibited the PMN-induced vasocontraction. Reproduced with permission from ref. *136*.

   In the study shown in Fig. 4, cat PMNs stimulated with fMLP or 0.9%NaCl were given either 500 nM SPM-5185 or SPM-5267. Only the active NO• donor (SPM-5185) blunted the PMN-induced cat coronary vasoconstriction. Similar results were obtained with SPM-5185 in dogs subjected to MI/R *(137,138)* who also showed clearly that the cardioprotective effect of SPM-5185 was due to inhibition of neutrophil-induced cardiac injury rather than to hemodynamic effects of the NO• donor. More recently, an S-nitrosated tissue plasminogen activator (NO•-tPA) was found to attenuate markedly myocardial reperfusion injury in the same model of feline MI/R as was used in the earlier NO• donor studies. This NO•-tPA also preserved coronary endothelial function (i.e., attenuated endothelial dysfunction, inhibited PMN adherence to the coronary vascular endothelium, and markedly blunted P selectin expression on the affected cat coronary endothelium) *(139)*. This particular formulation of an NO• donor coupled to a thrombolytic agent may be especially relevant during clinical cases of acute myocardial infarction, as the tPA may lyse the clot in the coronary artery thus instituting reperfusion, coupled with NO• to the tPA to preserve endothelial function, prevent PMN adherence, and markedly diminish reperfusion injury. Because NO• donors mediate angiogenesis *(140)*, an added benefit may be stimulation of coronary collaterals in the ischemic reperfused myocardium. Finally, NO• donors have been shown to suppress ischemic arrhythmias in pigs subjected to MI *(141)*, an effect that may contribute to the cardioprotective actions of NO•.

   In addition to myocardial ischemia/reperfusion, NO• donors have been shown to be useful in splanchnic ischemia (i.e. splanchnic artery occlusion reperfusion, SAO/R) and in total body ischemia/reperfusion (i.e., hemorrhage/reperfusion). In SAO/R in the cat, the NO• donor C87-3754 was shown to protect against the lethality of SAO/R. Survival rate increased significantly from 0% in untreated SAO/R cats to 75% in C87-3754 treated cats *(142)*. Moreover, the plasma activities of cathepsin D (a lysosomal protease acting as a marker for enhanced plasma proteolysis) and of a myocardial depressant factor (MDF) a cardiotoxic peptide *(143)*, were significantly diminished by the active NO• donor. A few years later, Gauthier et al. *(72)* reported that SNAP, but not its NO• depleted form, exerts important protective effects in a rat model of SAO/R. These beneficial effects included attenuating leukocyte–endothelium interaction at the microcirculatory level. SNAP, a well-known NO• donor, had previously been shown to have potent antineutrophil effects *(144)*, and to protect rats subjected to severe hemorrhage/reperfusion resulting in shock *(144)*. In hemorrhagic shock, SNAP increased survival from 0–88% and markedly attenuated PMN infiltration into intestinal tissue as well as preserving the mesenteric vascular endothelium. Additionally, NO• donors have been shown to moderate microvascular protein leakage in SAO/R in the rat *(146)*.

The central theme emerging from these studies with NO• donors is that (1) low doses of NO• donors, below those that produce large vasodilator effects, can be effective against reperfusion injury; and (2) the major mechanisms of the tissue protection of these agents in I/R are endothelial preservation and inhibition of leukocyte–endothelium interaction. These mechanisms are consistent with the effects observed with authentic NO• in ischemia/reperfusion *(147)*.

L-Arginine

The substrate for NO• biosynthesis, the amino acid L-arginine, has also been studied in different forms of reperfusion injury. L-arginine, but not its stereoisomer D-arginine, markedly attenuated myocardial necrosis in cats subjected to MI/R *(66)*. This report appeared simultaneously with a similar study in dogs *(148)*. In both cases, L-arginine was infused intravascularly just prior to reperfusion and continuing for several hours. In addition to the cardioprotection afforded by L-arginine, reduced cardiac MPO activity was observed, indicative of attenuated neutrophil infiltration into the reperfused myocardium. Both studies also showed coronary endothelial preservation by L-arginine, suggesting an effect on the vascular endothelium via generation of NO• synthesis. This beneficial effect probably is mediated by antineutrophil effects on the partially dysfunctional endothelium, since Pabla et al. *(149)* showed that L-arginine infused into isolated rat hearts perfused with PMNs protected cardiac contractility during ischemia/reperfusion, but did not protect in the absence of the neutrophils. Moreover, L-arginine has been shown to diminish the severity of ventricular arrhythmias in dogs experiencing acute myocardial ischemia *(150)*. Thus, L-arginine preserves the vascular endothelium, suppresses leukocyte–endothelial interaction, attenuates PMN infiltration, maintains cardiac integrity (i.e., reduces necrosis), preserves cardiac contractility, and moderates ventricular arrhythmias in the setting of myocardial ischemia/reperfusion.

In addition to myocardial ischemia/reperfusion, L-arginine infusion reduced ischemia-reperfusion of rabbit skeletal muscle *(151)*, rat liver *(152)*, or rat skin *(153)*. Thus, L-arginine exerts tissue protective effects in a wide variety of tissues when given parentally just before reperfusion. L-arginine also can be given orally. This has been shown to be effective in hypercholesterolemic rabbits by oral feeding of L-arginine *(154)*, which improved endothelial function and retarded atherogenesis over a 10-wk period. More recently, human subjects ingesting L-arginine orally for 6 mo experienced significantly improved coronary vascular endothelial function in association with reduced symptoms of coronary artery disease (Fig. 5) *(155)*. This type of result supports the value of chronically enhancing nitric oxide in coronary vascular disorders.

Peroxynitrite

NO• and superoxide can form the highly reactive species, peroxynitrite (ONOO⁻) *(156)*, which is cytotoxic at high concentrations *(157)*. Thus, peroxynitrite has been invoked as a mediator of the myocardial cell injury resulting from ischemia-reperfusion *(158,159)*. These investigations claim that 30–100 μM ONOO⁻ causes myocardial injury in isolated perfused

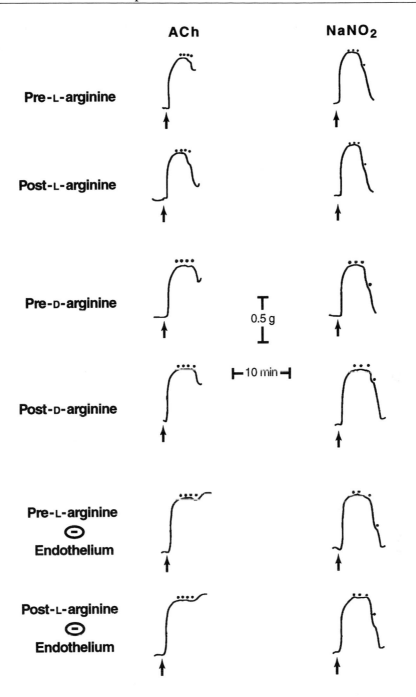

ACh **NaNO$_2$**

Pre-L-arginine

Post-L-arginine

Pre-D-arginine

0.5 g

Post-D-arginine

├─ 10 min ─┤

Pre-L-arginine
⊖
Endothelium

Post-L-arginine
⊖
Endothelium

Fig. 5. Representative recordings of rings isolated from cat left anterior descending coronary arteries undergoing 90 min of ischemia and 20 min of reperfusion. Rings were precontracted with 100 nM U-46619 (arrow), and the response to endothelium-dependent (100 nM acetylcholine, ACh) and endothelium-independent (100 μM NaNO•$_2$) vasodilators were measured prior to (Pre) and following (Post) a 3-min incubation with 3 mM L- or D-arginine or L-arginine with the endothelium removed. Dots indicate the addition of increasing log concentrations of ACh or NaNO•$_2$. L-arginine, but not D-arginine, preserved endothelium-dependent relaxation. Reproduced with permission from ref. 67.

rat hearts subjected to ischemia/reperfusion, and that nitrotyrosine, a purported "footprint" of peroxynitrite, is found in these rat hearts as evidence of the presence of peroxynitrite.

There are several serious problems with accepting peroxynitrite as a mediator of reperfusion injury. First, circulating levels of NO• are 1–10 nM/L (57) and ONOO$^-$ levels even at maximal iNOS activation are only in the low micromolar range (i.e., 0.4–5 µM) (160). These facts, coupled with the half-life of ONOO$^-$ of <1 s, render it highly unlikely to occur in vivo at concentrations above 1–2 µM. Peroxynitrite occurs in the ischemic-reperfused rat heart at concentrations of 100 nM (161). Second, NO• and superoxide form peroxynitrite only when they both exist at approx equimolar concentrations. When there is a significant imbalance between these two reactants, there is feedback inhibition of ONOO$^-$ formation (162). Third, one cannot directly measure peroxynitrite in vivo. One must resort to immunohistochemical measurement of the so-called "footprint" of ONOO$^-$, nitrotyrosine. Unfortunately, nitrotyrosine can be formed from a variety of substances other than ONOO$^-$, including chloride ions, hypochlorous acid, myeloperoxidase, and other nitrogenous radicals $(163,164)$. Fourth, physiologically relevant concentrations of ONOO$^-$ (i.e., in the range of 400 nM– 2 µM) actually protect against myocardial ischemia–reperfusion injury in the rat (165) and the cat (166). Moreover, these concentrations of ONOO$^-$ significantly attenuate leukocyte–endothelium interactions both in vitro and in vivo $(165,166)$. Fifth, ONOO$^-$ in vivo releases NO• in solution as a NO• donor (167). Thus, NO• can be transnitrosated onto carrier proteins in plasma, which acts as a NO• carrier, thus transporting and protecting the circulating NO• until it is released from the S-nitrosated carrier molecule (168). Stamler et al. have suggested that S-nitrosothiol protein adducts act as circulating carriers of NO• (169). This mechanism could explain the cytoprotective and beneficial effects of ONOO$^-$ in vivo. Thus, there is significant evidence currently available to question the role of peroxynitrite as a mediator of myocardial ischemia–reperfusion injury.

Ischemia-Reperfusion in NO• Gene-Deleted Mice

Two exciting new approaches to our understanding of the role of NO• in vascular disorders like ischemia-reperfusion is to employ specific gene-deleted mice and to transfect blood vessels with NO•-related genes (i.e., gene therapy). Although, these techniques are relatively difficult and few studies exist in the literature, they offer powerful insight into the regulatory role of NO• in physiological processes.

One such technique is that of gene deletion (i.e., knockout mice lacking the eNOS gene). This mouse has been described as hypertensive and lacks vascular responses to endothelium-dependent vasodilators (170). Using these mice, Moroi et al. (171) showed that they have a genetic disposition for intimal proliferation in large arteries that results in restricted luminal diameters and reduced blood flow. More recently, these eNOS deficient mice were shown to have an exacerbated degree of myocardial necrosis compared to wild-type mice subjected to the same MI/R protocol (172). Moreover, these eNOS deficient mice exhibited significantly high expression of P-selectin on their vascular endothelium. These findings add substantial weight to the physiologic role of endothelium-derived NO• in preventing leukocyte–endothelial interaction and in attenuating reperfusion injury.

The second new molecular approach is that of gene transfer to animals (i.e., gene therapy). Using this approach, one can locally inject a gene carried by a viral vector into an animal (i.e., gene transfection) enabling the gene to be expressed, and allowing one to turn on or off some physiologic process. In the case of the eNOS gene, von der Leyen et al. (173) utilizing a Sendai virus vector-transfected rat carotid arteries and found that this procedure markedly attenuated the intimal injury following balloon injury. Although this gene transfection has not been accomplished in myocardial ischemia, this represents an attractive target for future investigation.

The message thus far seems to be that loss of the gene for eNOS and thus reduced formation of endothelium derived-NO· is detrimental in vascular disorders including ischemia-reperfusion and restenosis. Conversely, gene transfection of eNOS and enhancement of NO· formation in these vascular disorders may be beneficial. The inescapable conclusion is that maintaining physiologic amounts of NO· from the endothelium at the blood–vascular interface is important and probably necessary for normal vascular function.

Inhibition of NO· Synthesis

Another approach to studying the effects of NO· in ischemia-reperfusion is to inhibit its synthesis by the use of inhibitors of nitric oxide synthase (NOS). The three isoforms of NOS (eNOS, nNOS, and iNOS) are reviewed elsewhere in this volume.

There have been a few studies employing NOS inhibitors in some form of myocardial hypoxia or ischemia. The earliest study was by Matheis et al. *(174)* in neonatal piglets subjected to hypoxia and reoxygenation. L-NAME given to the extracorporeal circuit afforded significant protection against reoxygenation injury to the myocardium over a 30-min period. However, the effect was not sustained postbypass. It is difficult to evaluate these results, as they were in neonates that were not subjected to ischemia per se, and no other NO·-related studies have been done in this model. In the other study in which a NOS inhibitor has been shown to be protective in MI/R was conducted in isolated perfused rabbit hearts *(175)*. L-NAME preserved mechanical function in these studies following 35 min of global ischemia and 30 min of reperfusion. The major effect was an increased pressure-rate-product in L-NAME-treated hearts. However, as L-NAME is a vasoconstrictor and is known to increase pressure, at the expense of blood flow, this effect may not ultimately prove to be beneficial in vivo. Moreover, L-arginine also protected but to a lesser degree. Finally, these hearts were perfused in the absence of leukocytes, thus eliminating a major potential site of NO· action in reperfusion injury *(175)*.

In contrast to these studies, two others show detrimental affects of NOS inhibitors in MI/R and related phenomena. Pabla et al. *(149)* employed isolated rat hearts perfused with PMNs. In these rat hearts, L-NAME exacerbated the contractile dysfunction observed following ischemia-reperfusion. Moreover, a NO·-donor promoted significant improvement in cardiac performance under the same conditions. Similarly, Duncker and Bache *(176)* showed that the NOS inhibitor, N^G-nitro-L-arginine aggravated myocardial hypoperfusion in the dog heart in the presence of a coronary artery stenosis probably due to its coronary constrictor effect. These latter two studies provide strong support for the key role of NO· in maintaining coronary perfusion and inhibiting neutrophil-induced myocardial injury following reperfusion of an ischemic coronary vasculature and are consistent with NO· having an important maintenance role in preserving vascular function in circulatory disorders like ischemia-reperfusion.

SUMMARY

Endothelium-derived NO· plays a pivotal role in the maintenance of vascular homeostasis in the setting of ischemia-reperfusion. This is particularly relevant in the myocardium, the splanchnic region, skeletal muscle, and the kidneys. This defensive multifaceted role of NO· includes preservation of endothelial function, prevention of platelet adhesion and aggregation, attenuation of leukocyte rolling, adherence, and transmigration across the endothelium, and the suppression of cell injury associated with reperfusion.

NO· is cytoprotective in reperfusion injury. There are a number of ways of augmenting NO· levels locally including the use of authentic NO· either as an inhaled gas or as a dissolved gas in solution, organic NO· donors, infusion or diet supplementation with L-arginine or BH_4 or its analogs, or NOS gene transfection. Reperfusion injury is usually aggravated by NOS inhibitors or in gene-deleted animals lacking eNOS. At physiologically achievable concentrations, peroxynitrite a product of NO• and superoxide radicals, actually protects in ischemia-reperfusion probably by transnitrosation of plasma proteins or nitrosothiols. The signaling mechanisms that mediate these important physiological effects of NO• are just being investigated and likely involve multiple pathways including NFκB, protein kinase C, mitogen-activated protein kinase and other mechanisms.

The remarkable effects of NO• in suppressing endothelial–leukocyte interactions is the crux of the cytoprotective actions of NO• in reperfusion injury, and is now widely accepted in this field.

REFERENCES

1. Hearse DJ. Reperfusion of the ischemic myocardium. J Mol Cell Cardiol 1977;9:605–616.
2. Rosenkranz ER, Buckberg GD. Myocardial protection during surgical coronary reperfusion. J Am Coll Cardiol 1983;1:1235–1246.
3. Braunwald E, Kloner RA. Myocardial reperfusion: a double-edged sword? J Clin Invest 1985;76: 1713–1719.
4. Bulkley GB. Mediators of splanchnic organ injury: overview and perspective. In: Marston A, Bulkley GB, Fiddian-Green RG, Haglund UH, eds. Splanchnic Ischemia and Multiple Organ Failure. Edward Arnold, London, 1989, pp. 183–194.
5. Tsao PS, Aoki N, Lefer DJ, Johnson G 3rd, Lefer AM. Time course of endothelial dysfunction and myocardial injury during myocardial ischemia and reperfusion in the cat. Circulation 1990;82: 1402–1412.
6. Ku DD. Coronary vascular reactivity after acute myocardial ischemia. Science 1982;218:576–578.
7. Mehta JL, Nichols WW, Donnelly WH, Lawson DL, Saldeen TG. Impaired canine coronary vasodilation response to acetylcholine and bradykinin after occlusion-reperfusion. Circ Res 1989;64:43–54.
8. Hayward R, Nossuli TO, Lefer AM. Heparinase III exerts endothelial and cardioprotective effects in feline myocardial ischemia-reperfusion injury. J Pharmacol Exp Ther 1997;283:1032–1038.
9. Tsao PS, Lefer AM. Time course and mechanism of endothelial dysfunction in isolated ischemic- and hypoxic-perfused rat hearts. Am J Physiol 1990;259:H1660–H1666.
10. Van Benthuysen KM, McMurtry IF, Horowitz LD. Reperfusion after acute coronary occlusion in dogs impairs endothelium-dependent relaxation to acetylcholine and augments contractile reactivity in vitro. J Clin Invest 1987;79:265–274.
11. Hayward R, Lefer AM. Time course of neutrophil-endothelial interaction in splanchnic artery ischemia-reperfusion. Am J Physiol 1998;275:H2080–H2086.
12. Lieberthal W, Wolf EF, Rennke HG, Valen CR, Levinsky NG. Renal ischemia and reperfusion impair endothelium-dependent vascular relaxation. Am J Physiol 1989;256:F894–F900.
13. Mayhan WG, Amundsen SM, Faraci FM, Heistad DD. Responses of cerebral arteries after ischemia and reperfusion in cats. Am J Physiol 1988;255:H879–H884.
14. Sternbergh WC, Makhoul RG, Adelman B. Nitric oxide-mediated, endothelium-dependent vasodilation is selectively attenuated in the postischemic extremity. Surgery 1993;114:960–967.
15. Viehman GE, Ma XL, Lefer DJ, Lefer AM. Time course of endothelial dysfunction and myocardial injury during coronary arterial occlusion. Am J Physiol 1991;261:H874–H881.
16. Arminger LC, Gavin JB. Changes in the microvasculature of ischemic and infarcted myocardium. Lab Invest 1975;33:51–56.
17. Lefer AM, Ma XL. Cytokines and growth factors in endothelial dysfunction. Crit Care Med 1993;21: S9–S14.
18. Lefer AM, Tsao P, Aoki N, Palladino MA Jr. Mediation of cardioprotection by transforming growth factor-β. Science 1990;249:61–64.
19. Jewett SL, Eddy LJ, Hochstein P. Is the autoxidation of catecholamines involved in ischemia-reperfusion injury? Free Rad Biol Med 1989;6:185–188.
20. Kontos HA, Wei EP, Ellis EF, Jenkins LW, Polvilshock JT, Rowe T, et al. Appearance of superoxide anion radical in cerebral extracellular space during increased prostaglandin synthesis in cats. Circ Res 1985;57:142–152.
21. Shlafer M, Myers C, Adkins S. Mitochondrial hydrogen peroxide generation and activities of glutathione peroxidase and superoxide dismutase following global ischemia. J Mol Cell Cardiol 1987; 19:1195–1206.
22. Ratych RE, Chunknyiska RS, Bulkley GB. The primary localization of free radical generation after anoxia/reoxygenation in isolated endothelial cells. Surgery 1987;102:122–131.

23. Grisham MB, Hernandez LA, Granger DN. Xanthine oxidase and neutrophil infiltration in intestinal ischemia. Am J Physiol 1986;251:G567–G574.

24. Zweier JL, Kuppasamy P, Lutty GA. Measurement of endothelial cell free radical generation: evidence for a central mechanism of free radical injury in post-ischemic tissue. Proc Natl Acad Sci USA 1988;85: 4046–4050.

25. Chambers DE, Parks DA, Patterson G, Roy R, McCord JM, Yoshida S, et al. Xanthine oxidase as a source of free radical damage in myocardial ischemia. J Mol Cell Cardiol 1985;17:145–152.

26. McCord JM. Oxygen-derived free radicals in postischemic tissue injury. N Engl J Med 1985;312: 159–163.

27. Bolli R, Patel BS, Jeroudi MO, Lai EK, McCay PB. Demonstration of free radical generation in "stunned" myocardium of intact dogs with the use of the spin trap α-phenyl N-tert-butyl nitrone. J Clin Invest 1988;82:476–485.

28. Zweier JL. Measurement of superoxide derived free radicals in the reperfused heart. J Biol Chem 1988;263:1353–1357.

29. Lamb FS, King CM, Harrell K, Burkel W, Webb RC. Free radical-mediated endothelial damage in blood vessels after electrical stimulation. Am J Physiol 1987;252:H1041–H1046.

30. Stewart DJ, Pohl U, Bassenge E. Free radicals inhibit endothelium-dependent dilation in the coronary resistance bed. Am J Physiol 1988;255:H765–H769.

31. Inauen W, Payne DK, Kvietys PR, Granger DN. Hypoxia/reoxygenation increases the permeability of endothelial cell monolayers: role of oxygen radicals. Free Radic Biol Med 1990;9:219–223.

32. Wu S, Nagashima T, Ikeda K, Kondoh T, Yamaguchi M, Tamaki N. The mechanism of free radical generation in brain capillary endothelial cells after anoxia and reoxygenation. Acta Neurochir 1997; 70(Suppl):37–39.

33. Michiels C, Arnould T, Houbion A, Remacle J. Human umbilical vein endothelial cells submitted to hypoxia-reoxygenation in vitro: amplification of free radicals, xanthine oxidase, and energy deficiency. J Cell Physiol 1992;153:53–61.

34. Razack S, D'Agnillo F, Chang TM. Crosslinked hemoglobin-superoxide dismutase-catalase scavenges free radicals in a rat model of intestinal ischemia-reperfusion injury. Artif Cells Blood Substit Immobil Biotechnol 1997;25:181–192.

35. Gryglewski RJ, Palmer RM, Moncada S. Superoxide anion is involved in the breakdown of endothelium-derived relaxing factor. Nature 1986;320:454–456.

36. Eppinger MJ, Jones ML, Deeb GM, Bolling SF, Ward PA. Pattern of injury and the role of neutrophils in reperfusion injury of rat lung. J Surg Res 1995;58:713–718.

37. Litt, MR, Jeremy RW, Weisman HF, Winkelstein JA, Becker LC. Neutrophil depletion limited to reperfusion reduces myocardial infarct size after 90 minutes of ischemia: evidence for neutrophil-mediated reperfusion injury. Circulation 1989;80:1816–1827.

38. Mullane KM, Read N, Salmon JA, Moncada S. Role of leukocytes in acute myocardial infarction in anesthetized dogs: relationship to myocardial salvage by anti-inflammatory drugs. J Pharmacol Exp Ther 1984;228:510–522.

39. Granger DN, Benoit, JN, Suzuki M, Grisham MB. Leukocyte adherence to venule endothelium during ischemia-reperfusion. Am J Physiol 1989;257:G683–G688.

40. Tsao PS, Ma X, Lefer AM. Activated neutrophils aggravate endothelial dysfunction after reperfusion of the ischemic feline myocardium. Am Heart J 1992;123:1464–1471.

41. Ma XL, Tsao PS, Viehman GE, Lefer AM. Neutrophil-mediated vasocontraction and endothelial dysfunction in low-flow perfusion-reperfused cat coronary artery. Circ Res 1991;69:95–106.

42. Brody HR, Persson U, Ballerman BJ, Brenner BM, Serhan CN. Leukotrienes stimulate neutrophil adhesion to mesangial cells: modulation with lipoxins. Am J Physiol 1990;259:F809–F815.

43. Karasawa A, Guo JP, Ma XL, Tsao PS, Lefer AM. Protective actions of a leukotriene B_4 antagonist in splanchnic ischemia and reperfusion in rats. Am J Physiol 1991;261:G191–G198.

44. Zimmerman BJ, Guillory DJ, Grisham MB, Gaginella TS, Granger DN. Role of leukotriene B_4 in granulocyte infiltration into the postischemic feline intestine. Gastroenterology 1990;99:1358–1364.

45. Zimmerman BJ, Granger DN. Reperfusion-induced leukocyte infiltration: role of elastase. Am J Physiol 1990;259:H390–H394.

46. Rice WG, Weiss SJ. Regulation of proteolysis at the neutrophil-substrate interface by secretory leukoprotease inhibitor. Science 1990;249:178–181.

47. Boudier C, Holle C, Bieth JG. Stimulation of the elastolytic activity of leukocyte elastase by leukocyte cathepsin G. J Biol Chem 1981;256:10,256–10,258.

48. Camussi G, Tetta C, Bussolino F, Baglioni. C. Tumor necrosis factor stimulates human neutrophils to release leukotriene B_4 and platelet-activating factor. Induction of phospholipase A2 and acetyl-CoA:

1-alkyl-sn-glycero-3-phosphocholine O_2-acetyl-transferase activity and inhibition by antiproteinase. Eur J Biochem 1989;182:661–666.

49. Ma XL, Weyrich AS, Krantz S, Lefer AM. Mechanisms of the cardioprotective actions of WEB-2170, a platelet activating factor antagonist, in myocardial ischemia and reperfusion. J Pharmacol Exp Ther 1992;260:1229–1236.

50. Delyani JA, Murohara T, Lefer. AM. Novel recombinant serpin, LEX-032, attenuates myocardial reperfusion injury in cats. Am J Physiol 1996;270:H881–H887.

51. Murohara T, Guo JP, Lefer AM. Cardioprotection by a novel recombinant serine protease inhibitor in myocardial ischemia and reperfusion injury. J Pharm Exp Ther 1995;274:1246–1253.

52. Hayward R, Lefer AM. Beneficial effects of LEX-032, a novel recombinant serpin, during splanchnic ischemia and reperfusion. Cardiovasc Pathobiol 1998;2:191–198.

53. Werns SW, Lucchesi BR. Free radicals and ischemic tissue injury. Trends Pharmacol Sci 1990;11: 161–166.

54. Tsao PS, Lefer AM. Recovery of endothelial function following myocardial ischemia and reperfusion in rats. J Vasc Med Biol 1991;3:5–10.

55. Ambrosio G, Becker LC, Hutchins GM, Weisman HF, Weisfeldt, ML. Reduction in experimental infarct size by recombinant human superoxide dismutase: Insights into the pathophysiology of reperfusion injury. Circulation 1986;74:1424–1433.

56. Bitterman H, Aoki N, Lefer AM. Anti-shock effects of human superoxide dismutase in splanchnic artery occlusion (SAO) shock. Proc Soc Exp Biol Med 1988;188:265–271.

57. Kelm M, Schrader J. Control of coronary vascular tone by nitric oxide. Circ Res 1990;66:1561–1575.

58. Guo JP, Murohara T, Buerke M, Scalia R, Lefer AM. Direct measurement of nitric oxide release from vascular endothelial cells. J Appl Physiol 1996;81:774–779.

59. Palmer RM, Ferrige AG, Moncada S. Nitric oxide release accounts for the biological activity of endothelium-derived relaxing factor. Nature 1987;327:524–526.

60. Moncada S, Palmer RM, Higgs EA. Biosynthesis of nitric oxide from L-arginine: a pathway for regulation of all function and communication. Biochem Pharmacol 1989;38:1709–1715.

61. Lefer AM, Lefer DJ. The role of nitric oxide and cell adhesion molecules on the microcirculation in ischaemia-reperfusion. Cardiovasc Res 1996;32:743–751.

62. Lefer DJ, Nakanishi K, Vinten-Johansen J, Ma XL, Lefer AM. Cardiac venous endothelial dysfunction after myocardial ischemia and reperfusion in dogs. Am J Physiol 1992;263:H850–H856.

63. Moncada S, Palmer RM, Higgs EA. Nitric oxide: physiology, pathophysiology, and pharmacology. Pharmacol Rev 1991;43:109–142.

64. Rees DD, Palmer RM, Schulz R, Hodson HF, Moncada S. Characterization of three inhibitors of endothelial nitric oxide synthase in vitro and in vivo. Br J Pharmacol 1990;101:746–752.

65. Davenpeck KL, Gauthier TW, Lefer AM. Inhibition of endothelial-derived nitric oxide promotes P-selectin expression and actions in the rat microcirculation. Gastroenterology 1994;107:1050–1058.

66. Ma XL, Weyrich AS, Lefer DJ, Lefer AM. Diminished basal nitric oxide release after myocardial ischemia and reperfusion promotes neutrophil adherence to coronary endothelium. Circ Res 1993;72:403–412.

67. Weyrich AS, Ma XL, Lefer AM. The role of L-arginine in ameliorating reperfusion injury after myocardial ischemia in the cat. Circulation 1992;86:279–288.

68. Kubes P, Suzuki M, Granger DN. Nitric oxide: an endogenous modulator of leukocyte adhesion. Proc Natl Acad Sci USA 1991;88:4651–4655.

69. Rubanyi GM, Vanhoutte PM. Superoxide anions and hyperoxia inactivate endothelium-derived relaxing factor. Am J Physiol 1986;250:H822–H827.

70. Tiefenbacher CP, Chilian WM, Mitchell M, DeFily DV. Restoration of endothelium-dependent vasodilation after reperfusion injury by tetrahydrobiopterin. Circulation 1996;94:1423–1429.

71. Kugiyama K, Yasue H, Okumura K, Ogawa H, Fujimoto K, Nakao K, et al. Nitric oxide activity is deficient in spasm arteries of patients with coronary spastic angina. Circulation 1996;94:266–272.

72. Gauthier TW, Davenpeck KL, Lefer AM. Nitric oxide attenuates leukocyte-endothelial interaction via P-selectin in splanchnic ischemia-reperfusion. Am J Physiol 1994;267:G562–G568.

73. Ignarro LJ, Buga GM, Wood KS, Byrns RE, Chaudhuri G. Endothelium-derived relaxing factor produced and released from artery and vein is nitric oxide. Proc Natl Acad Sci USA 1987;84:9265–9269.

74. Butcher EC. Leukocyte-endothelial cell recognition: three (or more) steps to specificity and diversity. Cell 1991;67:1033–1036.

75. Weyrich AS, Buerke M, Albertine KH, Lefer AM. Time course of coronary vascular endothelial adhesion molecule expression during reperfusion of the ischemic feline myocardium. J Leukoc Biol 1995;57:45–55.

76. Spertini O, Kansas GS, Munro JM, Griffin JD, Tedder TF. Regulation of leukocyte migration by activation of the leukocyte adhesion molecule-1 (LAM-1) selectin. Nature 1991;349:691–694.

77. Kishimoto TK, Jutila M, Berg EL, Butcher EC. Neutrophil MAC-1 and MEL-14 adhesion proteins inversely regulated by chemotactic factors. Science 1989;245:1238–1241.
78. Kubes P, Jutila M, Payne D. Therapeutic potential of inhibiting leukocyte rolling in ischemia/reperfusion. J Clin Invest 1995;95:2510–2519.
79. Kurose ID, Anderson C, Miyasaka M, Tamatani T, Paulson JC, Todd RF, et al. Molecular determinants of reperfusion-induced leukocyte adhesion and vascular protein leakage. Circ Res 1994;74:336–343.
80. Perry MA, Granger DN. Role of CD11/CD18 in shear rate-dependent leukocyte-endothelial cell interactions in cat mesenteric venules. J Clin Invest 1991;87:1798–1804.
81. Suzuki M, Inauen W, Kvietys PR, Grisham MB, Meininger C, Schelling ME, et al. Superoxide mediates reperfusion-induced leukocyte-endothelial cell interactions. Am J Physiol 1989;257:H1740–H1745.
82. Ma XL, Tsao PS, Lefer AM. Antibody to CD-18 exerts endothelial and cardiac protective effects in myocardial ischemia and reperfusion. J Clin Invest 1991;88:1237–1243.
83. Kuzume M, Nakano H, Yamaguchi M, Matsumiya A, Shimokohbe G, Kitamura N, et al. A monoclonal antibody against ICAM-1 suppresses hepatic ischemia-reperfusion injury in rats. Eur Surg Res 1997;29: 93–100.
84. Rabb H, Mendiola CC, Saba SR, Dietz JR, Smith CW, Bonventre JV, et al. Antibodies to ICAM-1 protect kidneys in severe ischemic reperfusion injury. Biochem Biophys Res Commun 1995;211:67–73.
85. Granger DN, Russell JM, Arfors KE, Rothlein R, Anderson DC. Role of CD18 and ICAM-1 in ischemia/reperfusion-induced leukocyte adherence and emigration in mesenteric venules. FASEB J 1991;5: A1753.
86. Ferrante RJ, Hobson RW 2nd, Miyasaka M, Granger DN, Druan WN. Inhibition of white blood cell adhesion at reperfusion decreases tissue damage in postischemic striated muscle. J Vasc Surg 1996;24: 187–193.
87. Ma XL, Lefer DJ, Lefer AM, Rothlein R. Coronary endothelial and cardiac protective effects of a monoclonal antibody to intercellular adhesion molecule-1 in myocardial ischemia and reperfusion. Circulation 1992;86:937–946.
88. Zhao ZQ, Lefer DJ, Sato H, Hart, KK, Jeffords PR, Vinten-Johansen J. Monoclonal antibody to ICAM-1 preserves postischemic blood flow and reduces infarct size after ischemia-reperfusion in the rabbit. J Leukoc Biol 1997;62:292–300.
89. Muller WA. The role of PECAM-1 (CD31) in leukocyte emigration: studies in vitro and in vivo. J Leukoc Biol 1995;57:523–528.
90. Wakelin MW, Sanz MJ, Dewar A, Albelda SM, Larkin SW, Boughton-Smith N, et al. An anti-platelet-endothelial cell adhesion molecule-1 antibody inhibits leukocyte extravasation from mesenteric microvessels in vivo by blocking the passage through the basement membrane. J Exp Med 1996;184: 229–239.
91. Scalia R, Lefer AM. In vivo regulation of PECAM-1 activity during acute endothelial dysfunction in the rat mesenteric microvasculature. J Leukoc Biol 1998;64:163–169.
92. Gumina RJ, Schultz JE, Yao Z, Kenny D, Warltier DC, Newman PJ, et al. Antibody to platelet/endothelial cell adhesion molecule-1 reduces myocardial infarct size in a rat model of ischemia-reperfusion injury. Circulation 1996;94:3327–3333.
93. Murohara T, Delyani JA, Albelda SM, Lefer AM. Blockade of platelet endothelial cell adhesion molecule-1 protects against myocardial ischemia and reperfusion injury in cats. J Immunol 1996;156: 3550–3557.
94. Davenpeck KL, Gauthier TW, Albertine KH, Lefer AM. Role of P-selectin in microvascular leukocyte-endothelial interaction in splanchnic ischemia-reperfusion. Am J Physiol 1994;267:H622–H630.
95. Biffl WL, Moore EE, Moore FA, Barnett, C. Nitric oxide reduces endothelial expression of intercellular adhesion molecule (ICAM)-1. J Surg Res 1996;63:328–332.
96. Hess DC, Zhao W, Carroll M, McEachin M, Buchanan K. Increased expression of ICAM-1 during reoxygenation in brain endothelial cells. Stroke 1994;25:1463–1467.
97. Kupatt, C, Weber C, Wolf DA, Becker BF, Smith TW, Kelly RA. Nitric oxide attenuates reoxygenation-induced ICAM-1 expression in coronary microvascular endothelium: role of NF-κB. J Mol Cell Cardiol 1997;29:2599–2609.
98. Gaboury JP, Anderson DC, Kubes P. Molecular mechanisms involved in superoxide-induced leukocyte-endothelial cell interactions in vivo. Am J Physiol 1994;266:H637–H642.
99. Suzuki M, Grisham M, Granger DN. Leukocyte-endothelial cell interactions: role of xanthine oxidase-derived oxidants. J Leukoc Biol 1991;50:488–494.
100. Mataki H, Inagaki T, Yokoyama M, Maeda S. ICAM-1 expression and cellular injury in cultured endothelial cells under hypoxia/reoxygenation. Kobe J Med Sci 1994;40:49–63.
101. Palluy O, Morliere L, Gris JC, Bonne C, Modat G. Hypoxia/reoxygenation stimulates endothelium to promote neutrophil adhesion. Free Rad Biol Med 1992;13:21–30.

102. Patel KD, Zimmerman GA, Prescott, SM, McEver RP, McIntyre TM. Oxygen radicals induce human endothelial cells to express GMP-140 and bind neutrophils. J Cell Biol 1991;112:749–759.

103. Murohara T, Parkinson JS, Waldman SA, Lefer AM. Inhibition of nitric oxide biosynthesis promotes P-selectin expression in platelets. Role of protein kinase C. Arterioscler Thromb Vasc Biol 1995;15: 2068–2075.

104. Geng JG, Bevilacqua MP, Moore KL, McIntyre TM, Prescott, SM, Kin JM, et al. Rapid neutrophil adhesion to activated endothelium mediated by GMP-140. Nature 1990;343:5757–5760.

105. Gopalakrishna R, Chen ZH, Gundimeda U. Nitric oxide and nitric oxide-generating agents induce a reversible inactivation of protein kinase C activity and portbol ester binding. J Biol Chem 1993;268: 27,180–27,185.

106. Takai Y, Kaibuchi K, Matsubara T, Nishizuka Y. Inhibitory action of guanosine 3', 5'-monophosphate on thrombin-induced phosphatidylinositol turnover and protein phosphorylation in human platelets. Biochem Biophys Res Commun 1981;101:61–67.

107. Scalia R, Murohara T, Delyani JA, Nossuli TO, Lefer AM. Myocardial protection by N,N,N-trimethyl-sphingosine in ischemia reperfusion injury is mediated by inhibition of P-selectin. J Leukoc Biol 1996; 59:317–324.

108. De Caterina R, Libby P, Peng HB, Thannickal VJ, Rajavashisth TB, Gimbrone MG Jr, et al. Nitric oxide decreases cytokine-induced endothelial activation. Nitric oxide selectively reduces endothelial expression of adhesion molecules and proinflammatory cytokines. J Clin Invest 1995;96:60–68.

109. Peng HB, Libby P, Liao JK. Induction and stabilization of IκBα by nitric oxide mediates inhibition of NF-κB. J Biol Chem 1995;270:14,214–14,219.

110. Spiecker M, Darius H, Kaboth K, Hübner F, Liao JK. Differential regulation of endothelial cell adhesion molecule expression by nitric oxide donors and antioxidants. J Leukoc Biol 1998;63:732–739.

111. Armstead VE, Minchenko AG, Schuhl RA, Hayward R, Nossuli TO, Lefer AM. Regulation of P-selectin expression in human endothelial cells by nitric oxide. Am J Physiol 1997;273:H740–H746.

112. Khan BV, Harrison DG, Olbrych MT, Alexander RW, Medford RM. Nitric oxide regulates vascular cell adhesion molecule-1 gene expression and redox-sensitive transcription events in human vascular endothelial cells. Proc Natl Acad Sci USA 1996;93:9114–9119.

113. Eppihimer MJ, Russell J, Anderson DC, Epstein CJ, Laroux S, Granger DN. Modulation of P-selectin expression in the postischemic intestinal microvasculature. Am J Physiol 1997;273:G1326–G1332.

114. Barnes PJ. Nuclear factor-κB. Int J Biochem Cell Biol 1997;29:867–870.

115. Blackwell TS, Christman JW. The role of nuclear factor-κB in cytokine gene regulation. Am J Respir Cell Mol Biol 1997;17:3–9.

116. Lander HM, Sehajpal P, Levine DM, Novogrodsky A. Activation of human peripheral blood mononuclear cells by nitric oxide-generating compounds. J Immunol 1993;150:1509–1516.

117. Fialkow L, Chan CK, Grinstein S, Downey GP. Regulation of tyrosine phosphorylation in neutrophils by the NADPH oxidase. Role of reactive oxygen intermediates. J Biol Chem 1993;268:17,131–17,137.

118. Schreck R, Alberman K, Baeuerle PA. Nuclear factor κB: an oxidative stress-response transcription factor of eukaryotic cells (a review). Free Radic Res Commun 1993;17:221–237.

119. Moine P, Shenkar R, Kaneko D, Le Tulzo Y, Abraham E. Systemic blood loss affects NF-κB regulatory mechanisms in the lungs. Am J Physiol 1997;273:L185–L192.

120. Aoki N, Johnson G 3rd, Lefer AM. Beneficial effects of two forms of NO• administration in feline splanchnic artery occlusion shock. Am J Physiol 1990;258:G275–G281.

121. Lefer AM, Barenholz Y. Pancreatic hydrolyses and the formation of a myocardial depressant factor in shock. Am J Physiol 1972;223:1103–1109.

122. Johnson G 3rd, Tsao PS, Lefer AM. Cardioprotective effects of authentic nitric oxide in myocardial ischemia with reperfusion. Crit Care Med 1991;19:244–252.

123. Brady AJ, Poole-Wilson PA, Harding SE, Warren JB. Nitric oxide production within cardiac myocytes reduces their contractility in endotoxemia. Am J Physiol 1992;263:H1963–H1966.

124. Balligand JL, Ungureanu D, Kelly RA, Kobzik L, Pimental D, Michel T, Smith TW. Abnormal contractile function due to induction of nitric oxide synthesis in rat cardiac myocytes follows exposure to activated macrophage-conditioned medium. J Clin Invest 1993;91:2314–2319.

125. Weyrich AS, Ma XL, Buerke M, Murohara T, Armstead VE, Lefer AM, et al. Physiological concentrations of nitric oxide do not elicit an acute negative inotropic effect in unstimulated cardiac muscle. Circ Res 1994;75:692–700.

126. Crystal GJ, Gurevicius J. Nitric oxide does not modulate myocardial contractility acutely in in situ canine hearts. Am J Physiol 1996;270:H1568–H1576.

127. Pennington DG, Vezeridis MP, Geffin G, O'Keefe DD, Lappas DG, Daggett, WM. Quantitative effects of sodium nitroprusside on coronary hemodynamics and left ventricular function in dogs. Circ Res 1979;45:351–359.

128. Hasebe N, Shen YT, Vatner SF. Inhibition of endothelium-derived relaxing factor enhances myocardial stunning in conscious dog. Circulation 1993;88:2862–2871.
129. Frostell C, Fratacci MD, Wain JC, Jones R, Zapol WM. Inhaled nitric oxide: a selective pulmonary vasodilator reversing hypoxic pulmonary vasocontraction. Circulation 1991;83:2038–2047.
130. Fox-Robichaud A, Payne D, Hasan SU, Ostrovsky L, Fairhead T, Reinhardt P, et al. Inhaled NO• as a viable antiadhesive therapy for ischemia/reperfusion injury of distal microvascular beds. J Clin Invest 1998;101:2497–2505.
131. Loscalzo J, Vaughan DE. Tissue plasminogen activator promotes platelet desegregation in plasma. J Clin Invest 1987;79:1749–1755.
132. Lefer AM, Lefer DJ. Therapeutic role of nitric oxide donors in the treatment of cardiovascular disease. Drugs Future 1994;19:665–672.
133. Johnson G 3rd, Tsao PS, Mulloy D, Lefer AM. Cardioprotective effects of acidified sodium nitrite in myocardial ischemia with reperfusion. J Pharmacol Exp Therap 1990;252:35–41.
134. Siegfried MR, Erhardt J, Rider R, Ma XL, Lefer AM. Cardioprotection and attenuation of endothelial dysfunction by organic nitric oxide donors in myocardial ischemia-reperfusion. J Pharmacol Exp Ther 1992;260:668–675.
135. Lefer AM, Siegfried MR, Ma XL. Protection of ischemia-reperfusion injury by sydnonimine NO• donors via inhibition of neutrophil-endothelium interaction. J Cardiovasc Pharmacol 1993;22: S27–S33.
136. Siegfried MR, Carey C, Ma XL, Lefer AM. Beneficial effects of SPM-5185, a cysteine-containing NO• donor in myocardial ischemia-reperfusion. Am J Physiol 1992;263:H771–H777.
137. Lefer DJ, Nakanishi K, Vinten-Johansen J. Endothelial and myocardial cell protection by a cysteine-containing nitric oxide donor after myocardial ischemia and reperfusion. J Cardiovasc Pharmacol 1993;22:S34–S43.
138. Lefer DJ, Nakanishi K, Johnston WE, Vinten-Johansen J. Antineutrophil and myocardial protecting actions of a novel nitric oxide donor after acute myocardial ischemia and reperfusion in dogs. Circulation 1993;88:2337–2350.
139. Delyani JA, Nossuli TO, Scalia R, Thomas G, Garvey DS, Lefer AM. S-nitrosylated tissue-type plasminogen activator protects against myocardial ischemia/reperfusion injury in cats: role of the endothelium. J Pharmacol Exp Ther 1996;279:1174–1180.
140. Ziche M, Morbidelli L, Masini E, Amerini S, Granger HJ, Maggi CA, et al. Nitric oxide mediates angiogenesis in vivo and endothelial cell growth and migration in vitro promoted by substance P. J Clin Invest 1994;94:2036–2044.
141. Wainwright CL, Martorana PA. Pirsidomine, a novel nitric oxide donor, suppresses ischemic arrhythmias in anesthetized pigs. J Cardiovasc Pharmacol 1993;22:S44–S50.
142. Carey C, Siegfried MR, Ma XL, Weyrich SA, Lefer AM. Antishock and endothelial protective actions of a NO• donor in mesenteric ischemia and reperfusion. Circ Shock 1992;38:209–216.
143. Lefer AM. Interaction between myocardial depressant factor and vasoactive mediators with ischemia and shock. Am J Physiol 1987;252:R193–R205.
144. Ma XL, Lefer AM, Zipkin RE. S-nitroso-N-acetylpenicillamine is a potent inhibitor of neutrophil-endothelial interaction. Endothelium 1993;1:31–39.
145. Symington PA, Ma XL, Lefer AM. Protective actions of S-nitroso-N-acetylpenicillamine (SNAP) in a rat model of hemorrhagic shock. Methods Find Exp Clin Pharmacol 1992;14:789–797.
146. Kurose I, Wolf R, Grisham MB, Granger DN. Modulation of ischemia/reperfusion-induced microvascular dysfunction by nitric oxide. Circ Res 1994;74:376–382.
147. Lefer AM, Lefer DJ. Pharmacology of the endothelium in ischemia-reperfusion and circulatory shock. Annu Rev Pharmacol Toxicol 1993;33:71–90.
148. Nakanishi K, Vinten-Johansen J, Lefer DJ, Zhao J, Fowler WC 3rd, McGee DS, et al. Intracoronary L-arginine during reperfusion improves endothelial function and reduces infarct size. Am J Physiol 1992;263:H1650–H1658.
149. Pabla R, Buda AJ, Flynn DM, Blesse SA, Shin AM, Curtis MJ, et al. Nitric oxide attenuates neutrophil-mediated myocardial contractile dysfunction after ischemia and reperfusion. Circ Res 1996;78:65–72.
150. Fei L, Baron AD, Henry DP, Zipes DP. Intrapericardial delivery of L-arginine reduces the increased severity of ventricular arrhythmias during sympathetic stimulation in dogs with acute coronary occlusion: nitric oxide modulates sympathetic effects on ventricular electrophysiological properties. Circulation 1997;96:4044–4049.
151. Huk I, Nanobashvili J, Neumayer C, Punz A, Mueller M, Afkhampour K, et al. L-arginine treatment alters the kinetics of nitric oxide and superoxide release and reduces ischemia/reperfusion injury in skeletal muscle. Circulation 1997;96:667–675.
152. Nilsson B, Yoshida T, Delbro D, Andius S, Friman S. Pretreatment with L-arginine reduces ischemia/reperfusion injury of the liver. Transplant Proc 1997;29:3111,3112.

22   Nitrovasodilators

John D. Horowitz

HISTORY

The term "nitrovasodilator" has come to be utilized to designate a chemically heterogeneous group of agents that are linked by the fact that they contain at least one biologically active nitric oxide (NO•) moiety, which is potentially released as NO•, and that their pharmacological effects include dilatation of vascular smooth muscle. Such agents include not only the organic nitrate esters, but also a wide variety of non-nitrate donors of NO•.

Initial reports of the vasodilator effects of the organic nitrates and their therapeutic utility extend back to the observations of Brunton in 1857 that the related compound amyl nitrite rapidly relieved anginal pain, but with relatively transient beneficial effects. Murrell *(1)* reported that sublingual nitroglycerin (glyceryl trinitrate, NTG) was useful for the treatment of episodes of angina pectoris; the 1% solution utilized also appeared to prevent attacks of angina over a moderate period of time.

Despite the rapid acceptance of the use of organic nitrates for the management of angina pectoris, it also became apparent that creating an optimal balance between excessive vasodilator response and eventual loss of clinical efficacy ("tolerance") presented potential problems. In the setting of NTG exposure in the munitions industry, there were reports, not only of headaches and flushing, but also of the development of immunity to these symptoms during continuous exposure to NTG *(2)*. Furthermore, reports of development of angina pectoris and occasionally of myocardial infarction in munitions workers during periods of nitrate withdrawal also appeared. In the clinical setting, initial reports of loss of nitrate effect were followed by a systematic investigation by Crandall and colleagues in 1931 demonstrating attenuation both of headaches and of hypotensive effects of nitrates *(3)*.

CHEMICAL STRUCTURE: AVAILABLE PREPARATIONS

Nitrovasodilators may be conventionally classified on the basis of the presence or absence of at least one organic nitrate ester group. However the structures of both nitrate-containing and other NO• donors are extremely heterogeneous and result in biologically important accessory actions for several such agents.

A comparison of chemical structures of a number of agents in current therapeutic use is provided in Fig. 1, whereas the major categories of nitrovasodilators under current or potential therapeutic development, together with currently available preparations, are summarized in Table 1. Some available intravenous formulations of NTG contain propylene glycol, which

From: *Contemporary Cardiology, vol. 4: Nitric Oxide and the Cardiovascular System*
Edited by: J. Loscalzo and J. A. Vita © Humana Press Inc., Totowa, NJ

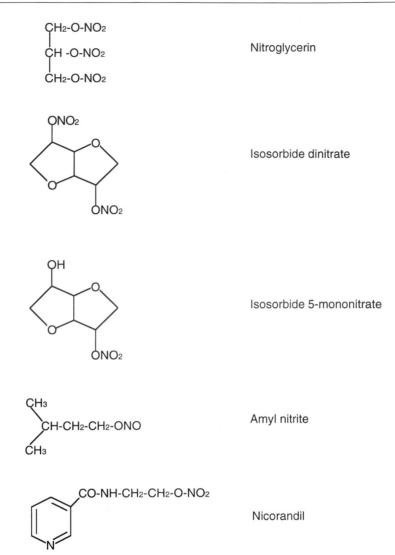

Fig. 1. Structures of various representative nitrovasodilators: Nitroglycerin (glyceryl trinitrate), isosorbide dinitrate, isosorbide 5-mononitrate, amyl nitrite, and nicorandil.

is potentially cardiotoxic, and which may have contributed to the previously reported interaction between high concentrations of intravenously infused NTG and heparin *(4)*. Propylene glycol-containing NTG preparations should probably not be utilized for intracoronary administration, regardless of prior dilution. Furthermore, because of the poor aqueous solubility of most organic nitrates, stock solutions of such agents for intravenous infusion contain high concentrations of alcohol, which occasionally may become clinically relevant, with infusion of nitrates at relatively high rates.

Intravenous infusion of organic nitrates, especially NTG, is complicated by the potential for significant adsorption of NTG onto plastic, particularly polyvinyl chloride *(5)*. Hence, utilization of specialized infusion apparatus with polyethylene tubing is essential to eliminate the possibility of marked, although variable, loss of infused nitrate. This problem is particularly important in the context of clinical attempts to optimize nitrate efficacy over relatively prolonged periods of time, which tend to require quite low rates of administration of nitrates *(6)*.

Nitrate preparations utilized for the relief of anginal attacks are administered sublingually, either as tablets or spray. Available preparations of NTG for sublingual administration range

Table 1
Major Categories of Nitrovasodilators
with Currently Available Preparations for Therapeutic Administration Where Relevant

Category	Preparations in widespread clinical use
Organic nitrites	
Amyl nitrite	—
Organic nitrates	Sublingual tablets or spray, buccal tablets,
Glyceryl trinitrate	Cutaneous ointment or transdermal discs,
(nitroglycerin)	intravenous injection
Isosorbide dinitrate	Sublingual tablets (including sustained release),
	intravenous injection
Isosorbide 5-mononitrate	Tablets (including sustained release)
Erythrityl tetranitrate	Sublingual and oral tablets
Pentaerythritol etranitrate	Tablets (including sustained release)
Organic nitrate/K_{ATP} agonist	
Nicorandil	Tablets
Substituted sydnonimines	
Molsidomine	Tablets
Nitroprusside	
Sodium nitroprusside	Intravenous injection

from 0.15–0.6 mg, whereas NTG spray administers 0.4 mg per spray. However, as individual responsiveness to nitrates varies widely, even in the absence of prior induction of tolerance, many patients may find that optimal therapeutic effects are achieved with considerably lower doses, necessitating sublingual administration of fragments of NTG tablets.

PHARMACOKINETICS AND BIOCHEMICAL PHARMACOLOGY

All nitrovasodilators are prodrugs, and their biological activity resides largely or entirely in the process of release of NO•. However, considerable uncertainty persists as to the precise mechanism(s) of bioconversion, or to their relationship to the resultant biological activity of the agents concerned; this reflects both difficulty in quantifying NO• generation in parallel with denitration of these compounds in biological systems, and the requirement for utilization of a gas chromatographic assay with electron-capture detection system in order to quantitate organic nitrate kinetics in vivo (7,8).

The majority of investigations of mechanisms of organic nitrate bioconversion have been performed with NTG. A number of aspects of this process remain controversial to some extent:

1. Does nonenzymatic denitration occur?
2. Which enzyme systems are involved, and are they equally effective in NO• generation?
3. To what extent is bioconversion sulfhydryl (SH) related?
4. Does end-product inhibition occur?

Although none of these controversies have been resolved totally to date, a number of aspects have been clarified in part (8) by recent investigations. As regards the issue of non-enzymatic release of NO•, it is clear that this occurs readily with most nonnitrate compounds, particularly in the presence of reducing agents. However, many such NO• donors are relatively stable; e.g., if sodium nitroprusside is protected from light, there is no detectable in vitro release of NO• (9). As regards organic nitrates, the evidence for occurrence of nonenzymatic bioconversion is limited to the observation that large concentrations of some (but not all) thiol compounds release NO• from NTG (10). However, the overwhelming evidence favors the hypothesis that bioconversion of organic nitrates in vivo is virtually entirely enzymatic

(8,11,12) and, indeed, that there may be a component of enzymatic bioconversion of some non-nitrate compounds *(11)*.

As regards the enzyme system(s) involved in bioconversion of organic nitrates, it is clear that multiple enzymes, some of which have not been fully characterized to date, are involved and that these vary considerably from tissue to tissue. Enzymatic denitration of organic nitrates, however, may under some circumstances induce primarily the formation of inorganic nitrite, which in turn is a poor vasodilator and probably does not yield significant quantities of any other activator of soluble guanylyl cyclase *(13)*. Overall, difficulties in understanding the relationship between nitrate bioconversion and biological effect include the following:

1. The fact that not all denitration reactions inevitably result in the release of NO•,
2. Difficulty in quantitation of NO• release in biological systems in association with enzymatic bioconversion, and
3. The possibility that bioconversion may vary between intact tissues and broken cell preparations.

In fact, studies in broken cell preparations are complicated by the potential under such circumstances for nonenzymatic bioconversion of nitrates in the presence of thiols, such as glutathione *(14)*, and critical fluctuation of bioconversion depending on the use of aerobic or anaerobic conditions *(15)*; it appears that a greater proportion of bioconversion in broken cell preparations is nonenzymatic than in intact cells *(12)*.

Because of the uncertain relationship between organic nitrate metabolism and nitrate (effectively NO•) response, the evaluation of this process should ideally involve assessment of the metabolizing system, kinetics of denitration, and continuous assessment of NO• release. No single study to date has achieved these objectives. Regarding the metabolizing enzymes, it appears that most tissues metabolize organic nitrates, and, therefore, the relevance of the enzyme system concerned relates in part to the probability that NO• will be generated in the immediate vicinity of a "target" organ, e.g., vascular smooth muscle, platelets, etc. Metabolism of orally administered nitrates within the liver is, therefore, predictably associated with some loss of biological activity within the systemic circulation.

It appears that the major enzyme system involved in the generation of NO• from organic nitrates is localized within cell membranes *(16)*. The microsomal protein concerned, with a molecular weight of about 160 kDa, exhibits a high rate of NO• generation (e.g., in bovine coronary artery smooth muscle cells), which is increased in the presence of increased thiol concentration. Although this enzyme has not been further characterized, a considerable body of information is available concerning the relative contributions of the cytochrome P450 system and various forms of the enzyme glutathione *S*-transferase (GST) in both denitration and NO• generation. Bennett and colleagues *(12)* have utilized the terms "mechanism-based" and "clearance-based" nitrate biotransformation to distinguish processes that lead to appreciable or minimal biological activity (in association with NO• generation), respectively; this is a useful concept, although it must be recalled that neither cytochrome P450 nor GST is likely to account for the majority of the biotransformation process.

There is considerable evidence that cytochrome P450 activity is associated with at least some mechanism-based bioconversion; although it also accounts for a component of hepatic presystemic nitrate inactivation *(17)*, the process has been shown to result in significant NO• release. Cytochrome P450, in association with reduced nicotinamide adenine dinucleotide phosphate (NADPH), has been shown to facilitate bioconversion of NTG in vascular smooth muscle microsomes *(18,19)*. Furthermore, the flavoprotein inhibitor diphenylene iodonium (DPI) has been shown to inhibit cDNA-expressed rat liver cytochrome P450 reductase, as well as reducing bioconversion of NTG in isolated aorta *(19)*. However, although DPI inhibits NTG-induced relaxation in some forms of vascular smooth muscle *(20)*, it is ineffective in others *(21)*, suggesting that NADPH–cytochrome P450 reductase is not uniformly involved in mechanism-based bioconversion.

A number of investigations have also implicated GST in the process of nitrate biotrans-formation. However, the role of GST in mechanism-based bioconversion is less clear-cut. On one hand, some investigators (22) have demonstrated only formation of nitrite (without detectable NO• release) as a result of the GST effect (in dog carotid artery); these results would imply that GST is involved entirely in clearance-based bioconversion. Other studies, however have found some evidence for involvement of GST both in formation of cyclic guanosine monophosphate (cGMP) and in vascular smooth muscle relaxation (23,24). More detailed studies have strongly suggested that GST is the major enzyme metabolizing NTG to yield NO• in human plasma (25), and that most vascular bioconversion of NTG in several preparations can be attributed to the mu isotype of GST (26,27).

Thus overall, it is clear that multiple enzyme systems are involved in nitrate biotransfor-mation, with regional variability not only of the enzymes involved but also of the efficiency of resultant NO• release. A final critical issue is the precise role played by thiol compounds in enzymatic biotransformation. Initially it was suggested that facilitation of guanylyl cyclase (GC) activation in the presence of some thiols might reflect formation of S-nitrosothiols, perhaps as an obligatory component of the sequence (14). However, formation of S-nitroso-thiols appears to account for only a minor component of nitrate effect, even in the presence of supplementary thiol sources (28). However, a series of experiments from Harrison's group indicate that a number of thiol agents potentiate, in a stereoselective manner, both the bio-conversion and the vasodilator effects of NTG, particularly in relatively small arteries (29,30). Both L-cysteine and N-acetylcysteine effects have been attributed primarily to resultant increased intracellular formation of glutathione (8). Intriguingly, it has also recently been shown that organic nitrates combined with cysteine are more effective than either NTG or isosorbide dinitrate in releasing NO• within arteries, suggesting a more critical level of involvement of thiols in the bioconversion process than in veins (31). In summary, a number of sulfhydryl (-SH)-containing compounds interact with bioconversion of organic nitrates and formation of NO• (as well as of S-nitrosothiols).

The pharmacokinetics of the nitrovasodilators are therefore of interest in particular as regards the relationship between regional denitration and regional NO• formation. Neverthe-less, there are important pharmacokinetic differences among the various organic nitrates, depending both on formation and on metabolism. A central aspect of the pharmacokinetics of organic nitrates is the presence of marked arteriovenous concentration gradients at steady state, reflecting continuous extraction and metabolism of parent drug by all vascular beds, although the extent of extraction varies (being approximately 60–70% across the femoral vascular bed and 17% across the lung) (32). Because of the facts that nitrates are prodrugs, and that the existence of arteriovenous concentration gradients, there is little purpose in util-izing venous plasma concentrations of nitrates as a measure of effect. Indeed, the possibility of measuring rates of bioconversion (either ratios of denitrated metabolite to the parent drug) or utilizing the magnitude of the arteriovenous gradient as a measure of drug bioconversion is also of only limited potential utility as a correlate of nitrate biochemical effect, as neither are necessarily related to NO• release to target tissues.

Nevertheless, both the bioconversion of organic nitrates and their conventional pharma-cokinetics are of some clinical relevance. Relevant aspects of the pharmacokinetics of some commonly utilized nitrates are summarized on Table 2. A common feature of all the com-monly utilized organic nitrates is a relatively high apparent volume of distribution, reflecting extensive tissue penetration. Despite this, clearance of all these agents is also high, with very short elimination half-lives, particularly for NTG. Hence, sustained therapeutic efficacy for all of these agents can be achieved only via controlled administration, e.g., via prolonged release from cutaneous patches (NTG) or by sustained release from orally administered tablets/capsules (e.g., ISDN [isosorbate dinitrate], IS5-MN [isosorbide-5-mononitrate]).

Table 2
Pharmacokinetics of Some Commonly Utilized Nitrate Preparations

Nitrate	Prep.	Major metabolite(s)	Pharmacokinetics		
			Bioavailability (%)	VD (L/kg)	$t_{1/2}$ (H)
Glyceryl trinitrate (nitroglycerin, (NTG)	i.v.	G 1,2-DN G 1,3-DN G 1-MN G 2-MN	<10	1.1	0.02
Isosorbide dinitrate (ISDN)	Oral	IS2-MN IS5-MN	25	3.5	1.2
Isosorbide 5-mononitrate (IS5-MN)	Oral	IS	>90	0.7	4.5
Nicorandil	Oral	SG86	75	1.4	1.0

VD = apparent volume of distribution (liters/kg); $t_{1/2}$ = elimination half-life (hours); G = glyceryl; IS = isosorbide; MN = mononitrate; DN = dinitrate; SG86 = N-(2-hydroxyethyl) nicorandil.

A number of other aspects of pharmacokinetics are of importance. As the process of denitration may release other nitrated metabolites (in, e.g., the cases of NTG, ISDN), these metabolites are themselves active (via further enzymatic denitration) (33) and tend to have more prolonged biological activity than the parent drug(s). There is also evidence that the specific metabolites produced vary with enzymatic systems involved, substrate concentration, and time; this has been investigated most extensively with NTG (12). Bennett and co-workers have demonstrated that glyceryl-1, 2-dinitrate (G-1,2-DN) is the major metabolite of NTG at relatively low (i.e., normal therapeutic) concentrations and that NTG biotransformation in the presence of hemoglobin (and the heme moiety of cytochrome P450) is also highly selective for G 1,2 DN, suggesting the presence of a second, low-affinity metabolic pathway that may exhibit increased activity following exposure to some enzyme inducers (18).

An interesting observation made in many relatively short-term pharmacokinetic studies is that of progressive reduction in nitrate clearance, manifest by increased plasma concentrations of the parent drugs within the first 24 h of drug administration (34–37). This observation relates in part to the various mechanisms contributing to the development of nitrate tolerance (vide infra), and has also raised the issue of inhibition of nitrate metabolism by endproducts, such as glyceryl dinitrate and/or NO* (38).

A final issue of critical pharmacokinetic importance relates to regional variability in extent of NO* formation from organic nitrates in the various major sites of nitrate effect, including endothelium, vascular smooth muscle, platelets, and myocardium. Although information is currently limited, available studies suggest that there is relatively limited bioconversion in the microvasculature (8,30), accounting for minimal arteriolar dilation response. Within the coronary circulation, it appears that the endothelium is a relatively minor site of NO* formation from nitrates (34), whereas most NO* effects on platelet function arise from nitrate biotransformation in plasma (25). However, small quantities of NO* formation from nitrates are detectable both in isolated endothelial cells and platelets (40).

A final issue relevant to the biochemical pharmacology and pharmacokinetics of the organic nitrates is to what extent release of oxygen-derived free radicals occurs as a component of nitrate biotransformation. This is discussed in association with the phenomenon of nitrate tolerance.

The "direct" NO* donor sodium nitroprusside (SNP), despite over 40 yr of clinical use, has not been studied adequately from a biochemical/pharmacokinetic point of view. However, it is clear that largely nonenzymatic formation of the cyanate and/or cyanide may occur, especially after prolonged infusion of high doses of SNP, resulting in potential toxicity *(41)*. Coadministration of hydroxycobalamin limits the risk of cyanide toxicity *(42)*.

PHARMACOLOGICAL EFFECTS

Vascular

The vasodilator effects of organic nitrates have long been considered to account for their anti-ischemic effects as well as their beneficial effects in patients with acute and chronic heart failure. However, the relationship between site(s) of vasodilator effect and specific therapeutic effect is complex, depending to some extent on the type of ischemic process. Overall, the major issue concerns the relative importance of peripheral vs. coronary vasodilator effects. However, the issue of relative potency within the various component vessels within both systemic and coronary circulations is also of clinical importance.

PERIPHERAL CIRCULATION

A number of investigations have provided evidence to suggest that the peripheral veins are most sensitive to acute organic nitrate administration *(43)*; however, the large arteries tend to be almost as responsive *(44)*. Detectable changes in peripheral resistance, reflecting arteriolar dilatation, tend to occur in response to nitrate doses approximately 10 times higher than those inducing effects on large arteries and veins. Hence, it is likely that therapeutic effects of nitrates may include improvement in left ventricular afterload achieved primarily by arterial dilatation with resultant changes in the reflected pulse wave; in the absence of arteriolar dilatation, such effects may be associated with only minimal changes in brachial arterial pressure *(45)*.

CORONARY CIRCULATION

Evaluation of nitrate effects on the coronary circulation may be performed either via systemic or direct intracoronary drug administration; the latter will minimize the potential for hypotension and secondary hemodynamic effects. In patients with stable angina pectoris, sublingual administration of NTG produced up to 40% increase in coronary artery diameter in normal vascular segments. Regions of coronary artery stenosis also dilated with NTG, although less than with native vessels. Maximal dilatation occurred in occluded arteries filled via bridging collateral vessels, suggesting a disproportionate effect on collateral blood flow *(46)*.

Intracoronary administration of NTG in doses as low as 5 µg produces marked coronary dilation *(47)*; selectivity for arteries filled via collaterals was again observed *(47,48)*.

A critically important issue is the effect of such agents on distribution of coronary blood flow relative to sites of possible or actual myocardial ischemia. Although a number of investigations have addressed this issue, perhaps the greatest contribution was made by Bache and colleagues *(49)* who studied the interaction between regional coronary perfusion, reactive hyperemia, and NTG therapy in a conscious dog model. Transient occlusion of the circumflex coronary artery in dogs with a residual circumflex stenosis resulted in underperfusion of the subendocardium during the postocclusive period. This maldistribution was partially corrected by NTG; it was suggested that NTG's effects in improving the subendocardial: subepicardial perfusion ratio might have reflected selective dilatation of penetrating arteries. It is also possible that the biochemical basis for augmented nitrate-mediated vasodilator effect in the presence of regional ischemia might be increased rates of denitration during hypoxia.

A related issue is whether the effects of organic nitrates in protecting subendocardial perfusion in ischemic zones and, thus, not exhibiting the phenomenon of coronary "steal" also apply in the presence of marked hypotension. Limited experimental data *(50,51)* indicate continued beneficial effect in some models. Finally, there are no definitive investigations to date concerning the effect of nonnitrate NO• donors (e.g., SNP, molsidomine, S-nitrosothiols) on regional coronary flow distribution during ischemia; concern has been expressed that because of their greater effects on arteriolar tone, these agents may be more prone to induce "steal" (8).

INTERACTIONS WITH ENDOTHELIUM

As the vascular endothelium represents the principal source of endogenous NO• formation within blood vessels, it is theoretically possible that incremental vascular responsiveness to organic nitrates might be affected by the extent of basal NO• release. Indeed, studies performed in isolated blood vessels from normal animals (52,53) indicate that endothelial removal results in not only a decrease in vascular cGMP content, but also a marked increase in apparent vascular responsiveness to exogenous NO• sources, such as NTG or SNP; similar effects resulted from inhibition of NOS.

An implication of these studies is that concentrations of superoxide anion within the normal endothelium are insufficient to constitute a critical limitation to nitrate response. On the other hand, endothelial injury promotes cyclic platelet thrombus formation, and this effect can be reversed by NTG; this beneficial action of NTG was potentiated by the thiol N-acetylcysteine (NAC) (58). In both normal subjects and patients with angina pectoris, there is evidence that organic nitrates inhibit ex vivo platelet aggregation (59,60) and prolong bleeding time (61). Effects of NTG on aggregation are dose related within conventional infusion regimens (62) and are incremental over the effects of aspirin (63,64).

The issue of apparent discrepancy between efficacy of nitrates in limiting aggregation in vivo and in vitro can be explained on the basis of a number of factors:

1. Maintenance of intracellular concentrations of reduced thiols critically modulating inhibition of aggregation (65) perhaps reflecting in part concomitant S-nitrosothiol formation.
2. The apparent potency of NO• donors to reverse platelet aggregation transiently enhanced in vitro at the time of initiation of aggregation, reflecting increased sensitivity of soluble guanylyl cyclase (sGC) to NO• (66).
3. Increased responsiveness to NO• donors when aggregation is induced by multiple agonists, as in vivo, rather than by a single agent (67).

The antiaggregatory effects of organic nitrates are of critical importance as regards their potential efficacy, both in the management of acute coronary syndromes (unstable angina pectoris and acute myocardial infarction) and also in the prevention of these conditions.

Myocardium

The major effects of organic nitrates on myocardial contractile performance would in most clinical settings reflect primarily nitrate-induced changes in regional myocardial ischemia. Hence, increases in left ventricular systolic function are usually secondary to the coronary and peripheral vasomotor effects of these agents. However, there is increasingly strong evidence that the direct effects of NO•, and, hence, of NO• donors, on contractility and on efficiency of myocardial oxygen utilization may also be of clinical importance.

There is evidence to suggest that NO• exerts a biphasic effect on contractile performance, with positive inotropic effects at very low concentrations and negative ones at higher concentrations (68), the latter effect partially reflecting interaction with β-adrenoceptor-mediated inotropic effects (possibly largely mediated by β_3-adrenoceptor stimulation [69]). Limited studies performed to date with organic nitrates (as distinct from nonnitrate NO• donors) also have demonstrated positive inotropic effects in vivo, which are not mediated by the process of coronary vasodilation or by changes in loading (70).

THERAPEUTIC UTILITY

Angina Pectoris

Angina pectoris, or symptomatic but potentially reversible myocardial ischemia, is relatively heterogeneous in origin. Clinical categories of angina are:

1. Classical ("exertional") angina, reflecting inadequacy of regional coronary perfusion induced in the presence of coronary stenosis in response to a temporary increase in myocardial oxygen requirement (e.g., exercise).
2. Mixed-pattern angina, reflecting a variable threshold for precipitation of ischemic symptoms owing to superimposed coronary stenoses and fluctuating adjacent coronary vasoconstriction.
3. Variant (Prinzmetal's) angina or precipitation of ischemia by purely coronary vasoconstriction (a relatively rare condition in Caucasians).
4. Unstable angina, in which myocardial ischemia is engendered by acute changes in coronary perfusion secondary to localized fissure/rupture of coronary atheromatous plaques and superimposed platelet aggregation and thrombus formation.
5. Angina decubitus, in which ischemia is precipitated in the recumbent position, primarily due to increased venous return in the presence of severely impaired left ventricular systolic function.

In view of this heterogeneity, potential efficacy (or otherwise) of organic nitrates reflects different aspects of nitrate pharmacotherapy depending on the cause of ischemia. For example, effects in exertional angina are likely a primary consequence of the peripheral vasodilator effects of these agents, perhaps particularly the effects on venous tone (although effects on arterial wave reflection may also be relevant); effects in mixed pattern and variant angina will be more closely related to effects on resting and elevated coronary vasomotor tone; efficacy in unstable angina will reflect changes in platelet aggregability as well as, possibly, regional coronary perfusion; and, finally, effects in angina decubitus may be mediated by changes in venous capacitance and efficiency of myocardial oxygen utilization. Hence, the clinical data available for evaluation of nitrate effects should be assessed according to the clinical anginal syndrome treated.

However, the mode of use of nitrates for the relief of acute episodes of angina in the various syndromes is independent of underlying cause. In all cases, choice of therapy is limited to preparations formulated for rapid systemic availability and, hence, rapid onset of action, such as sublingual NTG tablets or spray, or sublingual ISDN. In general, NTG is preferable to ISDN for relief of acute episodes of ischemia because of more rapid onset of effect. The choice between NTG tablets and spray is more difficult. NTG spray provides the advantage of a preparation that deteriorates minimally, and, thus, delivers a predictable dose of medication. Sublingual NTG tablets deteriorate markedly within several months of exposure to air, and, therefore, bottles should be replaced about every 3 mo once opened. On the other hand, there is marked interindividual variability in responsiveness to sublingual NTG, with many patients requiring very small doses (<0.1 mg) for relief of angina, and experiencing limiting symptoms (e.g., dizziness/headaches) with "standard" dosage; such individuals may find NTG tablets more suitable.

STABLE ANGINA

First, it should be recognized that sublingual nitrate therapy has a limited but important therapeutic role in prophylaxis of angina, despite the relatively short duration of action. When patients are able to predict the probable onset of angina with planned physical exercise or emotional stress, prophylactic use of short-acting nitrate preparations is very beneficial in these circumstances.

Efficacy of most currently available nitrate preparations for more prolonged prophylaxis of exertional angina has been evaluated extensively in clinical trials. The major issues that have dominated such investigations are:

1. Mode of evaluation of efficacy (e.g., treadmill exercise duration vs frequency of spontaneous ischemia).
2. Degree of efficacy during acute vs. chronic therapy (that is, potential for attenuation of effect due to onset of "nitrate tolerance").
3. Efficacy as monotherapy vs. incremental effect over other pharmacotherapies.

Of the various available organic nitrate preparations, NTG transdermal patches, ISDN, sustained-release isosorbide-5-mononitrate (ISMN), and nicorandil are most extensively used for stable angina. In each case, the process of developing optimal dosage regimens has been complicated by concerns about development of nitrate tolerance associated with continuous drug administration and by the relative difficulty in evaluating optimal dosage.

Clinical data with transdermal NTG patches initially suggested improvement in angina with continuous application over 24 h, but it rapidly became apparent that assessment of the benefit was complicated by the existence of a marked placebo effect. Furthermore, there was a strong suggestion that individual patients exhibited marked variability, both in initial and chronic responsiveness to NTG, with the result that a number of studies involved highly selected individuals. However, following reports of attenuation of NTG effect on exercise performance during chronic, continuous therapy, a large multicenter investigation of 562 patients on a wide range of doses of NTG revealed rapid and extensive loss of anti-ischemic effect (within 24 h) together with no evidence that a strategy of increasing NTG dosage would eventually result in achievement of a useful residual extent of efficacy. This has resulted in the almost universal (72) acceptance that intermittent application of NTG patches (e.g., for 12 of every 24 h) is the optimal method for achieving protection from ischemia with this delivery system. Indeed, there is now considerable evidence that such a strategy achieves long-term improvement of exercise tolerance (73,74); it appears that delivery of approx 0.6 mg/h of NTG is associated with optimal efficacy. The major residual concern about this, and indeed all intermittent nitrate delivery regimens, is not tolerance (which remains a minor problem), but the potential for development of rebound phenomena, an area of ongoing controversy (72–74) (see following).

A number of studies have been performed with ISDN, both in standard and sustained release formulations, in patients with stable angina pectoris. Standard formulations of ISDN provide appreciable plasma concentrations of the parent drug for up to 6 h. However, utilization of ISDN four times daily leads to induction of a considerable degree of tolerance (75). However, if ISDN (10–40 mg) is taken three times a day, with an eccentric dosing schedule incorporating a period of 14 h between two of the doses, there is limitation (but not elimination) of resultant tolerance (76). Sustained-release ISDN, given as single doses once a day, provides anti-ischemic effects for approx 12 h. It is unlikely that twice-daily administration of this preparation would avert the onset of tolerance.

IS5MN is available both in standard and sustained-release preparations. However, the majority of carefully controlled studies of anti-ischemic effect during acute and chronic dosing have been undertaken using sustained-release formulations, which provide for release of clinically relevant concentrations of IS5MN over a period of 12–16 h. A multicenter-controlled study evaluating the effects of 30–240 mg of IS5MN once daily in 313 patients with stable angina (77) over 42 d of treatment revealed that following initial dosing, there was significant prolongation of exercise duration (by 30–50 s) with all doses, together with efficacy over at least 12 h. By 42 d, there was no longer any prolongation of exercise duration with 30 and 60 mg/d, although benefits of 120 and 2540 mg remained statistically significant, indicating partial tolerance induction.

Less-extensive data are available to date regarding the efficacy of nicorandil in the prophylaxis of exertional angina. The majority of studies have utilized nicorandil doses of 10 mg or 20 mg twice daily. Investigations performed over periods of up to 7 wk have suggested that anti-anginal efficacy is comparable to that of β-adrenoceptor antagonists (78,79). Insuf-

Table 3
Categories of Pharmacotherapy Commonly Utilized
for In-Hospital Therapy of Patients with Unstable Angina Pectoris

Class	Agents	Evidence of efficacy
Cyclo-oxygenase inhibitor	Aspirin	No definite evidence of antianginal efficacy
		Limits rebound ischemia following heparin withdrawal
		Reduces incidence of long-term ischemia/ infarction
Heparin/ LMW heparins	Heparin (unfractionated)	Reduced risk of ongoing ischemia
	Enoxaparin	Reduced risk of ischaemia in short/medium term
	Fragmin	
Glycoprotcin IIb/IIIa antagonists	Abciximab	Short-term anti-ischemic effect
	Tirofiban	Reduced risk of infarction during coronary angioplasty
Organic nitrates	Intravenous NTG/ISDN	Reduced frequency of ischemia
	Cutaneous NTG/ oral ISDN	?
β-Adrenoceptor antagonists	Metoprolol	
	Atenolol	?
	Propranolol	
(Nondihydropyridine) calcium antagonists	Verapamil	Reduced risk of ongoing ischemia
	Diltiazem	

ficient clinical data arc available to determine to what extent induction of nitrate tolerance is associated with attenuation of therapeutic response to nicorandil during long-term use.

MIXED PATTERN AND VARIANT ANGINA

Both of these conditions are characterized by episodic increases in coronary vasomotor tone. Hence, sublingual nitrates are initially effective in relief of acute episodes of ischemia, including episodes of coronary spasm precipitated by provocative manoevres such as injection of ergonovine or acetylcholine (80). Occasionally, ergonovine injection may precipitate spasm resistant both to sublingual and intracoronary nitrate administration (81).

There are few controlled studies of treatment strategies for the prophylaxis of mixed pattern or variant angina pectoris. The latter condition tends to be associated with periods of activity and quiescence; hence, there is need for a large long-term study to evaluate optimal treatment methodology. In general, long-acting nitrates are coadministered with calcium antagonists, which may reduce the risk of "rebound" vasoconstriction during nitrate-free periods. As the maximal frequency of episodes of ischemia in variant angina is usually nocturnal (82), prophylactic nitrate administration regimens should emphasize the need for cover during this period.

UNSTABLE ANGINA

Although the pathogenesis of unstable angina is that of fissure or rupture of atheromatous plaques within the coronary circulation, probably preceded by local inflammatory change and followed by the development of local platelet aggregation and thrombus formation, the clinical course of the condition is extremely variable (83). In particular, the severity of initial ischemic symptoms, the evidence (or otherwise) of microinfarction of the myocardium on the basis of release of troponins into plasma, and the response to initial therapy all provide information as to the risk of medically intractable symptoms and/or development of acute myocardial infarction. Furthermore, current regimens for the management of unstable angina pectoris, regardless of the severity of the condition, involve various forms of polypharmacy, often making it difficult to evaluate the contribution of individual agents to resolution or continuation of ischemia. A summary of current perspectives in the initial management of unstable angina pectoris is provided in Table 3. It is important to emphasize that:

1. Efficacy of various agents may vary markedly according to the severity of the underlying condition *(84,85)*.
2. Although many reported clinical trials of anti-ischemic therapy in the past have utilized monotherapy with the investigated agents, most patients with unstable angina currently receive several agents during the inpatient phase, which almost inevitably will include low-dose aspirin, heparin, or a low-molecular-weight heparin analog, and some form of nitrate therapy.
3. There are a number of possible therapeutic goals, including suppression of acute ischemic symptoms (and thus removing the need for urgent coronary angioplasty or surgery), increasing safety during/following coronary angioplasty, and limitation of risk of long-term recurrence of ischemia; different agents may achieve different purposes in this regard.
4. Because occurrence of symptoms (or of asymptomatic ischemia) in patients with unstable angina pectoris is essentially independent of changes in heart rate and myocardial oxygen demand, there is need for 24-h protection against ischemia; hence, the potential development of tolerance with continuous organic nitrate therapy presents a particular problem with such agents; furthermore, unstable angina represents a major clinical risk scenario should sudden cessation of nitrate therapy induce "rebound" aggravation of ischemia.

Most clinical data as regards the acute-phase management of unstable angina pectoris with regimens including organic nitrates have utilized intravenously infused NTG. Although there is strong clinical evidence that such therapy suppresses ischemic symptoms in the short term *(6)*, a number of problems exist. These include the tendency of nitrates to adsorb onto plastics, particularly polyvinylchloride; hence, a specialized delivery system comprising a glass-bottle reservoir and polyethylene delivery tubing is optimal. Acute hemodynamic studies utilizing appropriate delivery systems have demonstrated that the threshold infusion rate for detectable effects of NTG in patients with angina pectoris is approx 5 µg/min *(86)*. Numerous studies have now demonstrated that infusion of NTG at rates only marginally higher than this is associated with the development of marked degrees of nitrate tolerance within 24 h *(87,88)*. Furthermore, sudden cessation of intravenous NTG administration has been associated with a high risk of clinically significant rebound ischemia *(89)*. Despite this, the majority of clinical studies investigating therapeutic efficacy of intravenous NTG have permitted infusion rates as high as 1000 µg/min *(6)*, and have not necessarily utilized transition to other nitrate delivery systems on cessation of intravenous NTG infusion. Hence, it is most unlikely that such regiments have achieved optimal therapeutic efficacy of the infused nitrate. It would appear optimal to utilize intravenous NTG infusion rates of ≤20 µg/min in the absence of coadministered agents limiting development of nitrate tolerance *(see* following). Notably, interpretation of the results of the only double-blind controlled study reported to date of nitrate vs. diltiazem pharmacotherapy for short-term management of unstable angina *(90)* must be limited by (1) lack of specifications of nonadsorbent delivery tubing, and (2) utilization of intravenous NTG infusion rates of ≥50 µg/min in most patients.

The coinfusion of NTG with the sulfhydryl agent *N*-acetylcysteine (NAC), which potentiates the systemic and coronary haemodynamic effects of NTG, and which may prevent nitrate tolerance *(see* following), has been associated with improved short-term efficacy of NTG *(91)*. Furthermore, long-term coadministration of NAC and NTG limits the risk of recurrence of angina in patients with unstable angina *(92)*.

DECUBITUS ANGINA

As indicated earlier, mechanisms of symptom development in patients with angina decubitus are similar to those in patients with severe congestive heart failure and paroxysmal nocturnal dyspnea. Therapy (including treatment with nitrates) is, therefore, primarily that for the underlying heart failure.

Acute Myocardial Infarction

An extensive body of experimental data has raised the possibility that nitrates may be effective as a component of initial pharmacotherapy of acute myocardial infarction. In fact, nitrates in non-Q-wave acute infarction; as in unstable angina pectoris, probably provide the major benefit by suppressing ongoing ischemia, reflecting both antiaggregatory and coronary hemodynamic effects.

Experimental studies of nitrate effect in models of acute infarction have generally been conducted in animals with persistently occluded infarct-related arteries (thus imitating circumstances associated with failed/nonattempted thrombolysis on coronary angioplasty. Under these conditions, beneficial effects of nitrates in the short term might result from improved collateral blood flow and from the systemic hemodynamic effects limiting afterload and ameliorating pulmonary edema. Experimental data strongly favor the use of relatively low doses of nitrates; infusion rates of NTG associated with 0–10% reduction in mean arterial pressure reduced infarct size in a conscious dog model, whereas higher doses had no beneficial effect (94).

Early clinical trials of nitrovasodilators in acute myocardial infarction (exclusively carried out in the absence of thrombolytic therapy) utilized both intravenous NTG and SNP (95). Although results of studies with SNP infusion tended to be inconclusive, the available data on NTG suggested a reduction of short-term mortality of approx 30%. However, two larger randomized studies, GISSI-3 and ISIS-4, performed during the thrombolytic era, have subsequently cast some doubt over the value of nitrate therapy.

The GISSI-3 study (96) involved a comparison of treatment with NTG, lisinopril, both, or neither within 24 h of the onset of symptoms, in a total of 19,394 patients. Initially, NTG was infused at a rate of 5 µg/min, but the rate was increased to induce a hypotensive response. After 24 h, the infusion was terminated and transdermal NTG (10 mg/24 h, with a nitrate-free period) was utilized for the remainder of the 6 wk of the trial. The results of the study showed a 12% (significant) reduction in mortality with lisinopril and a 6% (nonsignificant) reduction in mortality with NTG. Importantly, combined administration of lisinopril and NTG produced a 17% reduction in mortality, as against 9% with lisinopril alone. Thus, the results of the study raised the possibility of an incremental therapeutic effect with combined therapy.

The ISIS-4 study (97) randomized patients to potentially receive intravenous magnesium sulphate, and IS5MN, captopril alone, or in combination. Although captopril produced a small but significant reduction in 5-wk mortality, IS5MN was without significant effect. There was a marked reduction in mortality on the first day postinfarct ($p < 0.001$) with IS5MN. It is probable that the daily dose utilized (60 mg) was too small to have a sustained anti-ischemic effect in the majority of patients (77). Consistent with this, IS5MN failed to reduce the incidence of postinfarction angina.

A number of further important issues must be mentioned in association with current recommendations for nitrate therapy during the acute phase of myocardial infarction. First, nitrate efficacy may depend on the mode of therapy utilized. Specifically, nitrates may impair the thrombolytic efficacy of tissue plasminogen activator (98) while possibly increasing that of streptokinase (99). Data on the impact of acute nitrates on efficacy of primary angioplasty for infarction are lacking. Second, nitrate therapy, although effective in treating peri-infarction pulmonary edema, is generally safe; systemic hypotension is rare. Finally, there is some evidence that prolonged nitrate therapy may prevent the process of "remodeling," i.e., progressive deterioration of systolic function and enlargement of the left ventricle during the months following infarction. In view of the widely accepted role for therapy with angiotensin-converting enzyme (ACE) inhibitors in such patients, the critical issue is whether the effects of nitrates are incremental. Available data to date in postinfarct patients are largely confined to a double-blind placebo controlled study in 291 postinfarct patients; active treatment consisted of NTG patches delivering 0.4, 0.8, or 1.6 mg/h of NTG *(100)*. The results after 6 mo of treatment indicated that beneficial effects on left ventricular systolic function were observed only with the lowest NTG dose, and were most marked in patients with markedly depressed function at entry. The implications of these results on utilization of nitrates long-term postinfarct cannot be fully assessed without a larger investigation powered to evaluate the impact on clinical status/survival.

Congestive Heart Failure

Largely because of their effects in reducing venous return and limiting myocardial ischemia, many nitrovasodilators have been utilized in the short- and long-term management of congestive heart failure (CHF). In general, studies have provided evidence for good symptomatic improvement, but less clearcut evidence of impact on long-term outcome.

In patients with acute pulmonary edema, both reflecting acute myocardial ischemia and as a result of fluid overload in congestive cardiomyopathy, acute treatment with both sodium nitroprusside *(101)* and with organic nitrates (generally intravenous NTG or ISDN) *(102)* has been shown to improve both hemodynamics and clinical status rapidly in most cases. Although efficacy of nitrate therapy in the immediate management of CHF is comparable or superior to that of diuretic-based therapy *(102)*, two major problems have been found to limit efficacy in the long term: *de novo* nitrate resistance and nitrate tolerance. The majority of recent clinical studies have utilized nitrates in combination with other agents, in attempts to limit these problems; these investigations are discussed later in the chapter.

Two large long-term studies investigating (inter alia) the effects of long-term therapy with ISDN on outcome in patients with chronic CHF are of considerable importance. The V-HeFT I study utilized a combination of ISDN (administered four times daily) and hydralazine, and demonstrated that this regimen was associated with a survival benefit of borderline statistical significance relative to placebo therapy *(103)*. Subsequently the V-HeFT II study suggested that this ISDN–hydralazine combination was less effective than enalapril (20 mg/d) as regards survival, but that ISDN-hydralazine was more effective in improving exercise performance *(104)*. Unfortunately, both V-HeFT studies were somewhat undersized for assessment of drug effects on prognosis. Perhaps more importantly, these studies leave unanswered the issues of (1) whether or not the therapeutic effect of ISDN-hydralazine was mediated by the drug combination, or was either agent alone effective (an important question, given the high incidence of adverse effects with high dose hydralazine therapy), and (2) whether or not nitrate therapy might be combined effectively with ACE inhibitors, which are of proven benefit on prognosis in CHF.

On the basis of currently available data, therefore, organic nitrates may be regarded as first-line therapy for the management of cardiac acute pulmonary edema, except in the presence of cardiogenic shock. However, their role in the management of chronic CHF in the absence of ongoing ischemia is a secondary one. Perhaps the most useful role of long-term nitrate therapy in such patients is in prevention of nocturnal pulmonary edema; in such circumstances nitrates should be administered at night (e.g., IS5MN or transdermal NTG just before retiring).

Systemic Hypertension

Organic nitrate therapy has never been evaluated in the long-term management of hypertension. Doses of nitrates sufficient to lower brachial arterial pressure appreciably are usually sufficient to induce development of considerable nitrate tolerance. However, given the more recently appreciated effects of nitrates on left ventricular afterload, which are achieved largely via increases in arterial compliance and reduction in afterload, it is possible that nitrate therapy may improve clinical outcomes in hypertensive patients; this possibility merits clinical trial assessment.

In patients with hypertensive crises, SNP has a well-recognized clinical role in acute management. Infusion of SNP has the advantage of titrating blood pressure predictably to appropriate endpoints, with minimal risk of occurrence of hypotension *(103)*.

Peri-Intervention

In patients with acute ischemic syndromes who are to undergo urgent coronary revascularization, nitrate therapy is usually continued prior and throughout the procedure. Among the possible benefit of this strategy are prevention of withdrawal phenomena, reduced risk of coronary spasm during surgery or angioplasty, and of internal mammary artery constriction during surgery.

However, it is also possible that nitrate therapy prior to revascularization procedures may be beneficial via activation of the process of ischemic preconditioning *(104)*.

LIMITATION OF NITRATE EFFECT

As previously indicated, it has been apparent since the early experience of nitrate effects on workers in the munitions industry that the intensity of NTG-induced vasodilation may decrease during chronic exposure: this phenomenon has been designated nitrate tolerance. However, impairment of vascular and other responses to nitrovasodilators may also occur without prior exposure to these agents (i.e., *de novo* resistance may occur). Furthermore, decreased responsiveness during chronic nitrovasodilator exposure does not necessarily imply a reduction in NO• release nor in biochemical response to NO•. Several interacting mechanisms appear to account for *de novo* nitrate resistance and (acquired) nitrate tolerance.

Nitrate Resistance

As discussed earlier, there is evidence to suggest that endothelial integrity/disruption may modulate responsiveness to nitrovasodilators. Furthermore, endothelial "dysfunction" is characterized in part by diminution or absence of vasodilator responses to agents such as acetylcholine (ACh), which induce NO• release from endothelium *(54)*. However, information on determinants of responsiveness to exogenous NO• donors in conditions associated with endothelial "dysfunction" remains limited.

In patients with chronic CHF, a number of observations provide evidence for the occurrence of nitrate resistance. Armstrong et al. *(105)* reported that approx 30% of patients with heart failure failed to achieve a 25% reduction in mean pulmonary artery pressure despite infusion of NTG at very high rates. Similar findings were reported by other investigators *(106, 107)*. It was also noted that patients resistant to high doses of isosorbide dinitrate tended to have higher resting right atrial pressures than responders *(107)*. Although it was suggested initially that nitrate resistance might reflect the presence of high vasoconstrictor tone, no studies demonstrated such a mechanism. Recent investigations *(108,109)* have demonstrated that in patients with severe CHF there is also a reduction in arterial vasodilator response to infusion of NTG or SNP; again it is possible that reduced responsiveness to a "direct" NO• donor might reflect neurohumoral activation. However, it is also possible that this abnormality may reflect increased rates of NO• clearance in patients with CHF, perhaps by virtue of increased production of NO• via induction (iNOS), may result in decreased responsiveness of sGC to exogenous NO• donors *(109,110)*.

Furthermore, there is evidence that responsiveness to nitrovasodilators may be diminished in some circumstances in the absence of CHF. Cardillo and colleagues *(111)* demonstrated that normotensive black subjects have smaller forearm vasodilator responses to SNP than whites. Elevation of plasma triglyceride concentrations markedly diminished vasomotor responses to NTG *(112)*. Platelets from patients with stable angina pectoris show diminished antiaggregatory responses to NTG and SNP *(60,113)*.

These findings suggest that nitrate resistance is an important cause of reduced responsiveness to nitrovasodilators. At this stage, however, insufficient data are available as to the precise mechanism(s) of this phenomenon.

Nitrate Tolerance

Nitrate tolerance, defined on the basis of progressive attenuation of some or all responses to organic nitrates during chronic exposure, represents the major limiting factor to the therapeutic utility of nitrovasodilators. It is now clear that there is no single cause for nitrate tolerance, and, indeed, that there is not necessarily any diminution in NO$^\bullet$ effect in all cases. Conceptually, it is of some use to examine two major components of the problem:

1. "True tolerance": i.e., decreased activity of the NO$^\bullet$-cGMP biochemical "cascade."
2. "Pseudotolerance": i.e., activation of mechanisms in vivo that exert opposing pharmacological effects to those of NO$^\bullet$, thus limiting the net effect independent of any diminution of NO$^\bullet$ biochemical response. Thus, activation of vasoconstrictor mechanisms may obscure the vasodilator effect of NO$^\bullet$ donors.

It is likely that these two component mechanisms do not exist entirely in isolation from one another, but that they are responsible for somewhat different aspects of the clinical features associated with nitrate tolerance.

A further major problem concerns the extent to which mechanisms of nitrate tolerance may be elucidated by in vitro study, which may fail to observe the effects of changes in neurohumoral milieu during chronic exposure to nitrovasodilators in vivo. For these reasons, it appears that in vitro studies may provide misleading results under some circumstances.

The clinical features of nitrate tolerance may be very subtle; attenuation of nitrate-induced prolongation of exercise duration is rarely noted clinically. Indeed, clinical trials powered to detect onset of tolerance in patients with exertional angina generally require at least 100 subjects selected on the basis of stable exercise tolerance and good initial response to nitrates *(73,74,77)*, particularly as the development of tolerance does not necessarily imply total abolition of therapeutic effect.

More easily detectable clinically are those phenomena associated primarily with "pseudotolerance," i.e., the "zero-hour phenomenon" and other forms of rebound phenomena associated with nitrate withdrawal. It is emphasised that these phenomena may occur under circumstances (e.g., during intermittent nitrate administration) when "true" tolerance is minimised. The zero-hour phenomenon consists of unexpected impairment of exercise capacity during nitrate-free periods, e.g., just before application of transdermal nitrate patches in the morning. This has been observed in several *(73,114)*, but not all *(74)*, studies of intermittent administration of prophylactic nitrates. Related to the zero-hour phenomenon is the occurrence of anginal pain at rest during nitrate withdrawal, related to the phenomena originally described in munitions workers *(2)*. Sudden cessation of intravenous NTG infusion has been reported to induce exacerbation of ischemia in a high proportion of patients *(89)*. Similarly, applications of transdermal NTG for 12 h beginning in the morning appears to increase the risk of nocturnal angina while reducing risk of angina during the day *(115)*. On the other hand, it remains uncertain to what extent patients taking multiple prophylactic antianginal agents remain prone to aggravation of ischemia during nitrate-free periods.

Table 4
Postulated Mechanisms for Occurrence of Nitrate Tolerance/Pseudotolerance

Mechanism	Current status/comments
Impaired NO• release	Implies essentially nitrate-specific process: possibly SH related
Increased NO• inactivation	Prerequisite is increased formation of superoxide via angiotensin II. May lead to peroxynitrite formation.
Inactivation of sGC	Limited in vivo data
Increased production of vasoconstrictors	Probable major mechanism of pseudotolerance/rebound. However, it is a variable phenomenon Endothelin, catecholamines, angiotensin II may be involved.
Plasma volume expansion	Probably paraphenomenon

It is clear that no single mechanism accounts for the various components of tolerance in all patients. However, a number of categories of abnormality have been proposed, and may be summarized as outlined in Table 4. Of the five major areas of postulated mechanisms outlined, the largest body of experimental data until very recently have been concerned with the possibility that NO• formation is impaired, essentially via progressive decreases in extent of denitration. Thus, this hypothesized process is essentially nitrate specific. It was initially suggested by Needleman and coworkers (116) that nitrate tolerance was the result of vascular sulfhydryl (SH) depletion during chronic therapy. Although this postulate is supported by some data, such as the critical role of SH-containing compounds in nitrate biotransformation (8,11) and the formation of S-nitrosothiols as a component of the biotransformation "cascade" (11); other data are more equivocal. There are convincing data linking nitrate effect with extent of denitration (62), and a number of studies have suggested that onset of nitrate tolerance is associated with elevated plasma concentrations of nonmetabolized nitrate (34,117).

Similarly, impairment of nitrate bioconversion associated with tolerance development has been demonstrated in in vitro studies (37,118). On the other hand, one recent study could no reduction in NO• formation in the presence of in vivo induction of nitrate tolerance (119).

Data concerning the extent of association of generalized or localized SH depletion with induction of nitrate tolerance do not resolve to the issue of mechanism(s) of tolerance induction, as it is likely that SH depletion reflects, at least largely, the occurrence of oxidant stress. Furthermore, SH depletion is an inconstant finding (116,120,121) in models of nitrate tolerance, being best documented for low-molecular-weight thiols, such as cysteine and glutathione in platelets and plasma (122). Similarly, the extensive data concerning potentiation of nitrate responses and/or reversal of tolerance by SH-containing agents (discussed as follows) are nonspecific as regards mechanism of effect, as these agents are likely both to limit redox stress and facilitate nitrate bioconversion.

Specificity of nitrate-induced tolerance offers an important clue as to the involvement of nitrate-specific bioconversion processes in the genesis of tolerance. However, the various available studies very to some extent. Specifically, most investigations in which tolerance is induced in vitro indicate extensive crosstolerance between nitrates, but considerably lesser degrees of crosstolerance to SNP, molsidomine, and NO• (123). However, tolerance induction in vivo has been reported both as a relatively nitrate-specific phenomenon (124,125) and also under other circumstances associated with appreciable crosstolerance to "direct" NO• donors (126,127). It may, therefore, be concluded that the balance of evidence suggests that nitrate tolerance is generally associated with impaired nitrate bioconversion. Crosstolerance to non-nitrates, where present, implies the existence of other mechanisms, such as increased clearance of NO• and/or inactivation of sGC.

The most attractive mechanism postulated thus far to account for a second, non-nitrate-specific, site for nitrate tolerance is interaction of NO• with superoxide anion, with resultant

Table 5
Major Strategies Directed Toward Minimization of Tolerance Development

Strategy	Current status
Nitrates other than NTG	Possible that nicorandil and/or pentaerythrytyl tetranitrate may be less prone to tolerance induction.
Nonnitrates	Molsidomine and linsidomine appear relatively resistant to tolerance induction, as do *S*-nitrosothiols.
Nitrate-free intervals	Tolerance can be limited provided interval >10 h. However possible risk of "rebound"; lack of 24-h effect.
Sulfhydryl agents	*N*-Acetylcysteine potentiates nitrate effect and prevents tolerance in some models. ?Promise of nitrate/SH combinations.
ACE inhibitors	High-dose ACE inhibitors effective in some models—possibly via limitation of O_2^- formation.
Other agents	Limited data in support of hydralazine, carvedilol, angiostensin-receptor antagonists, and vitamins C and E.

formation of peroxynitrite, with less active vasodilator and some toxic effects. In an important study, Munzel and coworkers *(127)* induced tolerance to NTG in rabbits, and subsequently demonstrated impaired dilatation of aortae both to NTG and acetylcholine, consistent with diminished $NO^•$ release or effect. Simultaneously, vascular superoxide levels were elevated, and liposome-entrapped superoxide dismutase normalized responses to NTG and ACh. A number of subsequent findings engendered the hypothesis *(128)* that angiotensin II might initiate the cellular events leading to incremental superoxide generation, essentially via activation of NAD[P]H oxidase and protein kinase C *(129)*. On the other hand, investigations in patients with coronary artery disease (in the absence of heart failure) showed that continuous infusion of NTG at a rate of 0.5 µg/kg resulted in initial transient activation of neurohormonal mechanisms (increased plasma renin activity, plasma aldosterone and plasma vasopressin) but that this activation had disappeared prior to development of tolerance *(130)*. Furthermore, given the involvement of thiols in antioxidant mechanisms, it is possible that thiol depletion observed in some models of nitrate tolerance reflects increased superoxide formation.

It might, therefore, be suggested that apparent loss of tissue response to nitrates may involve three factors, alone or in combination:

1. Impairment of $NO^•$ release from organic nitrates ("site 1 tolerance" *[123]*).
2. Increased inactivation of $NO^•$ via superoxide, perhaps most relevant when there is increased activation of the renin-angiotensin system ("site 2 tolerance").
3. Increased vasoconstrictor tone (pseudotolerance) representing both the release of vasoconstrictors and potentiation of arterial responses to these agents.

Strategies for Optimization of the Effects of Nitrovasodilation

A large number of strategies have been devised for possible circumvention of the problem of tolerance. These are summarized in Table 5.

Use of Nitrates Other Than NTG

Although most current investigations suggest that all organic nitrates are potentially susceptible to induction of tolerance, it appears that the extent of this phenomenon may vary. Pentaerythrytyl tetranitrate displays minimal development of tolerance relative to NTG in some models, perhaps via less susceptibility to release of superoxide and resultant tissue thiol depletion *(131)*. It has also been suggested that nicorandil may exhibit decreased propensity toward tolerance induction, but, as tolerance is easily demonstrable in vitro *(132)*, this is likely to represent residual nitrate-independent vasodilator effect (via a K^+-channel opening), which may be less relevant to anti-ischemic effects.

NON-NITRATE SOURCES OF NO•

A number of non-nitrate NO• donors have been developed as potential antiischemic agents. Notable among these are molsidomine and linsidomine (substituted sydnonimines), which show diminished susceptibility to tolerance induction in most models *(123)*. However, it remains uncertain whether the anti-ischemic efficacy of such compounds is equivalent to that of organic nitrates.

NITRATE-FREE INTERVALS

There is now an extensive literature documenting that nitrate tolerance can be minimized by the use of dosing regimens that provide nitrate-free (or nitrate-poor) intervals of 10–12 h/d. Indeed, it is widely considered that this is the only unequivocally proven strategy for limitation of tolerance induction *(73,74,76,77)*. However, this is a far from perfect strategy, for several reasons. First, there is still some evidence of tolerance induction *(77)*. Second, intermittent nitrate administration may predispose toward the development of rebound syndromes *(89,115)* including the "zero hour" phenomenon *(73)*. Finally, as noted earlier, intermittent nitrate therapy (even excluding the possibility of rebound) is unsuitable for monotherapy of acute coronary syndromes such as unstable angina pectoris or acute myocardial infarction, where the risk of ischemia is not purely dependent on exercise-induced increased heart rate.

SH AGENTS

The possible use of SH-containing agents for limiting and/or reversing nitrate tolerance stems from the original observations of Needleman and coworkers *(116)* suggesting that nitrate tolerance reflected a state of SH depletion, and that it could be partially reversed by some SH agents. Furthermore, Ignarro and coworkers demonstrated subsequently that in broken cell preparations activation of sGC by organic nitrates was variably potentiated by SH-containing compounds and inhibited by ethacrynic acid, which decreases SH availability. It was also suggested that formation of *S*-nitrosothiols might represent an intermediate stage in sGC activation *(14)*. Finally, a series of experiments in patients undergoing cardiac catheterization revealed that the SH agent NAC potentiated NTG-induced systemic *(86)* and coronary *(133)* vasodilatation, and partially reversed nitrate tolerance in the systemic *(134)* and coronary *(135)* circulations. Furthermore, NAC markedly potentiated the effects of NTG in inhibiting platelet aggregation *(65)*.

In the past 15 years, a large number of studies have addressed the possible clinical significance of potentiation of nitrate effects by SH-containing agents. Although the majority of studies indicate that NAC (the most frequently utilized SH source) potentiates nitrate effects, results are conflicting as to whether it is also effective in both preventing and reversing tolerance induction in vivo. This may stem, in part, from the precise mechanism(s) of "tolerance" present: NAC may increase release of NO• from nitrates, and also reduce NO• clearance by superoxide anion, but there is little evidence that it interferes with the mechanisms underlying pseudotolerance. Recent in vitro studies also suggest that SH agents may be more effective in preventing rather than reversing SH depletion *(136)*.

In the clinical arena, there are somewhat conflicting data as regards the significance of incremental effects of NAC over nitrates in exertional angina *(137)*, unstable angina, and acute myocardial infarction (summarized in ref. *138*). The most consistent data are in patients with unstable angina pectoris, where both short-term *(139)* and long-term *(140)* beneficial effects on major cardiac events have been observed. Furthermore, studies in acute myocardial infarction demonstrate reduced redox stress and suggest improved hemodynamics with combined NTG–NAC therapy *(141)*. However, the extent to which these results may reflect antiaggregatory *(58,65)* rather than vascular nitrate–SH interactions is currently uncertain. Combined NTG–NAC therapy also shows promise in the management of pulmonary edema *(134,142–144)*.

A number of in vivo and in vitro studies have tested the hypothesis that the SH-containing angiotensin-converting enzyme (ACE) inhibitors captopril may potentiate nitrate effects and/or limit nitrate tolerance. However, there are insufficient data to evaluate whether the SH content of captopril may be relevant to any observed interactions (*see* following).

ACE INHIBITORS

Prevention of nitrate tolerance by non-SH–ACE inhibitors would support the postulated role of angiotensin II formation in the genesis of tolerance. Although some data support the concept that tolerance development can be retarded by high doses of ACE inhibitors *(145, 146)*, these results are not consistent in the clinical setting.

OTHER AGENTS

Hydralazine has been shown to limit nitrate tolerance in experimental models *(148,149)* by inhibiting NADH oxidase activation *(149)*. However, although this has been suggested as the basis for beneficial effect of combined therapy with ISDN and hydralazine in heart failure, a clinical trial found no evidence of beneficial interaction *(150)*.

Vitamin C (in high doses) has also been shown to have some effect in retarding nitrate tolerance development in arteries and platelets *(151)*. However, studies of the clinical consequences of this effect are currently lacking.

ADVERSE EFFECTS, INTERACTIONS AND CONTRAINDICATIONS

The common adverse effect of organic nitrate therapy is headache, due to dilatation of extracranial arteries. In some patients, this may limit the therapeutic utility of nitrates for both treatment and prophylaxis of angina, despite the use of very small doses of the drug. Systemic hypotension also is a relatively frequent complication of acute nitrate therapy, especially in the presence of previously reduced left ventricular filling pressure. Hence, nitrate use is relatively hazardous in the presence of right ventricular infarction, chronic pulmonary hypertension, and acute pulmonary embolism. There have also been occasional reports of precipitation of methemoglobinemia with very high doses of intravenous NTG.

As previously discussed, nitrate tolerance imposes limits to nitrate efficacy, whereas pseudotolerance may lead to a clinically significant rebound phenomenon, with the risk of aggravation of ischemia.

Organic nitrates have been implicated in a number of interactions of potential clinical significance. Inhibition of clinical efficacy of heparin appears to occur only with very high infusion rates of NTG *(4,152)*. Of more clinical relevance, however, is impairment of the thrombolytic efficacy of tissue-type plasminogen activator (t-PA) thrombolysis by concurrent NTG infusion, with associated reduction in plasma t-PA concentrations probably reflecting increases in clearance due to NTG *(153)*.

However, the interaction of most clinical significance involving organic nitrates is that involving inhibitors of cyclic GMP-specific phosphodiesterase, of which sildenafil is the prototype in clinical use. The vasodilator effects of all organic nitrates are markedly potentiated by sildenafil, and may result in severe and potentially fatal hypotension. Sildenafil should be regarded as absolutely contraindicated in patients taking nitrates for angina pectoris, whereas, conversely, the development of angina or acute infarction within 24 h of sildenafil ingestion is best managed without nitrates *(154)*.

FUTURE PERSPECTIVES
IN NITROVASODILATOR THERAPY

A number of distinct areas of developments can be discerned at this stage:

1. *New indications for nitrate therapy.* Nitrates have shown therapeutic promise in the management of a number of gastrointestinal (bleeding associated with portal hypertension, spasm of sphincter of Oddi, anal fissure) and obstetric (pre-eclampsia, preterm labor) conditions. However, clinical data are limited to date in these disorders; further investigation is required.

2. *Prevention of tolerance.* As outlined earlier, a large number of strategies are currently under investigation for limitation of tolerance development. Achievement of that aim offers the prospect of providing, via nitrovasodilator therapy, partial restoration of homeostasis in many cardiovascular ("NO•-deficient") disorders.

REFERENCES

1. Murrell W. Nitroglycerine as a remedy for angina pectoris. Lancet I 1879;80–1, 113–115, 151–152, 225–227, 642–646.
2. Ebright GE. The effects of nitroglycerin in those engaged in its manufacture. JAMA 1914;62:201–209.
3. Crandall LA, Leake CD, Loevenhart AS, Muehlberger CW. Acquired tolerance to and cross tolerance between the nitrous and nitric acid esters in sodium nitrite in man. J Pharmacol Exp Ther 1931;41: 103–112.
4. Col J, Col-Debeys C, Lavenne-Pardonge E, Meert P, Hericks L, Broze MC, et al. Propylene glycol-induced heparin resistance during nitroglycerin infusion. Am Heart. J 1985;110:171–173.
5. Roberts MS, Cossum PA, Galbraith AJ, Boyd GW. The availability of nitroglycerin from parenteral solutions. J Pharm Pharmacol 1980;32:237–244.
6. Horowitz JD. Role of nitrates in unstable angina pectoris. Am J Cardiol 1992;70:64B–71B.
7. Yap PS, McNiff EF, Fung H-L. Improved GLC determination of plasma nitroglycerin concentrations. J Pharm Sci 1978;67:582–584.
8. Harrison DG, Bates JN. The nitrovasodilators. New ideas about old drugs. Circulation 1993;87: 1461–1467.
9. Bates JN, Baker MT, Guerra R Jr, Harrison DG. Nitric oxide generation from nitroprusside by vascular tissue: evidence that reduction of the nitroprusside and cyanide loss are required. Biochem Pharmacol 1991;42:S157–S165.
10. Feelisch M, Noack E. Nitric oxide (NO) formation from nitrovasodilators occurs independently of hemoglobin or non-heme iron. Eur J Pharmacol 1987;142:465–469.
11. Fung H-L, Chung S-J, Bauer JA, Chong S, Kowaluk EA. Biochemical mechanism of organic nitrate action. Am J Cardiol 1992;70:4B–10B.
12. Bennett BM, McDonald BJ, Nigam R, Simon WC. Biotransformation of organic nitrates and vascular smooth muscle cell function. Trends Pharmacol Sci 1994;15:245–249.
13. Romanin C, Kukovetz WR. Guanylate cyclase activation by organic nitrates is not mediated via nitrite. J Mol Cell Cardiol 1988;20:389–396.
14. Ignarro LJ, Lippton H, Edwards JC, Baricos WH, Hyman AL, Kadowitz PJ, et al. Mechanism of vascular smooth muscle relaxation by organic nitrates, nitrites, nitroprusside and nitric oxide: evidence for the involvement of S-nitrosothiols as active intermediates. J Pharmacol Exp Ther 1981;218:739–749.
15. Bennett BM, McDonald BJ, St James MJ. Hepatic cytochrome P-450-mediated activation of rat aortic guanylyl cyclase by glyceryl trinitrate. J Pharmacol Exp Ther 1992;261:716–723.
16. Chung S-J, Fung H-L. Identification of the subcellular site for nitroglycerin metabolism to nitric oxide in bovine coronary smooth muscle cells. J Pharmacol Exp Ther 1990;253:614–619.
17. Servent D, Delaforge M, Ducrocq C, Mansuy D, Lenfant M. Nitric oxide formation during microsomal hepatic denitration of glyceryl trinitrate: involvement of cytochrome P-450. Biochem Biophys Res Commun 1989;163:1210–1216.
18. McDonald BJ, Bennett BM. Biotransformation of glyceryl trinitrate by rat aortic cytochrome P450. Biochem Pharmacol 1993;45:268–270.
19. McGuire JJ, Anderson DJ, McDonald BJ, Narayanasami R, Bennett BM. Inhibition of NADPH-cytochrome P450 reductase and glyceryl trinitrate biotransformation by diphenyleneiodonium sulfate. Biochem Pharmacol 1998;56:881–893.

20. McGuire JJ, Anderson DJ, Bennett BM. Inhibition of the biotransformation and pharmacological actions of glyceryl trinitrate by the flavoprotein inhibitor, diphenyleneiodonium sulfate. J Pharmacol Exp Ther 1994;271:708–714.

21. De la Lande IS, Philp T, Stafford I, Horowitz JD. Lack of inhibition of glyceryl trinitrate by diphenyleneiodonium in bovine coronary artery. Eur J Pharmacol 1996;314:347–350.

22. Kurz MA, Boyer TD, Whalen R, Peterson TE, Harrison DG. Nitroglycerin metabolism in vascular tissue: role of glutathione S-transferases and relationship between NO. and NO_2^- formation. Biochem J 1993;292:545–550.

23. Nigam R, Whiting T, Bennett BM. Effect of inhibitors of glutathione S-transferase on glyceryl trinitrate activity in isolated rat aorta. Can J Physiol Pharmacol 1993;71:179–184.

24. Simon WC, Anderson DJ, Bennett BM. Inhibition of the pharmacological actions of glyceryl trinitrate after the electroporetic delivery of a glutathione S-transferase inhibitor. J Pharmacol Exp Ther 1996; 279:1535–1540.

25. Chen LY, Mehta P, Mehta JL. Platelet inhibitory effect of nitroglycerin in platelet-rich plasma: relevance of glutathione-s-transferase in plasma. J Invest Med 1996;44:561–565.

26. Kenkare SR, Han C, Benet LZ Correlation of the response to nitroglycerin in rabbit aorta with the activity of the mu class glutathione S-transferase. Biochem Pharmacol 1994;16:2231–2235.

27. Nigam R, Anderson DJ, Lee SF, Bennett BM. Isoform-specific biotransformation of glyceryl trinitrate by rat aortic glutathione S-transferases. J Pharmacol Exp Ther 1996;279:1527–1534.

28. Chirkov YY, Gee DJ, Naujalis I, Sage RE, Horowitz JD. Reversal of ADP-induced platelet aggregation by S-nitrosothiols, nitroglycerine and nitroglycerine/N-acetylcysteine. Pharmacol Commun 1993;3: 97–105.

29. Sellke FW, Tomanrek RJ, Harrison DG. L-cysteine selectively potentiates nitroglycerin-induced dilation of small coronary microvessels. J Pharmacol Exp Ther 1991;258:365–369.

30. Kurz MA, Lamping KG, Bates JN, Eastham CL, Marcus ML, Harrison DG. Mechanisms responsible for the heterogeneous coronary microvascular response to nitroglycerin. Circ Res 1991;68:847–855.

31. Mulsch A, Bara A, Mordivintcev P, Vanin A, Busse R. Specificity of different organic nitrates to elicit NO formation in rabbit vascular tissues and organs in vivo. Br J Pharmacol 1995;116:2743–2749.

32. Armstrong PW, Moffat JA, Marks GS. Arterial-venous nitroglycerin gradient during intravenous infusion in man. Circulation 1982;66:1273–1276.

33. Haefeli WE, Gumbleton M, Benet LZ, Hoffman BB, Blaschke TF. Comparison of vasodilatory responses to nitroglycerin and its dinitrate metabolites in human veins. Clin Pharmacol Ther 1992;52:590–596.

34. Fung H-L. Pharmacokinetics of nitroglycerin and long-acting nitrate esters. Am J Med 1983;74:13–20.

35. Bergami A, Bernasconi R, Caccia S, Leopaldi D, Mizrahi J, Sardina M, et al. Pharmacokinetics of isosorbide dinitrate in healthy volunteers after 24-hours intravenous infusion. J Clin Pharmacol 1997; 37:828–833.

36. Wolf DL, Ferry JJ, Hearron AE, Froeschke MO, Luderer JR. The haemodynamic effects and pharmacokinetics of intravenous nicorandil in healthy volunteers. Eur J Clin Pharmacol 1993;44:27–33.

37. Feelisch M, Kelm M. Biotransformation of organic nitrates to nitric oxide by vascular smooth muscle and endothelial cells. Biochem Biophys Res Commun 1991;180:286–293.

38. Kojda G, Patzner M, Hacker A, Noack E. Nitric oxide inhibits vascular bioactivation of glyceryl trinitrate: a novel mechanism to explain preferential venodilatation of organic nitrates. Mol Pharmacol 1998;53:547–554.

39. Schror K, Forster S, Woditsch I. On-line measurement of nitric oxide release from organic nitrates in the intact coronary circulation. Naunyn Schmiedebergs Arch Pharmacol 1991;344:240–246.

40. Weber AA, Neuhaus T, Seul C, Dusing R, Schror K, Sachinidis A, et al. Biotransformation of glyceryl trinitrate by blood platelets as compared to vascular smooth muscle cells. Eur J Pharmacol 1996;309: 209–213.

41. Vesey CJ, Cole PV, Linnell JC, Wilson J. Some metabolic effects of sodium nitroprusside in man. Br Med J 1974;2:140–142.

42. Zerbe NF, Wagner BK. Use of vitamin B12 in the treatment and prevention of nitroprusside-induced cyanide toxicity. Crit Care Med 1993;21:465–467.

43. Bassenge E, Stewart DJ. Effects of nitrates in various vascular sections and regions. Z Kardiol 1986; 75:1–7.

44. Bassenge E, Zanzinger J. Nitrates in different vascular beds, nitrate tolerance, and interactions with endothelial function. Am J Cardiol 1992;70:23B–29B.

45. Kelly RP, Gibbs HH, O'Rourke MF, Daley JE, Mang K, Morgan JJ, et al. Nitroglycerin has more favourable effects on left ventricular afterload than apparent from measurement of pressure in a peripheral artery. Eur Heart J 1990;11:138–144.

46. Feldman RL, Pepine CJ, Curry RC Jr, Conti CR. Coronary arterial responses to graded doses of nitroglycerin. Am J Cardiol 1979;43:91–97.

47. Feldman RL, Marx JD, Pepine CJ, Conti CR. Analysis of coronary responses to various doses of intracoronary nitroglycerin. Circulation 1982;66:321–327.

48. Cohen MV, Downey JM, Sonnenblick EH, Kirk ES. The effects of nitroglycerin on coronary collaterals and myocardial contractility. J Clin Invest 1973;52:2836–2847.

49. Bache RJ, Ball RM, Cobb FR, Rembert JC, Greenfield JC Jr. Effects of nitroglycerin on transmural myocardial blood flow in the unanaesthetized dog. J Clin Invest 1975;55:1219–1228.

50. Fujita Y, Habazettl H, Corso CO, Messmer K, Yada T. Comparative effects of hypotension due to isoflurane, nitroglycerin, and adenosine on subendocardial microcirculation: observation of the in situ beating swine heart under critical stenosis. Anesthesiology 1997;87:343–353.

51. Wenzel V, Lidner KH, Mayer H, Lurie KG, Prengel AW. Vasopressin combined with nitroglycerin increases endocardial perfusion during cardiopulmonary resuscitation in pigs. Rescuscitation 1998;38: 13–17.

52. Jackson WF, Busse R. Elevated guanosine 3':5'-cyclic monophosphate mediates the depression of nitro-vasodilator reactivity in endothelium-intact blood vessels. Naunyn Schmiedebergs Arch Pharmacol 1991;344:345–350.

53. Moncada S, Rees DD, Schulz R, Palmer RM. Development and mechanisms of a specific supersensitivity to nitrovasodilators after inhibition of vascular nitric oxide synthesis in vivo. Proc Natl Acad Sci USA 1991;88:2166–2170.

54. Ludmer PL, Selwyn AP, Shook TL, Wayne RR, Mudge GH, Alexander RW, et al. Paradoxical vaso-constriction induced by acetylcholine in atherosclerotic coronary arteries. N Engl J Med 1986;315: 1046–1051.

55. Hampton JR, Harrison MJ, Honour AJ, Mitchell JR. Platelet behaviour and drugs used in cardiovas-cular disease. Cardiovasc Res 1967;1:101–106.

56. Schafer AI, Alexander RW, Handin RI. Inhibition of platelet function by organic nitrate vasodilators. Blood 1980;55:649–654.

57. Lam JY, Chesebro JH, Fuster V. Platelets, vasoconstriction, and nitroglycerin during arterial wall injury. A new antithrombotic role for an old drug. Circulation 1988;78:712–716.

58. Folts JD, Stamler J, Loscalzo J. Intravenous nitroglycerin infusion inhibits cyclic blood flow responses caused by periodic platelet thrombus formation in stenosed canine coronary arteries. Circulation 1991; 83:2122–2127.

59. Diodati J, Theroux P, Latour JG, Lacoste L, Lam JT, Waters D. Effects of nitroglycerin at therapeutic doses on platelet aggregation in unstable angina pectoris and acute myocardial infarction. Am J Cardiol 1990;66:683–688.

60. Chirkov YY, Naujalis JI, Sage RE, Horowitz JD. Antiplatelet effect of nitroglycerin in healthy subjects and in patients with stable angina pectoris. J Cardiovasc Pharmacol 1993;21:384–389.

61. De Caterina R, Lanza M, Manca G, Strata GB, Maffei S, Salvatore L. Bleeding time and bleeding: an analysis of the relationship of the bleeding time test with parameters of surgical bleeding. Blood 1994; 84:3363–3370.

62. Karlberg KE, Torfgard K, Ahlner J, Sylven C. Dose-dependent effect of intravenous nitroglycerin on platelet aggregation, and correlation with plasma glyceryl dinitrate concentration in healthy men. Am J Cardiol 1992;69:802–805.

63. Karlberg KE, Ahlner J, Henriksson P, Torfgard K, Sylven C. Effects of nitroglycerin on platelet aggregation beyond the effects of acetylsalicylic acid in healthy subjects. Am J Cardiol 1993;71:361–364.

64. Cockcroft JR, Ritter JM. Effects of aspirin and glyceryl trinitrate on bleeding time in man. Thromb Haemorrh Dis 1991;3:49–51.

65. Loscalzo J. N-acetylcysteine potentiates inhibition of platelet aggregation by nitroglycerin. J Clin Invest 1985;76:703–708.

66. Chirkov YY, Belushkina NN, Tyshchuk IA, Severina IS, Horowitz JD. Increase in reactivity of human platelet guanylate cyclase during aggregation potentiates the disaggregating capacity of sodium nitro-prusside. Clin Exp Pharmacol Physiol 1991;18:517–524.

67. Willoughby SR, Chirkova LP, Horowitz JD, Chirkov YY. Multiple agonist induction of aggregation: an approach to examine anti-aggregating effects in vitro. Platelets 1996;7:329–333.

68. Mohan P, Brutsaert DL, Paulus WJ, Sys SU. Myocardial contractile response to nitric oxide and cGMP. Circulation 1996;93:1223–1229.

69. Gauthier C, Leblais V, Kobzik L, Trochu JN, Khandoudi N, Bril A, et al. The negative inotropic effect of beta 3-adrenoceptor stimulation is mediated by activation of a nitric oxide synthase pathway in human ventricle. J Clin Invest 1998;102:1377–1384.

70. Preckel B, Kojda G, Schlack W, Ebel D, Kottenberg K, Noack E, et al. Inotropic effects of glyceryl trinitrate and spontaneous NO donors in the dog heart. Circulation 1997;96:2675–2682.
71. Reichek N, Priest C, Zimrin D, Chandler T, Sutton MS. Antianginal effects of nitroglycerin patches. Am J Cardiol 1984;54,1–7.
72. Klemsdal TO, Gjesdal K. Intermittent or continuous transdermal nitroglycerin: still an issue, or is the case closed? Cardiovasc Drug Ther 1996;10:5–10.
73. DeMots H, Glasser SP. Intermittent transdermal nitroglycerin therapy in the treatment of chronic stable angina. J Am Coll Cardiol 1989;13:786–795.
74. Parker JO, Amies MH, Hawkinson RW, Heilman JM, Hougham AJ, Vollmer MC, et al. Intermittent transdermal nitroglycerin therapy in angina pectoris. Clinically effective without tolerance or rebound. Minitran Efficacy Study Group. Circulation 1995:1368–1374.
75. Thadani U, Fung H-L, Darke AC, Parker JO. Oral isorbide dinitrate in angina pectoris: comparison of duration of action and dose-response relation during acute and sustained therapy. Am J Cardiol 1982; 49:411–419.
76. Parker JO, Farrell B, Lahey KA, Moe G. Effect of intervals between doses on the development of tolerance to isosorbide dinitrate. N Engl J Med 1987;316:1440–1444.
77. Chrysant SG, Glasser SP, Bittar N, Shahidi FE, Danisa K, Ibrahim R, et al. Efficacy and safety of extended-release isosorbide mononitrate for stable effort angina pectoris. Am J Cardiol 1993;72:1249–1256.
78. Meeter K, Kelder JC, Tijssen JG, Bucx JJ, Henneman JA, Kerker JP, et al. Efficacy of nicorandil versus propranolol in mild stable angina pectoris of effort: a long-term, double-blind, randomized study. J Cardiovasc Pharmacol 1992;20:S59–S66.
79. Di Somma S, Liguori V, Petitto M, Carotenuto A, Bokor D, de Divitiis O, et al. A double-blind comparison of nicorandil and metoprolol in stable effort angina pectoris. Cardiovasc Drugs Ther 1993;7:119–123.
80. Okumura K, Yasue H, Horio Y, Takaoka K, Matsuyama K, Kugiyama K, et al. Multivessel coronary spasm in patients with variant angina: a study with intracoronary injection of acetylcholine. Circulation 1988;77:535–542.
81. Babbitt DG, Perry JM, Forman MB. Intracoronary verapamil for reversal of refractory coronary vasospasm during percutaneous transluminal coronary angioplasty. J Am Coll Cardiol 1988;12:1377–1381.
82. Miwa K, Ingawa A, Miyagi Y, Nakagawa K, Inoue H. Alterations of autonomic nervous activity preceding nocturnal variant angina: sympathetic augmentation with parasympathetic impairment. Am Heart J 1998;135:762–771.
83. Bashour TT, Myler RK, Andreae GE, Stertzer SH, Clark DA, Ryan CJ. Current concepts in unstable angina pectoris. Am Heart J 1987;115:850–861.
84. No authors listed. A comparison of aspirin plus tirofiban with aspirin plus heparin for unstable angina. N Engl J Med 1998;338:1498–1505.
85. PRISM-Plus Investigators. Inhibition of the platelet glycoprotein IIb/III: a receptor with tirofiban in unstable angina and non-Q-wave myocardial infarction. N Engl J Med 1998;338:1488–1497.
86. Kern MJ, Ganz P, Horowitz JD, Gaspar J, Barry WH, Lorell BH, et al. Potentiation of the coronary vasoconstriction by beta-adrenergic blockade in patients with coronary artery disease. Circulation 1983;67:1178–1185.
87. Elkayam U, Kulick D, McIntosh N, Roth A, Hsueh W, Rahimtoola SH. Incidence of early tolerance to hemodynamic effects of continuous infusion of nitroglycerin in patients with coronary heart disease and heart failure. Circulation 1987;76:577–584.
88. Jugdutt BI, Warnica JW. Tolerance with low dose intravenous nitroglycerin therapy in acute myocardial infarction. Am J Cardiol 1989;64:581–587.
89. Figueras J, Lidon R, Cortadellas J. Rebound myocardial ischaemia following abrupt interruption of intravenous nitroglycerin infusion in patients with unstable angina at rest. Eur Heart J 1991;12:405–411.
90. Gobel EJ, Hautvast RW, van Gilst WH, Spanjaard JN, Hillege HL, De Jongste MJ, et al. Randomised, double-blind trial of intravenous diltiazem versus glyceryl trinitrate for unstable angina pectoris. Lancet 1995;346:1653–1657.
91. Horowitz JD, Henry CA, Syrjanen ML, Louis WJ, Fish RD, Smith TW, et al. Combined use of nitroglycerin and N-acetylcysteine in the management of unstable angina pectoris. Circulation 1988;77: 787–794.
92. Ardissino D, Merlini PA, Savonitto S, Demicheli G, Zanini P, Bertocchi F, et al. Effect of transdermal nitroglycerin or N-acetylcysteine, or both, in the long-term treatment of unstable angina pectoris. J Am Coll Cardiol 1997;29:941–947.
93. Jugdutt BI, Becker LC, Hutchins GM, Bulkley BH, Reid PR, Kallman CH. Effect of intravenous nitroglycerin on collateral blood flow and infarct size in the conscious dog. Circulation 1981;63:17–28.

94. Jugdutt BI. Myocardial salvage by intravenous nitroglycerin in conscious dogs: loss of beneficial effect with marked nitroglycerin-induced hypotension. Circulation 1983;68:673–684.

95. Yusuf S, Collins R, MacMahon S, Peto R. Effects of intravenous nitrates on mortality in acute myocardial infarction: an overview of the randomised trials. Lancet 1988;1:1088–1092.

96. No authors listed. GISSI-3: effects of lisinopril and transdermal glyceryl trinitrate singly and together on 6-week mortality and ventricular function after acute myocardial infarction. Gruppo Italiano per lo Studio della Sopravvivenza nell' infarto Miocardico. Lancet 1994;343:1115–1122.

97. ISIS-4 Collaborative Group. Fourth International Study of Infarct Survival. ISIS-4: a randomised factorial trial assessing early oral captopril, oral mononitrate, and intravenous magnesium sulphate in 58,050 patients with suspected acute myocardial infarction. Lancet 1995;345:669–685.

98. Nicolini FA, Ferrini D, Otani F, Galvani M, Ronchi A, Behrens PH, et al. Concurrent nitroglycerin therapy impairs tissue-type plasminogen activator-induced thrombolysis in patients with acute myocardial infarction. Am J Cardiol 1994;74:662–666.

99. Lee KJ, Horowitz JD, McKay WJ, Goble AJ. Myocardial salvage with steptokinase combined with nitroglycerine and verapamil in acute myocardial infarction. Int J Cardiol 1988;21:279–291.

100. Mahmarian JJ, Moye LA, Chinoy DA, Sequeira RF, Habib GB, Henry WJ, et al. Transdermal nitroglycerin patch therapy improves left ventricular function and prevents remodeling after acute myocardial infarction: results of a multicenter prospective randomised, double-blind, placebo-controlled trial. Circulation 1998;97:2017–2024.

101. Guiha NH, Gohn JN, Mikulic E, Franciosa JA, Limas CJ. Treatment of refractory heart failure with infusion of nitroprusside. N Engl J Med 1974;291:587–592.

102. Cotter G, Metzkor E, Kaluski E, Faigenberg Z, Miller R, Simovitz A, et al. Randomised trial of high-dose isosorbide dinitrate plus low-dose furosemide versus high-dose furosemide plus low-dose isosorbide dinitrate in severe pulmonary edema. Lancet 1998;351:389–393.

103. Gifford RW. The treatment of hypertensive emergencies. Am J Cardiol 1962;9:880–887.

104. Takano H, Tang X-L, Qiu Y, Guo Y, French BA, Bolli R. Nitric oxide donors induce late preconditioning against myocardial stunning and infarction in conscious rabbits via an antioxidant sensitive mechanism. Circ Res 1998;83:73–84.

105. Armstrong PW, Armstong JA, Marks GS. Pharmacokinetic-hemodynamic studies of intravenous nitroglycerin in congestive heart failure. Circulation 1980;62:160–166.

106. Packer M, Medina N, Yushak M, Lee WH. Hemodynamic factors limiting the response to transdermal nitroglycerin in severe chronic congestive heart failure. Am J Cardiol 1986;57:260–267.

107. Kulick D, Roth A, McIntosh N, Rahimtoola SH, Elkayam U. Resistance to isosorbide dinitrate in patients with severe chronic congestive heart failure: incidence and attempt at hemodynamic prediction. J Am Coll Cardiol 1988;12:1023–1028.

108. Katz SD, Rao R, Berman JW, Schwarz M, Demopoulos L, Bijou R, et al. Pathophysiological correlates of increased serum tumour necrosis factor in patients with heart failure. Relation to nitric oxide-dependent vasodilation in the forearm circulation. Circulation 1994;90:12–16.

109. Carville C, Adnot S, Sediame S, Benacerraf S, Castaigne A, Calvo F, et al. Relation between impairment in nitric oxide pathway and clinical status in patients with congestive heart failure. J Cardiovasc Pharmacol 1998;32:562–570.

110. Papapetropoulos A, Abou-Mohamed G, Marczin N, Murad F, Caldwell RW, Catravas JD. Down-regulation of nitrovasodilator-induced cyclic GMP accumulation in cells exposed to endotoxin or interleukin-1 beta. Br J Pharmacol 1996;118:1359–1366.

111. Cardillo C, Kilcoyne CM, Cannon RO, Panza JA. Attenuation of cyclic nucleotide-mediated smooth muscle relaxaton in blacks as a cause for racial differences in vasodilator function. Circulation 1999; 99:90–95.

112. Lundman P, Eriksson M, Schenck-Gustafsson K, Karpe F, Tornvall P. Transient triglyceridemia decreased vascular reactivity in young, healthy men without risk factors for coronary heart disease. Circulation 1997;96:3266–3268.

113. Chirkov YY, Chirkova LP, Horowitz JD. Suppressed anti-aggregating and cGMP-elevating effects of sodium nitroprusside in platelets from patients with stable angina pectoris. Naunyn Schmiedebergs Arch Pharmacol 1996;354:520–525.

114. Parker JD, Parker AB, Farrell B, Parker JO. Intermittent transdermal nitroglycerin therapy. Decreased anginal threshold during the nitrate-free interval. Circulation 1995;91:973–978.

115. Ferratini M, Pirelli S, Merlini P, Silva P, Pollavini G. Intermittent transdermal nitroglycerin monotherapy in stable exercise-induced angina, a comparison with a continuous schedule. Eur Heart J 1989; 10:998–1002.

116. Needleman P, Johnson EM Jr. Mechanism of tolerance development to organic nitrates. J Pharmacol Exp Ther 1973;184,709–715.
117. Torfgard K, Ahlner J, Axelsson KL, Norlander B, Bertler A. Tissue levels of glyceryl trinitrate and cGMP after in vivo administration in rat, and the effect of tolerance development. Can J Physiol Pharmacol 1991;69:1257–1261.
118. Slack CJ, McLaughlin BE, Brien JF, Marks GS, Nakatsu K. Biotransformation of glyceryl trinitrate and isosorbide dinitrate in vascular smooth muscle made tolerant to organic nitrates. Can J Physiol Pharmacol 1989;67:1381–1385.
119. Laursen JB, Mulsch A, Boesgaard S, Mordvintcev P, Trautner S, Gruhn N, et al. In vivo nitrate tolerance is not associated with reduced bioconversion of nitroglycerin to nitric oxide. Circulation 1996; 94:2241–2247.
120. Boesgaard S, Aldershvile J, Poulsen HE, Loft S, Anderson ME, Meister A. Nitrate tolerance in vivo is not associated with depletion of arterial or venous thiol levels. Circ Res 1994;74:115–120.
121. Haj-Yehia AI, Benet LZ. Dissociation of tissue thiols content from nitroglycerin-induced cyclic-3'5'-guanosine monophosphate and the state of tolerance in: in vivo experiments in rats. J Pharmacol Exp Ther 1995;273:94–100.
122. Fink B, Bassenge E. Unexpected tolerance devoid vasomotor and platelet actions of pentaerythrityl tetranitrate. J Cardiovasc Pharmacol 1997;30:831–836.
123. Henry PJ, Horowitz JD, Louis WJ. Nitroglycerin-induced tolerance affects multiple sites in the organic nitrate bioconversion cascade. J Pharmacol Exp Ther 1989;248:762–768.
124. Sutsch G, Kim JH, Bracht C, Kiowski W. Lack of cross-tolerance to short-term linsidomine in forearm resistance vessels and dorsal hand veins in subjects with nitroglycerin tolerance. Clin Pharmacol Ther 1997;62:538–545.
125. Du ZY, Buxton BF, Woodman OL. Tolerance to glyceryl trinitrate in isolated human internal mammary arteries. J Thorac Cardiovasc Surg 1992;104:1280–1284.
126. Laursen JB, Boesgaard S, Poulsen HE, Aldershvile J. Nitrate tolerance impairs nitric oxide-mediated vasodilation in vivo. Cardiovasc Res 1996;31:814–819.
127. Munzel T, Sayegh H, Freeman BA, Tarpey MM, Harrison DG. Evidence for enhanced vascular superoxide anion production in nitrate tolerance. A novel mechanism underlying tolerance and cross-tolerance. J Clin Invest 1995;95:187–194.
128. Munzel T, Kurz S, Heitzer T, Harrison DG. New insights into mechanisms underlying nitrate tolerance. Am J Cardiol 1996;77:24c–30c.
129. Munzel T, Harrison DG. Evidence for a role of oxygen-derived free radicals and protein kinase C in nitrate tolerance. J Mol Med 1997;75:891–900.
130. Munzel T, Heitzer T, Kurz S, Harrison DG, Luhman C, Pape L, et al. Dissociation of coronary vascular tolerance and neurohormonal adjustments during long-term nitroglycerin therapy in patients with stable coronary artery disease. J Am Coll Cardiol 1996;27:297–303.
131. Fink B, Bassenge E. Unexpected tolerance-devoid vasomotor and platelet actions of pentaerythrityl tetranitrate. J Cardiovasc Pharmacol 1997;30:831–836.
132. Henry PJ, Horowitz JD, Louis WJ. Nitrate tolerance induced by nicorandil or nitroglycerin is associated with minimal loss of nicorandil vasodilator activity. J Cardiovasc Pharmacol 1990;15:365–370.
133. Winniford MD, Kennedy PL, Wells PJ, Hillis LD. Potentiation of nitroglycerin-induced coronary dilatation by N-acetylcysteine. Circulation 1986;73:138–142.
134. Packer M, Lee WH, Kessler PD, Gottlieb SS, Medina N, Yushak M. Prevention and reversal of nitrate tolerance in patients with congestive heart failure. N Engl J Med 1987;317:799–804.
135. May DC, Popma JJ, Black WH, Schaefer S, Lee HR, Levine BD, et al. In vivo induction and reversal of nitroglyerin tolerance in human coronary arteries. N Engl J Med 1987;317:805–809.
136. Kearney MF, Brien JF, Marks GS, Lei H, Nakatsu K. Thiol agents separate nitric oxide formation from vasodilatation induced by glyceryl trinitrate. Drug Metab Dispos 1998;26:547–551.
137. Boesgaard S, Aldershvile J, Poulsen HE. Preventive administration of intravenous N-acetylcysteine and development of tolerance to isosorbide dinitrate in patients with angina pectoris. Circulation 1992; 85:143–149.
138. Horowitz JD. Thiol-containing agents in the management of unstable angina pectoris and acute myocardial infarction. Am J Med 1991;91:113S–117S.
139. Horowitz JD, Henry CA, Syrjanen ML, Louis WJ, Fish RD, Smith TW, et al. Combined use of nitroglycerin and N-acetylcysteine in the management of unstable angina pectoris. Circulation 1988;77: 787–794.
140. Ardissino D, Merlini PA, Savonitto S, Demicheli G, Zanini P, Bertocchi F, et al. Effect of transdermal nitroglycerin or N-acetylcysteine, or both, in the long-term treatment of unstable angina pectoris. J Am Coll Cardiol 1997;29:941–947.

141. Arstall MA, Yang J, Stafford I, Betts WH, Horowitz JD. N-acetylcysteine in combination with nitroglycerin and streptokinase for the treatment of evolving acute myocardial infarction. Safety and biochemical effects. Circulation 1995;92:2855–2862.

142. Ghio S, Poli A, Ferrario M, Campana C, Diotallevi P, Eleuteri E, et al. Haemodynamic effects of glyceryl trinitrate during continuous 24 hour infusion in patients with heart failure. Br Heart J 1994; 72:145–149.

143. Mehra A, Shotan A, Ostrzega E, Hsueh W, Vasquez-Johnson J, Elkayam U. Potentiation of isosorbide dinitrate effects with N-acetylcysteine in patients with chronic heart failure. Circulation 1994;89: 2595–2600.

144. Beltrame JF, Zeitz CJ, Unger SA, Brennan RJ, Hunt A, Moran JL, et al. Nitrate therapy is an alternative to furosemide/morphine therapy in the management of acute cardiogenic pulmonary edema. J Card Fail 1998;4:271–279.

145. Munzel T, Bassenge E. Long-term angiotensin-converting enzyme inhibition with high-dose enalapril retards nitrate tolerance in large epicardial arteries and prevents rebound coronary vasoconstriction in vivo. Circulation 1996;93:2052–2058.

146. Heitzer T, Just H, Brockhoff C, Meinertz T, Olschewski M, Munzel T. Long-term nitroglycerin treatment is associated with supersensitivity to vasoconstrictors in men with stable coronary artery disease: prevention by concomitant treatment with captopril. J Am Coll Cardiol 1998;31:83–88.

147. Parker JD, Parker JO. Effect of therapy with an angiotensin-converting enzyme inhibitor on hemodynamic and counter regulatory responses during continuous therapy with nitroglycerin. J Am Coll Cardiol 1993;21:1445–1453.

148. Bauer JA, Fung H-L. Concurrent hydralazine administration prevents nitroglycerin-induced hemodynamic tolerance in experimental heart failure. Circulation 1991;84:35–39.

149. Munzel T, Kurz S, Rajogopalan S, Thoenes M, Berrington WR, Thompson JA, et al. Hydralazine prevents nitroglycerin tolerance by inhibiting activation of a membrane-bound NADH oxidase. A new action for an old drug. J Clin Invest 1996;98:1465–1470.

150. Parker JD, Parker AB, Farrell B, Parker JO. The effect of hydralazine on the development of tolerance to continuous nitroglycerin. J Pharmacol Exp Ther 1997;280:866–875.

151. Bassenge E, Fink N, Skatchkov M, Fink B. Dietary supplement with vitamin C prevents nitrate tolerance. J Clin Invest 1998;102:67–71.

152. Berk SI, Grunwald A, Pal S, Bodenheimer MM. Effect of intravenous nitroglycerin on heparin dosage requirements in coronary artery disease. Am J Cardiol 1993;72:393–396.

153. Nicolini FA, Ferrini D, Ottani F, Galvani M, Ronchi A, Behrens PH, et al. Concurrent nitroglycerin therapy impairs tissue-type plasminogen activator-induced thrombolysis in patients with acute myocardial Infarction. Am J Cardiol 1994;74:662–666

154. Cheitlin MD, Hutter AM Jr, Brindis RG, Ganz P, Kaul S, Russel RO Jr, et al. Use of sildenafil (Viagra) in patients with cardiovascular disease. Technology and Practice Executive Committee. Circulation 1999;99:168–177.

23   S-Nitrosothiols

Jane A. Leopold and Joseph Loscalzo

Nitric oxide (NO$^\bullet$) is a heterodiatomic molecule that dynamically modulates physiological functions of the cardiovascular system. NO$^\bullet$ regulates vascular tone, inhibits vascular smooth muscle cell (VSMC) proliferation, serves as an antithrombotic agent, and mediates cardiac contractility. Under basal conditions, NO$^\bullet$ additionally reacts with thiols to form a singular class of NO$^\bullet$ adducts identified as S-nitrosothiols. These nitrosated thiol derivatives are a readily available, stable reservoir of NO$^\bullet$ in the circulation that do not require NO$^\bullet$ release to achieve biological activity, and may, in fact, possess greater biological effects than NO$^\bullet$ alone (1).

NO$^\bullet$ BIOCHEMISTRY

NO$^\bullet$ is formed via the five-electron oxidation of the terminal guanidino nitrogen atom of L-arginine, thereby converting this amino acid to L-citrulline (2,3) in a reaction catalyzed by the enzyme (family) nitric oxide synthase (NOS). NOS contains both flavin adenine dinucleotide and flavin mononucleotide (4) cofactors, requires nicotinamide adenine dinucleotide phosphate (NADPH) (3) and molecular oxygen (5) as cosubstrates, and utilizes a heme complex (6), reduced glutathione (7), and tetrahydrobiopterin (8) to facilitate its redox chemistry.

Nitric oxide synthase(s) exists as two main isoform classes: the constitutive enzyme (cNOS) identified in the endothelium (eNOS or *Nos3* gene product) and neuronal cells (nNOS or *Nos1* gene product); and the inducible enzyme (iNOS or *Nos2* gene product) present in smooth muscle cells (SMC), neutrophils, and macrophages following exposure to cytokines or bacterial endotoxin (9–11). cNOS activity is under the regulatory control of Ca^{2+} and calmodulin. Endothelial cell agonists such as acetylcholine or bradykinin stimulate inositol 1,4,5-trisphosphate production resulting in the release of intracellular Ca^{2+} stores (12). This transient increase in intracellular Ca^{2+} enhances the formation of a Ca^{2+}/calmodulin complex, which, in turn, activates cNOS. Once activated, cNOS generates low level of NO$^\bullet$ until Ca^{2+} levels are depleted (13–15). In this manner, cNOS rapidly modulates vascular tone in addition to serving as an effective neurotransmitter (16). In contrast, iNOS is regulated at the transcriptional level and may, therefore, require several hours to effect a physiological response (17). Concentrations of NO$^\bullet$ (per mole of enzyme per minute) generated by iNOS are substantially greater than those achieved by cNOS (18), and are potentially cytotoxic suggesting that iNOS may play an integral role in both the immune response (19) and apoptosis (20).

NO$^\bullet$, as a free radical gas, has a half-life of 3–5 s under physiological conditions. Once formed, the free radical NO$^\bullet$ rapidly diffuses across biological membranes where it may react with oxygen, hemoglobin, redox metals, and superoxide anion (21). In the presence of molecular oxygen, NO$^\bullet$ or an oxidized derivative thereof, NO$^+$ or N_2O_3, combines with thiols

From: *Contemporary Cardiology, vol. 4: Nitric Oxide and the Cardiovascular System*
Edited by: J. Loscalzo and J. A. Vita © Humana Press Inc., Totowa, NJ

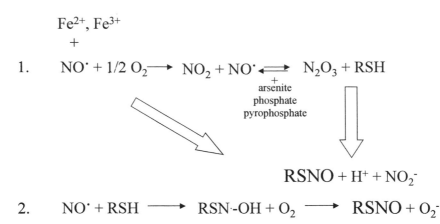

Fe^{2+}, Fe^{3+}
+

1. $NO^{\bullet} + 1/2\ O_2 \longrightarrow NO_2 + NO^{\bullet} \rightleftharpoons N_2O_3 + RSH$

+
arsenite
phosphate
pyrophosphate

$RSNO + H^+ + NO_2^-$

2. $NO^{\bullet} + RSH \longrightarrow RSN^{\cdot}-OH + O_2 \longrightarrow RSNO + O_2^-$

Fig. 1. *S*-nitrosothiol (RSNO) formation. RSNO formation results from the reaction of a thiol moiety with an oxidized derivative of $NO^{\bullet}$ with nitrosating capability, such as NO_2, N_2O_3, or $ONOO^-$. In the presence of iron (Fe^{2+}) or dinitrosyl iron complexes, this reaction is markedly enhanced; however, the bifunctional anions arsenite, phosphate, and pyrophosphate, diminish RSNO synthesis by promoting hydrolysis of the nitrosating species. In addition, $NO^{\bullet}$ may directly react with a reduced thiol group to form a novel intermediate, RSN-OH, which reacts with oxygen to form RSNO and superoxide anion.

to generate a unique class of $NO^{\bullet}$ adducts, identified as thionitrites or *S*-nitrosothiols (RSNOs) *(21)*. RSNOs exist as the predominant redox form of $NO^{\bullet}$ in plasma and further serve as a circulating pool of bioavailable $NO^{\bullet}$ *(22)*. RSNOs accumulate in acidic vesicles and release $NO^{\bullet}$ on exposure to an aqueous solution with a pH 7.0 *(23)*.

RSNO Formation

Nitrosation of low-molecular-weight thiols or cysteinyl side chains of proteins occurs in the aqueous phase to yield RSNOs. The formation of these compounds in biological systems is dependent on the presence of oxygen and is influenced by the relative concentrations of bioavailable $NO^{\bullet}$ and thiols as well as transition metal ions and oxygen-derived free radicals in the surrounding milieu *(24)*. The mechanism(s) by which RSNOs are synthesized have not yet been fully elucidated; however, evidence exists to suggest that $NO^{\bullet}$ may react directly, as well as indirectly, with thiol groups (Fig. 1)

RSNO formation occurs by the interaction of an oxidized derivative of $NO^{\bullet}$ with nitrosating capability, such as NO_2, $OONO^-$, or N_2O_3, with a thiol moiety *(25)*. RSNO production requires available oxygen, which, in turn, promotes the formation of these nitrosating species *(26)*. Under physiological conditions, N_2O_3 undergoes a reaction with the millimolar concentrations of intracellular glutathione that is kinetically preferred in that environment to that with water, thereby supporting the formation of RSNOs in biologic systems *(16,21,22)*. Under anerobic conditions, $NO^{\bullet}$ may also interact with thiols to yield reduced nitrogen species and the corresponding disulfide *(27)*.

The relative concentrations of inorganic anions present in the reaction environment additionally determine the extent of *S*-nitrosation of thiols. The bifunctional anions—arsenite, phosphate, and pyrophosphate—effectively inhibit *S*-nitrosation of low-molecular-weight thiols by 20–40%. These anions may limit RSNO synthesis by selectively promoting the catalytic hydrolysis of the nitrosating species, N_2O_3; however, the reduction of accessible N_2O_3 is insignificant compared to the observed inhibition of *S*-nitrosation, suggesting these anions diminish RSNO formation by an alternate mechanism *(28)*.

Optical and electron paramagnetic resonance studies have revealed that iron and dinitrosyl iron complexes play an integral role in the synthesis of RSNO compounds. In vitro, RSNO formation in aqueous solutions of cysteine or glutathione and gaseous NO• under aerobic conditions is markedly enhanced by the addition of Fe^{2+} to the reaction mixture and readily diminished by the selective Fe^{2+} chelator, o-phenanthroline. In the presence of Fe^{2+}, RSNO formation was additionally accompanied by the synthesis of dinitrosyl–iron complexes with thiol-containing ligands *(29)*. These dinitrosyl–iron complexes may, in turn, function as direct nitrosating species. In these complexes, each Fe^{2+} binds two NO• molecules and promotes their mutual oxidation-reduction with resultant formation of nitrous oxide and nitrosonium ions. These ions become available to *S*-nitrosate thiol-containing compounds and form RSNO *(30)*.

Kinetic analysis of RSNO formation has demonstrated that the reaction is first order with respect to oxygen concentration, second order with respect to NO• concentration, and requires a threshold concentration of thiols. The rate-limiting step appears to be the reaction of NO• with oxygen to form the main nitrosating species, N_2O_3, such that $RSH + N_2O_3$ yields $RSNO + NO_2^- + H^+$. Rate constants for this reaction for glutathione and human albumin are of the order of $3 \times 10^{-5}\ M^{-1}s^{-1}$ and $0.3 \times 10^{-5}\ M^{-1}s^{-1}$, respectively. The reaction rate of thiols with the nitrosating species, N_2O_3, is competitive with its rate of hydrolysis. Thus, a physiologic concentration of (intracellular) glutathione, the majority of N_2O_3 formed is utilized in the synthesis of *S*-nitrosoglutathione *(31)*.

It has been suggested further that at physiological concentrations, NO• may directly react with a reduced thiol to form a novel radical intermediate, RSN^-OH. Under aerobic conditions, oxygen serves as an electron acceptor and reacts with this intermediate to yield RSNO and superoxide anion which, in turn, reacts with NO• at a diffusion-limited rate to generate peroxynitrite *(32)*. The validity of these reactions has been confirmed in vitro by demonstrating that cysteine accelerates the decomposition of NO• under aerobic conditions to form *S*-nitrosocysteine. This reaction consumes oxygen with a 1:1 stoichiometry between molecular oxygen and NO• and results in the measurable production of hydrogen peroxide in the presence of Cu,Zn-superoxide dismutase (SOD). The formation of RSNO in this manner is additionally dependent on the relative concentrations of cysteine and NO•; the thiol concentration must exceed the concentration of NO• by 100-fold. Importantly, this reaction mechanism is only relevant at NO• concentrations of less than 50 μ*M*, suggesting that an NO_x-based mechanism for RSNO formation may become important at higher concentrations of NO• *(32)*.

RSNO Stability

Once formed, the stability of RSNOs is variable and dependent on temperature, pH, the presence of transition metals (*vide infra*), and the presence of oxygen and reactive oxygen species (ROS) *(33)*. The stability of RSNO had previously been attributed to the reduced capacity of the S–NO• bond to react with oxygen-derived free radicals; however, recent evidence has demonstrated RSNOs react with superoxide anion. This interaction may serve favorably to limit the overall biotoxicity of NO_x.

The relative stability of RSNOs under controlled physiological conditions has facilitated characterization of a number of naturally occurring and chemically synthesized RSNOs. For example, investigators have measured the half-life of *S*-nitroso-*N*-acetyl-D,L-pencillamine (SNAP) in solution and have found a wide range of values, from 1.15–4.6 h, owing to the presence of contaminating transition metal ions in the buffer *(23,34)*. In contrast, in the absence of light and contaminating transition metal ions, a crystalline form of SNAP has been synthesized, and its atomic structural coordinates determined *(35)*. It is important to note that it is not RSNO stability but the structure of the parent thiol from which the RSNO is formed that determines many of the compounds' biochemical properties. This point is best illustrated by the observation that the EC_{50} for vascular smooth muscle relaxation is 4.0 n*M* for *S*-nitrosogalactopyranose as compared to 220 n*M* for SNAP *(34)*. In addition, there is a discordance between RSNO stability and biological activity suggesting that hydrolytic decomposition of RSNOs with resulting NO_x release cannot adequately explain the biological properties of

Table 1
Mechanisms of RSNO Decomposition

Photolysis
Transition metal ions
S-transnitrosation reactions
Glutathione peroxidase
Superoxide anion

these compounds *(34)*. Instead, bioactivity may result from selective metabolism or the direct stereoselective action of some RSNOs.

Decomposition of RSNOs

RSNOs decompose by photolysis, transition metal ion-mediated catalysis, or via S-transnitrosation reactions if the resultant RSNO compound is more susceptible to decomposition by the aforementioned mechanisms than in the donor RSNO (*see* Table 1). As such, RSNOs remain stable under physiological conditions only in the absence of light and the presence of transition metal ion chelators. RSNO decomposition is achieved by homolytic cleavage of the S–N bond; however, there is evidence to suggest that heterolytic transfer of NO$^\bullet$ may play an equally, if not more important, role in RSNO breakdown *(21,36,37)*. It has been suggested further that RSNO decomposition may be directly enhanced by the enzyme glutathione peroxidase, even in the absence of thiol groups *(38)*.

Photolysis-mediated decomposition of RSNOs has been well described. Exposure to UV-visible light results in a homolytic cleavage of the S–N bond, thereby generating NO$^\bullet$ and a thiyl radical. Photolysis of S-nitrosoglutathione at 545 nm results in a quantum yield of 0.056 for NO$^\bullet$ and is best approximated by a first-order process with $k_{obs} = 4.9 \times 10^{-7} \mathrm{s}^{-1}$ *(39)*. Furthermore, the addition of photosensitizers, such as Rose Bengal, enhances the quantum yield for NO$^\bullet$ formation and thiyl radical production up to nine-fold *(40)*. In contrast, RSNO decomposition in the dark occurs relatively slowly, $t_{1/2} = 80$ h, and does not yield a thiyl radical intermediate as demonstrated by permitting S-nitrosoglutathione to decompose in the dark and monitoring the conversion to oxidized glutathione. In addition, the presence or absence of 5,5'-dimethyl-1-pyrroline-N-oxide, a thiyl radical trap, offered no difference in measurable oxidized glutathione indicating that RSNO decomposition does not occur via thiyl radical formation *(41)*. Recent observations have suggested that photolytic decomposition of RSNOs may additionally result in the formation of superoxide anion *(42)*.

The exact mechanism by which transition metal ions modulate RSNO breakdown remains undefined; however, the binding of copper ions to RSNOs is a prerequisite for augmented decomposition. Cu^+ is more efficient than Cu^{2+} at enhancing NO$^\bullet$ release, yet RSNO decomposition is not dependent on a Cu^{2+}/Cu^+ redox cycling mechanism or an intermediate thiyl radical. In vivo, amino acid and protein-bound Cu^{2+} are reduced by thiolate ion to Cu^+ which, in turn, enhances NO$^\bullet$ release from RSNOs *(43)*. The increased efficiency of RSNO decomposition mediated by Cu^+ compared with Cu^{2+} suggests that reducing agents such as ascorbate and α-tocopherol will enhance the breakdown of RSNOs by chemical reduction of contaminating metal ions *(41,44)*. In the presence of additional reducing equivalents, autoxidation of Cu^+ to Cu^{2+} may promote further NO$^\bullet$ release by generating superoxide anion *(41)*.

The importance of Cu^+ in RSNO decomposition has been demonstrated utilizing neocuproine, a specific inhibitor of Cu^+, to evaluate vasodilator responses to RSNOs in a rat isolated perfused tail artery model. Vessels were exposed to neocuproine prior to SNAP or S-nitrosoglutathione, or were treated with these agents concomitantly. Vasodilator responses to these RSNOs in either treatment regimen were significantly inhibited by the administration neocuproine, thereby demonstrating a role for Cu^+ in physiological RSNO decomposition and NO• release *(45)*.

S-transnitrosation reactions may enhance NO• release by forming an RSNO that is more readily susceptible to decomposition than the parent compound. This phenomenon has been demonstrated for the *S*-transnitrosation reaction that occurs between *S*-nitrosoglutathione and *N*-acetyl-D,L-penicillamine. Once formed, SNAP is more susceptible to transition metal ion-mediated breakdown than S-nitrosoglutathione *(41)*.

There exists evidence that NO• release from RSNOs may result from heterolytic NO^+ transfer and reductive activation to NO• as opposed to the decomposition of labile RSNOs. Utilizing spin-trapping experiments, it has been demonstrated in vivo that NO• is released from *S*-nitroso-albumin and *S*-nitrosoglutathione in a slow, but continuous, manner and is subsequently oxidized to NO_2^- in the absence of erythrocytes. Furthermore, the thiol groups of serum albumin and the antioxidant ascorbate appear to be the main plasma components that facilitate the release of NO• from these compounds *(46)*.

S-TRANSNITROSATION REACTIONS

Once formed, RSNOs participate in *S*-transnitrosation reactions that are of particular importance because thiols, such as glutathione and cysteinyl side chains of proteins, are present in abundant concentrations in mammalian cells. In a *S*-transnitrosation reaction, the NO• moiety is directly transferred from one intracellular thiol group to another; however, this reaction is complex and additionally generates several intermediate species that may include nitroxyl (NO^-) with subsequent formation of ammonia (NH_3), NO•, nitrous oxide (N_2O), and nitrite (NO_2^-) *(47)*. *S*-Transnitrosation reactions occur rapidly and in a pH-dependent manner as demonstrated utilizing chemically synthesized *S*-nitroso-glutathionyl-Sepharose 4B beads. In this system, NO• transfer to glutathione at 25°C increased concordant with pH; the initial rate of transfer was 0.53, 3.03, and 5.14 μ*M*/min at pH 5.0, 7.4, and 9.0, respectively *(48)*.

S-Transnitrosation reactions follow a second-order process with rate constants ranging from $3 \times 10^{-3}\ M^{-1}s^{-1}$ for the *S*-nitroso-L-cysteine/cysteine exchange reaction to $8 \times 10^{-3}\ M^{-1}s^{-1}$ for that between *S*-nitrosoglutathione/glutathione under aerobic conditions *(49)*. To resolve further the kinetics of *S*-transnitrosation reactions, differential optical absorption was employed. Utilizing this technique, it was demonstrated that the variability observed in rate constants was dependent on both the parent RSNO species and the thiol donor. For example, the k^2 ranged between 0.9 $M^{-1}s^{-1}$ for the reaction between *S*-nitrosoglutathione and *N*-acetyl-penicillamine and 279 $M^{-1}s^{-1}$ for the exchange between *S*-nitrosopenicillamine and glutathione. The physiological exchange between *S*-nitroso-albumin and plasma glutathione or cysteine was relatively slow with k_2 values measured at 3.2 and 9.1 $M^{-1}s^{-1}$, respectively; however, if *S*-nitrosocysteine served as the RSNO donor, this exchange reaction was significantly faster *(50)*.

S-transnitrosation reactions may also involve protein cysteinyl residues. The resulting *S*-nitrosoproteins that form can lead to significant changes in protein function (Table 2). This form of posttranslational modification of RSNO cell proteins can also lead to the rapid modulation of cell function and phenotype. For example, *S*-transnitrosation of the *N*-methyl-D-aspartate receptor in neurons results in functional inhibition of an excitatory response *(51)*. More likely, modification of the cysteinyl residue will alter cellular ion balance by modulating local plasma membrane channels, such as Ca^{2+}-dependent potassium channels *(52)*. This mechanism may additionally participate in the inhibition of glyceraldehyde-3-phosphate dehydrogenase, protein kinase C, and glutathione peroxidase activity *(53–55)*.

It has been suggested that *S*-transnitrosation reactions may effect a repair process of RSNO proteins by glutathione. Glutathione, which is present at millimolar concentrations in the cell cytoplasm, may facilitate unidirectional transfer (i.e., transnitrosation) of NO• from an RSNO donor, resulting in the formation of *S*-nitrosoglutathione. In experimental systems, *S*-nitrosoglutathione decays in the presence of glutathione to yield NO_2^-, peroxynitrite, or nitrous

Table 2
S-Nitroso Proteins in Mammalian Systems

Protein	Effect of S-nitrosation	Ref.
S-nitroso-albumin	NO• carrier	126
AP-1 (jun/fos)	Inhibition of AP-1-dependent transcription	127
Calpains	Inhibition of enzyme activity	128
Glyceraldehyde-3-phosphate dehydrogenase	NAD⁺-covalent modification	129
M2 muscarinic receptor	Disruption of receptor G protein	130
Alcohol dehydrogenase	Inhibition of enzyme activity	131
L-type calcium channel	Activation of $^I Ca^{2r}$	132
p21 (ras)	Triggering of guanine nucletotide exchange and p21 activation	133
ICE/CPP-32	Inhibition of enzyme activity/apoptosis	134
Caspases	Inhibition of enzyme activity	135
Factor XIII	Inhibition of enzyme activity	136
Creatinine kinase	Inhibition of enzyme activity	137
c-Jun N-terminal kinase 2 (JNK-2)	Inhibition of enzyme activity/apoptosis	138
Mitochondrial complex I	Inhibition of cell respiration	139
Ryanodine receptor	Activation of channel activity	140
Methionine adenosyltransferase	Inactivation of enzyme activity	141
Protein disulfide isomerase	Catalysis of transnitrosation	142

oxide depending on oxygen availability. In contrast, in cellular systems S-nitrosoglutathione subsequently undergoes either further reaction with glutathione or transition metal ion-mediated decomposition. In this manner, the NO• moiety is transferred from the parent RSNO and functional activity of NO• is restored. There is also some evidence to suggest that the enzyme γ-glutamyl transpeptidase enhances S-nitrosoglutathione breakdown thereby forming S-nitrosocysteinylglycine and glutamate. S-nitrosocysteinylglycine remains more susceptible to transition metal ion-dependent decomposition than S-nitrosoglutathione. These observations suggest that glutathione may serve as a competent thermodynamic sink for S-transnitrosation processes (41).

INTERACTION WITH SUPEROXIDE

Superoxide and reactive oxygen metabolites modulate S-nitrosation reactions by directly promoting the decomposition of RSNOs. The degree of oxidation of thiol groups is dependent on the relative concentrations of NO• and superoxide anion in the surrounding milieu. For example, glutathione, when exposed to the NO•-donor Et2NN(O)NONa, is exclusively nitrosated to form S-nitrosoglutathione; however, when superoxide anion is introduced into the system, there is a 95% reduction in nitrosation at equimolar concentrations of superoxide and NO•, which is reversed in the presence of SOD (56). Once formed, S-nitrosoglutathione reacts rapidly with superoxide anion to generate glutathione disulfide and equimolar quantities of nitrate and nitrite via an intermediate compound with strong oxidant properties as evidenced by its oxidation of dihydrorhodamine in the absence of apparent NO• production (57). Furthermore, when S-nitrosocysteine and S-nitrosoglutathione are exposed to superoxide anion, there is a time-dependent decomposition of both RSNOs with a resultant increase in nitrite/nitrate. This reaction proceeds with a second-order rate constant of $7.69 \times 10^4 \, M^{-1}s^{-1}$ and $1.28 \times 10^4 \, M^{-1}s^{-1}$ for S-nitrosocysteine and S-nitrosoglutathione, respectively, and a stoichiometric ratio of 1 mol RSNO per 2 mol superoxide anion. These slower reaction rates of superoxide anion with RSNOs, compared with NO•, support the hypothesis that transient formation of RSNOs in biological systems may protect NO• from its rapid destruction by superoxide anion (57,58). Decomposition of RSNO via superoxide anion is accompanied by the formation of peroxynitrite as superoxide mediated reduction of S-nitrosothiols yields NO•,

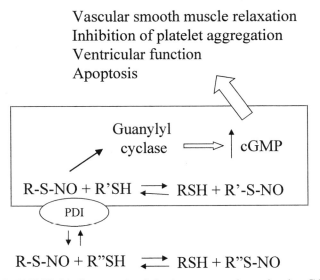

Fig. 2. *S*-nitrosothiols (RSNOs) influence physiologic responses by activating GC. RSNOs formed in the extracellular milieu activate intracellular GC to effect a response. This may be accomplished by several mechanisms: (1) thiol-*S*-nitrosothiol exchange reactions at the cell surface via protein disulfide isomerase (PDI), a homodimer that contains vicinal dithiols and catalyzes *S*-transnitrosation reactions; (2) the intracellular formation of RSNOs may facilitate signal transduction events; or (3) RSNO activation at the cell surface may result from a signal transduction event. In this manner, intracellular GC is activated and cGMP levels are increased. These events promote VSMC relaxation, inhibit platelet function, modulate ventricular function, and mediate apoptosis.

which freely reacts with a second superoxide anion molecule. *S*-nitrosothiol decomposition additionally occurs under anaerobic conditions in the presence of superoxide anion generators resulting in detectable NO• levels *(59)*.

Peroxynitrite oxidizes additional thiol groups through competing one- and two-electron pathways but quantitatively favors the two-electron pathway. In plasma, peroxynitrite induces the formation of a disulfide crosslinked protein that has been identified as a dimer of serum albumin. Peroxynitrite additionally mediates thiol group oxidation to form thiyl radicals, which is readily inhibited by $NaHCO_3$ and the antioxidant ascorbate. In the presence of iron-diethyldithiocarbamate, peroxynitrite enhances the formation of protein RSNOs. These observations suggest that $NaHCO_3$ promotes the one-electron thiol oxidation pathway by peroxynitrite resulting in the formation of RSNOs and thiyl radicals, which, in turn, are involved in reactions by which thiols are oxidized to disulfide compounds *(60)*.

Biological Actions

The biological effects of RSNOs closely resemble those of organic nitrosovasodilator compounds. In fact, RSNOs may function as intermediates in the metabolism of these agents by serving as extracellular transporters of NO• eventually liberating free NO_x in the circulation, whereas the thiol component of the compound influences biologic potency as well as tissue selectivity. The hemodynamic effects of RSNOs do not differ significantly from those of organic nitrosovasodilators and were found to be indistinguishable from nitroglycerin in a closed-chest cat model *(23)*. This observation is supported by the pharmacology of nitrosovasodilators: organic nitrates are metabolized via an enzymatic step that necessitates a thiol group, whereas inorganic nitrates, such as nitroprusside, release NO_x spontaneously *(61,62)*.

Like NO•, RSNOs stimulate guanylyl cyclase (GC) effecting a rise in intracellular cGMP levels *(23)* (Fig. 2). Thiol groups play a significant role in enzyme activation which is demonstrated by the metabolism of organic nitrate ester. This species has an absolute requirement for a thiol group to liberate NO_x efficiently and initiate enzyme activity. Thiol or heme groups augment $NO^{\bullet}$-mediated GC activation, whereas enzyme activation by nitrosyl-hemoglobin is enhanced only in the presence of thiol groups *(63)*. There exists further evidence to suggest a reversible activation of GC by thiol-oxidizing and reactive sulfide compounds *(63)*. These compounds induce a thiol–disulfide exchange reaction involving vicinal dithiol groups at the enzyme's active site and an additional thiol resulting in GC activation or inhibition depending on the redox potential of the specific reaction and the redox state of the enzyme's −SH groups *(64)*.

The biologic actions of RSNOs are illustrated further by examining the concept of tolerance to nitrates. There are several potential mechanisms put forth to explain this phenomenon, the simplest of which is reflex sodium and volume retention following prolonged nitrate administration. The increased volume of the extravascular compartment would dilute circulating nitrate concentrations and thereby attenuate vasodilator capacity *(65)*. An alternate explanation suggests that nitrate tolerance results from tissue depletion of thiols, which are required to convert organic nitrates to nitrite. A decreased supply of thiol groups would retard RSNO formation and subsequently diminish GC activation; however, investigators have failed to demonstrate a relationship between $NO^{\bullet}$ production and thiol depletion in endothelial cells exposed to thiol-depleting agents *(66,67)*. In a rat model, animals were treated with diethylmaleate to induce free thiol depletion or *N*-ethylmaleaimide to alkylate protein thiols prior to nitrate administration. Tolerance to nitrosovasodilators was not accompanied by diminished thiol reserves, nor did thiol modification of proteins support nitrate tolerance *(68)*. The observation that glutathione, which is incapable of entering cells in its reduced form, potentiates the nitrosovasodilator effects of nitroglycerin suggests that extracellular formation of RSNOs, as opposed to, or in addition to intracellular thiol depletion, promotes tolerance to nitrates *(69)*.

In vivo, RSNOs that possess biological activity similar to $NO^{\bullet}$ have been readily identified. These RSNO compounds activate GC as well as enhance vascular smooth muscle relaxation and platelet inhibition *(70)*. RSNOs may be synthesized from proteins bearing thiol functionalities, and these *S*-nitrosoproteins similarly retain $NO^{\bullet}$-like properties in addition have a prolonged half-life compared to free $NO^{\bullet}$ *(22)*. Plasma RSNOs reside primarily as *S*-nitrosoproteins, with *S*-nitroso serum albumin existing as the most abundant form. The single free cysteine of serum albumin, Cys_{34}, which is situated in a narrow crevice in close proximity to an anionic charge *(72)*, maintains an anomalously low pK, which makes it ideally suited to react with bioavailable NO^+. Human plasma accommodates approximately micromolar concentrations of RSNOs, of which 96% is protein bound and 82% of this pool is comprised of *S*-nitroso serum albumin. The importance of *S*-nitroso albumin as an endogenous vasodilator has been demonstrated in analbuminemic rats, which failed to sustain $NO^{\bullet}$-induced hypotension for the same duration as normal animals *(73)*.

$NO^{\bullet}$ additionally circulates in plasma bound to hemoglobin as *S*-nitrosohemoglobin. Electrospray ionization mass spectrometry has revealed that when hemoglobin is incubated with an equimolar concentration of RSNO, only a single $NO^{\bullet}$ molecule is added to hemoglobin at the beta-Cys_{93} site, despite the presence of three available cysteine residues *(74)*. Once exposed to hemoglobin, $NO^{\bullet}$ binds rapidly, $k = 0^7\ M^{-1}s^{-1}$, and with high affinity, $K_d = 10^{-5}s^{-1}$, to the heme iron of the protein. In the presence of oxygen, nitrosylhemoglobin is converted from a partially nitrosylated, deoxy state to *S*-nitrosohemoglobin. Under relatively anaerobic conditions, as seen in the microcirculation, NO^- is released and methemoglobin is formed. It is the ratio of $NO^{\bullet}$ and hemoglobin that ultimately determines the quantities of *S*-nitrosohemoglobin and methemoglobin formed *(75)*. *S*-nitrosohemoglobin, both cell free and intraerythrocytic, and *S*-nitrosomethemoglobin have been shown to influence physiological functions. For example, these agents both inhibit platelet aggregation; however, *S*-nitrosomethemoglobin elicits a more potent response. This observation suggests that the oxidation state of the heme moiety, and not cGMP levels, mediates the actions of *S*-nitrosohemoglobin *(76)*.

NO$^\bullet$ metabolism appears to be intimately related to thiol status. This concept was examined in a rat model where animals received a loading dose of glutathione or an inhibitor of glutathione synthesis, L-buthionine-[S,R]-sulfoximine. Plasma samples were then incubated with an NO$^\bullet$-donor. In these samples, low-molecular-weight RSNO formation peaked at 10 min, whereas while levels of nitrosylhemoglobin and NO$_x$ were detectable almost immediately, similarly peaked at 10 min, and had a half-life of 35 min. The absolute measurable levels of RSNOs in plasma were markedly elevated only in those animals that were administered a glutathione load. In vivo, maximum blood levels of nitrosylhemoglobin were achieved at 30 min and maintained a half-life of 100 min. Nitrosylhemoglobin formation was decreased significantly in animals that received a glutathione load and increased in animals treated with L-buthionine-[S,R]-sulfoximine *(77)*.

Whereas RSNOs circulate in abundance in plasma, the mechanism by which this extracellular pool of RSNOs influences activation of intracellular GC remains unknown. Several explanations have been offered to account for this observation, including RSNO participation in a signal transduction event on the cell surface, an *S*-transnitrosation reaction across the cell membrane, or the intracellular production of *S*-nitrosoproteins as a posttranslational modification, and, hence, a signal transduction event *(78)*. RSNOs, serving as NO$^\bullet$ donors, additionally influence other intracellular events such as apoptosis. In 3T3 fibroblasts exposed to *S*-nitrosoglutathione and SNAP, apoptosis, as confirmed by electron microscopy, DNA laddering, and propidium iodide staining, occurred commensurate with RSNO breakdown and NO$^\bullet$ release. Apoptosis was hindered by oxyhemoglobin, an NO$^\bullet$ scavenger, and the antioxidants, ascorbic acid and *N*-acetylcysteine *(79)*.

PHYSIOLOGIC AND PATHOPHYSIOLOGIC EFFECTS

RSNOs, as circulating stores of NO$^\bullet$, contribute significantly to physiological responses in the cardiovascular system. As such, RSNOs modulate vascular tone, myocardial contractility, and platelet function. In turn, deficiencies in thiol stores or RSNO formation contribute to several pathophysiologically relevant disorders distinguished by endothelial cell dysfunction and abnormalities in vascular tone. These syndromes may be recognized clinically as atherosclerosis, pulmonary hypertension, essential hypertension, and shock.

Physiologic Cardiovascular Effects

MYOCARDIAL PERFUSION

Initial characterization of GC activity revealed that nitrosovasodilator compounds may stimulate enzyme activity by first forming an intermediate RSNO species *(23)*. For example, in a bovine model, nitrosovasodilators, such as nitroglycerin and nitroprusside, effectively mediate GC activation but only in the presence of thiol groups. Direct administration of RSNOs produce a modest, albeit short-lived, decrease in systemic blood pressure *(23)*. These hemodynamic findings extend to the experience with *S*-nitroso-serum albumin. In a canine model, *S*-nitroso albumin administration affords a dose-dependent decrease in mean arterial pressure that is 7.5- and 10-fold less potent than that observed with nitroglycerin and *S*-nitroso-L-cysteine, respectively. In the coronary artery, *S*-nitroso albumin increases blood flow less effectively than does nitroprusside or *S*-nitroso-L-cysteine, but maintained a longer duration of action *(80)*.

RSNOs may afford protection from ischemia–reperfusion injury, as well. To evaluate the effect of RSNOs in this setting, SPM-5185, a cysteine-containing NO$^\bullet$ donor, was compared with SPM-5267, an analogue of the same molecule lacking the thiol moiety. Only the thiol-containing NO$^\bullet$ donor compound offered significant protection from myocardial reperfusion injury: in the control group, 38% of the area at risk exhibited cell death, whereas in the SPM-5185 treatment group, this area was reduced to 7% necrosis. Further evaluation of the left anterior descending coronary artery revealed that endothelial cell dysfunction was tempered by 50% as evidenced by decreased adherence of leukocytes and diminished production of superoxide anion. In addition, these beneficial effects occurred without an obligate increase in oxygen demand as determined by the pressure-rate index *(81)*.

VENTRICULAR FUNCTION

NO• and RSNOs play a complex role in the regulation of ventricular function. Under basal conditions, NO• mediates the ability of the vagus nerve to attenuate the positive inotropic response to β-adrenergic stimulation. In a closed-chest canine model, infusion of the β-adrenergic agonist dobutamine prior to bilateral vagus nerve stimulation results in a significant increase in peak + dP/dt; however, after nerve stimulation these responses are significantly diminished. Inhibitors of NOS reduce by approx 50% the vagal inhibitory effect over the positive inotropic response elicited by dobutamine, suggesting that NO• participates significantly in the regulation of myocardial autonomic responses *(82)*.

At the cellular level, RSNOs may modulate myocardial contractility by dynamically regulating the L-type Ca^{2+}-channel. Patch clamp studies utilizing ferret right ventricular myocytes exposed to RSNOs demonstrate enhanced L-type Ca^{2+}-channel activity. This effect is not dependent on kinase activation, phosphatase inhibition, alterations in cGMP levels, or cellular permeability. This channel is additionally activated by thiol oxidants and inhibited by thiol reductants, suggesting the presence of an allosteric thiol-containing redox switch on the channel *(83)*. In contrast, whole-cell patch recordings in human embryonic kidney cells utilizing barium as the charge carrier demonstrate only inhibition of L-type Ca^{2+}-channel activity in cells exposed to RSNOs. This effect is not influenced by methylene blue or 8-bromo-cGMP, suggesting that the mechanism of inhibition is independent of cGMP *(84)*.

In experimental congestive heart failure, RSNO compounds offer prolonged and more potent nitrosovasodilator activity when compared to nitroglycerin. Employing a two-way crossover design, rats were administered *S*-nitroso-*N*-D,L-penicillamine (SNP) and nitroglycerin infusions for 10 h. Although both drugs produced marked decreases in left ventricular end-diastolic pressure at the highest infusion rates, only SNP was effective at lower doses. Tolerance to nitroglycerin, but not SNAP, occurred over the 10-h infusion time. Moreover, animals that became tolerant to nitroglycerin continued to demonstrate a mean reduction of 24% in the left ventricular end-diastolic pressure once challenged with SNAP, suggesting that crossreactivity between these compounds does not occur *(85)*.

PLATELET INHIBITION

NO• and NO•-generating compounds such as RSNOs have been shown to inhibit epinephrine- and adenosine 5′-diphosphate-induced platelet aggregation. Nitroglycerin additionally promotes platelet disaggregation in conjunction with an increase in platelet cGMP *(86–88)*. Ex vivo platelet studies from patients who had previously received nitrate therapies have demonstrated an attenuation in platelet aggregation once thiol stores are repleted. This observation suggests that nitroglycerin may inhibit platelet function by modulating intracellular thiol stores and influencing RSNO formation *(89)*. RSNOs similarly inhibit platelet function by increasing cGMP levels. In human platelets, both NO• and RSNOs promote heme-dependent activation of soluble GC, suggesting further that nitrosovasodilators may mediate their antiplatelet effects via RSNO formation *(90)*.

RSNOs have been shown to potentiate further the antiplatelet effects of nitroglycerin efficiently. *N*-acetyl-L-cysteine reduced the IC_{50} for platelet inhibition by 50% while increasing the cGMP, but not cAMP, content of platelets fivefold. In the absence of *N*-acetyl-L-cysteine, nitroglycerin administration stimulated the synthesis of RSNOs as evidenced by a

Table 3
Pathophysiologic Disorders
Characterized by Diminished Bioavalable NO•

Atherosclerosis
Hyperhomocysteinemia
Pulmonary hypertension
Congestive heart failure
Essential hypertension
Restenosis
Diabetes mellitus
Hypercholesterolemia

marked decrease in platelet glutathione levels *(91)*. Glutathione, present in millimolar con
centrations in platelets, acts synergistically with nitrates to inhibit platelet function, an effect
that may be mediated by platelet glutathione-*S*-transferase. This enzyme catalyzes the inactivation of lipid hydroperoxides, which, in turn, inactivate NO• *(92)*. In addition, the enzyme
glutathione peroxidase may play a regulatory role in platelet function by promoting RSNO
decomposition and NO• release *(93)*. Hydrogen peroxide, in conjunction with RSNOs, has
been shown to inhibit platelet aggregation by a GC-dependent mechanism. The action of GC
appears to follow the occupation by NO• of the heme site in the enzyme *(94)*. Like endogenous RSNOs, synthetic RSNOs inhibit platelet function in a dose-dependent fashion. Platelet
aggregation is effectively inhibited by *S*-nitroso-*N*-acetyl-L-cysteine and *S*-nitroso-L-cysteine
with an IC_{50} of 4–10 μ*M* *(95)*.

The physiological relevance of RSNO-mediated inhibition of platelet aggregation has
been established in a canine model. Following intravenous administration of *S*-nitroso albumin, a dose-dependent increase in bleeding time occurred suggesting platelet dysfunction
(79). Platelet function was evaluated further utilizing a Folts model of cyclic flow responses.
Transient platelet-dependent thrombotic occlusion of a canine coronary artery was reversed
by infusions of RSNOs at concentrations that produced minimal or no effect on mean arterial
pressure *(96)*. These observations suggest that RSNOs possess potent antiplatelet properties
that may influence thrombus formation as well as tissue perfusion under basal conditions.

Pathophysiologic Cardiovascular Effects (Table 3)

ENDOTHELIAL DYSFUNCTION

Endothelial dysfunction, as occurs in the setting of hypercholesterolemia or frank atherosclerosis, is characterized by diminished synthesis of NO• concomitant with elevated levels
of superoxide anion and peroxynitrite formation. In addition, the oxidation of thiol groups
by ROS in the atheromatous milieu restricts the formation of protective RSNOs. Superoxide
anion has been implicated further in the aberrant response to vasodilating agents *(97)*. In thoracic
aortic rings that were exposed to L-cysteine and dithiothreitol, dose-dependent contraction
occurred in the presence of an intact endothelium, and this effect was reversed by pretreatment with superoxide dismutase. These observations suggest that NO• release, and RSNO production, is influenced by superoxide anion generation, potentially via autooxidation of the
thiol moiety *(98)*.

Hyperhomocysteinemia has been implicated as an independent risk factor for precocious
atherosclerosis and thrombosis *(99,100)*. Homocysteine may exert its atherogenic effects via
the formation of hydrogen peroxide and homocysteine thiolactone, which promote endothelial dysfunction *(101–104)*. The endothelium, in turn, modulates the toxic properties of homocysteine by releasing endothelium-derived NO• to *S*-nitrosate circulating homocysteine, thereby

rendering it nontoxic to the vessel wall. For example, aortic rings incubated with homocysteine and exposed to shear stress to stimulate NO• release generate S-nitrosohomocysteine. S-nitrosohomocysteine, in contrast to homocysteine, induces vasorelaxation and platelet inhibition without producing hydrogen peroxide. In vitro, prolonged exposure (>3 h) of endothelial cells to homocysteine results in impaired NO• production; however, if the exposure is brief (<15 min), S-nitrosohomocysteine is readily formed *(105)*. Moreover, homocysteine itself stimulates *Nos3* transcription and NOS activity in bovine aortic endothelial cells. In turn, elevated levels of NO• result in a time- and dose-dependent increase in RSNO production *(106)*; prolonged exposure to high concentrations of homocysteine, however, suppresses *Nos3* transcription. These observations suggest that there exists a dynamic balance between endothelial function and homocysteine levels such that once the ability of the endothelium to elaborate NO• is impaired by markedly elevated levels of homocysteine, protective RSNO formation is diminished and oxidative damage to the vessel wall is initiated *(105)*.

PULMONARY HYPERTENSION AND CHF

In the normal lung, NO• and RSNOs exist in abundance *(107)*. In the setting of pulmonary hypertension, endothelial cell dysfunction may potentiate further the hypoxic pulmonary vasoconstrictor response *(108)*. Therapeutic interventions with inhaled NO• have demonstrated benefit for those patients with primary pulmonary hypertension *(109)* and pulmonary hypertension related to congenital heart disease *(110)*. The formation of NO_2 gas, a limiting toxicity of this therapy, is believed to be ameliorated by thiol groups that form RSNOs in alveolar fluid *(107)*. In contrast, inhaled NO• has a potentially detrimental effect in patients with congestive heart failure (CHF), a disease in which pulmonary vascular resistance is often elevated. In this setting, patients with Class III or IV CHF who received inhaled NO• at 80 ppm for 10 min demonstrated a 31% decrease in pulmonary vascular resistance at the expense of a 23% increase in pulmonary artery wedge pressure. This effect was associated with a decrease in cardiac index and a rise in left ventricular end-diastolic filling pressures resulting in an adverse hemodynamic profile *(111)*.

VASCULAR INJURY

The response of the vessel wall to injury following atherosclerotic plaque rupture or percutaneous revascularization procedures may be manipulated pharmacologically by RSNOs. Utilizing a Folts model, in which damaged vessels support cyclic flow reductions and hence thrombus formation, stenosed vessels were treated with S-nitroso-albumin and cyclic flow reductions were quantified. Those vessels that were treated with S-nitroso-albumin, applied directly to the luminal surface for 60 s, demonstrated a 94% inhibition of cyclic flow reduction when compared to stenosed, untreated arteries, suggesting that RSNO treatment renders the vessel wall less thrombogenic *(112)*. Local administration of RSNOs following balloon angioplasty has been shown to attenuate intimal and medial proliferation and suggests a therapeutic role for these agents in preventing restenosis. In a rabbit model of bilateral femoral artery injury, those arteries treated with a polynitrosated S-nitroso-albumin demonstrated a 4.4-fold decrease in platelet aggregation and a reduction in intimal hyperplasia at 2 wk when compared to control arteries *(113)*.

HYPERTENSION

Hypertension has been associated with diminished production, as well as enhanced consumption, of NO• *(114)*. In this manner, RSNOs may offer therapeutic benefit as agents that supplement inadequate levels of NO•. S-Nitrosation of the antihypertensive agent captopril, to form S-nitroso-captopril, results in a compound that possesses vasodilatory and platelet inhibitory effects due to GC activation in addition to its angiotensin-converting enzyme inhibitory action *(115,115)*. If administered as a continuous infusion, the half-life of S-nitroso-captopril may be prolonged and extend its therapeutic window. As a thiol-containing compound, S-nitroso-captopril enhances NO$^•$ release from nitroglycerin and may offer resistance to superoxide anion-mediated inactivation *(117)*.

SHOCK

Circulatory collapse in the setting of overwhelming bacterial infection has been attributed to an overabundance of NO$^•$ in the vasculature *(118)*. Owing to the similarities between NO$^•$ and RSNOs, it has been suggested that RSNOs may additionally contribute to the hemodynamic effects of shock. To elucidate the role of RSNOs this setting, anesthetized rabbits were administered lipopolysaccharide to induce systemic hypotension. In this setting, cardiovascular collapse was accompanied by an increase in measurable NO$^•$ and RSNOs in plasma. This effect was reversed by methylene blue treatment which inhibited both GC activity and NO$^•$ and RSNO production *(119)*.

In states of bacterial sepsis, elevated levels of circulating NO$^•$ may modulate thiol levels by enhancing RSNO formation, which, in turn, may result in depletion of thiol stores available to detoxify reactive metabolites, including free radicals. For example, in an endotoxemic rat model, glutathione levels were markedly reduced following exposure to lipopolysaccharide. Reduced glutathione levels were restored only after the administration of an inhibitor of NOS. Further analysis with L-buthionine sulfoximine demonstrated that glutathione metabolism was significantly increased in animals exposed to lipopolysaccharide by an NO$^•$-mediated mechanism *(120)*.

SUMMARY

RSNOs are formed in vivo by the reaction of bioavailable NO$^•$ with sulfhydryl groups. These nitrosated thiol derivatives form from both low-molecular-weight thiols as well as proteins that possess thiol functionalities. RSNOs serve as a circulating reservoir of stable NO$^•$ and allow NO$^•$ to function in a paracrine fashion. These compounds further protect NO$^•$ from reactive oxygen species. RSNOs contribute significantly to the pharmacological and physiological responses of the cardiovascular system, including maintenance of vascular tone, the response of the vessel wall to injury, and inhibition of platelet aggregation. Owing to the broad range of actions of RSNO compounds, there exists the potential for further pharmacological manipulation of these physiological responses to ameliorate pathophysiologically relevant disorders characterized by NO$^•$ deficiency.

REFERENCES

1. Ignarro LJ. Nitric oxide. A novel signal transduction mechanism for trancellular communication. Hypertension 1990;16:477–483.
2. Palmer RM, Ashton DS, Moncada S. Vascular endothelial cells synthesize nitric oxide from L-arginine. Nature (Lond) 1988;333:664–666.
3. Nathan C. Nitric oxide as a secretory product of mammalian cells. FASEB J 1992;6:3051–3064.
4. Bredt DS, Ferris CS, Snyder SH. Nitric oxide synthase regulatory sites. J Biol Chem 1992;267: 10,976–10,981.
5. Leone AM, Palmer RM, Knowles RG, Francis PL, Ashton DS, Moncada S. Constitutive and inducible nitric oxide synthases incorporate molecular oxygen into both nitric oxide and citrulline. J Biol Chem 1991;266:23,790–23,795.
6. White KA, Marletta MA. Nitric oxide synthase is a cytochrome P-450 type hemoprotein. Biochemistry 1992;31:6627–6631.
7. Stuehr DJ, Kwon NS, Nathan CF. FAD and GSH participate in macrophage synthesis of nitric oxide. Biochem Biophys Res Commun 1990;168:558–565.
8. Tayeh MA, Marletta MA. Macrophage oxidation of L-arginine to nitric oxide, nitrite, and nitrate. Tetrahydrobiopterin is required as a cofactor. J Biol Chem 1989;264:19,654–19,658.

9. Drapier JC, Hibbs JB. Differentiation of murine macrophages to express nonspecific cytotoxicity for tumor cell results in L-arginine-dependent inhibition of mitochondrial iron-sulfur enzymes in the macrophage effector cells. J Immunol 1988;140:2829–2838.

10. Stuehr DJ, Marletta MA. Induction of nitrite/nitrate synthesis in murine macrophages by BCG infection, lymphokines or interferon. J Immunol 1987;139 518–525.

11. Ding AH, Nathan CF, Stuehr DJ. Release of reactive nitrogen intermediates and reactive oxygen intermediates from mouse peritoneal macrophages. J Immunol 1988;141:2407–2412.

12. Dinerman JL, Lowenstein CJ, Snyder SH. Molecular mechanisms of nitric oxide regulation. Circ Res 1993;73:217–222.

13. Bredt DS, Snyder SH. Isolation of nitric oxide synthase, a calmodulin-requiring enzyme. Proc Natl Acad Sci USA 1990;87:682–685.

14. Busse R, Mulsch A. Calcium-dependent nitric oxide synthesis in endothelial cytosol is mediated by calmodulin. FEBS Lett 1990;265:133–136.

15. Mayer B, Schmidt K, Humbert P, Bohme E. Biosynthesis of endothelium-derived relaxing factor: a cytosolic enzyme in porcine endothelial cells Ca2+-dependently converts L-arginine into an activator of soluble guanylyl cyclase. Biochem Biophys Res Commun 1989;164 678–685.

16. Ignarro LJ. Biological actions and properties of endothelium-derived nitric oxide formed and released from artery and vein. Circ Res 1989;65:1–21.

17. Xie QW, Cho HJ, Calaycay J, Mumford RA, Swiderek KM, Lee TD, et al. Cloning and characterization of inducible nitric oxide synthase from mouse macrophages. Science 1992;256:599–604.

18. Welch G, Loscalzo J. Nitric oxide and the cardiovascular system. J Cardiac Surg 1994;74:1121–1125.

19. Nathan C, Hibbs JB. Role of nitric oxide synthesis in macrophages antimicrobial activity. Curr Opin Immunol 1991;3:65–70.

20. Wang B, Lin PS, Tsao PS, Cooke JP. Nitric oxide induces regression: role of apoptosis. Circulation 1996;94:I-155.

21. Stamler JS, Singel DJ, Loscalzo J. Biochemistry of nitric oxide and its redox-activated forms. Science 1992;258:1898–1902.

22. Stamler JS, Jaraki O, Osborne J, Simon DI, Keaney JF Jr, Vita J, et al. Nitric oxide circulates in mammalian plasma primarily as an S-nitroso adduct of serum albumin. Proc Natl Acad Sci USA 1992; 89:7674–7677.

23. Ignarro LJ, Lipton H, Edwards JC, Baricos WH, Hyman AL, Kadowitz PJ, et al. Mechanism of vascular smooth muscle relaxation by organic nitrates, nitrites, nitroprusside and nitric oxide: evidence for the involvement of S-nitrosothiols as active intermediates. J Pharmacol Exp Ther 1981;218:739–749.

24. Ridd JH. Nitrosation. In: Williams DS, ed. Advances in Physical and Organic Chemistry, Vol. 16. Cambridge University Press, New York, 1978, pp. 1–214.

25. Oae S, Tukushine D, Kim YH. Novel method of activating thiols by their conversion into thionitrites with dinitrogen tetroxide. J Chem Soc Chem Commun 1977;407.

26. Saville B. A scheme for colorimetric determination of microgram amounts of thiols. Analyst 1958;83: 670–672.

27. van der Vliet A, 't Hoen PAC, Wong PSV, Bast A, Cross CE. Formation of S-nitrosothiols via direct nucleophilic nitrosation of thiols by peroxynitrite with elimination of hydrogen peroxide. J Biol Chem 1998;273:30,255–30,262.

28. Pryor WA, Church DF, Govindan CK, Crank G. Oxidation of thiols by nitric oxide and nitrogen dioxide: synthetic utility and toxicological implications. J Org Chem 1982;47:156–159.

29. DeMaster EG, Quast BJ, Mitchell RA. Inhibition of S-nitrosation of reduced glutathione in aerobic solutions of nitric oxide by phosphate and other inorganic anions. Biochem Pharmacol 1997;53:581–585.

30. Vanin AF, Malenkova IV, Serezhenkov VA. Iron catalyzes both decomposition and synthesis of S-nitrosothiols: optical and electron paramagnetic resonance studies. Nitric Oxide 1997;3:191–203.

31. Vanin AF. Dinitrosyl iron complexes and S-nitrosothiols are two possible forms for stabilization and transport of nitric oxide in biological systems. Biochemistry 1998;82–793.

32. Kharitonov VG, Sundquist AR, Sharma VS. Kinetics of nitrosation of thiols by nitric oxide in the presence of oxygen. J Biol Chem 1995;270:28,158–28,164.

33. Gow AJ, Buerk DG, Ischiropoulos H. A novel reaction mechanism for the formation of S-nitrosothiol in vivo. J Biol Chem 1997;272:2841–2845.

34. Stamler JS, Singel DJ, Loscalzo J. Biochemistry of nitric oxide and its redox-activated forms. Science 1992;258:1898–1902.

35. Matthews WR, Kerr SW. Biological activity of S-nitrosothiols; the role of nitric oxide. J Pharmacol Exp Ther 1993;267:1529–1537.

36. Field L, Dilts RV, Ravichandran B, Lenhart PG, Carnahan GE. An unusually stable thionitrite from N-acetyl-D,L-penicillamine; x-ray crystal and molecular structure of 2-(acetylamino)-2-carboxy-1,1-dimethylethyl thionitrite. J Chem Soc Perkin Trans 1978;I:249,250.

37. Williams DL. S-nitrosation and the reactions of S-nitroso-compounds. Chem Soc Rev 1985;14:171–196.

38. Girard P, Ptier P. NO, thiols and disulfides. FEBS Lett 1993;320:7,8.

39. Hou Y, Guo Z, Li J, Wang PG. Seleno compounds and glutathione peroxidase catalyzed decomposition of S-nitrosothiols. Biochem Biophys Res Commun 1996;228:88–93.

40. Sexton DJ, Muruganandam A, McKenney DJ, Mutus B. Visible light photochemical release of nitric oxide from _S_-nitrosoglutathione: potential photochemotherapeutic applications. Photochem Photobiol 1994;59:463–467.

41. Singh RH, Hogg N, Joseph J, Kalyanaraman B. Photosensitized decomposition of _S_-ntirosothiols and 2-methyl-2-nitrosopropane. Possible use for site-directed nitric oxide production. FEBS Lett 1995; 360:47–51.

42. Singh RH, Hogg N, Joseph J, Kalyanaraman B. Mechanism of nitric oxide release from S-nitroso-thiols. J Biol Chem 1996;271:18,596–18,603.

43. Zhelyaskov VR, Gee KR, Godwin DW. Control of NO concentration in solutions of nitrosothiol compounds by light. Photochem Photobiol 1998;67:282–288.

44. Dicks AP, Williams DL. Generation of nitric oxide from _S_-nitrosothiols using protein-bound Cu^{2+} sources. Chem Biol 1996;3:655–659.

45. De Man JG, De Winter BY, Moreels TG, Herman AG, Pelckmans PA. _S_-nitrosothiols and the nitrergic neurotransmitter in the rat gastric fundus: effect of antioxidants and metal chelation. Br J Pharmacol 1998;123:1039–1046.

46. Al-Sa'doni HH, Megson IL, Bisland S, Butler AR, Flitney FW. Neocuproine, a selective CU(I) chelator, and the relaxation of rat vascular smooth muscle by S-nitrosothiols. Br J Pharmacol 1997;121: 1047–1050.

47. Crow JP, Beckman JS. Reactions between nitric oxide, superoxide, and peroxynitrite: footprints of peroxynitrite in vitro. Adv Pharmacol 1995;34:17–433.

48. Koppenol WII. The centennial of the Fenton reaction. Free Rad Biol Med 1993;15:645–651.

49. Scorza G, Pietraforte D, Minetti M. Role of ascorbate and protein thiols in the release of nitric oxide from _S_-nitroso-albumin and _S_-nitroso-glutathione in human plasma. Free Radic Biol Med 1997;22:633–642.

50. Wong PS, Hyun J, Fukuto JM, Shirota FN, DeMaster EG, Shoeman DW. Reaction between _S_-nitrosothiols and thiols: generation of nitroxyl (HNO) and subsequent biochemistry. Biochemistry 1998;37: 5362–5371.

51. Liu Z, Rudd MA, Freedman JE, Loscalzo J. _S_-transnitrosation reactions are involved in the metabolic fate and biologic actions of nitric oxide. J Pharm Exp Ther 1998;284:526–534.

52. Hogg N, Singh RJ, Kalyanaraman B. The role of glutathione in the transport and catabolism of nitric oxide. FEBS Lett 1996;382:223–228.

53. Meyer DJ, Kramer H, Ozer N, Coles B, Ketterer B. Kinetics and equilibria of S-nitrosothiol-thiol exchange between glutathione, cysteine, penicillamines and serum albumin. FEBS Lett 1994;345: 177–180.

54. Lipton SA, Choi YB, Pan ZH, Lei SZ, Vincent Chen HS, Sucher NJ, et al. A redox based mechanism for the neuroprotective and neurodestructive effects of nitric oxide-related nitroso-compounds. Nature 1993;364:626–631.

55. Elliott S, Koliwad SK. Oxidant stress and endothelial membrane transport. Free Radic Biol Med 1995; 19:649–658.

56. Gopalakrishna R, Chen ZH, Gundimeda U. Nitric oxide and nitric oxide-generating donors induce a reversible activation of protein kinase C activity and phorbol ester binding. J Biol Chem 1993;268: 27,180–27,185.

57. Clancy RM, Levartovsky D, Lescynska-Piziak J, Yegudin J, Abramson SB. Nitric oxide reacts with intracellular glutathione and activates the hexose monophosphate shunt in human neutrophils: evidence for S-nitrosoglutathione as a bioactive intermediary. Proc Natl Acad Sci USA 1994;91:3680–3684.

58. Asahi M, Fujii J, Suzuki K, Seo HG, Kuzuya T, Hori M, et al. Inactivation of glutathione peroxidase by nitric oxide. Implication for cytotoxicity. J Biol Chem 1995;270:21,035–21,039.

59. Wink DA, Cook JA, Kim SY, Vodovotz Y, Pacelli R, Krishna MC, et al. Superoxide modulates the oxidation and nitrosation of thiols by nitric oxide-derived reactive intermediates. Chemical aspects involved in the balance between oxidative and nitrosative stress. J Biol Chem 1997;272:11,147–11,151.

60. Jourd'heuil D, Mai CT, Laroux FS, Wink DA, Grisham MB. The reaction of _S_-nitrosoglutathione with superoxide. Biochem Biophys Res Commun 1998;246:525–530.

61. Aleryani S, Milo E, Rose Y, Kostka P. Superoxide-mediated decomposition of biological S-nitroso-thiols. J Biol Chem 1998;273:6041–6045.

62. Trujillo M, Alvarez MN, Peluffo G, Freeman BA, Radi R. Xanthine oxidase-mediated decomposition of S-nitrosothiols. J Biol Chem 1998;273:7828–7834.

63. Scorza G, Minetti M. One-electron oxidation pathway of thiols by peroxynitrite in biological fluids: bicarbonate and ascorbate promote the formation of albumin disulphide dimers in human blood plasma. Biochem J 1998;329:405–413.

64. Newman CM, Warren JB, Taylor GW, Boebis AR, Davies DS. Rapid tolerance to the hypotensive effects of glyceryl trinitrate in the rat: prevention by N-acetyl-L- but not N-acetyl-D-cysteine. Br J Pharmacol 1990;99:825–829.

65. Bates NJ, Baker MT, Guerra R, Harrison DG. Nitric oxide generation from nitroprusside by vascular tissue. Evidence that reduction of the ntiroprusside anion and cyanide loss are required. Biochem Pharmacol 1991;42(Suppl):S157–S165.

66. Ignarro LF, Barry BK, Gruetter DV, Ohlstein EH, Gruetter CA, Kadowitz PJ, et al. Selective alterations in responsiveness of guanylate cyclase to activation by nitroso compounds during enzyme purification. Biochim Biophys Acta 1981;673:394–407.

67. Wu XB, Brune B, von Appen F, Ullrich V. Reversible activation of soluble guanylate cyclase by oxidizing agents. Arch Biochem Biophys 1992;294:75–82.

68. Upchurch GR Jr, Welch GN, Loscalzo J. The vascular biology of S-nitrosothiols, nitrosated derivatives of thiols. Vasc Med 1996;I:25–33.

69. Feelisch M, Noack EA, Schroder H. Explanation of the discrepancy between the degree of organic nitrate decomposition, nitrite formation and guanylate cyclase stimulation. Eur Heart J 1989;9(Suppl A): 57–62.

70. Murphy ME, Piper HM, Watanabe H, Sies H. Nitric oxide production by cultured aortic endothelial cells in response to thiol depletion and replenishment. J Biol Chem 1991;286:19,378–19,383.

71. Haj-Yehia AI, Benet LZ. In vivo depletion of free thiols does not account for nitroglycerin-induced tolerance: a thiol-nitrate interaction hypothesis as an alternative explanation for nitroglycerin activity and tolerance. J Pharmacol Exp Ther 1996;278:1296–1305.

72. Fung HL, Kowaluk CE, Hough K, Kakemi M. Mechanisms for the pharmacologic interaction of organic nitrates with thiols. Existence of an extracellular pathway for the reversal of nitrate vascular tolerance by N-acetylcysteine. J Pharmacol Exp Ther 1988;245:524–530.

73. Ignarro LJ, Kadowitz PJ, Baricos WH. Evidence that regulation of hepatic guanylate cyclase activity involves interactions between catalytic site SH groups and both substrate and activator. Arch Biochem Biophys 1981;208:75–86.

74. Stamler JS, Simon DI, Osborne JA, Mullins ME, Jaraki O, Michel T, et al. S-nitrosylation of proteins with nitric oxide: synthesis and characterization of biologically active compounds. Proc Natl Acad Sci USA 1992;89:444–448.

75. Zhang H, Means GE. S-nitrosation of serum albumin: spectrophotometric determination of its nitro-sation by simple S-nitrosothiols. Anal Biochem 1996;237:141–144.

76. Minamiyama Y, Takemura S, Inoue M. Albumin is an important vascular tonus regulator as a reservoir of nitric oxide. Biochim Biophys Res Commun 1996;225:112–115.

77. Ferranti P, Malorni A, Mamone G, Sannolo N, Marino G. Characterization of S-nitrosohemoglobin by mass spectrometry. FEBS Letts 1997;400:19–24.

78. Gow AJ, Stamler JS. Reactions between nitric oxide and hemoglobin under physiological conditions. Nature 1998;391:169–173.

79. Pawloski JR, Swaminathan RV, Stamler JS. Cell-free and erythrocytic S-nitrosohemoglobin inhibits human platelet aggregation. Circulation 1998;97:263–267.

80. Minamiyama Y, Takemura S, Inoue M. Effect of thiol status on nitric oxide metabolism in the circu-lation. Arch Biochem Biophys 1997;341:186–192.

81. Scharfstein JS, Keaney J, Slivka A, Welch GN, Vita JA, Stamler JS, et al. In vivo transfer of nitric oxide between a plasma protein-bound reservoir and low molecular weight thiols. J Clin Invest 1994;94: 1432–1439.

82. Zai A, Rudd MA, Ward AM, Loscalzo J. Cell-surface protein-disulfide isomerase catalyzes transnitro-sation and regulates intracellular transfer of nitric oxide. J Clin Invest 1999;103:393–399.

83. Khan S, Kayahara M, Joashi U, Mazarakis ND, Sarraf C, Edwards AD, et al. Differential induction of apoptosis in Swiss 3T3 cells by nitric oxide and the nitrosonium cation. J Cell Sci 1997;110:2315–2322.

84. Keaney JF Jr, Simon DI, Stamler JS, Janaki O, Scharfstein J, Vita JA, et al. NO forms an adduct with serum albumin that has endothelium-derived relaxing factor-like properties. J Clin Invest 1993;91: 1582–1589.

85. Seigfried MR, Carey C, Xin-Liang X, Lefer AM. Beneficial effects of SPM-5185, a cysteine-containing NO donor in myocardial ischemia-reperfusion. Am J Physiol 1992;32:H771–H777.

86. Hare JM, Keaney JF Jr, Balligand JL, Loscalzo J, Smith TW, Colucci WS. Role of nitric oxide in sympathetic parasympathetic modulation of myocardial contractility in normal dogs. J Clin Invest 1995;95: 360–366.

87. Campbell DL, Stamler JS, Strauss HC. Redox modulation of L-type calcium channels in ferret ventricular myocytes. Dual mechanism regulation by nitric oxide and S-nitrosothiols. J Gen Physiol 1996; 108:277–293.

88. Hu H, Chiamvimonvat N, Yamagishi T, Marban E. Direct inhibition of expressed cardiac L-type Ca^{2+}-channels by S-nitrosothiol nitric oxide donors. Circ Res 1997;81:742–752.

89. Bauer JA, Fung HL. Differential hemodynamic effects and tolerance properties of nitroglycerin and an S-nitrosothiol in experimental heart failure. J Pharmacol Exp Ther 1991;256:249–254.

90. Synek P, Rusanek K, Spanova H, Mlenjnkova M. The effect of ethanol and nitroglycerin on platelet aggregation. Act Nerv 1970;12:77–82.

91. Hampton JR, Harrison AJ, Honour AJ, Mitchell JR. Platelet behavior and drugs used in cardiovascular disease. Cardiovasc Res 1967;1:101–106.

92. Mellion BT, Ignarro LJ, Ohlstein EH, Pontecorvo EG, Hyman AI, Kadowitz PJ. Evidence for the inhibitory role of guanosine 3'5'-monophosphate in ADP-induced human platelet aggregation in the presence of nitric oxide and related nitrosovasodilators. Blood 1981;57:946–955.

93. Stamler J, Cunningham M, Loscalzo J. Reduced thiols and the effect of intravenous nitroglycerin on platelet aggregation. Am J Cardiol 1988;62:377–380.

94. Mellion BT, Ignarro LJ, Myers CB, Ohlstein EH, Ballot BA, Hyman AL, et al. Inhibition of human platelet aggregation by S-nitrosothiols. Heme-dependent activation of soluble guanylate-cyclase and stimulation of cyclic GMP accumulation. Mol Pharmacol 1983;23:653–664.

95. Loscalzo J. N-acetylcysteine potentiates inhibition of platelet aggregation by nitroglycerin. J Clin Invest 1985;76:703–708.

96. Loscalzo J, Freedman JE. Purification and characterization of human platelet glutathione-S-transferase. Blood 1986;67:1595–1599.

97. Freedman JE, Frei B, Welch GN, Loscalzo J. Glutathione peroxidase potentiates the inhibition of platelet function by S-nitrosothiols. J Clin Invest 1995;96:394–400.

98. Naseem KM, Chirico S, Mohammadi B, Bruckdorfer KR. The synergism of hydrogen peroxide with plasma S-nitrosothiols in the inhbition of platelet activation. Biochem J 1996;318:759–766.

99. Amano M, Takahashi M, Kosaka T, Kinoshita M. Differential inhibition of platelet aggregation and calcium mobilization by nitroglycerin and stabilized nitric oxide. J Cardiovasc Pharm 1994;24:860–866.

100. Keaney JF Jr, Stamler JS, Scharfstein JS, Loscalzo J. NO forms a stable adduct with serum albumin that has potent antiplatelet propertics in vivo. Clin Res 1992;40:194a.

101. Radi R, Beckman JS, Bush KM, Freeman BA. Peroxynitrite oxidation of sulfhydryls. The cytotoxic potential of superoxide and nitric oxide. J Biol Chem 1991;266:4244–4250.

102. Jia L, Furchgott RF. Inhibition by sulfhydryl compounds of vascular relaxation induced by nitric oxide and endothelium-derived relaxing factor. J Pharm Exp Ther 1993;267:371–378.

103. Clarke R, Daly L, Robinson K, Naughten E, Cahalane S, Fowler B, et al. Hyperhomocysteinemia: an independent risk factor for vascular disease. N Engl J Med 1991;324:1149–1155.

104. Manilow MR. Hyperhomocyst(e)inemia: a common and easily reversible risk factor for occlusive atherosclerosis. Circulation 1990;81:1149–1155.

105. Kang SS, Wong PWK, Cook HY, Norusis M, Messer JV. Protein-bound homocyst(e)ine: a possible risk factor for coronary artery disease. J Clin Invest 1986;77:1482–1486.

106. Refsum H, Helland S, Ueland PM. Radioenzyme determination of homocysteine in plasma and urine. Clin Chem 1985;31:624–628.

107. Spindel E, McCulley KS. Conversion of methionine to homocysteine thiolactone in liver. Biochim Biophys Acta 1974;343:687–691.

108. McCulley KS. Homocysteine metabolism in scurvy, growth and atherosclerosis. Nature 1971;231: 391,392.

109. Stamler JS, Osborne JA, Jaraki O, Rabbani LE, Mullins M, Singel D, et al. Adverse effects of homocysteine are modulated by endothelium-derived relaxing factor and related oxides of nitrogen. J Clin Invest 1993;91:308–318.

110. Upchurch GR Jr, Welch GN, Fabian AJ, Pigazzi A, Keaney JF Jr, Loscalzo J. Stimulation of endothelial nitric oxide production by homocysteine. Atherosclerosis 1997;132:177–185.

111. Gaston B, Reilly HM, Drazen JM, Fackler J, Ramdel P, Arnelle D, et al. Endogenous nitric oxides and bronchodilator S-nitrosothiols in human airways. Proc Natl Acad Sci USA 1993;90:10,956–10,961.

112. Loscalzo J. Endothelial dysfunction in pulmonary hypertension. N Engl J Med 1992;327:117–119.
113. Pepke-Zaba J, Higgenbottam TW, Dinh Xuan AT, Stone D, Wallwork J. Inhaled nitric oxide as a cause of selective pulmonary vasodilation in pulmonary hypertension. Lancet 1991;338:1173,1174.
114. Roberts JD Jr, Lang P, Bigatello LM, Vlahakes GJ, Zapol WM. Inhaled nitric oxide in congenital heart disease. Circulation 1993;87:447–453.
115. Loh E, Stamler JS, Hare JM, Loscalzo J, Colucci WS. Cardiovascular effects of inhaled nitric oxide in patients with left ventricular dysfunction. Circulation 1994;90:2780–2785.
116. Folts JD, Stamler JS, Keaney JF Jr, Loscalzo J. Coating stenosed intimally damaged dog coronary arteris with S-nitrosated albumin prevents platelet adhesion-aggregation and thrombus formation. Circulation 1994;90:I-345.
117. Marks DS, Vita JA, Folts JF, Welch GN, Loscalzo J. Inhibition of neointimal proliferation in rabbits following vascular injury by a single treatment with a protein adduct of nitric oxide. J Clin Invest 1995; 96:2630–2638.
118. Panza JA, Quyyumi AA, Brush JE Jr, Epstein SE. Abnormal endothelial-dependent vasorelaxation in patients with essential hypertension. N Engl J Med 1990;323:22–27.
119. Loscalzo J, Smick D, Andon N, Cooke J. S-nitrosocaptopril. 1. Molecular characterization and effects on the vasculature and on platelets. J Pharmacol Exp Ther 1989;249:726–729.
120. Schaffer JE, Lee F, Thompson S, Han B, Cooke J, Loscalzo J. The hemodynamic effects of S-nitroso-captopril in anesthetized dogs. J Pharmacol Exp Ther 1991;256:704–709.
121. Goldschmidt JE, Tallarida RJ. Pharmacological evidence that captopril possesses endothelium-derived relaxing factor properties. J Pharmacol Exp Ther 1991;256:1136–1145.
122. Kilbourn RG, Jurban A, Gross S, Griffith OW, Feldman PL, Wiseman J. Reversal of endotoxin-mediated shock by NG-methyl-L-arginine, an inhibitor of nitric oxide synthesis. Biochem Biophys Res Commun 1990;172:1132–1138.
123. Keaney JF Jr, Loscalzo J, Puyana JC, Francis S, Stamler J. Methylene blue reverses endotoxin-induced hypertension. Circ Res 1994;75:1121–1125.
124. Minamiyama Y, Takemura S, Koyama K, Yu H, Miyamoto M, Inoue M. Dynamic aspects of gluta-thione and nitric oxide metabolism in endotoxemic rats. Am J Physiol 1996;271:G575–G581.
125. Stamler JS, Simon DI, Osborne JA, Mullins ME, Jaraki O, Michel T, Singel DJ, Loscalzo J. S-nitro-sylation of proteins with nitric oxide: synthesis and characterization of biologically active compounds. PNAS 1992;89:444–448.
126. Stamler JS, Jaraki O, Osborne J, Simon DI, Keaney JF Jr, Vita J, Singel D, Valeri CR, Loscalzo J. Nitric oxide circulates in mammalian plasma primarily as an S-nitroso adduct of serum albumin. PNAS 1992; 89:7674–7677.
127. Tabuchi A, Sano K, Oh E, Tsuchiya T, Tsuda M. Modulation of AP-1 activity by nitric oxide in vitro: NO-mediated modulation of AP-1. FEBS Lett 1994;351:123–127.
128. Michetti M, Salomino F, Melloni E, Pontremoli S. Reversible inactivation of calpain isoforms by nitric oxide. BBRC 1994;207:1009–1014.
129. Brune B, Lapetina EG. Protein thiol modification of glyceraldehyde-3-phosphate dehydrogenase as a target for nitric oxide signalling. Genetic Engineer 1995;17;149–164.
130. Aronstam RS, Martin DC, Dennison RL, Cooley HG. S-nitrosylation of M2 muscarinic receptor thiols disrupts receptor-G-protein coupling. Ann NY Acad Sci 1995;757:215–7.
131. Gergel D, Cedarbaum AI. Inhibition of the catalytic activity of alcohol dehydrogenase by nitric oxide is associated with S-nitrosylation and the release of zinc. Biochemistry1996;35:16,186–16,194.
132. Campbell DL, Stamler JS, Strauss HC. Redox modulation of L-type calcium channels in ferret ventric-ular myocytes. Dual mechanism regulation by nitric oxide and S-nitrosothiols. J Gen Physiol 1996; 108:277–293.
133. Lander HM, Hajjar DP, Hempstead BL, Mizra UA, Chait BT, Campbell S, Quilliam LA. A molecular redox switch on p21 (ras). Structural basis for nitric oxide-p21 (ras) interaction. J Biol Chem 1997; 262:4223–4226.
134. Dimmeler S, Haendeler J, Nehls M, Zeiher AM. Suppression of apoptosis by nitric oxide via inhibition of interleukin-1β-converting enzyme (ICE)-like and cysteine protease protein (CPP)-32-like pro-teases. J Exp Med 1997;185:601–607.
135. Li J, Billiar TR, Talanian RV, Kim YM. Nitric oxide reversibly inhibits seven members of the caspase family via S-nitrosylation. BBRC 1997;240:419–424.
136. Catani MV, Bernassola F, Rossi A, Melino G. Inhibition of clotting factor XIII activity by nitric oxide. BBRC 1998;249:275–278.
137. Arstall MA, Bailey C, Gross WL, Bak M, Balligand JL, Kelly RA. Reversible S-nitrosation of crea-tinine kinase by nitric oxide in adult rat ventricular myocytes. J Mol Cell Cardiol 1998;30:979–988.

138. So HS, Pack RK, Kim MS, Lee SR, Jung BH, Chung SY, Jun CD, Chung HT. Nitric oxide inhibits c-jun N-terminal kinase 2 (JNK2) via S-nitrosylation. BBRC 1998;247:809–813.
139. Clementi E, Brown GC, Feelisch M, Moncada S. Persistant inhibition of cell respiration by nitric oxide: crucial role of S-nitrosylation of mitochondrial complex I and protective action of glutathione. PNAS 1998;95:7631–7636.
140. Xu L, Eu JP, Meissner G, Stamler JS. Activation of the cardiac calcium release channel (ryanodine receptor) by poly-S-nitrosylation. Science 1998;279:234–237.
141. Ruiz F, Corrales FJ, Miqueo C, Mato JM. Nitric oxide inactivates rat hepatic methionine adenosyl-transferase in vivo by S-nitrosylation. Hepatology 1998;28:1051–1057.
142. Zai A, Rudd MA, Scribner AW, Loscalzo J. Nitric oxide reacts with platelet-surface protein disulfide isomerase and inhibits platelet function. Circulation 1998;98:I–594.

24

Diazeniumdiolates (Formerly NONOates) in Cardiovascular Research and Potential Clinical Applications

Joseph E. Saavedra,
Anthony L. Fitzhugh, and Larry K. Keefer

INTRODUCTION

The Need for Compounds Allowing Controlled Release and Targeted Delivery of NO•

Nitric oxide (NO•) is a crucial messenger in biological systems. This simple diatomic molecule functions as an important protective, regulatory, and signaling agent involved in homeostatic regulation of blood pressure and platelet aggregation, neurotransmission, and immune response (1,2). The protective nature of NO• makes this compound an appealing therapeutic target to treat or prevent disorders characterized by NO• deficiency such as vasospasm and thrombosis. In fact, inhaled NO• gas produces selective pulmonary vasodilation and thus can be used to treat disorders such as adult respiratory distress syndrome (3,4). Administration of exogenous NO• by inhalation can be a successful way of reducing pulmonary vascular resistance in children with persistent pulmonary hypertension of the newborn (5,6).

NO• is a gas under standard temperature and pressure and it behaves as such in the lung; therefore, inhalation therapy is viable. However, because the lifetime of this compound is extremely short in vivo, a continuous delivery of the gas is necessary. Also, rebound hypoxemia may occur if treatment is stopped; this poses some serious limitations in inhalation therapy. Moreover, in probably all other biological functions, NO• is not a gas but a lipid soluble nonelectrolyte, and is so rapidly inactivated that it cannot function as a circulating hormone. Accordingly, the controlled delivery of NO• to a specific organ or cell type within the host remains a challenge. The objective, then, is to develop therapeutic strategies that sequester the NO• functionality into a chemically stable carrier that can be directed to the deficient site to carry out its effector functions without systemic consequences.

In order to discuss strategies for site-directed administration of NO•, it is important first to present some of the basic physical and chemical properties of this extraordinary free radical.

From: *Contemporary Cardiology, vol. 4: Nitric Oxide and the Cardiovascular System*
Edited by: J. Loscalzo and J. A. Vita © Humana Press Inc., Totowa, NJ

NO• AS A LEWIS ACID

NO•'s Reaction with Lewis Bases

The most important characteristic of NO•, at least for the purpose of preparing stable bio-logically active agents of the diazeniumdiolate class, is its Lewis acid property (7). Certain adducts of nucleophiles with NO• have been known for many years; however, their biological properties were not investigated until recently (8). It is the electron-acceptor quality of NO• that provides the rationale for the preparation of nonclassical NO•-releasing compounds. As a Lewis acid, NO• can react with a nucleophile (Nu−) in a 2:1 molar ratio to give the anionic species $NuN_2O_2^-$, as illustrated in Eq. 1.

$$Nu^- \ + \ 2NO \longrightarrow Nu-\overset{+}{N}\overset{\displaystyle O^-}{\underset{\displaystyle N-O^-}{\diagup}} \tag{1}$$

One such process that clearly depicts this chemistry is the reaction of sulfite ion $[(SO_3)^{-2}]$ with two molecules of NO• to give $(O_3SN_2O_2)^{-2}$ (7). This compound does not revert to NO• when dissolved in water but instead disproportionates to N_2O (9). Angeli's salt is prepared, not through a reaction of NO•, but by the nitration of hydroxylamine; however, structurally speaking, this compound is an oxygen adduct of NO• represented by the structure $(ON_2O_2)^{-2}$ (10). Like the sulfite analog, this compound disproportionates to N_2O, but at low concentra-tion it also yields significant amounts of NO• in neutral buffers. This spontaneous release of NO• under physiological conditions was confirmed by Vanin et al. (11), who discovered that administration of this compound produces NO• in vivo and exhibits vasorelaxant properties. Active acidic methylene groups react with NO• in the presence of base to give N-nitroso-hydroxylamines with the general structure $[R_2CH-N_2O_2^-]$; these are known as Traube com-pounds (12). Complexes of these structures may be considered as carbon/NO• adducts and are generally very stable; some are known to release NO• on enzymatic oxidation, however. Analogous NO• adducts may be obtained from oximes (13). Nucleophilic amines, on the other hand, form complexes (14), usually as stable white powders, that on dissolution release a nearly quantitative two molecules of NO• per [N(O)NO]− group (15).

Reaction with Nucleophilic Amines Leading to the Formation of NO•-Releasing Diazeniumdiolate Species

Amine/NO• complexes (substituted 1-amino diazen-1-ium-1,2-diolates) are normally made by exposing nucleophilic amines in ether, or other suitable solvent, to 5 atmospheres of NO• in the absence of air. The reaction proceeds according to Eq. 2, where one equivalent of amine reacts with two equivalents of NO• and a second amine molecule abstracts a proton from the initially formed complex, keeping the [N(O)NO]− group in its stable anionic form. The product precipitates as a white powder and is collected by suction filtration. These white powders may be stored under nitrogen at refrigerator temperatures, often for extended periods of time without decomposition. A cation exchange to the sodium salt may be easily performed (Eq. 3), not only to form a generally more stable salt, thereby increasing the shelf-life, but also as a ready "synthon" for further derivatization (16).

SPONTANEOUS RELEASE OF NO• FROM ANIONIC AMINE/NO• COMPLEXES

Many of the diazeniumdiolates derived from amine nucleophiles, when dissolved in buffers, blood, or cell culture medium, dissociate to regenerate NO•, with the amine molecule as the by-product (Eq. 4). Most of these compounds have a strong chromophore at 250 nm in the ultraviolet region, which serves as a convenient marker for their detection, quantifi-

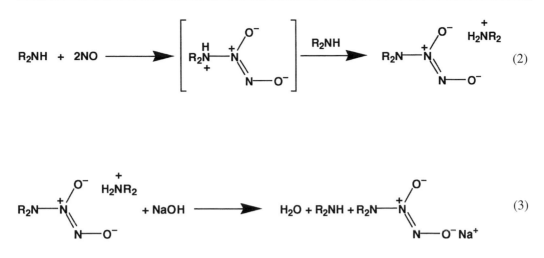

$$(2)$$

$$(3)$$

cation, and quality control. The dissociation of these anions to NO$^{\bullet}$ proceeds with simple first-order kinetics at pH 7.4, with half-lives ranging from 2 s *(17)* to 20 h at 37°C *(15)*.

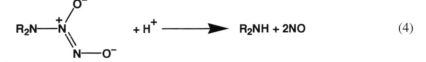

$$(4)$$

We have established that substituted 1-amino diazeniumdiolates are reliable sources of NO$^{\bullet}$ and that because of the vast differences in their half-lives they may be tailored to different biomedical applications. However, spontaneous, nearly quantitative NO$^{\bullet}$ release and variable rates of decomposition meet only some of the criteria needed when one is to decide where and how to use these diazeniumdiolates. Up to now, we have been referring to the amine nucleophile portion in general terms. However, as the NO$^{\bullet}$ is released from the diazeniumdiolate the nucleophile residue or byproducts thereof increase in concentration and will possibly have their own pharmacological or toxicological activity in addition to those of NO$^{\bullet}$. Therefore, an additional criterion in choosing compounds for NO$^{\bullet}$ generation is to consider as well the effects of the byproducts. The nucleophilic residues may be polyamines or simple primary or secondary amines including secondary amino acids.

NO$^{\bullet}$-RELEASING ZWITTERIONS DERIVED FROM POLYAMINES

In 1961, Drago and Karstetter *(18)* were the first to report the reaction of diamines, specifically *N,N'*-dimethylethylenediamine and piperazine, with NO$^{\bullet}$ to produce *inter*molecular salts. The *inter*molecular diazeniumdiolate adduct of the former is as formulated in structure **1**. Years later Hrabie et al. *(19)* began to study the reaction of polyamines with NO$^{\bullet}$ under conditions that would favor the formation of *intra*molecular salts, or zwitterions, with the general structure **2**.

In organic solvents, polyamines are very soluble compounds, in sharp contrast to many of the corresponding diazeniumdiolated zwitterions; accordingly, the zwitterions tend to precipitate rapidly, such that the reaction of NO$^{\bullet}$ with compounds containing multiple nitrogen atoms can often be limited to a single site. Numerous zwitterionic diamine, triamine, and polyamine/NO$^{\bullet}$ adducts were synthesized by placing the free bases under 5 atmospheres (atm) of NO$^{\bullet}$ in ether, tetrahydrofuran, or acetonitrile as the solvent. These white powders are usually stable indefinitely as solids in closed containers at freezer temperatures, but they release NO$^{\bullet}$ rapidly under acidic conditions and at slower rates in neutral solutions. In order to determine the effect of structure and/or nitrogen substitution on the rate of NO$^{\bullet}$ release, Hrabie and colleagues *(19)* conducted a systematic study of these adducts with the intent to

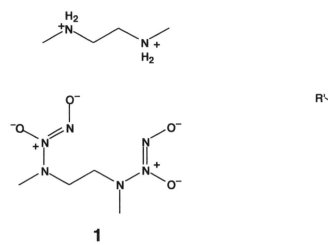

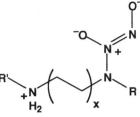

2a: R = R' = Me, x = 2
2b: R = R' = Me, x = 1
2c: R = R' = Et, x = 1
2d: R = Et, R' = H, x = 1

1

provide criteria for predictable, controlled release of NO•. These materials contain as much as 45% NO• by weight and most of them release two full equivalents of NO•, but the rates of decomposition vary considerably from one to another. The half-lives at room temperature in pH 7.4 buffered solution varied from 1.3 min for the adduct of N,N'-dimethylbutane-diamine, **2a**, to 56 h for that of diethylenetriamine, **3**, routinely called DETA/NO. In the diamine series **2** for any value of x separating the two nitrogen atoms, a small increase in the size of R resulted in a sharp increase in stability, whereas changes in R' resulted in relatively minor differences. For example, the half-life ($t_{1/2}$) of the N,N'- dimethylethylenediamine/NO• adduct, **2b**, was 36 min at pH 7.4 and 22°C but the diethyl analog, **2c**, increased to 5.6 h; however, relatively little change in the rate of decomposition was observed ($t_{1/2}$ = 5.45 h) with the monoethyl compound **2d**. In addition to the long-lived DETA/NO, **3**, two other triamine adducts were reported including the diazeniumdiolate from the biologically relevant spermi-dine with a half-life of close to 3 h. It was speculated that the exceptional and unexpected stability of the zwitterionic NO• adducts may be due to hydrogen bonding. As depicted in **3a**, hydrogen bonding in DETA/NO is thought to reduce the negative charge character of the diazeniumdiolate, which thus becomes more resistant to acid-catalyzed fragmentation.

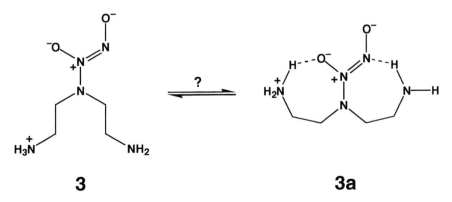

3   **3a**

The reaction of spermine, another important biomolecule, with NO• gave the diazeniumdi-olate in good yield. A single adduct was obtained in spite of the presence of four nitrogen atoms in the molecule and it was of comparable stability to the triamine analogue derived from spermidine. These studies have revealed some important aspects of the basic chemistry of polyamine-NO• interaction and structural features of the corresponding zwitterions. A salient discovery was the fact that NO• preferentially reacts with secondary amino groups even when more than one primary amino nitrogen is present in the same molecule. More importantly, this work has provided diazeniumdiolates of varied stability, an attribute that should facilitate the study of the effects of NO• on the vasculature or other tissues.

DIAZENIUMDIOLATES OF PRIMARY AND SECONDARY AMINES

Drago and Paulik *(14)* reported the reaction of diethylamine with NO• to obtain the diethylammonium salt of 1-(*N,N*-diethylamino)diazen-1-ium-1,2-diolate, $Et_2NH_2^+Et_2NN_2O_2^-$. The thrust of their work was to obtain additional evidence on the Lewis acid or electron pair acceptor property of NO•. This work was later extended to other primary and secondary amines *(18)*, and thus they came to establish these complexations as general reaction types between NO• and amine nucleophiles. Two preparative techniques were used to react these amines with NO•. One method simply required bubbling NO• into an ether solution of the desired substrate at −78°C, whereas the second procedure required high pressure in an autoclave. Both methods gave the same ammonium salt of the diazeniumdiolate, the latter providing higher yields. The ammonium salts were conveniently converted to more stable sodium salts with sodium ethoxide. Only symmetrical, unhindered amines, as large as di-n-hexylamine, were successfully converted to the corresponding diazeniumdiolates. In our laboratory, we have found that 5 atm of NO• is adequate for these reactions in acetonitrile–ether solutions even at room temperature. More than occasionally we have directly isolated the sodium salts of these diazeniumdiolates by reacting the amine with NO• in methanol–ether solutions in the presence of one equivalent of sodium methoxide.

Longhi and Drago *(20)* studied the interaction of $Et_2N-N_2O_2^-$ anion with several metal cations. Sodium, potassium and calcium complexes were formed, isolated and characterized. Evidence was presented regarding the formation of Co^{2+}, Ni^{2+}, Mn^{2+}, Fe^{2+} and Cr^{3+} complexes in solution. Christodoulou and coworkers *(21,22)* further investigated the interactions of the same diazeniumdiolate anion with different metal centers in nonaqueous solutions. In the case of Cu^{2+}, mixed-ligand complexes of various nuclearity were described.

X-ray diffraction studies of one of the isolated Cu^{2+} complexes, the mononuclear Cu(MeOH) $(Et_2NN_2O_2)_2$, **4**, demonstrated the planar, bidentate nature of the $N_2O_2^-$ functional group. The N–N linkage in the $N_2O_2^-$ group has double bond character while the $(Et_2)N-N$ linkage is a single bond, as is the N–O bond. Both oxygen atoms interact with the metal center. These studies indicate that diazeniumdiolates contain a bidentate chelating ligand found in the Z configuration. Crystallographic comparison of nitrogen diazeniumdiolates and other types of compound containing the $N_2O_2^-$ group, e.g., cupferron, Angeli's salt, and so forth, indicates that despite the diversity of substituents there is a remarkable degree of similarity in the structure of the $[N(O)NO]^-$ moieties.

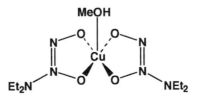

4

Studies of the diazeniumdiolation of primary amines have been reported *(18)*. t-Butylamine gave no adduct with NO•; methylamine formed a diazeniumdiolate but it was too unstable to be isolated. However, NO• complexes derived from n-propyl-, isopropyl-, isobutyl-, n-amyl- and cyclohexylamine were isolated and purified as either the ammonium or sodium salts. As was the case with secondary amines, increases in chain length result in augmented stability. Moreover, the branching of the chain or ring attachment provided even greater stability, as was the case for the isopropylamine and cyclohexylamine adducts. However, diazeniumdiolates of primary amines may not be very practical compounds as therapeutic NO• donors. These materials are unsafe to handle, as traces of base can catalyze the production of large amounts of nitrogen very quickly, creating a potentially explosive condition.

PHARMACOLOGICAL TARGETING OF NO• WITH DIAZENIUMDIOLATES—SYNTHETIC STRATEGIES

The anionic complexes discussed above decompose spontaneously at physiological pH, some of them at a very rapid rate. Thus, an important goal in our research is to deliver NO• to a prescribed site before it has a chance to decompose and without affecting other NO•-sensitive functions. By taking advantage of the remarkable chemical versatility of diazenium-diolates, we have developed three general strategies for targeting NO• delivery: (1) incorporation of the diazeniumdiolate functionality into polymeric matrices of different structural types; (2) prodrug design involving protection of the terminal oxygen, and (3) binding of a diazen-iumdiolate prodrug to a biomolecule or biocompatible molecule that tends to concentrate in the target tissue or cell type.

Polymer-Bound Diazeniumdiolates

We have incorporated the diazeniumdiolate functionality and compounds of structure $X\text{-}N_2O_2^-$, where X is an amino group, into polymeric matrices of different structural types *(23)*. Structures 5–7 depict the generalized polymer types considered in this investigation. As illustrated in structure **5**, a low-molecular-weight diazeniumdiolate may simply be incorporated as a blend or dispersion into a polymer matrix such as polyethylene glycol, polyure-thane, or polycaprolactone. These blends drastically alter the time course of NO• release and may provide a prolonged shelf life for the monomer. As represented in structure **6**, the diazeniumdiolate functionality may be covalently attached to a crosslinked polymer contain-ing pendant amino groups, whereas **7** illustrates that the [N(O)NO]⁻ group can be directly attached to the polymer backbone. Incorporation of the diazeniumdiolate functionality into stationary solids can control the rate of NO• release and concentrate it in the cells in closest proximity to the polymer surface.

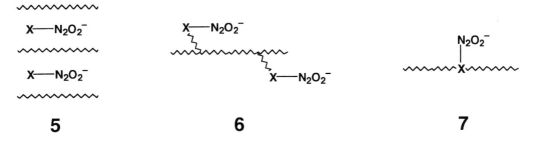

5   **6**   **7**

Prodrug Formation via O^2-Functionalization Chemistry

The incorporation of [N(O)NO]⁻ moieties into a stationary solid was designed to place the donor in close proximity to the target tissue. However, the prodrug approach provides a strategy that allows the diazeniumdiolate to move freely throughout the circulatory system without spontaneously dissociating. This can be effected by covalently attaching a protective group at the terminal oxygen, as in the conversion of **8** to **9** (Eq. 5). The ideal prodrug will not release NO• until it is metabolically reconverted to the anionic diazeniumdiolate, **8**. The possibility of doing this type of alkylation on diazeniumdiolates was reported by Longhi and

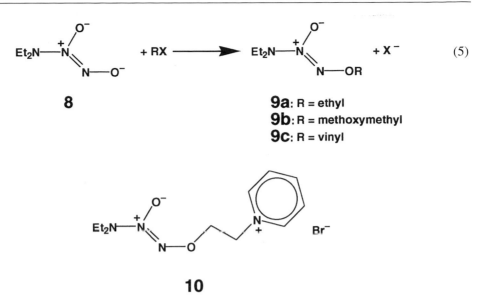

$$ \mathbf{8} \qquad\qquad \mathbf{9a}: \text{R = ethyl} $$
$$ \mathbf{9b}: \text{R = methoxymethyl} $$
$$ \mathbf{9c}: \text{R = vinyl} $$

10

Drago *(20)* in their study of NO⁺ complexes and by Reilly *(24)* in a patent dealing primarily with nitrosamine manufacture. Our laboratory advanced these early studies and established the O-alkylation of diazeniumdiolates as a general synthetic method.

Anions of structure **8** proved reactive toward alkyl halides, sulfate esters, and epoxides. The product **9**, as predicted, was very stable toward hydrolysis. For example, **9a** was stable indefinitely at pH 7.4; even heating at reflux for 18 h in 0.01 *M* hydrochloric acid resulted in only 32% decomposition. Even derivatives with labile protective groups, such as **9b** and **9c**, exhibited considerably more stability toward hydrolysis than the starting anion **8**. X-ray analysis was carried out on compound **10**, providing unambiguous information regarding the chemical connectivity and relative stereochemistry of the compound. The terminal oxygen (O^2) and not the interior one (O^1) was the site of alkylation, and the two oxygens bound to the nitrogens of the N—N bond had the *Z* (*cis*) configuration *(16)*.

Our preliminary studies on the O^2-alkylation of diazeniumdiolates provided valuable basic information on the reactivity of the anions toward various electrophiles, the stereochemistry of the products, and their stability in the absence of enzymes. Since then, studies have been aimed at the variation of both the protective group and the amine nucleophile in order to explore the full potential of **9** in a variety of pharmacological applications. Changes in the protective group at O^2 determine the conditions under which this group will be removed in order to generate the anion, and variations at the amine nucleophile end determine the velocity of NO⁺ release at the anionic stage. To illustrate these points we refer to an application of the prodrug approach developed by Makings and Tsien *(25)*. These authors prepared a series of compounds from **8** and various substituted derivatives of ortho-nitrobenzyl bromides. These new compounds were tailored to either permeate cell membranes or remain specifically trapped in the intercellular spaces resulting in prodrugs that were photochemically triggered NO⁺ donors. The prodrugs were biologically inert until photolyzed, whereupon a rapid release of NO⁺ took place. This technique involves the localized application of a O^2-substituted diazeniumdiolate into a specific location where it awaits focused illumination to trigger NO⁺ release.

We have reported a prodrug that is not hindered by the limitations of local or direct NO⁺ administration, but rather acts selectively in the liver after systemic administration *(26)*. This vinyl compound, **11**, was the best candidate in a series of O^2-alkylated prodrugs derived from the sodium salt of the pyrrolidine/NO⁺ complex ion, **12** (PYRRO/NO). The pyrrolidine complex was chosen for its ability to regenerate NO⁺ at a very fast rate ($t_{1/2}$ = 3 s at pH 7.4 and 37 °C)

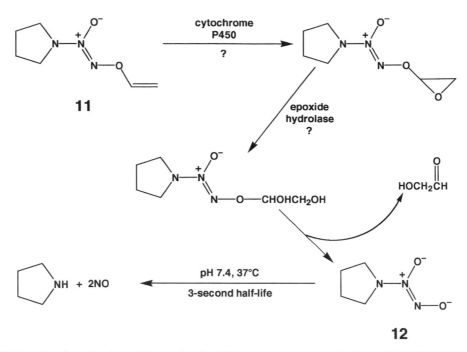

Fig. 1. Postulated mechanism of liver-selective NO˙ generation on metabolism of V-PYRRO/NO (**11**) (adapted from ref. *26*).

and thus avoid inducing systemic effects. The vinyl substituted diazeniumdiolate proved to be liver selective, where the released NO˙ resulted in an increase of cGMP levels that blocked tumor necrosis factor-α-induced apoptosis and toxicity in that organ without significant impact on the systemic blood pressure. The postulated mechanism of liver-selective NO˙ generation on metabolism of **11** is illustrated in Fig. 1.

Attachment of O^2-Substituted Polyfunctional Diazeniumdiolates to Other Bioactive Molecules

A third strategy, discussed here, takes advantage of the remarkable reactivity of the diazeniumdiolate functionality to complement and at times combine the prodrug and polymer-bound $[N(O)NO]^-$ approaches discussed earlier. The goal of this method is to develop an O^2-substituted diazeniumdiolate with a remote and reactive functionality that would enable a prodrug to bind to a substrate *(27)*. This functionality may be either nucleophilic or electrophilic in nature and the substrate may range from a simple low molecular weight drug or natural product to a peptide, protein, polysaccharide, or synthetic polymer.

Piperazine, a bifunctional base used medicinally for its anthelmintic properties, appears to us to be the ideal type of linker compound for this strategy. Early reports *(28)* of the high-pressure reaction of piperazine with NO˙ show that salts of diazeniumdiolated piperazines have been produced. We have used, with the aid of protection and deprotection techniques, one of piperazine's two nucleophilic nitrogen centers as a carrier for an O^2-protected diazeniumdiolate group, whereas the second nitrogen remains available for linking the diazeniumdiolated piperazine to a desired substrate. The emerging technology where the piperazine is used as a synthetic scaffold to affix the active diazeniumdiolate functionality is illustrated in Fig. 2.

N-Substituted piperazines are easily prepared and many of them are commercially available. For example, the reaction of 1-ethoxycarbonyl piperazine with NO˙ in the presence of sodium methoxide gives diazeniumdiolate **13** that in turn is blocked at the O^2-position by an

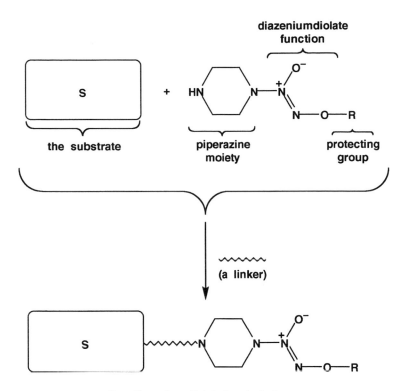

Fig. 2. Strategy by which biologically important substrates (S: a biocompatible polymer, drug, or natural product) can be converted to NO•-releasing agents through covalent attachment of diazeniumdiolated piperazine molecules. R is a group whose hydrolytic or metabolic removal allows NO• generation to begin.

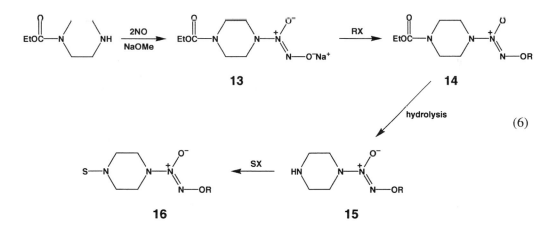

(6)

R group to give **14**. The base labile ethoxycarbonyl protective group of **14** is then removed to give a compound (**15**) containing a protected diazeniumdiolate functionality as well as a distal nucleophilic nitrogen. Piperazine **15** has provided a practical way to incorporate the NO•-releasing diazeniumdiolate group into other biologically relevant substrates (S), with the product having the general structure **16**. Among the substrates that have been linked to the diazeniumdiolate-containing molecule are a nonsteroidal anti-inflammatory agent, amino acids, polysaccharides, purine riboside derivatives, and polymers. This linker chemistry, as

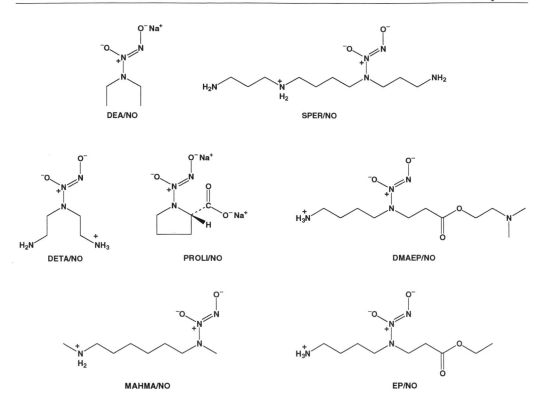

Fig. 3. Structures of diazeniumdiolates whose pharmacologic properties are discussed in the text (DEA, diethylamino; SPER, spermine).

illustrated in Eq. 6, may be very useful in the development of NO•-releasing diazeniumdiolates capable of receptor-mediated interactions that target specific sites of the anatomy.

DIAZENIUMDIOLATES AS CARDIOVASCULAR RESEARCH TOOLS

The diazeniumdiolates' ability to generate NO• in physiological media with a wide range of rates (2 s–20 h) makes them advantageous agents for studying many aspects of cardiovascular function. In one of the first such applications, DEA/NO and SPER/NO (structures shown in Fig. 3), two spontaneous NO•-releasers with 10-fold different NO• generation rates (<3 min and >30 min, respectively, at physiological pH and temperature) were administered intravenously to anesthetized rabbits to probe the effect of NO• generation rate on systemic blood pressure. The short-acting diazeniumdiolate had a duration of action closely mirroring that of sodium nitroprusside (SNP) in that the blood pressure reached its minimum within 1 min then rapidly recovered to baseline. The dose-response curve was virtually congruent with that of nitroprusside ion. By contrast, the long-acting diazeniumdiolate was much less potent when measured in terms of blood pressure drop at 1 min after injection, but generated significant hypotension even 30 min after bolus injection. These results demonstrated that the potency of NO•'s hemodynamic effects is primarily a function of the amount of NO• being generated at the relevant location in a given short interval of observation, persisting as long as NO• exposure continues but not longer *(29)*, as had been predicted based on in vitro studies with aortic rings *(9)*.

NO•'s antiplatelet effects followed a similar pattern. When the same two diazeniumdiolates were given intravenously to rabbits with blood samples being drawn 1 and 30 min after bolus administration, the short-acting compound displayed potent antiaggregatory activity at a dose (50 nmol/kg) at which aspirin was inactive when measured at 1 min postinjection, but insignificant activity at the 30-min time point. By contrast, a 10-fold higher molar dose of the compound with half-life greater than 30 min was less potent at the 1-min point than it was at 30 min after injection. Here again, the antithrombotic effect of the NO• donors in vivo correlated well with the rate of NO• generation seen in parallel work with simple buffers *(30)*, suggesting considerable promise for exploiting the diazeniumdiolates' predictability of NO• release rate in vivo for the design of improved pharmacologic agents.

A very different relationship between NO• generation rate and biological effect was seen in studies of vascular smooth muscle cell (VSMC) proliferation in vitro. When cultured rat aorta smooth muscle cells (SMC) were treated with the same two diazeniumdiolates mentioned previously plus others ranging in half-life up to 20 h, the compounds with the longest half-lives were the most potent antiproliferative agents. The results indicated that the compounds' effect on growth of these cells is reversible, such that a short but intense burst of NO• lasting only a small fraction of the observation period ceased to have lasting impact after the NO• source was exhausted, whereas spreading the same total molar dose of NO• more or less evenly throughout the entire observation period led to maximum effect. Indeed, complete inhibition of proliferation in these cells was observed during 6 d of continuous exposure to 0.1–0.5 mM DETA/NO (structure shown in Fig. 3) with no observable toxic consequences *(31)*.

The uncomplicated dissociation mechanism by which the diazeniumdiolates generate NO• makes them an important tool for checking conclusions derived from experiments with other NO• donors. A case in point is a recent study *(32)* of NO•'s role in macrophage-dependent oxidation of low-density lipoproteins (LDLs). When LDLs were incubated with activated murine macrophages, SNP was found to increase lipid hydroperoxide formation. By contrast, SPER/NO strongly inhibited lipid oxidation in this system. Many authors have used only nitroprusside, an NO• donor long valued as a rapidly acting hypotensive agent for its highly reliable and rapid conversion to NO• in the blood stream, to investigate the role of NO• in such toxic phenomena. However, nitroprusside's by-products of NO• release include both cyanide ion and iron species capable of generating highly oxidizing and toxic conditions in the cell *(33,34)*. The authors showed this phenomenon to be responsible for enhancement of LDL oxidation by nitroprusside in explaining why it served a prooxidant role, whereas SPER/NO and the other NO• donors employed were protective *(32)*.

The example of the previous paragraph illustrates the great importance of using considerable caution in interpreting results based on a single NO• donor, particularly nitroprusside. Each of the several classes of donor in common use today has its own strengths and limitations. Thus, it is generally advisable to confirm the results obtained with one class by performing parallel experiments with one or more additional classes; if divergent results of the type discussed are seen, additional study is required, but increasing confidence in a given conclusion is forthcoming as the number of different NO• donor classes giving similar results is increased.

EXPLOITING THE DIAZENIUMDIOLATES' CHEMICAL VERSATILITY IN DESIGNING POTENTIAL CLINICAL ADVANCES

Cerebral Vasospasm

The diazeniumdiolates' unique chemistry has allowed development of two different approaches to treatment of cerebral vasospasm. Reasoning that the potent vasodilatory properties of NO• should reverse the spasm, Pluta and colleagues infused DEA/NO into the carotid arteries of monkeys whose middle cerebral arteries were undergoing spasm *(35)*. By generating NO• as the compound passed the affected area, the vessel was successfully reopened. Unfortunately, however, the 2-min half-life of the drug allowed it to survive until reaching the systemic circulation, thereby lowering mean arterial pressure. To avoid this unwanted hemodynamic perturbation, the authors needed only to change to a shorter-lived diazeniumdiolate. By infusing PROLI/NO (Fig. 3) instead of DEA/NO under otherwise iden-tical conditions, the former drug's 2-s half-life reversed the vasospasm without observable systemic effects *(35)*.

In a very different approach to solving the same problem, Wolf and colleagues adminis-tered the 20-h half-life compound DETA/NO intrathecally to dogs at risk of developing spasms in their basilar arteries. By thus creating a reservoir of continuous NO˙ generation in the cisterna magna, dose-dependent reversal of vasospasm was achieved. No toxicity or other adverse physiological effects were observed *(36)*.

Selectively Dilating the Pulmonary Vasculature

Several groups have sought to build on the clinical utility of NO˙ inhalation therapy by administering nitrovasodilators as aerosols. The hypothesis has been that inhalation of par-ticles or solutions of longlasting NO˙ donor compounds would permit replacement of con-tinuous inhalation of NO˙ gas by intermittent dosage via inhaler.

This strategy was successfully applied in reducing pulmonary hypertension in monocro-taline-treated rats. Dosage with nebulized DETA/NO once each day for four consecutive days produced a lasting reduction of pulmonary vascular resistance without observable sys-temic hemodynamic effects *(37)*.

Interestingly, profound systemic hypotension was seen in sheep inhaling aerosols of the DETA/NO analog DEA/NO, which proved to be even less lung-selective than nitroprusside *(38)*. Brilli and coworkers *(39)* have shed light on the likely origins of the difference in selectivity between these two diazeniumdiolates by comparing analogs ethylputreanine/NO (EP/NO) and (2-dimethylamino)-ethylputreanine/NO (DMAEP/NO) (Fig. 3) with nitroprus-side in their ability to reduce U46619-induced pulmonary hypertension in pigs. DMAEP/NO was more effective at selectively reducing pulmonary vascular resistance relative to systemic vascular resistance than EP/NO after administration as an aerosol. Because the major struc-tural difference between these two diazeniumdiolates is the presence of a second ioniz-able amino group in DMAEP/NO that at physiological pH would make the overall molecule cationic, the authors attributed its lung selectivity to this structural feature *(39)*. It is notewor-thy that a similar relationship holds between DETA/NO and DEA/NO. The former is cationic and lung-selective *(37)*, whereas the latter is an obligatory anion at physiological pH and produces systemic consequences *(38)*. These mechanistic correlations should provide useful structure–activity insights as pharmacologists attempt to design improved NO˙ donors for treatment of pulmonary hypertension.

Inducing Penile Erection
by Regulating Cavernosal Blood Flow

Since the discovery that NO˙ is a prime mediator of relaxation in the corpus cavernosum that allows blood to flow into the penis, engorging it and producing an erection, considerable work has been done on the physiology of the erectile response. Some of that work has focused on the use of NO˙ donor drugs as potential treatments for impotence. Nitroglycerin and SNP, both of which are already approved for human use in other connections, have been the primary agents used until now, but both have produced undesirable systemic effects even when applied locally to the penis. This has not been the case in experiments with diazenium-diolates having solution half-lives of up to 15 min, however. Several such compounds have proven active at inducing erections in cats without perturbing systemic hemodynamics. More-over, they have been effective whether administered by intracorporal or intracavernosal injection. Interestingly, even PROLI/NO produced a lasting erection despite its 2-s half-life, suggesting that NO˙'s role is to initiate a chain of events that are in turn more important deter-minants of duration of action. These findings too could aid in design of improved clinical agents *(40)*.

Reducing the Risk of Thrombosis, Intimal Hyperplasia, Stenosis, and Restenosis Following Vascular Surgery

THROMBOSIS ACCOMPANYING VASCULAR GRAFT PLACEMENT

The demonstrated efficacy of diazeniumdiolates as agents for inhibiting platelet adhesion in vivo led to the hypothesis that their local application at the site of vascular graft placement would reduce the risk of thrombosis even in the absence of systemic anticoagulant administration. Initial experiments designed to test this possibility centered on infusion of diazeniumdiolate solutions through the walls of a specially designed polyester graft inserted into a plastic arteriovenous shunt connecting a baboon's femoral artery and vein. (Z)-1-{N-methyl-N-[6-(N-methylammoniohexyl)-amino]} diazen-1-ium-1,2-diolate (MAHMA/NO) (Fig. 3), with its 1-min half-life, inhibited platelet adhesion by 35% at an infusion rate of 1 nmol/min, but its 2-s analogue PROLI/NO was considerably more potent, producing 58% inhibition at one-fifth this molar infusion rate (17).

Although this local infusion strategy may offer some benefits for selected vascular surgery applications, a more satisfying clinical approach would involve incorporating the diazeniumdiolate into the graft itself, thereby eliminating the need for the infusion line and attendant hospitalization. This was achieved by crosslinking polyethylenimine onto commercial polytetrafluoroethylene grafts, then exposing them to NO• to introduce the diazeniumdiolate functional group. Insertion of these grafts into the baboon arteriovenous shunt system similarly led to dramatic reductions in platelet attachment over a 1-h observation period. Grafts emitting NO• at the rate of 1–2 nmol/min/mg remained patent, whereas control grafts coated with crosslinked polyethylenimine that had not been converted to its diazeniumdiolate form were essentially sealed with thrombus within an hour of graft placement (23,41). An alternate approach to diazeniumdiolating these grafts was provided by Pulfer and colleagues who embedded microspheres of the same crosslinked polyethylenimine diazeniumdiolate into the pores of the polytetrafluoroethylene fabric (42).

HEALING AFTER VASCULAR INJURY

Many vascular surgery applications, including angioplasty, stent deployment, and endarterectomy, are complicated by aberrant healing characterized by excessive proliferation and migration of VSMCs. Several groups have followed up the in vitro antiproliferative studies mentioned earlier by studying the utility of diazeniumdiolates in in vivo models of vascular injury. When PROLI/NO was administered via the boundary layer local infusion graft described in the previous section, dogs undergoing femoral artery endarterectomy immediately downstream from the polytetrafluoroethylene infusion device displayed significantly less SMC proliferation at the injury site 7 d after the surgery. PROLI/NO infused at an initial rate of 7 nmol/min reduced proliferation by 43% at the distal anastomosis and by 68% at the site of endarterectomy relative to the contralateral vessels infused with the carrier molecule proline instead of PROLI/NO. Of further note, blood flow measurements in treated versus control vessels were not significantly different, nor was any clinical side effect observed (43).

Yin and Dusting have used periadventitial application of diazeniumdiolates to achieve similar results (44). In a rabbit model of atheroma induction, these authors induced arterial lesions by placing a collar around the carotid artery; neointima formation after 14 d was reduced by 74% when the collars contained SPER/NO at an initial concentration of 1 mg/mL relative to contralateral control arteries whose collars contained the carrier molecular spermine at similar concentrations. There was no observable effect on blood pressure in these animals (44).

Chaux and colleagues observed similar results in vein grafts implanted in the arterial circulation. In experiments with hypercholesterolemic rabbits, jugular vein implants in the carotid artery were packed perivascularly with a biodegradable polymer containing SPER/

NO. Intimal thickening was reduced by more than 40% in treated grafts relative to controls at 28 d after surgery *(45)*.

Thromboresistant Blood Contact Surfaces

Availability of insoluble NO*-releasing polymers has allowed extension of these materials from the vascular graft coatings described earlier to other applications in which platelet attachment to blood contact surfaces is a problem. For example, blends of MAHMA/NO (Fig. 3) with polyurethane or polyvinyl chloride have been used to coat intravascular biosensors. These electrochemical probes are characterized by improved reliability and extended lifetime compared to controls whose surfaces emit no NO*; these findings were attributed to the marked reduction of platelet adhesion and activation seen at the surfaces, chemical events that progressively distort the analytical response *(46)*.

SUMMARY AND CONCLUSIONS

Although NO*'s electrophilicity is not among its most widely appreciated physicochemical attributes, it can nevertheless be exploited for the preparation of a wide variety of agents useful as storage and transport forms for this notoriously reactive bioregulatory species. Simply by exposing certain nucleophiles to NO* in anoxic media, a wide variety of diazeniumdiolate salts (compounds bearing an anionic [N(O)NO]⁻ function) have been prepared.

Many of these salts generate NO* spontaneously (i.e., without requiring redox activation) in physiological buffer at 37°C. Their half-lives for NO* release range from 2 s (for PROLI/NO, Fig. 3) to 20 h (for DETA/NO) among the anionic diazeniumdiolates characterized thus far. This has made them advantageous research tools, e.g., for probing the influence of exposure rate on the course of NO*-dependent physiological phenomena.

A further advantage is that these ions can be converted to prodrug forms by attaching protecting groups to their terminal oxygens. Depending on the structures of the ion and the protecting group, such derivatization can increase the half-life for NO* release from seconds or minutes to days or weeks, and can even render the diazeniumdiolate effectively stable at physiological pH. An example of such a diazeniumdiolate prodrug that circulates freely with little effect on systemic hemodynamics, but generates abundant NO* in the liver when the protecting group is efficiently cleaved by hepatic enzymes, is V-PYRRO/NO (Fig. 1).

Such organ-, cell-, or tissue-selective NO* delivery strategies represent a major focus of our current research. Diazeniumdiolated polymers that are insoluble in aqueous media can be used as thromboresistant coatings for blood contact surfaces. Local administration of fast-acting spontaneous NO* donors of the diazeniumdiolate series can be exploited to limit exposure to a particular vascular bed, such as the lung, the corpus cavernosum, or a spastic artery. Techniques employing piperazine as a linker for diazeniumdiolating proteins and other natural products (Fig. 2) should lead to means of capitalizing on the receptor-mediated interactions such biomolecules often display in targeting NO* to specific anatomic sites. Diazeniumdiolation of existing drugs may offer the advantages of a dual-function medicament in situations where concurrent generation of free NO* is of added benefit.

In sum, the exceptional chemical versatility of the diazeniumdiolates provides a unique opportunity for designing NO* delivery agents appropriate for an enormous variety of specific applications. Evidence accumulated thus far suggesting considerable clinical promise on the part of the diazeniumdiolates covers potential cardiovascular applications ranging from reversal of cerebral vasospasm, relief of pulmonary hypertension, regulation of cavernosal blood flow, and development of improved intravascular biosensors to methods for inhibiting thrombosis and hyperplasia during vascular surgery. Indeed, we believe the potential benefit of this technology is limited only by the imagination and ingenuity of the teams of chemists and clinicians who attempt to profit from it.

ACKNOWLEDGMENT

This project has been funded in part with federal funds from the National Cancer Institute under contract NO1-CO-5600.

REFERENCES

1. Marletta MA, Tayeh MA, Hevel JM. Unraveling the biological significance of nitric oxide. BioFactors 1990;2:219–225.
2. Ignarro LJ. Nitric oxide: a novel signal transduction mechanism for transcellular communication. Hypertension 1990;16:477–483.
3. Grover R, Murdoch I, Smithies M, Mitchell I, Bihari D. Nitric oxide during hand ventilation in patient with acute respiratory failure. Lancet 1992;340:1038,1039.
4. Adatia I, Thompson J, Landzberg M, Wessel DL. Inhaled nitric oxide in chronic obstructive lung disease. Lancet 1993;341:307,308.
5. Roberts JD, Polaner DM, Lang P, Zapol WM. Inhaled nitric oxide in persistent pulmonary hypertension of the newborn. Lancet 1992;340:818,819.
6. Goldman AP, Tasker RC, Haworth SG, Sigston PE, Macrae DJ. Four patterns of response to inhaled nitric oxide for persistent pulmonary hypertension of the newborn. Pediatrics 1996;98:706–713.
7. Drago RS. Reactions of nitrogen(II) oxide. In: Colburn CB, ed. Free Radicals in Inorganic Chemistry. American Chemical Society (Advances in Chemistry Series Number 36), Washington, DC, 1962, pp. 143–149.
8. Morley D, Keefer LK. Nitric oxide/nucleophile complexes: a unique class of nitric oxide-based vasodilators. J Cardiovasc Pharmacol 1993;22(Suppl 7):S3–S9.
9. Maragos CM, Morley D, Wink DA, Dunams TM, Saavedra JE, Hoffman A, et al. Complexes of 'NO with nucleophiles as agents for the controlled biological release of nitric oxide. Vasorelaxant effects. J Med Chem 1991;34:3242–3247.
10. Hope H, Sequeira MR. Angeli's salt. Crystal structure of sodium trioxodinitrate(II) monohydrate, $Na_2N_2O_3 \cdot H_2O$. Inorg Chem 1973;12:286–288.
11. Vanin AF, Vedernikov YI, Galagan ME, Kubrina LN, Kuzmanis YA, Kalvin'sh IY, et al. Angeli salt as a producer of nitrogen oxide in the animal organism. Biochemistry (Transl. Biokhimiya (Moscow)) 1990;55:1048–1052.
12. Traube W. Ueber Synthesen stickstoffhaltiger Verbindungen mit Hülfe des Stickoxyds. Liebigs Ann Chem 1898;300:81 128.
13. Danzig MJ, Martel RF, Riccitiello SR. A new reaction of oximes and nitric oxide. J Org Chem 1961;26: 3327–3331.
14. Drago RS, Paulik FE. The reaction of nitrogen(II) oxide with diethylamine. J Am Chem Soc 1960;82: 96–98.
15. Keefer LK, Nims RW, Davies KM, Wink DA. "NONOates" (1-substituted diazen-1-ium-1,2-diolates) as nitric oxide donors: convenient nitric oxide dosage forms. Methods Enzymol 1996;268:281–293.
16. Saavedra JE, Dunams TM, Flippen-Anderson JL, Keefer LK. Secondary amine/nitric oxide complex ions, $R_2N[N(O)NO]^-$. O-Functionalization chemistry. J Org Chem 1992;57:6134–6138.
17. Saavedra JE, Southan GJ, Davies KM, Lundell A, Markou C, Hanson SR, et al. Localizing antithrombotic and vasodilatory activity with a novel, ultrafast nitric oxide donor. J Med Chem 1996;39:4361–4365.
18. Drago RS, Karstetter BR. The reaction of nitrogen(II) oxide with various primary and secondary amines. J Am Chem Soc 1961;83:1819–1822.
19. Hrabie JA, Klose JR, Wink DA, Keefer LK. New nitric oxide-releasing zwitterions derived from polyamines. J Org Chem 1993;58:1472 1476.
20. Longhi R, Drago RS. Metal-containing compounds of the anion $(C_2H_5)_2NN_2O_2^-$. Inorg Chem 1963;2: 85–88.
21. Christodoulou D, George C, Keefer LK. An unusual bi-tri-binuclear sandwich complex formed in the reaction of $CuCl_2$ with the $Et_2N-N_2O_2^-$ ion. J Chem Soc, Chem Commun 1993;937–939.
22. Christodoulou D, Maragos CM, George C, Morley D, Dunams TM, Wink DA, et al. Mixed-ligand, non-nitrosyl Cu(II) complexes as potential pharmacological agents via NO release. In: Karlin KD, Tyeklár Z, eds. Bioinorganic Chemistry of Copper. Chapman & Hall, New York, 1993, pp. 427–436.
23. Smith DJ, Chakravarthy D, Pulfer S, Simmons ML, Hrabie JA, Citro ML, et al. Nitric oxide-releasing polymers containing the $[N(O)NO]^-$ group. J Med Chem 1996;39:1148–1156.
24. Reilly EL. Nitrosamine manufacture. U.S. Patent 3,153,094; 1964.

25. Makings LR, Tsien RY. Caged nitric oxide. Stable organic molecules from which nitric oxide can be photoreleased. J Biol Chem 1994;269:6282–6285.

26. Saavedra JE, Billiar TR, Williams DL, Kim Y-M, Watkins SC, Keefer LK. Targeting nitric oxide (NO) delivery *in vivo*. Design of a liver-selective NO donor prodrug that blocks tumor necrosis factor-α-induced apoptosis and toxicity in the liver. J Med Chem 1997;40:1947–1954.

27. Saavedra JE, Booth MN, Hrabie JA, Davies KM, Keefer LK. Piperazine as a linker for incorporating the nitric-oxide releasing diazeniumdiolate group into other biomedically relevant functional molecules. J Org Chem 1999;64:5124–5131.

28. Longhi R, Ragsdale RO, Drago RS. Reactions of nitrogen(II) oxide with miscellaneous Lewis bases. Inorg Chem 1962;1:768–770.

29. Diodati JG, Quyyumi AA, Keefer LK. Complexes of nitric oxide with nucleophiles as agents for the controlled biological release of nitric oxide: hemodynamic effect in the rabbit. J Cardiovasc Pharmacol 1993;22:287–292.

30. Diodati JG, Quyyumi AA, Hussain N, Keefer LK. Complexes of nitric oxide with nucleophiles as agents for the controlled biological release of nitric oxide: antiplatelet effect. Thromb Haemost 1993;70:654–658.

31. Mooradian DL, Hutsell TC, Keefer LK. Nitric oxide (NO) donor molecules: effect of NO release rate on vascular smooth muscle cell proliferation in vitro. J Cardiovasc Pharmacol 1995;25:674–678.

32. Hogg N, Struck A, Goss SPA, Santanam N, Joseph J, Parthasarathy S, et al. Inhibition of macrophage-dependent low density lipoprotein oxidation by nitric oxide donors. J Lipid Res 1995;36:1756–1762.

33. Bates JN, Baker MT, Guerra R Jr, Harrison DG. Nitric oxide generation from nitroprusside by vascular tissue. Evidence that reduction of the nitroprusside anion and cyanide loss are required. Biochem Pharmacol 1991;42:S157–S165.

34. Wink DA, Cook JA, Pacelli R, DeGraff W, Gamson J, Liebmann J, et al. The effect of various nitric oxide-donor agents on hydrogen peroxide-mediated toxicity: a direct correlation between nitric oxide formation and protection. Arch Biochem Biophys 1996;331:241–248.

35. Pluta RM, Oldfield EH, Boock RJ. Reversal and prevention of cerebral vasospasm by intracarotid infusions of nitric oxide donors in a primate model of subarachnoid hemorrhage. J Neurosurg 1997;87:746–751.

36. Wolf EW, Banerjee A, Soble-Smith J, Dohan FC Jr, White RP, Robertson JT. Reversal of cerebral vasospasm using an intrathecally administered nitric oxide donor. J Neurosurg 1998;89:279–288.

37. Hampl V, Tristani-Firouzi M, Hutsell TC, Archer SL. Nebulized nitric oxide/nucleophile adduct reduces chronic pulmonary hypertension. Cardiovasc Res 1996;31:55–62.

38. Adrie C, Ichinose F, Holzmann A, Keefer L, Hurford WE, Zapol WM. Pulmonary vasodilation by nitric oxide gas and prodrug aerosols in acute pulmonary hypertension. J Appl Physiol 1998;84:435–441.

39. Brilli RJ, Krafte-Jacobs B, Smith DJ, Roselle D, Passerini D, Vromen A, et al. Intratracheal instillation of a novel NO/nucleophile adduct selectively reduces pulmonary hypertension. J Appl Physiol 1997;83:1968–1975.

40. Hellstrom WJG, Wang R, Champion HC, Sikka SC, Keefer LK, Doherty P. Penile erection induced by transurethral administration of novel nitric oxide donors. J Androl 1997;18(Suppl):P-33 (abstr. 36).

41. Hanson SR, Hutsell TC, Keefer LK, Mooradian DL, Smith DJ. Nitric oxide donors: a continuing opportunity in drug design. Adv Pharmacol 1995;34:383–398.

42. Pulfer SK, Ott D, Smith DJ. Incorporation of nitric oxide-releasing crosslinked polyethyleneimine microspheres into vascular grafts. J Biomed Mater Res 1997;37:182–189.

43. Chen C, Hanson SR, Keefer LK, Saavedra JE, Davies KM, Hutsell TC, et al. Boundary layer infusion of nitric oxide reduces early smooth muscle cell proliferation in the endarterectomized canine artery. J Surg Res 1997;67:26–32.

44. Yin Z. L, Dusting GJ. A nitric oxide donor (spermine-NONOate) prevents the formation of neointima in rabbit carotid artery. Clin Exp Pharmacol Physiol 1997;24:436–438.

45. Chaux A, Ruan XM, Fishbein MC, Ouyang Y, Kaul S, Pass JA, et al. Perivascular delivery of a nitric oxide donor inhibits neointimal hyperplasia in vein grafts implanted in the arterial circulation. J Thorac Cardiovasc Surg 1998;115:604–614.

46. Espadas-Torre C, Oklejas V, Mowery K, Meyerhoff ME. Thromboresistant chemical sensors using combined nitric oxide release/ion sensing polymeric films. J Am Chem Soc 1997;119:2321,2322.

25 Inhaled Nitric Oxide Therapy for Acute Respiratory Failure

William E. Hurford and Warren M. Zapol

INHALED NO•—HYPOTHESES

Inhaled NO• is a Selective Pulmonary Vasodilator

Pulmonary hypertension and severe hypoxemia complicate the care of patients with such diseases as acute respiratory distress syndrome (ARDS). Numerous vasodilator therapies aimed at reducing pulmonary hypertension have been tested in these patients. All of the currently available intravenous vasodilators produce systemic vasodilation and hypotension at dosages sufficient to reduce the pulmonary artery pressure. In addition, intravenous infusions of systemic vasodilators, such as nitroprusside or prostacyclin (PGI_2), diffusely reverse hypoxic pulmonary vasoconstriction, creating ventilation-perfusion ($\dot{V}/\dot{Q}$) mismatch and markedly increasing venous admixture (1).

Inhaled NO• selectively vasodilates the pulmonary circulation (2,3). The use of this novel therapy as an adjunct in the treatment of ARDS has attracted immense interest. When administered by inhalation, NO• diffuses into the pulmonary vasculature of ventilated lung regions and reduces the pulmonary vasoconstrictor response to a variety of stimuli, including hypoxia (2,3). Administering NO• by inhalation distributes the gas predominantly to well-ventilated alveoli and not to collapsed or fluid-filled areas of the lung. In the presence of an increased vasomotor tone, selective vasodilation of well-ventilated lung regions diverts pulmonary artery blood flow toward these well-ventilated alveoli and often improves the matching of ventilation to perfusion (4). As a consequence, arterial oxygenation may improve dramatically when NO• is administered to patients with acute respiratory failure.

It remains unclear whether inhaled NO• has widespread clinical utility and safety in addition to its useful properties as a selective pulmonary vasodilator. Laboratory studies suggest that inhaled NO• has important effects in reducing some forms of lung and tissue injury. These effects include the ability to scavenge oxygen free radicals (5–9), reduce oxygen toxicity (10–12), inhibit platelet and leukocyte aggregation (13–15), and increase the oxygen affinity of sickle erythrocytes (16). If these effects are proven to be clinically significant and safe, early and continued therapy with inhaled NO• could potentially reduce the severity of some forms of lung injury.

EVALUATION OF INHALED NO• IN LABORATORY MODELS

Endotoxin Administration

The effects of inhaled NO• on endotoxin-induced pulmonary hypertension are complex. In a study by Weitzberg and colleagues, inhaled NO• at a concentration of 10 parts per million

From: *Contemporary Cardiology, vol. 4: Nitric Oxide and the Cardiovascular System*
Edited by: J. Loscalzo and J. A. Vita © Humana Press Inc., Totowa, NJ

(ppm) selectively decreased the acute pulmonary hypertension occurring at least 30 min after the intravenous administration of *Escherichia coli* endotoxin in anesthetized pigs *(17)*. Arterial oxygenation and pH were also improved during NO• inhalation. The early increase of pulmonary artery pressure (within 30 min after endotoxin administration) was unaffected by 10 ppm of inhaled NO•.

Ogura and coworkers reported that NO• inhalation 40 ppm decreased the late-phase pulmonary hypertension following the infusion of *E. coli* endotoxin in anesthetized swine *(18)*. NO• inhalation improved arterial oxygenation by redistributing blood flow from true shunt to ventilated lung regions as measured by the multiple inert gas elimination technique. The accumulation of pulmonary edema, as assessed by the blood-free wet-to-dry lung weight ratio, was decreased in animals breathing 40 ppm NO•. Dahm and coworkers similarly reported selective pulmonary vasodilation following NO• inhalation in an anesthetized swine endotoxemia model *(19)*.

Oleic Acid-Induced Lung Injury

A common animal model of ARDS is produced by intravenous injection of oleic acid. An injection of this 18-carbon unsaturated fatty acid produces a syndrome of acute endothelial and alveolar epithelial cell necrosis, resulting in proteinaceous alveolar edema that mimics the acute phase of ARDS. In a dog model of acute lung injury induced by oleic acid injections, Putensen and coworkers examined the role of NO• by giving inhaled NO• and/or intravenous N^G-monomethyl-L-arginine (L-NMMA), a nitric oxide synthase (NOS) inhibitor *(20)*. After the induction of lung injury, inhaled NO• at 40 ppm improved gas exchange by redistributing blood flow from shunting regions to lung units with a nearly ideal $\dot{V}/\dot{Q}$ ratio. The improvement of $\dot{V}/\dot{Q}$ matching and gas exchange was most pronounced when NO• was inhaled in the presence of a systemic infusion of L-NMMA. Systemic L-NMMA administration alone increased pulmonary and systemic vascular resistance, but did not affect $\dot{V}/\dot{Q}$ mismatching or gas exchange. Inhaled NO• reversed the pulmonary but not the systemic vasoconstriction caused by L-NMMA. This effect may be clinically important because the infusion of NOS inhibitors is being tested as a treatment for sepsis-induced hypotension *(21,22)*.

The effect of inhaled NO• on pulmonary vascular resistance (PVR) in a canine ARDS model was reported by Romand and coworkers *(22)*. NO• inhalation (up to 145 ppm) reduced hypoxic pulmonary vasoconstriction, but not the mild pulmonary hypertension (mean pulmonary artery pressure 23 mmHg) induced by oleic acid infusion. In a pig model of acute lung injury induced by oleic acid injection, Shah and colleagues *(23)* reported that inhaled NO• (10–80 ppm) reduced mean pulmonary artery pressure and shunt fraction in a concentration-dependent manner. Because almost the same dose of oleic acid (0.08–0.1 mL/kg) was used to induce acute lung injury in these studies, these varying results are most likely due to differences between the experimental species.

The degree of lung inflation may be an important determinant of the effects of inhaled NO•. Putensen and colleagues reported that the recruitment of lung units by the application of 10 cm H_2O continuous positive airway pressure (CPAP) augmented the improvement of oxygenation caused by inhaling 40 ppm NO• in anesthetized dogs with oleic acid-induced lung injury *(24)*. Application of CPAP converted shunting regions (shunt = $48 \pm 7\%$ (SD) of cardiac output) to regions with a more normal ratio $\dot{V}/\dot{Q}$. Inhaled NO• also selectively reduced the pulmonary artery pressure in this study, but the extent of pulmonary vasodilation was independent of the CPAP level.

Inhaled NO• mediates pulmonary vasodilation during lung injury by activating guanylyl cyclase (GC) and increasing cyclic guanosine-3',5'-monophosphate (cGMP) levels within pulmonary vascular smooth muscle. This increase is reflected by increased plasma cGMP concentrations. Rovira and coworkers studied a model of acute lung injury induced by bilateral lung lavage in anesthetized lambs *(25)*. When endogenous NO· production was inhibited by infusing N^G-nitro-L-arginine methyl ester (L-NAME), a consistent increase of aortic, as compared with pulmonary arterial plasma, cGMP concentration could be measured within 5 min of breathing 60 ppm NO·. Increased aortic plasma cGMP levels were associated with selective pulmonary vasodilation, reduced venous admixture, and an increased PaO_2. Levels of plasma cGMP returned to baseline within 10 min of discontinuing NO· breathing.

Inhalation Injury

The effect of inhaled NO· on lung injury caused by smoke inhalation has been studied in sheep *(26)*. Compared with air breathing controls, pulmonary artery hypertension was reduced and oxygenation was improved in sheep breathing 20 ppm NO· in the air for 48 h. There was no significant difference of lung wet-to-dry weight ratio, compliance, or histologic changes between the two groups. NO· inhalation neither improved nor worsened the tracheobronchial or alveolar pathologic changes occurring after inhalation injury.

Oxidant-Induced Acute Lung Injury

Oxygen-derived free radicals are important in the pathogenesis of ARDS and may contribute to leukocyte adherence and emigration and subsequent endothelial cell injury *(27)*. Depending on the species or model used, endogenous NO· appears to enhance *(28–31)* or attenuate *(32–34)* the acute inflammatory response.

Other Effects

NO· combines with reactive oxygen species to produce intermediates, such as the peroxynitrite anion, which can exacerbate cellular injury. Nozik and coworkers, e.g., reported that the administration of 1 mM L-arginine to isolated buffer-perfused rabbit lungs produced significant pulmonary hypertension and edema when the lungs were ventilated with 95% oxygen or in the presence of a H_2O_2 generating system *(35)*. This injury was attenuated by the administration of L-NAME or by pretreatment with catalase. The authors postulated that the administration of L-arginine increased the synthesis of NO· within the lungs, and that NO· reacted with H_2O_2 to cause lung injury via the syntheses of reactive intermediates.

NO· may also act as a superoxide scavenger. In the isolated buffer-perfused rabbit lung, Kavanagh and coworkers investigated the effects of inhaled NO· and endogenous NOS inhibition on oxidant-induced acute lung injury *(6)*. Superoxide radicals were produced by the combination of purine and xanthine oxidase. Pretreatment with inhaled NO· (90–120 ppm) prevented the increase of pulmonary artery pressure and capillary permeability as measured by the pulmonary capillary filtration coefficient. Inhibition of endogenous NOS by the infusion of L-NAME increased pulmonary vascular tone without affecting capillary permeability. In addition, Guidot and coworkers reported that inhaled NO· prevented neutrophil-mediated pulmonary edema in isolated rat lungs and speculated that NO· may have anti-inflammatory properties *(36)*. Although the mechanism by which inhaled NO· protected against lung injury is unclear, it may involve alterations in cellular cGMP levels and cytoskeletal changes.

Inhibition of cGMP-Specific Phosphodiesterases

The selectivity of inhaled NO· is primarily due to the inactivation of NO· by its rapid combination with hemoglobin within the pulmonary circulation *(37)*. Conceivably, pharmacological agents that potentiate and/or prolong the pulmonary vasodilator effects of inhaled NO· could reduce the effective dose of NO·, permit intermittent inhalation, and reduce the toxicity of prolonged exposures.

Zaprinast (M&B 22948; 2-o-propoxyphenyl-8-azapurin-6-one, Rhône-Poulenc Rorer, Dagenham, Essex, UK) is a type 5 phosphodiesterase (PDE) inhibitor that selectively inhibits the hydrolysis of cGMP with minimal effects on the breakdown of adenosine 3',5'-cyclic monophosphate (cAMP) *(38)*. Vasodilator responses to infusions of endothelium-dependent vasodilators and nitrosovasodilators are modified by zaprinast in newborn lambs *(39)* and in the isolated cat lobar artery *(40)*. Ichinose and coworkers investigated the effects of intravenously administered zaprinast on the pulmonary vasodilating effects of inhaled NO˙ in awake spontaneously breathing lambs with pharmacologically induced pulmonary hypertension *(41)*. The reduction of pulmonary vascular resistance was significantly greater during the zaprinast infusion. The duration of the vasodilator response to inhaled NO˙ was also markedly increased by the zaprinast infusion. Ichinose reported similar results in lambs with the inhalation of zaprinast and NO˙ *(42)*. Similar results have been reported in the ovine transitional circulation by Ziegler and coworkers *(43)*. Pilot studies in pediatric patients with pulmonary hypertension further suggest that phosphodiesterase inhibition with dipyridamole may augment the response to inhaled NO˙ and reduce the rebound pulmonary hypertension that sometimes accompanies with acute withdrawal of inhaled NO˙ therapy *(44)*. Additional preliminary studies in patients with pulmonary hypertension following mitral or aortic valve replacement suggest that the intravenous administration of dipyridamole (0.2 mg/kg) can augment the pulmonary vascular response to inhaled NO˙ *(45)*.

Combination of Inhaled NO˙ Therapy with Partial Liquid Ventilation

Perfluorocarbons (PFC) are inert liquids that have the ability to lower surface tension in surfactant-depleted lungs without being absorbed by the respiratory epithelium and can efficiently transport respiratory gases. Zobel and colleagues *(46)* demonstrated in piglets with acute lung injury induced by bilateral lung lavage that inhaled NO˙ (1–20 ppm) enhanced pulmonary gas exchange during partial liquid ventilation with perfluorocarbon. An additive effect of inhaled NO˙ and partial liquid ventilation on pulmonary gas exchange in an acute lung injury model has been confirmed by others *(47)*.

NO˙ in Poorly Ventilated Lung Regions

Hopkins and colleagues *(48)* studied the effects of NO˙ on gas exchange by selectively creating areas of shunt or areas of low $\dot{V}/\dot{Q}$ ratios. Inhaled NO˙ (80 ppm) reduced blood flow to shunting areas. In the areas with $\dot{V}/\dot{Q}$ inequality, NO˙ caused an inconsistent response. When the pulmonary vascular resistance of partially obstructed areas was decreased by NO˙ inhalation, $\dot{V}/\dot{Q}$ inequality increased, as the blood flow to a relative poorly ventilated area was increased by vasodilation. When NO˙ did not reach the lung distal to the partial obstruction, and thus did not alter local vascular resistance, $\dot{V}/\dot{Q}$ matching was improved. These results indicate that the effects of NO˙ on $\dot{V}/\dot{Q}$ mismatching are dependent on the distribution of NO˙ within lung regions. NO˙ can improve arterial oxygenation when it is administered to well-ventilated lung regions that are vasoconstricted. NO˙ can worsen oxygenation if it reaches and augments perfusion to poorly ventilated lung regions.

ADULT RESPIRATORY DISTRESS SYNDROME

Pathophysiology

Acute pulmonary hypertension consistently occurs in severe ARDS. The increased pulmonary artery pressure is independent of changes in cardiac output and persists after the correction of systemic hypoxemia *(49)*. The pulmonary vascular changes in ARDS are produced by a complex combination of direct lung injury (i.e., aspiration, trauma, infection), the consequences of the response to systemic inflammation (e.g., hypoxia, acidosis, release of cytokines and components of the complement system and the arachidonic acid pathway, as well as inhibitors of fibrinolysis), and the iatrogenic complications of intensive care therapy (e.g., oxygen toxicity and barotrauma). In severe ARDS, thromboembolic occlusion of the pulmonary vasculature is common (50).

Initial Clinical Studies

Rossaint and coworkers compared the effects of NO• inhalation (18 and 36 ppm) to intravenously infused prostacyclin in nine patients with ARDS (51). NO• selectively reduced mean pulmonary artery pressure (Fig. 1). Oxygenation improved due to decreased venous admixture (Q_{VA}/Q_t). Although an intravenous infusion of prostacyclin also reduced pulmonary artery pressure, the mean systemic arterial pressure and PaO$_2$ were decreased as the Q_{VA}/Q_t ratio increased. Multiple clinical studies have confirmed these findings (52–55).

Inhaling low concentrations of NO• effectively reduces pulmonary artery pressure and improves systemic oxygenation in many patients with ARDS. Inhaled NO• concentrations of <2 ppm have been reported to be effective (Fig. 2) (51,56–60). Even the low levels of NO• contaminating hospital air supplies (2–550 parts per billion [ppb]) have been reported to increase arterial oxygenation in patients receiving mechanical ventilation (61). Right ventricular ejection fraction may increase in some patients responding to inhaled NO•, suggesting that the observed decreases of pulmonary artery pressure may be hemodynamically important (62,63).

Although unproven, it is reasonable to speculate that decreasing pulmonary capillary pressure by breathing NO• may reduce the severity of lung injury in patients with ARDS. Benzing and coworkers (64) reported that breathing 40 ppm NO• decreased pulmonary capillary pressure and the pulmonary transvascular flux of albumin (an index of fluid efflux into the pulmonary interstitium). Similarly, Rossetti and coworkers, studying seven patients with ARDS who inhaled 15 and 25 ppm NO•, reported a reduction of pulmonary capillary pressure during NO• breathing. The reduction was primarily the result of a reduction in the resistance of pulmonary capillary and venous vessels (65). It is unclear if such changes are clinically significant or persist during long-term NO• therapy in unselected groups of patients with ARDS (66,67).

If inhaled NO• can improve the matching of ventilation to perfusion, it would be expected that V_D/V_T and PaCO$_2$ might decrease during NO• inhalation. Although most studies have reported no change of PaCO$_2$ during NO• inhalation, several studies have shown small but statistically significant decreases of V_D/V_T and PaCO$_2$ (58,62). These changes were too small to produce clinical important changes or permit minute ventilation to be reduced.

Variability of Response

Some patients do not respond to NO• inhalation with pulmonary vasodilation and improved oxygenation. In studies of critically ill patients with ARDS who were ventilated with inhaled NO• (<40 ppm), approx 35% of patients had minimal or no response to inhaled NO• (54,68–70). In addition, there is considerable interindividual and intraindividual variability to the response (71,72). Several hypotheses have been proposed to explain the mechanisms of nonresponsiveness. Manktelow and coworkers (54) and Krafft and colleagues (73) reported that ARDS patients without sepsis were more likely to respond to inhaled NO• than patients with septic shock. Holzmann and coworkers (74) tested the effects of sepsis on NO• hyporesponsiveness in an isolated lung model. They reported that hyporesponsivess was associated with decreased cGMP release, suggesting that the NO•–cGMP signal transduction pathway is downregulated in sepsis. This was attributable to increased PDE activity and, therefore, increased cGMP breakdown within the pulmonary vasculature. Inhibition of PDE activity with dipyridamole has been reported to augment the NO•-induced reduction of pulmonary vascular resistance (PVR) in pediatric patients with pulmonary hypertension (44) and in adult patients immediately following aortic or mitral valve replacement (45).

Other factors are undoubtedly important in determining responsiveness. In general, the baseline level of PVR appears to predict the magnitude of pulmonary vasoconstriction reversible

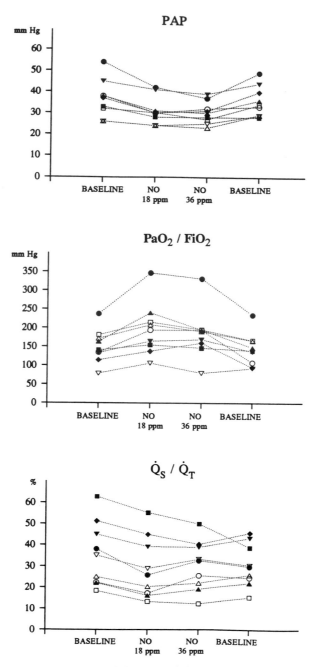

Fig. 1. Mean pulmonary artery pressure (PAP), arterial oxygenation efficiency (PaO$_2$/FiO$_2$), and venous admixture ($\dot{Q}_s/\dot{Q}_T$) during inhalation of 18 and 36 ppm NO$^\bullet$ in nine patients with ARDS. Solid symbols represent patients treated with extracorporeal membrane oxygenation (ECMO). Reproduced with permission from Roissaint et al. *(51)*.

by NO$^\bullet$ inhalation. Those with the greatest degree of pulmonary hypertension appear to respond best to NO$^\bullet$ inhalation (Fig. 3) *(59,60,68,75)*. The concomitant intravenous infusion of a novel vasoconstricting drug, almitrine, which increases the degree of hypoxic vasoconstriction in the lung, has been reported to enhance the beneficial effect of inhaled NO$^\bullet$ on PaO$_2$ *(76,77)*. The infusion of other vasoconstrictors, such as phenylephrine *(78)* and norepinephrine *(79)*, also augments the improvement of arterial oxygenation observed during NO$^\bullet$ therapy.

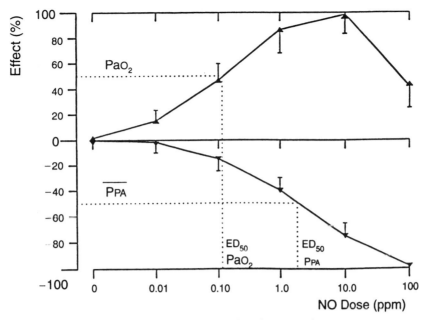

Fig. 2. Dose response of inhaled NO˙ for PaO_2 (upper) and mean pulmonary artery pressure (P_{PA}, lower). Values are means ± standard deviation of 12 patients with ARDS, expressed as percentage of maximal change. The estimated ED_{50} of NO˙ for the PaO_2 increase and for the pulmonary artery decrease are indicated above the x-axis. Reproduced with permission from Gerlach et al. (56).

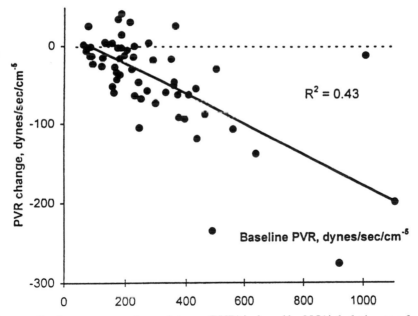

Fig. 3. Change of pulmonary vascular resistance (PVR) induced by NO˙ inhalation as a function of baseline PVR in patients with ARDS. The magnitude of the PVR decrease during NO˙ inhalation correlated with the patients' baseline PVR. Reproduced with permission from Bigatello et al. (68).

Combinations of various therapies with inhaled NO˙, such as the use of almitrine, as detailed earlier, and prone positioning that are aimed at improving the matching of pulmonary perfusion to ventilation may produce additive effects with NO˙ (80–82). The degree of response appears to depend on the stage of lung maturity (83), the extent of recruited (open) alveoli, and the pattern of mechanical ventilation (24.59,84).

Rebound Pulmonary Hypertension

In some cases, rapid withdrawal of inhaled NO$^\bullet$ therapy has been associated with the sudden worsening of hypoxemia and pulmonary hypertension *(56,68,85)*. This deterioration appears to be transient, but the hemodynamic consequences of this "rebound" may be catastrophic. The severity of the rebound may be minimized by transiently increasing the FiO$_2$, administering intravenous vasoactive agents as necessary, and avoiding sudden discontinuation of NO$^\bullet$ inhalation in patients with hemodynamic instability or severe hypoxemia. The mechanism for this acute pulmonary vasoconstriction is unknown and its occurrence in patients is unpredictable. It may be the result of reduced production of endogenous NO$^\bullet$ caused by inhaling high levels of exogenous NO$^\bullet$, a phenomenon known as product inhibition *(86–88)*. It could also be caused by enhanced release of vasoconstrictor substances by the pulmonary circulation or enhanced PDE activity. An infusion of the PDE inhibitor, dipyridamole, has been reported to attenuate the degree of rebound pulmonary hypertension observed after the withdrawal of inhaled NO$^\bullet$ from pediatric patients with pulmonary hypertension *(89)*.

Randomized Trials

Several randomized, double-blind studies of the efficacy of NO$^\bullet$ inhalation in patients with ARDS are currently underway. In a multicenter phase 2 trial, Dellinger and colleagues reported the effects of inhaled NO$^\bullet$ (0, 1.25, 5, 20, and 40 ppm) on 177 patients with nonseptic ARDS *(69)*. Sixty percent of patients receiving inhaled NO$^\bullet$ had at least a 20% improvement of PaO$_2$ after 4 h of treatment as compared to 24% of patients receiving placebo. The 28-d mortality rate of all patients was 30% and was unaffected by NO$^\bullet$ therapy. Subgroups receiving the same dose of NO$^\bullet$ for the treatment period consisted of 8–34 patients. This severely limited the power of the study. The mortality rates in the subgroups were not statistically different: 32% (7/22 patients) in the 1.25 ppm group, 24% (8/24 patients) in the 5 ppm group, 31% (9/29) in the 20 ppm group, 30% (8/27 patients) in the 40 ppm group, and 38% in the 80 ppm group. The ARDS patients who received 5 ppm NO$^\bullet$ appeared to have a more rapid resolution of their respiratory failure (Fig. 4). A randomized study reported by Troncy and associates *(67)* similarly found no significant difference between ARDS patients receiving inhaled NO$^\bullet$ and controls with regard to 30 d mortality or days of mechanical ventilation, but the small sample size (15 patients in each group) severely limited the power of the study to detect significant differences. A larger randomized, double-blind, multicenter phase 3 study investigating the long-term effects of 5 ppm inhaled NO$^\bullet$ on ARDS is currently in progress.

A European phase 3 trial studied 260 medical and surgical patients with acute lung injury *(70)*. A positive response was defined as an increase of PaO$_2$ > 25%. Sixty-six percent of the patients were responders, and the treatment was continued at the lowest effective dose of inhaled NO$^\bullet$ or placebo by random allocation for up to 30 d. A mortality rate of 45% in patients receiving inhaled NO$^\bullet$ treatment, 38% in placebo patients, and 45% in nonresponders was reported in an abstract presentation *(70)*. Complete results have not yet been published.

Effect of Inhaled NO$^\bullet$ on Outcome

Why have the currently published randomized studies failed to demonstrate a beneficial effect on inhaled NO$^\bullet$ on clinical outcome? Decreased pulmonary capillary pressure should decrease the extent of pulmonary edema, should improve lung compliance, and might improve resolution of lung injury. Improved oxygenation should permit a reduction of FIO$_2$ and airway pressure. If high airway pressures were being used, lower airway pressures could reduce barotrauma.

Proving such hypotheses is difficult. The pulmonary artery pressure is usually only moderately elevated in ARDS *(49)*. This degree of pulmonary hypertension is usually well tolerated, and few patients with ARDS die of acute pulmonary hypertension.

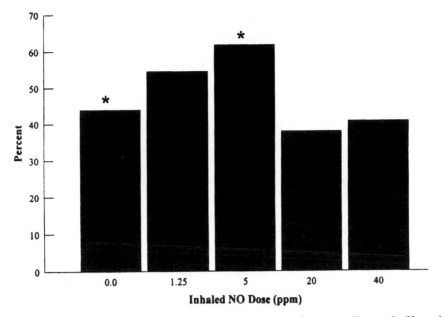

Fig. 4. Percentage of patients with ARDS in each dose group who were alive and off mechanical ventilation at d 28 following randomization to 0, 1.25, 5, 20, or 40 ppm NO• breathing. * = $P < 0.05$ for the difference between the 0-and 5-ppm groups. Reproduced with permission from Dellinger et al. *(69)*.

A worsened outcome might occur if NO•-induced improvements in oxygenation are offset by prematurely reducing the level of positive end-expiratory pressure (PEEP). Such reductions in PEEP can result in alveolar derecruitment and perhaps increased shear stress and barotrauma during mechanical ventilation *(90,91)*. Such premature derecruitment could explain the transitory nature of the improvement in PaO_2/FiO_2 noted in several prospective studies *(66,67,69)*.

Improvements in oxygenation alone may not be sufficient to alter the clinical outcome of a population of ARDS patients. The survival rate of patients with ARDS appears to depend more on the occurrence of sepsis and multiple organ failure than on gas exchange. The majority of ARDS patients die from severe sepsis or multiple organ failure rather than refractory hypoxemia *(92.93)*. It is unknown if patients with severe life-threatening hypoxemia would benefit from inhaled NO• because such patients have been excluded from prospective studies.

The effect of inhaled NO• varies among patients. Approximately 30–40% of patients fail to demonstrate a significant improvement in oxygenation or reductions of pulmonary artery pressure *(54,69)*. Nevertheless, such patients must be included in studies that place subjects in the experimental or placebo group on an "intention to treat" basis. In addition, protocols may select a single fixed dose to administer. Such designs assume that the dose–response relationship of inhaled NO• is similar among ARDS patients and over time. This may not be true *(94)*.

The beneficial effects of NO• inhalation may be offset by its toxic effects. Doses as high as 80 ppm have been evaluated in both pediatric and adult studies. In recent experimental studies of ischemia–reperfusion injury during lung transplantation, low doses of inhaled NO• were protective, but high doses were not *(95)*. Before such studies, it was not well appreciated that the beneficial effects of inhaled NO• could be lost at higher doses. The dose for NO• inhalation may therefore have a narrow therapeutic range. Small doses, e.g., 1–5 ppm, could be effective and improve survival; very low doses might be not effective; and larger doses could be toxic.

Finally, the patients included in studies of ARDS rarely have a single disease of uniform severity. This might increase the heterogeneity of response or benefit to NO•. The response to inhaled NO˙ may be confounded by many factors including sepsis, excessive endogenous NO˙ production, or a lack of endogenous production.

NEONATAL RESPIRATORY FAPILURE

Pathophysiology

At birth, there is a sustained decrease of PVR and an increase of pulmonary blood flow. If this does not occur, persistent pulmonary hypertension of the newborn (PPHN) may result. PPHN is characterized by an increased PVR and severe hypoxemia that is unresponsive to oxygen therapy. Extracorporeal membrane oxygenation (ECMO) is often used to support these infants; however, the anticoagulation and cannulation of large vessels required for ECMO are often associated with complications. It has been hypothesized that the endogenous pulmonary vascular production of NO˙ may be decreased and endothelin-1 production increased in PPHN *(96)*. Therefore, inhaled NO˙ might provide an effective therapy for these critically hypoxemic babies *(97,98)*.

Laboratory Studies

Laboratory studies have documented that inhaled NO˙ is an effective pulmonary vasodilator of the neonatal pulmonary circulation *(99–106)*. Zayek and coworkers studied the effects of inhaled NO˙ (6–100 ppm) in a model of PPHN created by prenatal ligation of the ductus arteriosus in lambs *(107)*. Inhaled NO˙ caused dose-dependent decreases of pulmonary artery pressure and PVR. NO˙ inhalation decreased right-to-left shunting of blood through the foramen ovale and increased PaO_2 and arterial oxygen saturation, whereas $PaCO_2$ was decreased. Systemic blood pressure was unaffected by breathing NO˙ *(107)*. Using this model, Zayek and coworkers subsequently documented an increased survival rate with NO˙ therapy *(108)*. Inhalation of NO˙ can also attenuate hypoxic pulmonary vascular remodeling of the pulmonary circulation *(109,110)*. Conceivably, inhaled NO˙ therapy might be used to limit the acute pulmonary vascular remodeling that accompanies neonatal pulmonary hypertension.

Clinical Studies

Several large randomized multicenter trials studying the effects of inhaled NO˙ in near-term and term newborn patients have been published *(111–116)*. In the majority of PPHN patients, NO˙ had beneficial effects on pulmonary hypertension and oxygenation and reduced the requirement for ECMO. Doses in excess of 30 ppm were rarely required in order to produce a maximal response *(115,117)*. The clinical response appeared most dramatic in those patients with the most severe hypoxemia *(118)*. In a follow-up of children who received inhaled NO˙ therapy for PPHN as a newborn, neurodevelopment, incidence of airway disease, and need for supplemental oxygen were comparable in both conventionally and ECMO-treated patients *(119,120)*. The mortality rate was quite low at 10–15% in these small series and clinical trials and appeared unaffected. In a retrospective cohort study of newborns with PPHN, inhaled NO˙ improved systemic oxygenation, reduced the necessity for ECMO, and decreased the incidence of subsequent chronic lung disease and intracranial hemorrhage *(121)*.

PRETERM NEONATES WITH RESPIRATORY DISTRESS SYNDROME

Respiratory distress syndrome (RDS), or hyaline membrane disease of the premature newborn, is characterized by surfactant deficiency or dysfunction, and in many cases, by pulmonary hypertension. Several clinical studies of inhaled NO˙ in premature newborns with RDS have been reported *(122–125)*. In general, oxygenation was improved by NO˙ breathing. Overall mortality has been unaffected. About 40–50% of patients did not respond to NO˙ inhalation and this remains an area for research. There is concern that an inhibitory effect of NO˙ on platelet aggregation might contribute to the occurrence of intracranial hemorrhages in these patients *(126)*. An increased rate of bleeding complications has not been noted in term infants, but sufficient data have not yet been published to confirm the safety of inhaled NO˙ therapy in premature newborns.

TOXICITY OF INHALED NO˙

The interest generated by reports of the successful therapeutic use of inhaled NO˙ is tempered by concerns over its toxicity *(127)*. High inhaled concentrations of NO˙ can cause acute pulmonary injury, methemoglobinemia, asphyxia, and death *(128–131)*. The US Occupational Safety and Health Administration has set a time-weighted average exposure limit of 25 ppm for NO˙ when breathed for 8 h/d in the workplace *(132)*. Few long-term toxicological studies of inhaled NO˙ have been conducted *(3)*. In a study of airway specimens from 24 infants who inhaled NO˙ for 1–4 d, no associated pulmonary toxicity was detected *(133)*.

Nitrogen Dioxide

In oxygen mixtures, NO˙ is oxidized to nitrogen dioxide (NO_2) *(131,134–139)*. NO_2 is cytotoxic and converted in aqueous solutions to nitric and nitrous acids. Occupational safety and health standards limit the NO_2 exposure of workers to 5 ppm *(132)*.

Inhaled NO_2 may remain in the lungs for prolonged periods of time because it reacts with water to produce nitric acid and undergoes irreversible reactive absorption by pulmonary epithelial lining fluid *(140)*. High levels (>10 ppm) of inhaled NO_2 have produced pulmonary edema, hemorrhage, changes in the surface tension of surfactant, reduced alveolar numbers, and death in experimental animals *(128,141–143)*. At inhaled concentrations as low as 2 ppm, alveolar cell hyperplasia, altered surfactant hysteresis, changes in the epithelium of the terminal bronchioles, and loss of epithelial cilia have been reported *(144,145)*. In humans, 2.3 ppm NO_2 increased alveolar permeability *(146)*. Airway responsiveness may be increased at inhaled NO_2 concentrations of <2 ppm *(144,147–149)*. The extent of conversion of NO˙ to NO_2 is determined by the concentrations of NO˙ and oxygen in the local environment, and is accelerated by increased NO˙ and oxygen concentrations *(131,134–139,150,151)*. The conversion rate of NO˙ to NO_2 follows second-order kinetics with respect to the NO˙ concentration and is described by the relationship *(134,150)*:

$$-d[\text{NO}^\bullet]/dt = k \cdot [\text{NO}^\bullet]^2 \cdot [\text{O}_2]$$

Because the oxygen concentration is typically much greater than the NO˙ concentration, it is assumed that the oxygen concentration remains constant. This formula also assumes that NO˙ is exclusively converted to NO_2. Glasson and Tuesday reported the value of k as 1.57×10^{-9} ppm^{-2}/min at 23°C and one atmosphere *(134)*. Under physical conditions similar to adult mechanical ventilation, Nishimura and coworkers reported a rate constant of 1.46×10^{-9} ppm^{-2}/min when NO˙ was mixed with nitrogen before entering the ventilator; the rate constant increased eightfold to 1.16×10^{-8} ppm^{-2}/min when NO˙ was mixed with air prior to introduction into the ventilator *(150)*. Aida and coworkers reported that the rate constant was smaller at 37°C than 25°C, but that it was not affected by humidity *(151)*. The residence time within mechanical ventilators depends on the minute ventilation and internal volume of the ventilator. Mechanical ventilators with a higher internal volume (e.g., Servo 900C) have a longer residence time and thus a greater delivered [NO_2] than those with a lower internal volume (e.g., Puritan-Bennett 7200ae) *(150)*.

A soda lime absorber can be used to remove NO_2 from the inspiratory gas *(135,152,153)*. The efficacy of soda lime varies with the preparation used and decreases with time *(154)*. The soda lime also absorbs NO˙ *(151)*. Adding a soda lime canister to the inspiratory limb of a breathing circuit may introduce other problems during mechanical ventilation, such as an increased resistance to breathing, difficulty in triggering the ventilator, increased compression volume, and an increased risk of leaks.

Nitrosylation of Metalloproteins

NO• forms complexes with transitional metal complexes, including those in metalloproteins, such as hemoglobin. In tissues, nitrosylation of iron-containing enzymes and iron–sulfur proteins of target cells may be responsible for the cytotoxic action of NO• generated by activated macrophages (155,156). High levels of intracellular NO• have been reported to cause DNA damage and mutations in human cell preparations (157). Damage to erythrocyte membranes may occur following long-term, low-level exposures. Oda and coworkers reported enlarged spleens and increased bilirubin levels, suggestive of increased erythrocyte turnover, in mice following 6 mo of exposure to 10 ppm NO• (158).

S-Nitrosation of thiols also occurs in vivo, and the resulting S-nitrosothiols have been identified in human airway lining fluid and in the plasma of patients inhaling NO• mixtures and also normal subjects (159). The formation of relatively stable iron–nitrosyl complexes and S-nitrosothiols may provide ways of tailoring the duration of action and transport properties of NO• and a means of detoxifying NO• in tissues (137,159).

Methemoglobinemia

NO• combines extremely rapidly with hemoglobin to form nitrosyl Fe(II)-hemoglobin (37, 160–167). The heme iron of the hemoglobin subsequently is oxidized from Fe^{2+} to Fe^{3+} (168).

Methemoglobinemia may occur if the production of Fe(III)-hemoglobin is increased or its reduction is diminished (169). Methemoglobin reductase contained within erythrocytes is the predominant mechanism for metabolizing methemoglobin. The activity of methemoglobin reductase may be decreased as a result of a hereditary deficiency and is normally low in newborn infants (169). Patients with decreased methemoglobin reductase activity may develop methemoglobinemia in the face of an increased rate of hemoglobin oxidation. Significant methemoglobinemia during NO• inhalation may occur, especially in newborns, but its incidence appears very low and related to the inhaled NO• dose (167,170). In a clinical study, Wessel and coworkers reported methemoglobin concentrations in excess of 5% in four of 123 pediatric patients who received inhaled NO• (171). In human adults (51,52,54,55, 68,75,172–174) and experimental animals (3,23,158,175,176), clinically significant methemoglobinemia is rare during exposure to NO• concentrations below <40 ppm. Normal methemoglobin levels are <2%; levels <5% do not require treatment. Increasing levels of methemoglobin during inhaled NO• therapy can usually be controlled by decreasing the dose of NO•. Methylene blue may be administered to treat severe methemoglobinemia. Because methylene blue may inhibit the activity of GC, methylene blue treatment could conceivably reduce or reverse the effects of inhaled NO•. Young and coworkers, however, reported that methylene blue did not inhibit the action of inhaled NO• in hypoxic sheep (177).

Peroxynitrite and Other Intermediates

In aqueous solutions, NO• reacts rapidly with $O_2^{•-}$ to form peroxynitrite ($OONO^-$) (127, 128,179). This species is a strong oxidant and catalyzes membrane lipid peroxidation and formation of nitrotyrosine residues in proteins. In plasma, NO• is eventually converted to nitrates and nitrites that are eliminated primarily by the kidney (175,180,181). It is unknown if the increased plasma nitrate and nitrite concentrations during inhaled NO• therapy have any deleterious effects.

Inhibition of Platelet Function

NO• inhibits platelet adhesion to endothelial cells and reverses platelet aggregation in vitro (182,183). These antiplatelet effects appear to be due to activation of GC and increased concentrations of cGMP within the platelet (184–187). Prolongation of the bleeding time during experimental NO• inhalation in rabbits (13) and human volunteers (188) has been reported. The clinical significance of this effect in humans is uncertain. In patients with ARDS, in vivo platelet aggregation and agglutination was decreased during NO˙ breathing at doses between 1 and 100 ppm. The effect on platelet function was not dose-dependent, however, and was not associated with a change in the bleeding time *(14)*.

DELIVERY AND MEASUREMENT

Adult Mechanical Ventilation

The simplest method to deliver NO˙ into a breathing circuit is to continuously administer NO˙ into the inspiratory limb *(75,189)*. The average delivered NO˙ concentration can be estimated from the flow rates of NO˙ and the inspiratory flow rate. Most adult mechanical ventilators have gas flow within the inspiratory limb only during the inspiratory phase. No gas flows in the inspiratory limb during exhalation. With such systems, the inspiratory circuit will fill with NO˙ that is continually delivered into the inspiratory limb during exhalation, and a high concentration of NO˙ (admixed with nitrogen) will be delivered to the patient at the beginning of each breath. In such systems, the delivered NO˙ concentration will also be affected by the inspiratory flow waveform, changes of minute ventilation, and by the site at which NO˙ is introduced into the breathing circuit.

If NO˙ is introduced into the Y-piece of the circuit *(14,77,190,191)*, the inspiratory limb will not fill with NO˙ during exhalation. Instead, the NO˙ will pass out the expiratory limb of the ventilator during exhalation. With this technique, it is not possible to measure the inspired NO˙ concentration; the dose can only be approximated by mathematical calculation. Again, changes of inspiratory flow or minute ventilation will alter the NO˙ concentration.

NO˙ has been administered directly into the endotracheal tube *(59,62)*. The problems associated with this technique are similar to NO˙ administered via the Y-piece. In addition, if the patient becomes apneic, the anoxic gas mixture (NO˙ in nitrogen) will continue to flow into the trachea and could asphyxiate the patient.

NO˙ may be selectively injected into the inspiratory limb of the ventilator circuit during the inspiratory phase of the ventilator cycle *(51,57–59)*. This has been accomplished by a nebulizer drive mechanism operating during inspiration. The gas supply to the nebulizer contains the NO˙ required to achieve the desired inhaled dose after mixing with gas delivered from the ventilator. Because the gas flow from the nebulizer is constant during inspiration, the technique will produce varying concentrations if the inspiratory flow pattern varies (e.g., pressure control ventilation) or tidal volume is variable (e.g., pressure support ventilation). The advantage of this system is that the residence time of NO˙ in an oxygen-containing gas mixture is reduced and the generation of NO_2 is minimized.

An alternative to the above techniques is to premix the NO˙ with nitrogen (or air) and introduce the gas mixture proximal to the gas inlet of the ventilator or breathing circuit *(68,150,153,171,174,176,191,192)*. The NO˙ dose remains constant throughout inspiration with this technique and is not affected by changes of minute ventilation or inspiratory flow waveform. The generation of NO_2 will be greater, however, in ventilators with large internal volumes *(150)*. The delivered NO˙ dose will also change when the FiO_2 setting on the ventilator is changed. This change can be easily regulated, however, by adjusting the concentration of NO˙ delivered to the ventilator.

Recently, microprocessor-controlled NO˙ delivery systems using precision solenoids have been developed. These devices mix nitrogen, oxygen, and NO˙ to achieve the desired NO˙ concentration and FiO_2, and can reliably deliver a constant and monitored NO˙ concentration during a wide variety of ventilatory patterns and gas flow rates *(193)*.

Pediatric Mechanical Ventilation

NO˙ can be titrated into the inspiratory limb of continuous flow mechanical ventilators such as those used in pediatrics (including high-frequency oscillators) *(194–196)*. Ideally, the NO$^\bullet$ should be administered near the outlet of the ventilator to permit adequate mixing of gases prior to inhalation by the patient. Once the desired NO$^\bullet$ concentration is established, the dose should remain constant provided that the total flow through the system is not changed. The NO_2 generation rate is low because the residence time of NO$^\bullet$ within such systems is short. The FiO_2 should be analyzed distal to the point of NO$^\bullet$ introduction into the system.

Manual Ventilators

For bag valve mask ventilators, NO$^\bullet$ can be mixed with oxygen and administered into the gas inlet port of the ventilator's reservoir (195). With such systems, the delivered NO$^\bullet$ concentration will change with changes of minute ventilation if the flow into the manual ventilator is less than the patient's minute ventilation. If the ventilator reservoir is not continuously flushed, the NO_2 concentration within the ventilator will increase. This may produce high levels of NO_2.

Spontaneous Ventilation

High-flow systems using tight-fitting masks have been used for brief inhalations of NO$^\bullet$ (171,197,198). Reservoir bags should be avoided with such systems because of the increased generation of NO_2 within the bag. Inhaled NO$^\bullet$ has also been administered by transtracheal catheters (199) or nasal cannulas (200). With such systems, however, the delivered dose varies widely with the ventilatory pattern of the patient and cannot easily be accurately analyzed.

Anesthesia Machines

The possible mixing sites in a standard anesthesia machine are at the flowmeter bank, the fresh gas flow outlet, and in the inspiratory limb of the circuit. Administration of NO$^\bullet$ directly into the trachea has also been reported, but this technique could asphyxiate an apneic patient. Constant flow rates of NO$^\bullet$ into the inspiratory limb of the circuit produce very wide and unpredictable variations of NO$^\bullet$ concentration because of the varying cyclic flow and mixing within the circuit. Administration of NO$^\bullet$ at the flowmeter bank or the fresh gas outlet produces more stable concentrations (201). Owing to the recirculation of gas within the circle system, it is prudent to maintain high fresh gas flow rates to reduce NO_2 concentrations and to minimize errors in gas mixing. The safety of NO$^\bullet$ passing through vaporizers and other components of the anesthesia machine is unstudied.

MEASUREMENT OF NO$^\bullet$ AND NO_2 CONCENTRATIONS

Chemiluminescence Monitors

Chemiluminescence techniques for the measurement of NO$^\bullet$ and NO_2 concentrations are well described for industrial and environmental monitoring (202,203). These techniques have been adapted for biomedical use. Sampled gas reacts with O_3^- to produce activated NO_2*. NO_2* reverts to the ground state by emitting electromagnetic radiation. The emitted radiation has a wavelength maximum of 1200 nm and is detected by a photomultiplier tube. To measure NO_2, it is first converted to NO$^\bullet$ in a thermal converter and then measured as before. The sum of the NO$^\bullet$ concentration measured with and without the converter is referred to as the NO_x. Most chemiluminescence analyzers measure NO$^\bullet$ and NO_x simultaneously and display [NO$^\bullet$], [NO_2], and [NO_x]. Quenching of the emitted photons is a potential problem (204–207). Quenching occurs when some of the NO_2* produced by ozonation of NO$^\bullet$ reverts to the ground state by reacting with other molecules (e.g., O_2, N_2, H_2O, CO_2). The greater the concentration of the quenching molecules, the lower will be the chemiluminescence signal. The effects of quenching can be corrected mathematically or avoided by calibrating the analyzer with the same concentration of gases that will be present in the analyzed sample.

Table 1
Clinical Indications for Inhaled NO•

Substantiated

Neonatal hypoxemic respiratory failure and persistent pulmonary hypertension of the newborn (PPHN) *(111,113,114,121)*

Assessment of pulmonary vascular reactivity in patients with pulmonary hypertension *(219,220)*

Investigational

Acute Respiratory Distress Syndrome (ARDS) *(69)*

Lung and cardiac transplantation *(221–225)*

Congenital and acquired heart disease *(154,171,197,226–231)*

Chronic pulmonary hypertension *(199,232–234)*

Chronic Obstructive Pulmonary Disease (COPD) *(235,236)*

Acute chest syndrome in sickle cell disease *(16)*

Bronchodilation *(237–240)*

Chemiluminescence analyzers, although highly accurate, precise, and sensitive, are large, expensive, and cumbersome to use.

Electrochemical Monitors

NO• and NO_2 concentrations may also be measured by electrochemical techniques. Electrochemical analyzers generate a potential difference from reactions of NO• or NO_2 within an electrolyte *(208)*. The resulting current is proportional to the NO• or NO_2 concentration of the sample. Electrochemical cells have been specifically designed for biomedical and clinical use. They are small, portable, rugged, and far less expensive than chemiluminescence analyzers *(209–214)*. The cells are affected by humidity and are pressure sensitive. The severity of these problems may be reduced by sampling the gas prior to humidification, using drying agents, and using sidestream sampling techniques.

Sampling Sites for Measurement of NO• And NO_2

Most NO• analyzers have slow response times and provide time weighted average measurements of NO• and NO_2 concentrations *(215,216)*. Rapid fluctuations of NO• or NO_2 concentrations will not be detected by such methods. Measurement of the NO• and NO_2 concentrations within the inspiratory limb of the ventilator circuit accurately reflects the NO• concentration delivered to the lungs. The NO• concentration has also been measured in intratracheal gas samples. The values derived from such samples are affected by changes of exhaled NO• concentrations and by the ventilatory pattern *(215)*. Rapid-response analyzers are currently available that can accurately record the rapid changes of NO• concentration occurring within a delivered or exhaled breath *(217)*.

THE FUTURE OF INHALED NO•

NO• inhalation has been used to reverse pulmonary hypertension and hypoxemia in thousands of patients for periods of days to months (Table 1). The intense interest in inhaled NO• is indicative of the great need for simple and effective therapies for such critically ill patients. The use of inhaled NO• to treat newborns and infants with hypoxemia respiratory failure and PPHN has been well substantiated by multiple randomized, multicenter, double-blind, placebo-controlled trials *(111,113,114,131,218)*. NO• inhalation therapy, in combination with conventional *(111,113)* or high-frequency oscillatory ventilation *(114)*, significantly reduces the need for ECMO, an expensive and invasive support procedure in newborn patients with hypoxic respiratory failure. In addition, inhaled NO• has been widely recommended to assess pulmonary vascular reactivity in patients with pulmonary hypertension *(219)*. A survey of long-term vasodilator treatment in patients with primary pulmonary hypertension reported that inhaled NO• was used as the primary vasodilator to test pulmonary vascular responsiveness in 32% of the responding tertiary hospitals in the United States *(220)*. The role of inhaled NO• continues to be investigated in patients receiving lung and cardiac transplants *(221– 225)*, or suffering from ARDS *(69)*, congenital and acquired heart disease *(154,171,197,226– 231)*, or chronic pulmonary hypertension *(199,232–234)*. In selected groups of such patients, inhaled NO• improves arterial oxygenation and selectively reduces pulmonary arterial hypertension. In sickle cell disease, inhaled NO• significantly shifts the blood O_2 dissociation curve to the left, returning it to toward normal, and may decrease the sickling of affected erythrocytes *(16)*. At this time, the use of inhaled NO• for such conditions remains investigational. It is uncertain whether NO• inhalation improves clinical outcome or survival rates in these conditions. What is currently clear, however, is that the study of the pulmonary effects of inhaled NO• has greatly expanded our knowledge of the physiology and pathophysiology of the pulmonary circulation and provides a new opportunity for designing effective novel therapies.

ACKNOWLEDGMENTS

Supported by United States Public Health Service grant HL-42397 (Dr. Zapol). The Massachusetts General Hospital has licensed a patent covering the use of NO• inhalation and has a right to receive royalties.

REFERENCES

1. Radermacher P, Santak B, Wust HJ, Tarnow J, Falke KJ. Prostacyclin for the treatment of pulmonary hypertension in the Adult Respiratory Distress Syndrome: effects on pulmonary capillary pressure and ventilation-perfusion distributions. Anesthesiology 1990;72:238–244.
2. Fratacci MD, Frostell CG, Chen TY, Wain JC Jr, Robinson DR, Zapol WM. Inhaled nitric oxide. A selective pulmonary vasodilator of heparin-protamine vasoconstriction in sheep. Anesthesiology 1991;75:990–999.
3. Frostell C, Fratacci MD, Wain JC, Jones R, Zapol WM. Inhaled nitric oxide. A selective pulmonary vasodilator reversing hypoxic pulmonary vasoconstriction. Circulation 1991;83:2038–2047.
4. Pison U, Lopez FA, Heidelmeyer CF, Roissant R, Falke KJ. Inhaled nitric oxide reverses hypoxic pulmonary vasoconstriction without impairing gas exchange. J Appl Physiol 1993;74:1287–1292.
5. Kanner J, Harel S, Granit R. Nitric oxide as an antioxidant. Arch Biochem Biophys 1991;289:130–136.
6. Kavanagh BP, Mouchawar A, Goldsmith J, Pearl RG. Effects of inhaled NO and inhibition of endogenous NO synthesis in oxidant-induced acute lung injury. J Appl Physiol 1994;76:1324–1329.
7. Clancy RM, Leszcyznska-Piziak J, Abramson SB. Nitric oxide, an endothelial cell relaxation factor, inhibits neutrophil superoxide anion production via a direct action on the NADPH oxidase. J Clin Invest 1992;90:1116–1121.
8. Hassoun PM, Yu FS, Zulueta JJ, White AC, Lanzillo JJ. Effect of nitric oxide and cell redox status on the regulation of endothelial cell xanthine dehydrogenase. Am J Physiol 1995;268:L809–L817.
9. Wink DA, Hanbauer I, Krishna MC, DeGraff W, Gamson J, Mitchell JB. Nitric oxide protects against cellular damage and cytotoxicity from reactive oxygen species. Proc Natl Acad Sci USA 1993;90: 9813–9817.
10. Nelin L, Dolinski S, Morrisey J, Dawson C. The effect of inhaled nitric oxide on survival of rats in oxygen. Am J Respir Crit Care Med 1995;151:A757.
11. Garat C, Adnot S, Reyaiguia S, Meignan M, Jayr C. Effect of inhaled nitric oxide on 100% oxygen induced lung injury in rats. Anesthesiology 1994;81:A1454.
12. Garat C, Adnot S, Rezaiguia S, Kouyoumdjian C, Meignan M, Jayr C. Effect of inhaled NO or treatment with L-NAME on 100% oxygen induced lung injury in rats. Am J Respir Crit Care Med 1995;151: A757.
13. Hiigman M, Frostell C, Arnberg H, Sandhagen B, Hedenstierna G. Prolonged bleeding time during nitric oxide inhalation in the rabbit. Acta Physiol Scand 1994;151:125–129.

14. Samama CM, Diaby M, Fellahi JL, Mdhafar A, Eyraud D, Arock M, et al. Inhibition of platelet aggregation by inhaled nitric oxide in patients with acute respiratory distress syndrome. Anesthesiology 1995;83:56–65.
15. May GR, Crook P, Moore PK, Page CP. The role of nitric oxide as an endogenous regulator of platelet and neutrophil activation within the pulmonary circulation of the rabbit. Br J Pharmacol 1991;102: 759–763.
16. Head CA, Brugnara C, Martinez-Ruiz R, Kacmarek RM, Bridges KR, Kuter D, et al. Low concentrations of nitric oxide increase oxygen affinity of sickle erythrocytes in vitro and in vivo. J Clin Invest 1997;100:1193–1198.
17. Weitzberg E, Rudehill A, Lundberg JM. Nitric oxide inhalation attenuates pulmonary hypertension and improves gas exchange in endotoxin shock. Eur J Pharmacol 1993;233:85–94.
18. Ogura H, Cioffi WG, Offner PJ, Jordan BS, Johnson AA, Pruitt BA Jr. Effect of inhaled nitric oxide on pulmonary function after sepsis in a swine model. Surgery 1994;116:313–321.
19. Dahm P, Blomquist S, Martensson L, Theme J, Zoucas E. Circulatory and ventilatory effects of intermittent nitric oxide inhalation during porcine endotoxemia. J Trauma 1994;37:769–777.
20. Putensen C, Rasanen J, Downs JB. Effect of endogenous and inhaled nitric oxide on the ventilation-perfusion relationships in oleic-acid lung injury. Am J Respir Crit Care Med 1994;150:330–336.
21. Klemm P, Thiemermann C, Winklmaier G, Martorana PA, Henning R. Effects of nitric oxide synthase inhibition combined with nitric oxide inhalation in a porcine model of endotoxin shock. Br J Pharmacol 1995;14:363–368.
22. Romand JA, Pinsky MR, Firestone L, Zar HA, Lancaster HR Jr. Effect of inhaled nitric oxide on pulmonary hemodynamics after acute lung injury in dogs. J Appl Physiol 1994;76:1356–1362.
23. Shah NS, Nakayama DK, Jacob TD, Nishio I, Imai T, Billiar TR, et al. Efficacy of inhaled nitric oxide in a porcine model of adult respiratory distress syndrome. Arch Surg 1994;129:158–164.
24. Putensen C, Rasanen J, Lopez FA, Downs JB. Continuous positive airway pressure modulates effect of inhaled nitric oxide on the ventilation-perfusion distributions in canine lung injury. Chest 1994;106: 1563–1569.
25. Rovira I, Chen TY, Winkler M, Kawai N, Bloch KD, Zapol WM. Effects of inhaled nitric oxide on pulmonary hemodynamics and gas exchange in an ovine model of ARDS. J Appl Physiol 1994;76: 345–355.
26. Ogura H, Cioffi WG Jr, Jordan BS, Okerberg CV, Johnson AA, Mason AD Jr, et al. The effect of inhaled nitric oxide on smoke inhalation injury in an ovine mode. J Trauma 1994;37:294–302.
27. Kubes P, Kanwar S, Niu X-F, Gaboury JP. Nitric oxide synthesis inhibition induces leukocyte adhesion via superoxide and mast cells. FASEB J 1993;7:1293–1299.
28. Hughes SR, Williams TJ, Brain SD. Evidence that endogenous nitric oxide modulates oedema formation induced by substance P. Eur J Pharmacol 1990;191:481–484.
29. Ialenti A, Ianaro A, Moncada S, Di Rosa RM. Modulation of acute inflammation by endogenous nitric oxide. Eur J Pharmacol 1992;211:177–182.
30. Mayhan WG. Role of nitric oxide in modulating permeability of hamster cheek pouch in response to adenosine 5'-diphosphate and bradykinin. Inflammation 1992;16:295–305.
31. Mulligan MS, Hevel JM, Marletta MA, Ward PA. Tissue injury caused by deposition of immune complexes is L-arginine dependent. Proc Natl Acad Sci USA 1991;88:6338–6342.
32. Boughton SN, Deakin AM, Whittle BJ. Actions of nitric oxide on the acute gastrointestinal damage induced by PAF in the rat. Ann NY Acad Sci 1992;664:126–139.
33. Hutcheson IR, Whittle BJ, Boughton-Smith N. Role of nitric oxide in maintaining vascular integrity in endotoxin-induced acute intestinal damage in the rat. Br J Pharmacol 1990;101:815–820.
34. Kubes P. Nitric oxide modulates epithelial permeability in the feline small intestine. Am J Physiol 1992;262:G1138–G1142.
35. Nozik ES, Huang Y-CT, Piantadosi CA. L-arginine enhances injury in the isolated rabbit lung during hyperoxia. Respir Physiol 1995;100:63–74.
36. Guidot DM, Repine MJ, Hybertson BM, Repine JE. Inhaled nitric oxide prevents neutrophil-mediated, oxygen radical-dependent leak in isolated rat lungs. Am J Physiol 1995;269:L2–L5.
37. Rimar S, Gillis CN. Selective pulmonary vasodilation by inhaled nitric oxide is due to hemoglobin inactivation. Circulation 1993;88:2884–2887.
38. Harris AL, Lemp BM, Bentley RG, Perrone MH, Hamel LT, Silver PJ. Phosphodiesterase isozyme inhibition and the potentiation by zaprinast of endothelium-derived relaxing factor and guanylate cyclase stimulating agents in vascular smooth muscle. J Pharmacol Exp Ther 1989;249:394–400.
39. Braner DAV, Fineman JR, Chang R, Soifer SJ. M&B 22948, a cGMP phosphodiesterase inhibitor, is a pulmonary vasodilator in lambs. Am J Physiol 1993;264:H252–H258.

40. McMahon TJ, Ignarro LJ, Kadowitz PJ. Influence of Zaprinast on vascular tone and vasodilator responses in the cat pulmonary vascular bed. J Appl Physiol 1993;74:1704–1711.

41. Ichinose F, Adrie C, Hurford WE, Zapol WM. Prolonged pulmonary vasodilator action of inhaled nitric oxide by Zaprinast in awake lambs. J Appl Physiol 1995;78:1288–1295.

42. Ichinose F, Adrie C, Hurford WE, Bloch KD, Zapol WM. Selective pulmonary vasodilation induced by aerosolized zaprinast. Anesthesiology 1998;88:410–416.

43. Ziegler JW, Ivy DD, Kinsella JP, Clark WR, Abman SH. Dypyridamole, a cGMP phosphodiesterase inhibitor, augments inhaled nitric oxide induced pulmonary vasodilation in the ovine transitional circulation. Pediatr Res 1994;90A:527.

44. Ivy DD, Ziegler JW, Kinsella JP, Wiggins JW, Abman SH. Hemodynamic effects of dipyridamole and inhaled nitric oxide in pediatric patients with pulmonary hypertension. Chest 1998;114:S17.

45. Fullerton DA, Jaggers J, Piedalue F, Grover FL, McIntyre RC Jr. Effective control of refractory pulmonary hypertension after cardiac operations. J Thorac Cardiovasc Surg 1997;113:363–368.

46. Zobel G, Urlesberger B, Dacar D, Rodl S, Reiterer F, Friehs I. Partial liquid ventilation combined with inhaled nitric oxide in acute respiratory failure with pulmonary hypertension in piglets. Pediatr Res 1997;41:172–177.

47. Houmes RJ, Hartog A, Verbrugge SJ, Bohm S, Lachmann B. Combining partial liquid ventilation with nitric oxide to improve gas exchange in acute lung injury. Intensive Care Med 1997;23:163–169.

48. Hopkins SR, Johnson EC, Richardson RS, Wagner H, De Rosa M, Wagner PD. Effects of inhaled nitric oxide on gas exchange in lungs with shunt or poorly ventilated areas. Am J Respir Crit Care Med 1997; 156:484–491.

49. Zapol WM, Snider MT. Pulmonary hypertension in severe acute respiratory failure. N Engl J Med 1977;296:476–480.

50. Zapol WM, Jones R. Vascular components of ARDS: clinical pulmonary hemodynamics and morphology. Am Rev Respir Dis 1987;136:471–474.

51. Rossaint R, Falke KJ, Lopez F, Slama K, Pison U, Zapol WM. Inhaled nitric oxide for the adult respiratory distress syndrome. N Engl J Med 1993;328:399–405.

52. Rossaint R, Gerlach H, Schmidt-Ruhnke H, Pappert D, Lewandowski K, Steudel JW, et al. Efficacy of inhaled nitric oxide in patients with severe ARDS. Chest 1995;107:1107–1115.

53. Hurford WE. Inhaled nitric oxide therapy. Curr Opin Anaesthesiol 1996;9:117–126.

54. Manktelow C, Bigatello LM, Hess D, Hurford WE. Physiologic detenninants of the response to inhaled nitric oxide in patients with the acute respiratory distress syndrome. Anesthesiology 1997;87:297–307.

55. Luhr O, Nathorst-Westfeltl U, Lundin S, Wickerls CJ, Stiernslrom H, Berggren L, et al. A retrospective analysis of nitric oxide inhalation in patients with severe acute lung injury in Sweden and Norway 1991–1994. Acta Anaesthesiol Scand 1997;41:1238–1246.

56. Gerlach H, Pappert D, Lewandowski K, Rossaint R, Falke KJ. Long-term inhalation with evaluated low doses of nitric oxide for selective improvement of oxygenation in patients with adult respiratory distress syndrome. Intensive Care Med 1993;19:443–449.

57. Puybasset L, Stewart T, Rouby JJ, Cluzel P, Mourgeon E, Belin MF, et al. Inhaled nitric oxide reverses the increase in pulmoniuy vascular resistance induced by permissive hypercapnia in patients with acute respiratory distress syndrome. Anesthesiology 1994;80:1254–1267.

58. Puybasset L, Rouby JJ, Mourgeon E, Stewart TE, Cluzel P, Arthaud M, et al. Inhaled nitric oxide in acute respiratory failure: dose-response curves. Int Care Med 1994;20:319–327.

59. Puybasset L, Rouby JJ, Mourgeon E, Cluzel P, Souhil Z, Law-Koune JD, et al. Factors influencing cardiopulmonary effects of inhaled nitric oxide in acute respiratory failure. Am J Respir Crit Care Med 1995;152:318–328.

60. Lowson SM, Rich GF, McArdle PA, Jaidev J, Morris GN. The response to varying concentrations of inhaled nitric oxide in patients with acute respiratory distress syndrome. Anesth Analg 1996;82:574–581.

61. Lee KH, Tan PS, Rico P, Delgado E, Kellum JA, Pinsky MR. Low levels of nitric oxide as contaminant in hospital compressed air: physiologic significance? Crit Care Med 1997;25:1143–1146.

62. Fierobe L, Brunet F, Dhainaut JF, Monchi M, Belghith M, Mira JP, et al. Effect of inhaled nitric oxide on right ventricular function in adult respiratory distress syndrome. Am J Respir Crit Care Med 1995; 151:1414–1419.

63. Rossaint R, Slama K, Steudel W, Gerlach H, Pappert D, Veit S, et al. Effects of inhaled nitric oxide on right ventricular function in severe acute respiratory distress syndrome. Intensive Care Med 1995; 21:197–203.

64. Benting A, Bräutigam P, Geiger K, Loop T, Beyer U, Moser E. Inhaled nitric oxide reduces pulmonary transvascular albumin flux in patients with acute lung injury. Anesthesiology 1995;83:1153–1161.

65. Rossetti M, Guenard H, Gabinski C. Effects of nitric oxide inhalation on pulmonary serial vascular resistances in ARDS. Am J Respir Crit Care Med 1996;154:1375–1381.

66. Michael JR, Barton RG, Saffle JR, Mone M, Markewitz BA, Hillier K, et al. Inhaled nitric oxide versus conventional therapy. Effect on oxygenation in ARDS. Am J Respir Crit Care Med 1998;157:1372–1380.

67. Troncy E, Collet JP, Shapiro S, Guimond JG, Blair L, Ducruet T, et al. Inhaled nitric oxide in acute respiratory distress syndrome: a pilot randomized controlled study. Am J Respir Crit Care Med 1998; 157:1483–1488.

68. Bigatello LM, Hurford WE, Kacmarek RM, Roberts JD Jr, Zapol WM. Prolonged inhalation of low concentrations of nitric oxide in patients with severe adult respiratory distress syndrome. Effects on pulmonary hemodynamics and oxygenation. Anesthesiology 1994;80:761–770.

69. Dellinger RP, Zimmerman JL, Taylor RW, Straube RC, Hauser DL, Criner GJ, et al. Effects of inhaled nitric oxide in patients with acute respiratory distress syndrome: results of a randomized phase II trial. Crit Care Med 1998;26:15–23.

70. Lundin S, Mang H, Smithies M, Stenquist O, Frostell C. Inhalation of nitric oxide in acute lung injury: preliminary results of a European multicenter study. Intensive Care Med 1997;23:S2.

71. Lundin S, Westfelt UN, Stenqvist O, Blomqvist H, Lindh A, Berggren L, et al. Response to nitric oxide inhalation in early acute lung injury. Intensive Care Med 1996;22,728–734.

72. Treggiari-Venzi M, Ricou B, Remand JA, Suter PM. The response to repeated nitric oxide inhaled is inconsistent in patients with acute respiratory distress syndrome. Anesthesiology 1998;88:634–641.

73. Krafft P, Fridrich P, Fitzgerald RD, Koc D, Steltzer H. Effectiveness of nitric oxide inhalation in septic ARDS. Chest 1996;109:486–493.

74. Holzmann A, Bloch KD, Sanchez LS, Filippov G, Zapol WM. Hyporesponsiveness to inhaled nitric oxide in isolated, perfused lungs from endotoxin-challenge rats. Am J Physiol 1996;271:L981–L986.

75. Young JD, Brampton WJ, Knighton JD, Finfer SR. Inhaled nitric oxide in acute respiratory failure in adults. Br J Anaesth 1994;73;499–502.

76. Payen DM, Gatecel C, Plaisance P. Almitrine effect on nitric oxide inhalation in adult respiratory distress syndrome. Lancet 1993;341:1164.

77. Wysocki M, Delclaux C, Roupie E, Langeron O, Liu N, Herman B, et al. Additive effect on gas exchange of inhaled nitric oxide and intravenous almitrine bismesylate in the adult respiratory distress syndrome. Intensive Care Med 1994;20:254–259.

78. Doering EB, Hanson CWI, Reily DJ, Marshall C, Marshall BE. Improvement in oxygenation by phenylephrine and nitric oxide in patients with adult respiratory distress syndrome. Anesthesiology 1997;87: 18–25.

79. Papazian L, Bregeon F, Gaillat F, Kaphan E, Thirion X, Saur P, et al. Does norepinephrine modify the effects of inhaled nitric oxide in septic patients with acute respiratory distress syndrome? Anesthesiology 1998;89:1089–1098.

80. Gillart T, Bazin JE, Cosserant B, Guelon D, Aigouy L, Mansoor O, et al. Combined nitric oxide inhalation, prone positioning and almitrine infusion improve oxygenation in severe ARDS. Can J Anaesth 1998; H45:402–409.

81. Jolliet P, Bulpa P, Ritz M, Ricou B, Lopez J, Chevrolet JC. Additive beneficial effects of the prone position, nitric oxide, and almitrine bismesylate on gas exchange and oxygen transport in acute respiratory distress syndrome. Crit Care Med 1997;25:786–794.

82. Papazian L, Bregeon F, Gaillat F, Thirion X, Gainnier M, Gregoire R, et al. Respective and combined effects of prone position and inhaled nitric oxide in patients with acute respiratory distress syndrome. Am J Respir Crit Care Med 1998;157:580–585.

83. Karamanoukian HL, Glick PL, Zayek M, Steinhom RH, Zwass MS, Fineman JR, et al. Inhaled nitric oxide in congenital hypoplasia of the lungs due to diaphragmatic hernia or oligohydramnios. Pediatrics 1994;94:715–718.

84. Hoehn T, Krause M, Hentschel R. High-frequency ventilation augments the effect of inhaled nitric oxide in persistent pulmonary hypertension of the newborn. Eur Respir J 1998;11:234–238.

85. Miller OI, Tang SF, Keech A, Celermajer DS. Rebound pulmoniuy hypertension on withdrawal from inhaled nitric oxide. Lancet 1995;346:51,52.

86. Assreuy J, Cunha FQ, Liew FY, Moncada S. Feedback inhibition of nitric oxide synthase activity by nitric oxide. Br J Pharmacol 1993;108:833–837.

87. Rengasamy A, Johns RA. Regulation of nitric oxide synthase by nitric oxide. Mol Pharmacol 1993;44: 124–128.

88. Kiff RJ, Moss DW, Moncada S. Effect of nitric oxide gas on the generation of nitric oxide by isolated blood vessels: implications for inhalation therapy. Br J Pharmacol 1994;113:496–498.

89. Ivy DD, Kinsella JP, Ziegler JW, Abman SH. Dipyridamole attenuates rebound pulmonary hypertension after inhaled nitric oxide withdrawal in postoperative congenital heart disease. J Thorac Cardiovasc Surg 1998;115:875–882.

90. Amato MBP, Barbas CSV, Medeiros DM, Magaldi RB, Schettino GP, Lorenzi-Filho G, et al. Effect of a protective-ventilation strategy on mortality in the acute respiratory distress syndrome. N Engl J Med 1998;338:347–354.

91. Lachmann B. Open up the lung and keep the lung open. Intensive Care Med 1992;17:375,376.

92. Montgomery AB, Stager MA, Carrico CJ, Hudson LD. Causes of mortality in patients with the adult respiratory distress syndrome. Am Rev Respir Dis 1985;132:485–489.

93. Suchyta MR, Clemmer TP, Elliott CG, Orme JFJ, Weaver LK. The adult respiratory distress syndrome. A report of survival and modifying factors. Chest 1992;101:1074–1079.

94. Gerlach M, Keh D, Gerlach H. Inhaled nitric oxide for the acute respiratory distress syndrome. Respir Care, in press, 1999.

95. Murakami S, Bacha EA, Herve P, Detruit H, Chapelier AR, Dartevelle PG, et al. Prevention of reperfusion injury by inhaled nitric oxide in lungs harvested from non-heart-beating donors. Ann Thorac Surg 1996;62:1632–1638.

96. Christou H, Adatia I, Van Marter LJ, Kane JW, Thompson JE, Stark AR, et al. Effect of inhaled nitric oxide on endothelin-1 and cyclic guanosine 5'-monophosphate plasma concentrations in newborn infants with persistent pulmonary hypertension. J Pediatar 1997;130:603–611.

97. Roberts JD, Polaner DM, Lang P, Zapol WM. Inhaled nitric oxide in persistent pulmonary hypertension of the newborn. Lancet 1992;340:818,819.

98. Kinsella JP, Neish SR, Shaffer E, Abman SH. Low-dose inhalation nitric oxide in persistent pulmonary hypertension of the newborn. Lancet 1992;340:819,820.

99. Roberts JD Jr, Chen TY, Kawai N, Wain J, Dupuy P, Shimouchi A, et al. Inhaled nitric oxide reverses pulmonary vasoconstriction in the hypoxic and acidotic newborn lamb. Circ Res 1993;72:246–254.

100. DeMarco V, Skimming J, Ellis TM, Cassin S. Nitric oxide inhalation. Effects on the ovine neonatal pulmonary and systemic circulations. Chest 1994;105:91S,92S.

101. Etches PC, Finer NN, Barrington KJ, Graham AJ, Chan WK. Nitric oxide reverses acute hypoxic pulmonary hypertension in the newborn piglet. Pediatr Res 1994;35:15–19.

102. Kinsella JP, Ivy DD, Abman SH. Inhaled nitric oxide improves gas exchange and lowers pulmonary vascular resistance in severe experimental hyaline membrane disease. Pediatr Res 1994;36:402–408.

103. Nelin LD, Moshin J, Thomas CJ, Sasidharan P, Dawson CA. The effect of inhaled nitric oxide on the pulmonary circulation of the neonatal pig. Pediatr Res 1994;35:20–24.

104. Skimming JW, DeMarco VG, Cassin S. The effects of nitric oxide inhalation on the pulmonary circulation of preterm lambs. Pediatr Res 1994;37:335–340.

105. Karamanoukian HL, Glick PL, Wilcox DT, Rossman JE, Holm BA, Morin FC 3rd. Pathophysiology of congenital diaphragmatic herni. VIIII: inhaled nitric oxide requires exogenous surfactant therapy in the lamb model of congenital diaphragmatic hernia. J Pediat Surg 1995;30:1–4.

106. Rosenberg AA, Kinsella JP, Abman SH. Cerebral hemodynamics and distribution of left ventricular output during inhalation of nitric oxide. Crit Care Med 1995;23:1391–1397.

107. Zayek M, Cleveland D, Morin FC 3rd. Treatment of persistent pulmonary hypertension in the newborn lamb by inhaled nitric oxide. J Pediatr 1993;122:743-750.

108. Zayek M, Wild L, Roberts JD, Morin FC 3rd. Effect of nitric oxide on the survival rate and incidence of lung injury in newborn lambs with persistent pulmonary hypertension. J Pediatr 1993;123:947–952.

109. Kouyoumdjian C, Adnot S, Levame M, Eddahibi S, Bousbaa H, Raffestin B. Continuous inhalation of nitric oxide protects against development of pulmonary hypertension in chronically hypoxic rats. J Clin Invest 1994;94:578–584.

110. Roberts JD Jr, Roberts CT, Jones RC, Zapol WM, Bloch KD. Continuous nitric oxide inhalation reduces pulmonary arterial structural changes, right ventricular hypertrophy, and growth retardation in the hypoxic newborn rat. Circ Res 1995;76:215–222.

111. The Neonatal Inhaled Nitric Oxide Study Group. Inhaled nitric oxide in full term and nearly full-term infants with hypoxic respiratory failure. N Engl J Med 1997;336:597–604.

112. The Neonatal Inhaled Nitric Oxide Study Group. Inhaled nitric oxide and hypoxic respiratory failure in infants with congenital diaphragmatic hernia. Pediatrics 1997;99:838–845.

113. Roberts JD Jr, Fineman JR, Morin FC 3rd, Shaul PW, Rimar S, Schreiber MD, et al. Inhaled nitric oxide and persistent pulmonary hypertension of the newborn. N Engl J Med 1997;336:605–610.

114. Kinsella JP, Truog WE, Walsh WF, Goldberg RN, Bancalari E, Mayock DE, et al. Randomized, multicenter trial of inhaled nitric oxide and high-frequency oscillatory ventilation in severe, persistent pulmonary hypertension of the newborn. J Pediatr 1997;131:55–62.

115. Lonnqvist PA. Inhaled nitric oxide in newborn and paediatric patients with pulmonary hypertension and moderate to severe impaired oxygenation: effects of doses of 3–100 parts per million. Intensive Care Med 1997;23:773–779.

116. Davidson D, Baarefield ES, Kattwinkel J, Dudell G, Damask M, Straube R, et al. Inhaled nitric oxide for the early treatment of persistent pulmonary hypertension of the term newborn: a randomized, double-masked, placebo-controlled, dose-response, multicenter study. The I-NO/PPHN Study Group. Pediatrics 1998;101:325–334.

117. Day RW, Guarin M, Lynch JM, Vernon DD, Dean JM. Inhaled nitric oxide in children with severe lung disease: results of acute and prolonged therapy with two concentrations. Crit Care Med 1996;24: 215–221.

118. Parker TA, Kinsella JP, Abman SH. Response to inhaled nitric oxide in persistent pulmonary hypertension of the newborn: relationship to baseline oxygenation. J Perinatol 1998;18:221–225.

119. Rosenberg AA, Kennaugh JM, Moreland SG, Fashaw LM, Hale KA, Torielli FM, et al. Longitudinal follow-up of a cohort of newborn infants treated with inhaled nitric oxide for persistent pulmonary hypertension. J Pediatr 1997;131:70–75.

120. Tang SF, Miller OI. Low-dose inhaled nitric oxide for neonates with pulmonary hypertension. J Paediatr Child Health 1996;32:419–423.

121. Hoffman GM, Ross GA, Day SE, Rice TB, Nelin LD. Inhaled nitric oxide reduces the utilization of extracorporeal membrane oxygenation in persistent pulmonary hypertension of the newborn. Crit Care Med 1997;25:352–359.

122. Abman SH, Kinsella JP, Schaffer MS, Wilkening RB. Inhaled nitric oxide in the management of a premature newborn with severe respiratory distress and pulmonary hypertension. Pediatrics 1993;92: 606–609.

123. Peliowski A, Finer NN, Etches PC, Tierney AJ, Ryan CA. Inhaled nitric oxide for premature infants after prolonged rupture of the membranes. J Pediatr 1995;126:450–453.

124. Skimming JW, Bender KA, Hutchison AA, Drummond WH. Nitric oxide inhalation in infants with respiratory distress syndrome. J Pediatr 1997;130:225–230.

125. Subhedar NV, Shaw NJ. Changes in oxygenation and pulmonary haemodynamics in preterm infants treated with inhaled nitric oxide. Arch Dis Child Fetal Neonatal Ed 1997;77:F191–F197.

126. Meurs KP, Rhine WD, Asselin JM, Durand DJ. Response of premature infants with severe respiratory failure to inhaled nitric oxide. Preemie NO Collaborative Group. Pediatr Pulmonol 1997;24: 319–323.

127. Gaston B, Drazen JM, Loscalzo J, Stamler JS. The biology of nitrogen oxides in the airway. Am J Respir Crit Care Med 1994;149:538–551.

128. Greenbaum R, Bay J, Hargreaves MD, et al. Effects of higher oxides of nitrogen on the anesthetized dog. Br J Anaesth 1967;39:393–404.

129. Stavert DM, Lehnert BE. Nitric oxide and nitrogen dioxide as inducers of acute pulmonary injury when inhaled at relatively high concentrations for brief periods. Inhal Toxicol 1990;2:53–67.

130. Clutton-Brock J. Two cases of poisoning by contamination of nitrous oxide with higher oxides of nitrogen during anaesthesia. Br J Anaesth 1967;39:388–392.

131. Austin AT. The chemistry of higher oxides of nitrogen as related to the manufacture, storage and administration of nitrous oxide. Br J Anaesth 1967;39:345–350.

132. Centers for Disease Control. Recommendations for occupational safety and health standard. MMWR 1988;37:21.

133. Hallman M, Bry K, Turbow R, Waffarn F, Lappalainen U. Pulmonary toxicity associated with nitric oxide in term infants with severe respiratory failure. J Pediatr 1998;132:827–829.

134. Glasson WA, Tuesday CS. The atmospheric thermal oxidation of nitric oxide. J Am Chem Soc 1963; 85:2901–2904.

135. Kain ML. Higher oxides of nitrogen in anaesthetic gas circuits. Br J Anaesth 1967;39,382–387.

136. Foubert L, Fleming B, Latimer R, et al. Safety guidelines for use of nitric oxide. Lancet 1992;339: 1615,1616.

137. Stamler JS, Singel DJ, Loscalzo J. Biochemistry of nitric oxide and its redox-activated forms. Science 1993;258:1898–1902.

138. Bouchet M, Renaudin MH, Raveau C, Mercier JC, Dehan M, Zupan V. Safety requirement for use of inhaled nitric oxide in neonates. Lancet 1993;341:968,969.

139. Miyamoto K, Aida A, Nishimura M, Nakano T, Kawakami Y, Ohmori Y, et al. Effects of humidity and temperature on nitrogen dioxide formation from nitric oxide. Lancet 1994;343:1099–1100.

140. Postlethwait EM, Langford SD, Bidani A. Kinetics of NO2 air space absorption in isolated rat lungs. J Appl Physiol 1992;73:1939–1945.

141. Freeman G, Crane SC, Furiosi NJ, Stephens RJ, Evans MJ, Moore WD. Covert reduction in ventilatory surface in rats during prolonged exposure to subacute nitrogen dioxide. Am Rev Respir Dis 1972;106: 563–579.

142. Shiel FO. Morbid anatomical changes in the lungs of dogs after inhalation of higher oxides of nitrogen during anaesthesia. Br J Anaesth 1967;39:413–424.

143. Williams RA, Rhoades RA, Adams WS. The response of lung tissue and surfactant to nitrogen dioxide exposure. Arch Intern Med 1971;l28:101–108.

144. Stephens RJ, Freeman G, Evans MJ. Early response of lungs to low levels of nitrogen dioxide. Arch Environ Health 1972;24:160–179.

145. Evans MJ, Stephens RJ, Cabral LJ, Freeman G. Cell renewal in the lungs of rats exposed to low levels of NO2. Arch Environ Health 1972;24:180–188.

146. Rasmussen TR, Kjaergaard SK, Tapp U, Pedersen OF. Delayed effects of NO2 exposure on alveolar permeability and glutathione peroxidase in healthy humans. Am Rev Respir Dis 1992;146:654–659.

147. Bylin G, Hedenstiema G, Lindvall T, Sundin B. Ambient nitrogen dioxide concentrations increase bronchial responsiveness in subjects with mild asthma. Eur Respir J 1988;1:606–612.

148. Frampton MW, Morrow PE, Cox C, Gibb FR, Speers DM, Utell MJ. Effects of nitrogen dioxide exposure on pulmonary function and airway reactivity in normal humana. Am Rev Respir Dis 1991;143: 522–527.

149. Morrow PE, Utell MJ, Bauer MA, Smeglin AM, Framton MW, Cox C, et al. Pulmonary performance of elderly normal subjects with chronic obstructive pulmonary disease exposed to 0.3 ppm nitrogen dioxide. Am Rev Respir Dis 1992;145:291–300.

150. Nishimura M, Hess D, Kacmarek RM, Ritz R, Hurford WE. Nitrogen dioxide production during mechanical ventilation with nitric oxide in adults. Effects of ventilator internal volume, air versus nitrogen dilution, minute ventilation, and inspired oxygen fraction. Anesthesiology 1995;82:1246–1254.

151. Aida A, Miyamoto K, Saito S, Nakano T, Nishimura M, Kawakami Y, et al. Effects of temperature and humidity on the stability of nitric oxide, and efficiency of soda lime as a selective absorber of nitrogen dioxide. Jpn J Thorac Dis 1995;33:306–311.

152. Dupuy PM, Shore SA, Drazen JM, Frostell C, Hill WA, Zapol WM. Bronchodilator action of inhaled nitric oxide in guinea pigs. J Clin Invest 1992;90:421–428.

153. Stenqvist O, Kjelltoft B, Lundin S. Evaluation of a new system for ventilatory administration of nitric oxide. Acta Anaesthesiol Scand 1993;37:687–691.

154. Pickett JA, Moors AH, Latimer RD, Mahmood N, Ghosh S, Oduro A. The role of soda lime during administration of inhaled nitric oxide. Br J Anaesth 1994;72:683–685.

155. Hibbs JB Jr, Taintor RR, Vavrin Z, Rachlin EM. Nitric oxide: a cytotoxic activated macrophage effector molecule. Biochem Biophys Res Commun 1988;157:87–94.

156. Stuehr DJ, Nathan CF. Nitric oxide: a macrophage product responsible for cytostasis and respiratory inhibition in tumor target cells. J Exp Med 1989;169:1543–1555.

157. Nguyen T, Brunson D, Crespi CL, Penman BW, Wishnok JS, Tannenbaum SR. DNA damage and mutation in human cells exposed to nitric oxide in vitro. Proc Natl Acad Sci USA 1992;89:3030–3034.

158. Oda H, Nogami H, Kisumoto S, Nakajima T, Kurata A. Long-term exposure to nitric oxide in mice. Nippon Eiseigaku Zasshi 1975;1:159.

159. Stamler JS, Jaraki O, Osborne J, Simon DI, Keaney J, Vita J, et al. Nitric oxide circulates in mammalian plasma primarily as an S-nitroso adduct of serum albumin. Proc Natl Acad Sci USA 1992;89:7674–7677.

160. Gibson QH, Roughton FJW. The kinetics and equilibria of the reactions of nitric oxide with sheep haemoglobin. J Physiol (Lond) 1957;136:507–526.

161. Toothill C. The chemistry of the in vivo reaction between hemoglobin and various oxides of nitrogen. Br J Anaesth 1967;39:405–412.

162. Kon K, Maeda N, Shiga T. Effect of nitric oxide on the oxygen transport of human erythrocytes. J Toxicol Environ Health 1977;2:1109–1113.

163. Azoulay E, Lachia L, Blayo MC, Pocidalo JJ. Methaemoglobinemia induced by nitric oxide in whole blood. Quantitative relationship. Toxicol Eur Res 1978;1:7–12.

164. Doyle MP, Pickering RA, DeWeert TM, Hoekstra JW, Pater D. Kinetics and mechanism of the oxidation of human doxyhemoglobin by nitrites. J Biol Chem 1981;256:12,393–12,398.

165. Maeda N, Imaizumi K, Kon K, Shiga T. A kinetic study on functional impairment of nitric oxide-exposed rat erythrocytes. Environ Health Perspec 1987;73:171–177.

166. Wennmalm A, Benthin G, Edlund A, Jungersten L, Kieler-Jensen N, Lundin S, et al. Metabolism and excretion of nitric oxide in humans. An experimental and clinical study. Circ Res 1993;73:1121–1127.

167. Iwamoto J, Krasney JA, Morin FC 3rd. Methemoglobin production by nitric oxide in fresh sheep blood. Respir Physiol 1994;96:273–283.

168. Curry S. Methemoglobinemia. Ann Emerg Med 1982;11:214–221.
169. Beutler E. Methemoglobinemia and sulfhemoglobinemia. In: Williams WJ, Beutler E, Erslev AJ, Rundles RW, eds. Hematology. McGraw-Hill, New York, 1977, pp. 291–494.
170. Young JD, Dyar O, Xiong L, Howell S. Methaemoglobin production in normal adults inhaling low concentrations of nitric oxide. Intensive Care Med 1994;20:581–584.
171. Wessel DL, Adatia I, Thompson JE, Hickey PR. Delivery and monitoring of inhaled nitric oxide in patients with pulmonary hypertension. Crit Care Med 1994;22,930–938.
172. von Nieding G, Wagner H, Kockeler H. Investigation of the acute effects of nitrogen monoxide on lung function in man. Staub-Reinhalt luft 1975;35:175–178.
173. Abman SH, Griebel JL, Parker DK, Schmidt JM, Swanton D, Kinsella JP. Acute effects of inhaled nitric oxide in children with severe hypoxemic respiratory failure. J Pediatr 1994;124:881–888.
174. McIntyre R, Moore F, Moore E, Piedalue F, Haenel J, Fullerton D. Inhaled nitric oxide variably improves oxygenation and pulmonary hypertension in patients with acute respiratory distress syndrome. J Trauma 1995;39:418–425.
175. Jacob TD, Nakayama DK, Seki I, Exler R, Lancaster JR Jr, Sweetland MA, et al. Hemodynamic effects and metabolic fate of inhaled nitric oxide in hypoxic piglets. J Appl Physiol 1994;76:1794–1801.
176. Channick RN, Newhart JW, Johnson FW, Moser KM. Inhaled nitric oxide reverses hypoxic pulmonary vasoconstriction in dogs. A practical nitric oxide delivery and monitoring system. Chest 1994;105:1842–1847.
177. Young JD, Dyar OJ, Xiong L, Zhang J, Gavaghan D. Effect of methylene blue on the vasodilator action of inhaled nitric oxide in hypoxic sheep. Br J Anaesth 1994;73:511–516.
178. Freeman B. Free radical chemistry of nitric oxide: looking at the dark side. Chest 1994;105:79S–84S.
179. Kooy NW, Royall JA. Agonist-induced peroxynitrite production from endothelial cells. Arch Biochem Biophysics 1994;310:352–359.
180. Westfelt UN, Benthin G, Lundin S, Stenqvist O, Wennmalm A. Conversion of inhaled nitric oxide to nitrate in man. Br J Pharmacol 1995;114:1621–1624.
181. Valvini EM, Young JD. Serum nitrogen oxides during nitric oxide inhalation. Br J Anaesth 1995;74. 338,339.
182. Mellion BT, Ignarro LJ, Ohlstein EH, Pontecorvo EG, Hyman AL, Kadowitz PJ. Evidence for the inhibitory role of guanosine 3'5'-monophosphate in ADP-induced human platelet aggregation in the presence of nitric oxide and related vasodilators. Blood 1981;57:946–955.
183. Radomski MW, Palmer RMJ, Moncada S. Endogenous nitric oxide inhibits human platelet adhesion to vascular endothelium. Lancet 1987;2:1057,1058.
184. Bassenge E. Antiplatelet effects of endothelium-derived relaxing factor and nitric oxide donors. Eur Heart J 1991;12:12–15.
185. Loscalzo J. Antiplatelet and antithrombotic effect of organic nitrates. Am J Cardiol 1992;70:18B–22B.
186. Radomski MW, Moncada S. Regulation of vascular homeostasis by nitric oxide. Thromb Haemost 1993;70:36–41.
187. Weber AA, Strobach J, Schror K. Direct inhibition of platelet function by organic nitrates via nitric oxide formation. Eur J Pharmacol 1993;247:29–37.
188. Högman M, Frostell C, Arnberg H, Hedenstierna G. Bleeding time prolongation and NO inhalation. Lancet 1993;341:1663–1665.
189. Watkins DN, Rankin JM, Clarke GM. Inhaled nitric oxide in severe acute respiratory failure—its use in intensive care and description of a delivery system. Anaesth Intens Care 1993;21:861–875.
190. Levy B, Bollaert PE, Bauer P, Nace L, Audibert G, Larcan A. Therapeutic optimization including inhaled nitric oxide in adult respiratory distress syndrome in a polyvalent intensive care unit. J Trauma 1995;38:370–374.
191. Putensen C, Rasanen J, Thomson MS, Braman RS. Method of delivering constant nitric oxide concentrations during full and partial ventilatory support. J Clin Monit 1995;11:23–31.
192. Tibballs J, Hochmann M, Carter B, Osborne A. An appraisal of techniques for administration of gaseous nitric oxide. Anaesth Intensive Care 1993;21:844–847.
193. Kirmse M, Hess D, Fujino Y, Kacmarek RM, Hurford WE. Delivery of inhaled nitric oxide using the Ohmeda I. NOvent delivery system. Chest 1998;113:1650–1657.
194. Miller OI, Celermajer DS, Deanfield JE, Macrae DJ. Guidelines for the safe administration of inhaled nitric oxide. Arch Dis Child 1994;70:F47–F49.
195. Betit P, Adatia I, Benjamin P, Thompson JE, Wessel DL. Inhaled nitric oxide: evaluation of a continuous titration delivery technique for infant mechanical and manual ventilation. Respir Care 1995;40: 706–715.

196. Skimming JW, Cassin S, Blanch PB. Nitric oxide administration using constant-flow ventilation. Chest 1995;108:1065–1072.
197. Roberts JD Jr, Lang P, Bigatello LM, Vlahakes GJ, Zapol WM. Inhaled nitric oxide in congenital heart disease. Circulation 1993;87:447–453.
198. Semigran MJ, Cockrill BA, Kacmarek R, Thompson BT, Zapol WM, Dec GW, et al. Hemodynamic effects of inhaled nitric oxide in heart failure. J Am Coll Cardiol 1994;24:982–988.
199. Snell GI, Salamonsen RF, Bergin P, Esmore DS, Khan S, Williams TJ. Inhaled nitric oxide used as a bridge to heart-lung transplantation in a patient with end-stage pulmonary hypertension. Am J Respir Crit Care Med 1995;151:1263–1266.
200. Hess D, Kacmarek R, Imanaka H, Bigatello L, Hurford W. Administration of inhaled nitric oxide by nasal cannula. Am J Respir Crit Care Med 1995;151:A44.
201. Grubb W, Putensen C, Thrush DR. Can nitric oxide be administered with a semiclosed anesthesia circuit? Anesthesiology 1994;81:A574.
202. Fontijin A, Sabadell AJ, Ronco RJ. Homogeneous chemiluminescent measurement of nitric oxide and ozone. Implications for continuous selective monitoring of gaseous air pollutants. Anal Chem 1970;42: 575–579.
203. Black F, Sigsby J. Chemiluminescent method for NO and NOx (NO + NO2) analysis. Environ Sci Technol 1974;8:149–152.
204. Matthews RD, Sawyer RF, Schefer RW. Interferences in chemiluminescent measurement of NO and NO_2 emissions from combustion systems. Environ Sci Technol 1977;12:1092–1096.
205. Zableiski MF, Seery DJ, Dodge LG. Influence of mass transport and quenching on nitric oxide chemiluminescent analysis. Environ Sci Technol 1984;l8:88–92.
206. Miller CC. Chemiluminescence analysis and nitrogen dioxide measurement. Lancet 1994;343:300,301.
207. Goldman AP, Macrae DJ. Nitrogen dioxide measurement in breathing systems. Lancet 1994;343:850.
208. Body SC, Hartigan PM, Shernan SK, Formanek V, Hurford WE. Nitric oxide: delivery, measurement, and clinical application. J Cardiothorac Vasc Anesth 1995;9:748–763.
209. Petros AJ, Cox PB, Bohn D. Simple method for monitoring concentration of inhaled nitric oxide. Lancet 1992;340:1167.
210. Mercier J, Zupan V, Deham M, Renaudin M, Bochet M, Raveau C. Device to monitor concentration of inhaled nitric oxide. Lancet 1993;342:431,432.
211. Petros AJ, Cox P, Bohn D. A simple method for monitoring the concentration of inhaled nitric oxide. Anaesthesia 1994;49:317–319.
212. Moutafis M, Hatahet Z, Castelain MH, Renaudin MH, Monnot A, Fischler M. Validation of a simple method assessing nitric oxide and nitrogen dioxide concentrations. Intensive Care Med 1995;21: 537–541.
213. Purtz EP, Hess D, Kacmarek RM. Evaluation of electrochemical nitric oxide analyzers suitable for use during mechanical ventilation. J Clin Monit 1997;13:25–34.
214. Etches PC, Harris ML, McKinley R, Finer NN. Clinical monitoring of inhaled nitric oxide: comparison of chemiluminescent and electrochemical sensors. Biomed Instrum Technol 1995;29:134–140.
215. Hess D, Kacmarek RM, Hurford WE. Inspired versus tracheal [NO]. Respir Care 1995;40.
216. Nishimura M, Tashiro C, Fujino Y, Imanaka H, Hess D, Kacmarek RM. Response of chemiluminescent analyzers on the measured value of nitric oxide (NO). Respir Care 1995;40:1186.
217. Imanaka H, Hess D, Kirmse M, Bigatello LM, Kacmarek RM, Steudel W, et al. Inaccuracies of nitric oxide delivery systems during adult mechanical ventilation. Anesthesiology 1997;86:676–688.
218. Clark R. CINGRI study. Pediatr Res, in press, 1999.
219. Fishman AP, McGoon MD, Chazova IE, Fedullo PF, Kneussel M, Peacock AJ, et al. Diagnosis and assessment of pulmonary hypertension. In: Rich S, ed. Executive Summary from the World Symposium—Primary Pulmonary Hypertension 1998, World Health Organization, Geneva, Switzerland. Available via the Internet (http://www.who.int/ncd/cvd/pph.html).
220. Robbins IM, Christman BW, Newman JH, Matlock R, Loyd JE. A survey of diagnostic practices and the use of epoprostenol in patients with primary pulmonary hypertension. Chest 1998;114:1269–1275.
221. Adatia I, Lillehei C, Arnold JH, Thompson JE, Palazzo R, Fackler JC, et al. Inhaled nitric oxide in the treatment of postoperative graft dysfunction after lung transplantation. Ann Thorac Surg 1994;57: 1311–1318.
222. Kieler-Jensen N, Ricksten SE, Stenqvist O, Bergh CH, Lindelov B, Wennmalm A, et al. Inhaled nitric oxide in the evaluation of heart transplant candidates with elevated pulmonary vascular resistance. J Heart Lung Transplant 1994;13:366–375.
223. Adatia I, Perry S, Landzberg M, Moore P, Thompson JE, Wessel DL. Inhaled nitric oxide and hemodynamic evaluation of patients with pulmonary hypertension before transplantation. J Am Coll Cardiol 1995;25:1656–1664.

224. Date H, Triantafillou AN, Trulock EP, Pohl MS, Cooper JD, Patterson GA. Inhaled nitric oxide reduces human lung allograft dysfunction. J Thorac Cardiovasc Surg 1996;111:913–919.

225. Auler JO Jr, Carmona M, Bocchi E, Bacal F, Fiorelli A, Stolf N, et al. Low doses of inhaled nitric oxide in heart transplant recipients. J Heart Lung Transplant 1996;15:443–450.

226. Allman K, Young J, Carapiet D, Stevens J, Ostman-Smith I, Archer L. Effects of oxygen and nitric oxide in oxygen on pulmonary arterial pressures of children with congenital cardiac defects. Pediatr Cardiol 1996;17:246–250.

227. Berner M, Berghetti M, Spahr-Schopfer I, Oberhansli I, Friedli B. Inhaled nitric oxide to test the vasodilator capacity of the pulmonary vascular bed in children with long-standing pulmonary hypertension and congenital heart disease. Am J Cardiol 1996;77:532–535.

228. Roze JC, Storme L, Zupan V, Morville P, Dinh-Xuan AT, Mercier JC. Echocardiographic investigation of inhaled nitric oxide in newborn babies with severe hypoxaemia. Lancet 1994;344:303–305.

229. Goldman AP, Delius RE, Deanfield JE, de Leval MR, Sigston PE, Macrae DJ. Nitric oxide might reduce the need for extracorporeal support in children with critical postoperative pulmonary hypertension. Ann Thorac Surg 1996;62:750–755.

230. Rich GF, Murphy GD Jr, Roos CM, Johns RA. Inhaled nitric oxide: selective pulmonary vasodilation in cardiac surgical patients. Anesthesiology 1993;78:1028–1035.

231. Fullerton DA, Jones SD, Jaggers J, Piedalue F, Grover FL, McIntyre RC Jr. Effective control of pulmonary vascular resistance with inhaled nitric oxide after cardiac operation. J Thorac Cardiovasc Surg 1996;111:753–762.

232. Channick RN, Newhart JW, Johnson FW, Williams PJ, Auger WR, Fedullo PF, et al. Pulsed delivery of inhaled nitric oxide to patients with primary pulmonary hypertension: an ambulatory delivery system and initial clinical tests. Chest 1996;109:1545–1549.

233. Channick RN. Chronic use of inhaled nitric oxide for pulmonary hypertension. Respir Care, in press, 1999.

234. Goldman AP, Pees PG, Macrae DJ. Is it time to consider domiciliary nitric oxide? Lancet 1995;345: 199,200.

235. Yoshida M, Taguchi O, Gabazza EC, Kobayashi T, Yamakami T, Kobayashi H, et al. Combined inhalation of nitric oxide and oxygen in chronic obstructive pulmonary disease. Am J Respir Crit Care Med 1997;155:526–529.

236. Roger N, Barbera JA, Roca J, Rovira I, Gomez FP, Rodriguez-Roisin R. Nitric oxide inhalation during exercise in chronic obstructive pulmonary disease. Am J Respir Crit Care Med 1997;156:800–806.

237. Högman M, Frostell CG, Hedenstrom H, Hedenstierna G. Inhalation of nitric oxide modulates adult human bronchial tone. Am Rev Respir Dis 1993;148:1474–1478.

238. Sanna A, Kurtansky A, Veriter C, Stanescu D. Bronchodilator effect of inhaled nitric oxide in healthy men. Am J Respir Crit Care Med 1994;150:1702–1704.

239. Kacmarek RM, Ripple R, Cockrill BA, Bloch KJ, Zapol WM, Johnson DC. Inhaled nitric oxide: a bronchodilator in mild asthmatics with methacholine-induced bronchospasm. Am J Respir Crit Care Med 1996;153:128–135.

240. Pfeffer KD, Ellison G, Robertson D, Day RW. The effect of inhaled nitric oxide in pediatric asthma. Am J Respir Crit Care Med 1996;153:747–751.

26 Antioxidants and Endothelium-Derived Nitric Oxide Action

Annong Huang and John F. Keaney, Jr.

NITRIC OXIDE: AUTOCRINE AND PARACRINE FUNCTIONS

In 1980, Furchgott and Zawadzki demonstrated the release of an endothelium-derived relaxing factor in isolated rabbit aorta with exposure to acetylcholine (ACh) (1). This factor has subsequently been identified as nitric oxide (NO•) (2) or a closely related redox form of NO• (3). It is now known that NO• is synthesized enzymatically from L-arginine and O_2 by a family of FAD- and FMN-containing enzymes, the nitric oxide synthases (NOSs), that require NADPH and tetrahydrobiopterin (BH_4) as cofactors (4). As a class of enzymes, the NOSs appear ubiquitous and have been identified in a number of mammalian cell types and tissues including endothelium (5), epithelium (6), neurons skeletal muscle (8), ventricular myocardium (9), and cytokine-stimulated inflammatory cells (10,11).

The widespread distribution of NOS enzymes is concordant with the role for NO• in an ever-increasing number of important cellular and tissue functions. In the heart, NO• is involved in parasympathetic control of myocardial contractility (12,13). Macrophage antimicrobial activity against fungal, protozoal, and bacterial pathogens is also mediated, in part, by NO• (14). In the brain, NO• mediates the action of glutamate acting on the N-methyl-D-aspartate (NMDA) receptor (15) and may also be involved in the control of aggression (16). At the molecular level, NO• has been implicated in the regulation of intracellular iron (17), the control of mitochondrial oxygen consumption (18), and the modulation of basic signaling pathways such as protein kinase C (PKC) activity (19). Thus, the production of NO• is ubiquitous in mammalian tissues and NO• acts as an important autocrine and paracrine mediator of cellular function.

One important function mediated by NO• is the local control of vascular homeostasis. In endothelial cells, NO• is normally produced by the endothelial isoform of NOS (eNOS) that is derived from the NOS3 gene (20). Unlike other NOS isoforms, eNOS is acylated and targeted to specialized invaginations of the plasmalemma termed caveolae (21,22). The interaction of eNOS with the "scaffolding" domain of caveolin-I (23) renders the enzyme catalytically inactive (24). In the presence of calcium, eNOS interacts with calmodulin permitting electron flow through the enzyme and the oxidation of L-arginine to form L-citrulline and NO• (24). The endothelial production of NO• is crucial in the control of vascular tone (25), blood pressure (25–27), and platelet adhesion to the endothelial surface (28).

Two principal mechanisms have been identified that are responsible for the biologic action of NO•. The first is binding NO• to the heme moiety of soluble guanylyl cyclase (sGC) producing an abrupt increase in intracellular 3',5'-cyclic guanosine monophosphate (cGMP) (29). This activation of GC appears critical for NO•-mediated vasodilation (30,31) and platelet inhibition (31,32). Under aerobic conditions, NO• can form oxides of nitrogen that react

From: *Contemporary Cardiology, vol. 4: Nitric Oxide and the Cardiovascular System*
Edited by: J. Loscalzo and J. A. Vita © Humana Press Inc., Totowa, NJ

with biologic thiols to form *S*-nitrosothiols *(3,33)*. This chemistry facilitates NO• activation of potassium channels *(34)* and calcium channels *(35,36)* as well as NO•-mediated modulation of hemoglobin oxygen affinity *(37)*.

Abnormalities of the NO• pathway are common features of many conditions that are manifested as vascular diseases. Defective NO•-mediated platelet inhibition has been associated with spontaneous arterial thrombosis *(38)*. NO•-mediated arterial relaxation is impaired in patients with atherosclerosis *(39)*, diabetes *(40)*, and hypertension *(41)*. These defects in the NO• pathway typically precede the clinical manifestations of vascular disease. For example, offspring of patients with coronary atherosclerosis demonstrate impaired NO• bioactivity *(42)*, as do individuals with risk factors for coronary artery disease (CAD) such as cigarette smoking *(43)*, advanced age *(44,45)*, and increased cholesterol *(44,45)*. In fact, impaired bioactivity of endothelium-derived NO• is so prevalent as an early feature of clinical vascular disease, it may be considered a premorbid condition that ultimately contributes to the clinical manifestations of CAD *(46,47)*.

OXIDATIVE STRESS IMPAIRS NO• ACTION

One important mechanism of impaired NO• action that we will discuss in great detail is excess oxidative stress. However, before we entertain any discussion of this term a few words pertaining to its definition are in order. As a descriptive term, it is woefully imprecise. Nevertheless, this term has received general acceptance as a reference to a wide range of damaging biochemical processes that occur in the course of oxidative metabolism in biologic systems. In this chapter, we use the definition first proposed by Helmut Sies *(48)*—that "oxidative stress" is an imbalance between oxidants and antioxidants in favor of the former. According to this definition, increased oxidative stress may result from either an excess of oxidants or a decrease in the availability of antioxidants. It is from this perspective that we will discuss the interaction between oxidative stress and NO• action. We will specifically focus on biologically relevant sources of oxidative stress with a primary emphasis on the vasculature.

SOURCES OF OXIDATIVE STRESS

Reactive Oxygen Species

As their name implies, all reactive oxygen species (ROS) are derived from oxygen, an obligate component of eukaryotic organisms. In its ground state, molecular oxygen is a diradical containing two unpaired electrons with parallel spins. In this state, any reaction of oxygen with a spin-paired substance will yield another diradical, thus, there is little stabilization energy to drive such reactions. As a consequence of this molecular orbital structure, ground-state oxygen is rather unreactive toward spin-paired species. In contrast, molecular oxygen reacts readily with other radicals (which have a single, unpaired electron) because electron spins will match 50% of the time producing a chemical bond that stabilizes two previously unpaired electrons.

The reactivity of molecular oxygen with spin-paired coreactants may be enhanced through several means. For example, the absorption of energy sufficient to promote one of the two unpaired electrons to a different orbital results in the formation of singlet oxygen. This chemical species is highly reactive toward spin-paired compounds, although its relevance for oxidative stress in biologic systems remains controversial *(49)*. Partial reduction of molecular oxygen also removes the spin restriction on its reactivity. A superoxide anion results from the addition of one electron to molecular oxygen as shown in reaction **1**. The entire spectrum of ROS can then be derived from sequential reduction of superoxide to yield hydrogen peroxide (H_2O_2), and finally, hydroxyl radical as outlined in reaction **1**.

$$O_2 + e\text{-} \Rightarrow O_2^{\bullet-} + e\text{-} \Rightarrow H_2O_2 + e\text{-} \Rightarrow {}^{\bullet}OH \qquad (1)$$

Superoxide

The reduction of molecular oxygen may arise as a result of leakage from the electron transport chain *(50)* or through the action of various oxidase enzymes such as xanthine oxidase *(51)*, cyclooxygenase *(52)*, lipoxygenase *(52)*, NADH oxidase *(53)* or NADPH oxidase *(54)*, and others. There is considerable evidence that superoxide is produced by a number of cell types during the course of normal oxidative metabolism. Neuronal cells *(55)*, inflammatory cells *(56)*, and fibroblasts *(57)* are all known to produce superoxide in vitro. In the vasculature, superoxide production has been detected in cultured endothelial cells *(58)*, smooth muscle cells (SMC) *(59)*, and monocytes *(60)*. Specific pathologic conditions such as inflammation *(56)*, diabetes *(61)*, hypertension *(62)*, and atherosclerosis *(63,64)*, are also characterized by an increased flux of superoxide.

In order to understand the oxidative stress induced by superoxide, one must consider the consequences of its increased flux in biologic tissues. In rats, chronic inhibition of Cu,Zn–SOD (superoxide dismutase) leads to an increased flux of superoxide that is associated with enhanced lipid peroxidation in vivo *(65)*. The precise mechanism for this observation is not entirely clear. In vitro, superoxide alone is unable to initiate lipid peroxidation *(66)*. Superoxide-mediated lipid peroxidation is completely dependent on a source of metal ions *(66,67)* or NO• *(67)*. The former facilitates the formation of hydroxyl radical (*see* following), whereas the latter leads to formation of peroxynitrite, a potent oxidant.

Peroxynitrite

Superoxide and NO• react readily in a diffusion-limited reaction ($k = 1.9 \times 10^{10} M^{-1}/s$) *(68)* to form peroxynitrite as depicted in reaction **2** *(69,70)*.

$$O_2^- + NO^• \Rightarrow O\text{-}O\text{-}N\text{=}O^- \tag{2}$$

$$H^+ + O\text{-}O\text{-}N\text{=}O^- \Rightarrow HO\text{-}O\text{-}N\text{=}O \tag{3}$$

This reaction is physiologically relevant as it is known to occur in vivo *(71,72)* and it has important implications for the propagation of oxidative stress. Peroxynitrite is rapidly protonated at physiologic pH according to reaction **3**, forming peroxynitrous acid, a potent oxidant *(73)*. This oxidant is quite promiscuous it can transfer oxygen atoms *(73)*, oxidize protein tyrosine residues *(74,75)* oxidize sulfhydryls *(76)*, and initiate lipid peroxidation *(77)*. Thus, peroxynitrite formation represents an important means of propagating superoxide-mediated oxidative stress.

Hydrogen Peroxide and Hydroxyl Radical

There are two principal mechanisms for the formation of hydrogen peroxide (H_2O_2) in biologic systems. The first involves a two-electron reduction of molecular oxygen as has been described for a number of enzymes including xanthine oxidase *(78)*, NADH oxidase *(79)*, and neuronal nitric oxide synthase (nNOS) *(80)*. The second and perhaps, most relevant means of H_2O_2 generation in vivo is the dismutation of superoxide either spontaneously or through the action of SOD *(78)*.

Once formed, H_2O_2 participates in two major oxidation reactions relevant to biologic systems. In the first of these reactions, H_2O_2 may oxidize sulfur atoms to the corresponding sulfoxide via S_N2 reaction of the sulfur with the O-O bond of H_2O_2 *(81)*. Similarly, H_2O_2 may oxidize reduced thiols to the corresponding disulfide or sulfenic acid *(81)*. The latter action of H_2O_2 may, in part, be responsible for the signaling functions that have been associated with cellular H_2O_2 production *(82)*. Alternatively, superoxide-derived H_2O_2 may promote one-electron oxidation reactions indirectly through the superoxide-driven Fenton reaction depicted in reactions **4–6**.

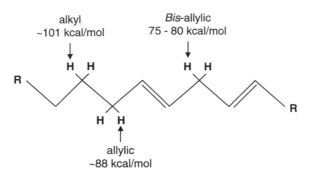

Fig. 1. Diagram of carbon–hydrogen bonds and bond dissociation energies in polyunsaturated fatty acid hydrocarbon backbone. Bond dissociation energies are derived from Koppenol *(254)*.

$$2O_2^{\cdot-} + 2H^+ \Rightarrow H_2O_2 + O_2 \tag{4}$$

$$H_2O_2 + H^+ + Fe^{2+} \Rightarrow OH^\cdot + H_2O + Fe^{3+} \tag{5}$$

$$O_2^{\cdot-} + Fe^{3+} \Rightarrow O_2 + Fe^{2+} \tag{6}$$

This process involves the dismutation of superoxide to H_2O_2 followed by the reduction of H_2O_2 to the hydroxyl radical ($^\cdot$OH) via the Fenton reaction, as shown in reactions **5** and **6**. Because superoxide can also reduce ferric iron to the ferrous state (as shown in reaction **6**), only catalytic amounts of iron are required for the formation of OH$^\cdot$ from $O_2^{\cdot-}$. Hydroxyl radical is extremely unstable (half-life approx 10^{-9} s) and a potent one-electron oxidant that will react indiscriminately with any adjacent molecule to extract a hydrogen atom *(81)*. Fenton chemistry has been implicated in a number of biologically important oxidation processes including protein oxidation *(83)* and lipid peroxidation *(81)*.

Lipid Peroxidation

In biologic systems, one common target for one-electron oxidation reactions is hydrogen abstraction from lipids found in membranes and lipoproteins. Phospholipids and cholesteryl esters that contain polyunsaturated fatty acids represent attractive targets for oxidizing species. This is due to the relatively low-bond dissociation energy for *bis*-allylic methylene carbon–hydrogen bonds (75–80 kcal/mol) compared to the corresponding monoallylic (approx 88 kcal/mol) and alkyl (101 kcal/mol) bonds *(84)* (Fig. 1). One-electron oxidation leads to the formation of a carbon-centered radical (Fig. 2) that may initiate the chain reaction of lipid peroxidation via the formation of alkoxyl (LO$^\cdot$) and lipid peroxyl radicals (LOO$^\cdot$) and the accumulation of lipid hydroperoxides (LOOH), as shown in Fig. 2.

The accumulation of lipid hydroperoxides in biological membranes and lipoproteins is not without consequence. LOOHs have similar chemical characteristics as H_2O_2 and generally participate in two-electron oxidation reactions such the oxidation of methionine to the sulfoxide *(85)*. Another important aspect of LOOHs is their breakdown into reactive aldehyde species *(86)*. In particular, LOOHs from lipoproteins and membranes are subject to decomposition into a range of reactive aldehydes such as malondialdehyde and 4-hydroxynonenal. These aldehydes react with a number of species including lysine groups to form Schiff bases that may covalently modify proteins *(87)*.

Other Sources of Oxidative Stress

Without question, there are many other sources for oxidative stress in biologic systems, many of which are beyond the scope of this discussion. At sites of inflammation, neutrophils secrete myeloperoxidase, a heme enzyme that produces a number of oxidizing species includ-

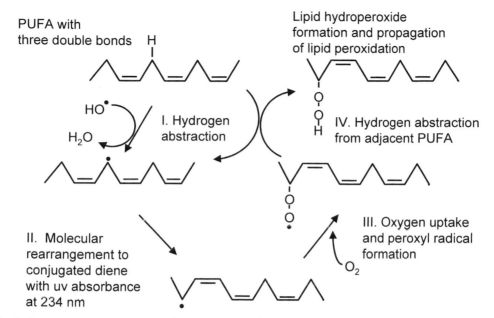

Fig. 2. Schematic representation of lipid peroxidation in polyunsaturated fatty acids (PUFAs). In this scheme, a prototypical PUFA with three double bonds undergoes one-electon oxidation (I) by a prototypical one electron oxidant (in this case hydroxyl radical) leading to molecular rearrangement and the formation of a conjugated diene (II) with a carbon-centered radical. This carbon-centered radical spontaneously combines with O_2 to form a lipid peroxyl radical (III) that abstracts hydrogen atoms from an adjacent PUFA (IV) and propagates the chain reaction of lipid peroxidation. Adapted from ref. *87* with permission.

ing hypochlorous acid (HOCl) and tyrosyl radical *(88,89)*. Emerging evidence also indicates that reactive nitrogen species such as nitrogen dioxide ($NO_2^\bullet$) or nitryl chloride ($CL-NO_2$) may form as a consequence of peroxidase-catalyzed oxidation of nitrite *(90)* or the reaction of nitrite with HOCL *(91)*. Thus, the sources of oxidative stress discussed in this chapter should by no means be considered exhaustive.

ANTIOXIDANTS AND NO° ACTION
Antioxidant Overview

The human body is endowed with a number of antioxidant defense mechanisms (Table 1). In general, the endogenous antioxidants can be divided into three major groups. The first, enzymatic antioxidants, represents the main form of intracellular antioxidant defense, and examples include SOD, catalase, and glutathione peroxidase. The second, nonenzymatic protein antioxidants, are primarily found in plasma and are represented by proteins such as transferrin, haptoglobin, and albumin. Finally, the nonenzymatic, low-molecular-weight antioxidants are found in plasma, other extracellular fluids, intracellular fluids, and lipoproteins and membranes. These nonenzymatic, low-molecular-weight antioxidants can be further subdivided into water-soluble and lipid-soluble antioxidants. Common examples of water-soluble antioxidants are ascorbic acid (vitamin C), glutathione, and uric acid. The lipid-soluble antioxidants are localized mainly to membranes and lipoproteins and include compounds such as α-tocopherol (the biologically and chemically most active form of vitamin E), β-carotene, and ubiquinol-10. These three main types of endogenous antioxidants all combine to provide protection against free radical species generated during normal oxidative metabolism and other oxidative insults. In the following pages, we discuss the role of these antioxidant species in the modulation of NO° action.

Table 1
Antioxidants in Human Blood Plasma

Antioxidant	Plasma or serum concentrations
Protein antioxidants	
Enzymatic	
CuZn-Superoxide dismutase (endothelium-derived)	5–20 IU/mL
Catalase	Not detectable
Glutathione peroxidase	0.4 U/mL
Nonenzymatic (binding of metal ions or metal ion-complexes)	
Albumin	50 g/L
Haptoglobin	0.5–3.6 g/L
Transferrin	1.8–3.3 g/L
Hemopexin	0.6–1.0 g/L
Ceruloplasmin	0.18–0.4 g/L
Lactoferrin	0.0002 g/L
Low-molecular-weight antioxidants	
Water-soluble	
Uric acid	160–450 μM
Ascorbic acid (vitamin C)	30–150 μM
Thiols (nonalbumin)	50–100 μM
Bilirubin	5–20 μM
Lipid-soluble (lipoprotein-associated)	
Vitamin E ($\alpha + \gamma$-tocopherol)	15–40 μM
Ubiquinol-10	0.4–1.0 μM
β-carotene (provitamin A)	0.3–0.6 μM
Lycopene	0.5–1.0 μM

Adapted from ref. 87 with permission.

Enzymatic Antioxidants

SUPEROXIDE DISMUTASE

Among the biological free-radical species, superoxide is perhaps the most important with respect to NO· signaling. As discussed earlier, superoxide and NO· react readily to form peroxynitrite as depicted in reaction 2 (69,70). Like NO·, peroxynitrite also activates the soluble form of guanylyl cyclase (92,93) although it does so much less effectively than NO· (93). Therefore, any interaction between NO· and superoxide effectively reduces the biologic activity of NO· that stems from changes in cellular cGMP. Because the reaction of NO· and superoxide is so facile, and many cells produce superoxide constitutively (58), it follows that the relative flux of either species in a given tissue should modulate the biologic activity of NO·. Available data supports this contention, Rubanyi and Vanhoutte demonstrated that SOD augments the endothelium-derived NO· response to ACh (Fig. 3) (94). In addition, the exposure of unstimulated endothelial cells to SOD produced relaxation of the bioassay ring, suggesting that basal endothelial superoxide production modulates endothelium-derived NO· action (94). Similar findings have been observed independently by other groups in superfused bioassay systems (95,96).

Vascular tissue contains considerable intra- and extracellular SOD activity as protection against superoxide leakage from normal oxidative metabolism (97). As a result, vascular SOD activity exerts considerable influence over the local activity of endothelium-derived NO· (98–100) and NO·-dependent vasodilators (99). Cultured endothelial cells exposed to diethyl-dithiocarbamate (DDC), a copper chelator that inhibits copper–zinc SOD (101), produce less

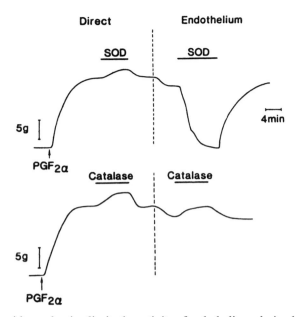

Fig. 3. Ambient superoxide production limits the activity of endothelium-derived nitric oxide. Tracings demonstrate tension in a bioassay ring contracted with 4 µM prostaglandin $F_{2\alpha}$ that is superfused with the effluent from an endothelialized arterial segment. In the top tracing, SOD (150 U/mL) applied directly to the bioassay ring has no effect but produces profound relaxation when applied to the endothelium, indicating that superoxide modulates the activity of endothelium-derived NO˙. In the lower tracing, application of catalase has no effect. Reprinted with permission from ref. *94*.

NO˙-mediated arterial relaxation than untreated cells despite similar production of inactive nitrogen oxides *(99)*. Similarly, DDC-treated bovine coronary arteries demonstrate impaired NO˙-mediated relaxation to ACh, or the NO˙-dependent vasodilators nitroprusside or nitroglycerin *(98)*. These data suggest that intact SOD activity is required for normal NO˙-mediated arterial relaxation, although the capacity of DDC to scavenge NO˙ through the formation of Fe(DDC)$_2$ and Fe(DDC)$_3$ complexes *(102)* makes interpretation of such experiments difficult. In this context, the rat model of dietary copper-deficiency merits some consideration. In vivo, the activity of copper–zinc SOD is dependent on the copper content of the enzyme *(103)* and rats rendered copper-deficient demonstrate impaired copper–zinc SOD activity *(65,104)*, an increased vascular superoxide flux *(65)* and impaired NO˙-mediated arterial relaxation *(65,105)*. Taken together, available evidence indicates that NO˙ bioactivity is modulated by the balance between NO˙ production and the local flux of superoxide.

Excessive vascular superoxide has been implicated in abnormal endothelium-derived NO˙ action in a number of disease states including hypercholesterolemia *(63)*, atherosclerosis *(106)*, hypertension *(107)*, and diabetes mellitus *(108,109)*. In hypercholesterolemic rabbits, blood vessels produce excess superoxide compared to normal controls *(63,64,110)* and dietary treatment of hypercholesterolemia normalizes both the vascular superoxide flux and the bioactivity of endothelium-derived NO˙ *(111)*. In light of such observations, one might predict that increasing vascular SOD activity should result in improved NO˙ bioactivity in disease states characterized by excess superoxide. Available data support this contention; atherosclerotic rabbits treated for 1 wk with polyethylene glycolated-SOD demonstrate increased vascular SOD activity and improved NO˙-mediated arterial relaxation to ACh compared to untreated animals *(112)* (Fig. 4). Similarly, acute treatment of arterial segments from atherosclerotic rabbits with liposome-encapsulated SOD also improves NO˙-mediated arterial relaxation *(106)*. The extent to which SOD manipulation restores endothelium-derived NO˙

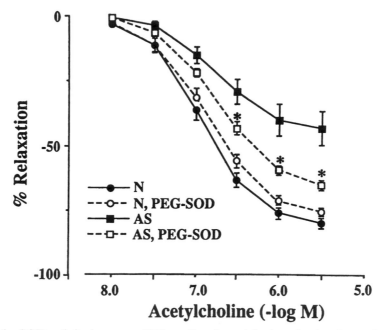

Fig. 4. Vascular SOD activity increases NO•-mediated arterial relaxation in atherosclerotic rabbits. Rabbits were fed either a normal diet (N) or an atherosclerotic diet (AS) containing 1% cholesterol for 4 mo. Half the animals in each dietary group were treated with polyethylene-glycolated super-oxide dismutase (PEG-SOD) for 1 wk before assessment of NO•-mediated arterial relaxation. Treat-ment with PEG-SOD improved NO•-mediated arterial relaxation induced by ACh in animals on the AS diet, but had no effect in normal animals. *$P < 0.05$ vs. PEG-SOD untreated animals. Reprinted with permission from ref. *112*.

bioactivity in hypercholesterolemia and atherosclerosis is highly dependent on the disease stage. Early stages of pathology tend to respond to SOD *(106,112)*, whereas advanced athero-sclerosis is largely insensitive to the status of vascular SOD activity *(113)*. Human studies have not demonstrated improved endothelium-derived NO• action with SOD treatment, presumably due to the limited access of SOD to the vascular wall *(114)*.

The impairment of NO• bioactivity in diabetes has also been linked, in part, to excess vascular superoxide. Diabetes is characterized by high levels of glucose, a monosaccharide with an α-hydroxyaldehyde structure that is subject to enediol rearrangement and the forma-tion of an enediol radical anion *(115)*. A general feature of enediol radical anions is the reduction of molecular oxygen to form superoxide *(115)*. Consistent with this known chemis-try, isolated rabbit arterial segments exposed to pathophysiologic levels of glucose (44 m*M*) demonstrate impaired NO•-mediated arterial relaxation to ACh that is normalized by SOD *(108)*. Autoxidation of glucose, however, does not provide a complete explanation for the effects of hyperglycemia on NO•-mediated arterial relaxation. Isolated arteries from chemi-cally induced diabetic rats *(109,116)* and rabbits *(108)* are characterized by impaired NO•-mediated arterial relaxation even under normal glucose conditions, and this defect is partially restored by SOD. One putative mechanism for this observation is increased superoxide pro-duction in the vascular wall such as that observed in the diabetic rat *(117)*, although the precise source of this increased superoxide flux is currently under investigation.

Hypertension is rapidly emerging as yet another vascular disease that has been linked to excess vascular oxidative stress. Early evidence for superoxide involvement in the pathogen-esis of hypertension was largely indirect. Hypertensive rats treated with SOD demonstrated a marked reduction in arterial pressure that is not observed with normal rats, prompting speculation that superoxide may have impaired the bioactivity of basal endothelial NO•

release leading to hypertension *(118)*. In light of recent observations that mice lacking eNOS are hypertensive *(27,119)*, and that some forms of hypertension are characterized by excess vascular superoxide *(107)*, such speculation would now seem justified. In particular, there is now strong evidence that hypertension mediated by angiotensin II involves some component of oxidative stress manifested by an increased ambient vascular flux of superoxide. Rats subjected to a 5-d infusion of angiotensin II demonstrate an increase in steady-state vascular superoxide leading to impaired NO•-mediated arterial relaxation that is mitigated, in part, by liposome-encapsulated SOD *(62)*. This phenomenon is specific to angiotensin II-mediated hypertension as equivalent increases in blood pressure due to chronic norepinephrine infusion are not characterized by an increase in vascular superoxide *(107)*. This effect of angiotensin II is due to induction of an NADH/NADPH oxidase activity in vascular smooth muscle cells (VSMC) *(62,120)* and liposome-encapsulated SOD lowers blood pressure in angiotensin II-treated animals *(107)*. In patients with essential hypertension, the situation appears more complex. Infusion of SOD has no effect on NO•-mediated arterial relaxation in response to ACh *(114)*, perhaps because of the limited access of SOD to the vascular wall.

Although there is consensus that ambient levels of vascular superoxide are an important determinant of NO• bioactivity, considerable debate remains as to the source of superoxide in the normal and diseased vascular wall. Staining of fixed normal rabbit arterial segments with nitroblue tetrazolium localizes superoxide generating activity to the endothelial and adventitial layers of the vascular wall *(121,122)*. Studies of cultured endothelial cells suggest that an NADH oxidoreductase is the principal source of superoxide *(123)*. In contrast, aortic adventitia principally contains an NADPH oxidoreductase activity *(121)* as well as a number of known NADPH oxidase subunits including p22phox, gp91phox, p47phox, and p67phox *(122)*. Other potential sources of superoxide such as cyclooxygenase *(52)*, lipoxygenase *(52)*, and xanthine oxidase *(124)* do not contribute importantly to vascular superoxide under resting conditions.

Sources of vascular superoxide appear more diverse under pathologic conditions. Xanthine oxidase has been implicated as an important source of superoxide with hypercholesterolemia. In isolated segments of cholesterol-fed rabbit aorta, the increased steady-state flux of superoxide is abrogated with endothelial denudation or oxypurinol, an inhibitor of xanthine oxidase *(63)*. Consistent with this observation, hypercholesterolemic patients treated with oxypurinol demonstrate a partial improvement in NO•-mediated arterial relaxation *(125)*. Although one could speculate from these data that hypercholesterolemia may upregulate endothelial xanthine oxidase activity *(63)*, other animal work indicates that hypercholesterolemia may be associated with increased circulating levels of xanthine oxidase that may bind to the vascular endothelium *(126)*. The precise role of circulating xanthine oxidase in human pathology remains to be determined.

One unique twist in the balance between superoxide and NO• is the observation that all NOS isoforms are capable of reducing molecular oxygen to produce superoxide. This was initially described for brain NOS under conditions where the L-arginine concentration is limiting *(127)*. Similar findings have also been reported for isolated eNOS *(128,129)* and cultured endothelial cells deprived of L-arginine *(130)*. These findings may have particular relevance for hypercholesterolemia-induced vascular superoxide generation as endothelial cells exposed to low-density lipoprotein (LDL) exhibit enhanced superoxide anion generation from eNOS *(131)*.

Combined evidence from biochemical, cell culture, and animal studies clearly indicates that the bioactivity of endothelium-derived NO• is highly dependent on the local availability of superoxide. In the setting of vascular diseases such as hypercholesterolemia, atherosclerosis, diabetes, and hypertension, the vascular levels of superoxide have an even more profound influence on NO• bioactivity, as the superoxide flux appears increased. Further work is needed to define precisely the role and contribution of superoxide to the modulation of NO• action.

In addition, more investigation will be required to identify the exact sources of excess superoxide anion and the signals involved in its generation.

CATALASE

Unlike superoxide, H_2O_2 does not react appreciably with $NO^•$ in any direct manner. As a consequence, the local concentration of H_2O_2 does not appear to modulate the action of $NO^•$ to the same degree as superoxide. That is not to say that H_2O_2 has no influence on $NO^•$ bioactivity; under specific conditions H_2O_2 does adversely affect $NO^•$-mediated arterial relaxation. In cat cerebral arterioles, transient exposure to physiologically relevant concentrations of H_2O_2 (0.1–3 μM) impaired $NO^•$-mediated arterial relaxation in response to ACh, sodium nitroprusside, or authentic $NO^•$, and this effect was reversed by SOD and catalase *(132)*. Similarly, cultured endothelial cells exposed to H_2O_2 demonstrate impaired $NO^•$ production even after all residual H_2O_2 is removed *(133)*. There are two potential mechanisms to explain the effect of H_2O_2 on $NO^•$ production. The first involves H_2O_2-mediated oxidation of intracellular thiols *(81)* that are required for normal endothelial $NO^•$ production *(134,135)*. Alternatively, H_2O_2 treatment of endothelial cells is associated with tyrosine phosphorylation of eNOS that results in a 50% reduction in its specific activity *(136)*. Catalase will prevent the effect of H_2O_2 in all of these experiments with an H_2O_2 challenge. In the absence of an H_2O_2-induced stress, however, endothelial cell catalase activity does not seem to be required for normal $NO^•$ production *(99)*.

GLUTATHIONE PEROXIDASE

Although H_2O_2 is subject to reduction by either catalase or glutathione peroxidase, organic hydroperoxides are detoxified principally by enzymes of the glutathione peroxidase family. This is a family of selenocysteine-containing proteins that reduce H_2O_2 and lipid hydroperoxides to their corresponding alcohols using glutathione as a source of reducing equivalents. This function of glutathione peroxidase may be relevant for $NO^•$ bioactivity, as organic hydroperoxides are an important source of lipid peroxyl radicals that combine readily with $NO^•$ (rate constant of $1–3 \times 10^9$ M^{-1}/s) *(137)* leading to the formation of peroxynitrite *(137)* or lipid peroxynitrite derivatives *(67,138)*. This reaction between $NO^•$ and lipid peroxyl radicals is thought to underlie observations that $NO^•$ inhibits lipid peroxidation in cells *(139)* and lipoproteins *(140)*. The role of peroxyl radicals in modulating $NO^•$ bioactivity, however, has not been studied in great detail. Rabbit arteries exposed to the model organic hydroperoxides, cumene hydroperoxide, or *tert*-butyl hydroperoxide demonstrate an abrupt increase in tension and a reduction in smooth muscle cell cGMP production, suggesting an acute loss of endothelium-derived $NO^•$ action *(141)*. Platelet aggregation involves the consumption of oxygen *(142)*, the production of ROS, and the formation of lipid hydroperoxides *(143)*. Observations that $NO^•$-mediated inhibition of platelet aggregation is potentiated by glutathione peroxidase suggests that reduction of lipid hydroperoxides enhances $NO^•$ bioactivity *(144)*.

The role of glutathione peroxidase in modulating $NO^•$ bioactivity is not restricted to the reduction of organic hydroperoxides. The reduction of H_2O_2 by glutathione peroxidase proceeds in the presence of either authentic glutathione or S-nitroso-glutathione and, with the latter, $NO^•$ is liberated *(144)*. Recent data indicate that this phenomenon is not specific for either glutathione peroxidase or S-nitroso-glutathione. A number of selenium-containing compounds such as selenocystine and selenocystamine also catalyze the decomposition of several different S-nitrosothiols resulting in the liberation of $NO^•$ *(145)*. Moreover, the decomposition of S-nitroso-glutathione by glutathione peroxidase does not appear to require the presence of any peroxide *(145)*. Thus, glutathione peroxidase may modulate the bioactivity of $NO^•$ either through the reduction of organic hydroperoxides or the decomposition of endogenous S-nitrosothiols resulting in the liberation of $NO^•$.

There is also a role for $NO^•$ in the modulation of glutathione peroxidase activity. $NO^•$ has been reported to inactivate bovine glutathione peroxidase in a dose- and time-dependent manner

(146). Subsequent studies have demonstrated that peroxynitrite (in the absence of glutathione) inactivates glutathione peroxidase through the oxidation of selenocysteine *(147)*. The relevance of such findings for events in vivo, however, remains to be determined, as glutathione peroxidase actually functions as a peroxynitrite reductase in the presence of glutathione *(148)*.

Lipid-Soluble, Low-Molecular-Weight Antioxidants

Lipid peroxidation is an important source of oxidative stress. This is particularly true with atherosclerotic vascular disease and its associated conditions such as hypercholesterolemia, diabetes, and hypertension. Atherosclerosis is associated with LDL deposition and lipid peroxidation in the subintimal space of the arterial wall (for review, *see* refs. *48* and *150*). This accumulation of oxidized-LDL (ox-LDL) in the arterial wall has a number of important implications for NO· bioactivity. For example, ox-LDL stimulates the recruitment of intimal monocytes and macrophages to the arterial wall leading to the release of ROS that, as discussed before, may impair NO· bioactivity *(94,95)*. Formation of ox-LDL may also reduce the availability of NO· through its cytotoxic effects against endothelial cells *(149)*. The process of lipid peroxidation in LDL also has profound effects on the release of NO· from endothelial cells. Normal arteries acutely exposed to ox-LDL demonstrate impaired endothelium-derived NO·-mediated arterial relaxation *(150–152)*. Potential mechanisms for these observations include direct chemical inactivation of NO· *(153)*, impairment of G-protein-mediated signal transduction *(150,152,154)* and inhibition of guanylyl cyclase *(155)*.

Given the potential for lipid peroxidation to impair NO· bioactivity in the setting of vascular disease, it is reasonable to speculate that reducing vascular lipid peroxidation by bolstering antioxidant defenses should improve NO· bioactivity. In the following sections, the evidence to support an effect of vascular antioxidant status on endothelium-derived NO· is reviewed. Particular attention is directed at the vascular wall antioxidant status, as this is the principal site of vascular pathology.

α-Tocopherol and β-Carotene

Lipid-soluble, low-molecular-weight antioxidants inhibit lipid peroxidation *(156)*, although the activity of β-carotene in this regard is controversial *(157,158)*. In order to evaluate the role of lipid-soluble antioxidants in modulating NO· bioactivity in atherosclerosis, we examined the effects of α-tocopherol and β-carotene on endothelial vasodilator dysfunction in a cholesterol-fed rabbit model. Consumption of a 1% cholesterol diet in rabbits is typically associated with marked impairment in endothelium-dependent, NO·-mediated arterial relaxation *(159)*. We found that cholesterol-fed rabbits supplemented with β-carotene or α-tocopherol demonstrated normal NO·-mediated arterial relaxation in response to ACh and A23187 *(160)* (Fig. 5). This effect on NO·-mediated arterial relaxation could not be explained by any effects of antioxidants on lipoprotein profiles or the extent of atherosclerosis *(160)*. Similar findings have been reported in the coronary *(161)* and carotid *(162)* arteries of cholesterol-fed rabbits as well as the aorta of rats fed a high-fat diet *(163)*. In hypercholesterolemic rats, a combined deficiency of α-tocopherol and selenium, an essential cofactor for glutathione peroxidase, is associated with NO·-mediated arterial relaxation *(164)*. Taken together, these data indicate that antioxidant protection in vivo is important in maintaining normal NO· bioactivity in the setting of hypercholesterolemia and atherosclerosis.

Lipid-soluble antioxidants such as α-tocopherol localize mainly to membranes and lipoproteins where they serve to limit lipid peroxidative damage *(165)*. Because LDL oxidation produces impaired NO· bioactivity, and α-tocopherol can inhibit ex vivo LDL oxidation *(166)*, one might speculate that lipid-soluble antioxidants may preserve NO· bioactivity through decreased oxidative modification of LDL. To address this issue, we treated cholesterol-fed rabbits with two different dietary regimens of α-tocopherol *(167)*. As expected, the lowest dose of α-tocopherol (110 IU/d) reversed the effect of cholesterol feeding on NO·-mediated

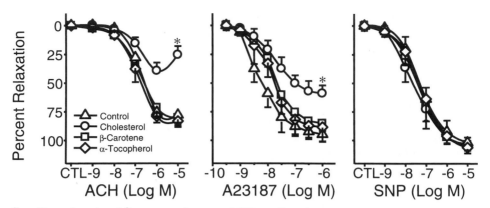

Fig. 5. α-Tocopherol and β-carotene improve NO•-mediated arterial relaxation in cholesterol-fed rabbits. Aortic rings from rabbits fed chow (△), 1% cholesterol (○), 1% cholesterol with β-carotene (□), and 1% cholesterol with α-tocopherol (◇) were exposed to increasing concentrations of ACh (A), calcium ionophore A23187 (B), or SNP (C). NO•-mediated arterial relaxation to ACh and A23187 was impaired in cholesterol-fed rabbits, whereas α-tocopherol- or β-carotene-treated animals demonstrated normal arterial relaxation. *$p < 0.001$ compared to chow-fed animals. Reprinted with permission from ref. *160.*

arterial relaxation and protected LDL from copper-mediated oxidation ex vivo *(167).* In contrast, a 10-fold greater dose of α-tocopherol (1100 IU/d) actually worsened NO• bioactivity despite continued protection of LDL against ex vivo copper-mediated oxidation *(167).* Thus, antioxidant protection of LDL is not sufficient to preserve NO•-mediated bioactivity in the setting of cholesterol feeding.

Although α-tocopherol is an efficient scavenger of lipid peroxyl radicals, it is now clear that lipid peroxidation in the vascular wall does occur in the presence of α-tocopherol during atherosclerosis *(168).* It is possible, therefore, that α-tocopherol may preserve NO• bioactivity by preventing the deleterious effects of ox-LDL on vascular cells. There is now considerable evidence to suport this contention. Isolated arterial segments from α-tocopherol-deficient animals demonstrate impaired NO•-mediated arterial relaxation after exposure to ox-LDL *(151).* Arterial segments derived from animals supplemented with α-tocopherol, however, exhibit a marked resistance to endothelial dysfunction from ox-LDL *(151).* The same holds true for isolated endothelial cells in culture *(169).* This impairment of NO•-mediated arterial relaxation by ox-LDL results from PKC stimulation, a known consequence of ox-LDL exposure to vascular tissue *(170).* Incorporation of α-tocopherol into endothelial cells prevents PKC stimulation by ox-LDL (Fig. 6), thereby preserving NO•-mediated arterial relaxation *(151).* A similar effect on PKC activity has been observed with α-tocopherol incorporation into smooth muscle cells *(171)* and platelets *(172).*

The role of α-tocopherol in preserving NO• bioactivity is not limited to models of atherosclerosis. Diabetes mellitus is another chronic disease that involves hyperglycemia, increased oxidative stress *(173),* and impaired NO•-mediated arterial relaxation *(40,108).* Chronic treatment of streptozotocin-induced diabetic rats with vitamin E preserves NO•-mediated arterial relaxation in isolated aorta *(174–176)* and perfused coronary arteries *(177),* but not in mesenteric arteries *(178).* There is also some role for vitamin E in preserving NO• action in the absence of vascular disease. Vitamin E-deprived rats demonstrated impaired NO•-mediated arterial relaxation that appears to result from an increase in vascular superoxide *(179).*

PROBUCOL

Probucol, a cholesterol-lowering compound, is a dimer of the common antioxidant butylated hydroxytoluene containing two phenolic hydroxy groups providing for efficient hydrogen atom donation and antioxidant activity. Being lipid-soluble, probucol is transported in

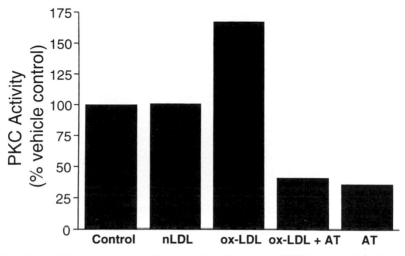

Fig. 6. Endothelial cell incorporation of α-tocopherol prevents PKC stimulation due to oxidized LDL Human aortic endothelial cells were loaded with α-tocopherol (AT) or vehicle for 3 d, washed, and incubated with oxidized LDL (ox-LDL; 300 µg/mL), native LDL (nLDL; 300 µg/mL), or media alone (control) for 4 h. Cells were then washed three times with Hank's balanced salt solution and PKC activity determined with an *in situ* assay *(255)* normalized to control conditions. Reproduced from ref. *151* by copyright permission of the American Society for Clinical Investigation.

plasma primarily in lipoproteins *(180)* and does accumulate in the vascular wall *(64,181)*. Probucol inhibits LDL oxidation in a number of oxidizing systems *(180,182)*, principally as a consequence of the LDL–probucol content *(183)*. On a molar basis, probucol has only one-third the lipid peroxyl radical scavenging activity of α-tocopherol *(184)*, and it unequivocally inhibits atherosclerosis in hypercholesterolemic rabbits *(181,185,186)*, but not mouse models of atherosclerosis *(187)*.

The effect of probucol on endothelium-derived NO• action has been examined in cholesterol-fed *(164,188)* and LDL receptor-deficient *(189)* rabbits. In these studies, probucol treatment did not significantly alter plasma cholesterol, but did prevent the increase in plasma *(188,190)* and aortic lipid peroxides *(164)* associated with cholesterol feeding. Probucol treatment was associated with preserved NO• bioactivity as assessed by endothelium-dependent arterial relaxation in response to ACh or A23187 *(64)*. In normocholesterolemic animals, probucol did not alter NO• bioactivity *(188)*, suggesting that this effect of probucol is specific for mechanisms that depend on increased oxidative stress. This contention is supported by observations that probucol treatment of rabbits with alloxan-induced diabetes is also associated with improved NO• bioactivity as determined by endothelium-dependent arterial relaxation *(108)*.

Other studies have shed light on the mechanism of probucol action in cholesterol-fed rabbits. Probucol treatment is associated with a reduction in the vascular flux of superoxide *(64,190)* that is known to accompany cholesterol feeding in rabbits *(63)* (Fig. 7). This reduction in vascular superoxide inhibits lipid peroxidation *(64,190)* and lysophosphatidylcholine *(64)* accumulation in the arterial wall, two phenomena that have been associated with reduced NO• bioactivity *(65,154)*. In these models of hypercholesterolemia, probucol treatment had no significant effect on the extent of intimal proliferation or arterial cholesterol content (two indices for the extent of atherosclerosis) *(64)*.

HUMAN STUDIES

Human studies of lipid-soluble antioxidants and NO• bioactivity have been both sparse and mixed. Hypercholesterolemic patients treated with vitamin E (400 IU/d) or probucol

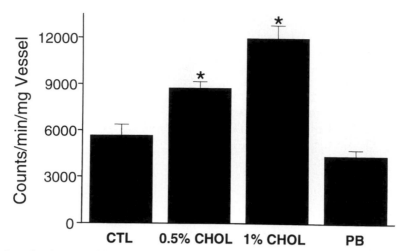

Fig. 7. Probucol reduces ambient vascular superoxide in cholesterol-fed rabbits. Segments of thoracic aorta were harvested from animals fed diets consisting of standard chow (CTL), chow with 0.5% cholesterol (0.5% CHOL), chow with 1% cholesterol (1% CHOL), or chow with 1% cholesterol and 1% probucol (PB). Vessel copper–zinc SOD activity was inhibited by incubating vessels with diethyldithiocarbamate for 30 min and prior to the assessment of superoxide using lucigenin chemiluminescence. * $P < 0.05$ vs CTL by analysis of variance (ANOVA). Reproduced from ref. *164* by copyright permission of the American Society for Clinical Investigation.

(500 mg/d) for a period of 8 wk did not demonstrate any improvement in NO•-mediated arterial relaxation of forearm resistance vessels *(191)*. Similarly, Gilligan and colleagues treated hypercholesterolemic patients with a cocktail of vitamin E (800 IU/d), vitamin C (1000 mg/d), and β-carotene (30 mg/d) for 1 mo and found no effect on resistance vessel NO•-mediated arterial relaxation *(192)*. Similar results have been reported in vitamin E-treated patients that had recently suffered a myocardial infaction *(193)*.

Recent reports with antioxidants and NO•-mediated arterial relaxation in conduit arteries have been more positive. Postmenopausal women treated with estrogen demonstrate an improvement in NO•-dependent, flow-mediated dilation of the brachial artery *(194)* and a similar effect has been observed with α-tocopherol (800 IU/d) *(195)*. Abnormally high remnant lipoprotein levels are associated with impaired NO•-bioactivity in the brachial artery that is improved with α-tocopherol supplementation *(196)*. In patients with coronary spastic angina, NO•-mediated arterial relaxation in the coronary artery is impaired but can be normalized by treatment with α-tocopherol *(197)*. Thus, studies of human conduit arteries indicate that there is a salutory effect of α-tocopherol that normalizes NO• bioactivity.

Recent data also indicate that lipid-soluble antioxidants may act synergistically with cholesterol reduction therapy. Neunteufl and colleagues found that treatment of hypercholesterolemic patients with a combination of α-tocopherol (300 IU/d) and a cholesterol-lowering drug (simvastatin) over 4 wk provided an additional benefit over and above that of simvastatin alone *(198)*. In studies of the coronary circulation, Anderson and coworkers found that probucol improved NO•-mediated arterial relaxation in patients treated with the lipid-lowering drug lovastatin compared with the combination of cholestryramine and lovastatin *(199)*. These observations suggest that the effect of lipid-soluble antioxidants on NO• bioactivity in patients may depend, in part, on the cholesterol status of these patients.

Water-Soluble, Low-Molecular-Weight Antioxidants

Although it is clear that the cellular and vascular wall content of lipid-soluble antioxidants is an important component of vascular antioxidant protection, it is important to realize that these lipid-soluble compounds represent only part of the cellular antioxidant defenses. The remainder of cellular antioxidant protection is provided by the water-soluble antioxidants. The main water-soluble antioxidants in cells and tissues are glutathione (GSH) and ascorbic acid. GSH is present in plasma at very low concentrations (<0.3 μM) *(200)*, whereas GSH concentrations within the cell cytosol range from 1–5 mM *(201)*. Vitamin C is normally present at concentrations of 30–150 μM in plasma *(87)* and, like GSH, is present within the cell at concentrations up to 5 mM *(202)*. There is considerable evidence that both vitamin C and GSH are strictly required for normal cellular function. For example, all cells appear to demonstrate the active transport and/or synthesis of both GSH and vitamin C. Animals deprived or depleted of either vitamin C or GSH become morbid and die *(203,204)*. In light of the critical role of both vitamin C and GSH for intracellular redox state, it is not surprising that both species could have important implications for NO• bioactivity.

GLUTATHIONE

Considerable controversy exists over the role of intracellular GSH in the action and metabolism of NO• elaborated from endothelial cells. Early studies with the inducible isoform of NOS (iNOS) suggested that GSH was required as a cofactor for NO• production *(205)*. Similar studies in endothelial cells produced mixed results. Hecker and colleagues found that bradykinin-induced release of NO• from cultured bovine endothelial cells was impaired by alkylating thiols with *N*-ethylmaleimide (NEM) or oxidizing intracellular thiols with 2,2'-dithiodipyridine (DTDP) *(206)*. Although these findings were consistent with a role for GSH in eNOS activity, treatment with DTDP was not associated with a demonstrable reduction in endothelial cell GSH *(206)*, suggesting that the level of intracellular thiols per se is not important in the release of NO•. The oxidation state of critical thiols involved in Ca^{2+} homeostasis was proposed as an alternative factor responsible for the effects of NEM and DTDP *(206)*. Other studies with cultured porcine *(207)* or bovine *(99)* endothelial cells failed to demonstrate a correlation between thiol depletion and NO• production. Taken together, these studies provided no clear evidence that GSH is required for the production of bioactive NO•.

One important consideration in such studies may be the species from which cells were derived. In this regard, Ghigo and colleagues *(134)* used human umbilical vein endothelial cells to study the effect of thiol manipulation on endothelial cell NO• production. These investigators reduced intracellular GSH levels with 1-chloro-2,4 dinitrobenzene (CDNB), a compound that forms a covalent complex with GSH through glutathione-S-transferase activity. Treatment of endothelial cells with CDNB was associated with a dose-dependent reduction of both cellular GSH and NO• production *(134)*. Conversely, bolstering cellular GSH with glutathione monoethyl ester enhanced NO• production that was strongly correlation with cellular GSH ($r = .992$).

Recent human studies support a role for GSH in the bioactivity of endothelium derived NO•. Patients with CAD are known to demonstrate impaired NO•-mediated arterial relaxation in the conduit arteries of the coronary *(39)* and brachial *(208)* circulation. Manipulation of intracellular GSH levels in such patients appears to alter NO•-mediated arterial relaxation. Specifically, CAD patients treated with L-2-oxo-4-thiazolidine carboxylate, a compound that selectively increases intracellular GSH *(209,210)*, produced improved endothelium-dependent NO•-mediated arterial relaxation in the brachial artery *(211)* (Fig. 8). This effect was specific for the endothelium as nitroglycerin-mediated arterial relaxation was unaffected. Thus, there appears to be some role for intracellular GSH in the control of NO• bioactivity, at least in the setting of a known impairment in NO•-mediated arterial relaxation.

The precise mechanism(s) by which intracellular GSH may modulate the production and/or bioactivity of NO• is not yet clear. Isolated enzyme preparations of both neuronal *(212,213)* and iNOS *(205)* demonstrate optimal enzymatic activity in the presence of GSH. With nNOS, this enhanced activity is associated with the direct binding of thiol compounds to the heme moiety in a manner that is facilitated by BH_4 *(214)*. Another potential role of GSH may be

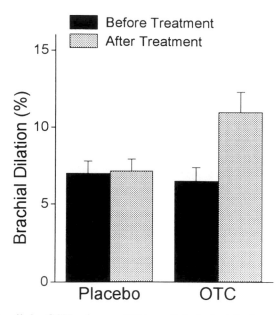

Fig. 8. Increasing intracellular GSH enhances NO·-mediated arterial relaxation in the brachial artery of patients with CAD. Patients with established CAD were randomized to receive L-2–oxo-4–thiazolidine carboxylate (OTC) or placebo. Both before and 4 h after treatment NO·-mediated arterial relaxtion was assessed in the brachial artery using vascular ultrasound. The effect of OTC was significant by repeated measures ANOVA ($P < 0.005$). Reproduced from ref. *211* by copyright permission of the American Society for Clinical Investigation.

to prevent inactivation of NOS that likely results from the formation of peroxynitrite during simultaneous generation of NO· and superoxide by the enzyme *(215)*.

The antioxidant activity of GSH may also indirectly influence the enzymatic activity of NOS. The NOS cofactor, BH_4, is readily oxidized, and thiol compounds have been shown to protect BH_4 from oxidation *(216,217)*. Moreover, endothelial L-arginine transport is sensitive to adequate intracellular GSH levels *(218)*. The potential effect(s) of intracellular GSH on cellular NOS cofactor levels has important implications for NO· production as a relative lack of either BH_4 *(80)* or L-arginine *(127,130)* reduces enzymatic efficiency and stimulates NOS-mediated oxidant production, particularly superoxide *(129)*.

Another consideration for the role of GSH in NO· bioactivity relates to *S*-nitrosothiols. Once formed, NO· can combine with oxygen to form oxides of nitrogen that react with biologic thiols to form *S*-nitrosothiols *(219)*, compounds that possess bioactivity reminiscent of authentic NO· *(3,220)*. The relative abundance of GSH among intracellular thiol species available for *S*-nitrosothiol formation renders the formation of S-nitroso-glutathione (GSNO) kinetically feasible *(221,222)* and GSNO formation has been implicated in cellular functions such as neutrophil glucose metabolism and oxidant production *(223)*. To the extent that GSNO formation contributes to NO· bioactivity—admittedly a matter of some controversy—intracellular GSH levels may modulate the extent of GSNO formation. Thus, there are many potential mechanisms through which GSH has the potential to modulate NO· bioactivity.

Other Thiols

There is considerable evidence linking biologic thiols to the action of endothelium-derived NO·. The synthetic thiol, *N*-acetylcysteine, increases intracellular glutathione concentrations and potentiates platelet inhibition by endothelium-derived NO· *(224)*. Furthermore, vasodilation due to flow-mediated endothelial NO· release is also potentiated by reduced thiol *(225)*. Albumin, the most abundant source of thiol in plasma *(226)*, also forms adducts

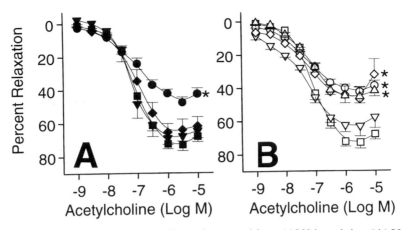

Fig. 9. Ascorbic acid fails to prevent the effect of superoxide on NO• bioactivity. (**A**) Vessels were contracted with phenylephrine (1 μM) and NO• bioactivity assayed as relaxation in response to ACh in the presence of no additions (■), superoxide from 200 μM pyrogallol (●), 200 μM pyrogallol with 300 IU/mL SOD (◆), or 300 IU/mL SOD alone (▼). (**B**) Vessels were contracted and NO• bioactivity assayed as relaxation to ACh in the presence of no additions (□), 200 μM pyrogallol (○), or 200 μM pyrogallol with 0.1 (△), 1.0 (◇), or 10 (▽) mM ascorbic acid. *$P < 0.05$ vs. no additions only by two-way ANOVA.

with nitrogen oxides and these adducts possess NO• bioactivity *(220,227)*. Moreover, the biologic half-life of these adducts exceeds that of authentic NO• *(3)*. Thus it is conceivable that thiols may promote adduct formation with nitrogen oxides and may, in this manner, promote the bioactivity of NO•. The biologic relevance of such adduct formation, however, remains to be determined.

Ascorbic Acid

Among the most effective water-soluble antioxidants in human tissues and extracellular fluids is ascorbic acid *(228)*. Ascorbic acid is an extremely versatile antioxidant and that effectively scavenges a wide variety of radical species and oxidants, including superoxide, H_2O_2, aqueous peroxyl radicals, hydroxyl radicals, HOCl, and singlet oxygen *(229–232)*.

The effect of ascorbic acid on NO•-mediated arterial relaxation has been examined in human subjects with impaired NO• bioactivity. Ting and colleagues found that NO•-mediated forearm blood flow responses to methacholine were enhanced with a concomitant infusion of ascorbic acid in patients with type II diabetes *(233)* or hypercholesterolemia *(234)*. In chronic smokers with impaired NO•-mediated arterial relaxation, Heitzer and co-workers found that an acute arterial infusion of ascorbic acid normalized NO•-mediated forearm blow flow responses to ACh *(235)*. Similar results have been reported in the brachial arteries of patients with heart failure *(236)* and hypertension *(237)*.

The specific mechanisms responsible for the effect of ascorbic acid on NO• bioactivity remain under investigation. Given that ascorbic acid is a potent scavenger of superoxide *(229)*, and superoxide is a major mechanism of impaired NO• bioactivity (*see* earlier), many have speculated that ascorbic acid improves NO• bioactivity through superoxide scavenging *(233–236)*. Recent studies suggest this line of reasoning may be too simplistic. In isolated arterial segments, superoxide from a variety of sources will readily impair NO•-mediated arterial relaxation and this effect is reversed by physiologic concentrations (approx 1–3 μM) of SOD *(94–96,238)*. In contrast, physiologic concentrations of ascorbic acid (<10 mM) fail to inhibit the impairment of NO• bioactivity by superoxide in isolated arterial segments *(238)* (Fig. 9). Competing reactions with disparate kinetics provide a plausible explanation for such observations. The bimolecular rate constant for the reaction of superoxide with ascorbate is

$2.7 - 3.3 \times 10^5\ M^{-1}s^{-1}$ *(229,239)*, approximately 10^5-fold less than the rate at which super-oxide reacts with either SOD ($2 \times 10^9\ M^{-1}s^{-1}$) *(78)* or NO$^\bullet$ ($1.9 \times 10^{10}\ M^{-1}s^{-1}$) *(68)*. In order for ascorbic acid to compete effectively with NO$^\bullet$ for superoxide, the concentration of ascor-bic acid must exceed that of NO$^\bullet$ by a factor of 10^5. Considering that NO$^\bullet$ has been detected at concentrations of approx $0.1–1.0\ \mu M$ adjacent to endothelial cells in culture *(240)* and in rabbit aorta *(241)*, one would predict that a concentration of $10^5 \times (0.1 - 1.0)\ \mu M \cong 10 - 100\ mM$ ascorbic acid is required to prevent the interaction of NO$^\bullet$ and superoxide. This value is in excellent agreement with recent experimental data *(238)* and far exceeds what would be considered physiologically relevant ($<10\ mM$). Thus, although ascorbic acid is an efficient scavenger of superoxide, the *rate* of this reaction is insufficient to compete effectively with NO$^\bullet$ for superoxide at anything less than supraphysiologic concentrations.

There is data to suggest that physiologically relevant concentrations of ascorbic acid have important implications for NO$^\bullet$ bioactivity. We have examined the effect of oral ascorbic acid administration on NO$^\bullet$-mediated arterial relaxation in patients with documented CAD and impaired NO$^\bullet$ bioactivity *(242)*. In these patients, a single oral dose of ascorbic acid (2 g) reversed enhanced brachial artery NO$^\bullet$-mediated arterial relaxation over 2 h in association with an increase in plasma ascorbate that remained within the normal range ($46–114\ \mu M$) *(242)*. The same population treated chronically with 500 mg/d of ascorbic acid over 30 d also demonstrated enhanced NO$^\bullet$-mediated arterial relaxation *(243)*. In light of these data, it is unlikely that ascorbic acid modulates NO$^\bullet$-mediated arterial relaxation simply through super-oxide scavenging.

Although currently there is no consensus on the precise mechanisms responsible for the effect of ascorbic acid on NO$^\bullet$ bioactivity, several actions of ascorbic acid merit consid-eration in this regard. In its capacity as an intracellular antioxidant, ascorbic acid can both spare and substitute for GSH and vice versa *(203,204,244)*. Therefore, ascorbic acid could influence NO$^\bullet$ bioactivity through mechanisms described for GSH. In addition, ascorbic acid increases the efficiency of nNOS directly, in a manner similar to GSH *(213)*. Finally, ascorbic acid also accelerates the release of NO$^\bullet$ from GSNO *(245)*, providing yet another mechanism to modulate NO$^\bullet$ bioactivity.

Hydroxyl Radical Scavengers

Hydroxyl radical has been implicated in tissue damage resulting from reperfusion injury and inflammation *(56)*, and may be present in atherosclerotic lesions *(246)*. However, the direct effects of hydroxyl radical in the action and metabolism of NO$^\bullet$ are relatively unknown. Some of this ignorance is undoubtedly due to the difficulty with quantifying and inhibiting hydroxyl radical-mediated reactions. With a one electron reduction potential of approx -2300 mV, hydroxyl radical is the most oxidizing species known and readily reacts with most adjacent species *(247)*. These chemical properties essentially exclude the existence of "specific" inhibitors for hydroxyl radical-mediated oxidations. In fact, the very chemical nature of hydroxyl radical dictates that almost all compounds, to some extent, are hydroxyl radical "scavengers." Therefore, an important parameter to consider is the rate at which a compound reacts with hydroxyl radical. Secure evidence for a hydroxyl radical-mediated process requires inhibition of this process by at least three distinct hydroxyl radical "scavengers" (e.g., mannitol, dimethyl thiourea, dimethylsulfoxide) *in a rank order that mirrors the known reaction rates of these compounds with hydroxyl radical (248)*. There are very few (if any) studies in the NO$^\bullet$ literature that can meet such a standard.

Data documenting an important biologic interaction between hydroxyl radical and NO$^\bullet$ are, at best, indirect. Rat lingual arteries exposed to a flux of hydroxyl radicals demonstrate impaired endothelium-dependent relaxation *(249)*. Whether this observation is due to the chemical reaction between NO$^\bullet$ and hydroxyl radical remains to be determined. In diabetic rats, defective NO$^\bullet$-mediated relaxation in mesenteric arteries is improved with either dimethylthiourea, a hydroxyl radical scavenger *(250)* or diethylenetriamine pentaacetic acid (DTPA), a metal ion chelator *(251)*. In diabetic patients, specific iron chelation with deferrioxamine improves NO˙-mediated arterial relaxation *(252)*. Although all of these studies are consistent with a role for hydroxyl radicals in causing impaired NO˙ bioactivity, these data must be interpreted with some caution. For example, a singular observation with DTPA or deferrioxamine alone does not prove a role of hydroxyl radical, as iron alone impairs the bioactivity of NO˙ *(95)*. Dimethylthiourea, a widely employed "specific" hydroxyl radical scavenger, also binds metal ions *(253)*, further complicating the interpretation of these studies. Thus, there is no secure data suggesting that hydroxyl radical plays an important role in the modulation of NO˙ bioactivity within the cardiovascular system.

SUMMARY

NO˙ is an important component of vascular homeostasis, and abnormal NO˙ bioactivity has been implicated in a number of disease states with important public health implications. One clear mechanism of impaired NO˙ bioactivity in vascular disease is excess vascular oxidative stress. There is now a wealth of developing data that manipulation of vascular antioxidant status has considerable influence on the biologic activity of endothelium-derived NO˙. In remains to be seen if this influence can be exploited in a manner that favorably alters the course of human disease.

ACKNOWLEDGMENTS

Dr. Keaney is supported by grants from the American Heart Association and the National Institutes of Health (HL59346:HL55854:and HL58976), and also received a Clinical Investigator Development Award (HL03195) from the National Institutes of Health.

REFERENCES

1. Furchgott, RF, Zawadzki, JV The obligatory role of endothelial cells in the relaxation of arterial smooth muscle by acetylcholine. Nature 1980;288:373–376.
2. Ignarro, LJ, Buga GM, Wood KS, Byrns RE, Chaudhuri, G. Endothelium-derived relaxing factor produced and released from artery and vein is nitric oxide. Proc Natl Acad Sci USA 1987;84:9265–9269.
3. Stamler JS, Singel DJ, Loscalzo J. Biochemistry of nitric oxide and its redox-activated forms. Science 1992;258:1898–1902.
4. Stuehr DJ. Structure-function aspects in the nitric oxide synthases. Ann Rev Pharmacol Toxicol 1997; 37:339–359.
5. Lamas S, Marsden PA, Li GK, Tempst P, Michel T. Endothelial nitric oxide synthase: molecular cloning and characterization of a distinct constitutive enzyme isoform. Proc Natl Acad Sci USA 1992; 89:6348–6352.
6. Kobzik L, Bredt DS, Lowenstein CJ, Drazen J, Gaston B, Sugarbaker D, et al. Nitric oxide synthase in human and rat lung: immunocytochemical and histochemical localization. Am J Respir Cell Mol Biol 1993;9:371–377.
7. Bredt DS, Hwang PM, Snyder SH. Localization of nitric oxide synthase indicating a neural role for nitric oxide. Nature 1990;347:768–770.
8. Kobzik L, Reid MB, Bredt DS, Stamler JS. Nitric oxide in skeletal muscle. Nature 1994;372:546–548.
9. de Belder AJ, Radomski MW, Why HJ, Richardson PJ, Bucknall CA, Salas E, et al. Nitric oxide synthase activities in human myocardium. Lancet 1993;341:84–85.
10. Mannick JB, Asano K, Izumi K, Kieff E. Nitric oxide produced by human B lymphocytes inhibits apoptosis and Epstein-Barr virus reactivation. Cell 1994;79:1137–1146.
11. Stuehr DJ, Cho HJ, Kwon NS, Weise MF, Nathan CF. Purification and characterization of the cytokine-induced macrophage nitric oxide synthase: an FAD- and FMN-containing flavoprotein. Proc Natl Acad Sci USA 1991;88:7773–7777.

12. Hare JM, Keaney JF Jr, Balligand JL, Loscalzo J, Smith TW, Colucci WS. Role of nitric oxide in parasypathetic modulation of Beta-adrenergic myocardial contractility in normal dogs. J Clin Invest 1995;95:360–366.
13. Keaney JF Jr, Hare JM, Balligand JL, Loscalzo J, Smith TW, Colucci WS. Inhibition of nitric oxide synthase augments myocardial contractile responses to β-adrenergic stimulation. Am J Physiol 1996; 271:H2646–H2652.
14. Nathan CF, Hibbs JB Jr. Role of nitric oxide synthesis in macrohage antimicrobial activity. Curr Opin Immunol 1991;3:65–70.
15. Bredt DS, Snyder SH. Nitric oxide mediates glutamate-linked enhancement of cGMP levels in the cerebellum. Proc Natl Acad Sci USA 1989;86:9030–9033.
16. Demas GE, Eliasson MJ, Dawson RM, Dawson FL, Kriegsfeld LJ, Nelson RJ, et al. Inhibition of neuronal nitric oxide synthase increases aggressive behavior in mice. Mol Med 1997;3:610–616.
17. Pantopoulos K, Hentze MW. Nitric oxide signaling to iron-regulatory protein: direct control of ferritin mRNA translation and transferrin receptor mRNA stability in transfected fibroblasts. Proc Natl Acad Sci USA 1995;92:1267–1271.
18. Shen W, Hintze TH, Wolin MS. Nitric oxide: an important signaling mechanism between vascular endothelium and parenchymal cells in the regulation of oxygen consumption. Circulation 1995;92: 3505–3512.
19. Gopalakrishna R, Chen ZH, Gundimeda U. Nitric oxide and nitric oxide-generating agents induce a reversible inactivation of protein kinase C activity and phorbol ester binding. J Biol Chem 1993;268: 27,180–27,185.
20. Michel T, Feron O. Nitric oxide synthases: which, where, and why. J Clin Invest 1998;100:2146–2152.
21. Shaul PW, Smart EJ, Robinson LJ, German Z, Yuhanna IS, Ying Y, et al. Acylation targets endothelial nitric-oxide synthase to plasmalemmal caveolae. J Biol Chem 1996;271:6518–6522.
22. Garcia-Cardena G, Oh P, Liu J, Schnitzer JE, Sessa WC. Targeting of nitric oxide synthase to endo-thelial cell caveolae via palmitoylation: implications for nitric oxide signaling. Proc Natl Acad Sci USA 1996;93:6448–6453.
23. Couet J, Li S, Okamoto T, Ikezu T, Lisanti MP. Identification of peptide and protein ligands for the caveolin-scaffoliding domain. Implications for the interaction of caveolin with caveolae-associated proteins. J Biol Chem 1997;272:6525–6533.
24. Michel JB, Feron O, Sase K, Prabhakar P, Michel T. Caveolin versus calmodulin. counterbalancing allosteric modulators of endothelial nitric oxide synthase. J Biol Chem 1997;272:25,907–25,912.
25. Lefroy DC, Crake T, Uren NG, Davies GJ, Maseri A. Effect of inhibition of nitric oxide synthesis on epicardial coronary artery caliber and coronary blood flow in humans. Circulation 1993;88:43–54.
26. Rees DD, Palmer RM, Moncada S. Role of endothelium-derived nitric oxide in the regulation of blood pressure. Proc Natl Acad Sci USA 1989;86:3375–3378.
27. Huang PL, Huang Z, Mashimo H, Bloch KD, Moskowitz MA, Bevan JA, et al. Hypertension in mice lacking the gene for endothelial nitric oxide syntase. Nature 1995;377:239–242.
28. Azuma H, Ishikawa M, Sekizaki S. Endothelium-dependent inhibition of platelet aggregation. Br J Pharmacol 1986;88:411–415.
29. Arnold WP, Mittal CK, Katsuki S, Murad F. Nitric oxide activates guanylate cyclase and increases guanosine 3',5'-cyclic monophosphate levels in various tissue preparations. Proc Natl Acad Sci USA 1977;74:3203–3207.
30. Ignarro LJ, Burke TM, Wood KS, Wolin MS, Kadowitz PJ. Association between cyclic GMP accu-mulation and acetylcholine-elicited relaxation of bovine intrapulmonary artery. J Pharmacol Exp Ther 1984;228:682–690.
31. Moro MA, Russell RJ, Cellek S, Lizasoain I, Su Y, Darley-Usmar VM, et al. cGMP mediates the vascular and platelet actions of nitric oxide: confirmation using an inhibitor of the soluble guanylyl cyclase. Proc Natl Acad Sci USA 1995;93:1480–1485.
32. Radomski MW, Palmer RM, Moncada S. The role of nitric oxide and cGMP in platelet adhesion to the vascular endothelium. Biochem Biophys Res Commun 1987;148:1482–1489.
33. Wink DA, Darbyshire JF, Nims RW, Saavedra JE, Ford PC. Reactions of the bioregulatory agent nitric oxide in oxygenated aqueous media: determination of the kinetics for oxidation and nitrosation by intermediates generated in the NO/O2 reaction. Chem Res Toxicol 1993;6:23–27.
34. Bolotina VM, Najibi S, Palacino JJ, Pagano PJ, Cohen RA. Nitric oxide directly activates calcium-dependent potassium channels in vascular smooth muscle. Nature 1994;368:850–853.
35. Xu L, Eu JP, Meissner G, Stamler JS. Activation of the cardiac calcium release channel (ryonadine receptor by poly-S-nitrosylation. Science 1998;279:234–237.

36. Campbell DL, Stamler JS, Strauss HC. Redox modulation of L-type calcium channels in ferret ventricular myocytes. Dual mechanism regulation by nitric oxide and S-nitrosothiols. J Gen Physiol 1996; 108:277–293.

37. Stamler JS, Jia L, Eu JP, McMahon TJ, Demchenko IT, Bonoventura J, et al. Blood flow regulation by S-nitrosohemoglobin in the physiological oxygen gradient. Science 1997;276:2034–2037.

38. Freedman JE, Loscalzo J, Benoit SE, Valeri CR, Barnard MR, Michelson AD. Decreased platelet inhibition by nitric oxide in two brothers with a history of arterial thrombosis. J Clin Invest 1996;97: 979–987.

39. Ludmer PL, Selwyn AP, Shook TL, Wayne RR, Mudge GH, Alexander RW, et al. Paradoxical vasoconstriction induced by acetylcholine in atherosclerotic coronary arteries. N Engl J Med 1986;315: 1046–1051.

40. Nitenberg A, Valensi P, Sachs R, Dali M, Aptecar E, Attali JR. Impairment of coronary vascular reserve and ACh-induced coronary vasodilation in diabetic patients with angiographically normal coronary arteries and normal left ventricular systolic function. Diabetes 1993;42:1017–1025.

41. Panza JA, Casino PR, Kilcoyne CM, Quyyumi AA. Role of endothelium-derived nitric oxide in the abnormal endothelium-dependent vascular relaxation of patients with essential hypertension. Circulation 1993;87:1468–1474.

42. Clarkson P, Celermajer DS, Powe AJ, Donald AE, Henry RMA, Deanfield JE. Endothelium-dependent dilatation is impaired in young healthy subjects with a family history of premature coronary disease. Circulation 1997;96:3378–3383.

43. Kugiyama K, Yasue H, Ihgushi M, Motoyama T, Dawano H, Inobe Y, et al. Deficiency in nitric oxide bioactivity in epicardial coronary arteries of cigarette smokers. J Am Coll Cardiol 1996;28:1161–1167.

44. Celermajer DS, Sorensen KE, Bull C, Ribinson J, Deanfield JE. Endothelium-dependent dilation in the systemic arteries of asymptomatic subjects relates to coronary risk factors and their interaction. J Am Coll Cardiol 1994;24:1468–1474.

45. Vita JA, Treasure CB, Nabel EG, McLenachan JM, Fish RD, Yeung AC, et al. Coronary vasomotor response to acetylcholine relates to risk factors for coronary artery disease. Circulation 1990;81:491–497.

46. Levine GN, Keaney JF Jr, Vita JA. Cholesterol reduction in cardiovascular disease. Clinical benefits and possible mechanisms. N Engl J Med 1995;332:512–521.

47. Diaz M, Frei B, Vita JA, Keaney JF Jr. Antioxidants and atherosclerotic heart disease. N Engl J Med 1997;337:408–416.

48. Sies H. Hydroperoxides and thiol oxidants in the study of oxidative stress in intact cells and organs. In: Sies H, ed. Oxidative Stress. Academic Press, London, 1985, pp. 73–91.

49. Kehrer JP, Smith CV. Free radicals in biology: sources, reactivities, and roles in the etiology of human diseases. In: Frei B, ed. Natural Antioxidants in Human Health and Disease. Academic Press, San Diego, 1994, pp. 25–62.

50. Boveris A, Cadenas E. Mitochondrial production of superoxide anions and its relationship to the antimycin insensitive respiration. FEBS Lett 1975;54:311–314.

51. Storch J, Ferber E. Detergent-amplified chemiluminescence of lucigenin for determination of superoxide anion production by NADPH oxidase and xanthine oxidase. Anal Biochem 1988;169:262–267.

52. Kukreja RC, Kontos HA, Hess ML, Ellis EF. PGH synthase and lipoxygenase generate superoxide in the presence of NADH or NADPH. Circ Res 1986;59:612–619.

53. Geiss D, Schlze HU. Isolation and chemical composition of the NADH:semidehydroascorbate oxidoreductase rich membranes from rat liver. FEBS Lett 1975;60:374–379.

54. Babior BM, Curnutte JT, McMurrich BJ. The particulate superoxide-forming system from human neutrophils. Properties of the system and further evidence supporting its participation in the respiratory burst. J Clin Invest 1976;58:989–996.

55. Daval JL, Ghersi-Egea JF, Oilet J, Koziel V. A simple method for evaluation of superoxide radical production in neual cells under varous culture conditions: application to hypoxia. J Cereb Blood Flow Metab 1995;15:71–77.

56. Fantone JD, Ward PA. Role of oxygen-derived free radicals and metabolites in leukocyte-dependent inflammatory reactions. Am J Pathol 1982;107:397–403.

57. Meier B, Cross AR, Hancock JR, Kaup JF, Jones OT. Identification of a superoxide-generating NADPH-oxidase system in human fibroblasts. Biochem J 1991;275:241–245.

58. Rosen GM, Freeman BA. Detection of superoxide generated by endothelial cells. Proc Natl Acad Sci USA 1984;81:7269–7273.

59. Heinecke JW, Baker L, Rosen H, Chait A. Superoxide mediated modification of low density lipoprotein by human arterial smooth muscle cells in culture. J Clin Invest 1986;77:757–761.

60. Hiramatsu K, Rosen H, Heinecke JW, Wolfbauer G, Chait A. Superoxide initiates oxidation of low density lipoprotein by human monocytes. Arteriosclerosis 1986;7:55–60.
61. Mullarkey CJ, Edelstein D, Brownlee M. Free radical generation by early glycation products: a mechanism for accelerated atherogenesis in diabetes. Biochem Biophys Res Commun 1990;173:932–939.
62. Rajagopalan S, Kurz S, Munzel T, Tarpey M, Freeman BA, Griendling KK, et al. Angiotensin II-mediated hypertension in the rat increases vascular superoxide production via membrane NADH/HADPH oxidase activation. Contribution to alterations of vasomotor tone. J Clin Invest 1996;97:1916–1923.
63. Ohara Y, Peterson TE, Harrison DG. Hypercholesterolemia increases endothelial superoxide anion production. J Clin Invest 1993;91:2546–2551.
64. Keaney JF Jr, Xu A, Cunningham D, Jackson T, Frei B, Vita JA. Dietary probucol preserves endothelial function in cholesterol-fed rabbits by limiting vascular oxidative stress and superoxide generation. J Clin Invest 1995;95:2520–2529.
65. Lynch SM, Frei B, Morrow JD, Roberts LJ II, Xu A, Jackson T, et al. Vascular superoxide dismutase deficiency impairs endothelial vasodilator function through direct inactivation of nitric oxide and increased lipid peroxidation. Arterioscler Thromb Vasc Biol 1997;17:2975–2981.
66. Lynch SM, Frei B. Mechanisms of copper-and iron-dependent oxidative modification of human low-density lipoprotein. J Lipid Res 1993;34:1745–1753.
67. Rubbo H, Radi R, Trujillo M, Telleri R, Kalyanaraman B, Barnes S, et al. Nitric oxide regulation of superoxide and peroxynitrite-dependent lipid peroxidation. Formation of novel nitrogen-containing oxidized lipid derivatives. J Biol Chem 1994;269:26,066–26,075.
68. Kissner R, Nauser T, Bugnon P, Lye PG, Koppenol WH. Formation and properties of peroxynitrite as studied by laser flash photolysis, high-pressure stopped-flow technique, and pulse radiolysis. Chem Res Toxicol 1997;10:1285–1292.
69. Beckman JS, Beckman TW, Chen J, Marshall PA, Freeman BA. Apparent hydroxyl radical production by peroxynitrite: implications for endothelial injury from nitric oxide and superoxide. Proc Natl Acad Sci USA 1990;87:1620–1624.
70. Saran M, Michel C, Bors W. Reaction of NO with O2–. Implications for the action of endothelium-derived relaxing factor (EDRF). Free Radic Res Commun 1990;10:221–226.
71. Leeuwenburgh C, Hansen P, Shaish A, Holloszy JO, Heinecke JW. Markers of protein oxidation by hydroxyl radical and reactive nitrogen species in tissues of aging rats. Am J Physiol 1998;274: R453–R461.
72. Ischiropoulos H, Zhu L, Beckman JS. Peroxynitrite formation from macrophage-derived nitric oxide. Arch Biochem Biophys 1992;298:446–451.
73. Beckman JS, Crow JP. Pathological implications of nitric oxide superoxide, and peroxynitrite formation. Biochem Soc Trans 1993;21:330–334.
74. Landino LM, Crews BC, Timmons MD, Morrow JD, Marnett LJ. Peroxynitrite, the couling product of nitric oxide and superoxide, activates prostaglandin biosynthesis. Proc Natl Acad Sci USA 1996;93: 15,069–15,074.
75. Ischiropoulos H, Zhu L, Chen J, Tsai M, Martin JC, Smith CD, et al. Peroxynitrite-mediated tyrosine nitration catalyzed by superoxide dismutase. Arch Biochem Biophys 1992;298:431–437.
76. Moreno JJ, Pryor WA. Inactivation of a-1-proteinase inhibitor by peroxynitrite. Chem Res Toxicol 1992;5:425–431.
77. Graham A, Hogg N, Kalyanaraman B, O'Leary V, Darley-Usmar V, Moncada S. Peroxynitrite modification of low-density lipoprotein leads to recognition by the macrophage scavenger receptor. FEBS Lett 1993;330:181–185.
78. Fridovich I. Superoxide radical: an endogenous toxicant. Ann Rev Pharmacol Toxicol 1983;23:239–257.
79. Thannickal VJ, Fanbur BL. Activation of an H2O2–generating NADH oxidase in human lung fibroblasts by transforming growth factor Beta-1. J Biochem 1995;270:30,334–30,338.
80. Heinzel B, John M, Klatt P, Bohme E, Mayer B. Ca2+/calmodulin-dependent formation of hydrogen peroxide by brain nitric oxide synthase. Biochem J 1992;281:627–630.
81. Pryor WA. Free radicals and lipid peroxidation: what they are and how they got that way. In: Frei B, ed. Natural Antioxidants in Human Health and Disease. Academic Press, San Diego, 1993, pp. 1–19.
82. Lander HM. An essential role for free radicals and derived species in signal transduction. FASEB J 1997;11:118–124.
83. Stadtman ER. Role of oxidized amino acids in protein breakdown and stability. Methods Enzymol 1995;258:379–393.
84. Wagner BA, Buettner GR, Burns CP. Free radical-mediated lipid peroxidation in cells: oxidizability is a function of cell lipid bis-allylic hydrogen content. Biochemistry 1994;33:4449–4453.

85. Garner B, Waldeck AR, Witting PK, Rye KA, Stocker R. Oxidation of high density lipoproteins. II. Evidence for a direct reduction of lipid hydroperoxides by methionine residues of apolipoproteins AI and AII. J Biol Chem 1998;273:6088–6095.

86. Esterbauer H, Jürgens G, Quehenberger O, Koller E. Autooxidation of human low density lipoprotein: loss of polyunsaturated fatty acids and vitamin E and generation of aldehydes. J Lipid Res 1987;28:495–509.

87. Keaney JF Jr, Frei B. Antioxidant protection of low-density lipoprotein and its role in the prevention of atherosclerotic vascular disease. In: Frei B, ed. Natural Antioxidants in Human Health and Disease. Academic Press, San Diego, 1994, pp. 303–352.

88. Heinecke JW, Li W, Francis GA, Goldstein JA. Tyrosyl radical generated by myeloperoxidase catalyzes the oxidative cross-linking of proteins. J Clin Invest 1993;91:2866–2872.

89. Heinecke JW. Pathways for oxidation of low density lipoprotein by meloperoxidase: tyrosyl radical reactive aldehydes, hypochlorous acid, and molecular chlorine. Biofactors 1997;6:145–155.

90. van der Vliet A, Eiserich JP, Halliwell B, Cross CE. Formation of reactive nitrogen species during peroxidase-catalyzed oxidation of nitrite. J Biol Chem 1997;272:7617–7625.

91. Eiserich JP, Cross CE, Jones AD, Halliwell B, van der Vliet A. Formation of nitrating and chlorinating species by reaction of nitrite with hypocholorous acid. J Biol Chem 1996;271:19,199–19,208.

92. Mayer B, Schrammel A, Klatt P, Koesling D, Schmidt K. Peroxynitrite-induced accumulation of cyclic GMP in endothelial cells and stimulation of purified soluble guanylyl cyclase. Dependence on glutathione and possible role of S-nitrosation. J Biol Chem 1995;270:17,355–17,360.

93. Tarpey MM, Beckman JS, Ischiropoulos H, Gore JZ, Brock TA. Peroxynitrite stimulates vascular smooth muscle cell cyclic GMP synthesis. FEBS Lett 1995;364:314–318.

94. Rubanyi GM, Vanhoutte PM. Superoxide anions and hyperoxia inactivate endothelium-derived relaxing factor. Am J Physiol 1986;250:H822–H827.

95. Gryglewski RJ, Palmer RM, Moncada S. Superoxide anion is involved in the breakdown of endothelium-derived vascular relaxing factor. Nature 1986;320:454–456.

96. Ignarro LJ, Byrns RE, Buga GM, Wood KS, Chaudhuri G. Pharmacological evidence that endothelium-derived relaxing factor is nitric oxide: use of pyrogallol and superoxide dismutase to study endothelium dependent and nitric oxide elicited vascular smooth muscle relaxation. J Pharmacol Exp Ther 1988;244:181–189.

97. Stralin P, Karlsson K, Johansson BO, Marklund SL. The interstitium of the human arterial wall contains very large amounts of extracellular superoxide dismutase. Arterioscler Thromb Vasc Biol 1995;15:2032–2036.

98. Omar HA, Cherry PD, Mortelliti MP, Burke-Wolin T, Wolin MS. Inhibition of coronary artery superoxide dismutase attenuates endothelium-dependent and -independent nitrovasodilator relaxation. Circ Res 1991;69:601–608.

99. Mugge A, Elwell JK, Peterson TE, Harrison DG. Release of intact endothelium-derived relaxing factor depends on endothelial superoxide dismutase activity. Am J Physiol 1991;260:C219–C225.

100. Abrahamsson T, Brandt U, Marklund SL, Sjoqvist PO. Vascular bound recombinant extracellular superoxide dismutase type C protects against the detrimental effects of superoxide radicals on endothelium-dependent arterial relaxation. Circ Res 1992;70:264–271.

101. Heikkila RE, Cohen G. The inactivation of copper-zinc superoxide dismutase by diethyldithiocarbamate. In: Superoxide and Superoxide Dismutases. Academic Press, New York, 1977, pp. 367–373.

102. Mulsch A, Mordvintcev P, Bassenge E, Jung F, Clement B, Busse R. In vivo spin trapping of glyceryl trinitrate-derived nitric oxide in rabbit blood vessels and organs. Circulation 1995;92:1876–1882.

103. McCord JM, Crapo JD, and Fridovich I. Superoxide dismutase assays: a review of methodology. In: Michelson AM, McCord JM, Fridovich I, eds. Superoxide and Superoxide Dismutases. Academic Press, New York, 1977, pp. 11–17.

104. Sarvazyan N, Askari A, Klevay LM, Huang WH. Role of intracellular SOD in oxidant-induced injury to normal and copper-deficient cardiac myocytes. Am J Physiol 1995;268:H1115–H1121.

105. Schuschke DA, Ree MW, Saari JT, Miller FN. Copper deficiency alters vasodilation in the rat cremaster muscle microcirculation. J Nutr 1992;122:1547–1552.

106. White CR, Brock TA, Chang LY, Crapo J, Briscoe P, Ku D, et al. Superoxide and peroxynitrite in atherosclerosis. Proc Natl Acad Sci USA 1994;91:1044–1048.

107. Laursen JB, Rajagopalan S, Galis Z, Tarpey M, Freeman BA, Harrison DG. Role of superoxide in angiotensin II-induced but not catecholamine-induced hypertension. Circulation 1997;95:588–593.

108. Tesfamariam B, Cohen RA. Free radicals mediate endothelial cell dysfunction caused by elevated glucose. Am J Physiol 1992;263:H321–H326.

109. Hattori Y, Kawasaki H, Abe K, Kanno M. Superoxide dismutase recovers altered endothelium-dependent relaxation in diabetic rat aorta. Am J Physiol 1991;261:H1086–H1094.

110. Mugge A, Brandes RP, Boger RH, Dwenger A, Bode-Boger S, Kienke S, et al. Vascular release of superoxide radicals is enhanced in hypercholesterolemic rabbits. J Cardiovasc Pharmacol 1994;24:994–998.

111. Ohara Y, Peterson TE, Sayegh HS, Subramanian RR, Wilcox JN, Harrison DG. Dietary correction of hypercholesterolemia in the rabbit normalizes endothelial superoxide production. Circulation 1995; 92:898–903.

112. Mugge A, Elwell JH, Peterson TE, Hofmeyer TG, Heistad DD, Harrison DG. Chronic treatment with polyethylene-glycolated superoxide dismutase partially restores endothelium-dependent vascular relaxations in cholesterol-fed rabbits. Circ Res 1991;69:1293–1300.

113. Kagota S, Yamaguchi Y, Shinozuka K, Kunitomo M. Mechanisms of impairment of endothelium-dependent relaxation to acetylcholine in Watanabe heritable hyperlipidemic rabbit aortas. Clin Exp Pharmacol Physiol 1998;25:104–109.

114. Garcia CE, Kilcoyne CM, Cardillo C, Cannon RO, Quyyumi AA, Panza JA. Evidence that endothelial dysfunction in patients with hypercholesterolemia is not due to increased extracellular nitric oxide breakdown by superoxide anions. Am J Cardiol 1995;76:1157–1161.

115. Wolff SP, Dean RT. Glucose autoxidation and protein modification. Their potential role of autoxidative glycosylation in diabetes. Biochem J 1987;245:243–250.

116. Pieper GM, Gross G. Oxygen-derived free radicals abolish endothelium-dependent relaxation in diabetic rat aorta. Am J Physiol 1988;255:H825–H833.

117. Pieper GM. Oxidative stress in diabetic blood vessels. FASEB J 1995;9:A891.

118. Nakazono K, Watanabe N, Matsuno K, Sasaki J, Sato T, Inoue M. Does superoxide underlie the pathogenesis of hypertension? Proc Natl Acad Sci USA 1991;88:10,045–10,048.

119. Shesely EG, Maeda N, Kim HS, Desai KM, Krege JH, Laubach VE, et al. Elevated blood pressures in mice lacking endothelial nitric oxide synthase. Proc Natl Acad Sci USA 1996;93:13,176–13,181.

120. Griendling K, Minieri CA, Ollerenshaw JD, Alexander RW. Angiotensin II stimulates NADH and NADPH oxidase activity in cultured vascular smooth muscle cells. Circ Res 1994;74:1141–1148.

121. Pagano PJ, Ito Y, Tornheim K, Gallop P, Tauber AI, Cohen RA. An NADPH oxidase superoxide generating system in rabbit aorta. Am J Physiol 1995;268:H2274–H2280.

122. Pagano PJ, Clark J, Cifuentes-Pagano ME, Clark SM, Callis GM, Quinn MT. Localization of a constitutively active, phagocyte-like NADPH oxidase in rabbit aortic adventitia: enhancement by angiotensin II. Proc Natl Acad Sci USA 1997;94:14,483–14,488.

123. Mojazzab H, Kaminski PM, Wolin MS. NADH oxidoreductase is a major source of superoxide anion in bovine coronary artery endothelium. Am J Physiol 1994;266:H2568–H2572.

124. Paler-Martinez A, Panus PC, Chumley PH, Ryan US, Hardy MM, Freeman BA. Endogenous xanthine oxidase does not significantly contribute to vascular endothelial production of reactive oxygen species. Arch Biochem Biophys 1994;311:79–85.

125. Cardillo C, Kilcoyne CM, Cannon RO III, Quyyumi AA, Panza JA. Xanthine oxidase inhibition with oxypurinol improves endothelial vasodilator function in hypercholesterolemic but not in hypertensive patients. Hypertension 1997;30:57–63.

126. White CR, Darley-Usmar V, Berrington WR, McAdams M, Gore JZ, Thompson JA, et al. Circulating plasma xanthine oxidase contributes to vascular dysfunction in hypercholesterolemic rabbits. Proc Natl Acad Sci USA 1996;93:8745–8749.

127. Pou S, Pou WS, Bredt DS, Snyder SH, Rosen GM. Generation of superoxide by purified brain nitric oxide synthase. J Biol Chem 1992;267:24,173–24,176.

128. Kurz S, Kent JD, Venema RC, Harrison DG. Differences in flavin-based superoxide production by the endothelial and neuronal NO synthases. Circulation 1996;94:I-2.

129. Vasquez-Vivar J, Kalyanaraman B, Martasek P, Hogg N, Masters BS, Karoui H, et al. Superoxide generation by endothelial nitric oxide synthase: the influence of cofactors. Proc Natl Acad Sci USA 1998;95:9220–9225.

130. Xia Y, Dawson VL, Dawson TM, Snyder SH, Zweier JL. Nitric oxide synthase generates superoxide and nitric oxide in arginine-depleted cells leading to peroxynitrite-mediated cell injury. Proc Natl Acad Sci USA 1996;93:6770–6774.

131. Pritchard KA Jr, Groszek L, Smalley DM, Sessa WC, Wu M, Villalon P, et al. Native low-density lipoprotein increases endothelial cell nitric oxide synthase generation of superoxide anion. Circ Res 1995;77:510–518.

132. Wei EP, Kantos HE. H2O2 and endothelium-dependent cerebral arteriolar dilation. Implications for the identity of endothelium-derived relaxing factor generated by acetylcholine. Hypertension 1990;16: 162–169.

133. Marczin N, Ryan US, Catravas JD. Effects of oxidant stress on endothelium-derived relaxing factor-induced and nitrovasodilator-induced cGMP accumulation in vascular cells in culture. Circ Res 1992; 70:326–340.
134. Ghigo D, Alessio P, Foco A, Bussolino F, Costamagna D, Heller R, et al. Nitric oxide synthesis is impaired in glutathione depleted human umbilical vein endothelial cells. Am J Physiol 1993;265: C728–C732.
135. Marczin N, Ryan US, Catravas JD. Sulfhydryl-depleting agents, but not deferoxamine, modulate EDRF action in cultured pulmonary arterial cells. Am J Physiol 1993;265:L220–L227.
136. Garcia-Cardena G, Fan R, Stern DF, Liu J, Sessa WC. Endothelial nitric oxide synthase is regulated by tyrosine phosphorylation and interacts with caveolin-1. J Biol Chem 1996;271:27,237–27,240.
137. Padmaja S, Huie RE. The reaction of nitric oxide with organic peroxyl radicals. Biochem Biophys Res Commun 1993;195:539–544.
138. Rubbo H, Parthasarathy S, Barnes S, Kirk M, Kalyanaraman B, Freeman BA. Nitric oxide inhibition of lipoxygenase-dependent liposome and low-density lipoprotein oxidation: termination of radical chain propagation reactions and formation of nitrogen-containing oxidized lipid derivatives. Arch Biochem Biophys 1995;324:15–25.
139. Wink DA, Hanbauer I, Krishna MC, DeGraff W, Gamson J, Mitchell JB. Nitric oxide protects against cellular damage and cytotoxicity from reactive oxygen species. Proc Natl Acad Sci USA 1993;90: 9813–9817.
140. Hogg N, Kalyanaraman B, Joseph J, Struck A, Parthasarathy S. Inhibition of low-density lipoprotein oxidation by nitric oxide. Potential role in atherogenesis. FEBS Lett 1993;334:170–174.
141. Zembowicz A, Hatchett RJ, Jakubowski AM, Gryglewski RJ. Involvement of nitric oxide in the endothelium-dependent relaxation induced by hydrogen peroxide in rabbit aorta. Br J Pharmacol 1993;110: 151–158.
142. Murer EH. Release reaction and energy metabolism in blood platelets with special reference to the burst in oxygen uptake. Biochim Biophys Acta 1968;162:320–326.
143. Okuma M, Steiner M, Baldini MG. Studies on lipid peroxides in platelets. II. Effect of aggregating agents and platelet antibody. J Lab Clin Med 1971;77:728–742.
144. Freedman JE, Frei B, Welch GN, Loscalzo J. Glutathione peroxidase potentiates the inhibition of platelet function by S-nitrosothiols. J Clin Invest 1995;96:394–400.
145. Hour Y, Guo Z, Li J, Wang PG. Seleno compounds and glutathione peroxidase catalyzed decomposition of s-nitrosothiols. Biochem Biophys Res Commun 1996;228:88–93.
146. Asahi M, Fujii J, Suzuki K, Seo HG, Kuzura T, Hori M, et al. Inactivation of glutathione peroxidase by nitric oxide. Implication for cytotoxicity. J Biol Chem 1995;270:21,035–21,039.
147. Asahi M, Fujii J, Takao T, Kuzuya T, Hori M, Shimonishi Y, et al. The oxidation of selenocysteine is involved in the inactivation of glutathione peroxidase by nitric oxide donor. J Biol Chem 1997;272: 19,152–19,157.
148. Sies H, Sharov VS, Klotz LO, Briviba K. Glutathione peroxidase protects against peroxynitrite-mediated oxidations. A new function for selenoproteins as peroxynitrite reductase. J Biol Chem 1997;272: 27,812–27,817.
149. Nègre-Salvayre A, Pieraggi MT, Mabile L, Salvayre R. Protective effect of 17-beta-estradiol against the cytotoxicity of minimally oxidized LDL to cultured bovine aortic endothelial cells. Atherosclerosis 1993;99:207–217.
150. Kugiyama K, Kerns SA, Morrisett JD, Roberts R, Henry PD. Impairment of endothelium-dependent arterial relaxation by lysolecithin in modified low-density lipoproteins. Nature 1990;344:160–162.
151. Keaney JF Jr, Guo Y, Cunningham D, Shwaery GT, Xu A, Vita JA. Vascular incorporation of α-tocopherol prevents endothelial dysfunction due to oxidized LDL by inhibiting protein kinase C stimulation. J Clin Invest 1996;98:386–394.
152. Tanner FC, Noll G, Boulanger CM, Luscher TF. Oxidized low density lipoproteins inhibit relaxations of porcine coronary arteries. Role of scavenger receptor and endothelium-derived nitric oxide. Circulation 1991;83:2012–2020.
153. Chin JH, Azhar S, Hoffman BB. Inactivation of endothelium-derived relaxing factor by oxidized lipoproteins. J Clin Invest 1992;89:10–18.
154. Flavahan NA. Atherosclerosis or lipoprotein-induced endothelial dysfunction: potential mechanisms underlying reduction in A2RF/nitric oxide activity. Circulation 1992;85:1927–1938.
155. Schmidt K, Klatt P, Graier WF, Kostner GM, Kukovetz WR. High-density lipoprotein antagonizes the inhibitory effects of oxidized low-density lipoprotein and lysolecithin on soluble guanylate cyclase. Biochem Biophys Res Commun 1992;182:302–308.

156. Esterbauer H, Striegl G, Puhl H, Oberreither S, Rotheneder M, el-Saadani M, et al. The role of vitamin E and carotenoids in preventing oxidation of low density lipoprotein. Ann NY Acad Sci 1989;570: 254–267.

157. Jialal I, Norkus EP, Cristol L, Grundy SM. Beta-carotene inhibits the oxidative modification of low density lipoprotein. Biochim Biophys Acta 1991;1086:134–138.

158. Gaziano JM, Hatta A, Flynn M, Johnson EJ, Krinsky NI, Ridker PM, et al. Supplementation with beta-carotene in vivo and in vitro does not inhibit low density lipoprotein (LDL) oxidation. Atherosclerosis 1995;112:187–195.

159. Verbeuren TJ, Jordaens FH, Zonnekeyn LL, VanHove CE, Coene MC, Herman AG. Effect of hyper-cholesterolemia on vascular reactivity in the rabbit. Circ Res 1986;58:553–564.

160. Keaney JF Jr, Gaziano JM, Xu A, Frei B, Curran-Celantano J, Shwaery GT, et al. Dietary antioxidants preserve endothelium-dependent vessel relaxation in cholesterol-fed rabbits. Proc Natl Acad Sci USA 1993;90:11,880–11,884.

161. Andersson TLG, Matz J, Ferns GA, Änggård EE. Vitamin E reverses cholesterol-induced endothelial dysfunction in the rabbit coronary circulation. Atherosclerosis 1994;111:39–45.

162. Stewart-Lee AL, Forster LA, Nourooz-Zadeh J, Ferns GA, Änggård EE. Vitamin E protects against impairment of endothelium-mediated relaxations in cholesterol-fed rabbits. Arterioscler Thromb 1994; 14:494–499.

163. Lutz M, Cortez J, Vinet R. Effects of dietary fats, alpha-tocopherol and beta-carotene supplementation on aortic ring segment responses in the rat. Int J Vitam Nutr Res 1995;65:225–230.

164. Raij L, Jagy J, Coffee K, DeMaster EG. Hypercholesterolemia promotes endothelial dysfunction in vitamin E- and selenium-deficient rats. Hypertension 1993;22:56–61.

165. Stocker R, Frei B. Endogenous antioxidant defences in human blood plasma. In: Sies H, ed. Oxidative Stress: Oxidants and Antioxidants. Academic Press, London, 1991, pp. 213–243.

166. Dieber-Rotheneder M, Puhl H, Waeg H, Striegl G, Esterbauer H. Effect of oral supplementation with D-alpha-tocopherol on the vitamin E content of human low density lipoproteins and resistance to oxidation. J Lipid Res 1991;32:1325–1332.

167. Keaney JF Jr, Gaziano JM, Xu A, Frei B, Curran-Celentano J, Shwaery GT, et al. Low-dose α-toco-pherol improves and high-dose α-tocopherol worsens endothelial vasodilator function in cholesterol-fed rabbits. J Clin Invest 1994;93:844–851.

168. Suarna C, Dean RT, May J, Stocker R. Human atherosclerotic plaque contains both oxidized lipids and relatively large amounts of α-tocopherol and ascorbate. Arterioscler Thromb Vasc Biol 1995;15: 1616–1624.

169. Jay MT, Chirico S, Siow RC, Bruckdorfer KR, Jacobs M, Leake DS, et al. Modulation of vascular tone by low density lipoproteins: effects on L-arginine transport and nitric oxide synthesis. Exp Physiol 1997;82:349–360.

170. Sugiyama S, Kugiyama K, Ohgushi M, Fujimoto K, Yasue H. Lysophosphatidylcholine in oxi-dized low-density lipoprotein increases endothelial susceptibility to polymorphonuclear leukocyte-induced endothelial dysfunction in porcine coronary arteries: role of protein kinase C. Circ Res 1994; 74:565–575.

171. Boscoboinik D, Szewczyk A, Hensey C, Azzi A. Inhibition of cell proliferation by α-tocopherol. J Biol Chem 1991;266:6188–6194.

172. Freedman JE, Farhat JH, Loscalzo J, Keaney JF Jr. α-Tocopherol inhibits aggregation of human platelets by a protein kinase C-dependent mechanism. Circulation 1996;94:2434–2440.

173. Gopaul NK, Änggård EE, Mallet AI, Betteridge DJ, Wolff SP, Nourooz-Zadeh J. Plasma 8-epi-PGF2alpha levels are elevated in individuals with non-insulin dependent diabetes mellitus. FEBS Lett 1995;368:225–229.

174. Keegan A, Walbank H, Cotter MA, Cameron NE. Chronic vitamin E treatment prevents defective endothelium-dependent relaxation in diabetic rat aorta. Diabetologia 1995;38:1475–1478.

175. Karasu C, Ozansoy G, Bozkurt O, Erdogan D, Omeroglu S. Changes in isoprenaline-induced endo-thelium-dependent and -independent relaxations of aorta in long-term STZ-diabetic rats: reversal effect of dietary vitamin E. Gen Pharm 1997;29:561–567.

176. Karasu C, Ozansoy G, Bozkurt O, Erdogan D, Omeroglu S. Antioxidant and triglyceride-lowering effects of vitamin E associated with the prevention of abnormalities in the reactivity and morphology of aorta from streptozotocin-diabetic rats. Antioxidants in Diabetes-Induced Complications (ADIC) Study Group. Metabolism 1997;46:872–879.

177. Rosen P, Ballhausen T, Stockklauser K. Impairment of endothelium dependent relaxation in the diabetic rat heart: mechanisms and implications. Diabetes Res Clin Pract 1996;31(Suppl):S143–S155.

178. Palmer AM, Thomas CR, Gopaul N, Dhir S, Änggård EE, Poston L, et al. Dietary antioxidant supplementation reduces lipid peroxidation but impairs vascular function in small mesenteric arteries of the streptozotocin-diabetic rat. Diabetologia 1998;41:148–156.

179. Davidge ST, Ojimba J, Mclaughlin MK. Vascular function in the vitamin E-deprived rat: an interaction between nitric oxide and superoxide anions. Hypertension 1998;31:830–835.

180. Marshall FN. Pharmacology and toxicology of probucol. Artery 1982;10:7–21.

181. Shaish A, Daugherty A, O'Sullivan F, Schonfeld G, Heinecke JW. Beta-carotene inhibits atherosclerosis in hypercholesterolemic rabbits. J Clin Invest 1995;96:2075–2082.

182. Parthasarathy S, Young SG, Witztum JL, Pittman RC, Steinberg D. Probucol inhibits oxidative modification of low density lipoprotein. J Clin Invest 1986;77:641–644.

183. Barnhart RL, Busch SJ, Jackson RL. Concentration-dependent antioxidant activity of probucol in low density lipoproteins in vitro: probucol degradation precedes lipoprotein oxidation. J Lipid Res 1989;30: 1703–1710.

184. Pryor WA, Cornicelli JA, Devall LJ, Tait BA, Trivedi BK, Witiak DT, et al. A rapid screening test to determine the antioxidant potencies of natural and synthetic antioxidants. J Org Chem 1993;58: 3521–3532.

185. Carew TE, Schwenke DC, Steinberg D. Antiatherogenic effect of probucol unrelated to its hypocholesterolemic effect: evidence that antioxidants in vivo can selectively inhibit low density lipoprotein degradation in macrophage-rich fatty streaks and slow the progression of atherosclerosis in the Watanabe heritable hyperlipidemic rabbit. Proc Natl Acad Sci USA 1987;84:7725–7729.

186. Kita T, Nagano Y, Yokode M, Ishii K, Kume N, Ooshima A, et al. Probucol prevents the progression of atherosclerosis in Watanabe heritable hyperlipidemic rabbit, an animal model for familial hypercholesterolemia. Proc Natl Acad Sci USA 1987;84:5928–5931.

187. Zhang SH, Reddick RL, Avdievich E, Surles LK, Jones RG, Reynolds JB, et al. Paradoxical enhancement of atherosclerosis by probucol treatment in apolipoprotein E-deficient mice. J Clin Invest 1997;99: 2858–2866.

188. Simon BC, Haudenschild CC, Cohen RA. Preservation of endothelium-dependent relaxation in atherosclerotic rabbit aorta by probucol. J Cardiovasc Pharmacol 1993;21:893–901.

189. Hoshida S, Yamashita N, Igarashi J, Aoki K, Kuzuya T, Hori M. Long-term probucol treatment reverses the severity of myocardial injury in watanabe heritable hyperlipidemic rabbits. Arterioscler Thromb Vasc Biol 1997;17:2801–2807.

190. Inoue N, Ohara Y, Fukai T, Harrison DG, Nishida K. Probucol improves endothelial-dependent relaxation and decreases vascular superoxide production in cholesterol-fed rabbits. Am J Med Sci 1998; 315:242–247.

191. McDowell I, Brennan GM, McEneny J, Young IS, Nicholls DP, McVeigh GE, et al. The effect of probucol and vitamin E treatment on the oxidation of low-density lipoprotein and forearm vascular responses in humans. Eur J Clin Invest 1994;24:759–765.

192. Gilligan DM, Sack MN, Guetta V, Casino PR, Quyyumi AA, Rader DJ, et al. Effect of antioxidant vitamins on low density lipoprotein oxidation and impaired endothelium-dependent vasodilation on patients with hypercholesterolemia. J Am Coll Cardiol 1994;24:1611–1617.

193. Elliott TG, Barth JD, Mancini J. Effects of vitamin E on endothelial function in men after myocardial infarction. Am J Cardiol 1995;76:1188–1190.

194. Lieberman EH, Gerhard MD, Uehata A, Walsh BW, Selwyn AP, Ganz P, et al. Estrogen improves endothelium-dependent, flow mediated vasodilation in post menopausal women. Ann Intern Med 1994; 121:936–941.

195. Koh KK, Blum A, Hathaway L, Mincemoyer R, Csako G, Waclawiw MA, Panza JA, Cannon RO 3rd. Vascular effects of estrogen and vitamin E therapies in postmenopausal women. Circulation 1999;100: 1851–1857.

196. Kugiyama K, Motoyama T, Doi H, Kawano H, Hirai N, Soejima H, Miyao Y, Takazoe K, Moriyama Y, Mizuno Y, Tsunoda R, Ogawa H, Sakamoto T, Sugiyama S, Yasue H. Improvement of endothelial vasomotor dysfunction by treatment with alpha-tocopherol in patients with high remnant lipoproteins levels. J Am Coll Cardiol 1999;33:1512–1518.

197. Motoyama T, Kawano H, Kugiyama K, Hirashima O, Ohgushi M, Tsunoda R, Moriyama Y, Miyao Y, Yoshimura M, Ogawa H, Yasue H. Vitamin E administration improves impairment of endothelium-dependent vasodilation in patients with coronary spastic angina. J Am Coll Cardiol 1998;32:1672–1679.

198. Neunteufl T, Kostner K, Katzenschlager R, Zehetgruber M, Maurer G, Weidinger FF. Additional benefit of vitamin E supplementation to simvistatin therapy on vasoreactivity of the brachial artery of hypercholesterolemic men. J Am Coll Cardiol 1998;32:711–716.

199. Anderson TJ, Meredith IT, Yeung AC, Frei B, Selwyn AP, Ganz P. The effect of cholesterol-lowering and antioxidant therapy on endothelium-dependent coronary vasomotion. N Engl J Med 1995;332:488–493.
200. Wendel A, Cikryt P. The level and half-life of glutathione in human plasma. FEBS Lett 1980;120: 209–211.
201. Bray TM, Taylor CG. Tissue glutathione, nutrition, and oxidative stress. Can J Physiol Pharmacol 1993;71:746–751.
202. Bergsten P, Yu R, Kehrl J, Levine M. Ascorbic acid transport and distribution in human B lymphocytes. Arch Biochem Biophys 1994;317:208–214.
203. Martensson J, Han J, Griffith EW, Meister A. Glutathione ester delays the onset of scurvy in ascorbate-deficient guinea pigs. Proc Natl Acad Sci USA 1993;90:317–321.
204. Martensson J, Meister A. Glutathione deficiency decreases tissue ascorbate levels in newborn rats: ascorbate spares glutathione and protects. Proc Natl Acad Sci USA 1991;88:4656–4660.
205. Stuehr DJ, Kwon NS, Nathan CF. FAD and GSH participate in macrophage synthesis of nitric oxide. Biochem Biophys Res Commun 1990;168:558–565.
206. Hecker M, Seigle I, Macarthur H, Sessa WC, Vane JR. Role of intracellular thiols in release of EDRF from cultured endothelial cells. Am J Physiol 1992;262:H888–H896.
207. Murphy ME, Piper HM, Watanabe H, Sies H. Nitric oxide production by cultured aortic endothelial cells in response to thiol depletion and replenishment. J Biol Chem 1991;266:19,378–19,383.
208. Celermajer DS, Sorensen KE, Gooch VM, Spiegelhalter DJ, Miller OI, Sullivan ID, et al. Non-invasive detection of endothelial dysfunction in children and adults at risk of atherosclerosis. Lancet 1992;340: 1111–1115.
209. Williamson JM, Meister A. Stimulation of hepatic glutathione formation by administration of L-2-oxo-thiazolidine-4-carboxylate: a 5-oxo-L-prolinase substrate. Proc Natl Acad Sci USA 1981;78:936–939.
210. Boesgaard S, Aldershvile J, Poulsen HE, Loft S, Anderson ME, Meister A. Nitrate tolerance in vivo is not associated with depletion of arterial or venous thiol levels. Circ Res 1994;74:115–120.
211. Vita JA, Frei B, Holbrook M, Gokce N, Leaf C, Keaney JF Jr. L-2-Oxothiazolidine-4-carboxylic acid revereses endothelial dysfunction in patients with coronary artery disease. J Clin Invest 1998;101: 1408–1414.
212. Komori Y, Hyun J, Chiang K, Fukuto JM. The role of thiols in the apparent activation of rat brain nitric oxide synthase (NOS). J Biochem 1995;117:923–927.
213. Hofmann H, Schmidt HH. Thiol dependence of nitric oxide synthase. Biochemistry 1995;34:13,443–13,452.
214. Gorren AC, Schrammel A, Schmidt K, Mayer B. Thiols and neuronal nitric oxide synthase: complex formation, competitive inhibition, and enzyme stabilization. Biochemistry 1997;36:4360–4366.
215. Hobbs AJ, Fukoto JM, Ignarro LJ. Formation of free nitric oxide from L-arginine by nitric oxide synthase: direct enhancement of generation by superoxide dismutase. Proc Natl Acad Sci USA 1994; 91:10,992–10,996.
216. Howells DW, Hyland K. Direct analysis of tetrahydrobiopterin in ceribrospinal fluid by high-performance liquid chromatography with redox electrochemistry: prevention of autoxidation during storage and analysis. Clin Chim Acta 1987;167:23–30.
217. Heales S, Hyland K. Determination of quinonoid dihydrobiopterin by high-performance liquid chromatrography and electrochemical detection. J Chromatogr 1989;494:77–85.
218. Patel JM, Abeles AJ, Block ER. Nitric oxide exposure and sulfhydryl modulation alter L-arginine transport in cultured pulmonary artery endothelial cells. Free Radic Biol Med 1996;20:629–637.
219. Wink DA, Nims RW, Darbyshire JF, Christodoulou D, Hanbauer I, Cox GW, et al. Reaction kinetics for nitrosation of cysteine and glutathione in aerobic nitric oxide solutions at neutral pH Insights into the fate and physiological effects of intermediates generated in the NO/O2 reaction. Chem Res Toxicol 1994;7:519–525.
220. Keaney JF Jr, Simon DI, Stamler JS, Jaraki O, Scharfstein J, Vita JA, et al. NO forms an adduct with serum albumin that has endothelium-derived relaxing factor-like properties. J Clin Invest 1993;91: 1582–1589.
221. Kharitonov VG, Sundquist AR, Sharma VS. Kinetics of nitrosation of thiols by nitric oxide in the presence of oxygen. J Biol Chem 1995;270:28,158–28,164.
222. Singh RJ, Hogg N, Joseph J, Kalyanaraman B. Mechanism of nitric oxide relase from S-nitrosothiols. J Biol Chem 1996;271:18,596–18,603.
223. Clancy RM, Levartovsky D, Leszczynska-Piziak J, Yegudin J, Abramson SB. Nitric oxide reacts with intracellular glutathione and activates the hexose monophosphate shunt in human neutrophils: evidence for S-nitrosoglutathione as a bioactive intermediary. Proc Natl Acad Sci USA 1994;91: 3680–3684.

224. Stamler JS, Mendelsohn ME, Amarante P, Smick D, Andon N, Davies PF, et al. N-acetylcysteine potentiates platelet inhibition by endothelium-derived relaxing factor. Circ Res 1989;65:789–795.

225. Cooke JP, Stamler J, Andon N, Davies PF, McKinley G, Loscalzo J. Flow stimulates endothelial cells to release nitrovasodilator that is potentiated by reduced thiol. Am J Physiol 1990;259:H804–H812.

226. Jocelyn PC. Thiols and disulfides in blood. In: Biochemistry of the SH Group. Academic Press, London, 1972, pp. 240–260.

227. Zhang YY, Xu A, Nomen M, Walsh M, Keaney JF Jr, Loscalzo J. Nitrosation of tryptophan residue(s) in serum albumin and model dipeptides: biochemical characterization and bioactivity. J Biol Chem 1996;271:14,271–14,279.

228. Frei B, Stocker R, Ames BN. Antioxidant defenses and lipid peroxidation in human blood plasma. Proc Natl Acad Sci USA 1988;85:9748–9752.

229. Nishikimi M. Oxidation of ascorbic acid with superoxide anion generated by the xanthine-xanthine oxidase system. Biochem Biophys Res Commun 1975;63:463–468.

230. Bodannes RS, Chan PC. Ascorbic acid as a scavenger of singlet oxygen. FEBS Lett 1979;105:195,196.

231. Halliwell B, Wasil M, Grootveld M. Biologically significant scavenging of the myeloperoxidase-derived oxidant hypochlorous acid by ascorbic acid. Implications for antioxidant protection in the inflamed rheumatoid joint. FEBS Lett 1987;213:15–17.

232. Frei B, England L, Ames BN. Ascorbate is an outstanding antioxidant in human blood plasma. Proc Natl Acad Sci USA 1989;86:6377–6381.

233. Ting HH, Timimi FK, Boles KS, Creager SJ, Ganz P, Creager MA. Vitamin C improves endothelium-dependent vasodilation in patients with non-insulin-dependent diabetes mellitus. J Clin Invest 1996;97:22–28.

234. Ting HH, Timimi FK, Haley EA, Roddy MA, Ganz P, Creager MA. Vitamin C improves endothelium-dependent vasodilation in forearm resistance vessels of humans with hypercholerolemia. Circulation 1997;95:2617–2622.

235. Heitzer T, Just H, Munzel T. Antioxidant vitamin C improves endothelial dysfunction in chronic smokers. Circulation 1996;94:6–9.

236. Hornig B, Arakawa N, Kohler C, Drexler H. Vitamin C improves endothelial function of conduit arteries in patients with chronic heart failure. Circulation 1998;97.363–368.

237. Taddei S, Virdis A, Ghiadoni L, Magagna A, Salvetti A. Vitamin C improves endothelium-dependent vasodilation by restoring nitric oxide activity in essential hypertension. Circulation 1998;97:2222–2229.

238. Jackson TS, Xu A, Vita JA, Keaney JF Jr. Ascorbic acid prevents the interaction of nitric oxide and superoxide only at very high physiologic concentrations. Circ Res 1998;83:916–922.

239. Gotoh N, Niki E. Rates of interactions of superoxide with vitamin E, vitamin C, and related compounds as measured by chemiluminescence. Biochim Biophys Acta 1992;1115:201–207.

240. Blatter LA, Taha Z, Mesaros S, Shacklock PS, Wier WG, Malinski T. Simultaneous measurements of Ca2+ and nitric oxide in bradykinin-stimulated vascular endothelial cells. Circ Res 1995;76:922–924.

241. Malinski T, Taha Z, Grunfeld S, Patton S, Kapturczak M, Tomboulian P. Diffusion of nitric oxide in the aorta wall monitored in situ by porphyrinic microsensors. Biochem Biophys Res Commun 1993;193:1076–1082.

242. Levine GN, Frei B, Koulouris SN, Gerhard MD, Keaney JF Jr, Vita JA. Ascorbic acid reverses endothelial dysfunction in patients with coronary artery disease. Circulation 1996;96:1107–1113.

243. Gokce N, Keaney JF Jr, Frei B, Holbrook M, Olesiak M, Zachariah BJ, et al. Long-term ascorbic acid administration reverses endothelial vasomotor dysfunction in patients with coronary artery disease. Circulation 1999;99:3234–3240.

244. Jain A, Martensson J, Mehta T, Krauss AN, Auld PA, Meister A. Ascorbic acid prevents oxidative stress in glutathione-deficient mice: effects on lung type 2 cell lamellar bodies, lung survactant, and skeletal muscle. Proc Natl Acad Sci USA 1992;89:5093–5097.

245. Kashiba-Iwatsuki M, Yamaguchi M, Inoue M. Role of ascorbic acid in the metabolism of S-nitroso-glutathione. FEBS Lett 1996;389:149–152.

246. Smith C, Mitchinson MJ, Aruoma OI, Halliwell B. Stimulation of lipid peroxidation and hydroxyl radical generation by the contents of human atherosclerotic lesions. Biochem J 1992;286:901–905.

247. Buettner GR. The pecking order of free radicals and antioxidants: lipid peroxidation, alpha-tocopherol, and ascorbate. Arch Biochem Biophys 1993;300:535–543.

248. Halliwell B, Gutteridge JMC. Role of free radicals and catalytic metal ions in human disease. Methods Enzymol 1990;186:1–85.

249. Sasaki H, Okabe E. Modification by hydroxyl radicals of functional reactivity in rabbit lingual artery. Jpn J Pharm 1993;62:305–314.

250. Dai FC, Diederich A, Skopec J, Diederick D. Diabetes-induced endothelial dysfunction in strepto-zotocin-treated rats: role of prostaglandin endoperoxides and free radicals. J Am Soc Neph 1993;4: 1327–1336.
251. Pieper GM, Langenstroer P, Siebeneich W. Diabetic-induced endothelial dysfunction in rat aorta: role of hydroxyl radicals. Cardiovasc Res 1997;34:145–156.
252. Nitenberg A, Paycha F, Ledoux S, Sachs R, Attali JR, Valensi P. 1998; Coronary artery responses to physiological stimuli are improved by deferoxiamine but not by L-arginine in non-insulin-dependent diabetic patients with angiographically normal coronary arteries and no other risk factors. Circulation 1998;97:736–743.
253. Varma SD, Shen X, Logman W. Copper catalyzed oxidation of ascorbate: chemical and ESR studies. Lens Eye Tox Res 1990;7:49–66.
254. Koppenol WH. Oxyradical reactions: from bond-dissociation energies to reduction potentials. FEBS Lett 1990;264:165–167.
255. Williams B, Schrier RW. Characterization of glucose-induced in situ protein kinase C activity in cultured vascular smooth muscle cells. Diabetes 1992;41:1464–1472.

27 Coating Arterial and Blood-Contacting Surfaces with NO˙-Donating Compounds

John D. Folts and Joseph Loscalzo

INTRODUCTION

Acutely Damaged Arteries with Loss of Protective Endothelial NO˙

Platelet activity is known to enhance the progression of coronary atherosclerosis and to precipitate platelet-mediated coronary thrombosis and acute ischemic events (1). Over the past 30 years, considerable research has been conducted to examine ways by which to inhibit abnormal platelet interaction with acutely damaged arterial walls, stents, and synthetic arterial grafts (1–3). These interactions contribute to the development of atherosclerosis, arterial thrombosis, and restenosis from intimal hyperplasia after interventional procedures, such as angioplasty or atherectomy, and also leads to failure of synthetic vascular grafts (4,5).

Loss of NO˙-Donating Endothelium

The main problem associated with atherosclerosis, angioplasty, vascular grafts, and stents is the lack or dysfunction of the normal protective endothelial layer that lines arterial walls when they are healthy. This layer of endothelial cells (EC) secretes a variety of protective substances that inhibit platelet adhesion, aggregation, and thrombus formation on the normal wall. One of the key substances normally released by ECs is endothelium-derived relaxing factor (EDRF) or a form of nitric oxide (NO˙)(6). NO˙ released luminally inhibits the interaction of circulating platelets with the damaged vessel wall. Both endogenous and exogenous NO˙ or NO˙ donating compounds inhibit platelet adhesion (7,8) and aggregation (9–11). NO˙ inhibits platelet and leukocyte adhesion and aggregation (heterotypic aggregates), as well as leukocyte migration into arterial walls (12–14). NO˙ (15,16) and NO˙-donating compounds, such as nitroglycerin (17) and sodium nitroprusside (18) given intravenously, specifically inhibit platelet interactions with damaged and stenosed canine coronary arteries. In addition, NO˙ relaxes vascular smooth muscle cells (VSMCs) and inhibits VSMC proliferation (19). Furthermore, NO˙-generating compounds potentiate the activity of thrombolytic factors to provide further protection against vascular thrombotic occlusion (20). These beneficial effects of NO˙ are lost, however, when endothelial function is impaired in chronic atherosclerotic lesions and in acutely induced lesions, such as those caused by balloon angioplasty (21). Injury to the endothelial layer causes it to have procoagulant instead of anticoagulant properties and to express vasoactive molecules, cytokines, and growth factors (22). If an artery has too long a section of arterial damage for effective dilation, or if it is aneurysmal, there is a need for synthetic vascular grafts, using Gore-Tex or other synthetic material. These grafts do not have

From: *Contemporary Cardiology, vol. 4: Nitric Oxide and the Cardiovascular System*
Edited by: J. Loscalzo and J. A. Vita © Humana Press Inc., Totowa, NJ

an endothelial layer when they are surgically inserted *(2)*. Over time, they develop an endothelial lining, which provides reasonable protection against thrombosis. However, vascular grafts are not effective at diameters less than 3 mm in diameter because they become occluded with intimal hyperplasia and thrombotic material *(2)*.

CURRENT INTERVENTIONAL TREATMENTS
FOR NARROWED AND DAMAGED CORONARY ARTERIES

Coronary Angioplasty/Atherectomy

Gruentzig in 1979 initiated a nonsurgical method of dilating narrowed coronary arteries using percutaneous transluminal coronary angioplasty, or PTCA *(22a)*. This technique employed a specially designed inflatable but nondistensible balloon-tipped catheter to dilate discrete coronary arterial stenoses. This treatment provided immediate relief of ischemic symptoms by providing a larger arterial lumen and increased coronary blood flow. However, the acute arterial damage produced by dilating or enlarging a narrowed artery, whether by angioplasty balloon, atherectomy, or laser, leads to two new problems. First, the acute injury to the narrowed artery causes significant intimal and medial damage, with dissection of the arterial wall and loss of or damage to the endothelial cells that are the source of EDRF or NO•. This leads to the deposition of platelets and neutrophils on the damaged surface and acute thrombotic occlusion can result. Vasospasm due to the loss of EC-derived NO•, as well as prostacyclin, and the presence of vasoconstrictors released from platelets and dysfunctional ECs can also occur and acutely narrow the artery. This effect is somewhat attenuated in patients by nitrate use. Second, the acute injury provokes a variety of normal and abnormal healing responses and inflammatory responses leading to neointimal hyperplasia, vascular remodeling, and restenosis *(23)*. The severity of these abnormal responses is directly related to the degree of arterial injury *(24)*.

Antiplatelet Therapy for Preventing
Acute Arterial Thrombosis and Restenosis after Angioplasty

Owing to the important role of platelet adhesion, aggregation, and growth factor release on the acutely damaged arterial surface (with the loss of functional endothelial cells and the NO• they release), platelet inhibitors have been utilized to limit thrombosis and restenosis. However, neither aspirin, aspirin plus dipyridamole, sulotroban, warfarin, ticlopidine, fish oil, nor angiotensin-converting enzyme inhibition with fosinopril produced a significant decrease in restenotic narrowing of dilated arteries after angioplasty *(25,26)*. New, very potent antiplatelet agents are now available and are being tested. However, with more potent antiplatelet and anticoagulant agents, like hirudin, the risk of excessive bleeding following the procedure increases. In addition to platelet inhibitors, a variety of other systemic treatments have been tried to reduce the incidence of intimal hyperplasia and restenosis after vascular injury produced by angioplasty. These include steroids, cyclosporin A, antineoplastics such as vincristine or actinomycin, or heparin *(23)*. The problem in finding a suitable platelet inhibitor may be that a very high concentration is needed systemically to have a major effect locally at the site of arterial damage. Thus, there is great interest in local delivery of substances with antiplatelet, anticoagulant, and antineoplastic properties. One of the substances that would be very beneficial to apply locally would be a NO• donor.

Endovascular Stents

In an effort to maintain arterial patency and maintain high blood flow after PTCA, endovascular stents were developed *(27)*. Stents are metal coils or slotted tubes that can be deployed in areas of stenosis by angioplasty balloons; after the balloon is expanded, the stent remains in place to limit arterial recoil and hold the area of arterial stenosis open. However, stents produce increased arterial wall damage, and by their very nature they are thrombogenic; thus, they produce new stimuli for thrombosis and restenosis. Metallic coronary stents were introduced to overcome two major limitations of balloon angioplasty: acute periprocedural vessel closure often related to dissection and intimal tears, which complicates 2–3% of attempts *(27–29)*, and chronic restenosis, which limits long-term patency in 20–50% of patients *(30)*. When angioplasty balloon dilation results in acute vessel closure, patients are placed in immediate peril of death (2–8%), myocardial infarction (20–30%), or need for emergency coronary bypass surgery (25–35%) *(29,30)*. Because of their ability to seal intimal tears, stents offer an attractive way to deal with threatened or abrupt vessel closure *(31)*. Stents can also rapidly and successfully restore luminal patency in 95% of patients with localized coronary dissections and threatened acute closure *(31)*.

However, metallic stents are very thrombogenic and more likely to thrombose than an angioplastied artery. In addition, as the stent provides continuous pressure on the arterial wall and is a foreign substance, it may cause further vascular injury and enhance the restenotic process, thereby reducing the lumen diameter. With time the stent becomes covered with neointima and moderately functional endothelial cells, which makes the surface less thrombogenic. In 1994 systemic anticoagulant therapy was of limited value in preventing early thrombosis and late (2–6 mo) restenosis after stenting or angioplasty *(32)*. Recent studies with the antiplatelet combination of aspirin and ticlopidine have shown significant reductions in the incidence of cardiac events and hemorrhagic complications *(33)*. Thus, although the stent maintains a large lumen initially, many of the same problems occur after stent placement as after angioplasty, i.e., the loss or lack of functional endothelial cells, exposure of thrombogenic subendothelial structures, platelet adherence, and release of growth factors, intimal hyperplasia, and loss of lumen. These are all related in part to the loss of NO• present on the normal luminal surface.

Synthetic Vascular Grafts

If an artery has too long a section of arterial damage for effective dilation, or if it is aneurysmal, synthetic Dacron (Dupont, Wilmington, DE) and other graft materials have been used to replace or bypass diseased arteries. However, the synthetic material, being foreign and devoid of endothelial cells and the NO• they produce, also provides a thrombogenic surface *(34,35)*. This attracts platelets and leukocytes, leading to thrombosis and intimal hyperplasia. This response is not a major problem with large-diameter grafts (8–20 mm in diameter) but is significant for small-diameter grafts between 2–6 mm in diameter *(2)*. The usual antiplatelet/anticoagulant therapy has been of limited success for maintaining the lumen of small-diameter vascular grafts (2–6 mm in diameter) *(34,35)*.

AN ALTERNATIVE TO SYSTEMIC ANTIPLATELET THERAPY: LOCAL COATING OF THROMBOGENIC SURFACES

Systemically administered pharmaceutical agents have diminished but not prevented the thrombosis and intimal hyperplasia that occurs in arteries further damaged by angioplasty, stent deployment, or insertion of synthetic vascular grafts. One reason may be that the dose needed when given systemically to provide sufficient drug concentration at the targeted site is too high. Very potent platelet inhibitors and anticoagulants are available, but at high systemic doses they cause excessive bleeding. If a potent protective coating containing drugs capable of inhibiting thrombosis and intimal hyperplasia could be delivered locally to the site of arterial damage or stent deployment, there would be much less of a systemic effect. In addition, high local concentrations of agents could be achieved. Furthermore, with local delivery, prolonged administration or high residence time of drug may be achieved. Thus, platelet deposition at the injured site could be significantly reduced by a high local concentration. Recently, a variety of devices have become available for delivering a potentially protective substance locally to acutely damaged arterial walls *(36)*.

Coating Endovascular Stents

Coronary stenting, while helping to maintain a larger lumen, suffers somewhat from the same two problems as that of the mechanically balloon-dilated coronary artery, which are the potential for early subacute thrombosis and restenosis. However, a stent offers a unique opportunity for local drug delivery, since the stent will be placed in very intimate contact with the acutely injured arterial wall and interfaces with the blood. In addition, a heavy protective coating can be applied prior to use. A number of attempts have been made to apply polymer coatings to stents. Polymer coating of the Wall® stent (Schneider, Minneapolis, MN) with cross-linked methane (Biogold) decreased early thrombosis of stents placed in pigs by 38% compared with uncoated stents. However, neointimal hyperplasia was not significantly reduced by this polymer coating *(37)*.

Intracoronary luminal irradiation with low-dose [^{192}Ir] or [^{90}Sr] reduced neointima formation in normolipemic pigs when administered for 20 min prior to stenting with a tantalum (Cordis Corp., Miami, FL) stent. The pigs were given heparin for the procedure and aspirin 325 mg/day for 28 d. At sacrifice, the luminal area of stented arteries was significantly increased and the neointimal area was significantly reduced with either form of radiation treatment compared to control, untreated stented arteries *(38)*. A drawback of this form of therapy is that radioactive ribbons must be properly positioned in the artery for 20–30 min before the stent is deployed *(38)*. Since stent deployment must often be performed under emergency conditions, the time delay attendant to this procedure may present a problem.

Another approach to coating stents in order to make them less thrombogenic is to "seed" or coat the stent with genetically engineered ECs. Using retroviral-mediated gene transfer, the gene for human tissue-type plasminogen activator (t-PA) was inserted into cultured sheep ECs *(39)*. These ECs will then release PGI$_2$, NO$^{\bullet}$, and high concentrations of t-PA. However, these cells do not stick to bare metal stents; therefore, the application of a substrate or "glue" is necessary before cell seeding *(39)*. Dichek and colleagues used a fibronectin substrate to "glue" or stick the ECs to the stent, which may have been a poor choice since the fibronectin "glue" is itself thrombogenic *(39)*. If some seeded ECs are released from the stent, a fibronectin-coated surface will remain that may be more thrombogenic than the bare stent itself. In vivo studies with the coating of genetically altered ECs placed on stents has been disappointing possibly for these reasons *(39)*. In addition, maintaining the viability of living ECs on the stent and their ability to make NO$^{\bullet}$ prior to use will be difficult.

A different approach to coating stents employs a fibrin film soaked in heparin that is then used as a circumferential coating on a tantalum stent. This coated stent was compared to an identical stent coated with a medical-grade polyurethane *(40)*. These stents were placed in pig coronary arteries that had no previous angioplasty or other injury. Heparin was given only during the procedure and no antiplatelet agents or anticoagulants were given following the procedure. After 28 d, the pigs were sacrificed and the stented arteries examined. The fibrin–heparin-coated stents had three total thrombotic occlusions out of 34 implanted stents at 48 h. Six of 12 polyurethane-coated stents were thrombosed at 48 h. The polyurethane-coated stents had marked neointimal thickening, and most stents were essentially occluded. In the fibrin–heparin coating group, there was less neointimal hyperplasia and the lumen reduction was less than 50% in most of the pigs; in addition, all arteries were patent *(40)*. Thus, the fibrin-heparin coating appeared to be better than the polyurethane coating in this model. Preliminary studies with a heparin-coated Benestent in patients also showed that the heparin-coated stent significantly decreased early thrombotic closure compared to an uncoated stent *(41)*. There was, however, no significant reduction in restenosis.

Coating of Synthetic Grafts

Artificial surfaces in contact with blood quickly develop a coating of adsorbed plasma protein that governs subsequent interaction with blood cells. This initial protein adsorption occurs within seconds, before the blood platelets and other cellular components reach the arterial surface *(2,42,43)*. Much research has focused on the role of the most prevalent plasma proteins. Albumin is the most abundant protein in serum, and albumin coating has been used to make synthetic surfaces more thromboresistant *(44–46)*. By contrast, polymer surfaces coated with fibrinogen, another abundant protein in serum, promotes platelet activation and presents a very thrombogenic surface *(42)*. Thus, the initial protein layer adsorbed to the polymer surface is very important in determining the thrombogenicity of that surface *(43)*.

Many interesting attempts have been made in the last 35 years to develop and apply protective antithrombogenic coatings to synthetic vascular grafts and other polymers exposed to blood *(2,47,48)*. In the 1960s, Whiffen and colleagues coated polycarbonate rings with colloidal graphite first, and when it had dried, they then added a dip coating of benzalkonium chloride and implanted them in dogs *(49)*. The implanted rings were found to take up heparin from the circulation that bound to the benzalkonium chloride layer and, thus, rendered the surface more thromboresistant *(4–9)*. These investigators then used a graphite coating followed by a second coating of benzalkonium chloride, followed again by a third layer of heparin purposely added prior to implantation. This coating was then denoted the *G*raphite *B*enzalkonium chloride *H*eparin or GBH surface. This GBH antithrombotic surface was used on an experimental hinged-leaf prosthetic mitral valve that was surgically implanted successfully in 86 patients with mitral valve disease *(50)*.

A number of studies dating back to 1969 have also shown that preadsorption of albumin to an artificial surface reduces platelet adhesion and aggregation *(42,43)*. Albumin contains no peptide sequences known to interact with blood cell membrane glycoproteins or enzyme receptors in the coagulation cascade and, thus, appears to provide a less thrombogenic surface. Many investigators have examined the effects of albumin adsorption and immobilization on the blood compatibility of polymer surfaces *(51–53)*.

Covalently bound conjugates of albumin and heparin were prepared as compounds that might improve the blood compatibility of polymer surface. The reduction in platelet adhesion on Biomer® polyvinyl chloride or silastic or glass surfaces treated with albumin–heparin conjugates was approximately 40% *(54)*. The effect of a heparin-coated surface on platelet adhesion and aggregation is inconsistent. Compared with control materials, heparin coatings have been shown both to increase *(55,56)* and decrease *(57,58)* platelet adhesion. Heparin coatings were least effective on small-diameter <4 mm grafts *(45,49,57)*.

SYSTEMIC USE OF NO· DONORS

NO· donors have been used to reduce platelet deposition and intimal proliferation following angioplasty. In the porcine carotid model, Groves and colleagues found reduced platelet thrombus formation after systemic administration of 3-morpholinosydnonimine (SIN-1), a spontaneous NO· donor and molsidomine metabolite *(59)*. Administration of this agent increased template bleeding time and platelet cyclic guanosine monophosphate (cGMP). The ACCORD trial also suggests that NO· donors might be beneficial following balloon angioplasty in patients *(60)*. In this trial, demonstration of SIN-1 acutely and molsidomine over the subsequent 6 mo significantly improved the restenosis rate compared with a diltiazem control. Oral L-arginine, the precursor of NO·, has also been shown to decrease intimal hyperplasia in rabbit aorta *(61)* and rat carotid artery *(62)*, and von der Leyen and colleagues showed that transfection of the constitutive endothelial NO· synthase (eNOS) gene in a rat carotid injury model *(63)* partially inhibited neointimal proliferation 2 wk after injury.

Coating Surfaces with NO• Donors

Recently Pulfer and colleagues have incorporated NO•-releasing crosslinked polyethel-eneimine microspheres into vascular grafts. Scanning electron microscopic analysis showed the microspheres entrapped in the pores of the vascular graft; these microspheres were designed to release 10 nmol NO•/mg with a half-life of 51 h *(64)*. This shows that NO•-releasing parti-cles can be incorporated into the pores of vascular grafts to deliver therapeutic amounts of NO• for the prevention of thrombosis and restenosis. Smith and colleagues incorporated the [N(O)NO•] group into polymeric matrices that can be used for altering the time course of NO• release *(65)*. The crosslinked poly-(ethylenimine) that has been exposed to NO• inhibited the in vitro proliferation of rat aorta smooth muscle cells when added as a powder to a culture medium. It also showed potent antiplatelet activity when coated on a normally thrombogenic vascular graft situated in an intravenous shunt in a baboon's circulatory system *(65)*. The assump-tion in the previous studies is that NO• inhibits platelet and leukocyte adhesion and aggrega-tion and inhibits smooth muscle proliferation and migration, and, thus, inhibits thrombosis and restenosis *(11–15)*.

Albumin has been used for coating vascular grafts to "passivate" surfaces in contact with blood and, thus, minimize surface-induced platelet activation *(52,66)*. Albumin reduces both the number of adherent platelets and the extent of platelet activation on the albumin-adsorbed surface *(52)*. Serum albumin can be modified to bear a covalently linked S-NO• functional group that manifests nitrovasodilation and platelet inhibitory properties *(67)*. In addition, bovine serum albumin (BSA) has been chemically modified so that the molar ratio of S-NO• to albumin is greater than 1:1 *(68)*. This modification produces a polynitrosated albumin (pS-NO•-BSA), which can be applied locally to foreign surfaces or to severely damaged arterial walls to make them less thrombogenic *(68–70)*. Among the most stable NO• donating com-pounds are the *S*-nitroso-thiols, such as *S*-nitrosated albumin *(67)*. S-Nitroso-thiols serve as carriers in the mechanism of action of EDRF by stabilizing the labile NO• *(67)*. In the dog, nitrosated albumin has been shown to inhibit in vivo platelet aggregation when given sys-temically *(71)* or locally *(70)*. It would seem reasonable that local delivery of an NO•-like species (pS-NO•-BSA) to restore or replace the relative deficiency of EDRF observed with dysfunctional, acutely damaged endothelium could modulate the effect of vascular injury and potentially reduce platelet aggregation and reduce intimal proliferation after angioplasty or stent deployment. This has been examined in several recent studies, where platelets were exposed to collagen or other coated surfaces.

Effect of pS-NO•-BSA Coating on Platelet Adhesion and Surface Activation

It has been postulated that the presence of NO• from healthy endothelial cells inhibits the attachment and spreading of platelets on normal arterial walls. In several experiments, plate-lets were placed in a chamber and directly visualized by video-enhanced light microscopy over time. Dog platelets exposed to glass, BSA-coated glass, or pS-NO•-BSA-coated glass behaved quite differently. There was a 50–70% reduction in platelet attachment and surface activation to a pS-NO•-BSA-coated surface when compared to BSA alone *(72)*. This sug-gests that the NO• can diffuse from the pS-NO•-BSA coating and inhibit platelet adhesion and activation in a time span of 60 min *(72)*.

There has been considerable recent interest in loading a drug onto a stent to limit early thrombogenicity and late neointima formation *(73)*. Drugs may be released by diffusion methods or during polymer breakdown. A variety of coatings, including fibrin, heparin, and multiple polymers containing drugs, have been tried (*see* ref. *73* for a recent review). Some coatings reduced early thrombosis and other coatings inhibited neointimal proliferation and restenosis, but none were very effective at both *(73)*.

We performed a study in which Palmaz–Schatz stents were coated with pS-NO•-BSA. Several questions needed to be answered. (1) Could stents be coated with pS-NO•-BSA? (2) Would the coating survive a week's shelf life? (3) Would the coating release NO•? Stents were dip-coated with pS-NO•-BSA and placed in the dark for 1 wk. They were then compared to untreated, bare stents for their ability to release NO•. To test whether NO• would be released, a bioassay was used. Coated and bare stents were placed in pig platelet-rich plasma (PRP) for 2 min and then removed. When the platelets were assayed for platelet cGMP levels, the level was more than twice as high in the PRP that had been exposed to a pS-NO•-BSA-coated stent compared to a bare stent (72). Because NO• is known to elevate platelet cGMP levels, this study led to several conclusions. Apparently the coating, dry and placed in the dark, survived for a week and NO• was able to elute off the stent and to diffuse into the platelets in platelet-rich plasma and raise the GMP levels. This suggests that pS-NO•-BSA might be placed on stents and used for local delivery of NO•.

Several groups have exposed coated stents to radiolabeled platelets to measure the extent of early platelet deposition. Heparin coating was tested in a rat arteriovenous shunt model. Early accumulation of radiolabeled platelets was significantly reduced on a heparin-coated stent compared to a bare stent (74). However, when the coated stents were implanted into pig coronary arteries, there was no decrease in intimal proliferation in the group with heparin-coated stent compared to a bare stent. Thus, there was no reduction in restenosis with the heparin coating (74).

In another study, Palmaz–Schatz stents coated with pS-NO•-BSA were compared to bare stents deployed in anesthetized pigs in six pairs of carotid arteries. Autologous [In^{III}]-labeled platelets were circulated in the pigs for 2 h. The average platelet deposition was four times higher on the bare, uncoated stents compared to the paired, coated stents (72). Thus the pS-NO•-BSA coating significantly retarded early platelet deposition (72). Because NO• has also been shown to inhibit SMC proliferation and migration, it would seem reasonable to test a NO• coating on an implanted stent over time. With inhibition of platelet deposition, and also inhibition of SMC involvement, a NO•-coated stent may reduce neointimal hyperplasia.

In eight pigs pS-NO•-BSA-coated Palmaz–Schatz stents were deployed in the carotid artery, with a matched bare stent placed in the contralateral carotid artery under sterile conditions. The pigs were given 5 mg/kg of aspirin for the first 5 d after stenting and no other treatment for the remaining 23 d. After 28 d, the pairs of stents were removed and examined histologically. The pS-NO•-BSA-coated stents had a 40% reduction in neointimal area compared to bare stents (72). There was also a statistically significant reduction in average neointimal thickness (72) (Fig. 1). Thus it appears that a pS-NO•-BSA-coated stent offers promise for further studies to inhibit early thrombosis and late restenosis.

Acute removal of the endothelium is a potent stimulus for thrombosis and neointimal proliferation (68). Thus, studies have been done applying NO•-donating substances directly to experimentally denuded arterial endothelial surfaces to determine if restenosis can be inhibited. One way to test the coating of damaged arterial walls is the direct application of pS-NO•-BSA to the angioplastied femoral arteries of anesthetized rabbits. After angioplasty of each femoral artery, one is exposed and coated with BSA prepared for nitrosation (pS-BSA) but without NO• incorporation. The other femoral artery is coated with chemically modified BSA (pS-NO•-BSA) that does contain NO•. The rabbits were then allowed to recover for 14 d. The artery receiving pS-NO•-BSA had a significantly larger lumen $0.86 \times 10^5 \, \mu M^2$ compared to the control $0.31 \times 10^5 \, \mu M^2$ ($p = 0.01$) and the treated arteries had 81% less neointimal area ($p = 0.02$) (68) (Fig. 2).

In these studies the pS-NO•-BSA also significantly inhibited radiolabeled platelet binding to the damaged arterial surface compared to control surfaces. Finally, when the arteries treated with pS-NO•-BSA were exposed to platelets for 1 min, they increased platelet cGMP levels more than fourfold compared to control, untreated arteries. Thus, the pS-NO•-BSA

A PSNO-BSA COATED STENT   **B** UNCOATED STENT

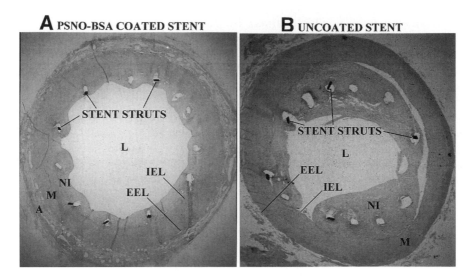

Fig. 1. The effect of pS-NO•-BSA on neointimal proliferation 28 d after stent deployment in the pig artery. (**A**) pSNO-BSA-coated stent. (**B**) Uncoated, control stent. L, lumen; IEL, internal elastic lamina; EEL, external elastic lamina; NI, neointima; M, media.

reacted in a similar fashion when the NO• donor was applied to implanted stents and when it was applied directly to damaged rabbit arteries.

SUMMARY

Loss of or dysfunctional ECs provide a thrombogenic surface. This surface permits platelet adhesion, activation, aggregation, and release of a variety of substances including platelet-derived growth factors. Synthetic vascular graft material is devoid of ECs when first inserted and is, thus, also thrombogenic until an endothelial layer grows over the exposed surface. A variety of coatings have been tried on vascular grafts and metallic stents to reduce thrombosis and restenosis. Coatings that provide a release of NO• appear to be promising.

NO• is known to inhibit platelets at least in part by diffusing into the cells and stimulating guanylyl cyclase (GC), which raises the concentration of platelet cGMP *(15)*. This elevation of cGMP inhibits the increase in cytosolic-free calcium produced by many of the input stimuli known to activate platelets. Elevated platelet cGMP also decreases the intracellular cytosolic calcium required for the triggering of actin and myosin interactions in the platelet cytoskeleton. By lowering the level of cytosolic calcium, it takes a much stronger stimulus to activate platelets. The inhibitory response of platelets is mediated by NO• binding to the heme iron of soluble guanylyl cyclase (sGC), which activates the enzyme and leads to the conversion of guanosine 5'-triphosphate to cyclic guanosine 3',5'-monophosphate (cGMP) *(75–77)*. cGMP regulates receptor-mediated Ca^{2+} influx and mobilization in platelets, which are necessary for platelet activation. The increase in cGMP reduces the platelet cytosolic calcium concentration *(78)*; it appears that cGMP is a more potent inhibitor of Ca^{2+} influx than of Ca^{2+} mobilization in platelets *(79)*.

In conclusion, the *S*-nitrosated albumin coatings are significantly more potent than an albumin coating in inhibiting platelet surface activation, adhesion, and aggregation on collagen-coated and glass surfaces. The albumin coating is also avid for metal stent surfaces and significantly reduced platelet attachment to the surface during an initial 2-h perfusion period in vivo. The application of pS-NO•-BSA to angioplastied rabbit femoral arteries for 15 min significantly reduces acute platelet accumulation and intimal hyperplasia. These results are

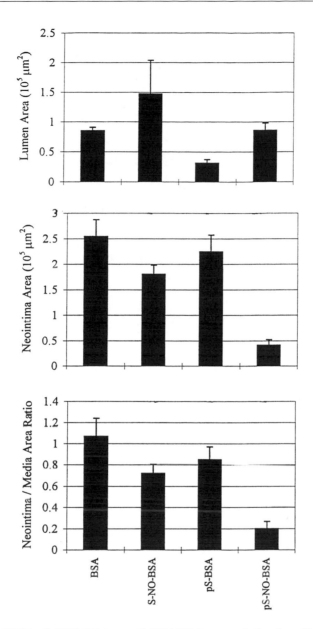

Fig. 2. The effect of BSA, S-NO•-BSA, or pS-NO•-BSA on neointimal proliferation 14 d after balloon injury of rabbit femoral artery. Neointimal proliferation is reported as the lumen area (**A**), the absolute neointimal area (**B**), and as a ratio of neointima/media (**C**) in three to six segments from each artery.

probably due to the mild antiadhesive properties of albumin combined with the more potent antiplatelet effects of NO•. By preventing early platelet attachment and activation to the thrombogenic surface, a *S*-nitrosated albumin coating may reduce the incidence of acute thrombosis and restenosis following angioplasty or stent placement.

REFERENCES

1. Vogel JH. On passivation and stenosis: Restenosis in coronary artery disease and percutaneous transluminal coronary angioplasty. Am J Cardiol 1987;60:68B–69B.

2. Leonard EF, Turitto VT, Vroman L, eds. Blood in Contact with Natural and Artificial Surfaces. New York Academy of Sciences, New York, 1987.

3. Fuster V, Stein B, Halperin JL, Chesebro JH. Antithrombotic therapy in cardiac disease: an approach based on pathogenesis and risk stratification. Am J Cardiol 1990;65:38C–44C.

4. Hennekens CH, Burin JE, Sandercock P, Collins R, Peto R. Aspirin and other antiplatelet agents in the secondary and primary prevention of cardiovascular disease. Circulation 1989;80:749–756.

5. Faxon DP, ed. Practical Angioplasty. Raven Press, New York, 1993.

6. Palmer RM, Ashton DS, Moncada S. Vascular endothelial cells synthesize nitric oxide from L-arginine. Nature 1988;333:664–666.

7. Groves PH, Penny WJ, Cheadle HA, Lewis MJ. Exogenous nitric oxide inhibits in vivo platelet adhesion following balloon angioplasty. Cardiovasc Res 1992;26:615–619.

8. Radomski MW, Palmer RM, Moncada S. Endogenous nitric oxide inhibits human platelet adhesion to vascular endothelium. Lancet 1987;2:1057,1058.

9. Lam JY, Chesebro JH, Fuster V. Platelets, vasoconstriction and nitroglycerin during arterial wall injury. A new antithrombotic role of an old drug. Circulation 1988;78:712–716.

10. DeCaterina R, Giannessi D, Bernini W, Lazzerini G, Mazzone A, Lombardi M. In vivo actions of organic nitrates on platelet function in humans. Z Kardiol 1989;78:56–60.

11. Azuma H, Ishikawa M, Sekizaki S. Endothelium-dependent inhibition of platelet aggregation. Br J Pharmacol 1986;88:411–415.

12. Garg UC, Hassid A. Nitric oxide-generating vasodilators and 8-bromo-cyclic guanosine monophosphate inhibit mitogenesis and proliferation of cultured rat vascular smooth muscle cells. J Clin Invest 1989;83:1774–1777.

13. Kubes P, Suzuki M, Granger DN. Nitric oxide: an endogenous modulator of leukocyte adhesion. Proc Natl Acad Sci USA 1991;88:4651–4655.

14. Radomski MW, Palmer RM, Moncada S. An L-arginine/nitric oxide pathway present in human platelets regulates aggregation. Proc Natl Acad Sci USA 1990;87:5193–5197.

15. Radomski MW, Palmer RM, Moncada S. Comparative pharmacology of endothelium-derived relaxing factor, nitric oxide and prostacyclin in platelets. Br J Pharmacol 1987;92:181–187.

16. Stamler JS, Loscalzo J. The antiplatelet effects of organic nitrates and related nitroso-compounds in vitro and in vivo and their relevance to cardiovascular disorders. J Am Coll Cardiol 1991;18:1529–1536.

17. Folts JD, Stamler JS, Loscalzo J. Intravenous nitroglycerin infusion inhibits cyclic blood flow responses caused by periodic platelet thrombus formation in stenosed canine coronary arteries. Circulation 1991;83: 2122–2127.

18. Rovin JD, Stamler JS, Loscalzo J, Folts JD. Sodium nitroprusside, an endothelium relaxing factor congener, increases platelet cyclic GMP levels and inhibits epinephrine-exacerbated in vivo platelet thrombus formation in stenosed canine coronary arteries. J Cardiovasc Pharmacol 1993;22:626–631.

19. Vita JA, Keaney JF, Loscalzo J. Endothelial dysfunction in vascular disease. In: Loscalzo J, Creager MA, Dzau VJ, eds. Vascular Medicine: A Textbook of Vascular Biology and Diseases. Little, Brown, Boston, MA, 1996, pp. 245,246.

20. Korbut R, Lidbury PS, Vane JR. Prolongation of fibrinolytic activity of tissue plasminogen activator by nitrovasodialators. Lancet 1990;335:669.

21. Chester AH, O'Neil GS, Moncada S, Tadjkarimi S, Yacoub MH. Low basal and stimulated release of nitric oxide in atherosclerotic epicardial coronary arteries. Lancet 1990;336:897–900.

22. Ross R. Atherosclerosis—an inflammatory disease. N Engl J Med 1999;340:115–126.

22a. Gruentzig AR, Senning A, Siegenthaler WE. Nonoperative dilatation of coronary-artery stenosis: percutaneous transluminal coronary angioplasty. N Engl J Med 1979;301:61–68.

23. Jonasson L, Holm J, Hansson GK. Cyclosporin A inhibits smooth muscle proliferation in the vascular response to injury. Proc Natl Acad Sci USA 1988;85:2303–2306.

24. Gravanis MB, Roubin GS. Histopathologic phenomena at the site of percutaneous transluminal coronary angioplasty: the problem of restenosis. Hum Pathol 1989;20:477–485.

25. Schwartz L, Lesperance J, Bourassa MG, Eastwood C, Kazim F, Arafah M, et al. The role of antiplatelet agents in modifying the extent of restenosis following percutaneous transluminal coronary angioplasty. Am Heart J 1990;119:232–236.

26. Desmet W, Vrolix M, DeScheerder I, VanLierde J, Willems JL, Piessens J. Angiotensin-converting enzyme inhibition with fosinopril sodium in the prevention of restenosis after coronary angioplasty. Circulation 1994;89:385–392.

27. Ruygrok PN, Serruys PW. Intracoronary stenting: from concept to custom. Circulation 1996;94:882–890.

28. Goldberg S, Savage MP, Fischman DL. Coronary artery stents. Lancet 1995;345:1523,1524.

29. DeFeyter PJ, DeJaegere PP, Murphy ES, Serruys PW. Abrupt coronary artery occlusion during percutaneous transluminal coronary angioplasty. Am Heart J 1992;123:1633–1642.

30. Hirshfeld JW Jr, Schwartz JS, Jugo R, MacDonald RG, Goldberg S, Savage MP, et al. Restenosis after coronary angioplasty: a multivariate statistical model to relate lesion and procedure variables to restenosis. J Am Coll Cardiol 1991;18:647–656.

31. Roubin GS, Cannon AD, Agrawal SK, Macander PJ, Dean LS, Baxley WA, et al. Intracoronary stenting for acute and threatened closure complicating percutaneous transluminal coronary angioplasty. Circulation 1992;85:916–927.

32. Fischman DL, Leon MB, Baim DS, Schatz RA, Savage MP, Penn I, et al. A randomized comparison of coronary-stent placement and balloon angioplasty in the treatment of coronary artery disease. N Engl J Med 1994;331:496–501.

33. Schomig A, Neumann F, Kastrati A, Schuhlen H, Blasini R, Hadamitzky M, et al. A randomized comparison of antiplatelet and anticoagulant therapy after the placement of coronary artery stents. N Engl J Med 1996;334:1084–1089.

34. Veith FJ, Gupta SK, Ascer I. Six-year multicenter comparison of autologous vein and expanded PTFE grafts in infrainguinal reconstruction. J Vasc Surg 1986;3:104–107.

35. Christenson JT, Al-Huneidi W, Owunwanne A. Early platelet deposition and distribution in various graft materials. Surg Res Com 1987;1·151–158.

36. Lincoff AM, Topol EJ, Ellis SG. Local drug delivery for the prevention of restenosis. Fact, fancy, and future. Circulation 1994;90:2070–2084.

37. Van Der Giessen WJ, Van Beusekom HM, Van Houten CD, Van Woerkens LJ, Verdouw PD, Serruys PW. Coronary stenting with polymer-coated and uncoated self-expanding endoprotheses in pigs. Coron Artery Dis 1992;3:631–640.

38. Waksman R, Robinson KA, Crocker IR, Gravanis MB, Palmer SJ, Wang C, et al. Intracoronary radiation before stent implantation inhibits neointima formation in stented porcine coronary arteries. Circulation 1995;92:1383–1386.

39. Dichek DA, Neville RF, Zwiebel JA, Freeman SM, Leon MB, Anderson WF. Seeding of intravasculara stents with genetically engineered endothelial cells. Circulation 1989;80:1347–1353.

40. Holmes DR Jr, Camrud AR, Jorgenson MA, Edwards WD, Schwartz RS. Polymeric stenting in the porcine coronary artery model: differential outcome of exogenous fibrin sleeves versus polyurethane-coated stents. J Am Coll Cardiol 1994;24:525–531.

41. Hardhammar PA, van Beusekom HM, Emanuelsson HU, Hofma SH, Albertsson PA, Verdouw PD, Boersma E, Serruys PW, van der Giessen WJ. Reduction in thrombotic events with heparin-coated Palmaz-Schatz stents in normal porcine coronary arteries. Circulation 1996;93:423–430.

42. Park K, Mosher DF, Cooper SL. Acute surface-induced thrombosis in the canine ex vivo model: importance of protein composition of the initial monolayer and platelet activation. J Biomed Mater Res 1986;20·589–612.

43. Brash JL. Protein interactions with artificial surfaces. In: Salzman EW, ed. Interaction of the Blood with Natural and Artificial Surfaces. Marcel Dekker, New York, 1981, p. 37.

44. Brynda E, Houska M, Pokorna Z, Cepalova NA, Moiseev YV, Kalal J. Irreversible adsorption of human serum albumin onto polyethylene film. J Bioeng 1978;2:411–418.

45. Ihlenfeld JV, Cooper SL. Transient in vivo protein adsorption onto polymeric biomaterials. J Biomed Mater Res 1979;13:577–591.

46. Ishikawa Y, Sasakawa S, Takase M, Osada Y. Effect of albumin immobilization by plasma polymerization on platelet reactivity. Thromb Res 1984;35:193–202.

47. Mustard JF, Groves HM, Kinlough-Rathbone RL, Packham MA. Thrombogenic and nonthrombogenic biological surfaces. In: Leonard EF, Turitto VT, Vroman L, eds. Blood in Contact with Natural and Artificial Surfaces. NY Academy of Sciences, New York, 1987, pp. 12–21.

48. Salzman EW, ed. Interaction of the Blood with Natural and Artificial Surfaces. Marcel Dekker, New York, 1981.

49. Whiffen JD, Gott VL. In vivo adsorption of heparin by graphite-benzalkonium surfaces. Surgery 1965; 121:287–290.

50. Gott VL, Daggett RL, Young WP. Development of a carbon-coated, central hinging, bileaflet valve. Ann Thorac Surg 1989;48:S28–S30.

51. Mohammad SF, Olsen DB. Immobilized albumin-immunoglobulin G for improved hemocompatibility of biopolymers. ASAIO Trans 1989;35:384–387.

52. Riccitelli SD, Schlatterer RG, Hendrix JA, Williams GB, Eberhart RC. Albumin coatings resistant to shear-induced desorption. Trans Am Soc Artif Intern Organs 1985;31:250–256.

53. Ryu G, Han D, Kim Y, Min B. Albumin immobilized polyurethane and its blood compatibility. ASAIO J 1992;38:M644–M648.

54. Hennink WE, Dost L, Feijen J, Kim SW. Interaction of albumin-heparin conjugate preadsorbed surfaces with blood. Trans Am Soc Artif Intern Organs 1983;29:200–205.

55. Salzman EW, Merrill EW, Binder F, Wolf CW, Ashford TP, Austen WG. Protein-platelet interaction on heparinized surfaces. J Biomed Mater Res 1969;3:69–81.
56. Goosen MF, Sefton MV. Heparin styrene-butadiene-styrene elastomers. J Biomed Mater Res 1979;13: 347–364.
57. Larsson R, Eriksson JC, Lagergren H, Olsson P. Platelet and plasma coagulation compatibility of heparinized and sulphated surfaces. Thromb Res 1979;15:157–167.
58. Rembaum A, Yen SP, Ingram J, Newton JF, Hu CL, Frasher WG, et al. Platelet adhesion to heparin bonded and heparin free surfaces. Biomater Med Devices Artif Organs 1973;1:99–119.
59. Groves PH, Lewis MJ, Cheadle HA, Penny WJ. SIN-1 reduces platelet adhesion and platelet thrombus formation in a porcine model of balloon angioplasty. Circulation 1993;87:590–597.
60. Lablanche JM, Grollier G, Lusson JR, Bassand JP, Drobinski G, Bertrand B, et al. Effect of the direct nitric oxide donors linsidomine and molsidomine on angiographic restenosis after coronary balloon angioplasty. The ACCORD study. Circulation 1997;95:83–89.
61. McNamara DB, Bedi B, Aurora H, Tena L, Ignarro LJ, Kadowitz PJ, et al. L-arginine inhibits balloon catheter-induced intimal hyperplasia. Biochem Biophys Res Commun 1993;193:291–296.
62. Taguchi J, Junichi A, Takuwa Y, Kurokawa K. L-Arginine inhibits neointimal formation following balloon injury. Life Sci 1993;53:387–392.
63. von der Leyen HE, Gibbons GH, Morishita R, Lewis NP, Zhang L, Nakajima M, Gene therapy inhibiting neointimal vascular lesion: in vivo transfer of endothelial cell nitric oxide synthase gene. Proc Natl Acad Sci USA 1995;92:1137–1141.
64. Pulfer SK, Ott D, Smith DJ. Incorporation of nitric oxide-releasing crosslinked polyethyleneimine microspheres into vascular grafts. J Biomed Mater Res 1997;37:182–189.
65. Smith DJ, Chakravarthy D, Pulfer S, Simmons ML, Harabie JA, Citro ML, et al. Nitric oxide releasing polymers containing the [N(O)NO•]-group. J Med Chem 1996;39:1148–1156.
66. Amiji M, Park H, Park K. Study on the prevention of surface induced platelet activation by albumin coating. J Biomater Sci Polymer 1992;3:375–388.
67. Stamler JS, Simon DI, Osborne JA, Mullins ME, Jaraki O, Michel T, et al. S-nitrosylation of proteins with nitric oxide: synthesis and characterization of biologically active compounds. Proc Natl Acad Sci USA 1992;89:444–448.
68. Marks DS, Vita JA, Folts JD, Keaney JF Jr, Welch GN, Loscalzo J. Inhibition of neointimal proliferation in rabbits after vascular injury by a single treatment with a protein adduct of nitric oxide. J Clin Invest 1995;96:2630–2638.
69. Folts JD. Coating Palmaz-Schatz stents with a unique NO• donor reduces the need for post-procedure anticoagulation when placed in pig carotid arteries. J Invest Med 1995;43:476A.
70. Folts JD, Keaney JF Jr, Loscalzo J. Local delivery of nitrosated albumin to stenosed and damaged coronary arteries inhibits platelet deposition and thrombosis. J Am Coll Cardiol 1995;Special Edition: 377A.
71. Keaney JF Jr, Stamler JS, Scharfstein J, Folts JD, Loscalzo J. NO• forms a stable adduct with serum albumin that has potent antiplatelet properties in vivo. Clin Res 1992;40:194A.
72. Maalej N, Albrecht R, Loscalzo J, Folts JD. The potent platelet inhibitory effect of S-nitrosated albumin coating of artificial surfaces. J Am Coll Cardiol 1999;33:1408–1414.
73. Bertrand OF. Biocompatibility aspects of new stent technology. J Am Coll Cardiol 1998;32:562–571.
74. De Scheerder IK. Wang K, Wilczek K, Meuleman D, Van Amsterdam R, Vogel G, et al. Experimental study of thrombogenicity and foreign body reaction induced by heparin-coated coronary stents. Circulation 1997;95:1549–1553.
75. Loscalzo J. N-Acetylcysteine potentiates inhibition of platelet aggregation by nitroglycerin. J Clin Invest 1985;76:703–708.
76. Keaney JF Jr, Simon DI, Stamler JS, Jaraki O, Scharfstein J, Vita JA, et al. NO• forms an adduct with serum albumin that has endothelium-derived relaxing factor-like properties. J Clin Invest 1993;91: 1582–1589.
77. Mellion BT, Ignarro LJ, Ohlstein EH, Pontecorvo EG, Hyman AL, Kadowitz PJ. Evidence for the inhibitory role of guanosine 3',5'-monophosphate in ADP-induced human platelet aggregation in the presence of nitric oxide and related vasodilators. Blood 1981;57:946–955.
78. Nakashima S, Tohmatsu T, Hattori H, Okano Y, Nozawa Y. Inhibitory action of cyclic GMP on secretion, polyphosphoinositide hydrolysis and calcium mobilization in thrombin stimulated human platelet. Biochem Biophys Res Commun 1986;135:1099–1104.
79. Morgan RO, Newby AC. Nitroprusside differentially inhibits ADP-stimulated calcium influx and mobilization in human platelets. Biochem J 1989;258:447–454.

28   Gene Therapy and Nitric Oxide

Heiko E. von der Leyen

GENERAL PRINCIPLES OF GENE THERAPY

The development of in vivo gene transfer technology has created a powerful new tool for the study of diseases by providing methods to overexpress or to inhibit specific local factors that are believed to contribute to a pathological process. In addition, this technology provides the opportunity for the development of novel therapeutic strategies such as gene replacement, gene correction, or gene augmentation paving the way for gene therapy as a therapeutic option for many diseases *(1,2)*. The recombinant DNA "breakthrough" has provided us with a new and powerful approach to the questions that have intrigued and plagued humans for centuries *(3)*. This paradigmatic shift in medicine led to a change of the view of pathophysiology from a more biochemical interpretation to the recognition of disease as a molecular event on the level of gene expression *(4,5)*. New therapeutic approaches are moving from biochemically designed pharmaceuticals to genetically engineered tools for the treatment of diseases. The elucidation of molecular and cellular pathobiological processes of diseases has depended on (1) in vitro cell culture experiments, (2) studies of gene expression in experimental animal models or human specimens using Northern blot, reverse transcription-polymerase chain reaction (RT-PCR), or *in situ* hybridization, and (3) the development of transgenic animal models and the use of homologous recombination.

To improve the efficiency of gene transfer, a number of alternatives to the classical precipitation techniques (calcium phosphate or diethylaminoethyl-dextran (DEAE)-polymer; *[6]*) have recently been developed (Table 1). The encapsulation of the DNA of interest in artificial lipid membranes (liposomes) resulted in a higher efficiency of gene transfer in certain cell types *(7)*. Microinjection has been successfully used to introduce purified recombinant proteins, neutralizing antibodies, and competitor oligonucleotides into cells, allowing a critical examination of the role of specific gene products in the acquisition of a variety of defined phenotypic features that can be assayed at the single-cell level *(8,9)*. The intramuscular injection of plasmid DNA into skeletal muscle resulted in transient expression of a foreign gene in different skeletal myotubes *(10)*. By extending direct gene injection to the heart muscle, the expression of a reporter gene was demonstrated for up to 4 wk after the initial injection *(11)*. Furthermore, expression of injected genes can be targeted to specific cell types in vivo (e.g., cardiac muscle cells) and can be modulated by the hormonal status of the animal *(12)*. Another approach for gene delivery consists in viral vectors or fusigenic liposomes that have recently been used in growing numbers to express exogenous genes in vivo *(13,14)*. Effective therapy by in vivo delivery of DNA requires efficient delivery, long-term maintenance of the DNA that is delivered, and physiological levels of expression of the therapeutic gene. Full level of physiologically controlled expression can be obtained after transfer of intact genes or fragments

From: *Contemporary Cardiology, vol. 4: Nitric Oxide and the Cardiovascular System*
Edited by: J. Loscalzo and J. A. Vita © Humana Press Inc., Totowa, NJ

Table 1
Experimental Gene Transfer Methods

Viral mediated	Retrovirus
	Adenovirus
	Replication deficient
	Adenoviral coat/transferrin-polylysin
	Adeno-associated virus (AAV)
	Lentivirus
Lipid mediated	Liposomes
	Cationic lipososmes
Fusigenic liposome mediated	Sendai virus (HVJ)-liposomes
Other methods	Microinjection
	Microparticle bombardment
	Myoblast implantation

of DNA hundreds of kilobases in size, as has been demonstrated by the transfer of yeast artificial chromosomes into transgenic mice *(15,16)*. Long-term maintenance of input DNA could be achieved if the DNA carried replication origins, a centromere, and telomeres to allow maintenance and segregation in mammalian cells *(17)*. These features could be combined as a mammalian artificial chromosome that would confer full levels of controlled expression as well as being maintained in any cell into which it was introduced *(18)*. In vivo gene transfer techniques for cardiovascular applications include:

1. Viral gene transfer, such as retrovirus or adenovirus;
2. Liposomal gene transfer with cationic liposomes (e.g., Lipofectin®, Gibco-BRL, Gaithersburg, MD);
3. Fusigenic liposomes using Sendai virus (HVJ; hemagglutinating virus of Japan) complexed with liposomes; and
4. Direct (micro)injection including myoblast implantation.

The recent development of efficient gene transfection procedures together with the arsenal of recombinant DNA technology has led to the application of transient or stable expressions of genes to study disease processes. In particular, this technique is useful for the characterization of locally expressed genes that have been postulated to play autocrine and/or paracrine roles in pathophysiology. Current approaches for experimental gene transfer include the application of oligonucleotides or recombinant DNA for gene replacement, gene inhibition or gene augmentation (Table 2).

The study of nitric oxide (NO•) has so many facets that it is uniting many sections of medicine like neuroscience, physiology, and immunology. NO• functions both as a signaling molecule in endothelial and nerve cells as well as a killer molecule by activated immune cells. Its ubiquitous distribution in the body and its multiple roles have influenced our understanding of how cells communicate and protect themselves *(19–21)*. The recent cloning and characterization of the different isoforms of the nitric oxide synthases (NOS) paved the way for integration of the various aspects of NOS gene transfer into current concepts of therapeutic gene transfer *(22–24)*. In this chapter I will review genetic engineering techniques such as transfer of antisense oligonucleotides or DNA expression vectors that were designed to modify the action of NOS and to elucidate the multiple aspects of the physiological as well as pathophysiological roles of NO•.

Vascular remodeling usually represents an adaptive process that occurs in response to long-term changes in hemodynamic and humoral conditions. It may subsequently contribute to the pathophysiology of vascular diseases *(25)*. The active process of vascular remodeling involves changes in several cellular processes including cell growth, cell death, cell migra-

Table 2
Molecular Approach to Cardiovascular Disease

1. Define pathobiological mediators by mRNA analysis
   • PCR
   • Northern blot
   • *In situ* hybridization
2. Simulate pathological conditions
   • Gene transfer of putative mediators
   • Antisense inhibition of putative mediators
   • Transgenic animals
3. Novel therapies
   • Gene augmentation
   • Antisense or decoy strategies
   • Gene replacement

Table 3
Genetic Engineering Approaches to Study NO•

"Gain of function": plasmid vector	*"Loss of function": antisense oligonucleotide*

Overexpression of NOS *(50)*
   Intracellular and extracellular action,
    autocrine and paracrine effect
	Inhibition of transcription and/or translation *(71)*
	   Intracellular action

tion, and extracellular matrix production or degradation. As illustrated in Table 3, the transfer of plasmid DNA (or gene) into cells or tissue in vivo to overexpress an isoform of nitric oxide sythase may subsequently result in increased nitric oxide production ("gain of function"). In fact, the role of a specific autocrine or paracrine factor in the (patho)biological adaptation of specific organ systems can be determined by genetic engineering studies resulting in obvious potential for the treatment of diseases. Another molecular approach is to *inhibit* the function of the gene for a specific NOS isoform by the application of antisense oligonucleotides ("loss of function"). Oligonucleotides could be employed as therapeutic agents that exert their molecular actions intracellularly either at the translational or transcriptional level *(26–28)*. Antisense oligonucleotides can bind specific mRNA and block ribosomal translocation, thereby inhibiting translation. The antisense DNA:mRNA duplex is also rapidly degraded by RNase H *(29)*.

IN VITRO STUDIES ON THE EFFECT
OF OVEREXPRESSION OF THE NOS GENE

NO• has been shown to inhibit vascular smooth muscle cell (VSCM) proliferation and migration in vitro and has been postulated to be an important mediator in vascular remodeling *(19,20,23,30)*. Endothelium-derived relaxing factor (EDRF) was first described by Furchgott and Zawadzki *(31)* and later identified as NO• *(32,33)*. In vitro studies by several research groups demonstrated overexpression of NOS in cultured cells using adenovirus-mediated gene transfer *(34,35)*. Expression of recombinant endothelial cell-type NOS (NOS III) in cultured SMCs resulted in inhibition of serum-stimulated DNA synthesis and cell proliferation *(35)*. These results are supporting the findings of Garg and Hassid *(30)*, who reported inhibition of mitogenesis and proliferation of cultured rat VSMCs by an NO• donor in vitro. A different approach was taken by Channon et al. *(34)* who used the neuronal isoform of NOS (nNOS; NOS I) for gene transfer experiments. Using an adenoviral vector, these authors characterized their vector in human cultured endothelial as well as SMCs and documented high-level expression after transfection. After nNOS transfection in VSMCs, nNOS activity was physiologically regulated and of a magnitude comparable to native ecNOS (NOS III) in endothelial cells. Thus, different isoforms of NOS seem to be versatile and efficient tools for gene transfer with widespread potential therapeutic applications.

Recently, it was demonstrated that NO$^{\bullet}$ inhibited migration of mitogen-stimulated VSMCs in vitro *(36)*. Stimulation of SMCs of guinea pig coronary artery by platelet-derived growth factor (PDGF)-BB retarded paxillin mobility (mobility shift) in sodium dodecyl sulfate-polyacrylamide gel electrophoresis (SDS-PAGE) in a time-dependent manner. This effect may be due to tyrosine phosphorylation of paxillin. Transfer of ecNOS (NOS III) gene by replication deficient recombinant adenovirus in VSMCs inhibited PDGF-BB stimulated mobility shift and tyrosine phosphorylation of paxillin *(37)*. In addition, tyrosine phospho-rylation of focal adhesion kinase (FAK) was inhibited. Considering the importance of FAK and paxillin in cell migration and proliferation, it was suggested from this gene transfer study that the FAK–paxillin pathway is a target for NO$^{\bullet}$ action to inhibit VSMC migration and proliferation *(37)*.

Gene transfer of inducible nitric oxide synthase (iNOS) using a retroviral vector demon-strated significant protein expression in endothelial cells as well as SMCs in vitro *(38)*. In SMCs, NO$^{\bullet}$ synthesis after iNOS transfection was dependent on exogenous tetrahydrobiop-terin (BH$_4$) *(39)*. Unstimulated VSMCs do not synthesize BH$_4$. Recently, it was shown in NIH 3T3 cells constitutively expressing recombinant human iNOS that iNOS subunits dimerize to form an active enzyme, and that BH$_4$ plays a critical role in promoting dimerization in intact cells *(39)*. A human expression plasmid encoding guanosine triphosphate (GTP) cyclohydrolase I (GTPCH), the rate-limiting enzyme for BH$_4$ biosynthesis, was successfully cotransfected with iNOS into SMCs to reconstitute iNOS activity *(40)*. Thus, even if it is synthesized in neighboring cells, GPTCH gene transfer could be used to deliver a cofactor to targeted cells and may augment the production of NO$^{\bullet}$ after iNOS gene transfer.

One mechanism by which NO$^{\bullet}$ may prevent intimal hyperplasia is protection of the endo-thelium and promotion of its regeneration. Tzeng et al. *(41)* constructed an adenoviral vector containing the inducible isoform of NOS (iNOS; NOS II) and transfected cultured sheep arterial endothelial cells. The increased NO$^{\bullet}$ production after transfection did not affect the viability of the endothelial cells, and prolonged exposure to NO$^{\bullet}$ did not induce apoptosis of endothelial cells. Instead, NO$^{\bullet}$ inhibited lipopolysaccharide-induced apoptosis by reducing caspase-3-like protease activity *(41)*.

Recent experiments support a protective effect of NO$^{\bullet}$ against superoxide radicals in endo-thelial cells exposed to oxidized low-density lipoprotein (LDL) *(42,43)*. Growing evidence suggests that atherosclerosis is an inflammatory disease, and that monocyte adherence to the endothelium represents the earliest vessel wall abnormality occuring within 1 wk of a high cholesterol diet in experimental animals *(44)*. Superoxide radicals may play a pivotal role in early atherosclerotic lesion formation. Besides shear stress and diethylenetriamine (DETA) NONOate (a NO$^{\bullet}$ donor), preliminary data showed that iNOS gene transfer reduced oxygen radical production in vitro *(45)*. Thus, it appears that iNOS gene transfer may provide a potentially powerful tool to modify vascular homeostasis beyond simple modulation of vaso-motion *(46)*. Increased availability of NO$^{\bullet}$ within the vascular wall may counteract the detri-mental effects of superoxide radicals and may reduce the degree of endothelial activation and dysfunction *(42,43)*.

IN VIVO STUDIES: OVEREXPRESSION OF THE NOS GENE

Overexpression of ecNOS (NOS III)

Injury to the endothelium plays an essential role in the "response to injury" hypothesis *(44)* and EDRF/NO$^{\bullet}$ has an important regulatory function in maintaining vascular homeo-stasis *(47)*. It was hypothesized that the loss of NO$^{\bullet}$ production and bioactivity might explain the fact that diverse pathological conditions such as hypercholesterolemia, hypertension,

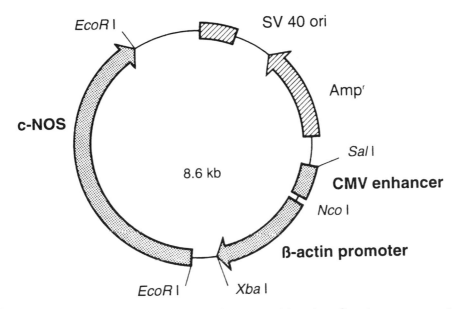

Fig. 1. Example of an ecNOS (*NOS3*) expression vector driven by a β-actin promoter and CMV enhancer *(50)*.

diabetes, and cigarette smoking are all considered risk factors for atherosclerosis *(46)*. Experimental studies have shown that vascular injury induces local expression of mitogens and chemotactic factors mediating neointimal lesion formation with subsequent vascular dysfunction. NO• has been shown to inhibit VSMC proliferation and migration in vitro and has been postulated to be an important local factor in vascular remodeling *(30,43,48,49)*.

To determine the effect of overexpression of the constitutive isoform of NOS (endothelial type NOS (ecNOS); NOS III), I constructed a NOS expression vector (Fig. 1) in which the ecNOS cDNA was controlled by a *CAG* promoter (cytomegalovirus CMV-IE enhancer sequence connected to a modified [AG] chicken β-actin promoter), rabbit β-globin gene sequences including a polyadenylation signal, and a SV40 *ori* in a pUC13 vector *(50)*. In vivo transfection of this construct using fusigenic liposomes *(51)* into balloon-injured rat carotid arteries not only restored NO• production within the vessel wall, but also significantly increased the vascular reactivity of the vessel *(50)*. Furthermore, ecNOS transgene expression resulted in a 70% inhibition of neointima formation after balloon injury (Fig. 2). Four complementary experimental methods were used to verify successful in vivo ecNOS gene transfer into the vessel wall:

1. Transgene protein expression was documented by Western blot;
2. Localization of enzyme expression in the vessel wall was verified by *in situ* histochemical staining using the nicotinamide adenine dinucleotide phosphate (NADPH) diaphorase assay;
3. Enzymatic activity of the transgene product was confirmed by measurement of increased NO• generation from transfected vessel segments using the chemiluminescence methods; and
4. Biological effectiveness of the transgene product was assessed by changes in vascular reactivity induced by the increased local generation of NO•, thereby potentially counterbalancing vasospasm induced by vascular injury.

In addition, at d 4 after ecNOS transfection, a significant decrease in DNA synthesis as measured by BrdUrd incorporation in ecNOS transfected vessels was demonstrated *(50)*. Given that the activation of mitogenic factors characterizing the cellular processes essential for lesion formation occurs within the first few of days after injury *(52)*, the characterization of transgene expression was focused during the same period. It has been shown that interventions

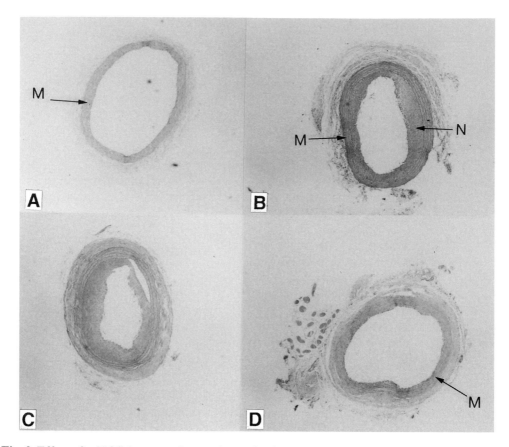

Fig. 2. Effect of ecNOS (or control vector) transfection on neointima formation in balloon-injured rat carotid arteries. Representative cross-sections (×25) from rat carotid arteries are shown: (**A**) uninjured, (**B**) injured untreated, (**C**) injured with control vector transfection, (**D**) injured with ecNOS transfection. M = media, N = neointima. Reprinted with permission of ref. *(50)*.

that inhibit cell proliferation and/or cell migration during this initial acute phase prevent neointima formation at least 2 wk after injury *(53–55)* . Thus, in vivo ecNOS gene transfer in the rat carotid injury model was a "proof of concept" that vascular-derived NO• plays an important role in modulating vascular remodeling. For the first time, this study documented therapeutic effects utilizing direct in vivo gene transfer of a cDNA encoding a functional enzyme. In fact, ecNOS gene transfer may be useful for gene therapy of neointimal hyperplasia and associated local vasospasm thereby modulating vascular remodeling *(56)*.

By using adenovirus-mediated gene transfer, Janssens et al. *(57)* extended the previously described genetic engineering strategy and demonstrated successful transfer of the gene encoding human endothelial NOS to balloon-injured rat carotid arteries. Transgene expression was demonstrated in 30% of medial SMCs and foci of adventitial cells. These effects were associated with increased local NO• production and restoration of cyclic guanosine monophosphate (cGMP) levels to those observed in uninjured vessels. Neointimal surface area after balloon injury was reduced by 70% compared to control injured arteries *(57)*. The same group also reported successful adenoviral gene transfer of ecNOS in pig coronary arteries *(58)*.

In extending their in vitro studies, Kullo et al. *(59)* showed a diminished contractile response as well as enhanced endothelium-dependent relaxation at d 4 after in vivo gene transfer of ecNOS in rabbit carotid arteries. Endothelium-specific transgene expression was confirmed by staining for β-galactosidase in *LacZ*-transduced arteries as well as ecNOS specific immunoreactivity in ecNOS transfected arteries. The results of these studies suggest that vascular ecNOS gene therapy may extend our therapeutic arsenal for the treatment of vasospasm and endothelial dysfunction (59,60).

In an ex vivo study, a recombinant ecNOS expression vector was successfully transferred to large canine cerebral arteries by adenovirus-mediated gene transfer via the cerebrospinal fluid (61). Functional expression of ecNOS resulted in increased basal production of cGMP with a subsequent reduction in receptor-mediated contractile response and enhancement of endothelium-dependent relaxation. The perivascular application via cerebrospinal fluid with subsequent expression of recombinant ecNOS in cerebral arteries may represent a potentially feasible therapeutic approach alleviating vasospastic conditions (60,61). Incubation of rabbit carotid arteries (62) or porcine coronary arteries (63) in organ culture with a replication-deficient adenovirus carrying the cDNA for ecNOS augmented vasorelaxation in response to stimuli that release NO•. Gene transfer in organ culture resulted in ecNOS transgene expression preferentially in adventitial cells, suggesting that adventitial gene transfer may be sufficient to alter vasomotor tone (62).

In applying these gene transfer studies in organ culture, Cable et al. (64) transduced human saphenous veins with an adenovirus vector encoding bovine ecNOS and demonstrated functional expression of recombinant NOS in vein grafts. Using fusigenic liposomes constructed by encapsulation of ecNOS plasmid into HVJ-liposomes, Matsumoto et al. (65) transfected vein grafts and showed ecNOS expression mainly in medial SMCs and adventitial cells at 4 d after transfection. In vein grafts under poor runoff conditions, intimal thickness at 4 wk after implantation was significantly reduced by ecNOS gene transfer. Thus, NOS gene transfer in saphenous vein grafts may provide a genetic engineering tool to reduce the risk of graft vasculopathy by providing increased vascular NO• production.

Overexpression of iNOS

Transfection of iNOS in vivo completely prevented myointimal thickness of porcine arteries induced by balloon catheter injury (38), demonstrating similar results as obtained with ecNOS gene transfer in experimental vascular balloon injury. So far, it is unclear whether iNOS or ecNOS gene transfer is more advantageous. Future studies will have to answer this question.

The alloimmune response in the rat aortic allograft model with subsequent endothelial dysfunction and injury results in the exposure of the underlying VSMCs to mitogenic factors with subsequent neointimal lesion formation (66). The development of allograft arteriosclerosis induced a sustained intramural expression of iNOS in rejecting aortic allografts (67). Interestingly, overexpression of an adenoviral vector encoding iNOS in the aortic grafts effectively inhibited intimal hyperplasia both in the presence and absence of cyclosporin A (67). Thus, overexpression of iNOS may allow iNOS expression to continue in the face of high cyclosporin and steroid doses, resulting in a suppression of allograft arteriosclerosis.

INHIBITION OF NO• PRODUCTION BY GENETIC ENGINEERING

Oxidant stress is—at least in some cell systems—accompanied by the induction of inducible NOS (iNOS), increased production of NO•, and impaired cell viability. With the description of a hypoxia-responsive element on the iNOS gene, a novel pathway for the activation of the iNOS gene was described (68). In BSC-1 kidney tubular epithelial cells, selective inhibition of iNOS using phosphorothioate-modified antisense oligonucleotides dramatically improved BSC-1 cell viability after oxidant stress (69). By inhibiting the hydrogen peroxide-induced elevation of NO• release, epithelial cells were rescued by reducing a possible detrimental effect of NO• or NO•-derived radicals.

Differences in the pathophysiological role of NO• in different cell types may be explained by a tissue-specific transcriptional regulation of the iNOS promoter/enhancer as reported recently in SMCs and macrophages (70). Cartwright et al. (71) generated a murine macrophage cell line expressing a 500-base pair (bp) sequence from iNOS in either the antisense or sense orientation, driven by the SV40 promoter/enhancer region. Adhesion of the antisense macrophage cell line A10 to cytokine-stimulated murine endothelial cells was significantly higher than adhesion of the sense cell lines. There was a negative correlation between the amount of NO• produced and the level of adhesion indicating an antiadhesive role of NO•.

By using antisense oligonucleotides in vivo, acute renal failure in rats subjected to renal ischemia was attenuated suggesting direct evidence for the cytotoxic effects of iNOS in the course of ischemic renal failure (72). The need to target the proximal tubular epithelium, the site of preferential injury in the acute ischemia–reperfusion model, seems to pose certain advantages for applying antisense oligonucleotides, as substantial accumulation of systemically injected phosphorothioate oligonucleotides by the kidney, and especially by the proximal tubular epithelium, has been demonstrated (73).

GENETIC ENGINEERING OF NOS IN THE PULMONARY SYSTEM

In cultured rat pulmonary artery SMCs, the NOS gene was induced in response to lipopolysaccharide and cytokines. Preincubation of the cells in the presence of an antisense oligonucleotide to the first 18 bases after the initiation codon of iNOS mRNA caused an significant decrease in cytokine-induced nitrite/nitrate production in a concentration-dependent manner (74).

In contrast to the in vitro experiments with pulmonary artery SMCs, pulmonary gene transfer in vivo with delivery of recombinant ecNOS adenovirus may be achieved by a single-dose aerosolization. This method enabled diffuse transduction of bronchial and alveolar epithelial cells and vascular adventitial and endothelial cells, thereby mediating increased NO• production (75). During acute hypoxia, this local overexpression of ecNOS in rat lungs significantly influenced pulmonary artery pressure and total pulmonary resistance without effecting systemic hemodynamics. Thus, aerosolized ecNOS gene transfer can act as a selective pulmonary vasodilator. The technique may represent an attractive therapeutical approach to treat patients with pulmonary hypertension, and serve as an extension of the already established therapeutical inhalation of NO• (76).

TRANSGENIC ANIMALS WITH A DISRUPTED NOS GENE

Transgenic mice with a disruption of the NOS gene represent a valuable tool to study the functional role of NOS in various (patho)physiological conditions. Gödecke et al. (77) constructed a knockout mouse with a defective ecNOS gene (disruption of the NADPH binding site) for a specific analysis of ecNOS in the cardiovascular system. Acute inhibition of ecNOS revealed that NO• has an important function in setting the basal coronary artery tone as well as participation in recative hyperemia and the response to acetylcholine (ACh). The hemodynamic analysis in ecNOS–/– knockout mice with chronic dysfunction of ecNOS showed no changes in basal coronary flow and reactive hyperemia suggesting the activation of compensatory mechanisms (77). The lack of eNOS during ACh-induced coronary vasodilation was compensated for by an elevated release of prostaglandins, in ecNOS–/– hearts. Huang et al. (78) found hypertension in mice lacking the gene for ecNOS and demonstrated lack of acetylcholine response in isolated aortic segments of ecNOS–/– mice. These conflicting data may indicate that the signal transduction pathway and mediators involved in the vascular response are different in large conduit vessels or small resistance vessels, respectively.

As just discussed, alloimmune injury to the donor vasculature is involved in accelerated graft arterioclerosis after transplantation. Inducible NOS seems to play a protective role in transplant arteriosclerosis, as iNOS–/– knockout mice display a significant increase in severity and frequency of intimal thickening in response to alloimmune injury in a heterotopic cardiac transplant model (79).

Table 4
Potential Clinical Applications of NOS Gene Transfer

Disease	NO• effect	Genetic engineering approach
Vasospastic disorders		
Prinzmetal angina	Vasodilation	NOS overexpression
Vascular proliferation	Antiproliferative effect	NOS overexpression
Restenosis		
Vein graft failure		
Atherosclerosis		
Transplant vasculopathy		
Vascular access (hemodialysis)		
Pulmonary hypertension	Pulmonary vasodilation	NOS overexpression
Septicemia	Vasodilation	Inhibition of NOS (antisense)

Table 5
Current Problems in Gene Therapy

Low efficiency
Delivery system
Inactivation or silencing of transgene
Toxicity
Identification of appropriate targets
Human application

Wound Healing and iNOS Knockout Mouse

Increased synthesis of the bioregulatory molecule NO• is reported to be a part of the cellular and biochemical events activated during wound repair *(80)*. In extending the series of pathophysiological studies in iNOS–/– knockout mice, Yamasaki et al. *(81)* demonstrated that the closure rate of excisional wounds was delayed by about 30% in iNOS knockout mice. Transient iNOS expression achieved with adenoviral-mediated iNOS gene transfer using a simple, brief exposure to low-titer virus was adequate to reverse the delayed wound closure in the iNOS-deficient mice *(81)*.

Together with data showing that in the process of vessel wall atherogenesis, the expression of iNOS was suppressed with continuation of a chronic inflammatory process *(82)*. The foregoing results in iNOS deficient mice support the hypothesis that an increase in NO• production resulting from upregulation of iNOS expression may be an important part of an endogenous physiological repair mechanism.

POTENTIAL THERAPEUTIC APPLICATIONS OF NOS GENE TRANSFER

Potential applications for in vivo gene therapy using NOS overexpression or inhibition may cover a broad range of vascular or inflammatory disorders. The evaluation of gene therapy for cardiovascular disease are now entering the stage of clinical pilot studies (phase II). Table 4 summarizes potential areas for NOS gene therapy. Despite the rapid progress of genetic engineering techniques, technical problems in the application of gene transfer to the clinical area remain to be addressed (Table 5). However, given the recent rapid progress in technology development and gene transfer, the application of NOS gene therapy will almost certainly bring new benefits to the treatment of specific diseases.

REFERENCES

1. Hawkins JW. A brief history of genetic therapy: gene therapy, antisense technology, and genomics. In: Wickstrom E, ed. Clinical Trials of Genetic Therapy with Antisense DNA and DNA Vectors. Marcel Dekker, New York, 1998, pp. 1–38.
2. von der Leyen H, Mann MJ, Dzau VJ. Gene therapy of cardiovascular disorders. In: Alexander RW, Schlant RC, Fuster V, eds. Hurst's The Heart. McGraw-Hill, New York, 1998, pp. 213–225.
3. Berg P. Dissections and reconstructions of genes and chromosomes. Science 1981;213:296–303.
4. Katz AM. Molecular biology in cardiology, a paradigmatic shift. J Mol Cell Cardiol 1988;20:355–366.
5. Dzau VJ, Gibbons GH, Cooke JP, Omoigui N. Vascular biology and medicine in the. 1990s: scope, concepts, potentials, and perspectives. Circulation 1993;87:705–719.
6. Sambrook J, Fritsch EF, Maniatis T, eds. Molecular Cloning. 2nd Ed. Cold Spring Harbor Laboratory Press, Cold Spring Harbor, New York, 1989, pp. 16.1–16.81.
7. Felgner PL, Gader TR, Holm M, Roman R, Chan HW, Wenz M, Northrop JP, Ringold GM, Danielsen M. Lipofection: a highly efficient, lipid mediated DNA-transfection procedure. Proc Natl Acad Sci USA 1987;84:7413–7417.
8. Capecchi M. High efficiency transformation by direct microinjection of DNA into mammalian cells. Cell 1980;22:479–488.
9. Adams BA, Tanabe T, Mikami A, Numa S, Beam KG. Intramembrane charge movement restored in dysgenic skeletal muscle by injection of dihydropyridine receptor cDNAs. Nature 1990;346:569–572.
10. Wolff JA, Malone RW, Williams P, Chong W, Acsadi G, Jani A, Felgner PL. Direct gene transfer into mouse muscle in vivo. Science 1990;247:1465–1468.
11. Lin H, Parmacek MS, Morle G, Bolling S, Leiden JM. Expression of recombinant genes in myocardium in vivo after direct injection of DNA. Circulation 1990;82:2217–2221.
12. Kitsis RN, Buttrick PM, McNally EM, Kaplan ML, Leinwand LA. Hormonal modulation of a gene injected into rat heart *in vivo*. Proc Natl Acad Sci USA 1991;88:4138–4142.
13. Nabel EG, Plautz G, Nabel GJ. Site-specific gene expression in vivo by direct gene transfer into the arterial wall. Science 1990;249:1285–1288.
14. Morishita R, Gibbons GH, Ellison KE, Nakajima M, von der Leyen H, Zhang L, Kaneda Y, Dzau VJ. Intimal hyperplasia after vascular injury is inhibited by antisense cdk 2 kinase oligonucleotides. J Clin Invest 1994;93:1458–1464.
15. Peterson KR, Clegg CH, Huxley C, Josephson BM, Haugen HS, Furukawa T, Stamatoyannopoulos G. Transgenic mice containing a 248-kb yeast artificial chromosome carrying the human beta-globin locus display proper developmental control of human globin genes. Proc Natl Acad Sci USA 1993;90: 7593–7597.
16. Schedl A, Montoliu L, Kelsey G, Schutz G. A yeast artificial chromosome covering the tyrosinase gene confers copy number-dependent expression in transgenic mice. Nature 1993;362:258–261.
17. Brown WR. Mammalian artificial chromosomes. Curr Opin Gene Dev 1992;2:479–486.
18. Huxley C. Mammalian artificial chromosomes: a new tool for gene therapy. Gene Ther 1994;1: 7–12.
19. Gibaldi M. What is nitric oxide and why are so many people studying it ? J Clin Pharmacol 1993;33: 488–496.
20. Änggård E. Nitric oxide: mediator, murderer, and medicine. Lancet 1994;343:1199–1206.
21. Schmidt HH, Walter U. NO at work. Cell 1994;78:919–925.
22. Lamas S, Marsden PA, Li GK, Tempst P, Michel T. Endothelial nitric oxide synthase: molecular cloning and characterization of a distinct constitutive enzyme isoform. Proc Natl Acad Sci USA 1992;89: 6348–6352.
23. Nathan C, Xie QW. Nitric oxide synthases: roles, tolls, and controls. Cell 1994;78:915–918.
24. Lowenstein CJ, Glatt CS, Bredt DS, Snyder SH. Cloned and expressed macrophage nitric oxide synthase contrasts with the brain enzyme. Proc Natl Acad Sci USA 1992;89:7611–6715.
25. Gibbons GH, Dzau VJ. The emerging concept of vascular remodeling. N Engl J Med 1994;330:1431–1438.
26. Davis AR. Current potential of antisense oligonucleotides as therapeutic drugs. Trends Cardiovasc Med 1994;4:51–55.
27. Phillips MI, Gyurko R. Antisense oligonucleotides: new tools for physiology. News Physiol Sci 1997; 12:99–105.
28. Flanagan WM, Wagner RW. Potent and selective gene inhibition using antisense oligodeoxynucleotides. Mol Cell Biochem 1997;172:213–225.
29. Colman A. Antisense strategies in cell and developmental biology. J Cell Sci 1990;97:399–409.

30. Garg UC, Hassid A. Nitric oxide-generating vasodilators and 8-bromo-cyclic guanosine monophosphate inhibit mitogenesis and proliferation of cultured rat vascular smooth muscle cells. J Clin Invest 1989;83: 1774–1777.
31. Furchgott RF, Zawadzki JV. The obligatory role of endothelial cells in the relaxation of arterial smooth muscle by acetylcholine. Nature 1980;288:373–376.
32. Palmer RM, Ferrige AG, Moncada S. Nitric oxide release accounts for the biological activity of endothelium-derived relaxing factor. Nature 1987;327:524–526.
33. Ignarro LJ. Endothlium-derived nitric oxide: actions and properties. FASEB J 1989;3:31–36.
34. Channon KM, Blazing MA, Shetty GA, Potts KE, George SE. Adenoviral gene transfer of nitric oxide synthase: high level expression in human vascular cells. Cardiovasc Res 1996;32:962–972.
35. Kullo IJ, Schwartz RS, Pompili VJ, Tsutsui M, Milstien S, Fitzpatrick LA, Katusic ZS, O'Brien T. Expression and function of recombinant endothelial NO synthase in coronary artery smooth muscle cells. Arterioscler Thromb Vasc Biol 1997;17:2405–2412.
36. Dubey RK, Jackson EK, Lüscher TF. Nitric oxide inhibits angiotensin II-induced migration of rat aortic smooth muscle cell. Role of cyclic-nucleotides and angiotensin1 receptors. J Clin Invest 1995;96: 141–149.
37. Fang S, Sharma RV, Bhalla RC. Endothelial nitric oxide synthase gene transfer inhibits platelet-derived growth factor-BB stimulated focal adhesion kinase and paxillin phosphorylation in vascular smooth muscle. Biochem Biophys Res Commun 1997;236:706–711.
38. Tzeng E, Shears LL, Robins PD, Pitt BR, Geller DA, Watkins SC, Simmons RL, Billiar TR. Vascular gene transfer of the human inducible nitric oxide synthase: characterization of activity and effects on myointimal hyperplasia. Mol Med 1996;2:211–225.
39. Tzeng E, Billiar TR, Robbins PD, Loftus M, Stuehr DJ. Expression of human inducible nitric oxide synthase in a tetrahydrobiopterin (H4B)-deficient cell line: H4B promotes assembly of enzyme subunits into an active dimer. Proc Natl Acad Sci USA 1995;92:11,771–11,775.
40. Tzeng E, Yoncyama T, Hatakeyama K, Shears LL, Billiar TR. Vascular inducible nitric oxide synthase gene therapy: requirement for guanosine triphosphate cyclohydrolase I. Surgery 1996;120:315–321.
41. Tzeng E, Kim YM, Pitt BR, Lizonova A, Kovesdi I, Billiar TR. Adenoviral transfer of the inducible nitric oxide synthase gene blocks endothelial cell apoptosis. Surgery 1997;122:255–263.
42. Tsao PS, McEvoy LM, Drexler H, Butcher EC, Cooke JP. Enhanced endothelial adhesiveness in hypercholesterolemia is attenuated by L-arginine. Circulation 1994;89:2176–2182.
43. De Caterina R, Libby P, Peng HB, Thannickal J, Rajavashisth TB, Gimbrone MA, Shin WS, Liao JK. Nitric oxide decreases cytokine-induced endothelial activation. Nitric oxide selectively reduces endothelial expression of adhesion molecules and proinflammatory cytokines. J Clin Invest 1995;96:60–68.
44. Ross R. The pathogenesis of atherosclerosis: a perspective for the 1990s. Nature 1993;362:801–809.
45. Buitrago R, von der Leyen H, Tsao PS, Mann MJ, Gibbons GH, Cooke JP, Dzau VJ. Superoxide generation from endothelial cells exposed to oxidized LDL can be reduced by nitric oxide synthase gene transfer in vitro (abstract). Circulation 1995;92:I–364.
46. Harrison DG. Cellular and molecular mechanisms of endothelial cell dysfunction. J Clin Invest 1997; 100:2153–2157.
47. Vane JR, Änggård EE, Botting RM. Regulatory functions of the vascular endothelium. N Engl J Med 1990;323:27–36.
48. Mooradian DL, Hutsell TC, Keefer LK. Nitric oxide (NO) donor molecules: effect of NO release rates on vascular smooth muscle cell proliferation in vitro. J Cardiovasc Pharmacol 1995;25:674–678.
49. Tsao PS, Wang B, Buitrago R, Shyy JY, Cooke JP. Nitric oxide regulates monocyte chemotactic protein–1. Circulation 1997;96:934–940.
50. von der Leyen HE, Gibbons GH, Morishita R, Lewis NP, Zhang L, Nakajima M, Kaneda Y, Cooke JP, Dzau VJ. Gene therapy inhibiting neointimal vascular lesion: In vivo transfer of endothelial-cell nitric oxide synthase gene. Proc Natl Acad Sci USA 1995;92:1137–1141.
51. Mann MJ, Morishita R, Gibbons GH, von der Leyen HE, Dzau VJ. DNA transfer into vascular smooth muscle using fusigenic Sendai virus (HVJ)-liposomes. Mol Cell Biochem 1997;172:3–12.
52. Clowes AW, Clowes MM, Reidy MA. Smooth muscle growth in the absence of endothelium. Lab Invest 1983;49.
53. Simons M, Edelman ER, DeKeyser JL, Langer R, Rosenberg RD. Antisense c-myb oligonucleotides inhibit intimal arterial smooth muscle cell accumulation in vivo. Nature 1992;359:67–70.
54. Morishita R, Gibbons GH, Ellison KE, Nakajima M, Zhang L, Kaneda Y, Ogihara T, Dzau VJ. Single intraluminal delivery of antisense cdc2 kinase and proliferating-cell nuclear antigen oligonucleotides results in chronic inhibition of neointimal hyperplasia. Proc Natl Acad Sci USA 1993;90:8474–8478.

55. Mann MJ, Gibbons GH, Kernoff RS, Diet FD, Tsao PS, Cooke JP, Kaneda Y, Dzau VJ. Genetic engineering of vein grafts resistant to atherosclerosis. Proc Natl Acad Sci USA 1995;92:4502–4506.

56. Dzau VJ, Horiuchi M. In vivo gene transfer and gene modulation in hypertension research. Hypertension 1996;28:1132–1137.

57. Janssens S, Flaherty D, Nong Z, Varenne O, van Pelt N, Haustermans C, Zoldhelyi P, Gerard R, Collen D. Human endothelial nitric oxide synthase gene transfer inhibits vascular smooth muscle cell proliferation and neointima formation after balloon injury in rats. Circulation 1998;97:1274–1281.

58. Varenne O, Pislaru S, Gillijns H, Van Pelt N, Gerard RD, Zoldhelyi P, Van de Werf F, Collen D, Janssens SP. Local adenovirus-mediated transfer of human endothelial nitric oxide synthase reduces luminal narrowing after coronary angioplasty in pigs. Circulation 1998;98:919–926.

59. Kullo IJ, Mozes G, Schwartz RS, Gloviczki P, Tsutsui M, Katusic ZS, O'Brien T. Enhanced endothelium-dependent relaxations after gene transfer of recombinant endothelial nitric oxide synthase to rabbit carotid arteries. Hypertension 1997;30:314–320.

60. Kullo IJ, Mozes G, Schwartz RS, Gloviczki P, Crotty TB, Barber DA, Katusic ZS, O'Brien T. Adventitial gene transfer of recombinant endothelial nitric oxide synthase to rabbit carotid arteries alters vascular reactivity. Circulation 1997;96:2254–2261.

61. Chen AF, O'Brien T, Tsutsui M, Kinoshita H, Pompili VJ, Crotty TB, Spector DJ, Katusic ZS. Expression and function of recombinant endothelial nitric oxide synthase gene in canine basilar artery. Circ Res 1997;80:327–335.

62. Ooboshi H, Chu Y, Rios CD, Faraci FM, Davidson BL, Heistad DD. Altered vascular function after adenovirus-mediated overexpression of endothelial nitric oxide synthase. Am J Physiol 1997;273(1 Pt 2): H265–H270.

63. Cable DG, O'Brien T, Kullo IJ, Schwartz RS, Schaff HV, Pompili VJ. Expression and function of a recombinant endothelial nitric oxide synthase gene in porcine coronary arteries. Cardiovasc Res 1997; 35:553–559.

64. Cable DG, O'Brien T, Schaff HV, Pompili VJ. Recombinant endothelial nitric oxide synthase-transduced human saphenous veins: gene therapy to augment nitric oxide production in bypass conduits. Circulation 1997;96:II-173–II-178.

65. Matsumoto T, Komori K, Yonemitsu Y, Morishita R, Sueishi K, Kaneda Y, Sugimachi K. Hemagglutinating virus of Japan-liposome-mediated gene transfer of endothelial cell nitric oxide synthase inhibits intimal hyperplasia of canine vein grafts under conditions of poor runoff. J Vasc Surg 1998;27:135–144.

66. Davis SF, Yeung AC, Meredith IT, Charbonneau F, Ganz P, Selwyn AP, Anderson TJ. Early endothelial dysfunction predicts the development of transplant coronary artery disease at 1 year posttransplant. Circulation 1996;93:457–462.

67. Shears LL, Kawaharada N, Tzeng E, Billiar TR, Watkins SC, Kovesdi I, Lizonova A, Pham SM. Inducible nitric oxide synthase suppresses the development of allograft arteriosclerosis. J Clin Invest 1997;100:2035–2042.

68. Melillo G, Musso T, Sica A, Taylor LS, Cox GW, Varesio L. A hypoxia-responsive element mediates a novel pathway of activation of the inducible nitric oxide synthase promoter. J Exp Med 1995;182: 1683–1693.

69. Peresleni T, Noiri E, Bahou WF, Goligorsky MS. Antisense oligodeoxynucleotides to inducible NO synthase rescue epithelial cells from oxidative stress injury. Am J Physiol 1996;270:F971–F977.

70. Kolyada AY, Savikovsky N, Madias NE. Transcriptional regulation of the human iNOS gene in vascular-smooth-muscle cells and macrophages: evidence for tissue specificity. Biochem Biophys Res Commun 1996;220:600–605.

71. Cartwright JE, Johnstone AP, Whitley GSJ. Inhibition of nitric oxide synthase by antisense techniques: investigations of the roles of NO produced by murine macrophages. Br J Pharmacol 1997;120:146–152.

72. Noiri E, Peresleni T, Miller F, Goligorsky MS. In vivo targeting of inducible NO synthase with oligodeoxynucleotides protects rat kidney against ischemia. J Clin Invest 1996;97:2377–2383.

73. Rappaport J, Hanss B, Kopp JB, Copeland TD, Bruggeman LA, Coffman TM, Klotman PE. Transport of phosphorothioate oligonucleotides in kidney: implications for molecular therapy. Kidney Int 1995; 47:1462–1469.

74. Thomae KR, Geller DA, Billiar TR, Davies P, Pitt BR, Simmons RL, Nakayama DK. Antisense oligodeoxynucleotide to inducible nitric oxide synthase inhibits nitric oxide synthesis in rat pulmonary artery smooth muscle cells in culture. Surgery 1993;114:272–277.

75. Janssens SP, Bloch KD, Nong Z, Gerard RD, Zoldhelyi P, Collen D. Adenoviral-mediated transfer of the human endothelial nitric oxide synthase gene reduces acute hypoxic pulmonary vasoconstriction in rats. J Clin Invest 1996;98:317–324.

76. Pepke-Zaba J, Higgenbottam TW, Dinh-Xuan AT, Stone D, Wallwork J. Inhaled nitric oxide as a cause of selective pulmonary vasodilatation in pulmonary hypertension. Lancet 1991;338:1173,1174.

77. Gödecke A, Decking UK, Ding Z, Hirchenhain J, Bidmon HJ, Gödecke S, Schrader J. Coronary hemodynamics in endothelial NO synthase knockout mice. Circulation 1998;82:186–194.

78. Huang PL, Huang Z, Mashimo H, Bloch KD, Moskowitz MA, Bevan JA, Fishman MC. Hypertension in mice lacking the gene for endothelial nitric oxide synthase. Nature 1995;377:239–242.

79. Koglin J, Glysing-Jensen T, Mudgett JS, Russell ME. Exacerbated transplant arteriosclerosis in inducible nitric oxide-deficient mice. Circulation 1998;97:2059–2065.

80. Schaffer MR, Tantry U, Gross SS, Wasserberg HL, Barbul A. Nitric oxide regulates wound healing. J Surg Res 1996;63:237–240.

81. Yamasaki K, Edington HD, McClosky C, Tzeng E, Lizonova E, Kovesdi I, Steed DL, Billiar TR. Reversal of impaired wound repair in iNOS-deficient mice by topical adenoviral-mediated iNOS gene transfer. J Clin Invest 1998;101:967–971.

82. Hamilton TA, Major JA, Chisolm GM. The effects of oxidized low density lipoproteins on inducible mouse macrophage gene expression are gene and stimulus dependent. J Clin Invest 1995;95:2020–2027.

29

Nitric Oxide and Tissue Preservation in Transplantation

David J. Pinsky and David M. Stern

VASCULAR HOMEOSTASIS IN ORGAN TRANSPLANTATION

Overview of Current Heart and Lung Preservation Strategies

In order to transfer a solid organ from a donor to a recipient, there is an obligate period during which the donor organ must be detached from its native blood supply. This period of ischemia followed by reperfusion, which occurs on reestablishment of blood flow, can wreak havoc on the cells within the organ that are critical to its intrinsic functions, as well as on the cells comprising the blood vessels that supply the organ. Primary graft nonfunction occurs in over 10% of cardiac transplant operations and over 30% of lung transplant operations (1–3), percentages that are unacceptably high given that patient survival is absolutely dependent on immediate function of the transplanted heart or lungs. Over the past several decades, as organ transplantation has become a realistic option with which to treat patients with end-stage pulmonary or cardiac disease, there have been a number of advances in the methods used to preserve these vulnerable organs during the period of transport between donor and recipient. Several strategies initially emerged to protect posttransplant organ function, such as the use of slow-drip infusions of various oxygenated solutions, but these were cumbersome and of equivocal benefit, and were dropped in favor of a simpler approach of infusing and immersing the organ in a hypothermic preservation solution. Initial preservation solutions focussed on the need to maintain proper electrolyte and osmolar composition of the organ preservation solution. In terms of vulnerable organs such as the heart or lungs, this permitted ex vivo survival of the organ to a sufficient degree to make transplantation feasible. For hearts, the acceptable duration of preservation is considered to be within a 6-h window from harvest, and for lungs, which are even more vulnerable to reperfusion injury, the window is even shorter. These time-related considerations place significant logistical burdens on the transplantation team, and limit organ traffic to a regional organ sharing network. Even when the heart, lung, or heart–lung block are "optimally preserved" for limited durations, primary graft failure occasionally and inexplicably occurs, with devastating consequences for the recipient.

There are numerous cell types that are transplanted in a solid organ, such as the heart or lungs, including the "functioning" cells, such as the alveolar pneumocytes in the lungs or cardiac myocytes in the heart; passenger cells, such as assorted leukocyte populations; and cells of the vascular wall. As all nucleated cells express major histocompatibility complex (MHC) class I molecules, and many express class II molecules, each of these cell populations may be targeted for rejection over the course of time during which a transplanted organ resides within a mismatched recipient. Owing to the hurried logistics of organ retrieval and brief

From: *Contemporary Cardiology, vol. 4: Nitric Oxide and the Cardiovascular System*
Edited by: J. Loscalzo and J. A. Vita © Humana Press Inc., Totowa, NJ

viable ex vivo organ preservation window, in heart and lung transplantation, there is insufficient time for extensive immunological cross-matching of donor and recipient. Rather, simple issues of organ size and ABO (blood type) compatibility are ensured, and the organ is implanted. Therefore, only retrospective analyses are available by which to study the effect of transplanting mismatched organs. Retrospective analysis of a large series of patients who have received cardiac grafts has shown that the degree of long-term organ survival is inversely related to the degree of human leukocyte antigen (HLA) disparity between donor and recipient *(4)*. Therefore, strategies that might permit a considerably longer ex vivo window might indirectly improve organ survival by permitting more extensive donor–recipient crossmatching.

Another interesting observation made in the study by Opelz et al. *(4)* was that prolonged ischemic times were associated with poorer long-term prognoses. The influence of ischemic time on long-term graft survival was dose-dependent, i.e., cold preservation durations of 4 h fared worse than 2, preservation durations of 6 h fared worse than 4, and so on. The negative impact of prolonged ischemic times was observed as late as 3 yr following transplantation and was statistically independent of other risk factors, including the degree of HLA disparity that the study was originally designed to evaluate. As vascular disease in the graft is the most significant limitation to long-term survival (outside of infection risk), these provocative data suggest that organ preservation somehow disrupts early graft vascular function, which increases the long-term risk for the graft. These data compel one to examine carefully the role of the vasculature in graft failure.

Endothelial Barrier Function

Endothelial cells, which line all blood vessels and comprise capillaries in their entirety, are far more than simple structural components of the vessel wall. They exhibit a distinctive phenotype that serves to maintain vascular homeostasis under quiescent conditions, but when perturbed, modulate this phenotype rapidly and actively. From a teleological point of view, endothelial cells presumably modulate their phenotype to enhance survival of an organism; for instance, under conditions of stress or infection, they increase their expression of leukocyte adhesion receptors to call in inflammatory cells to stave off the infection, and perhaps become more procoagulant to trigger a thrombotic nidus that begins the process of walling off an infected focus. However, under conditions of severely interrupted blood flow, such as occur during organ transplantation, modulation of the endothelial phenotype becomes maladaptive.

Although many think of endothelial cells as forming an impermeable barrier, this is not really the case. Rather, endothelial cells tightly apposed to each other present a barrier that is "selectively permeable," i.e., one characterized by restricted diffusion. This means that, under quiescent conditions, the diffusion of macromolecules is restricted according to size: larger molecules, with larger Stokes' radii, pass less freely than do smaller molecules. Under ischemic or hypoxic conditions, barrier function breaks down. Changes occur in the actin-based cytoskeleton, and the lateral margins of endothelial cells retract from one another. This opens up large gaps through which both water and macromolecules can freely pass, without restriction based on size, charge, or lipophilicity. In fact, the movement of macromolecules across such a disrupted barrier is no longer driven by simple diffusion, but, rather, convection and mass transport become dominant modes of solute transport. In physiological terms, the vasculature becomes "leaky," and tissue edema occurs as the capillary filtration coefficients increase to the point where egress of fluids and macromolecules from the vessel exceeds the capacity of the lymphatic system to return the fluid to the central venous capacitance reservoir.

One of the chief mechanisms by which hypoxia disrupts endothelial barrier function is by reducing cyclic nucleotide levels in the endothelial cells. This eventuates in disruption of the actin-based cytoskeleton leading to loss of barrier function. Both cyclic adenosine monophosphate (cAMP) and nitric oxide/cyclic guanosine monophosphate (NO•/cGMP) are critical

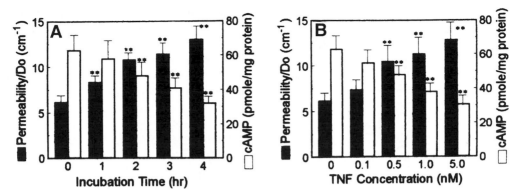

Fig. 1. Effect of TNF on the barrier function and cAMP levels of endothelial cell monolayers. (**A**) Dependence on incubation time. Endothelial cells were incubated for the indicated times with TNF (5 nM), and diffusion of ^{3}H-inulin across the monolayer and intracellular cAMP levels were assessed as permeability coefficients (P/D$_0$, cm^{-1}; higher values represent increased monolayer permeability). (**B**) Dependence on TNF concentration. ECs were incubated for 4 h with the indicated concentration of TNF-α, and diffusion of ^{3}H-inulin across the endothelial cell monolayer and intracellular cAMP levels were assessed. Adapted from ref. *(6)*.

pathways by which endothelial cells maintain their quiescent phenotype. Hypoxia, by reducing adenylyl cyclase activity and therefore cAMP synthesis, causes intracellular cAMP levels to plummet *(5,6)*. A similar decline in cAMP levels and increased permeability is seen following exposure of endothelial monolayers to the proinflammatory cytokine tumor necrosis factor (TNF) *(6)* (Fig. 1). During reoxygenation or reperfusion, reactive oxygen intermediates such as hydrogen peroxide increase endothelial cell phosphodiesterase activity (PDE), contributing to a further intracellular decline of cAMP *(7)*. Although during the ischemic period of lung preservation, NO· levels are relatively well maintained, during reperfusion, these levels plummet, owing to rapid quenching by superoxide generated in the reperfusion microenvironment *(8,9)* (Fig. 2). Using a bioassay for nitric oxide in which the presence of nitric oxide is detected by the ability of endothelial cells to inhibit platelet aggregation in response to thrombin challenge, it is clear that hypoxic/reoxygenated cells produce less "bioavailable" NO· than their normoxic counterparts. Addition of an agent that catalyzes the dismutation of superoxide (superoxide dismutase [SOD]) to the reoxygenated cells restores bioavailable NO· levels toward normal, helping illustrate how superoxide generated by the reoxygenated cells is responsible for quenching of bioavailable NO· *(8)* (Fig. 3). These studies have tremendous implications for a number of vascular homeostatic perturbations, including permeability changes as well as others described shortly. In terms of permeability changes, diminished NO· levels would be expected to increase permeability because of NO·'s barrier-maintaining properties *(10,11)*.

Antithrombotic Properties of the Vasculature

Because of the necessity for blood to flow, maintenance of blood fluidity is of utmost importance under homeostatic conditions. The blood vessel wall plays a key role in preventing intravascular thrombosis, by both preventing a nidus of thrombus formation and promoting rapid degradation of thrombus that has formed. Although one might think that the antithrombotic state of a quiescent vessel is absolute in reality, even under normal conditions there are minute quantities of fibrin that are continually formed and at the same time lysed. This observation is based on the detection of small amounts of fibrin degradation products even in normal humans subjects *(12)*. The antithrombotic mechanisms of the vasculature are multiple, and chiefly orchestrated by the endothelium. The endothelium is, first, a nonwetting physical

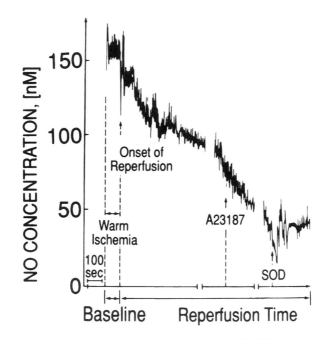

Fig. 2. Effect of lung ischemia and reperfusion on nitric oxide (NO˙) levels. Amperogram (current-concentration versus time) recorded in vivo with a porphyrinic microsensor placed on the surface of a transplanted lung. During warm ischemia, the period of time during which the donor lung is being sewn into place but during which the pulmonary artery remains crossclamped, exhibits relatively constant levels of NO˙, but immediately on reestablishment of blood flow (removal of the crossclamp), NO˙ levels plummet, despite topical addition of the calcium ionophore A23187. Superoxide dismutase (SOD) modestly restores measurable NO˙ levels. Adapted from ref. *(9)*.

barrier that prevents the intravascular luminal contents from making physical contact with the subjacent basement membrane, rich with collagen and tissue factor. Therefore, the loss of NO˙ or cyclic nucleotide levels that may cause a retraction of the lateral margins of endothelial cells may disrupt this physical barrier to contact. This is one way in which NO˙ can serve to prevent intravascular thrombosis. Endothelial cells also have a marked anticoagulant phenotype, expressing molecules such as thrombomodulin (a transmembrane protein that accelerates the conversion of inactive protein C to active protein C) and various heparan sulfates. Exposure of cells to hypoxia causes a downregulation of thrombomodulin expression at both the mRNA and protein levels; this downregulation can be prevented by restoring cyclic nucleotide levels toward normal. Other important vascular properties that prevent thrombus formation are endogenous fibrinolytic mechanisms, with tissue-type plasminogen activator (t-PA) released in the vicinity of an inflamed vessel to counterbalance the prevailing prothrombotic milieu. In fact, under hypoxic conditions, as PAI-1 expression increases in mononuclear phagocytes recruited to an ischemic region, there is inhibited expression of endogenous tissue-type and urokinase-type plasminogen activators *(13)*. These observations highlight the delicate balance between prothrombotic and antithrombotic forces acting within the blood vessel wall.

Another important mechanism by which NO˙ may maintain the normal antithrombotic vascular phenotype is by inhibiting the aggregation of platelets (*see* Fig. 3). Inhibiting the aggregation of platelets is an important way by which NO˙ prevents the amplification of thrombosis, because aggregating platelets obstruct the vascular lumen and provide the stroma on which nascent thrombus can form and the surface phospholipids on which many of the clotting reactions take place. In addition to these properties, the vasodilatory properties of NO˙

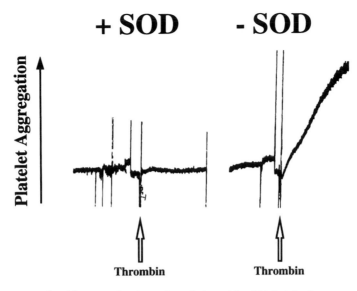

Fig. 3. Platelet aggregation bioassay for detecting nitric oxide. (**Right**) In the presence of hypoxic/reoxygenated endothelial cells, platelets aggregate rapidly in response to thrombin challenge. (**Left**) In the presence of the same hypoxic/reoxygenated endothelial cells, but with addition of SOD to reduce ambient superoxide levels, the platelets fail to aggregate in response to an identical thrombin challenge. NO·, produced by the endothelial cells, remains bioavailable because of reduced ambient superoxide levels, and is responsible for inhibiting platelet aggregation in response to thrombin (Left). Adapted from ref. *(9)*.

inhibit thrombosis by enhancing regional blood flow and thereby reducing the local accumulation of activated clotting factors.

When an organ is subjected to oxygen deprivation or ischemia, a number of vascular derangements occur that promote the accrual of thrombus. Arguably among the first of these prothrombotic triggers is the release of the von Willebrand factor (vWF) from preformed storage pools within endothelial cell Weibel–Palade bodies. The von Willebrand factor, which exists as a large multimeric protein, contributes to the adhesion of platelets and fibrinogen to the vessel wall. Endothelial cells exposed to hypoxia (independent of reoxygenation) exhibit Weibel–Palade body exocytosis, a process that is calcium-dependent *(14)*. This in vitro observation was shown to be relevant in the setting of hypothermic cardiac preservation in humans by studies in which blood was sampled from the coronary sinus immediately prior to and immediately after a period of aortic cross-clamping during cardiac surgery. These studies showed that the hypothermic preservation period was associated with an increase in vWF levels in the coronary sinus effluent (Fig. 4). Immunoelectrophoresis demonstrated that this vWF existed primarily as very high molecular weight multimers, and this observation served as presumptive evidence for the coronary endothelial origin of the vWF because vWF from the stimulatable storage pool tends to be of higher molecular weight than that which is constitutively secreted. Furthermore, simultaneously obtained peripheral blood samples failed to demonstrate a significant increase in vWF levels, suggesting that the increased vWF did not emanate from the stimulatable storage pool in platelets as an artifact of cardiopulmonary bypass.

The secretion of vWF by the process of Weibel–Palade body exocytosis may be directly influenced by ambient NO· levels, and is therefore relevant to the role of NO· as an inhibitor of intravascular thrombosis. In preliminary studies performed in our laboratory, we have demonstrated that the nitric oxide donor 3-morpholinosydnonimine (SIN-1) or the cGMP analog 8-bromo-cGMP caused a reduction in hypoxia-mediated vWF release from endothelial cells

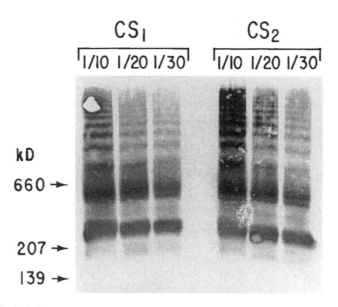

Fig. 4. Weibel–Palade body release during human cardiac surgery. Coronary sinus blood was sampled at the start (CS_1) and conclusion (CS_2) of the ischemic period (aortic cross-clamping). vWF immunoelectrophoresis of a representative sample of CS_1 and CS_2 blood from the same patient (dilution factors are indicated). There is an increase in high molecular weight multimers detected in the CS_2 samples. Adapted from ref. *(14)*.

(15). Presumably, this effect is due to an attenuation of the hypoxia-mediated rise in intracellular calcium levels in endothelial cells, as pharmacological stimulation of the NO•/cGMP pathway inhibited this rise simultaneous with the inhibition of Weibel–Palade body exocytosis. This observation is corroborated by in vivo studies in the enteric microcirculation in which inhibition of endothelial-derived nitric oxide was shown to promote P-selectin expression (and, hence, Weibel–Palade body exocytosis *[16]*).

Vasodilation

Although it is impossible to say which of the various vascular homeostatic properties are of paramount importance, the ability of a graft to preserve blood flow is of critical and immediate importance to graft survival. Because a transplanted organ is denervated at the instant of harvest, local vasoregulatory mechanisms are the key modulators of vasomotor tone during the earliest stages following reimplantation. Endothelial cells are the chief vascular cells that regulate vasomotion, with subjacent vascular smooth muscle cells being subservient effector cells. NO•, produced in large quantities by quiescent endothelial cells to maintain a certain level of vasodilation in the organ prior to harvest, is deficient in the transplanted organ. Direct measurements with a porphyrinic microsensor clearly reveal this, and provide evidence that the loss of bioavailable NO• is due to its quenching by superoxide generated by reperfusion *(8.9)*. The sources for this superoxide are multiple, but clearly involve both recruited inflammatory cells (particularly neutrophils) and the reperfused endothelial cells themselves. Thus, reperfusion may be thought of as an NO• deficiency state, and, not surprisingly, cGMP levels are reduced during reperfusion as well due to loss of stimulation by NO• of soluble guanylyl cyclase in effector cells such as vascular smooth muscle cells (VSMCs). This deficiency of the NO•/cGMP pathway strongly contributes to the apparent "vasoconstriction" of reperfusion. In addition to the loss of vascular tone caused by the lack of bioavailable NO•, it is very likely that there could be a concomitant derangement in cardiac mechanical function, as the heart normally produces vast quantities of NO• in response to mechanical perturbations during the cardiac cycle *(17)*.

cAMP is also a critical modulator of smooth muscle cell (SMC) relaxation, acting by stimulating the cAMP-dependent protein kinase (PKA) within cells to promote vasodilation. During the course of lung preservation, cAMP levels were noted to decline. The reason for this decline is likely to be twofold: in the case of endothelial cells, hypoxia decreases the activity of adenylyl cyclase, both under basal as well as under beta-adrenergic receptor complex-stimulated conditions (5); and, VSMCs subjected to hypoxic conditions demonstrated reduced cAMP levels, not because of decreased adenylyl cyclase activity, but rather, because of increased activity of types III and IV PDEs (18). The increase in cAMP-PDE may, thus, be responsible for increasing cAMP catabolism under hypoxic conditions. Therefore, as vascular organs represent a composite of many cell types, including endothelial cells and SMCs, it is likely that both decreased synthesis of cAMP and augmented catabolism of cAMP by specific PDEs cause a preservation-related decline in cAMP levels measured in the whole organ (19). The decline in cAMP levels contributes to vascular dysfunction, including vasoconstriction following transplantation, which can be reversed by adding membrane-permeable cAMP analogs or specific PDE inhibitors to the transplant preservation solution (18).

Nonadhesivity of the Vascular Wall for Leukocytes

Under quiescent conditions, the vascular wall is relatively nonadhesive for circulating leukocytes, with differing vascular segments (such as postcapillary venules) presenting different phenotypes to various leukocyte populations, promoting or restricting leukocyte adhesion, diapedesis, and subsequent emigration to the abluminal space. There are numerous redundant leukocyte adhesion receptor mechanisms, which accounts for the fact that mice deficient in only a single adhesion receptor, such as P-selectin, do not exhibit a complete absence of leukocyte adhesion to activated endothelium. Rather, these mice exhibit a delayed response to inflammatory stimuli, with leukocytes entering inflamed tissue at delayed time points (20). Other intact adhesion receptors, such as E-selectin, ICAM-1, PAF, and others, can still function and substitute for the limiting receptor. For the purposes of organ transplantation, however, as initial leukocyte recruitment causes a logarithmic amplification in inflammatory events (including further adhesion receptor expression, complement activation, and more accumulation of leukocytes), inhibiting even a single adhesion receptor can have a beneficial impact on organ survival.

NO• produced by endothelium is one particularly potent mechanism by which the endothelium maintains its relatively nonadhesive state for circulating neutrophils. Under experimental conditions in which NO• synthesis is blocked with a competitive nitric oxide synthase (NOS) inhibitor, P-selectin expression is augmented. In preliminary studies, we have shown that the inhibition of P-selectin expression by NO• under conditions of hypoxia is caused by a subdued calcium flux in endothelial cells, which suppresses the calcium-dependent exocytosis of Weibel–Palade bodies, the storage reservoir for membrane-bound P-selectin in endothelial cells. In the heart, NO• donors potently inhibit leukosequestration following ischemia (21,22). In intestinal ischemia and reperfusion, it is also apparent that NO• is a potent anti-adhesive force for circulating neutrophils (16).

PRESERVATION AND REPERFUSION
INJURY OF TRANSPLANTED ORGANS

Role of Cytokines, Leukocytes
and their Adhesion Receptors, and Complement

The cytokine milieu following organ transplantation recapitulates virtually all inflammatory mechanisms seen in an infectious process, and teleologically may be thought of as "maladaptive inflammation," which was not directly subjected to evolutionary pressures or modification. The triggers for this inflammation are multifactorial, and include the activation

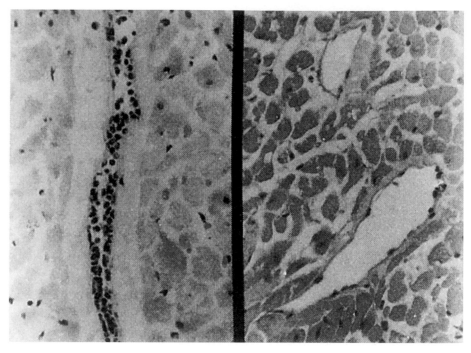

Fig. 5. Neutrophil recruitment to the newly reperfused rat cardiac isograft. (**Left**) Early neutrophil recruitment to the endovascular wall. Neutrophil recruitment is significantly attenuated if the graft had been preserved in a preservation solution containing a nitric oxide donor but otherwise transplanted under identical conditions (**Right**). Adapted from ref. *(8)*.

of hypoxia-responsive genes, such as interleukins-1, -6, and -8 (IL) *(23–27)*; adhesion receptor expression, which occurs due to activation of *de novo* transcription and translation of new adhesion receptor molecules at the endothelial surface (such as E-selectin and ICAM-1); adhesion receptor expression from preformed storage pools (P-selectin), which is triggered by calcium flux and reactive oxygen species; and activation of both the complement and coagulation cascades, which further amplify the proinflammatory posttransplant vascular milieu. In the setting of lung transplantation, even in an isogeneic model (i.e., one in which there is no genetic disparity between donor and recipient), complement activation occurs locally and its inhibition can be beneficial for organ function *(28)*. Taken together, these processes contribute to early recruitment of neutrophils to the reperfused graft (Fig. 5).

P-selectin expression is a critical mechanism of leukocyte recruitment following hypothermic cardiac *(14)* or lung preservation *(29)*. Mice deficient in the P-selectin gene are significantly protected from cardiac or pulmonary ischemia-reperfusion injury, and administration of a functionally blocking anti-P-selectin antibody just prior to reperfusion confers significant protection against primary graft failure for both the heart and the lungs *(14,29)*. As P-selectin expression may be inhibited by NO$^\bullet$ donors, this may explain a potential mechanism for the therapeutic benefit of these agents in the setting of organ transplantation. In the heart and lungs, ICAM-1 expression is also a critical mechanism responsible for leukocyte accumulation and early graft damage, a mechanism which is amplified tremendously by the local (*de novo*) synthesis of IL-1. In the mouse heart transplant model, it is clear that ICAM-1 can actually autoinduce its own expression in the transplanted vasculature as well as in organs remote from the site of transplantation *(30)*. This ICAM-1-dependent autoinduction of ICAM-1 occurs via an IL-1 intermediary, as shown in experiments in which administration of an IL-1 receptor antagonist can block ICAM-1-induced ICAM-1 expression on graft and remote organ vessels *(30)*.

How does this activation of inflammation damage the newly reperfused graft? Neutrophils stiffen during the process of activation and significantly contribute to capillary plugging, which impedes the forward flow of blood. In addition, they release a veritable arsenal of toxic compounds, such as cytotoxic lysosomal enzymes, including elastase; the metalloproteases collagenase and gelatinase; neutral proteases; and heparatinase *(31)*. Recruited neutrophils are also activated by cytokines and chemotaxins to undergo a respiratory burst, which elicits a sudden release of toxic reactive oxygen metabolites such as superoxide anion, chloramine, hypochlorous acid, hydroxyl radical, and hydrogen peroxide *(31)*. In addition, collateral tissue damage is caused by deposition of the membrane attack complex (C5b-9) on cells in an antigen-independent manner, i.e., graft vessels and tissue stroma are damaged without targeted specificity *(28)*.

Reactive Oxygen and Nitrogen Species in the Reperfusion Milieu

Of specific importance in understanding graft damage during reperfusion is the fact that reactive oxygen and reactive nitrogen intermediates are formed in abundance in the reperfusion milieu. Superoxide (O_2^-) combines with NO˙ in one of the fastest chemical reactions known (rate constant on the order of $6 \times 10^9 \, \mathrm{mol^{-1}/s}$) to produce peroxynitrite, OONO⁻. The fate of peroxynitrite depends on the chemical vicinity in which it is generated; it may become protonated, followed by isomerization to form a proton and nitrate, or it may undergo homolytic cleavage to form hydroxyl radical (OH˙) and nitrogen dioxide free radical ($NO_2^˙$) or heterolytic cleavage to nitronium cation (NO_2^+) and hydroxide anion (OH⁻). Three of these cleavage products (OH˙, $NO_2^˙$, and NO_2^+) are among the most reactive and damaging species in biological systems.

ROLE OF NO˙ IN ORGAN
PRESERVATION FOR TRANSPLANTATION

Endothelial Cells as a Transplantation Paradigm

All vascular organs contain an abundance of endothelial cells. It is estimated that up to 40% of the parenchymal mass of the lungs is comprised of endothelial cells *(32)*, and up to 10% of the parenchymal mass of the heart is comprised of endothelial cells in close proximity to all myocytes. It is therefore instructive to consider how endothelial cells behave in a simplified "ischemic" environment. Although hypoxia only simulates a single component of ischemia, it is a useful paradigm by which to gain insights into mechanisms of vascular dysfunction following transplantation. Endothelial cells, under quiescent conditions, synthesize NO˙ in response to mechanical perturbation or in response to the occupancy of specific receptors, such as bradykinin, histamine, or thrombin. Each of these stimuli triggers a brisk rise in intracellular calcium within the endothelial cell, which can promote shape change and the translocation of Weibel–Palade bodies to the cellular surface. Endothelial cells subjected to a period of oxygen deprivation behave similarly, as do endothelial cells reperfused in the setting of organ transplantation. As described in detail earlier, the result of preservation and transplantation is a remarkable shift of the endothelial phenotype from one that maintains an intact vascular barrier to one that does not, from a cell that is relatively nonadhesive for circulating neutrophils to one that is, from one that exhibits an antithrombotic phenotype to one that exhibits a prothrombotic phenotype, and from one that liberates NO˙ to promote relaxation of subjacent smooth muscle cells and inhibits platelet aggregation and leukocyte adhesion to one in which (in the setting of reperfusion) bioavailable NO˙ is scarce. Taken together, all of these perturbations in normal vascular homeostatic mechanisms contribute to primary graft failure or to organ dysfunction during the critical early stages after organ transplantation.

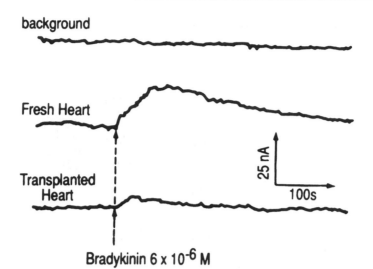

Fig. 6. Measurement of endocardial NO$^{\bullet}$ with a porphyrinic sensor. After baseline stabilization (top), $6 \times 10^{-6}\,M$ bradykinin was applied and NO$^{\bullet}$ release continuously monitored by amperometry at constant potential of 0.63 V. The middle and bottom tracings represent those from a fresh rat heart or those from a transplanted cardiac isograft shortly after reperfusion. Although the endocardium of a preserved/transplanted heart generates an analytic signal following bradykinin challenge, it is significantly less than that of a freshly explanted heart. Adapted from ref. *(8)*.

Deficient NO$^{\bullet}$ and Cyclic Nucleotide Second Messengers Contribute to Primary Graft Failure

There is some very direct evidence that NO$^{\bullet}$ and its second messenger cGMP play an important role in maintaining vascular homeostasis specifically in the setting of organ transplantation. First, direct measurements with a porphyrinic microsensor demonstrate that under reperfusion conditions, NO$^{\bullet}$ levels decline rapidly and are considerably lower than in either the nontransplanted heart *(8)* (Fig. 6) or lungs *(9)* (*see* Fig. 2). In the rat model of heterotopic cardiac transplantation in which a vascularized cardiac graft is placed in the abdomen of a strain-matched recipient, it is clear that repleting deficient NO$^{\bullet}$/cGMP second messenger pathways ameliorates posttransplant graft dysfunction, defined as graft survival *(8)*. Not only does incorporation of the amino acid precursor of NO$^{\bullet}$ (L-arginine) into the cardiac preservation solution improve graft survival, but NO$^{\bullet}$ donors (nitroglycerin or sodium nitroprusside) do, as well. In contrast and completely consistent with these results, inhibition of NO$^{\bullet}$ synthesis with a molar excess of the L-arginine analog N^{G}-monomethyl-L-arginine (L-NMMA) abrogates the beneficial effects of L-arginine on both graft blood flow and graft survival. The improvement in graft function with agents that stimulated the NO$^{\bullet}$/cGMP pathway was dose-dependent, and was associated with parallel improvements in graft blood flow, as measured by the entrapment of latex microspheres (Fig. 7). In addition, nitroglycerin was shown in this model to have a significant early inhibitory effect on graft neutrophil accumulation. Similarly, in the lungs the addition of nitrovasodilators such as nitroglycerin to the preservation solution was shown to have significant beneficial effects on posttransplant gas exchange as well as pulmonary hemodynamics *(33)* (Fig. 8).

When the mechanism by which NO$^{\bullet}$ acts to improve organ preservation was probed further, it became apparent that stimulation of the cGMP-dependent protein kinase was critical for successful organ function following transplantation in a highly stringent rat orthotopic left lung transplant model *(9)*. 8-Br-cGMP, a membrane-permeable, nonhydrolyzable analog of cGMP that can activate the cGMP-dependent protein kinase in a relatively specific fashion (500 times more potent for the cGMP-dependent protein kinase than for the cAMP-depen-

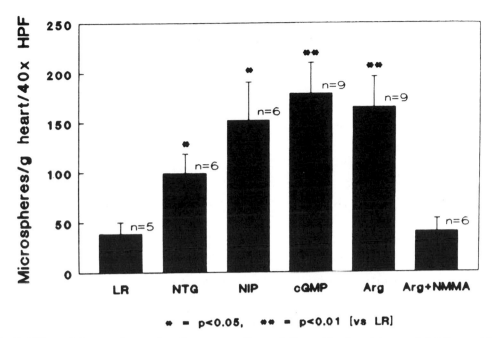

Fig. 7. Effect of the supplementing the preservation solution with stimulators or inhibitors of the NO•/cGMP pathway on graft blood flow. Blood flow to transplanted hearts was evaluated by injecting 10 μm latex microspheres into the donor aortic root, followed by quantification of entrapped microspheres. Stimulation of the NO•/cGMP pathway was associated with higher blood flows in cardiac grafts. In contrast, antagonism of this pathway was associated with lower blood flows. Endothelium independent vasodilators [nitroglycerin, NTG; nitroprusside NIP), a cGMP analogue (8-Br-cGMP, cGMP), and L-arginine (Arg)] all enhanced preservation, whereas a fivefold molar excess of N^G-monomethyl-L-arginine (L-NMMA) antagonized the beneficial action of L-arginine. Adapted from ref. (8).

dent protein kinase), caused a dose-dependent enhancement of lung preservation. Because 8-Br-cGMP does not interact with the allosteric binding sites on the cGMP-regulated cAMP PDEs, it is unlikely that the beneficial effects of 8-Br-cGMP could be explained by bolstering cAMP levels. In addition, in the setting of lung preservation, augmenting endogenous cGMP levels by inhibiting endogenous cGMP catabolism using the type V (cGMP-specific) PDE inhibitor zaprinast significantly improved lung graft survival. Although a membrane permeable cGMP analog (8-Br-cGMP) likewise improved lung preservation, these effects could be inhibited when the 8-Br-cGMP was combined with a pharmacological agent that inhibited the activity of the cGMP-dependent protein kinase. Taken together, these data point to a critical intermediary role (in NO•'s beneficial effects on organ preservation) of stimulation of the cGMP-dependent protein kinase.

One of the critical observations we made in terms of mechanisms of organ preservation was first elucidated in the context of studies on the effect of nitroglycerin on lung preservation. It had long been assumed that rapid delivery of a hypothermic preservation solution was critical for subsequent organ function, and that the more rapid (and homogeneous) this delivery, the better the preservation. This had been accepted as one of the tenets of organ preservation, and seemed so obvious as to never have been scrupulously examined. However, during the course of our studies with nitroglycerin, in which we used a potent direct-acting vasodilating agent (hydralazine) as a control, we were struck by an apparent discrepancy. During the infusion of the hypothermic preservation solution, hydralazine caused the lowest pulmonary vascular resistance (33). We termed this phenomenon "harvest pulmonary vascular resistance," to differentiate it from the vascular resistance that was measured following

A   **B**

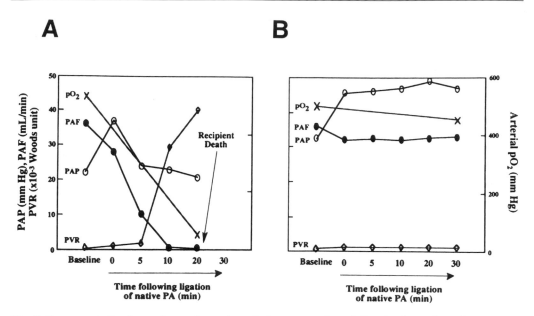

Fig. 8. Representative hemodynamic tracing of a lung transplant following hypothermic preservation for 6 h in Euro-Collins solution (Baxter Healthcare, Deerfield, IL) alone (**Left**) or Euro-Collins solution supplemented with nitroglycerin (**Right**) after the native lung was removed from the pulmonary circulation. PAP = mean pulmonary arterial pressure (mmHg); PAF = pulmonary arterial flow (mL/min); PVR = pulmonary vascular resistance ($\times 10^{-3}$ Woods unit). Adapted from ref. *(33)*.

transplantation of the donor organ. Although it too lowered harvest pulmonary vascular resistance, nitroglycerin was not as effective in this regard as hydralazine. However, grafts preserved with nitroglycerin fared far better than those preserved with hydralazine. Although subsequent experiments did show that harvest pulmonary vascular resistance was not unimportant, it appeared to be by far the least important parameter we could measure in terms of predicting subsequent graft function. Further study revealed that additional properties of nitroglycerin were critical to improved graft function, and these included its ability to attenuate graft platelet and leukocyte accumulation (Fig. 9). As discussed before, these are also known properties of NO• on endothelial cells in vitro, again proving the usefulness of the endothelial cell paradigm. Taken together, these studies show that harvest vasodilation is either unimportant or of only modest importance in graft preservation for transplantation.

Role of NO• in Rejection

Although NO• plays an important role in stabilizing vascular function during the vulnerable period immediately after transplantation, longer studies in various transplantation models demonstrate that across an allogeneic barrier, NO• synthesized by the inducible isoform of NOS contributes to cellular graft rejection. In the heart *(34,35)*, between the third and tenth day following transplantation across an allogeneic barrier, there is a marked increase in iNOS mRNA and protein in grafted tissue. Although this is predominantly localized to recruited mononuclear phagocytes, in the heart, cardiac myocytes themselves produce iNOS. As the iNOS produced within cardiac myocytes and adjacent cells can be toxic to these cells, both by inhibiting mitochondrial respiration as well as by promoting apoptosis *(36,37)*, it is apparent that graft damage may occur. Proof that the production of NO• by iNOS is toxic to the graft in allogeneic transplantation comes from data from two different laboratories in which inhibition of NO• production was shown to either retard or diminish objective indices of cardiac allograft rejection *(34,35)*. In the lungs, there is also substantial evidence for iNOS induction during acute rejection, both at the level of iNOS mRNA and activity *(38)*, as well by the detec-

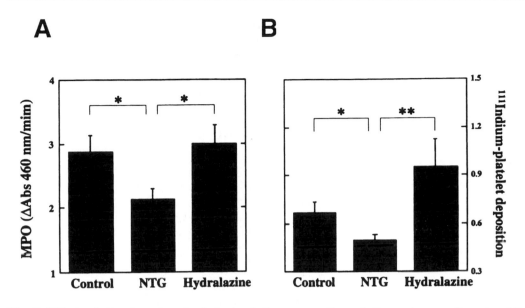

Fig. 9. Effects of nitroglycerin or hydralazine in the preservation solution on lung graft neutrophil and platelet accumulation. (**A**) Myeloperoxidase activity (MPO; ΔAbs 460 nm/min) is shown as a measure of graft neutrophil accumulation. (**B**) [111]Indium-labeled platelet accumulation is expressed as the ratio of graft radioactivity to blood radioactivity. Adapted from ref. *(33)*.

tion of increased NO• in the exhaled air of recipients rejecting lung allografts *(39)*. The significance of iNOS induction in lung allograft rejection is suggested by data demonstrating improvement in functional and histological parameters of lung rejection with iNOS inhibition using aminoguanidine *(40)*.

The role of NO• in transplant rejection is, however, not so simple. As is the case for inhaled NO• (*see* following), even in rejection NO• plays a dichotomous role. In contrast to the exacerbating role of iNOS in acute rejection, iNOS appears to inhibit the late development of allograft arteriopathy. When iNOS-deficient hearts were transplanted into recipient mice across an allogeneic barrier, the iNOS null hearts exhibited worse allograft arteriopathy *(41)*. In skin allografts, the lack of iNOS does not appear to influence the kinetics of the rejection process in vivo, although in vitro studies demonstrated increased capacity of iNOS-deficient splenocytes to proliferate to produce interferon-gamma, IL-2, and IL-12 in response to allogeneic stimulation *(42)*.

In the setting of lung transplantation, the production of NO• may play a role against the development of obliterative bronchiolitis, as was demonstrated in a heterotopic rat tracheal allograft model in which L-arginine supplementation reduced obliterative histological changes *(43)*. In this same study, treatment with aminoguanidine (to inhibit iNOS) was associated with enhanced proliferation of alpha-smooth muscle actin-immunoreactive cells and increased intensity of obliterative bronchiolitis early after transplantation. As obliterative bronchiolitis is the most important noninfectious long-term complication of lung transplantation in humans, these data deserve some note. These data show how iNOS induction may be at once both toxic to an allograft, contributing to cell damage and accelerating or exacerbating allograft rejection, yet at the same time protective by reducing the long-term consequences of obliterative vascular or bronchiolar remodeling.

Dichotomous Effects of Inhaled NO• in Lung Preservation for Transplantation

If reperfusion represents an NO• deficiency state, which it does by dint of the lack of bioavailable NO• caused by quenching by superoxide on reperfusion, then it seems logical that the administration of NO• could restore this deficiency, and hence ameliorate graft dysfunction. In cardiac or lung transplantation, supplementing a preservation solution with NO• donors does have a salutary vascular effect on reperfusion *(8,9,33,44)*. The lack of NO• may be especially critical in the setting of lung transplantation because the lung represents a vast excretory organ for NO•, with large quantities of NO• being exhaled with every breath. In the setting of lung transplantation, intubation facilitates studies of the direct inhalational administration of NO• gas. In the lungs, we hypothesized that this would replete the NO• "deficiency" state and, hence, improve vascular function. The data, however, did not support this hypothesis. Again using an orthotopic, isogeneic lung transplant model in rats, NO• was administered (65 ppm, monitored by chemiluminescence) to recipients at the time of reperfusion. These data demonstrated no improvement in graft function (arterial oxygenation, pulmonary vascular resistance after transplantation) or graft survival, even though in this same model distal stimulation of the NO•/cGMP conferred significant graft functional and survival advantage compared with an untreated control transplant group. Subsequently, other investigators have confirmed the beneficial effects of inhaled NO• given to the lung transplant donor *(45)*.

More recent data help us to account for this seeming paradox, i.e., that NO• inhaled at the time of reperfusion confers no benefit *(46,47)*. For these experiments, NO• was administered to the lung transplant donor at the time of lung harvest. In contrast to inhaled NO• given at the time of reperfusion, inhaled NO• given to the lung transplant donor conferred significant functional and survival advantages. We hypothesized that the formation of reactive nitrogen intermediates, due to the supply of inhaled NO• given in the setting of reperfusion, was causing a deleterious effect on graft function that could not be overcome by the potential beneficial vascular homeostatic effects that might otherwise have been conferred by the exogenous NO•. To prove this hypothesis, we indirectly monitored the production of peroxynitrite in the sections of lung tissue (caused by the interaction of NO• and superoxide, as described earlier). These studies were performed using an antibody that recognizes nitrosated tyrosine residues. These preliminary data demonstrated that, although freshly harvested lungs or those provided with inhaled NO• only at the time of harvest exhibited little evidence of protein nitrosation, lungs exposed to NO• in the setting of reperfusion exhibited extensive and diffuse nitrotyrosine staining, presumptive evidence for the formation of peroxynitrite. These data go a long way toward explaining why, in a setting in which ROS are scarce (remote from the immediate transplant setting) inhaled NO• has reported beneficial effects. The setting in which NO• is given by inhalation is, therefore, a critical component of its effects.

These provocative data lead to another question of seeming contradiction: if inhaled NO• confers no benefit on reperfusion, why does L-arginine supplementation appear to be beneficial? The answer to this, albeit somewhat speculative, may lie in the fact that NOS, itself an oxidoreductase, can not only produce NO• but, in the absence of substrate (L-arginine), may also produce superoxide. It is likely that provision of excess substrate in the form of L-arginine may have two parallel beneficial effects: it may reduce ambient superoxide concentrations by inhibiting superoxide formation by NOS, and it may promote the formation of NO•. In this setting, the relative lack of superoxide may tip the balance in favor of NO•'s beneficial vascular homeostatic effects.

SUMMARY

The preservation of solid organs for transplantation brings about changes in the endothelial phenotype during the preservation period that result in severe perturbations of vascular function after transplantation. These include changes in endothelial barrier properties, increases in leukocyte adhesion receptor expression, and changes in endogenous cyclic nucleotide levels in endothelial and VSMCs. When oxygen and leukocytes are reintroduced at the time of reestablishment of blood flow, additional vascular mechanisms of graft dysfunction are brought into play. ROS quench available NO•, whose levels plummet. Leukocytes are recruited by a large number of proinflammatory cytokines, and the expression of leukocyte adhesion receptors on the endothelial surface is increased by local autoregulatory amplification mechanisms. In addition to these cellular processes, cell and subcellular fragments activate the complement cascade, which further promote tissue damage by indiscriminate deposition of membrane attack complexes and by further amplifying neutrophil recruitment through the release of chemotaxins. Finally, thrombotic processes, including both humoral and platelet components, are activated, further plugging microvascular lumina and impeding the return of blood flow to the newly transplanted organ.

How does NO• fit into this maelstrom? NO• possesses many properties that promote restoration of a quiescent vascular phenotype. When NO• is abundant, endothelial barrier function is maintained, platelet aggregation is inhibited, leukocyte adhesion receptor expression and graft leukostasis are quelled, and vasodilation is promoted. These serve to promote vascular homeostasis and help maintain the viability of an organ's parenchymal or functional cells during the highly vulnerable reperfusion period. On the other hand, data are emerging to suggest that the pendulum may swing too far, in that excessively abundant NO• in the setting of reperfusion and superoxide may be deleterious to the graft, perhaps due to the formation of highly reactive peroxynitrite. Once the acute reperfusion milieu has subsided, NO• takes on another role, i.e., that of an immunosuppressive adjunct that may promote inflammation and rejection, yet that may inhibit delayed vascular or bronchiolar remodeling. These are some of the seeming paradoxical actions of NO• in the setting of organ transplantation for which further study is clearly warranted.

ACKNOWLEDGMENTS

The preparation of this chapter was supported by the US Public Health service (HL55397 and HL60900 to D.J.P., and HL40527 and PERC to D.M.S.). Dr. Pinsky completed this chapter during his tenure as an Established Investigator of the American Heart Association.

REFERENCES

1. Hosenpud JD, Bennett LE, Keck BM, Fiol B, Novick RJ. The Registry of the International Society for Heart and Lung Transplantation: fourteenth official report—1997. J Heart Lung Transp 1997;16:691–712.
2. Christie JD, Bavaria JE, Palevsky HI, Litzky L, Blumenthal NP, Kaiser LR, et al. Primary lung graft failure following lung transplantation. Chest 1998;114:51–60.
3. Schulman LL. Perioperative mortality and primary graft failure. Chest 1998;114:7,8.
4. Opelz G, Wujciak T. The influence HLA compatibility on graft survival after heart transplantation. N Engl J Med 1994;330:816–819.
5. Ogawa S, Koga S, Kuwabara K, Brett J, Morrow B, Morris SA, et al. Hypoxia-induced increased permeability of endothelial monolayers occurs through lowering of cellular cAMP levels. Am J Physiol 1992;262:C546–C554.
6. Koga S, Morris S, Ogawa S, Liao H, Bilezikian JP, Chen G, et al. TNF modulate endothelial properties by decreasing cAMP. Am J Physiol 1995;268:C1104–C1113.
7. Suttorp N, Weber U, Welsch T, Schudt C. Role of phosphodiesterases in the regulation of endothelial permeability in vitro. J Clin Invest 1993;91:1421–1428.
8. Pinsky DJ, Oz MC, Koga S, Taha Z, Broekman MJ, Marcus AJ, et al. Cardiac preservation is enhanced in a heterotopic rat transplant model by supplementing the nitric oxide pathway. J Clin Invest 1994;93: 2291–2297.
9. Pinsky DJ, Naka Y, Chowdhury NC, Liao H, Oz MC, Michler RE, et al. The nitric oxide/cyclic GMP pathway in organ transplantation: cricital role in successful lung preservation. Proc Natl Acad Sci USA 1994;91:12,086–12,090.
10. Kubes P, Granger DN. Nitric oxide modulates microvascular permeability. Am J Physiol 1992;262: H611–H615.

11. Kurose I, Wolf R, Grisham MB, Granger DN. Effects of an endogenous inhibitor of nitric oxide synthesis on postcapillary venules. Am J Physiol 1995;268:H2224–H2231.

12. Nossel HL. Relative proteolysis of the fibrinogen B beta chain by thrombin and plasmin as a determinant of thrombosis. Nature 1981;291:165–167.

13. Pinsky DJ, Liao H, Lawson CA, Yan S-F, Chen J, Carmeliet P, et al. Coordinated induction of plasminogen activator inhibitor-1 (PAI-1) and inhibition of plasminogen activator gene expression by hypoxia promotes pulmonary vascular fibrin deposition. J Clin Invest 1998;102:919–928.

14. Pinsky DJ, Naka Y, Liao H, Oz MC, Wagner DD, Mayadas TN, et al. Hypoxia-induced exocytosis of endothelial cell Weibel-Palade bodies. A mechanism for rapid neutrophil recruitment after cardiac preservation. J Clin Invest 1996;97:493–500.

15. Liao H, Heath M, Pinsky DJ. Stimulation of the NO/cGMP pathway reduces hypoxia-induced endothelial P-selectin expression: a mechanism whereby nitrosovasodilators reduces neutrophil adhesion. Circulation 1996;94:I–634.

16. Davenpeck KL, Gauthier TW, Lefer AM. Inhibition of endothelial-derived nitric oxide promotes P-selectin expression and actions in the rat microcirculation. Gastroenterology 1994;107:1050–1058.

17. Pinsky DJ, Patton S, Mesaros S, Brovkovych V, Kubaszewski E, Grunfeld S, et al. Mechanical transduction of nitric oxide synthesis in the beating heart. Circ Res 1997;81:372–379.

18. Pinsky D, Oz M, Liao H, Morris S, Brett J, Sciacca R, et al. Restoration of the cAMP second messenger pathway enhances cardiac preservation for transplantation in a heterotopic rat model. J Clin Invest 1993; 92:2994–3002.

19. Naka Y, Roy DK, Liao H, Chowdhury NC, Michler RE, Oz MC, et al. cAMP-mediated vascular protection in an orthotopic rat lung transplantation model. Insights into the mechanism of action of prostaglandin E1 to improve lung preservation. Circ Res 1996;79:773–783.

20. Mayadas TN, Johnson RC, Rayburn H, Hynes RO, Wagner DD. Leukoctye rolling and extravasation are severely compromised in P selectin-deficient mice. Cell 1993;74:541–554.

21. Lefer DJ, Nakanishi K, Johnston WE, Vinten-Johansen J. Antineutrophil and myocardial protecting actions of a novel nitric oxide donor after acute myocardial ischemia and reperfusion in dogs. Circulation 1993;88:2337–2350.

22. Ma XL, Weyrich AS, Lefer DJ, Lefer AM. Diminished basal nitric oxide release after myocardial ischemia and reperfusion promotes neutrophil adherence to coronary endothelium. Circ Res 1993;72: 403–412.

23. Yan S-F, Zou YS, Mendelsohn M, Gao Y, Naka Y, Pinsky D, et al. Nuclear factor interleukin-6 motifs mediate tissue-specific gene transcription in hypoxia. J Biol Chem 1997;272:4287–4294.

24. Yan S-F, Tritto I, Pinsky D, Liao H, Huang J, Fuller G, et al. Induction of Interleukin-6 (IL-6) by hypoxia in vascular cells: central role of the binding site for nuclear factor-IL-6. J Biol Chem 1995;270: 11,463–11,471.

25. Oz MC, Liao H, Naka Y, Seldomridge A, Becker DN, Michler RE, et al. Ischemia-induced interleukin-8 release after human heart transplantation. A potential role for endothelial cells. Circulation 1995;92: II-428–II-432.

26. Karakurum M, Shreeniwas R, Chen J, Pinsky D, Yan SD, Anderson M, et al. Hypoxic induction of interleukin-8 gene expression in human endothelial cells. J Clin Invest 1994;93:1564–1570.

27. Shreeniwas R, Koga S, Karakurum M, Pinsky D, Kaiser E, Brett J, et al. Hypoxia-mediated induction of endothelial cell interleukin-1 alpha. An autocrine mechanism promoting expression of leukocyte adhesion molecules on the vessel surface. J Clin Invest 1992;90:2333–2339.

28. Naka Y, Marsh HC, Scesney SM, Oz MC, Pinsky DJ. Complement activation as a cause for primary graft failure in an isogeneic rat model of hypothermic lung preservation and transplantation. Transplantation 1997;64:1248–1255.

29. Naka Y, Toda K, Kayano K, Oz MC, Pinsky DJ. Failure to express the P-selectin gene or P-selectin blockade confers early pulmonary protection after lung ischemia or transplantation. Proc Natl Acad Sci USA 1997;94:757–761.

30. Wang CY, Naka Y, Liao H, Oz MC, Springer TA, Gutierrez-Ramos J-C, et al. Cardiac graft intercellular adhesion molecule-1 (ICAM-1) and interleukin-1 expression mediate primary isograft failure and induction of ICAM-1 in organs remote from the site of transplantation. Circ Res 1998;82:762–772.

31. Weiss SJ. Tissue destruction by neutrophils. N Engl J Med 1989;320:365–376.

32. Crapo JD, Barry BE, Gehr P, Bachofen M, Weibel ER. Cell number and cell characteristics of the normal human lung. Am Rev Respir Dis 1982;125:740–745.

33. Naka Y, Chowdhury NC, Liao H, Roy DK, Oz MC, Michler RE, et al. Enhanced preservation of orthotopically transplanted rat lungs by nitroglycerin but not hydralazine. Requirement for graft vascular homeostasis beyond harvest vasodilation. Circ Res 1995;76:900–906.

34. Yang X, Chowdhury N, Cai B, Brett J, Marboe C, Sciacca RR, et al. Induction of myocardial nitric oxide synthase by cardiac allograft rejection. J Clin Invest 1994;94:714–721.

35. Worrall NK, Lazenby WD, Misko TP, Lin TS, Rodi CP, Manning PT, et al. Modulation of in vivo alloreactivity by inhibition of inducible nitric oxide synthase. J Exp Med 1995;181:63–70.

36. Szabolcs MJ, Ravalli S, Minanov O, Sciacca RR, Michler RE, Cannon PJ. Apoptosis and increased expression of inducible nitric oxide synthase in human allograft rejection. Transplantation 1998;65: 804–812.

37. Szabolcs M, Michler RE, Yang X, Aji W, Roy D, Athan E, et al. Apoptosis of cardiac myocytes during cardiac allograft rejection. Relation to induction of nitric oxide synthase. Circulation 1996;94:1665–1673.

38. Worrall NK, Boasquevisque CH, Misko TP, Sullivan PM, Ferguson TB Jr. Inducible nitric oxide synthase is expressed during experimental acute lung allograft rejection. J Heart Lung Transplant 1997; 16:334–339.

39. Mizuta T, Fujii Y, Minami M, Tanaka S, Utsumi T, Kosaka H, et al. Increased nitric oxide levels in exhaled air of rat lung allografts. J Thorac Cardiovasc Surg 1997;113:830–835.

40. Worrall NK, Boasquevisque CH, Botney MD, Misko TP, Sullivan PM, Ferguson TB Jr, et al. Inhibition of inducible nitric oxide synthase ameliorates functional and histological changes of acute lung allograft rejection. Transplantation 1997;63:1095–1101.

41. Koglin J, Glysing-Jensen T, Mudgett JS, Russell ME. Exacerbated transplant arteriosclerosis in inducible nitric oxide-deficient mice. Circulation 1998;97:2059–2065.

42. Casey JJ, Wei XQ, Orr DJ, Gracie JA, Huang FP, Bolton EM, et al. Skin allograft rejection in mice lacking inducible nitric oxide synthase. Transplantation 1997;64:589–593.

43. Kallio EA, Koskinen PK, Aavik E, Vaali K, Lemstom KB. Role of nitric oxide in experimental obliterative bronchiolitis (chronic rejection) in the rat. J Clin Invest 1997;100:2984–2994.

44. Naka Y, Chowdhury NC, Oz MC, Smith CR, Yana OJ, Michler RE, et al. Nitroglycerin maintains graft vascular homeostasis and enhances preservation in an orthotopic rat lung transplant model. J Thorac Cardiovasc Surg 1995;109:206–211.

45. Fujino S, Nagahiro I, Triantafillou AN, Boasquevisque CH, Yano M, Patterson GA. Inhaled nitric oxide at the time of harvest improves early lung allograft function. Ann Thorac Surg 1997;63:1383–1389.

46. Naka Y, Roy DK, Smerling AJ, Michler RE, Smith CR, Stern DM, et al. Inhaled nitric oxide fails to confer the pulmonary protection provided by distal stimulation of the nitric oxide pathway at the level of cyclic guanosine monophosphate. J Thorac Cardiovasc Surg 1995;110:1434–1441.

47. Naka Y, Liao H, Pinsky DJ. Paradoxical improvement in lung graft function by simultaneously inhibiting endogenous nitric oxide synthesis and butressing cGMP levels. Circulation 1998;98(17):I–265.

30

L-Arginine
Its Role in Cardiovascular Therapy

Andrew J. Maxwell and John P. Cooke

INTRODUCTION

A deficiency of nitric oxide (NO•) production and/or activity contributes to the patho-physiology and progression of a number of disorders or metabolic conditions associated with cardiovascular disease. Atherosclerosis and conditions predisposing to atherosclerosis (such as hypertension, hypercholesterolemia, tobacco use, estrogen deficiency, and age) are each associated with impaired endothelium-dependent vasodilation (1–10). Endothelium-dependent vasodilation is also attenuated in individuals suffering from such diverse diseases as renal insufficiency, heart failure, pulmonary hypertension, and in such conditions as ischemia-reperfusion, transplant vasculopathy, and restenosis. The mechanisms underlying endothelial impairment are also varied. These include degradation of NO• (because of vascular generation of superoxide anion); inhibition of NO• synthesis (by endogenous antagonists of nitric oxide synthase [NOS]); alterations in NOS structure or function; reduced availability of the NO• precursor or NOS cofactors; and/or attenuated expression of NOS. Some of these disorders (hypercholesterolemia, tobacco use, and coronary and peripheral arterial disease) manifest an endothelial vasodilator dysfunction that is clearly responsive to administration of L-arginine, whereas in other disorders (such as long-standing hypertension or diabetes mellitus) the benefit of L-arginine is less clear.

Accumulating evidence indicates that in those disorders where administration of L-arginine restores endothelium-dependent vasodilation, improvements can be seen in regional blood flow and arterial vasomotor tone, associated with beneficial extravascular effects on platelet and leukocyte reactivity, and fibrinogenolysis. Clinical benefits of L-arginine administration have been observed in systemic and pulmonary hypertension (6,11–16), coronary and peripheral arterial disease (4,17–23), heart failure (24–28), transplant vasculopathy (29,30), renovascular disease (31–33), Raynaud's phenomenon (34,35), erectile dysfunction (36,37), and in pre-eclampsia and placental insufficiency (38–40). Furthermore, an extensive number of animal studies shown beneficial effects of L-arginine in the settings of atherosclerotic plaque formation (41–43), restenosis (44–46), and reperfusion injury following tissue ischemia (47–55). In most of these disorders the therapeutic effect of L-arginine is caused by its metabolism by NOS.

However, some effects of L-arginine on the cardiovascular system may be independent of its conversion to NO•. Exogenous L-arginine is known to enhance wound healing (56), immunomodulation (57), and hepatic metabolism (58,59), as well as somatic and cellular growth (60,61). Part of the biologic action of L-arginine is due to the fact that it is a highly

From: *Contemporary Cardiology, vol. 4: Nitric Oxide and the Cardiovascular System*
Edited by: J. Loscalzo and J. A. Vita © Humana Press Inc., Totowa, NJ

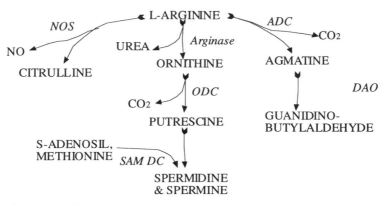

Fig. 1. The major metabolic pathways for L-arginine involve primarily the conversion to citrulline by nitric oxide synthase (NOS), conversion to ornithine by arginase, and conversion to agmatine by arginine decarboxylase (ADC). DAO; diamine oxidase, ODC; ornithine decarboxylase, SAM; S-adenosylmethionine decarboxylase.

basic molecule. In high doses, L-arginine may induce an endothelium-independent vasodilation possibly by depolarizing endothelial cells *(62,63)*. The guanidino group on L-arginine is a potential electron acceptor that may be able to participate directly in scavenging highly destructive superoxide anions *(64)*. The highly basic nature of L-arginine also appears to be greatly responsible for its properties as a hormone secretogogue *(65,66)*. L-Arginine stimulates the release of growth hormone, catecholamines, insulin, glucagon, and other hormone secretion in a dose-dependent manner. The effects of these hormones may contribute to the effects of L-arginine on cardiovascular function and structure. Another NO•-independent mechanism by which L-arginine affects the cardiovascular system is by its participation as a precursor to pyrimidines *(67)*, polyamines, and in the synthesis of tissue matrix proteins such as collagen *(68)* (Fig. 1). Polyamines play an important role in promoting cellular proliferation, tissue growth, and differentiation *(69)*. The tissue matrix proteins are central to the appropriate healing of injured tissue. Finally, L-arginine participates as a nutrient contributing to the production of most proteins. These other metabolic pathways of L-arginine also contribute to cardiovascular homeostasis particularly in angiogenesis and following vascular injury.

However, the weight of the evidence indicates that most of the beneficial effects of L-arginine in cardiovascular disease are due to its conversion to NO•. Initially, there was skepticism that administration of L-arginine could enhance NO• synthesis. This skepticism was based on in vitro observations of the enzyme kinetics of NOS. These studies indicated that intracellular stores of L-arginine are more than adequate to saturate the enzyme under physiologic conditions *(70)*. Nevertheless, a plethora of animal and human studies have revealed that endothelial vasodilator dysfunction is remediable by L-arginine. Furthermore, the enhancement by L-arginine of endothelial function is associated with evidence of increased NO• synthesis. The efficacy of supplemental L-arginine in cardiovascular diseases is understandable in light of recent evidence that a number of diseases are associated with an arginine-deficiency state; either relative or absolute *(71)*. One reason for a relative arginine deficiency is the presence of the competitive inhibitor, asymmetric dimethylarginine (ADMA). This competitive inhibitor of NOS is probably responsible for the endothelial dysfunction in most disorders that are responsive to L-arginine. However, in some disorders, such as heart failure, plasma levels of L-arginine are less than half that of healthy controls suggesting an absolute L-arginine deficiency *(72)*. In fact, an argument can be made based on nitrogen balance studies that even healthy individuals, particularly those on a vegetarian diet, may be L-arginine deficient *(73–75)*. To summarize, a wealth of evidence now indicates that administration of the NO• precursor may be a useful adjunct to other cardiovascular therapies. This chapter details the pharmacology, biology and clinical effects of L-arginine in cardiovascular health and disease.

BIOLOGY

Evidence for NO•-Dependent Action of L-Arginine

Shortly after the discovery that L-arginine was the precursor of NO•, L-arginine administration was shown to improve NO•-dependent endothelium-mediated vasodilation in cardiovascular disease *(76–78)*. Cooke and colleagues fed a normal or hypercholesterolemic diet to New Zealand white rabbits for 10 wk *(79)*. Subsequently, the animals were anesthetized for studies of hind-limb blood flow. Intra-arterial infusions of acetylcholine induced (ACh) dose-dependent vasodilation that was attenuated in the hypercholesterolemic animals. Infusions of L-arginine (but not D-arginine or saline) augmented hind-limb blood flow responses to ACh in the hypercholesterolemic animals. Thoracic aortae were then removed from these animals for in vitro studies *(80)*. Thoracic aortae obtained from hypercholesterolemic animals receiving the saline infusion manifested an impairment of endothelium-dependent vasorelaxation in response to ACh. By contrast, those animals that received L-arginine exhibited a normalization of endothelium-dependent vasorelaxation. Moreover, this effect was stereospecific as the enantiomer, D-arginine, had no effect on endothelium-dependent vasodilation *(79,81)*. Subsequently, in various animal models of hypercholesterolemia and atherosclerosis, as well as in individuals with atherosclerosis, supplemental L-arginine has been shown to increase NO• production as measured directly by chemiluminescence during ex vivo vascular ring studies *(13,82,83)*, by measurement of platelet cGMP *(84)*, or by urinary nitrate excretion *(23)*. These studies indicate that the bioavailability of L-arginine to NOS is rate limiting to NO• production, particularly in diseases whereby NO• production is decreased.

The Arginine Paradox

After the endothelial isoform of NOS (eNOS) was purified and characterized, enzyme kinetic studies raised questions regarding previous observations that L-arginine could restore endothelial vasodilator function. Pollock, Förstermann, and colleagues demonstrated that the half-saturating L-arginine concentration (K_m) for purified eNOS in vitro is 2.9 μM/L *(70)*. Others also demonstrated values for the K_m below 10 μM *(85,86)*. In cultured endothelial cells, intracellular concentrations of L-arginine have been reported in the range of 100–800 μM/L *(87–89)*, whereas in freshly isolated endothelial cells, intracellular concentrations of L-arginine have been reported as high as 2000 μM/L *(89)*. Furthermore, the intracellular L-arginine concentration can vary widely without affecting NO• production much *(87,90)*. Assuming that the values for the K_m and intracellular arginine levels reflect the in vivo conditions, eNOS should be saturated and additional L-arginine should not increase activity further *(91)*. Indeed, most investigators have reported little or no effect of exogenous L-arginine on endothelial vasodilator function in normal animals and healthy individuals.

Nevertheless, the weight of the evidence now strongly supports the notion that exogenous L-arginine enhances vascular NO• synthesis, particularly in hypercholesterolemia and atherosclerosis. Animal studies and clinical investigations are surprisingly concordant in demonstrating that exogenously administered L-arginine reverses endothelial vasodilator dysfunction in hypercholesterolemia and atherosclerosis. These beneficial effects are not mimicked by D-arginine, and are associated with the expected increases in urinary cGMP and nitrate.

At present, there is little doubt that exogenously administered L-arginine drives NO• production by endothelial cells. Multiple theories have been put forth to explain this puzzle. One consideration is that the "functional K_m" in intact cells is higher than that of the purified enzyme *(90)*. Whatever the underlying mechanism(s) is, it must explain how the availability

Table 1
Possible Mechanisms Underlying the Arginine Paradox

Alterations of arginine availability
    Reduced activity/expression of cationic amino acid transporter (CAT 1)
    Compartmentalization of arginine, CAT 1 and NOS
    Inhibition of intracellular L-arginine synthesis by L-glutamine
Inhibition of NOS signal cascade
    Inhibition of signal transduction by L-glutamine
Inhibition of NOS
    Competitive inhibition by ADMA or other inhibitors
    Decreased activity/expression of DDAH
    Feedback inhibition by endogenous NO•
Alterations in NOS
    Reduced NOS expression
    Reduced dimerization
    Aberrant palmitoylation, myristolation, or phosphorylation
    Reduced generation of the cofactor tetrahydrobiopterin (BH_4)
Inadequate plasma supply of L-arginine
    Dietary arginine deficiency
    Increased activity/expression of arginase or arginine decarboxylase
    Decreased renal tubular reuptake of L-arginine

of L-arginine is rate limiting. Table 1 lists possible mechanisms that make L-arginine rate limiting to endothelium-derived nitric oxide (EDNO) production.

Paradigms to Resolve the Paradox

ALTERATIONS IN L-ARGININE AVAILABILITY

Vane and colleagues demonstrated that cultured endothelial cells could recycle L-arginine from L-citrulline *(92,93)*. In addition to raising the possibility that this reaction could, in essence, provide a renewable source of intracellular L-arginine, it also raised the possibility that inhibition of this reaction may result in intracellular depletion of L-arginine during sustained EDNO production. Indeed these investigators found that the L-citrulline to L-arginine cycle could be inhibited by the presence of L-glutamine and this was associated with decreased EDNO production *(92–94)*. Labeling experiments demonstrated that L-glutamine at physiologic levels could inhibit arginosuccinate synthetase *(92)*. These investigators concluded that, in the presence of glutamine, intracellular L-arginine availability can become rate limiting in the formation of EDNO during prolonged production. Thus, by this model, one might conclude that exogenous L-arginine may replenish intracellular stores under these conditions. However, in these experiments, the levels of intracellular L-arginine in the depleted state were still in excess of the K_m of eNOS. Therefore, L-glutamate inhibition of L-arginine synthesis does not adequately explain the paradox.

Arnold et al. further investigated the ability of L-glutamine to inhibit EDNO production *(95)*. They found that physiologic plasma levels of L-glutamine affected EDNO production differently depending on the signal cascade activated. Whereas L-glutamine markedly inhibited EDNO release following receptor-mediated stimuli (bradykinin, adenosine diphosphate [ADP], ACh), the amino acid enhanced EDNO release following application of receptor-independent calcium-ionophore A23187. In these studies, intracellular L-arginine was not affected nor was the K_m of eNOS. The application of exogenous L-arginine was able to restore EDNO production without affecting intracellular L-glutamine levels. Taken together, these finding suggest that L-glutamine inhibits the receptor-mediated activation of NOS by an unknown mechanism, which can be reversed by exogenous L-arginine. These findings suggest that elevations in intracellular concentrations of L-glutamine may be a potential mechanism for the rate limitation of exogenous L-arginine in certain disease states.

Another hypothesis that would explain the paradox is that, in endothelial cells, the intracellular stores of L-arginine are sequestered, making them unavailable to eNOS whereas extracellular L-arginine transported into cells is preferentially delivered to eNOS *(96)*. eNOS has been shown to colocalize to cell-membrane proteins known as caveolin that are within membrane-bound structures known as caveolae *(97)*. Therefore, eNOS is potentially sequestered from intracellular L-arginine stores; intracaveolar L-arginine concentrations are not known.

Therefore, the source of L-arginine transport into caveoli may determine the rate of EDNO production. L-Arginine transport across membranes is mediated by several independent transport systems but the most important transport system into endothelial cells is the system y^+ *(98,99)*. The transport proteins for the y^+ transport system are the high-affinity cationic arginine transporters (CAT-1 and CAT-2B) *(100,101)*. McDonald and colleagues demonstrated colocalization of CAT-1 arginine transporter with membrane-bound eNOS within these caveolae *(96)*. The close association of eNOS and CAT-1 with the cell membrane suggests a mechanism for direct delivery of extracellular L-arginine to eNOS, negating the importance of intracellular L-arginine concentrations. In this paradigm, extracellular L-arginine concentrations determine the rate of transport and availability of L-arginine to eNOS. Therefore, depressed plasma concentrations of L-arginine as well as depressed activity of CAT-1 become potential mechanisms further limiting the rate of EDNO production in pathologic states.

Because of this caveolar sequestration, transport of L-arginine into caveolae may be rate limiting to EDNO production in certain conditions. This is particularly important if exogenous L-arginine concentration is a determinant of transport rate. Indeed, this may be the case particularly at higher plasma L-arginine concentrations. Factors that affect the rate of transport of L-arginine in endothelial cells include membrane potential, the presence of endotoxin, the concentrations of potassium ion, L-arginine, other cationic amino acids, glucose, and insulin *(98)*. The velocity of L-arginine transport is affected by the membrane potential. Zharikov and colleagues have demonstrated that hypoxia-induced membrane depolarization is responsible for reduced L-arginine transport in porcine pulmonary endothelial cells *(102)*. Conversely, adenosine stimulates L-arginine transport into endothelial and smooth muscle cells (SMCs) and does so by interacting with the A_2-purinoreceptor, which causes a rapid and transient hyperpolarization *(103,104)*. Vascular L-arginine transport can also be stimulated by inflammatory mediators. Endotoxin stimulates both the y^+ and B^{0+} transport systems through an autocrine pathway that involves the cytokines tumor necrosis factor (TNF) and interleukin-1 (IL-1) *(105,106)* and requires *de novo* RNA and protein synthesis *(107)*.

Glucose, insulin, and the diabetic state influence L-arginine transport. Acutely, glucose stimulates L-arginine transport, whereas insulin induces a protein synthesis-dependent stimulation of L-arginine transport. On the other hand, in the face of long-standing hyperglycemia, insulin downregulates elevated L-arginine transport *(108)*. Cultured umbilical veins from diabetic patients demonstrate an increased rate of L-arginine transport with a concomitant elevation in basal NO• activity *(109)*. By contrast, oxidized lipoprotein inhibits arginine transport via the high-affinity cationic amino acid transporter *(110)*. Concordant with this observation is the finding that oxidized low-density lipoprotein (LDL) inhibits L-arginine transport into platelets *(110)*. Thus, many pathologic conditions alter L-arginine transport potentially making it the rate-limiting step in EDNO production in these conditions. Alterations in L-arginine transport could underlie the arginine paradox.

In addition to the high-affinity, saturable y^+ system, L-arginine transport into human vascular cells is mediated by a nonsaturable component *(109)*. In addition, in the porcine pulmonary artery another (sodium-dependent) transport system has been identified (B^{0+}) *(99)*, although another group of investigators have identified only one population of L-arginine transporter with a K_m of 130 μM [98]). At physiologic concentrations, approx 70% of L-arginine is transported by y$^+$ transport system. However, at higher concentrations (1 mM) in human endothelium, 70% of the total L-arginine transported bypasses the y$^+$ system via the nonsaturable component (109). Thus, exogenous administration of L-arginine may increase availability of L-arginine to eNOS in conditions where the y$^+$ transport system is rate limiting.

INHIBITION OF eNOS

Another putative mechanism for the rate limitation of EDNO production by exogenous L-arginine has been provided by the work of Vallance and Moncada (111). These investigators characterized the physiologic effects of an endogenous inhibitor of NOS, asymmetric dimethylarginine (ADMA). They observed that patients with renal failure exhibit plasma levels of ADMA that are high enough to induce vasoconstriction of vascular rings in vitro (111). In guinea pigs, systemic infusion of ADMA (to attain ADMA levels similar to those observed in renal failure) results in a modest increase in blood pressure, whereas in normal individuals, infusions of ADMA into the brachial artery causes vasoconstriction and reduction in forearm blood flow. These observations suggest that ADMA may contribute to the hypertension observed in renal failure.

ADMA is degraded by the enzyme dimethylarginine dimethylaminohydrolase (DDAH). Inhibition of DDAH induces a gradual vasoconstriction in isolated vascular rings, which is reversible by exogenous L-arginine (112). This observation suggests that ADMA is continuously produced in sufficient levels to antagonize NOS, and its effects can be competitively reversed by exogenous L-arginine. In conditions where ADMA is elevated, its effect on eNOS appears to provide a satisfactory explanation of the arginine paradox.

ADMA is known to be elevated in atherosclerosis and in hypercholesterolemia (113,114) and in heart failure (72). The two- to threefold elevation of plasma ADMA that is observed in patients with hypercholesterolemia and/or atherosclerosis is physiologically significant. Faraci and Heistad found that concentrations of ADMA at these levels inhibit endothelium-dependent relaxation of basilar arteries in the rat and rabits (115a). Added to crude purified preparations of eNOS, ADMA in a physiological/pathophysiological range (1–10 μM) induces a dose-dependent inhibition of NO$^•$ synthesis (116). Indeed, plasma levels of ADMA correlate better with the magnitude of endothelial dysfunction than does LDL cholesterol in young hypercholesterolemic subjects (115). Furthermore, preliminary observations from our laboratory indicate that intracellular levels of ADMA in endothelial cells may be an order of magnitude greater than plasma levels. This is consistent with the alterations observed in L-arginine and ADMA transport. Using the erythrocyte as a model for L-arginine transport into vascular cells (116), the V_{max} of system y$^+$ L-arginine transport was examined in patients with uremia (117). In this model, L-arginine transport in uremic patients was higher than in healthy controls. Consistent with this finding the intracellular concentrations of L-arginine as well as NG-mono-methyl-L-arginine (L-NMMA) were significantly higher in this population. A similar finding has been demonstrated in erythrocytes of patients with heart failure (72). Indeed, endothelial cells and macrophages appear to have an inducible transporter (by cytokines and lipopoly-saccharides [LPS]) of mono- and dimethylarginines that allow for higher intracellular concentrations (118). Alternatively, the increased levels of ADMA in endothelial cells may be due to increased synthesis or reduced intracellular degradation of ADMA within the endothelial cell. Preliminary studies from our laboratory suggest that oxidized lipoprotein or cytokines reduce the activity of DDAH in endothelial cells, in association with an increase in ADMA released into the medium. This finding implies that hypercholesterolemia may induce endothelial dysfunction in part by interfering with the degradation of ADMA.

ALTERATIONS IN NOS

Whereas ADMA may belie the rate limitation of L-arginine in many vascular conditions associated with atherosclerosis, conformational changes in eNOS resulting in loss of affinity for L-arginine may be responsible in other conditions. Loss of affinity for L-arginine (and consequently an elevation in K_m) was first proposed by Pritchard and colleagues as the mechanism of the loss of EDNO activity in hypercholesterolemia (119). They observed that cultured endothelial cells exposed to native LDL cholesterol for several days began to generate superoxide anion. The generation of superoxide anion was blunted by the administration of L-arginine, or by treatment of the cell with an antagonist of eNOS. One explanation of this apparent paradox is that LDL may induce a conformational change in eNOS such that it still continues to receive electrons from reduced nicotinamide adenine dinucleotide phosphate (NADPH) but instead it donates them to its other substrate, O_2, to generate superoxide anion. In this case, exogenous L-arginine may effectively compete with molecular oxygen as a substrate, whereas administration of NOS antagonist may block electron transfer to molecular oxygen or L-arginine.

A similar scenario occurs during the reperfusion period following ischemia. Activated eNOS may quickly deplete local stores of L-arginine. In this substrate-depleted environment, eNOS may undergo a conformational change so as to preferentially generate superoxide anion (120). In this setting, it is possible that increases in local L-arginine concentrations may favor the dimer conformation of NOS. Indeed, L-arginine is known to stabilize the NOS dimer. In the absence of L-arginine, the monomer conformation is favored. The NOS monomer cannot synthesize NO*, but instead is capable of generating superoxide anion. Other alterations in eNOS reducing its affinity for L-arginine are likely as well. For example, insufficient availability of eNOS cofactors such as BH_4 may lead to decreased affinity and reduced EDNO production. However, it is unknown whether supplemental L-arginine is capable of overcoming an alteration in eNOS such as this to restore EDNO activity (121).

Evidence for Actions Independent of NO*

L-arginine also has effects on the cardiovascular system that are independent of the NOS system. Part of the biologic action of L-arginine is attributable to its highly basic nature. As such, it may contribute to the depolarization of vascular cell membranes thereby directly affecting vasomotor tone (62,63). For example, Rhodes and colleagues demonstrated that infusions of other cationic amino acids produce a vasodilatory response similar to that of L-arginine and, in fact, the D-isomers of these amino acids produced an even greater vasodilatory response than that of the L-isomer (62). A similar finding was demonstrated earlier by Thomas et al. (63). This mechanism may explain the observation in one study in which L-arginine was shown to cause vasodilation in endothelium-denuded aortic rings ex vivo (122). In addition to depolarizing cell membranes, it is conceivable that the positively charged amino acid may interact with negatively charged molecules such as heparin, which may alter blood coagulability (similar to protamine, which has a very high arginine content) (123,124).

The highly basic nature of L-arginine also appears to be responsible for its properties as a hormone secretagogue, which also has NO*-independent cardiovascular effects (65,66). L-Arginine stimulates insulin and glucagon release in a dose-dependent manner. Insulin and glucagon are each vasodilators, whereas insulin and glucagon have opposing effects on lipid and carbohydrate metabolism. The mechanism of insulin release appears to partly involve the generation of NO* and is partly the result of a direct depolarization of the islet cell plasma membrane by the positively charged amino acid (66). In this respect, L-arginine has the strongest insulinogenic effect of all the amino acids and its activity is equivalent to the infusion of all 10 dietary essential amino acids (125). The significance of the insulin-mediated effects of L-arginine on vascular function have been demonstrated by Giugliano and colleagues who found that if insulin and glucagon release are blocked by octreotide, the hemodynamic effects of high dose intravenous L-arginine are reduced (126).

By virtue of its ability to stimulate insulin and glucagon release, L-arginine, or perhaps more accurately the lysine/arginine ratio, has been shown by some investigators to have an effect on enzymes responsible for cholesterol synthesis and metabolism in healthy animals.

Work by Sanchez and Hubbard has demonstrated that altering the arginine/lysine ratio in the diet in favor of L-arginine increases the plasma insulin/glucagon ratio *(127)*. Insulin increases whereas glucagon decreases gene expression and activity of HMG-CoA reductase, the enzyme that regulates the rate-limiting step in cholesterol biosynthesis *(128)*. Indeed, HMG-CoA reductase activity is significantly greater in animals fed soy protein, which has a high arginine/lysine ratio, compared with those fed casein. The addition of L-arginine to a casein diet can increase HMG-CoA reductase activity by 67% *(129)*. Alternatively, supplementing a soy diet with L-lysine reduces activity of the enzyme by 16%. A high arginine/lysine ratio also stimulates the activities of cholesterol 7 alpha-hydroxylase, and cholesterol O-acyltransferase (ACATase) as well as hepatic apo B and apo E receptor activity resulting in higher fecal bile acid and steroid secretion *(130–132)*. These opposing effects of insulin and glucagon caused by an alteration in the arginine/lysine ratio translate into little or no observable effect on lipoprotein profile in clinical studies. Consequently, it is unlikely that the cardiovascular effects of L-arginine are attributable to an effect on lipid profile. Part of the effect on cholesterol metabolism may be the result of an NO•-dependent effect on apo B metabolism within lipoproteins *(133)*. In vitro studies on liver cell cultures demonstrate a dose-dependent reduction in apo B on the addition of NO• donors. As expected by this mechanism, addition of L-arginine to cell culture also reduced apo B levels. These effects on cholesterol metabolism are likely irrelevant to the antiatherogenic effects of L-arginine, as serum cholesterol levels are unchanged by L-arginine administration in most clinical studies.

In addition to stimulating insulin release, L-arginine has an effect on the peripheral sensitivity of tissues to insulin that is not known to be NO•-dependent *(134)*. This effect may have a particular impact in patients who are insensitive to insulin (non-insulin-dependent diabetics and obese patients) who demonstrate a loss of insulin-mediated vasodilation. L-Arginine (0.52 mg/kg/min) improves insulin sensitivity in both groups as well as in healthy controls with a concomitant improvement in insulin-mediated vasodilation in the two patient groups *(134)*.

Some investigators have proposed that L-arginine may have antioxidant properties. Wascher and colleagues have demonstrated that D- and L-arginine are equally effective at attenuating the reduction of electron acceptors by highly destructive superoxide anion in a cell-free environment *(64)*. Similarly, in isolated autooxidation systems, L-arginine (0.5–1 mmol) decreased the rate of superoxide formation by 17% *(135)*. It has been postulated that the guanidino group of L-arginine is capable of accepting the radical electron *(136)*. In contrast to the cell-free environment, incubation of endothelial cells with L-arginine, but not D-arginine, diminishes the amount of superoxide anion release and NO• degradation in a concentration-dependent manner *(64)*. This effect not only protects the longevity of NO• but also helps prevent copper-induced lipid peroxidation *(135,136)*. In rabbit thoracic aorta, lipid peroxidation can be inhibited by L-arginine (although this effect may be mediated by the conversion of L-arginine to NO•) *(137)*. By contrast, no antioxidant effect of L-arginine was observed in a cell-free system where superoxide anion was generated by xanthine oxidase *(83)*. Similarly, copper-mediated oxidation of LDL cholesterol was not inhibited by L-arginine in vitro. However, NO• is known to inhibit the generation of superoxide anion by NADPH oxygenase *(138)*. Inhibition of NOS removes the braking effect of NO• on oxidative enzymes, with a resulting increase in cellular generation of superoxide anion (*vide infra*). These actions of the L-arginine/NOS may explain the NO•-dependent modulation of oxidative stress in endothelial cells *(139,140)*.

OTHER NO•-INDEPENDENT ACTIONS ON THE CARDIOVASCULAR SYSTEM

Several other NO•-independent actions of L-arginine on the cardiovascular system have been recognized. Higashi et al. demonstrated the effect of L-arginine to reduce serum angiotensin converting enzyme activity thereby reducing angiotensin II levels by 35% *(141)*. These investigators concluded that this mechanism was partly responsible for the antihypertensive effect of L-arginine. Another NO•-independent mechanism by which L-arginine affects the cardiovascular system is by its participation as a precursor in a variety of metabolic pathways that may play an important role in cardiovascular homeostasis particularly in angiogenesis and following vascular injury. Animal studies reveal that L-arginine supplementation enhances collagen deposition and increases wound healing *(142–144)*. The mechanism of healing is likely multifactorial, involving enhanced vasodilation, allowing greater delivery of oxygen and nutrients as well as enhanced vascular permeability, enhanced immune function of *in situ* macrophages, increased secretion of growth hormone, and possibly the induced production of growth factors *(145)*. In addition, L-arginine is a precursor for both proline and hydroxyproline. Thus, increased L-arginine availability may enhance collagen synthesis *(68,146)*. L-Arginine is also a precursor to pyrimidines and polyamines *(67)*. Polyamines play an important role in promoting cellular proliferation, tissue growth, and differentiation *(69)*, whereas the tissue matrix proteins are central to the appropriate healing of injured tissue. Finally, by enhancing NO• synthesis, L-arginine may induce angiogenesis. All of these roles of L-arginine may contribute along with the beneficial effects of enhanced NO• production in tissue repair following balloon or other vascular injury.

APPLICATION IN CARDIOVASCULAR HEALTH AND DISEASE

Endothelial Vasodilator Dysfunction

Endothelial vasodilator dysfunction associated with a loss of EDNO activity occurs with all major risk factors for atherosclerosis as well as in association with certain drugs such as cyclosporin A. Exogenous L-arginine has been shown to reverse this dysfunction in humans and animal models in many of these settings. The ability to enhance vasodilator function has physiologic consequences. For instance, high-dose L-arginine has been shown to increase cerebral blood flow in humans. When measured by transcranial Doppler, mean cerebral blood flow velocity increases about 18% following L-arginine infusion *(147)*. L-Arginine (500 mg/kg iv) increased whole-brain blood flow by approx 10% as assessed by positron emission tomography (PET) scan. This increase in blood flow occurred selectively in the gray matter, and was not related to growth hormone or insulin release *(148)*. Other physiologic consequences of enhanced vasodilator function are discussed in sections on specific diseases.

We and others have shown that oral L-arginine improves or completely reverses endothelium-dependent vasodilator dysfunction in thoracic aorta, coronary, cerebral arteries, and hind-limb microvasculature of various animal models of hypercholesterolemia *(43,79,80,82, 149–156)*. These studies on the effects of L-arginine on endothelial vasodilator function have been extended to hypercholesterolemic humans. An intravenous infusion of L-arginine (30 g) acutely restores endothelium-dependent vasodilation in the forearm vasculature of hypercholesterolemic subjects *(2)*. Similarly, L-arginine infusion restores the responsiveness of the coronary microvasculature to ACh in individuals with coronary artery disease *(1)*. Clarkson and coworkers have shown that 21 g/d of oral L-arginine given to hypercholesterolemic young adults (ages 19–40 yr) for 4 wk doubled plasma arginine levels and significantly improved brachial artery flow-mediated vasodilation without affecting lipid levels *(3)*. Similar findings have been observed by other investigators *(157–159)* including a study demonstrating restoration of endothelial function in small peripheral arteries *(160)*. There is remarkable uniformity in the literature with respect to the beneficial effect of L-arginine in hypercholesterolemic humans, although there is one report each of no response of L-arginine *(161)*, a response only in men *(158)*, or a nonstereospecific response *(162)*. Preliminary evidence from our clinical laboratory reveals that administration of a food bar enriched with L-arginine (in combination with other substances that either enhance synthesis or prevent the destruction of EDNO) can reverse vasodilator dysfunction in hypercholesterolemic individuals *(163)*. This means of L-arginine delivery may prove to be a rational way to provide the amount of L-arginine required to produce a biologic effect.

Hypertension is associated with endothelial vasodilator dysfunction. In individuals with long-standing essential hypertension, it appears that the vasodilator dysfunction results from a defect in the NOS pathway, which precedes the onset of hypertension *(164)*. The ability of L-arginine to restore endothelial dysfunction in this setting is controversial. In various animal models of systemic hypertension, oral L-arginine in doses as low as 1 g/kg/d has been shown to restore endothelium-dependent vasodilator function *(165,166)*. By contrast, supplemental dietary L-arginine for 1–7 d in individuals with essential hypertension did not have any measurable effects on hemodynamics, nor did it to restore vasodilator dysfunction *(167)*. More recently, L-arginine has been shown to reverse the endothelial dysfunction associated with borderline hypertension *(168)*. In the setting of pulmonary hypertension there is also an endothelial vasodilator dysfunction that may contribute to the abnormal pulmonary vascular reactivity and structural changes *(169)*. In animal models of pulmonary hypertension, intravenous L-arginine restores pulmonary endothelial vasodilator function *(170,171)*. In advanced pulmonary hypertension, there appears to be reduced expression of eNOS, which would imply a defect that may not be responsive to L-arginine. The effects of L-arginine on endothelial function in these settings is likely responsible for antihypertensive effects of L-arginine discussed later.

In animal models of tobacco use, chronic nicotine administration enhances vasoconstriction to noradrenaline and reduces vasorelaxation to ACh. These effects are thought to be caused by an attenuation of EDNO production. Addition of L-arginine, but not D-arginine, to aortic strips ex vivo taken from animals exposed to nicotine reverses these effects of nicotine *(172)*. In animal studies investigating the effects of second-hand smoking, chronic exposure to tobacco smoke also produces an endothelial vasodilator dysfunction. The thoracic aorta from rabbits exposed for 10 wk to cigarette smoke demonstrated reduced vasorelaxation to ACh *(173)*. L-Arginine supplementation for the duration of tobacco smoke exposure prevented this dysfunction. In humans, long-term smoking is associated with impaired endothelial vasodilator function of epicardial conductance vessels regardless of the presence or absence of atherosclerotic lesions *(174)*. Similarly, smoking impairs endothelium-dependent vasodilation of the brachial artery, an effect which is partially reversed by administration of L-arginine *(174a)*.

Diabetic patients demonstrate both an endothelium-dependent and independent vasodilator impairment *(175)*. Indeed, diabetic patients often demonstrate a paradoxical vasoconstriction to ACh in the coronary circulation *(176)*. Because intravenous L-arginine modestly reduces blood pressure in insulin-dependent diabetics in association with an increase in plasma cyclic guanosine monophosphate (cGMP) *(7)*, an enhancement of EDNO production and restoration of endothelial function in this population would be anticipated. In one animal study, the administration of L-arginine to aortic rings taken from genetically diabetic rabbits restored endothelium-dependent vasodilation *(177)*. This effect was not observed, however, in the microcirculation of diabetic hamsters *(178)* suggesting that the effects may be localized to certain vascular beds. In one study, oral L-arginine improved systemic endothelium-dependent vasodilator dysfunction in streptozotocin-treated rats *(179,180)* but had no effect on cerebral vasodilator dysfunction *(181)*. Degradation of NO• by oxygen-derived free radicals undoubtedly plays a significant role in endothelial vasodilator dysfunction in diabetes as demonstrated by the work of Tesfamariam and colleagues. Rings of aorta from rabbits incubated in a solution of high glucose concentration demonstrate impairment of endothelium-dependent relaxation to ACh *(182)*. The impairment is preventable by coincubation with superoxide dismutase (SOD), catalase, deferoxamine, or allopurinol and does not occur in aortae from probucol-fed rabbits. Similarly, exposure of aortic segments to elevated glucose or to xanthine oxidase causes a significant increase in release of immunoreactive prostanoids. These data indicate that the endothelial cell dysfunction caused by elevated glucose is mediated by free radicals that are likely generated through the increased cyclooxygenase catalysis occurring in the endothelium. Treatment with antioxidants protects against impaired endothelium-dependent relaxations caused by elevated glucose.

The effects of L-arginine on vasodilator function in humans with diabetes parallel the animal studies. Nitenberg and colleagues have recently shown that intraarterial administration of L-arginine could not reverse the abnormal response to a cold pressor test or to increased blood flow in diabetes (183). These findings are consistent with those found in the forearm of insulin-dependent diabetic patients whereby the response to ACh was not enhanced by local infusions of L-arginine (10 g) (184). One potential reason for this lack of effect is that, in long-standing diabetes, altered neurotransmission is an important determinant of vascular reactivity (185). The long-term benefit of L-arginine on vascular function remains to be studied. Short-term therapy with L-arginine may play a role in restoring vascular function in gestational diabetes, however, where the dysfunction appears to be limited to the endothelium (186).

L-Arginine can reverse the adverse effects of acute hyperglycemia on vascular function. Acute hyperglycemia is known to increase vascular tone in normal humans and this is presumably through an oxygen free radical-mediated pathway (187). Infusion of NOS inhibitor mimics the effect of hyperglycemia suggesting that the observed effects are due to reduced NO$^\bullet$ activity. Giugliano and colleagues (187) induced acute hyperglycemia in 12 healthy subjects with the use of an artificial pancreas. After 30 min of hyperglycemia, blood pressure increased and leg blood flow was shown to be decreased. Infusion of L-arginine (30 g) but not D-arginine or L-lysine completely reverses these hemodynamic changes (187).

Just as acute hyperglycemia causes vasoconstriction, insulin mediates vasodilation in healthy subjects. Therefore, patients who are insensitive to insulin (non-insulin-dependent diabetics and obese patients) demonstrate a loss of insulin-mediated vasodilation. L-Arginine (0.52 mg/kg/min) improved insulin sensitivity in both groups as well as in healthy control subjects (134). This intervention resulted in an improvement in insulin-mediated vasodilation in the two patient groups. This finding is consistent with those of Paolisso and colleagues who described an increase in insulin-mediated glucose uptake following L-arginine (30 g iv) (188).

A selective endothelium dependent vasodilator dysfunction has been correlated to age independent of other risk factors for cardiovascular disease (10,189). With respect to the coronary circulation, Zeiher and colleagues observed that hypercholesterolemia and advanced age selectively impair endothelium-mediated relaxation of the coronary microvasculature in response to ACh, whereas endothelial dysfunction is restricted to epicardial arteries in age-matched normocholesterolemic patients with evidence of coronary atherosclerosis and/or hypertension (189). Zeiher found that n-acetylcysteine (an antioxidant), but not L-arginine, reversed this age-induced endothelial dysfunction. By contrast, Chauhan and colleagues found that L-arginine reversed age-induced endothelium-dependent vasodilator dysfunction of the coronary arteries (10).

Certain drugs decrease NO$^\bullet$ production and, as a consequence may cause an endothelial vasodilator dysfunction. It is interesting to note that many established anti-inflammatory drugs lower NO$^\bullet$ activity by inhibiting the expression of iNOS. Salicylates are scavengers of NO$^\bullet$ (190). Methotrexate blocks the synthesis of tetrahydrobiopterin (BH$_4$), one of the essential cofactors of NOS. Although methotrexate improves inflammatory disease symptoms, a relative deficiency of BH$_4$ has been speculated to contribute to vascular disease (121, 191,192). Endothelial dysfunction secondary to cyclosporin A appears to be specific to the bradykinin and substance P activation pathways of NOS as the ACh-activation pathway and the receptor-independent action of calcium ionophore is unaffected (193). It is thought that the lipophilic nature of cyclosporin A allows integration into cell membranes where signal transduction can be disrupted. Despite an alteration at this level, intravenous L-arginine given to dogs treated with cyclosporin A was able to restore pulmonary endothelial vasodilatory responses to substance P and bradykinin *(194)*. Likewise, oral and intraperitoneal doses of L-arginine reversed the effects of cyclosporin A on endothelium-dependent vasomotor dysfunction in rats *(195,196)*.

Chronic use of organic nitrates also leads to an endothelial vasodilator dysfunction, an effect that occurs concomitant with nitrate tolerance *(197)*. Current evidence indicates that the endothelial vasodilator dysfunction and the tolerance to exogenous NO• donors may be caused by excessive generation of superoxide anion *(197,198)*. In hypercholesterolemic rabbits treated with nitroglycerin patches, an endothelial vasodilator dysfunction and resistance to nitrates are observed after 3 d of treatment, as demonstrated by studies of isolated ring of thoracic aorta in vitro *(198)*. This abnormality appears to be due to excessive generation of superoxide anion by the endothelium as sensitivity to nitrates is restored by endothelial denudation. The endothelial alteration appears to be mediated by nitroglycerin-induced neurohumoral activation; coadministration of the angiotensin II receptor antagonist losartan attenuates nitroglycerin-induced endothelial dysfunction and "tolerance" *(198)*. In addition, it is possible that nitroglycerin may induce an alteration of L-arginine metabolism in the vessel wall *(199)*. Two case reports have documented a reversal of nitrate tolerance in humans with administration of L-arginine *(200)*.

Atherogenesis

Since 1992 when Cooke and colleagues first published evidence that chronic administration of supplemental dietary L-arginine reduces atherogenesis in fat-fed rabbits *(150)*, a number of studies have confirmed that administration of the NO• precursor inhibits atherogenesis in a variety of animal models *(41,42,201)*, whereas inhibition of NOS accelerates atherogenesis *(83,202)*. L-Arginine inhibits atherosclerotic lesion growth by virtue of its effects on multiple key processes in atherogenesis. Important among these are the ability of L-arginine to reduce superoxide activity, decrease the adhesiveness of monocytes for endothelial cells, decrease platelet reactivity, and participate in antithrombosis.

REDUCTION IN SUPEROXIDE FORMATION

Supplementation with L-arginine reduces the endothelial generation of superoxide anion by at least two mechanisms. By increasing the production of NO•, L-arginine inhibits oxidative enzyme activity. NO• is known to inhibit the production of superoxide anion by NADPH oxygenase as well as xanthine oxidase *(138,203)*. NO• might inhibit NADPH oxygenase by interacting with critical sulfhydryl groups or with the heme moiety of NADPH oxygenase. Furthermore, it is now known that NOS can generate superoxide anion *(204)*. In its monomer form, NOS cannot produce NO• *(205)*, but can still transfer electrons to molecular oxygen to generate superoxide anion. By stabilizing the dimer form of NOS, L-arginine reduces the elaboration of superoxide anion by NOS *(119,120)*. These mechanisms may underlie the observation that supplemental L-arginine reduces vascular generation of superoxide anion in the hypercholesterolemic rabbit thoracic aorta. The L-arginine-induced reduction in vascular generation of superoxide anion has important biological ramifications for monocyte adhesion as discussed shortly.

MONOCYTE ADHESION

The L-arginine/NOS pathway has a critical role with respect to monocyte adhesion. The effects of NO• on determinants of monocyte adherence may explain in part the beneficial function of L-arginine in the animal model of hypercholesterolemia. Thoracic aortae harvested from hypercholesterolemic rabbits demonstrated an enhanced adhesiveness for monocytes; this effect of hypercholesterolemia was abrogated by supplementation with L-arginine

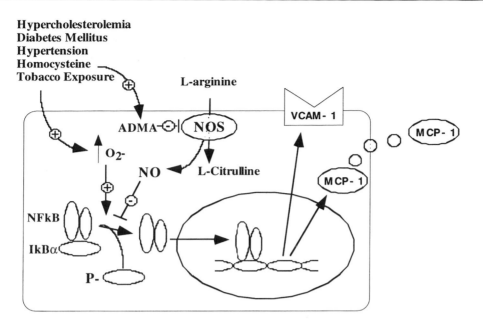

Fig. 2. Schematic of oxidant-sensitive gene expression regulated by NO•. A number of metabolic disorders (hypercholesterolemia, hypertension, hyperhomocysteinemia, and tobacco exposure) are known to induce endothelial elaboration of superoxide anion (O_2^-) and reduce synthesis and/or bioactivity of nitric oxide (NO•). This oxidative stress causes phosphorylation, ubiquination, and degradation of IκB$_\alpha$, permitting NFκB to translocate to the nucleus. There, NFκB activates a number of genes participating in atherogenesis, including vascular cell adhesion molecule (VCAM-1) and monocyte chemotactic peptide (MCP-1).

(81,83,206). In dogs, addition of L-arginine to coronary artery strips incubated with neutrophils reversed the degree of adhesion and the associated coronary vasodilatory dysfunction *(81).* This effect was not reproduced by D-arginine.

The effect of L-arginine appears to be through NO•-dependent inhibition in the expression of adhesion molecules and chemokines. When human umbilical vein cells grown in culture were incubated with L-arginine for 24 h, the expression of intercellular adhesion molecule-1 (ICAM-1) was reduced *(207).* Incubation of this monolayer with human monocytes resulted in a reduction in endothelial cell–monocyte adhesion. In addition to suppressing the expression of adhesion molecules and chemokines, NO• also appears to interfere acutely with adhesion signaling. Bath and colleagues have observed that NO• donors rapidly inhibit monocyte adhesion to endothelial cells, an effect that may be mediated by cGMP *(208).*

NO• inhibits the expression of adhesion molecules and chemokines by reducing vascular generation of superoxide anion. Reduced synthesis of NO• is associated with increased endothelial elaboration of superoxide anion, which triggers the expression of oxidant-sensitive genes (Fig. 2). The effect of oxidative stress is mediated by redox-responsive transcriptional proteins such as NFκB (nuclear factor κB) *(139,140,209).* Normally, NFκB circulates in the cytoplasm, bound to its inhibitor IκB$_\alpha$. Under conditions of oxidative stress, IκB$_\alpha$ becomes phosphorylated, ubiquinated, and degraded, leaving NFκB free to translocate to the nucleus. There, NFκB binds to *cis*-activating elements of the promoter region for genes encoding adhesion molecules (e.g., vascular cell adhesion molecule [VCAM]) and chemokines (e.g., monocyte chemoattractant peptide [MCP-1]) that participate in monocyte recruitment and infiltration. NO• blocks this redox-responsive transcription pathway by turning off the generation of superoxide anion. NO• also enhances the expression of IκB$_\alpha$ *(210).*

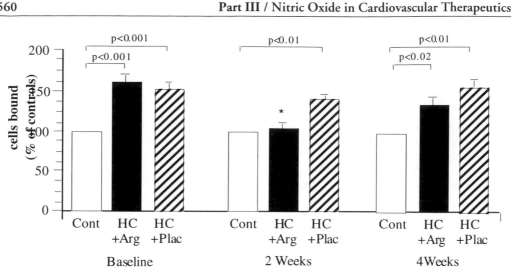

Fig. 3. Histogram demonstrating effects of oral L-arginine on mononuclear cell adhesiveness. Mononuclear cells isolated from hypercholesterolemic humans exhibit a greater adhesiveness for cultured endothelial cells at baseline. After 2 wk of L-arginine (8.4 g/d), monocyte adhesiveness was normalized (2-wk timepoint). After 2 wk of withdrawal from L-arginine, the adhesiveness of mononuclear cells from these hypercholesterolemic subjects is once again increased. Values represent mean ± SEM. *; $p < 0.05$ vs baseline value. From ref. *211*, used with permission.

Endothelial cells exposed to arginine-deficient medium for 24 h become more adhesive for human monocytes, an effect that is dose-dependently reversed by L-arginine *(208)*. The effect of L-arginine to reduce endothelial adhesiveness is blocked by antagonism of NOS.

In hypercholesterolemic patients, we found that dietary supplementation with 8.4 g/d of L-arginine over 2 wk normalized the adhesiveness of mononuclear cells (*[211]*, Fig. 3). More recently, we have observed by fluorescence-activated cell sorter (FACS) analysis that it is the adhesiveness of the monocytes and T-lymphocytes that is attenuated by L-arginine *(114)*. As with hypercholesterolemia, tobacco use is associated with an increase in the adhesiveness of monocytes for endothelium; supplemental L-arginine reverses this abnormality *(9)*.

ANTITHROMBOSIS

The administration of L-arginine also affects thrombosis. This is secondary to its ability to decrease platelet aggregation and inhibit the processes leading to fibrin formation. In hypercholesterolemic humans as well as in others with risk factors for atherosclerosis *(212,213)*, platelets are hyperaggregable. This may be because of an enhanced sensitivity of platelets to agonists in these individuals. In the rabbit model of hypercholesterolemia, supplemental L-arginine reduces platelet aggregation *(84)*. This finding has been extended into humans whereby hypercholesterolemic individuals given 8.4 g/d of dietary L-arginine for 2 wk demonstrated a reduction in platelet hyperaggregability in response to collagen stimulation *(214)*. Interestingly, this decrease in hyperaggregability persisted for 2 wk after discontinuing L-arginine therapy. L-Arginine inhibits platelet aggregation in healthy individuals as well *(215)*. The effect on ADP-stimulated platelet aggregation is related to plasma arginine level achieved (>300 μM). In three in vivo studies, an L-arginine infusion (30 g over 30 min) decreased adenosine-diphosphate (ADP)-stimulated platelet aggregation, to 32–50% of control value within 15 min *(126,216,217)*. There was no effect on collagen-stimulated platelet aggregation, which is consistent with the findings of Vallance and colleagues who showed no effect of EDNO on collagen-stimulated platelet aggregation in healthy humans ex vivo *(218)*.

The antiplatelet effect of L-arginine appears to be mediated by enhanced platelet cGMP production and inhibition of thromboxane B_2 formation *(219)*. Although the endothelial isoform of NOS is present in platelets in small amounts, it is probably not completely responsible for the L-arginine-induced increase in platelet cGMP *(220)*. Endothelium-derived NO• in the microvasculature may play a greater role in modulating platelet cGMP and reducing platelet reactivity. Platelets passing through the coronary microvasculature of the isolated perfused heart manifest an increase in intraplatelet cGMP. This effect is markedly enhanced by coadministration of ACh, which stimulates endothelial (but not platelet) NOS activity *(221)*. These effects are abrogated by NOS inhibitors. In vitro administration of supraphysiologic concentrations of L-arginine to platelet-rich plasma enhances platelet cGMP levels and causes a reduction in platelet thromboxane formation. The effect on platelet aggregation in one clinical study cited earlier was associated with a 43% increase in platelet cGMP *(216)*. The effect on cGMP levels is reversed by preincubation with NOS inhibitors demonstrating NO• dependency. It is interesting to note that polyamine metabolic products of L-arginine (putrescine, spermidine, and spermine) also have antiplatelet effects similar to L-arginine in normal and diabetic rats *(222)*. These findings suggest that there may also be an NO•-independent antiplatelet effect of L-arginine in antithrombosis.

L-Arginine has also been shown to inhibit the processes leading to fibrin formation and platelet-fibrin interaction and accelerate fibrin degradation in humans *(223)*. Recently, L-arginine has been shown in vitro to accelerate tPA-induced plasmin generation and thus augment fibrinogenolysis *(224)*. L-Arginine binds to plasminogen (probably at kringle 5) stimulating its conversion to plasmin with subsequent enhancement of fibrinogenolysis. This effect resulted in an acceleration of the early stages of clot lysis, although eventually clot lysis was equal in control groups as well. This finding is consistent with the findings in vivo in patients with peripheral arterial disease discussed shortly *(225)*. Additionally, when L-arginine is given in high doses (30 g iv), it lowers blood viscosity *(126)*. This effect is likely mediated by insulin because simultaneous administration of octreotide to inhibit endogenous insulin release prevents this effect. Furthermore, in diabetic patients, L-arginine infusion lowered blood viscosity and this effect was significantly amplified after an 8-wk treatment with metformin, which increases the peripheral sensitivity to insulin *(226)*. These studies indicate L-arginine may also act as an antithrombotic agent beyond its antiplatelet effects.

PLAQUE FORMATION AND REGRESSION

By virtue of its ability to reduce superoxide activity, inhibit monocyte adhesion and reduce thrombosis, chronic supplementation of L-arginine inhibits the progression of aortic and coronary artery atherosclerotic plaque formation (*[41,43,82,150–152,206,227,228]*, Fig. 4). In one particular study, the effects of L-arginine were compared to those of lovastatin *(42)*. In that study, L-arginine restored EDNO activity, prevented an increase in superoxide free radical production and slowed the progression of intimal lesion formation. In contrast, the cholesterol-lowering therapy lovastatin also reduced intimal proliferation but not to the extent of L-arginine. Furthermore, lovastatin failed to increase EDNO activity, enhanced the activity of superoxide radical production, and failed to restore endothelium-dependent vasodilator dysfunction.

In one study, this beneficial effect of dietary L-arginine was observed in male, but not female, hypercholesterolemic rabbits *(152)*. However, this gender difference was not found in a murine model of hypercholesterolemia in which the LDL receptor was disrupted by homologous recombination. Regardless of gender, dietary L-arginine prevented intimal lesions and xanthoma formation that otherwise occurs when these mice are fed a high-fat diet *(41)*. The reduction in atherosclerotic burden appears to be due to a reduction in both monocyte accumulation and in myointimal cell proliferation *(201)*. Immunohistochemical detection of 5-bromo-2'deoxyuridine (BrdU) incorporation demonstrated a 33% reduction in the proliferation rate of myointimal cells, whereas antibody staining demonstrated a 85% reduction in monocyte accumulation in L-arginine-treated animals. In this study, intimal/medial ratio of the L-arginine group was reduced about 63%.

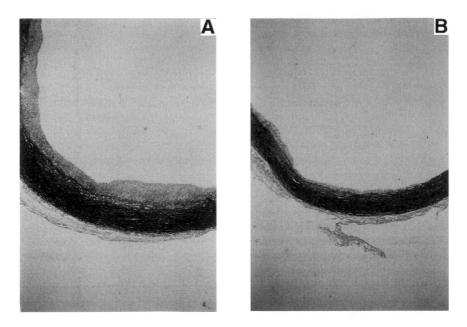

Fig. 4. Microphotograph of thoracic aortae from hypercholesterolemic rabbits. New Zealand White rabbits were fed a 1.0% cholesterol diet for 10 wk. Half of the animals also received oral supplementation of L-arginine. After 10 wk the aortae were harvested for histomorphometry. Those animals receiving vehicle (left) demonstrated impaired endothelium-dependent vasodilation and lesions that involved 75% of the surface area of the thoracic aorta. By contrast (right), hypercholesterolemic rabbits receiving L-arginine supplementation exhibited normalized endothelium-dependent vasodilation, and reduced lesion surface area (about 25%).

L-Arginine may have a beneficial effect on pre-existing lesions as well. New Zealand White rabbits fed a high-cholesterol diet for 10 wk develop atherosclerotic lesions that cover about 30% of the surface area of their aorta. If they continue on this diet for an additional 13 wk, the lesions progress to involve 57% of the surface area. By contrast, progression of the lesions is halted in rabbits fed a high-cholesterol diet that is supplemented with dietary L-arginine. Indeed, in a subset of these animals in which L-arginine persistently improved endothelial vasodilator dysfunction, an impressive regression of lesions was observed, with a final lesion surface area of only 5% *(43)*.

RESTENOSIS

Because NO$^{•}$ inhibits vascular smooth muscle proliferation and monocyte recruitment, enhancement of vascular NO$^{•}$ activity may be beneficial in the prevention of restenosis following balloon angioplasty. Intravenous L-arginine (0.5 g/kg/d) initiated 2 d prior to and continued 2 wk following balloon injury to the thoracic aorta of normocholesterolemic rabbits reduced intimal proliferation by 39% *(46)*. In a similar model, 4 wk of oral L-arginine therapy (2.25% in the drinking water) improved endothelium-dependent vasodilation to ACh and reduced intimal lesion area from 0.43 ± 0.08 to 0.24 ± 0.02 mm^2 *(229)*. In the hypercholesterolemic rabbit model of balloon injury, oral L-arginine improved endothelium-dependent vasodilation and reduced neointimal lesion area from 0.69–0.34 mm^2) *(230)*. This was associated with a significant reduction in monocyte recruitment to the area of balloon injury. In a recent study in heritable hyperlipidemic rabbits, L-arginine significantly reduced the extent of neointimal lesion formation following balloon injury, however, L-arginine reduced the endothelium-dependent inhibition of platelet aggregation and attenuated the vasodilator function of the injured vessel *(45)*. The authors of this study suggest that the detrimental effect on endothelial vasodilator function may be related to the ongoing hyperlipidemia and the presence of lipids in the vascular wall in their model. This effect may also be caused by an effect of oxidized LDL to inhibit L-arginine uptake and NOS expression in platelets *(110)*. More recently, Schwarzacher and colleagues have found that local delivery of L-arginine to the vessel wall could similarly reduce restenosis *(44)*. Using a drug-delivery balloon, local administration of L-arginine was observed to increase NO• production in the rabbit iliac artery for up to 1 wk following the injury, and reduced intimal thickening at 4 wk following balloon angioplasty *(44)*. This study suggests that a single intramural delivery of L-arginine is sufficient to enhance EDNO production for a sufficient amount of time to inhibit restenosis.

Arginine supplementation has also been shown to inhibit intimal proliferation in vein grafts. Intimal proliferation is responsible for early stenoses in more than 30% of peripheral vein grafts within a year of placement. In the experimental model, L-arginine inhibits intimal thickness by 47% in vein grafts implanted in the position of the carotid artery *(231)*. This effect of L-arginine was somewhat reduced if the rabbits were made hypercholesterolemic (24% reduction in intimal thickness) *(151)*. BrdU incorporation experiments demonstrated less SMC proliferation in the L-arginine treated animals *(232)*. Likewise, the vasorelaxation of venous rings to ACh remained intact in the supplemented animals. The mechanism by which L-arginine reduces intimal hyperplasia may be by inhibiting the expression of hyaluronan synthase-1 *(233)*. Normally, within 7 d of implantation there is about a 20-fold rise in the expression of this enzyme, which is responsible for making hyaluronan, a key component of the extracellular matrix. L-Arginine supplementation reduces the expression to less than a fivefold increase.

To date, there have been no studies demonstrating an inhibition or regression of plaque formation, an effect on venous engraftments, nor on the extent of restenosis following angioplasty in humans using supplemental L-arginine. However, investigators have demonstrated an effect on the key processes of human atherosclerosis as discussed previously.

ANGIOGENESIS

There is a significant heterogeneity between patients in their angiogenic response to obstructive vascular disease. Some individuals develop an exuberant network of collateral vessels, proving them with a "biologic bypass" that reduces symptomatology. Other individuals are less fortunate. Recent insights into the regulation of angiogenesis have permitted pioneering efforts to induce therapeutic angiogenesis in patients with peripheral arterial disease (PAD) or coronary artery disease (CAD). Preliminary studies indicate that administration of angiogenic factors (e.g. vascular endothelial growth factor [VEGF] or basic fibroblast growth factor [FGF]) may improve collateral circulation in atherosclerotic obstructive disease. NO• may play an important role in this process *(234)*. In endothelial cell culture, FGF upregulates the expression of eNOS and increases the elaboration of NO• while concurrently inducing tubule formation. FGF-induced tubule formation is mimicked by NO• donors and blocked by NOS antagonists *(235)*. In other studies, Substance P, transforming growth factor β_1 and VEGF all have been shown to increase the expression of eNOS and NO• elaboration, as well as to induce tubule formation (in vitro) or angiogenesis (in vivo) *(236)*. The angiogenic effects of these factors are antagonized or abolished by NOS antagonists. Indices of capillary formation and blood flow are enhanced by L-arginine in animal models of hind-limb ischemia, whereas the angiogenic response to ischemia is markedly inhibited in the eNOS knockout mouse *(237)*.

Coronary Artery Disease

By virtue of its ability to restore vasodilation and slow the progression of atherosclerosis, L-arginine may be of particular therapeutic value in patients with CAD. These patients often have a paradoxical vasoconstrictor response to ACh *(238)*. Systemic infusion of L-arginine reverses this vasoconstrictor response *(239,240)*. Furthermore, Drexler and colleagues have shown that in patients with angiographically demonstrated coronary artery disease undergoing coronary artery catheterization, a single intravenous infusion of L-arginine (30 g) normalizes coronary blood flow response to the endothelium-dependent vasodilator, ACh *(1)*. In patients with angina and normal coronary arteriograms (syndrome X), there is an endothelial vasodilator dysfunction of the microvasculature *(241)*, as evidenced by reduced coronary blood flow response to ACh *(242)*. This abnormality is reversed by intravenous infusion of L-arginine. However, when CAD is associated with hypertension, the endothelial vasodilator dysfunction does not appear to be reversible with L-arginine *(239)* consistent with other studies in hypertensive patients. In young men with documented CAD, an endothelial vasodilator dysfunction of the brachial artery also exists. L-Arginine improves brachial artery flow-mediated vasodilation and, in addition, inhibits monocyte adhesion to endothelial cells in this population *(20)*.

These beneficial effects of L-arginine on coronary vasculature have functional consequences. Concomitant with the reversal of endothelial vasodilator dysfunction in patients with coronary artery disease, L-arginine (30 g) modestly lowers mean arterial pressure (approx 5 mmHg), reduces total peripheral resistance (by approx 16%), increases cardiac output (by 11%) and plasma cGMP (by 12%) *(4)*. Recently, Lerman and colleagues demonstrated an impressive effect of dietary L-arginine on coronary vasomotor function in patients with significant CAD *(243)*. Oral L-arginine (9 g/d for 6 mo) improved coronary blood flow response to intracoronary ACh by 150%. This was associated with a decrease in plasma endothelin levels and an improvement in patient's symptoms scores.

Ceremuzynski and colleagues have recently demonstrated an increase in exercise capacity following oral L-arginine in patients with stable angina pectoris *(244,245)*. Patients included in this study all had documented CAD and a history of transmural myocardial infarction. Following 3 d of oral L-arginine (2 g t.i.d.), exercise time during a standardized treadmill protocol (Modified Bruce) was significantly increased (531 ± 195 to 700 ± 173 s, $p < 0.0002$). Along with the increased walking time was an increase in maximum work load (6.4 ± 2 to 7.4 ± 3 metabolic equivalents [METS], $p < 0.006$). Furthermore, the degree of maximum ST segment depression (summed for all leads) was less than before treatment. This study demonstrated that even moderate supplementation with oral L-arginine can reduce myocardial ischemia and improve cardiovascular activity in patients with stable angina.

Peripheral Arterial Disease

L-Arginine may have therapeutic utility in peripheral arterial disease (PAD) as well. In patients with severe PAD, intravenous L-arginine has been shown to improve limb blood flow *(23)*. A single intravenous dose of L-arginine (30 g over 60 min) enhanced femoral artery blood flow (42% increase). The increase in limb blood flow was associated with an elevation of urinary cGMP and nitrate excretion rate consistent with an L-arginine-induced enhancement of EDNO synthesis. The effect of L-arginine infusion on limb blood flow was equal to that of intravenous prostaglandin E_1 (29% increase, $p < 0.05$) in the same study. Furthermore, studies from the same group of investigators in Hannover, Germany, indicate that daily intravenous administration of arginine for two weeks enhances walking distance in patients with intermittent claudication *(246)*.

L-Arginine has also been shown to improve symptoms in patients with less severe PAD. Daily infusions of L-arginine (12.6 g) for 7 d increased calf blood flow and transcutaneous oxygen saturation, improved walking distance, shortened the time period to recovery from pain, and reduced platelet aggregation and clot lysis time *(225,246)*. The enhancement in blood flow has been extended to the microvascular circulation as well. Thirty grams of intravenous L-arginine was able to enhance calf muscle blood flow from 1.7 ± 0.1 to 2.2 ± 0.2 mL/min/100 g at 80 min following infusion *(22)*. There was no effect from 8 g of iv L-arginine in this time period, however. Preliminary evidence from our clinical laboratory suggests that administration of an L-arginine-enriched food bar can increase walking distance and quality of life in these patients (Cooke and colleagues, unpublished observations).

Patients with PAD have hyperaggregable platelets *(212,213)*. Consistent with observations in other patient populations, daily infusions of L-arginine (60 mmol) reduced ADP-induced platelet aggregation and shortened euglobin clot lysis time in subjects with PAD *(225)*. These antithrombotic effects of L-arginine may add to its vasodilatory effect to enhance overall walking ability and quality of life in this population.

Systemic Hypertension

By virtue of its ability to enhance vasodilation, L-arginine can lower blood pressure. The major mechanism is likely via the enhancement of EDNO *(247–249)*. In addition, L-arginine reduces serum angiotensin-converting enzyme activity and serum angiotensin II without affecting plasma renin activity, and these effects may contribute to the hypotensive effect of L-arginine *(141)*. In normotensive individuals, intravenous L-arginine causes modest effects on blood pressure. Giugliano and colleagues conducted a dose response study and found that blood pressure changes were linearly correlated with dose of L-arginine up to 3 g *(250)*. Multiple studies have shown that high doses (approx 30 g) of intravenous L-arginine cause a similar decrease in blood pressure to that of 3 g (approx 5–10 mmHg) *(126,215,247,249,251–257)*.

Because it has a modest effect on blood pressure, L-arginine may be adjunctive therapy in certain types of hypertensive disorders. In various animal models of systemic hypertension, oral L-arginine reduced or normalized blood pressure *(258–261)*. Specifically, oral L-arginine prevented salt-sensitive *(258,259)* and mineralocorticoid–salt (DOCA) hypertension *(261)* in rats. In several studies in spontaneously hypertensive rats however, oral L-arginine failed to lower blood pressure *(165,259,262)*, although it did prevent hypertension-induced cardiac hypertrophy in these animals *(262)*. In contrast, in animals with salt-sensitive hypertension, chronic oral supplementation with L-arginine prevented the salt-induced increase in blood pressure and drop in renal blood flow *(263)*. Oral L-arginine also prevented adrenocorticotropic hormone (ACTH)-induced hypertension and did so partly by lowering serum cortisone levels *(260)*. In contrast, dexamethasone-induced hypertension was not altered with L-arginine treatment *(264)*, suggesting that ACTH-induced hypertension is not simply a glucocorticoid-mediated process. Intravenous L-arginine lowered blood pressure in the rat model of pre-eclampsia *(265)* and surgical coarctation *(266)*. In another model of hypertension induced by lead, EDNO activity has been shown to be reduced and free radical activity increased *(267)*. Infusion of L-arginine causes a rise in urinary NO_x levels and a fall in blood pressure to normal. Interestingly, there is some evidence that part of the blood pressure effects of L-arginine are mediated by NO•-modulation of the baroreceptor reflex *(268)*. Cervical and aortic sympathetic nerve activity decreased along with mean arterial pressure following L-arginine infusion in anesthetized rabbits. This effect was not seen with D-arginine.

Similar to the animal models, in the clinical setting, L-arginine reduces blood pressure in only some forms of hypertension. Dietary L-arginine for 1–7 d in individuals with long-standing essential hypertension did not have any measured effects on hemodynamics *(167)*. However, oral L-arginine (2 g t.i.d.) was able to lower blood pressure in newly diagnosed borderline hypertensive individuals within 1 wk of therapy *(168)*. In responsive individuals, intravenous L-arginine (20–30 g infused over 30 min), causes a slight reduction in arterial pressure (5–10 mmHg), and reduces renovascular resistance *(269)*, although this is diminished in salt-sensitive hypertension after salt loading *(11)*. These findings were corroborated in a recent study on hypertensive African-Americans *(13)*. L-Arginine infusion (500 mg/kg) caused a 12-mmHg drop in mean arterial pressure in salt-sensitive individuals but only a 4 mmHg drop in insensitive individuals. However, the increase in effective renal plasma flow observed in normotensive controls was blunted in salt-resistant individuals and even more so in salt-sensitive individuals. Part of the reason for the diminished effect may be due to an increased production of ADMA following salt loading *(270)*. Concomitant with the reduction in hypertension is an improvement in ventricular ejection fraction *(271)* and increased cardiac output, urine output, and natriuresis *(249,272)*. The effect of intravenous L-arginine on blood pressure has led to its study during repair of coarctation *(257)*. Three adults undergoing coarctation repair received 10–20 g L-arginine during surgery, which resulted in desired reductions in mean arterial pressure of 5–20 mmHg during and immediately following surgery.

PULMONARY HYPERTENSION

Just as in systemic hypertension, patients with pulmonary hypertension manifest an endothelial vasodilator dysfunction that may contribute to the abnormal pulmonary vascular reactivity and structural changes *(169)*. In animal models of pulmonary hypertension, intravenous L-arginine reduces pulmonary pressure and reduced mortality *(170,173,273)*. Specifically, in a rat model of pulmonary hypertension induced by chronic hypoxia or by injection of monocrotaline, concomitant daily injections of L-arginine nearly abolished the development of pulmonary hypertension and the associated structural changes of the pulmonary arteries and right ventricle *(274)*.

Just as in systemic hypertension, the clinical setting of the pulmonary hypertension and the mechanism of the defect in the vasodilation are a major factors determining the effectiveness of L-arginine as a therapy. Adults with primary pulmonary hypertension or pulmonary hypertension secondary to myocardial disease demonstrate a reduced expression of NOS *(275)* as opposed to newborns with persistent pulmonary hypertension, which demonstrates a relative arginine deficiency *(276,277)*. Acute administration of intravenous L-arginine to adults with primary or secondary pulmonary hypertension reduces pulmonary pressure *(15)*. However, only patients with certain forms of secondary pulmonary hypertension exhibit substantial pulmonary vasodilation in response to intravenous L-arginine that is comparable to the response observed with the therapeutic use of prostacyclin *(278)*. In patients with primary pulmonary hypertension or pulmonary hypertension secondary to systemic sclerosis, intravenous L-arginine reduces systemic vascular resistance but, at best, transiently and minimally reduces pulmonary vascular resistance *(4,16,278,279)*. L-Arginine may have greater therapeutic effects in these settings if started before pulmonary hypertension progresses to significant pulmonary vascular disease. L-Arginine has been used to treat persistent pulmonary hypertension of the newborn. McCaffrey and colleagues treated five newborns with 500 mg/kg *(14)*. Ninety minutes after infusion there was a rise in P_aO_2 from 37–84 mmHg. There was a reduction in the oxygenation index in four of five of the newborns that persisted over 5 h and there were no adverse effects of therapy. Whereas short-term studies in humans with pulmonary hypertension have had disappointing results, these findings may have profound implications for the long-term use of L-arginine to prevent structural changes in such conditions as primary pulmonary hypertension and congenital heart disease.

TRANSPLANT VASCULOPATHY

In heart transplant patients, there is an endothelial vasodilator dysfunction in allograft coronary arteries *(29)*. These individuals have a coronary blood flow response to ACh that is about 50% of normal. The cause is probably multifactorial and includes hyperlipidemia, immune mediators, reperfusion injury, infection, and even cyclosporin A. An intravenous infusion of L-arginine (30 g) normalizes endothelium-dependent vasodilation in these patients *(29)*. When intracoronary L-arginine is given in combination with the endothelial agonist, substance P, there is an associated increase in left ventricular contractile performance *(30)*. These investigators were also interested in the physiologic significance of elevated iNOS content within the myocardium. Despite increased iNOS found on biopsy, there was no effect of direct L-arginine infusion on contractile performance in the absence of agonist. Furthermore, dietary L-arginine has been shown to reduce myointimal hyperplasia without affecting T-lymphocyte and macrophage infiltration in allograft coronary arteries in a rabbit cardiac transplant model *(227)*. Dietary L-arginine has also been shown to reverse coronary and pulmonary endothelial dysfunction caused by cyclosporin A as described previously *(194,196)*.

HEART FAILURE

In patients with congestive heart failure (CHF), there appears to be a generalized reduction in endothelium-dependent vasodilation and these patients have reduced peripheral blood flow at rest and during exercise *(280–282)*. Intravenous administration of L-arginine improves endothelial vasodilator function in this setting as evidenced by an increase in forearm blood flow response to ACh and reactive hyperemia *(23–26,281)*. Intravenous L-arginine also decreased systemic vascular resistance and mean arterial pressure while concomitantly increasing ventricular stroke volume and cardiac output in patients with heart failure secondary to CAD *(283)*. However, in one study in this population, oral administration of L-arginine (20 g/d for 28 d) did not improve vasodilator function *(28)*. Despite this report, another study in patients with heart failure showed that oral L-arginine (5.6–12.6 g/d) taken for 6 wk increased forearm blood flow in response to exercise *(27)*. In addition, these patients demonstrated an improved functional status with an increased walking distance and improved scores on the Living With Heart Failure questionnaire. There are no data presented on the difference in response of these two doses. Oral L-arginine also improved arterial compliance and reduced circulating endothelin levels. Interestingly, in patients progressing to cor pulmonale secondary to chronic obstructive pulmonary disease with renal vasoconstriction, L-arginine (20 g iv) had no effect at increasing intrarenal blood flow, suggesting a disturbance in the NOS pathway that is different from those seen in other forms of heart failure *(284)*.

ISCHEMIA/REPERFUSION

There is growing evidence that L-arginine may play a therapeutic role in tissue preservation during reperfusion following a period of hypoxia. Animal studies of cerebral, myocardial, hepatic, and other tissue ischemia/reperfusion generally show a benefit from administration of L-arginine (either iv or po) but not D-arginine. With respect to cerebral ischemia/reperfusion, L-arginine increased regional blood flow and reduced infarct size in areas of cerebral artery ligation in the rat model of focal cerebral ischemia *(285)*. If ischemia persisted to 20 min, L-arginine had no effect unless the animals were pretreated with N^G-nitro-L-arginine (L-NNA) *(51)*. This finding suggests that NO• may play a cytotoxic role in the ischemic or early reperfusion phase of ischemia/reperfusion. A similar finding occurred in hypertensive rats made globally ischemic *(286)*. In the rat model of traumatic brain injury, cerebral blood flow is significantly reduced within moments of injury. Administration of L-arginine (100 mg/kg) alone or in combination with SOD 5 minutes after injury, however, prevented a reduction in cerebral blood flow *(287)*. In a rat model of thrombotic occlusion, however, L-arginine failed to improve regional blood flow *(288)*. Similarly, in the cat model of global ischemia (temporary ligation of subclavian and brachiocephalic arteries with hemorrhagic hypotension), L-arginine failed to reduce neurological deficit scores and injury area *(289)*. Finally, in the gerbil model of cerebral ischemia, L-arginine (at doses of 1, 10, and 100 mg/kg before and after occlusion) failed to lessen hippocampal neuronal cell death and, in fact, L-NNA prevented cell death, suggesting an adverse role of NO• in hippocampal ischemia *(290)*. Nevertheless, the eNOS-deficient mouse manifests greater ischemic brain injury than normal animals, indicating that eNOS plays a protective role in ischemic brain injury *(291,292)*.

With respect to cardiac ischemia/reperfusion, such as that occurring with coronary occlusion, there is a ventricular dysfunction with an associated endothelial vasodilator dysfunction.

In this setting, intravenous L-arginine increases NOS activity *(50,293,294)* and reduces levels of soluble adhesion molecules, lipid peroxidation, and neutrophil accumulation *(48, 295)*. Increased NO• production during reperfusion appears to inhibit endothelin-1 (ET-1) release *(296)*. ET-1 release caused cell necrosis and a 25-fold extracellular release of L-arginine. These combined actions of supplemental L-arginine are likely responsible for the observed reduction in infarct size *(55,297,298)* and improved recovery of cardiac function *(50,295)*. One study in the isolated rabbit heart, however, showed a negative effect of exogenously applied L-arginine *(299)*. In dogs with acute coronary occlusion, intrapericardial administration of L-arginine was able to reduce the severity of ventricular arrhythmias *(300)*. Because of its ability to reduce the effective refractory period of the cardiac cell, the effect of L-arginine on cardiac rhythm appears to be via NO• modulation of sympathetic input.

Skeletal muscle may also benefit from L-arginine during periods of ischemia. L-Arginine infusion (4 mg/kg/min) during and after 6 min of hind-limb ischemia prevented a decline in EDNO levels to undetectable levels and attenuated a rise in superoxide release following reperfusion *(120)*. Consistent with the hypothesis that NOS loses its affinity for L-arginine under unfavorable conditions, the increase in superoxide in untreated animals appeared to be secondary to calcium-dependent eNOS activity.

L-Arginine has been studied in liver ischemia/reperfusion as well *(52,301,302)*. L-Arginine (540 mg/kg iv) given 1 h before and again during and after clamping of the hepatic hilum attenuated the rise in malondialdehyde content, aspartate transaminase and lactate dehydrogenase levels *(303,304)*. In addition, hepatic cellular integrity, glycogen content, and the rate of apoptosis was significantly better in the treated animals. Finally, overall survival was better at 7 d following ischemia.

These beneficial effects of L-arginine on ischemia/reperfusion have important implications in cardioplegic arrest, organ transplantation, and other surgeries involving periods of ischemia. Just as in cardiac ischemia/reperfusion secondary to coronary occlusion, cardio-pulmonary bypass is associated with a ventricular dysfunction and endothelial vasodilator dysfunction despite the use of cardioplegia and hypothermia *(305,306)*. In the isolated working rat heart model of cardioplegic arrest, exogenously applied L-arginine considerably improved the recovery of cardiac mechanical function and coronary flow rate when given in the reperfusate after hypothermic ischemia *(54,307)*. Hiramatsu and colleagues investigated the effect of L-arginine added to cardioplegic solution in neonatal lambs *(308,309)*. In these experiments, they examined the role of EDNO by adding either 10 mmol/L of D-arginine or 10 mmol/L of L-arginine to cardioplegia in isolated, blood-perfused neonatal lamb hearts having 2 h of cold cardioplegic ischemia. At 30 min of reperfusion, the L-arginine group showed a significantly improved recovery in left ventricular systolic function, diastolic function, coronary blood flow, endothelial function, and myocardial oxygen consumption compared with the control groups as those groups with D-arginine added to cardioplegia solution.

This protective effect extends to the rat model of transplantation *(310)*. L-Arginine given during reperfusion improves coronary endothelium-dependent vasodilation with recovery of systolic and diastolic function during early reperfusion. Similarly, in the rabbit model of lung transplantation, the addition of L-arginine or pentoxyfylline during reperfusion prevented pulmonary endothelial dysfunction *(311)*. These studies have also been extended to the setting of liver transplantation *(53)*. In the same way, L-arginine may beneficially impact skin flap survival as well. Exogenous administration of L-arginine to experimental tissue flaps increased the blood flow to the periphery of the flap *(312)*. Despite demonstrating evidence of oxidative tissue damage, the L-arginine-treated flaps had a greater length of survival. In a similar study, L-arginine administration decreased neutrophil infiltration and flap necrosis *(313)*. L-Arginine in combination with iloprost also reduced distal necrosis following reperfusion *(314)*. Other combinations that demonstrated increased survival are L-arginine with TGF-β and L-arginine with growth hormone *(315)*.

ERECTILE DYSFUNCTION

With the emerging body of evidence indicating the involvement of the NO• pathway in multiple aspects of the penile erectile response, the use of L-arginine supplementation is a promising therapy in erectile dysfunction. In animals and humans it appears that erectile function is dependent on intact systems of NO• generation within the cavernosum endothelium, the nonadrenergic, noncholinergic (NANC) nerves terminating within the penis, and centrally within the paraventricular nucleus (PVN) of the hypothalamus, which may be a center of arousal *(316)*. This concept is supported by the finding that the NOS inhibitor, L-nitroarginine methyl ester (L-NAME), ablates erectile response *(317)*. In addition, several risk factors for erectile dysfunction, including age *(317)*, smoking *(318)*, diabetes *(319)*, hypertension, atherosclerosis, and hypogonadism are associated with reduced EDNO production, further supporting its important role in erectile dysfunction. In particular, age has been shown in the rat to be associated with inhibition of penile NOS activity and a reduction in the content of penile NOS isoforms *(317)*.

To examine the role of EDNO in the normal penile erection, Kim and colleagues isolated corpus cavernosus strips and mounted these in an organ bath *(320)*. After precontraction with norepinephrine, electrical field stimulation (EFS) was performed. In the presence of L-nitroarginine, relaxation to EFS was attenuated. L-Arginine was capable of reversing the attenuated response to EFS unless the strips were deendothelialized. These results support the involvement of the EDNO in corpus cavernosus relaxation.

Local neuronal NO• also plays an important role. Several risk factors for erectile dysfunction have been shown to decrease nitrergic nerve activity. nNOS enzyme content (measured by Western blot) is reduced to 35% of controls in the rat penis following castration/adrenalectomy *(321)*. Along with the fall in nNOS level is a 55% reduction in NOS activity and a significant loss of erectile function following EFS. Similar to the studies in rats, human penile erectile function is mediated by NO• generated in response to NANC neurotransmission *(322)*. Strips of human corpus cavernosus mounted in an organ bath relaxed to EFS. This effect was blocked by NOS inhibitors and methylene blue, an inhibitor of guanylate cyclase. The relaxation was not influenced by atropine, however, suggesting that the source of NO• was not endothelial. Although this study demonstrated the presence of NANC innervation of the human penis, there is no data demonstrating the relative involvement of NANC-derived NO• vs. EDNO in erectile function nor the level at which dysfunction occurs in functional abnormalities in humans. Simonsen et al. found that NANC innervation of small penile arteries (200–700 µm diameter) within the cavernosa is responsible for vasorelaxation *(323)*. These nerve terminals contain NO• as well as another factor, the production of which is resistant to NOS inhibition.

Central NO• activity is also important for control of penile erection. Injections of dopamine receptor agonists, oxytocin, and other substances into the lateral ventricles or the PVN caused both erections and yawning *(316)*. These substances all increase NO• production within the PVN. Furthermore, these behaviors were abolished by injections of NOS inhibitors into the lateral ventricles, whereas NO• donors reproduced the behavior. The central role of NO• is cGMP-independent, as it could not be prevented by inhibitors of guanylate cyclase. Interestingly, NOS mRNA expression within the PVN of impotent rats is about half that of sexually potent rats *(324)*.

Therapy to restore NOS activity and erectile function in the animal model has involved L-arginine supplementation as well as gene therapy. Oral administration of L-arginine (2.25% in drinking water) for 8 wk to aged rats resulted in an increase in penile tissue levels of L-arginine, an increase in NOS activity and a complete reversal of erectile dysfunction *(37)*. In one small clinical study of 20 impotent men involving a placebo controlled, crossover design, L-arginine in small doses (2.8 g/d for 2 wk) subjectively restored erectile function as well as vaginal penetration ability in 6 of 15 patients completing the study *(36)*. This effect was not reported during the placebo phase.

RENAL INSUFFICIENCY

Dietary intervention with L-arginine has resulted in improved renal hemodynamics in a number of experimental renovascular diseases, such as those caused by subtotal nephrectomy, diabetic nephropathy, cyclosporin A administration, salt-sensitive hypertension, ureteral obstruction, puromycin amino-nucleoside nephrosis, kidney hypertrophy resulting from high-protein feeding, glomerular thrombosis resulting from administration of lipopolysaccharide, thrombotic thrombocytopenic purpura and hemolytic uremic syndrome, and even loss of function secondary to the normal aging process *(67,325,326)*.

With respect to uremia, L-arginine was as effective as captopril at ameliorating glomerular capillary hypertension *(327)*, and normalizing creatinine clearance *(328)*. At the doses of L-arginine required to lower blood pressure, renal blood flow was improved and the associated renal dysfunction was reversed or prevented *(166,258,261,265)*. When renal failure is myoglobin-induced, L-arginine (150 mg/kg/min) can restore renal blood flow and creatine clearance *(329)*. Oral L-arginine (1.6 g/kg/d) has also been shown to decrease preglomerular resistance and restore glomerular hemodynamic response to glycine infusion (NO$^•$-mediated renal vasodilation) *(195,330)*. At least part of the effects of L-arginine on renal blood flow are mediated through sympathetic neuronal mechanisms, as the effect of L-arginine to enhance renal blood flow was abolished in sympathetically denervated rats *(331)*.

In the rat model of subtotal nephrectomy, a high-protein diet leads to loss of NO$^•$ activity, renal hypertrophy, and glomerulosclerosis. Much of the loss of NO$^•$ results from a loss of inducible NOS (iNOS) content *(332)*. When supplemented with L-arginine (1% in drinking water) renal hypertrophy was decreased *(333)*.

In the rat model of cyclosporin nephrotoxicity, tubulointerstitial injury, macrophage infiltration, and progressive interstitial fibrosis occurs secondary to accelerated apoptosis and ischemia *(334)*. In a similar model, in addition to the aforementioned findings, arteriopathy and plasma renin levels were significantly less in the treated animals *(335)*. L-Arginine supplementation in this model reduces tubulointerstitial apoptosis and a reduction in interstitial fibrosis. The effect on L-arginine on renal function was greater than that of allopurinol given to reduce the formation of oxygen radicals *(336)*.

L-Arginine has been administered to patients with end-stage renal disease during dialysis. These individuals demonstrate an endothelial dysfunction that is likely caused by the accumulation of plasma levels of ADMA *(111,337)*. Hand and colleagues have recently demonstrated that hemodialysis reverses the endothelial dysfunction associated with renal failure *(33)*. Similarly, administration of intravenous L-arginine, but not D-arginine, reversed the vasodilator dysfunction without the need for dialysis.

L-Arginine has been used in other settings involving compromised kidney function. L-Arginine has been used to reverse the antinatiuretic effect of cyclosporin in renal transplant patients. In this study, L-arginine infusion (50–150 mg/kg/h) increased renal plasma flow, glomerular filtration rate, naturesis, and kaliureisis *(338)*.

RAYNAUD'S PHENOMENON

Raynaud's phenomenon associated with occlusive arterial disease is due to normal fluctuations in vessel tone superimposed on fixed lesions *(339,340)*. Raynaud's phenomenon may also be secondary to changes in rheologic properties of blood. Cold agglutinins, cryoproteins, or hyperviscosity due to other disorders of serum proteins may induce intermittent ischemia of the digits in the absence of vasospasm. When Raynaud's phenomenon occurs in the absence of organic arterial disease, it is thought to be due to digital artery vasospasm. This entity is known as Raynaud's disease *(339,340)*.

That at least some cases of Raynaud's disease may have a mechanism common to that of coronary vasospasm is underscored by the observation that patients with variant angina have a higher incidence of Raynaud's disease *(341)*. There are differences, however, between coronary and digital arteries in the determinants of vasomotion. Unlike the coronary arteries, α-adrenergic contraction predominates over β-adrenergic relaxation in limb arteries. The limb vessels are richly innervated by sympathetic fibers and are highly responsive to changes in sympathetic tone. Both α_1- and α_2-adrenergic subtypes are present on the postjunctional smooth muscle and initiate contraction when stimulated *(342)*.

Although aberrant sympathetic activity contributes greatly to the pathophysiology of Raynaud's phenomenon and disease, the actions of platelets are also important. Aggregating platelets contract human digital arteries in vitro by releasing serotonin and thromboxane A_2 *(343)*. Each of these vasoconstrictors makes approximately equal contributions to the vasoconstriction induced by platelet aggregation in these vessels. Serotonin may contribute to the vasoconstriction induced by environmental cooling, as the latter is partly reversed with blockade of serotonergic receptors *(344)*. The effect of L-arginine to inhibit platelet aggregation makes it a potential therapy in patients with these maladies.

In reality the utility of L-arginine in patients with Raynaud's phenomenon is mixed. In one study, patients with Raynaud's phenomenon secondary to systemic sclerosis demonstrated enhanced cutaneous vasodilation *(34)*. In this study, 12 patients were given oral L-arginine (8 g/d) for 1 mo. Following therapy there was an increase in digital vasodilation following warming and an increase in plasma levels of tissue-type plasminogen activator. In a similar study in patients with primary Raynaud's phenomenon, 8 g/d of oral L-arginine did not restore the abnormal vasodilator response to ACh *(35)*. This study underscores the minor contribution of abnormal EDNO production in the pathophysiology of Raynaud's. Neither study examined the effect of L-arginine on platelet activity in this disease.

CONCLUSION

Most of the known cardiovascular effects of L-arginine are exerted via its conversion to NO• by NOS. There are, however, NO•-independent actions of L-arginine that contribute to its beneficial action on the cardiovascular system. Accumulating evidence indicates that supplemental administration of L-arginine is sufficient to restore EDNO production in many disorders in which EDNO activity is reduced. A greater understanding of the pathophysiology of these disorders has helped to provide hypotheses to explain the paradox of supplemental L-arginine. Regardless of the mechanism, L-arginine may become a useful therapeutic approach to many cardiovascular disorders. The development of methods of practical L-arginine delivery in the quantities required will likely accelerate its acceptance in routine clinical practice.

REFERENCES

1. Drexler H, Zeiher AM, Meinzer K, Just H. Correction of endothelial dysfunction in coronary microcirculation of hypercholesterolaemic patients by L-arginine. Lancet 1991;338:1546–1550.
2. Creager MA, Gallagher SJ, Girerd XJ, Coleman SM, Dzau VJ, et al. L-arginine improves endothelium-dependent vasodilation in hypercholesterolemic humans. J Clin Invest 1992;90:1248–1253.
3. Clarkson P, Adams MR, Powe AJ, Donald AE, McCredie R, Robinson J, et al. Oral L-arginine improves endothelium-dependent dilation in hypercholesterolemic young adults. J Clin Invest 1996;97: 1989–1994.
4. Böger RH, Mugge A, Bode-Böger SM, Heinzel D, Hoper MM, Frolich JC. Differential systemic and pulmonary hemodynamic effects of L-arginine in patients with coronary artery disease or primary pulmonary hypertension. Int J Clin Pharmacol Ther 1996;34:323–328.
5. Malczewska-Malec M, Goldsztajn P, Kawecka-Jaszcz K, Czarnecka D, Siedlecki A, Siemienska T, et al. Effects of prolonged L-arginine administration on blood pressure in patients with essential hypertension (EH). Agents Actions 1995;45(Suppl):157–162.

53. Ferraresso M, Burra P, Cadrobbi R, Calabrese F, Pettenazzo E, Sarzo G, et al. Protective effect of L-arginine on liver ischemia-reperfusion injury. Transplant Proc 1997;29:393,394.
54. Amrani M, Gray CC, Smolenski RT, Goodwin AT, London A, Yacoub MH. The effect of L-arginine on myocardial recovery after cardioplegic arrest and ischemia under moderate and deep hypothermia. Circulation 1997;96:II-274–II-279.
55. Zhu B, Sun Y, Sievers RE, Glantz SA, Chatterjee K, Parmley WW. L-arginine decreases infarct size in rats exposed to environmental tobacco smoke. Am Heart J 1996;132:91–100.
56. Barbul A, Rettura G, Levenson SM, Seifter E. Arginine: a thymotropic and wound-healing promoting agent. Surg Forum 1997;28:101–103.
57. Park KG, Hayes PD, Garlick PJ, Sewell H, Eremin O. Stimulation of lymphocyte natural cytotoxicity by L-arginine. Lancet 1991;337:645,646.
58. Imler M, Ruscher H, Peter B, Kurtz D, Stahl J. [Action of arginine in a recurrent hepatic coma complicating a feminizing tumor of the adrenal cortex with hepatic metastases]. Sem Hop 1973;49:3183–3190.
59. Batshaw ML, Wachtel RC, Thomas GH, Starrett A, Brusilow SW. Arginine-responsive asymptomatic hyperammonemia in the premature infant. J Pediatr 1984;105:86–91.
60. Bellone J, Bartolotta E, Cardinale G, Arvat E, Cherubini V, Aimaretti G, et al. Low dose orally administered arginine is able to enhance both basal and growth hormone-releasing hormone-induced growth hormone secretion in normal short children. J Endo Invest 1993;16:521–525.
61. Brittenden J, Heys SD, Eremin O. L-arginine and malignant disease: a potential therapeutic role? Eur J Surg Oncol 1994;20:189–192.
62. Rhodes P, Barr CS, Struthers AD. Arginine, lysine and ornithine as vasodilators in the forearm of man. Eur J Clin Invest 1996;26:325–331.
63. Thomas G, Hecker M, Ramwell PW. Vascular activity of polycations and basic amino acids: L-arginine does not specifically elicit endothelium-dependent relaxation. Biochem Biophys Res Commun 1989;158:177–180.
64. Wascher TC, Posch K, Wallner S, Hermetter A, Kostner GM, Graier WF. Vascular effects of L-arginine: anything beyond a substrate for the NO-synthase? Biochem Biophys Res Commun 1997;234:35–38.
65. Korbonits M, Trainer PJ, Fanciulli G, Oliva O, Pala A, Dettori A, et al. L-arginine is unlikely to exert neuroendocrine effects in humans via the generation of nitric oxide. Eur J Endo 1996;135:543–547.
66. Blachier F, Mourtada A, Sener A, Malaisse WJ. Stimulus-secretion coupling of arginine-induced insulin release. Uptake of metabolized and nonmetabolized cationic amino acids by pancreatic islets. Endocrinology 1989;124:134–141.
67. Reyes AA, Karl IE, Klahr S. Role of arginine in health and in renal disease. Am J Physiol 1994;267:F331–F346.
68. Kirk SJ, Hurson M, Regan MC, Holt DR, Wasserkrug HL, Barbul A. Arginine stimulates wound healing and immune function in elderly human beings. Surgery 1993;114:155–160.
69. Pegg AE, McCann PP. Polyamine metabolism and function. Am J Physiol 1982;243:C212–C221.
70. Pollock JS, Forstermann U, Mitchell JA, Warner TD, Schmidt HH, Nakane M, et al. Purification and characterization of particulate endothelium-derived relaxing factor synthase from cultured and native bovine aortic endothelial cells. Proc Natl Acad Sci USA 1991;88:10,480–10,484.
71. Visek WJ. Arginine and disease states. J Nutr 1985;115:532–541.
72. Hanssen H, Brunini TM, Conway M, Banning AP, Roberts NB, Ellory JC, et al. Increased L-arginine transport in human erythrocytes in chronic heart failure. Clin Sci (Colch) 1998;94:43–48.
73. FAO/WHO/UNU. Energy and Protein Requirements. Technical Report Series. WHO, Geneva, Switzerland, 1985.
74. Walser M. Urea cycle disorders and other hereditary hyperammonemic syndromes. In: Stanbury JB, Wyngaarden JB, Fredrickson DS, Goldstein JL, Brown MS, eds. The Metabolic Basis of Inherited Disease. McGraw-Hill, New York, 1983, pp. 402–438.
75. Visek WJ. Arginine needs, physiological state and usual diets. A reevaluation. J Nutr 1986;116:36–46.
76. Aisaka K, Gross SS, Griffith OW, Levi R. NG-methylarginine, an inhibitor of endothelium-derived nitric oxide synthesis, is a potent pressor agent in the guinea pig: does nitric oxide regulate blood pressure in vivo? Biochem Biophys Res Commun 1989;160:881–886.
77. Aisaka K, Gross SS, Griffith OW, Levi R. L-arginine availability determines the duration of acetylcholine-induced systemic vasodilation in vivo. Biochem Biophys Res Commun 1989;3:710–717.
78. Rees DD, Palmer RM, Moncada S. Role of endothelium-derived nitric oxide in the regulation of blood pressure. Proc Natl Acad Sci USA 1989;86:3375–3378.

79. Girerd XJ, Hirsch AT, Cooke JP, Dzau VJ, Creager MA. L-arginine augments endothelium-dependent vasodilation in cholesterol- fed rabbits. Circ Res 1990;67:1301–1308.

80. Cooke JP, Andon NA, Girerd XJ, Hirsch AT, Creager MA. Arginine restores cholinergic relaxation of hypercholesterolemic rabbit thoracic aorta. Circulation 1991;83:1057–1062.

81. Sato H, Zhao ZQ, Vinten-Johansen J. L-Arginine inhibits neutrophil adherence and coronary artery dysfunction. Cardiovasc Res 1996;31:63–72.

82. Singer AH, Tsao PS, Wang BY, Bloch DA, Cooke JP. Discordant effects of dietary L-arginine on vascular structure and reactivity in hypercholesterolemic rabbits. J Cardiovasc Pharmacol 1995;25:710–716.

83. Tsao PS, McEvoy LM, Drexler H, Butcher EC, Cooke JP. Enhanced endothelial adhesiveness in hypercholesterolemia is attenuated by L-arginine. Circulation 1994;89:2176–2182.

84. Tsao PS, Theilmeier G, Singer AH, Leung LL, Cooke JP. L-arginine attenuates platelet reactivity in hypercholesterolemic rabbits. Arterioscl Thromb 1994;14:1529–1533.

85. Liu J, Garcia-Cardena G, Sessa WC. Palmitoylation of endothelial nitric oxide synthase is necessary for optimal stimulated release of nitric oxide: implications for caveolae localization. Biochemistry 1996;35:13,277–13,281.

86. Palmer RM, Moncada S. A novel citrulline-forming enzyme implicated in the formation of nitric oxide by vascular endothelial cells. Biochem Biophys Res Commun 1989;158:348–352.

87. Baydoun AR, Emery PW, Pearson JD, Mann GE. Substrate-dependent regulation of intracellular amino acid concentrations in cultured bovine aortic endothelial cells. Biochem Biophys Res Commun 1990;73:940–948.

88. Gold ME, Bush PA, Ignarro LJ. Depletion of arterial L-arginine causes reversible tolerance to endothelium-dependent relaxation. Biochem Biophys Res Commun 1989;164:714–721.

89. Hecker M, Mitchell JA, Harris HJ, Katsura M, Thiemermann C, Vane JR. Endothelial cells metabolize NG-monomethyl-L-arginine to L-citrulline and subsequently to L-arginine. Biochem Biophys Res Commun 1990;167:1037–1043.

90. Arnal JF, Munzel T, Venema RC, James NL, Bai CL, Mitch WE, et al. Interactions between L-arginine and L-glutamine change endothelial NO production. An effect independent of NO synthase substrate availability. J Clin Invest 1995;95:2565–2572.

91. Förstermann U, Closs EI, Pollock JS, Nakane M, Schwartz P, Gath I, et al. Nitric oxide synthase isozymes. Characterization, purification, molecular cloning, and functions. Hypertension 1994;23: 1121–1131.

92. Sessa WC, Hecker M, Mitchell JA, Vane JR. The metabolism of L-arginine and its significance for the biosynthesis of endothelium-derived relaxing factor: L-glutamine inhibits the generation of L-arginine by cultured endothelial cells. Proc Natl Acad Sci USA 1990;87:8607–8611.

93. Hecker M, Sessa WC, Harris HJ, Anggard EE, Vane JR. The metabolism of L-arginine and its significance for the biosynthesis of endothelium-derived relaxing factor: cultured endothelial cells recycle L-citrulline to L-arginine. Proc Natl Acad Sci USA 1990;87:8612–8616.

94. Swierkosz TA, Mitchell JA, Sessa WC, Hecker M, Vane JR. L-glutamine inhibits the release of endothelium-derived relaxing factor from the rabbit aorta. Biochem Biophys Res Commun 1990;172: 143–148.

95. Arnold WP, Mittal CK, Katsuki S, Murad F. Nitric oxide activates guanylate cyclase and increases guanosine 3':5'-cyclic monophosphate levels in various tissue preparations. Proc Natl Acad Sci USA 1977;74:3203–3207.

96. McDonald KK, Zharikov S, Block ER, Kilberg MS. A caveolar complex between the cationic amino acid transporter 1 and endothelial nitric-oxide synthase may explain the "arginine paradox." J Biol Chem 1997;272:31,213–31,216.

97. Garcia-Cardena G, Oh P, Liu J, Schnitzer JE, Sessa WC. Targeting of nitric oxide synthase to endothelial cell caveolae via palmitoylation: implications for nitric oxide signaling. Proc Natl Acad Sci USA 1996;93:6448–6453.

98. Zharikov SI, Block ER. Characterization of L-arginine uptake by plasma membrane vesicles isolated from cultured pulmonary artery endothelial cells. Biochim Biophys Acta 1998;1369:173–183.

99. Greene B, Pacitti AJ, Souba WW. Characterization of L-arginine transport by pulmonary artery endothelial cells. Am J Physiol 1993;264:L351–L356.

100. Kavanaugh MP. Voltage dependence of facilitated arginine flux mediated by the system y+ basic amino acid transporter. Biochemistry 1993;32:5781–5785.

101. Wang H, Kavanaugh MP, North RA, Kabat D. Cell-surface receptor for ecotropic murine retroviruses is a basic amino-acid transporter [see comments]. Nature 1991;352:729–731.

102. Zharikov SI, Herrera H, Block ER. Role of membrane potential in hypoxic inhibition of L-arginine uptake by lung endothelial cells. Am J Physiol 1997;272:L78–L84.

103. Sobrevia L, Yudilevich DL, Mann GE. Activation of A2-purinoceptors by adenosine stimulates L-arginine transport (system y+) and nitric oxide synthesis in human fetal endothelial cells. J Physiol (Lond) 1997;499:135–140.

104. Sobrevia L, Mann GE. Dysfunction of the endothelial nitric oxide signalling pathway in diabetes and hyperglycaemia. Exp Physiol 1997;82:423–452.

105. Cendan JC, Moldawer LL, Souba WW, Copeland EM, Lind DS. Endotoxin-induced nitric oxide production in pulmonary artery endothelial cells is regulated by cytokines. Arch Surg 1994;129:1296–1300.

106. Cendan JC, Souba WW, Copeland EM, Lind DS. Cytokines regulate endotoxin stimulation of endothelial cell arginine transport. Surgery 1995;117:213–219.

107. Lind DS, Copeland EM 3rd, Souba WW. Endotoxin stimulates arginine transport in pulmonary artery endothelial cells. Surgery 1993;114:199–205.

108. Sobrevia L, Nadal A, Yudilevich DL, Mann GE. Activation of L-arginine transport (system y+) and nitric oxide synthase by elevated glucose and insulin in human endothelial cells. J Physiol (Lond) 1996;490:775–781.

109. Sobrevia L, Cesare P, Yudilevich DL, Mann GE. Diabetes-induced activation of system y+ and nitric oxide synthase in human endothelial cells: association with membrane hyperpolarization. J Physiol (Lond) 1995;489:183–192.

110. Chen LY, Mehta P, Mehta JL. Oxidized LDL decreases L-arginine uptake and nitric oxide synthase protein expression in human platelets: relevance of the effect of oxidized LDL on platelet function. Circulation 1996;93:1740–1746.

111. Vallance P, Leone A, Calver A, Collier J, Moncada S. Accumulation of an endogenous inhibitor of nitric oxide synthesis in chronic renal failure. Lancet 1992;339:572–575.

112. MacAllister RJ, Parry H, Kimoto M, Collier J, Moncada S. Regulation of nitric oxide synthesis by dimethylarginine dimethylaminohydrolase. Br J Pharmacol 1996;119:1–8.

113. Bode-Böger SM, Boger RH, Kienke S, Junker W, Frolich JC. Elevated L-arginine/dimethylarginine ratio contributes to enhanced systemic NO production by dietary L-arginine in hypercholesterolemic rabbits. Biochem Biophys Res Commun 1996;219:598–603.

114. Chan JR, Boger RH, Bode-Boger SM, Tangphao O, Tsao PS, Blaschke TF, et al. Restoration of L-arginine/ADMA ratio normalizes mononuclear leukocyte adhesiveness in hypercholesterolemic humans. Arterioscler Thromb Vasc Biol, in press.

115. Böger R, Bode Böger SM, Szuba A, Tsao PS, Chan JR, Tangphao O, et al. Asymmetric Dimethylarginine (ADMA): a novel risk factor for endothelial dysfunction. Its role in hypercholesterolemia. Circulation 1998;98:1842–1847.

115a. Faraci FM, Brian JE Jr, Heistad DD. Response of cerebral blood vessels to an endogenous inhibitor of nitric oxide synthase. Am J Physiol 1995;269:H1522–H1527.

116. MacAllister RJ, Fickling SA, Whitley GS, Vallance P. Metabolism of methylarginines by human vasculature; implications for the regulation of nitric oxide synthesis. Br J Pharmacol 1994;112:43–48.

117. Mendes Ribeiro AC, Hanssen H, Kiessling K, Roberts NB, Mann GE, Ellory JC. Transport of L-arginine and the nitric oxide inhibitor NG-monomethyl-L-arginine in human erythrocytes in chronic renal failure. Clin Sci (Colch) 1997;93:57–64.

118. Bogle RG, MacAllister RJ, Whitley GS, Vallance P. Induction of NG-monomethyl-L-arginine uptake: a mechanism for differential inhibition of NO synthases? Am J Physiol 1995;269:C750–C756.

119. Pritchard KA Jr, Groszek L, Smalley DM, Sessa WC, Wu M, Villalon P, et al. Native low-density lipoprotein increases endothelial cell nitric oxide synthase generation of superoxide anion. Circ Res 1995;77:510–518.

120. Huk I, Nanobashvili J, Neumayer C, Punz A, Mueller M, Afkhampour K, et al. L-arginine treatment alters the kinetics of nitric oxide and superoxide release and reduces ischemia/reperfusion injury in skeletal muscle. Circulation 1997;96:667–675.

121. Stroes E, Kastelein J, Cosentino F, Erkelens W, Wever R, Koomans H, et al. Tetrahydrobiopterin restores endothelial function in hypercholesterolemia. J Clin Invest 1997;99:41–46.

122. Schini VB, Vanhoutte PM. L-arginine evokes both endothelium-dependent and -independent relaxations in L-arginine-depleted aortas of the rat. Circ Res 1991;68:209–216.

123. Fromm JR, Hileman RE, Caldwell EE, Weiler JM, Linhardt RJ. Differences in the interaction of heparin with arginine and lysine and the importance of these basic amino acids in the binding of heparin to acidic fibroblast growth factor. Arch Biochem Biophys 1995;323:279–287.

124. Liu Z, Perlin AS. Regioselectivity in the sulfation of some chemically-modified heparins, and observations on their cation-binding characteristics. Carb Res 1992;236:121–133.

125. Fajans SS, Floyd JC Jr, Knopf RF, Conn FW. Effect of amino acids and proteins on insulin secretion in man. Recent Prog Horm Res 1967;23:617–662.

126. Giugliano D, Marfella R, Verrazzo G, Acampora R, Coppola L, Cozzolino D, et al. The vascular effects of L-arginine in humans. The role of endogenous insulin. J Clin Invest 1997;99:433–438.
127. Sanchez A, Hubbard R. Dietary protein modulation of serum cholesterol: the amino acid connection. In: Freidman M, ed. Absorption and Utilization of Amino Acids. CRC Press, New York, 1990, pp. 247–273.
128. Ness GC, Zhao Z, Wiggins L. Insulin and glucagon modulate hepatic 3-hydroxy–3-methylglutaryl-coenzyme A reductase activity by affecting immunoreactive protein levels. J Biol Chem 1994;269: 29,168–29,172.
129. Kritchevsky XX. Dietary protein and atherosclerosis. In: Freidman M, ed. Absorption and Utilization of Amino Acids. CRC Press, New York, 1990, pp. 235–245.
130. Sirtori CR, Galli G, Lovati MR, Carrara P, Bosisio E, Kienle MG. Effects of dietary proteins on the regulation of liver lipoprotein receptors in rats. J Nutr 1984;114:1493–1500.
131. Barth CA, Pfeuffer M. Dietary protein and atherogenesis. Klin Wochenschr 1988;66:135–143.
132. Kritchevsky D. Protein and atherosclerosis. J Nutr Sci Vitaminol (Tokyo) 1990;36(Suppl 2):S81–S86.
133. Kurowska EM, Carroll KK. Hypocholesterolemic properties of nitric oxide. In vivo and in vitro studies using nitric oxide donors. Biochim Biophys Acta 1998;1392:41–50.
134. Wascher TC, Graier WF, Dittrich P, Hussain MA, Bahadori B, Wallner S, et al. Effects of low-dose L-arginine on insulin-mediated vasodilatation and insulin sensitivity. Eur J Clin Invest 1997;27:690–695.
135. Miliutina NP, Ananian AA, Shugalei VS. [Antiradical and antioxidant effect of arginine and its action on lipid peroxidation in hypoxia]. Biull Eksp Biol Med 1990;110:263–265.
136. Philis-Tsimikas A, Witztum JL. L-arginine may inhibit atherosclerosis through inhibition of LDL oxidation. Circulation 1995;92:I422–I443.
137. Xiong Y, Li YJ, Deng HW. Protection of l-arginine against oxygen free radicals-injured rabbit aortic endothelium. Chung Kuo Yao Li Hsueh Pao 1994;15:119–123.
138. Clancy RM, Leszczynska P, Piziak J, Abramson SB. Nitric oxide, an endothelial cell relation factor, inhibits neutrophil superoxide anion production via a direct action of NADPH oxidase. J Clin Invest 1992;90:1116–1121.
139. Peng HB, Libby P, Liao JK. Induction and stabilization of I kappa B alpha by nitric oxide mediates inhibition of NF-kappa B. J Biol Chem 1995;270:14,214–14,219.
140. Tsao PS, Wang B, Buitrago R, Shyy JY, Cooke JP. Nitric oxide regulates monocyte chemotactic protein–1. Circulation 1997;96:934–940.
141. Higashi Y, Oshima T, Ono N, Hiraga H, Yoshimura M, Watanabe M, et al. Intravenous administration of L-arginine inhibits angiotensin-converting enzyme in humans. J Clin Endocrinol Metab 1995;80: 2198–2202.
142. Barbul A, Fishel RS, Shimazu S, Wasserkrug HL, Yoshimura NN, Tao RC, et al. Intravenous hyper-alimentation with high arginine levels improves wound healing and immune function. J Surg Res 1985; 38:328–334.
143. Nirgiotis JG, Hennessey PJ, Andrassy RJ. Effects of an arginine-free enteral diet on wound healing and immune function in the postsurgical rat. J Ped Surg 1991;26:936–941.
144. Seifter E, Rettura G, Barbul A, Levenson SM. Arginine: an essential amino acid for injured rats. Surgery 1978;84:224–230.
145. Barbul A, Rettura G, Levenson SM, Seifter E. Wound healing and thymotropic effects of arginine: a pituitary mechanism of action. Am J Clin Nutr 1983;37:786–794.
146. Heys SD, Gough DB, Park KGM, Eremin O. L-arginine: clinical practice and potential applications. In: Eremin O, ed. L-Arginine: Biological Aspects and Clinical Applications. Chapman & Hall, Austin, TX, 1997, pp. 115–157.
147. Micieli G, Bosone D, Costa A, Cavallini A, Marchesselli S, Pompeo F, et al. Opposite effects of L-arginine and nitroglycerin on cerebral blood velocity: nitric oxide precursors and cerebral blood velocity. J Neurol Sci 1997;150:71–75.
148. Reutens DC, McHugh MD, Toussaint PJ, Evans AC, Gjedde A, Meyer E, et al. L-arginine infusion increases basal but not activated cerebral blood flow in humans. J Cereb Blood Flow Metab 1997; 17:309–315.
149. Cooke JP, Dzau J, Creager A. Endothelial dysfunction in hypercholesterolemia is corrected by L-arginine. Basic Res Cardiol 1991;86(Suppl 2):173–181.
150. Cooke JP, Singer AH, Tsao P, Zera P, Rowan RA, Billingham ME. Antiatherogenic effects of L-arginine in the hypercholesterolemic rabbit. J Clin Invest 1992;90:1168–7112.
151. Davies MG, Dalen H, Kim JH, Barber L, Svendsen E, Hagen PO. Control of accelerated vein graft atheroma with the nitric oxide precursor: L-arginine. J Surg Res 1995;59:35–42.

152. Jeremy RW, McCarron H, Sullivan D. Effects of dietary L-arginine on atherosclerosis and endothelium-dependent vasodilatation in the hypercholesterolemic rabbit. Response according to treatment duration, anatomic site, and sex. Circulation 1996;94:498–506.

153. Randall MD, Ujiie H, Griffith TM. L-arginine reverses the impairment of nitric oxide-dependent collateral perfusion in dietary-induced hypercholesterolaemia in the rabbit. Clini Sci (Colch) 1994; 87:53–59.

154. Rossitch E Jr, Alexander ED, Black PM, Cooke JP. L-arginine normalizes endothelial function in cerebral vessels from hypercholesterolemic rabbits. J Clin Invest 1991;87:1295–1299.

155. Schuschke DA, Miller FN, Lominadze DG, Feldhoff RC. L-arginine restores cholesterol-attenuated microvascular responses in the rat cremaster. Int J Microcirc Clin Exp 1994;14:204–211.

156. Kuo L, Davis MJ, Cannon MS, Chilian WM. Pathophysiological consequences of atherosclerosis extend into the coronary microcirculation. Restoration of endothelium-dependent responses by L-arginine. Circ Res 1992;70:465–476.

157. Clarkson PB, Lim PO, MacDonald TM. Influence of basal nitric oxide secretion on cardiac function in man. Br J Clin Pharmacol 1995;40:299–305.

158. Chowienczyk PJ, Watts GF, Cockcroft JR, Brett SE, Ritter JM. Sex differences in endothelial function in normal and hypercholesterolaemic subjects. Lancet 1994;344:305,306.

159. Stroes ES, Koomans HA, de Bruin TW, Rabelink TJ. Vascular function in the forearm of hypercholesterolaemic patients off and on lipid-lowering medication. Lancet 1995;346:467–471.

160. Goode GK, Heagerty AM. In vitro responses of human peripheral small arteries in hypercholesterolemia and effects of therapy. Circulation 1995;91:2898–2903.

161. Wennmalm A. Endothelial nitric oxide and cardiovascular disease. J Int Med 1994;35:317–327.

162. Casino PR, Kilcoyne CM, Quyyumi AA, Hoeg JM, Panza JA. Investigation of decreased availability of nitric oxide precursor as the mechanism responsible for impaired endothelium-dependent vasodilation in hypercholesterolemic patients. J Am Coll Cardiol 1994;23:844–850.

163. Maxwell AJ, Anderson B, Cooke JP. Endothelial dysfunction in hypercholesterolemia is reversed by a nutritional product designed to enhance nitric oxide activity. Cardiovasc Drugs Ther, in press.

164. Taddei S, Virdis A, Mattei P, Ghiadoni L, Sudano I, Salvetti A. Defective L-arginine-nitric oxide pathway in offspring of essential hypertensive patients. Circulation 1996;94:1298–1303.

165. Kitazono T, Faraci FM, Heistad DD. L-arginine restores dilator responses of the basilar artery to acetylcholine during chronic hypertension. Hypertension 1996;27:893–896.

166. Hayakawa H, Hirata Y, Suzuki E, Kimura K, Kikuchi K, Nagano T, et al. Long-term administration of L-arginine improves nitric oxide release from kidney in deoxycorticosterone acetate-salt hypertensive rats. Hypertension 1994;23:752–756.

167. Hind JM, Doodson AC. Oral L-arginine supplementation has no effect on cardiovascular responses to lower body negative pressure in man. Clin Auton Res 1994;4:293–297.

168. Rosano GM, Panina G, Cerquetani E, Leonardo F, Pelliccia F, Bonfigli B, et al. L-arginine improves endothelial function in newly diagnosed hypertensives. J Am Coll Cardiol 1998;31:262A (abstract).

169. Adnot S, Raffestin B, Eddahibi S, Braquet P, Chabrier PE. Loss of endothelium-dependent relaxant activity in the pulmonary circulation of rats exposed to chronic hypoxia. J Clin Invest 1991;87: 155–162.

170. Fineman JR, Chang R, Soifer SJ. L-Arginine, a precursor of EDRF in vitro, produces pulmonary vasodilation in lambs. Am J Physiol 1991;261:H1563–H1569.

171. Eddahibi S, Adnot S, Carville C, Blouquit Y, Raffestin B. L-arginine restores endothelium-dependent relaxation in pulmonary circulation of chronically hypoxic rats. Am J Physiol 1992;263:L194–L200.

172. Hui S, Mei Q, Qiu B. Effects of chronic nicotine ingestion on pressor response to N omega-nitro-L-arginine methyl ester and ex vivo concentration and relaxation response of aorta to L-arginine. Pharmacol Res 1997;36:451–456.

173. Hutchison SJ, Reitz MS, Sudhir K, Sievers RE, Zhu BQ, Sun YP, et al. Chronic dietary L-arginine prevents endothelial dysfunction secondary to environmental tobacco smoke in normocholesterolemic rabbits. Hypertension 1997;29:1186–1191.

174. Zeiher AM, Schachinger V, Minners J. Long-term cigarette smoking impairs endothelium-dependent coronary arterial vasodilator function. Circulation 1995;92:1094–1100.

174a. Thorne S, Mullen MJ, Clarkson P, Donald AE, Deanfield JE. Early endothelial dysfunction in adults at risk from atherosclerosis: different responses to L-arginine. J Am Coll Cardiol 1998;32:110–116.

175. Watts GF, O'Brien SF, Silvester W, Millar JA. Impaired endothelium-dependent and independent dilatation of forearm resistance arteries in men with diet-treated non-insulin-dependent diabetes: role of dyslipidaemia. Clin Sci (Colch) 1996;91:567–573.

176. Nitenberg A, Ledoux S, Attali JR, Valensi P. [Response of the coronary arteries to cold test and flow velocity increase is improved by deferoxamine but not by L-arginine in diabetic patients]. Arch Mal Coeur Vaiss 1997;90:1037–1041.

177. Pieper GM, Siebeneich W, Moore-Hilton G, Roza AM. Reversal by L-arginine of a dysfunctional arginine/nitric oxide pathway in the endothelium of the genetic diabetic BB rat. Diabetologia 1997; 40:910–915.

178. Mayhan WG, Patel KP, Sharpe GM. Effect of L-arginine on reactivity of hamster cheek pouch arterioles during diabetes mellitus. Int J Microcirc Clin Exp 1997;17:107–112.

179. Pieper GM, Peltier BA. Amelioration by L-arginine of a dysfunctional arginine/nitric oxide pathway in diabetic endothelium. J Cardiovasc Pharmacol 1995;25:397–403.

180. Pieper GM, Siebeneich W, Dondlinger LA. Short-term oral administration of L-arginine reverses defective endothelium-dependent relaxation and cGMP generation in diabetes. Eur J Pharmacol 1996; 317:317–320.

181. Mayhan WG, Didion SP, Patel KP. L-Arginine does not restore dilatation of the basilar artery during diabetes mellitus. J Cereb Blood Flow Metab 1996;16:500–506.

182. Tesfamariam B, Cohen RA. Free radicals mediate endothelial cell dysfunction caused by elevated glucose. Am J Physiol 1992;263:H321–H326.

183. Nitenberg A, Paycha F, Ledoux S, Sachs R, Attali JR, Valensi P. Coronary artery responses to physiological stimuli are improved by deferoxamine but not by L-arginine in non-insulin-dependent diabetic patients with angiographically normal coronary arteries and no other risk factors. Circulation 1998;97:736–743.

184. MacAllister RJ, Calver AL, Collier J, Edwards CM, Herreros B, Nussey SS, et al. Vascular and hormonal responses to arginine: provision of substrate for nitric oxide or non-specific effect? Clin Sci (Colch) 1995;89:183–190.

185. Makimattila S, Mantysaari M, Groop PH, Summanen P, Virkamaki A, Schlenzka A, et al. Hyperreactivity to nitrovasodilators in forearm vasculature is related to autonomic dysfunction in insulin-dependent diabetes mellitus. Circulation 1997;95:618–625.

186. Knock GA, McCarthy AL, Lowy C, Poston L. Association of gestational diabetes with abnormal maternal vascular endothelial function. Br J Obstet Gynaecol 1997;104:229–234.

187. Giugliano D, Marfella R, Coppola L, Verrazzo G, Acampora R, Giunta R, et al. Vascular effects of acute hyperglycemia in humans are reversed by L-arginine. Evidence for reduced availability of nitric oxide during hyperglycemia. Circulation 1997;95:1783–1790.

188. Paolisso G, Tagliamonte MR, Marfella R, Verrazzo G, D'Onofrio F, Giugliano D. L-arginine but not D-arginine stimulates insulin-mediated glucose uptake. Metabolism 1997;46:1068–1073.

189. Zeiher AM, Drexler H, Saurbier B, Just H. Endothelium-mediated coronary blood flow modulation in humans. Effects of age, atherosclerosis, hypercholesterolemia, and hypertension. J Clin Invest 1993; 92:652–662.

190. Grisham MB, Miles AM. Effects of aminosalicylates and immunosuppressive agents on nitric oxide-dependent N-nitrosation reactions. Biochem Pharmacol 1994;47:1897–1902.

191. Cosentino F, Katusic ZS. Tetrahydrobiopterin and dysfunction of endothelial nitric oxide synthase in coronary arteries. Circulation 1995;91:139–144.

192. Schaffner A, Blau N, Schneemann M, Steurer J, Edgell CJ, Schoedon G. Tetrahydrobiopterin as another EDRF in man. Biochem Biophys Res Commun 1994;205:516–523.

193. Balligand JL, Godfraind T. Endothelium-derived relaxing factor and muscle-derived relaxing factor in rat aorta: action of cyclosporin A. J Cardiovasc Pharmacol 1991;17:S213–S221.

194. Mathieu P, Carrier M, Dupuis J, Ryan J, Pelletier LC. L-arginine prevents cyclosporin A-induced pulmonary vascular dysfunction. Ann Thorac Sur 1997;64:414–420.

195. Gallego MJ, Lopez Farre A, Riesco A, Monton M, Grandes SM, Barat A, et al. Blockade of endothelium-dependent responses in conscious rats by cyclosporin A: effect of L-arginine. Am J Physiol 1993; 264:H708–H714.

196. Kim HS, Kim DH, Kang SW, Choi H, Lee HY, Han DS, et al. L-arginine restores suppressed acetylcholine-induced endothelium-dependent vascular relaxation in cyclosporine A-treated rats. Transplant Proc 1996;28:1372–1374.

197. Harrison DG, Kurz MA, Quillen JE, Sellke FW, Mugge A. Normal and pathophysiologic considerations of endothelial regulation of vascular tone and their relevance to nitrate therapy. Am J Cardiol 1992;70:11B–17B.

198. Munzel T, Sayegh H, Freeman BA, Tarpey MM, Harrison DG. Evidence for enhanced vascular superoxide anion production in nitrate tolerance. A novel mechanism underlying tolerance and cross-tolerance. J Clin Invest 1995;95:187–194.

199. Abou-Mohamed G, Kaesemeyer WH, Papapetropoulos A, Catravas JD, Caldwell RW. Nitroglycerin (NTG) but not sodium nitroprusside (SNP), increases aortic ring cGMP levels via an L-arginine dependent and L-NAME sensitive pathway. FASEB J 1995;9:A327.

200. Kaesemeyer WH, Abou-Mohamed G, Crute TD, Caldwell RW. Nitrates supplemented with L-arginine for the reversal and treatment of nitrate tolerance: two case reports. Appl Cardiopulm Physiol 1997; 1–8.

201. Böger RH, Bode-Böger SM, Kienke S, Stan AC, Nafe R, Frolich JC. Dietary L-arginine decreases myointimal cell proliferation and vascular monocyte accumulation in cholesterol-fed rabbits. Atherosclerosis 1998;136:67–77.

202. Cayatte AJ, Palacino JJ, Horten K, Cohen RA. Chronic inhibition of nitric oxide production accelerates neointima formation and impairs endothelial function in hypercholesterolemic rabbits. Arterioscl Thromb 1994;14:753–759.

203. Houston M, Chumley P, Radi R, Rubbo H, Freeman BA. Xanthine oxidase reaction with nitric oxide and peroxynitrite. Arch Biochem Biophys 1998;355:1–8.

204. Pou S, Pou WS, Bredt DS, Snyder SH, Rosen GM. Generation of superoxide by purified brain nitric oxide synthase. J Biol Chem 1992;267:24,173–24,176.

205. Klatt P, Pfeiffer S, List BM, Lehner D, Glatter O, Bachinger HP, et al. Characterization of heme-deficient neuronal nitric-oxide synthase reveals a role for heme in subunit dimerization and binding of the amino acid substrate and tetrahydrobiopterin. J Biol Chem 1996;271:7336–7442.

206. Wang BY, Singer AH, Tsao PS, Drexler H, Kosek J, Cooke JP. Dietary arginine prevents atherogenesis in the coronary artery of the hypercholesterolemic rabbit. J Am Coll Cardiol 1994;23:452–458.

207. Adams MR, Jessup W, Hailstones D, Celermajer DS. L-arginine reduces human monocyte adhesion to vascular endothelium and endothelial expression of cell adhesion molecules. Circulation 1997;95: 662–668.

208. Bath PM. The effect of nitric oxide-donating vasodilators on monocyte chemotaxis and intracellular cGMP concentrations in vitro. Eur J Clin Pharmacol 1993;45:53–58.

209. Tsao PS, Buitrago R, Chan JR, Cooke JP. Fluid flow inhibits endothelial adhesiveness. Nitric oxide and transcriptional regulation of VCAM-1. Circulation 1996;94:1682–1689.

210. Marui N, Offermann MK, Swerlick R, Kunsch C, Rosen CA, Ahmad M, et al. Vascular cell adhesion molecule-1 (VCAM-1) gene transcription and expression are regulated through an antioxidant-sensitive mechanism in human vascular endothelial cells. J Clin Invest 1993;92:1866–1874.

211. Theilmeier G, Chan JR, Zalpour C, Anderson B, Wang BY, Wolf A, et al. Adhesiveness of mononuclear cells in hypercholesterolemic humans is normalized by dietary L-arginine. Arteriosc Thromb Vasc Biol 1997;17:3557–3564.

212. Ichiki K, Ikeda H, Haramaki N, Ueno T, Imaizumi T. Long-term smoking impairs platelet-derived nitric oxide release. Circulation 1996;94:3109–3114.

213. Cadwgan TM, Benjamin N. Evidence for altered platelet nitric oxide synthesis in essential hypertension. J Hypertens 1993;11:417–420.

214. Wolf A, Zalpour C, Theilmeier G, Wang BY, Ma A, Anderson B, et al. Dietary L-arginine supplementation normalizes platelet aggregation in hypercholesterolemic humans. J Am Coll Cardiol 1997;29: 479–485.

215. Adams MR, Forsyth CJ, Jessup W, Robinson J, Celermajer DS. Oral L-arginine inhibits platelet aggregation but does not enhance endothelium-dependent dilation in healthy young men. J Am Coll Cardiol 1995;26:1054–1061.

216. Bode-Böger SM, Böger RH, Creutzig A, Tsikas D, Gutzki FM, Alexander K, et al. L-arginine infusion decreases peripheral arterial resistance and inhibits platelet aggregation in healthy subjects. Clin Sci (Colch) 1994;87:303–310.

217. Marietta M, Facchinetti F, Neri I, Piccinini F, Volpe A, Torelli G. L-arginine infusion decreases platelet aggregation through an intraplatelet nitric oxide release. Thromb Res 1997;88:229–235.

218. Vallance P, Benjamin N, Collier J. The effect of endothelium-derived nitric oxide on ex vivo whole blood platelet aggregation in man. Eur J Clin Pharmacol 1992;42:37–41.

219. Bode-Böger SM, Boger RH, Galland A, Frolich JC. Differential inhibition of human platelet aggregation and thromboxane A2 formation by L-arginine in vivo and in vitro. Naunyn Schmiedebergs Arch Pharmacol 1998;357:143–150.

220. Michel T, Smith TW. Nitric oxide synthases and cardiovascular signaling. Am Coll Cardiol 1993;72: 33C–38C.

221. Pohl U, Busse R. EDRF increases cyclic GMP in platelets during passage through the coronary vascular bed. Circ Res 1989;65:1798–1803.

222. Mendez JD, Zarzoza E. Inhibition of platelet aggregation by L-arginine and polyamines in alloxan treated rats. Biochem Molec Biol Int 1997;43:311–318.

223. Dambisya YM, Lee TL. A thromboelastography study on the in vitro effects of L-arginine and L-NG-nitro arginine methyl ester on human whole blood coagulation and fibrinolysis. Blood Coag Fibrin 1996;7:678–683.

224. Udvardy M, Posan E, Palatka K, Altorjay I, Harsfalvi J. Effect of L-arginine on in vitro plasmin-generation and fibrinogenolysis. Thromb Res 1997;87:75–82.

225. Gryglewski RJ, Grodzinska L, Kostka-Trabka E, Korbut R, Bieroon K, Goszcz A, et al. Treatment with L-arginine is likely to stimulate generation of nitric oxide in patients with peripheral arterial obstructive disease. Wien Klin Wochenschr 1996;108:111–116.

226. Marfella R, Acampora R, Verrazzo G, Ziccardi P, De Rosa N, Giunta R, et al. Metformin improves hemodynamic and rheological responses to L-arginine in NIDDM patients. Diabetes Care 1996;19:934–939.

227. Lou H, Kodama T, Wang YN, Katz N, Ramwell P, Foegh ML. L-arginine prevents heart transplant arteriosclerosis by modulating the vascular cell proliferative response to insulin-like growth factor-I and interleukin–6. J Heart Lung Transplant 1996;15:1248–1257.

228. Katan MB, Vroomen LH, Hermus RJ. Reduction of casein-induced hypercholesterolaemia and atherosclerosis in rabbits and rats by dietary glycine, arginine and alanine. Atherosclerosis 1982;43:381–391.

229. Hamon M, Vallet B, Bauters C, Wernert N, McFadden EP, Lablanche JM, et al. Long-term oral administration of L-arginine reduces intimal thickening and enhances neoendothelium-dependent acetylcholine-induced relaxation after arterial injury. Circulation 1994;90:1357–1362.

230. Wang BY, Candipan RC, Arjomandi M, Hsiun PT, Tsao PS, Cooke JP. Arginine restores nitric oxide activity and inhibits monocyte accumulation after vascular injury in hypercholesterolemic rabbits. J Am Coll Cardiol 1996;28:1573–1579.

231. Davies MG, Kim JH, Dalen H, Makhoul RG, Svendsen E, Hagen PO. Reduction of experimental vein graft intimal hyperplasia and preservation of nitric oxide-mediated relaxation by the nitric oxide precursor L-arginine. Surgery 1994;116:557–568.

232. Okazaki J, Komori K, Kawasaki K, Eguchi D, Ishida M, Sugimachi K. L-arginine inhibits smooth muscle cell proliferation of vein graft intimal thickness in hypercholesterolemic rabbits. Cardiovasc Res 1997;36:429–436.

233. Dattilo JB, Dattilo MP, Crane JT, Yager DR, Makhoul RG. The nitric oxide precursor L-arginine reduces expression of hyaluronan synthase in experimental vein bypass grafts. J Surg Res 1998;74:39–42.

234. Pipili-Synetos E, Sakkoula E, Maragoudakis ME. Nitric oxide is involved in the regulation of angiogenesis. Br J Pharmacol 1993;108:855–857.

235. Papapetropoulos A, Garcia-Cardena G, Madri JA, Sessa WC. Nitric oxide production contributes to the angiogenic properties of vascular endothelial growth factor in human endothelial cells. J Clin Invest 1997;100:3131–3139.

236. van der Zee R, Murohara T, Luo Z, Zollmann F, Passeri J, Lekutat C, et al. Vascular endothelial growth factor/vascular permeability factor augments nitric oxide release from quiescent rabbit and human vascular endothelium. Circulation 1997;95:1030–1037.

237. Murohara T, Asahara T, Silver M, Bauters C, Masuda H, Kalka C, et al. Nitric oxide synthase modulates angiogenesis in response to tissue ischemia. J Clin Invest 1998;101:2567–2578.

238. Quyyumi AA, Dakak N, Andrews NP, Husain S, Arora S, Gilligan DM, et al. Nitric oxide activity in the human coronary circulation. Impact of risk factors for coronary atherosclerosis. J Clin Invest 1995;95:1747–1755.

239. Hirooka Y, Egashira K, Imaizumi T, Tagawa T, Kai H, Sugimachi M, et al. Effect of L-arginine on acetylcholine-induced endothelium-dependent vasodilation differs between the coronary and forearm vasculatures in humans. J Am Coll Cardiol 1994;24:948–955.

240. Otsuji S, Nakajima O, Waku S, Kojima S, Hosokawa H, Kinoshita I, et al. Attenuation of acetylcholine-induced vasoconstriction by L-arginine is related to the progression of atherosclerosis. Am Heart J 1995;129:1094–1100.

241. Lekakis J, Papamichael C, Agrios N, Vemmos A, Voutsas S, Stamatelopoulos S, et al. Peripheral vascular endothelial dysfunction in patients with microvascular angina pectoris. J Am Coll Cardiol 1997;29:175A.

242. Egashira K, Hirooka Y, Kuga T, Mohri M, Takeshita A. Effects of L-arginine supplementation on endothelium-dependent coronary vasodilation in patients with angina pectoris and normal coronary arteriograms. Circulation 1996;94:130–134.

243. Lerman A, Burnett JC Jr, Higano ST, McKinley LJ, Holmes DR Jr. Long-term L-arginine supplementation improves small-vessel coronary endothelial function in humans. Circulation 1998;97:2123–2128.

244. Ceremuzynski L, Chamiec T, Herbaczynska-Cedro K. Effect of supplemental oral L-arginine on exercise capacity in patients with stable angina pectoris. Am J Cardiol 1997;80:331–333.

245. Ceremuzynski L, Tomasz C, Herbaczynska-Cedro K. L-arginine improves exercise capacity in patients with stable angina. J Am Coll Cardiol 1997;29:157A.

246. Böger R, Bode-Böger SM, Thiele W, Alexander K, Frolich JC. Biochemical evidence for impaired nitric oxide synthesis in patients with peripheral arterial occlusive disease. Circulation 1998;95:2068–2074.

247. Mehta S, Stewart DJ, Levy RD. The hypotensive effect of L-arginine is associated with increased expired nitric oxide in humans. Chest 1996;109:1550–1555.

248. Bijlsma JA, Rabelink AJ, Kaasjager KA, Koomans HA. L-arginine does not prevent the renal effects of endothelin in humans. J Am Soc Nephrol 1995;5:1508–1516.

249. Hishikawa K, Nakaki T, Tsuda M, Esumi H, Ohshima H, Suzuki H, et al. Effect of systemic L-arginine administration on hemodynamics and nitric oxide release in man. Jpn Heart J 1992;33:41–48.

250. Giugliano D, Marfella R, Verrazzo G, Acampora R, Nappo F, Ziccardi P, et al. L-arginine for testing endothelium-dependent vascular functions in health and disease. Am J Physiol 1997;273:E606–E612.

251. Harima A, Shimizu H, Takagi H. Analgesic effect of L-arginine in patients with persistent pain. Eur Neuropsychopharmacol 1991;1:529–533.

252. Nakaki T, Hishikawa K, Suzuki H, Saruta T, Kato R. L-arginine-induced hypotension. Lancet 1990; 336:696.

253. Kanno K, Hirata Y, Emori T, Ohta K, Eguchi S, Imai T, et al. L-arginine infusion induces hypotension and diuresis/natriuresis with concomitant increased urinary excretion of nitrite/nitrate and cyclic GMP in humans. Clin Exp Pharmacol Phys 1992;19:619–625.

254. Hishikawa K, Nakaki T, Suzuki H, Kato R, Saruta T. Role of L-arginine-nitric oxide pathway in hypertension. J Hypertens 1993;11:639–645.

255. Hishikawa K, Nakaki T, Suzuki H, Saruta T, Kato R. L-arginine-induced hypotension. Lancet 1991; 337:683,684.

256. Laghi Pasini F, Frigerio C, Blardi P, Domini L, De Giorgi L, Borgogni G, et al. Evidence of an adenosine-dependent mechanism in the hypotensive effect of L-arginine in man. Clin Exp Pharmacol Physiol 1995;22:254–259.

257. Petros AJ, Hewlett AM, Bogle RG, Pearson JD. L-arginine-induced hypotension. Lancet 1991;337: 1044,1045.

258. Chen PY, St. John PL, Kirk KA, Abrahamson DR, Sanders PW. Hypertensive nephrosclerosis in the Dahl/Rapp rat. Initial sites of injury and effect of dietary L-arginine supplementation. Lab Invest 1993; 68:174–184.

259. Chen PY, Sanders PW. L-arginine abrogates salt-sensitive hypertension in Dahl/Rapp rats. J Clin Invest 1991;88:1559–1567.

260. Turner SW, Wen C, Li M, Whitworth JA. L-arginine prevents corticotropin-induced increases in blood pressure in the rat. Hypertension 1996;27:184–189.

261. Laurant P, Demolombe B, Berthelot. Dietary L-arginine attenuates blood pressure in mineralocorticoid-salt hypertensive rats. Clin Exp Hypertens 1995;17:1009–1024.

262. Matsuoka H, Nakata M, Kohno K, Koga Y, Nomura G, Toshima A. Chronic L-arginine administration attenuates cardiac hypertrophy in spontaneously hypertensive rats. Hypertension 1996;27:14–18.

263. Tomohiro A, Kimura S, He H, Fujisawa Y, Nishiyama A, Kiyomoto K, et al. Regional blood flow in Dahl-Iwai salt-sensitive rats and the effects of dietary L-arginine supplementation. Am J Physiol 1997; 272:R1013–R1019.

264. Li M, Fraser T, Wang J, Whitworth JA. Dexamethasone-induced hypertension in the rat: effects of L-arginine. Clin Exp Pharmacol Physiol 1997;24:730–732.

265. Helmbrecht GD, Farhat MY, Lochbaum L, Brown HE, Yadgarova KT, Eglinton GS, et al. L-arginine reverses the adverse pregnancy changes induced by nitric oxide synthase inhibition in the rat. Am J Obstet Gynecol 1996;175:800–805.

266. Pucci ML, Dick LB, Miller KB, Smith CJ, Nasjletti A. Enhanced responses to L-arginine in aortic rings from rats with angiotensin-dependent hypertension. J Pharmacol Exp Therap 1995;274:1–7.

267. Ding Y, Vaziri ND, Gonick HC. Lead-induced hypertension. II. Response to sequential infusions of L-arginine, superoxide dismutase, and nitroprusside. Environ Res 1998;76:107–113.

268. Jimbo M, Suzuki H, Ichikawa M, Kumagai K, Nishizawa M, Saruta T. Role of nitric oxide in regulation of baroreceptor reflex. J Auton Nerve Sys 1994;50:209–219.

269. Higashi Y, Oshima T, Sasaki N, Ishioka N, Nakano Y, Ozono R, et al. Relationship between insulin resistance and endothelium-dependent vascular relaxation in patients with essential hypertension. Hypertension 1997;29:280–285.

270. Matsuoka H, Itoh S, Kimoto M, Kohno K, Tamai O, Wada Y, et al. Asymmetrical dimethylarginine, an endogenous nitric oxide synthase inhibitor, in experimental hypertension. Hypertension 1997;29: 242–247.

271. Haulica I, Cosovanu A, Ungureanu G, Zaharia D, Baltatu O, Boisteanu D. Cardiovascular effects of L-arginine as physiological precursor of nitric oxide. Rom J Int Med 1994;32:195–201.

272. Pedrinelli R, Ebel M, Catapano G, Dell'Omo G, Ducci M, Del Chicca M, et al. Pressor, renal and endocrine effects of L-arginine in essential hypertensives. Eur J Clin Pharmacol 1995;48:195–201.

273. Wideman RF Jr, Kirby YK, Ismail M, Bottje WG, Moore RW, Vardeman RC. Supplemental L-arginine attenuates pulmonary hypertension syndrome (ascites) in broilers. Poult Sci 1995;74:323–330.

274. Mitani Y, Maruyama K, Sakurai M. Prolonged administration of L-arginine ameliorates chronic pulmonary hypertension and pulmonary vascular remodeling in rats. Circulation 1997;96:689–697.

275. Giaid A, Saleh D. Reduced expression of endothelial nitric oxide synthase in the lungs of patients with pulmonary hypertension. N Engl J Med 1995;333:214–221.

276. Vosatka RJ, Kashyap S, Trifiletti RR. Arginine deficiency accompanies persistent pulmonary hypertension of the newborn. Biol Neonate 1994;66:65–70.

277. Castillo L, DeRojas-Walker T, Yu YM, Sanchez M, Chapman TE, Shannon D, et al. Whole body arginine metabolism and nitric oxide synthesis in newborns with persistent pulmonary hypertension. Pediatr Res 1995;38:17–24.

278. Stewart DJ. Endothelial dysfunction in pulmonary vascular disorders. Arzneimittel-Forschung 1994; 44:451–454.

279. Baudouin SV, Bath P, Martin JF, Du Bois R, Evans TW. L-arginine infusion has no effect on systemic haemodynamics in normal volunteers, or systemic and pulmonary haemodynamics in patients with elevated pulmonary vascular resistance. Br J Clin Pharmacol 1993;36:45–49.

280. Katz SD, Krum H, Khan T, Knecht M. Exercise-induced vasodilation in forearm circulation of normal subjects and patients with congestive heart failure: role of endothelium-derived nitric oxide. J Am Coll Cardiol 1996;28:585–590.

281. Takeshita A, Hirooka Y, Imaizumi T. Role of endothelium in control of forearm blood flow in patients with heart failure. J Cardiac Fail 1996;2:S209–S215.

282. Drexler H, Hayoz D, Munzel T, Hornig B, Just H, Brunner HR, et al. Endothelial function in chronic congestive heart failure. Am J Cardiol 1992;69:1596–1601.

283. Koifman B, Wollman Y, Bogomolny N, Chernichowsky T, Finkelstein A, Per G, et al. Improvement of cardiac performance by intravenous infusion of L-arginine in patients with moderate congestive heart failure. J Am Coll Cardiol 1995;26:1251–1256.

284. Howes TQ, Keilty SE, Maskrey VL, Deane CR, Baudouin SV, Moxham J. Effect of L-arginine on renal blood flow in normal subjects and patients with hypoxic chronic obstructive pulmonary disease. Thorax 1996;51:516–519.

285. Morikawa E, Moskowitz MA, Huang Z, Yoshida T, Irikura K, Dalkara T. L-arginine infusion promotes nitric oxide-dependent vasodilation, increases regional cerebral blood flow, and reduces infarction volume in the rat. Stroke 1994;25:429–435.

286. Sadoshima S, Nagao T, Okada Y, Fujii K, Ibayashi S, Fujishima M. L-arginine ameliorates recirculation and metabolic derangement in brain ischemia in hypertensive rats. Brain Res 1997;744: 246–252.

287. DeWitt DS, Smith TG, Deyo DJ, Miller KR, Uchida T, Prough DS. L-arginine and superoxide dismutase prevent or reverse cerebral hypoperfusion after fluid-percussion traumatic brain injury. J Neurotrauma 1997;14:223–233.

288. Prado R, Watson BD, Zhao W, Yao H, Busto R, Dietrich WD, et al. L-arginine does not improve cortical perfusion or histopathological outcome in spontaneously hypertensive rats subjected to distal middle cerebral artery photothrombotic occlusion. J Cereb Blood Flow Metab 1996;16:612–622.

289. Kirsch JR, Bhardwaj A, Martin LJ, Hanley DF, Traystman RJ. Neither L-arginine nor L-NAME affects neurological outcome after global ischemia in cats. Stroke 1997;28:2259–2264.

290. Nakagomi T, Kanemitsu H, Takagi K, Morikawa E, Kirino T, Tamura A. Effect of L-arginine and NG-nitro-L-arginine on delayed neuronal death in the gerbil hippocampus. Neurol Res 1997;19:426–430.

291. Huang Z, Huang PL, Ma J, Meng W, Ayata C, Fishman MC, et al. Enlarged infarcts in endothelial nitric oxide synthase knockout mice are attenuated by nitro-L-arginine. J Cereb Blood Flow Metab 1996;16: 981–987.

292. Samdani AF, Dawson TM, Dawson VL. Nitric oxide synthase in models of focal ischemia. Stroke 1997;28:1283–1288.

293. Wang QD, Morcos E, Wiklund P, Pernow J. L-arginine enhances functional recovery and Ca2+-dependent nitric oxide synthase activity after ischemia and reperfusion in the rat heart. J Cardiovasc Pharmacol 1997;29:291–296.

294. Wang P, Zweier JL. Ischemic preconditioning decreases nitric oxide (NO) formation and NO mediated injury in the postischemic heart. Circulation 1997;96:I–72.

295. Li XS, Uriuda Y, Wang QD, Norlander R, Sjoquist PO, Pernow J. Role of L-arginine in preventing myocardial and endothelial injury following ischaemia/reperfusion in the rat isolated heart. Acta Physiol Scand 1996;156:37–44.

296. Brunner F, Leonhard B, Kukovetz WR, Mayer B. Role of endothelin, nitric oxide and L-arginine release in ischaemia/reperfusion injury of rat heart. Cardiovasc Res 1997;36:60–66.

297. Weyrich AS, Ma XL, Lefer AM. The role of L-arginine in ameliorating reperfusion injury after myocardial ischemia in the cat. Circulation 1992;86:279–288.

298. Nakanishi K, Vinten-Johansen J, Lefer DJ, Zhao Z, Fowler WC, McGee DS, et al. Intracoronary L-arginine during reperfusion improves endothelial function and reduces infarct size. Am J Physiol 1992;263:H1650–H1658.

299. Takeuchi K, Takashima K, Suzuki S, Fukui K. [Basic amino acid, L-arginine aggravates ischemia-reperfusion injury]. Nippon Kyobu Geka Gakkai Zasshi 1996;44:155–161.

300. Fei L, Baron AD, Henry DP, Zipes DP. Intrapericardial delivery of L-arginine reduces the increased severity of ventricular arrhythmias during sympathetic stimulation in dogs with acute coronary occlusion: nitric oxide modulates sympathetic effects on ventricular electrophysiological properties. Circulation 1997;96:4044–4049.

301. Burra P, Ferraresso M, Cadrobbi R, Calabrese F, Crdin R, Parnigotto A, et al. Effect of L-arginine and oligotide on liver ischemia-reperfusion injury. Transplant Proc 1997;29:2992,2993.

302. Shiraishi M, Kusano T, Aihara T, Ikeda Y, Koyama Y, Muto Y. Protection against hepatic ischemia/reperfusion injury by exogenous L-arginine. Transplant Proc 1996;28:1887,1888.

303. Calabrese F, Valente M, Pettenazzo E, Ferraresso M, Burra P, Cadrobbi R, et al. The protective effects of L-arginine after liver ischaemia/reperfusion injury in a pig model. J Pathol 1997;183:477–485.

304. Shiraishi M, Hiroyasu S, Nagahama M, Miyaguni T, Higa T, Tomori H, et al. Role of exogenous L-arginine in hepatic ischemia-reperfusion injury. J Surg Res 1997;69:429–434.

305. Hiramatsu T, Forbess JM, Miura T, Roth SJ, Cioffi MA, Mayer JE Jr. Effects of endothelin-1 and L-arginine after cold ischemia in lamb hearts. Ann Thorac Surg 1997;61:36–40.

306. Duke T, South M, Stewart A. Altered activation of the L-arginine nitric oxide pathway during and after cardiopulmonary bypass. Perfusion 1997;12:405–410.

307. Stowe DF, Boban M, Roerig DL, Chang D, Palmisano BW, Bosnjak ZJ. Effects of L-arginine and N omega-nitro-L-arginine methyl ester on cardiac perfusion and function after 1-day cold preservation of isolated hearts. Circulation 1997;95:1623–1634.

308. Hiramatsu T, Forbess JM, Miura T, Mayer JE Jr. Effect of L-arginine cardioplegia on recovery of neonatal lamb hearts after 2 hours of cold ischemia. Ann Thorac Surg 1995;60:1187–1192.

309. Hiramatsu T, Forbess JM, Miura T, Mayer JE Jr. Effects of L-arginine and L-nitro-arginine methyl ester on recovery of neonatal lamb hearts after cold ischemia. Evidence for an important role of endothelial production of nitric oxide. J Thorac Cardiovasc Surg 1995;109:81–86.

310. Szabo G, Bahrle S, Dengler TJ, Batkai S, Vahl CF, Hagl S. [Reducing perfusion damage after heart transplantation with the nitric oxide donor L-arginine]. Langenbecks Arch Chir Supplement Kongressbd 1997;114:7–10.

311. Normandin L, Herve P, Brink C, Chapelier AR, Dartevelle PG, Mazmanian GM. L-arginine and pentoxifylline attenuate endothelial dysfunction after lung reperfusion injury in the rabbit. The Paris-Sud University Lung Transplant Group. Ann Thorac Surg 1995;60:646–650.

312. Um SC, Suzuki S, Toyokuni S, Kim BM, Tanaka T, Hiai H, et al. Involvement of nitric oxide in survival of random pattern skin flap. Plast Reconstr Surg 1998;101:785–792.

313. Cordeiro PG, Mastorakos DP, Hu QY, Kirschner RE. The protective effect of L-arginine on ischemia-reperfusion injury in rat skin flaps. Plastic Reconst Surg 1997;100:1227–1233.

314. Ercocen AR, Apaydin I, Emiroglu M, Gultan SM, Ergun H, Yormuk E. The effects of L-arginine and iloprost on the viability of random skin flaps in rats. Scand J Plast Reconstr Surg Hand Surg 1998;32:19–25.

315. Walls CM, Gregory CR, Beck LS, Cooke JP, Griffey SM, Kass PH. Effects of growth factors and L-arginine on ischemic skin flaps in rats. Vet Surg 1995;24:484–491.

316. Melis MR, Argiolas A. Role of central nitric oxide in the control of penile erection and yawning. Prog Neuropsychopharmacol Biol Psych 1997;21:899–922.

317. Garban H, Vernet D, Freedman A, Rajfer J, Gonzalez-Cadavid N. Effect of aging on nitric oxide-mediated penile erection in rats. Am J Physiol 1995;268:H467–H475.

318. Xie Y, Garban H, Ng C, Rajfer J, Gonzalez-Cadavid NF. Effect of long-term passive smoking on erectile function and penile nitric oxide synthase in the rat. J Urol 1997;157:1121–1126.

319. Vernet D, Cai L, Garban H, Babbitt ML, Murray FT, Rajfer J, et al. Reduction of penile nitric oxide synthase in diabetic BB/WORdp (type I) and BBZ/WORdp (type II) rats with erectile dysfunction. Endocrinology 1995;136:5709–5717.

320. Kim YC, Davies MG, Hagen PO, Carson CC. Experimental evidence for endothelium dependent relaxation and neuronal nitric oxide in corpus cavernosum. Yonsei Med J 1994;35:308–313.

321. Penson DF, Ng C, Rajfer J, Gonzalez-Cadavid NF. Adrenal control of erectile function and nitric oxide synthase in the rat penis. Endocrinology 1997;138:3925–3932.

322. Kimura K, Takahashi M, Naroda T, Iriguchi H, Miyamoto T, Kawanishi Y, et al. [The relaxation of human corpus cavernosum caused by nitric oxide]. Nippon Hinyokika Gakkai Zasshi 1993;84: 1660–1664.

323. Simonsen U, Prieto D, Delgado JA, Hernandez M, Resel L, Saenz de Tejada I, et al. Nitric oxide is involved in the inhibitory neurotransmission and endothelium-dependent relaxations of human small penile arteries. Clin Sci (Colch) 1997;92:269–275.

324. Benelli A, Bertolini A, Poggioli R, Cavazzuti E, Calza L, Giardino L, et al. Nitric oxide is involved in male sexual behavior of rats. Eur J Pharmacol 1995;294:505–510.

325. Luscher TF, Bock HA. The endothelial L-arginine/nitric oxide pathway and the renal circulation. Klin Wochenschr 1991;69:603–609

326. De Nicola L, Minutolo R, Bellizzi V, Andreucci M, La Verde A, Cianciaruso B. Enhancement of nitric oxide synthesis by L-arginine supplementation in renal disease: is it good or bad? Miner Electrolyte Metab 1997;23:144–150.

327. Katoh T, Takahashi K, Klahr S, Reyes AA, Badr KF. Dietary supplementation with L-arginine ameliorates glomerular hypertension in rats with subtotal nephrectomy. J Am Soc Nephrol 1994;4: 1690–1694.

328. Ashab I, Peer G, Blum M, Wollman Y, Chernihovsky T, Hassner A, et al. Oral administration of L-arginine and captopril in rats prevents chronic renal failure by nitric oxide production. Kidney Int 1995;47:1515–1521.

329. Wakabayashi Y, Kikawada R. Effect of L-arginine on myoglobin induced acute renal failure in the rabbit. Am J Physiol 1996;270:F784–F789.

330. De Nicola L, Thomson SC, Wead LM, Brown MR, Gabbai FB. Arginine feeding modifies cyclosporine nephrotoxicity in rats. J Clin Invest 1993;92:1859–1865.

331. Kumagai K, Suzuki H, Ichikawa M, Jimbo M, Murakami M, Ryuzaki M, et al. Nitric oxide increases renal blood flow by interacting with the sympathetic nervous system. Hypertension 1994;24:220–226.

332. Aiello S, Noris M, Remuzzi G. Nitric oxide synthesis and L-arginine in uremia. Miner Electrolyte Metab 1997;23:151–156.

333. Reyes AA, Klahr S. Dietary supplementation of L-arginine ameliorates renal hypertrophy in rats fed a high-protein diet. Proc Soc Exp Biol Med 1994;206:157–161.

334. Thomas SE, Andoh TF, Pichler RH, Shankland SJ, Couser WG, Bennett WM, et al. Accelerated apoptosis characterizes cyclosporine-associated interstitial fibrosis. Kidney Int 1998;53:897–908.

335. Yang CW, Kim YS, Kim J, Kim YO, Min SY, Choi EJ, et al. Oral supplementation of L-arginine prevents chronic cyclosporine nephrotoxicity in rats. Exp Nephrol 1998;6:50–56.

336. Assis SM, Monteiro JL, Seguro AC. L-Arginine and allopurinol protect against cyclosporine nephrotoxicity. Transplantation 1997;63:1070–1073.

337. MacAllister RJ, Rambausek MH, Vallance P, Williams D, Hoffmann KH, Ritz E. Concentration of dimethyl-L-arginine in the plasma of patients with end-stage renal failure. Nephr Dialys Transplant 1996;11:2449–2452.

338. Andres A, Morales JM, Praga M, Campo C, Lahera V, Garcia-Robles R, et al. L-arginine reverses the antinatriuretic effect of cyclosporin in renal transplant patients. Nephrol Dialys Transplant 1997;12: 1437–1440.

339. Creager MA, Halperin JL, Coffman, JD. Vasospastic diseases. In: Loscalzo J, Creager MA, Dzau VJ, eds. The Textbook of Vascular Medicine. Little Brown, Boston, 1992, pp. 975–1010.

340. Coffman JD, Davies WT. Vasospastic disease: a review. Prog Cardiovasc Dis 1975;18:123–146.

341. Robertson D, Oates JA. Variant angina and Raynaud's phenomenon. Lancet 1978;1:452.

342. Flavahan NA. Human postjunctional alpha 1 and alpha 2-adrenoceptors: differential distribution in arteries of the limbs. J Pharmacol Exp Ther 1986;241:361–365.

343. Moulds RF, Iwanov V, Medcalf RL. The effects of platlet-derived contractile agents on human digital arteries. Clin Sci 1984;66:443–451.

344. Coffman JD, Cohen RA. Serotoninergic vasoconstriction in human fingers during reflex sympathetic responses to cooling. Am J Physiol 1988;254:H889–H893.

Index